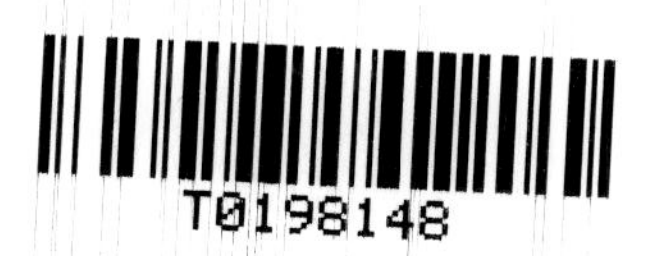

KLAUS and FANAROFF'S CARE *of the* HIGH-RISK NEONATE

KLAUS and FANAROFF'S

CARE of the HIGH-RISK NEONATE

Seventh Edition

Avroy A. Fanaroff, MD, FRCP, FRCPCH
Professor Emeritus
Department of Pediatrics and Neonatology in Reproductive Biology
Case Western Reserve University School of Medicine;
Eliza Henry Barnes Chair in Neonatology
Department of Pediatrics
University Hospitals Rainbow Babies & Children's Hospital
Cleveland, Ohio

Jonathan M. Fanaroff, MD, JD, FAAP, FCLM
Professor
Department of Pediatrics
Case Western Reserve University School of Medicine;
Director, Rainbow Center for Pediatric Ethics
University Hospitals Rainbow Babies & Children's Hospital
Cleveland Medical Center
Cleveland, Ohio

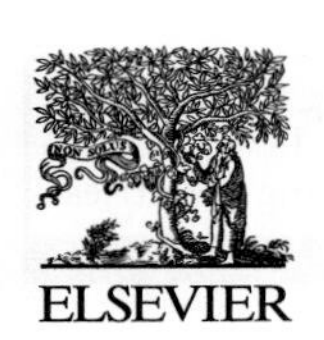

ELSEVIER

3251 Riverport Lane
St. Louis, Missouri 63043

KLAUS AND FANAROFF'S CARE OF THE HIGH-RISK NEONATE,
SEVENTH EDITION
ISBN: 978-0-323-60854-1

Library of Congress Cataloging-in-Publication Data or Control Number : 2019947133

Content Strategist: Sarah Barth
Content Development Specialist: Angie Breckon
Publishing Services Manager: Shereen Jameel
Project Manager: Rukmani Krishnan
Design Direction: Bridget Hoette

Printed in the United States of America

Last digit is the print number: 9 8 7 6 5 4 3 2 1

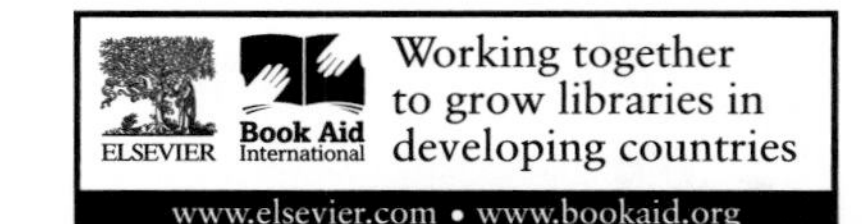

To all students of perinatology; our patients and their parents; Roslyn and Kristy, Mason, Cole, and Brooke Fanaroff; Peter, Jodi, Austin, and Morgan Tucker; and Amanda, Jason, Jackson, and Raya Hirsh

LIST OF CONTRIBUTORS

David H. Adamkin, MD
Professor of Pediatrics
Division of Neonatal Medicine
Department of Pediatrics
University of Louisville School of Medicine
Louisville, Kentucky

Sanjay Ahuja, MD, MSc
Associate Professor
Department of Pediatrics
Case Western Reserve University School of Medicine
Director, Hemostasis and Thrombosis Center
University Hospitals Rainbow Babies & Children's Hospital
Cleveland, Ohio

Namasivayam Ambalavanan, MBBS, MD
Professor, Departments of Pediatrics, Pathology, and Cell, Developmental, and Integrative Biology
Co-Director, Division of Neonatology
University of Alabama at Birmingham
Birmingham, Alabama

Felicia L. Bahadue, MD
Assistant Professor
Department of Obstetrics, Gynecology, and Reproductive Sciences
University of Miami
Miami, Florida

Sheila C. Berlin, MD
Associate Professor and Vice Chair
Department of Radiology
University Hospitals of Cleveland
Director of Pediatric CT
Department of Radiology
University Hospitals Rainbow Babies & Children's Hospital
Cleveland, Ohio

Mary Ann Blatz, DNP, RNC-NIC, IBCLC
Advanced Practice Nurse
NICU Nursing Research & Development
Neonatal Intensive Care Unit
University Hospitals Rainbow Babies & Children's Hospital
University Hospitals of Cleveland Medical Center
Cleveland, Ohio

Michael Caplan, MD
Chairman
Department of Pediatrics
NorthShore University HealthSystem
Evanston, Illinois
Clinical Professor of Pediatrics
University of Chicago
Pritzker School of Medicine
Chicago, Illinois

Waldemar A. Carlo, MD
Edwin M. Dixon Professor of Pediatrics
Co-Director, Division of Neonatology
University of Alabama at Birmingham
Birmingham, Alabama

Moira A. Crowley, M.D.
Associate Professor, Pediatrics
Case Western Reserve University School of Medicine
Director, Neonatal ECMO Program
Director, Neonatal Consultative Services
Co-Medical Director, Neonatal Intensive Care Unit
University Hospitals Rainbow Babies & Children's Hospital
Cleveland, Ohio

Clifford L. Cua, MD
Associate Professor of Clinical Pediatrics
Nationwide Children's Hospital
Columbus, Ohio

Ankita P. Desai, MD
Assistant Professor
Medical Director of Antimicrobial Stewardship
Fellowship Program Director
Pediatric Infectious Diseases
University Hospitals Rainbow Babies & Children's Hospital
Cleveland, Ohio

Michael Dingeldein, MD
Assistant Professor of Surgery
Pediatric Surgery
University Hospitals Rainbow Babies & Children's Hospital
Cleveland, Ohio

Avroy A. Fanaroff, MD, FRCP, FRCPCH
Professor Emeritus
Department of Pediatrics and Neonatology in Reproductive Biology
Case Western Reserve University School of Medicine;
Eliza Henry Barnes Chair in Neonatology
Department of Pediatrics
University Hospitals Rainbow Babies & Children's Hospital
Cleveland, Ohio

Jonathan M. Fanaroff, MD, JD, FAAP, FCLM
Professor of Pediatrics
Department of Pediatrics
Case Western Reserve University School of Medicine
Director, Rainbow Center for Pediatric Ethics
University Hospitals Rainbow Babies & Children's Hospital
Cleveland Medical Center
Cleveland, Ohio

Kimberly S. Gecsi, MD
Associate Professor
Reproductive Biology
Case Western Reserve University
Residency Program Director
Obstetrics and Gynecology
University Hospitals MacDonald Women's Hospital
Cleveland, Ohio

Amy E. Heiderich, MD
Neonatal-Perinatal Medicine Fellow
New York Presbyterian Hospital-Morgan Stanley Children's Hospital
Columbia University Medical Center
New York, New York

Terrie Eleanor Inder, MBChB, MD
Chair, Department of Pediatric Newborn Medicine
Brigham and Women's Hospital
Professor of Pediatrics
Mary Ellen Avery Professor in the field of Newborn Medicine
Harvard Medical School
Boston, Massachusetts

Kimberly A. Kripps, MD
University of Colorado Denver, Anschutz Medical Campus
Department of Pediatrics, Section of Genetics and Metabolism
Aurora, Colorado

Tina A. Leone, MD
Associate Professor of Pediatrics
Columbia University, Vagelos College of Physicians and Surgeons
New York, New York

Ethan G. Leonard, MD, FAAP, FIDSA
Chief Medical Officer and Vice Chair for Clinical Operations
Associate Professor of Pediatrics
University Hospitals Rainbow Babies and Children's Hospital
Case Western Reserve University School of Medicine
Cleveland, Ohio

John Letterio, MD
Professor of Pediatrics: Chief, Pediatric Hematology Oncology
University Hospitals Rainbow Babies & Children's Hospital
Cleveland, Ohio

Tom Lissauer, MB BChir, FRCPCH
Honorary Consultant Pediatrician
Consultant Pediatric Program Director in Global Health
Imperial College London
London, United Kingdom

M. Jeffrey Maisels, MB, BCh, DSc
Professor
Department of Pediatrics
Oakland University William Beaumont School of Medicine
Director, Academic Affairs
Department of Pediatrics
Beaumont Children's Hospital
Royal Oak, Michigan

Jaime Marasch, PharmD, BCPS
Clinical Pharmacist Specialist, Neonatal Intensive Care Unit
University Hospitals Rainbow Babies and Children's Hospital
Cleveland, Ohio

Richard J. Martin, M.B.B.S.
Professor, Pediatrics, Reproductive Biology, and Physiology & Biophysics
Case Western Reserve University School of Medicine
Drusinsky/Fanaroff Professor in Neonatology
Director, Neonatal Research
Rainbow Babies & Children's Hospital
Cleveland, Ohio

Lillian G. Matthews, PhD
Department of Pediatric Newborn Medicine
Brigham and Women's Hospital
Harvard Medical School
Boston, Massachusetts

Shawn E. McCandless, MD
Professor
University of Colorado Denver, Anschutz Medical Campus
Department of Pediatrics, Section of Genetics and Metabolism
Aurora, Colorado

Jacquelyn D. McClary, PharmD, BCPS
Clinical Pharmacist Specialist, Neonatal Intensive Care Unit
University Hospitals Rainbow Babies & Children's Hospital
Cleveland, Ohio

Scott T. McEwen, MD, PhD
Assistant Professor, Pediatrics
University of Minnesota Medical School
Division of Pediatric Nephrology
University of Minnesota Masonic Children's Hospital
Minneapolis, Minnesota

Jennifer McGuirl, DO, MBE
Attending Neonatologist
Pediatrics
Brigham and Women's Hospital
Instructor
Pediatrics
Harvard Medical School
Boston, Massachusetts

Mariana L. Meyers, MD
Assistant Professor
Director of Fetal MRI
Pediatric Radiology
University of Colorado Denver School of Medicine
Children's Hospital Colorado
Colorado Fetal Care Center
Aurora, Colorado

Peter D. Murray, MD, MSM
Assistant Professor of Pediatrics
University of Virginia School of Medicine
Department of Pediatrics, Division of Neonatology
Charlottesville, Virginia

Vijayalakshmi Padmanabhan, MBBS, MD, MPH
Associate Professor
Department of Pathology
Division of Cytopathology
Baylor College of Medicine
Houston, Texas

Mary Elaine Patrinos, MD
Assistant Professor
Pediatrics
Case Western Reserve University School of Medicine
University Hospitals Rainbow Babies and Children's Hospital
Cleveland, Ohio

Allison H. Payne, MD, MS
Assistant Professor
Pediatrics/Neonatology
University Hospitals Rainbow Babies & Children's Hospitals/Case Western Reserve University
Cleveland, Ohio

Christina M. Phelps, MD
Assistant Professor of Clinical Pediatrics
Nationwide Children's Hospital
Columbus, Ohio

Richard A. Polin, MD
Professor of Pediatrics
Director, Division of Neonatology and Perinatology
Department of Pediatrics
Columbia University
Vagelos College of Physicians and Surgeons
New York, New York

Paula G. Radmacher, MSPH, PhD
Associate Professor
Division of Neonatal Medicine
Neonatal Nutrition Research Laboratory
Department of Pediatrics
University of Louisville School of Medicine
Louisville, Kentucky

Sheri Ricciardi, OTR/L, CNT, NTMTC
Board Certified Neonatal Therapist
Developmental Specialist
Neonatal Intensive Care Unit
University Hospitals Rainbow Babies & Children's Hospital
University Hospitals of Cleveland Medical Center
Cleveland, Ohio

Ricardo J. Rodriguez, MD, FAAP
Neonatology
Cleveland Clinic Children's Hospital
Associate Professor
Pediatrics
Cleveland Clinic Lerner College of Medicine at CWRU
Cleveland, Ohio

Gautham K. Suresh, MD
Professor of Pediatrics
Section of Neonatology
Baylor College of Medicine
Houston, Texas

Philip T. Thrush, MD
Assistant Professor of Pediatrics
Northwestern University Feinberg School of Medicine
Ann & Robert H. Lurie Children's Hospital of Chicago
Chicago, Illinois

Beth A. Vogt, MD
Associate Professor, Pediatrics
The Ohio State University College of Medicine
Division of Nephrology
Nationwide Children's Hospital
Columbus, Ohio

Kristin C. Voos, MD
Associate Professor
Department of Pediatrics, Division of Neonatology
Case Western Reserve University School of Medicine
Director of Family Integrated Care Neonatal Intensive Care Unit
University Hospitals Rainbow Babies & Children's Hospitals
Cleveland, Ohio

Jon F. Watchko, MD
Professor of Pediatrics, Obstetrics, Gynecology, and Reproductive Sciences
University of Pittsburgh School of Medicine
Pittsburgh, Pennsylvania

Deanne Wilson-Costello, MD
Professor of Pediatrics
Division of Neonatology
University Hospitals Rainbow Babies & Children's Hospital
Cleveland, Ohio

PREFACE

It is with a deep sense of sadness that we report the death of our mentor, original author, and source of inspiration for this book, Marshall H. Klaus, M.D. He was a pioneer in the field of neonatal perinatal medicine, an incredibly kind and caring human being, and the perfect role model for a budding neonatologist. An original thinker, he was unafraid to challenge dogma, and through his research, writing, and teaching dramatically changed delivery room and neonatal intensive care units by opening these formerly sacrosanct areas to parents and families. He and his colleague John H. Kennell developed the concepts of family-centered care long before the term had been coined. Before that, he had discovered the lipid structures in surfactant and was a superb neonatal pulmonary physiologist. He was an emeritus author in the sixth edition, and this edition carries on his plea for humane care, promoting human milk, and support of the family. He is missed, but his messages will not be forgotten, and Jon and I cherish the wonderful years we had together with Marshall and his superb mentorship, which we have attempted to pass on to subsequent generations of neonatal trainees.

We are extremely proud and deeply grateful to the many contributors who have enabled us to present the seventh edition of *Klaus and Fanaroff's Care of the High-Risk Neonate*. Much has changed since the first edition was published 45 years ago, and so too has the book changed. This edition has had perhaps the most radical changes, with new chapters reflecting important advances in quality- and evidence-based medicine; a new chapter on genetics, inborn errors of metabolism and neonatal screening; a chapter on family-centered care and another on understanding the science of developmental care. We have been fortunate to add leading authorities on these important topics.

They say every baby is a miracle. Some, however, face unusually long odds, from difficult pregnancies, to harrowing births, to births at the limits of viability.

How to support the best possible outcome using evidence-based medicine, quality improvement programs, and best practices remains the abiding theme of this book. Our aim is to present all these factors in a user-friendly manner. We have stuck with the format of including editorial comments within the text and new material in the form of clinical cases with questions.

This book would not have come to fruition without the superb in-house editing of Bonnie Siner, R.N. Bonnie, you are the best, and we are eternally grateful to you for your assistance. We recognize and thank Angie Breckon from Elsevier for her guidance and assistance, and of course we thank the authors and commenters who gave of their time and expertise so that we are all better informed. Finally, we thank you the reader for all you do to support babies and families during an incredibly difficult and challenging time in their lives.

Avroy A. Fanaroff, MD, FRCP, FRCPCH
Jonathan M. Fanaroff, MD, JD, FAAP, FCLM

CONTENTS

APPENDIXES

Patient Safety, Quality, and Evidence-Based Medicine

Vijayalakshmi Padmanabhan, Gautham K. Suresh

Health care is viewed as a system, a network of interdependent components working together to accomplish a specific aim, which is to meet the needs of patients, families, and communities while constantly improving its performance. The quality of health care is defined as "the degree to which health services for individuals and populations increase the likelihood of desired health outcomes and are consistent with current professional knowledge."[1,2] A medical error is the failure of a planned action to be completed as intended, or the use of a wrong plan to achieve an aim, and an adverse event is defined as an injury resulting from a medical intervention. Unfortunately, as noted in numerous research studies and in the Institute of Medicine (IOM) reports in 2000 and 2001,[2,3] the US healthcare delivery system does not consistently provide high-quality care to all patients and populations, deficiencies in the quality of health care are highly prevalent,[4,5] and numerous patients suffer from preventable harm due to medical errors.

> **EDITORIAL COMMENT:** The Institute of Medicine report concluded that up to 98,000 people die each year as a result of preventable medical errors. The report was discussed not only in medical journals but also in lay journals and news media. One especially vivid analogy came from safety researcher Dr. Lucian Leape, who stated that this was the equivalent of three jumbo jet crashes every 2 days.

Ideally, units caring for neonates should monitor the care they provide and continuously improve the quality and safety of the care provided, both to improve clinical outcomes and to avoid medical errors and preventable adverse events. Examples of errors and adverse events noted in neonatal intensive care are shown in Box 1.1. To ensure high-quality and safe care with the best possible outcomes, each neonatal unit should have a framework to assess, monitor, and improve the quality of care provided, both generally and for neonates with specific conditions. Such a framework can be developed using Donabedian's triad and the IOM's six domains of quality.

DONABEDIAN'S TRIAD AND THE INSTITUTE OF MEDICINE'S SIX DOMAINS OF QUALITY

In the 1960s, Donabedian proposed that the domains of quality of care are structure, process, and outcomes.[6–8] Structure includes the environment in which care is provided; the facilities, equipment, services, and manpower available for care; the qualifications, skills, and experience of the healthcare professionals; and other characteristics of the hospital or system providing care. Examples of structural measures for a neonatal unit include space per patient, the layout of the unit, the nurse–patient ratio, the availability of imaging facilities around the clock, the types of respiratory equipment used, and the level of training and skills of the health professionals working in the unit and subspecialists available for consultation.

The process consists of the activities and steps involved and the sequence of these steps when patients receive health care. It refers to the content of care, i.e., how the patient was moved into, through, and out of the healthcare system and the services that were provided during the care episode. In a neonatal unit, the process of each aspect of care received by each infant can be analyzed and improved. For example, the processes of delivery room stabilization, neonatal transport, admission to the neonatal unit, performance of an invasive procedure, clinical rounds, and discharge home can all be studied and improved. Process measures of quality can be developed and monitored, such as the percentage of personnel performing hand hygiene prior to patient contact, percentage of eligible infants stabilized on continuous positive airway pressure (CPAP) at birth, the percentage of infants in whom the examination for retinopathy of prematurity (ROP) is performed on time, the efficiency with which a neonate is transported from a referring hospital, and the time taken to administer the first dose of antibiotic to infants with suspected sepsis.

Outcomes are consequences to the health and welfare of individuals and society, or, alternatively, the measured health status of the individual or community. Outcomes of care have also been defined as "the results of care…(which) can encompass biologic changes in disease, comfort, ability for self-care, physical function and mobility, emotional and intellectual performance, patient satisfaction, and self-perception of health, health knowledge and compliance with medical care, and functioning within family, job, and social role." For Newborn Intensive Care Unit (NICU) patients and their parents, examples of outcome measures are mortality rate, the frequency of chronic lung disease (CLD), percentage of very-low-birth-weight (VLBW) infants developing ROP, the number of nosocomial blood stream infections per 1000 patient days, the percentage of NICU survivors that are developmentally normal, and parental satisfaction with the care of their baby.

BOX 1.1 Errors and Adverse Events in Neonatal Care[15]

- Intra tracheal administration of enteral feeds
- Intravenous lipid given through orogastric/nasogastric tube
- Hundred-fold overdose of insulin
- Administration of fosphenytoin instead of hepatitis B vaccine
- Subtherapeutic dose of penicillin for Group B Streptococcal infection given for 3 days before discovery
- Infusion of total daily intravenous fluids over 1–2 hours
- Intravenous administration of lidocaine instead of saline flush
- "Stat" blood transfusion took 2.5 hours
- Antibiotic given 4 hours after ordering
- Delay of greater than an hour in obtaining intravenous dextrose to treat hypoglycemia
- Medications given to the wrong patient
- Infant fed breastmilk of wrong mother
- Medications with adverse side effects:
  - Benzyl alcohol (gasping, intraventricular hemorrhage, and death)
  - Chloramphenicol (gray baby syndrome)
  - Tetracyclines (yellow-stained teeth)
  - Intravenous vitamin E (liver failure and death)

Other Errors

- Consent for a blood transfusion obtained from wrong infant's parent
- Infant falls from weighing scale, incubator, and swing
- Failure of supply of compressed air throughout neonatal intensive care unit
- Incubator drawn toward magnetic resonance imaging machine requiring four security guards to pull it away

Six domains of quality were described by the IOM in 2001 in the report "Crossing the Quality Chasm."[2] These domains of care include safety, timeliness, effectiveness, efficiency, equity, and patient-centeredness (these can be remembered by the acronym STEEEP). A neonatal unit should try to provide care optimally in all these domains. Safety of care provided is a high-priority domain that deserves separate emphasis and is defined as freedom from accidental injury (avoiding harm to patients from the care that is intended to help them). Timeliness is providing care within an optimal range of time, without delays and unnecessary waits, and also without undue haste for patients, their families, and health professionals. Effectiveness is the provision of healthcare interventions supported by high-quality evidence to all eligible patients. Efficiency is avoiding waste, including avoiding intervention in those in whom it is unlikely to be beneficial, and waste of equipment, supplies, ideas, and energy. Equity is provision of care that does not vary based on a patient's personal characteristics such as gender, ethnicity, geographic location, and socioeconomic status. Patient-centered care is the provision of care that is respectful of, and responsive to, an individual neonate's family preferences, needs, and values, and ensuring that the family's values are incorporated into clinical decisions.

CLINICAL MICROSYSTEMS AND HOW TO ASSESS AND MONITOR THE QUALITY OF CARE PROVIDED

A clinical microsystem can be defined as the combination of a small group of people who work together on a regular basis to provide care and the subpopulation of patients who receive that care.[9] Each neonatal unit is a functioning clinical microsystem with the patient at the center and the physicians, nurses, respiratory therapists, and other professionals working with the patient and the family. It is the place where quality, safety, outcomes, satisfaction, and staff morale are created. Multiple microsystems are nested within a mesosystem (departments such as the pediatric department, or service lines such as women and children's services), and multiple mesosystems are in turn components of a larger entity—the macrosystem or the larger organization. This macrosystem is embedded in the environment—the community, healthcare market, health policy, and the regulatory milieu. Assessment and monitoring of the quality of care provided in a neonatal unit will ultimately be shaped by the organizational culture and the environment.

Each neonatal unit should establish a set of indicators that measure the quality of neonatal care provided. The exact indicators to measure can be determined using the frameworks of the Donabedian triad and the IOM's quality domains. Local priorities, local patterns of practice, ease of access to data, and resources required to collect, analyze, and display data, etc., will also play a role in determining the measures that are established to indicate the quality of neonatal care. The quality indicators collected can be used for (1) comparison, and (2) improvement.

Quality Indicators for Comparative Performance Measures

Comparator indicators can used to compare a unit's clinical performance (and not process measures) against the quality indicators of other similar units, national benchmarks, or targets. To make the comparisons valid, these data should be risk adjusted using statistical methods to differentiate intrinsic heterogeneity among patients (e.g., comorbid conditions, severity of underlying disease) and institutions (e.g., available hospital personnel and resources). With risk adjustment, an outcome can be better ascribed to the quality of clinical care provided by health professionals and system, and help evaluate interinstitutional variations.

A wide variation in neonatal process measures and neonatal outcomes that persists after risk adjustment is noted in published studies of comparator quality indicators from several neonatal networks.[11–14] Persistence of the variation after risk adjustment suggests that the observed differences in outcomes are the result of the quality of care provided to the patients and that the units with the poorer clinical outcomes have room to improve their quality of care. When quality indicators are monitored—although there is often a time lag between the events being measured and the analysis, display, and comparison of the data—the discrepancy between an individual unit's performance and the comparators can be used to motivate change and launch improvement projects around specific topics. Quality indicators may also be used by regulators and payors to rank hospitals and neonatal units (sometimes publicly) according to the quality of care they provide (their performance), withhold payments, and provide incentive payments. They may also be used by families of patients, when choice is feasible (for example, in an antenatally diagnosed fetal anomaly), to choose the neonatal unit where their infant will receive care. Many neonatal networks, such as the Vermont Oxford Network (VON), the Pediatrix neonatal database, and the Canadian Neonatal Network, collect predefined data items from member neonatal units and provide reports to these units that include quality indicators. For example, the VON provides member units each quarter and each year a report that includes, among others, their rates of ventilation, postnatal steroid use, surfactant use, inhaled nitric oxide use, pulmonary air leak, bronchopulmonary dysplasia (BPD), ROP, and mortality.

One of the most important subset of quality indicators is that of patient safety events. A variety of medical errors and adverse events related to neonatal care have been described in the literature.[15–17] Each neonatal unit should monitor medical errors and adverse events. These patient safety events are most commonly identified through reporting by health professionals involved in or witnessing the event. Although reporting is convenient and requires minimal resources,[18] other methods to identify patient safety events include the use of trigger tools, chart review, random safety audits, mortality and morbidity meetings, autopsies, and review of patient family complaints or medical-legal cases.[18,19] However, these methods do not yield a true rate of these events and therefore cannot be used to evaluate a unit's performance against comparators. The ideal method to identify patient safety events is prospective surveillance,[20] as it yields accurate rates and can be used for comparison. However, it is not widely used, as it is laborious and requires many resources.

Quality Indicators for Improvement

These indicators are usually a combination of outcome measures and process measures and are used to monitor the progress of a specific quality improvement (QI) project. They are collected in real time and used by QI teams (see below) to monitor the progress of the project, identify unintended consequences, and draw inferences about the effects of their attempts to make change. Ideally, these data should be disaggregated as much as possible (not lumped together) and displayed over time (with time on the x-axis and the indicator on the y-axis) in the form of either run charts or statistical process control charts, as displayed in Fig. 1.1.

WHY IS QUALITY IMPROVEMENT IMPORTANT IN NEONATAL CARE?

Published literature on wide variations in neonatal process measures and neonatal morbidity that persists after risk adjustment[11–14] suggests that the observed differences in

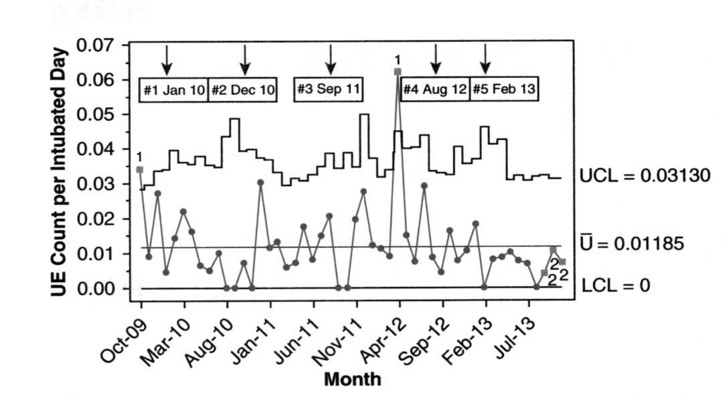

Fig. 1.1 Example of statistical process control chart. (From Merkel L, Beers K, Lewis MM, Stauffer J, Mujsce DJ, Kresch MJ. Reducing unplanned extubations in the NICU. *Pediatrics.* 2014;133(5):e1367–e1372.)

outcomes are the result of the quality of care provided to the patients, that a significant proportion of neonates managed in NICUs suffer from preventable morbidity, and that the units with the poorer clinical outcomes have opportunities to improve their quality of care. A particular concern is the high incidence in VLBW infants of morbidities such as CLD, necrotizing enterocolitis, ROP, periventricular-intraventricular hemorrhage, and other conditions that often result in major long-term medical and neurodevelopmental morbidity, require chronic complex care, and are associated with high healthcare and societal costs. Despite significant advances in neonatal care over time and a decrease in frequency in some neonatal units, these conditions continue to occur in high-risk infants, and demonstrate significant variation in frequency across units despite adjustment for confounding factors (suggesting that a proportion of these conditions is preventable). Neonatal health outcomes are influenced by a variety of endogenous and exogenous factors such as birth weight, gestation, obstetric management during delivery, resuscitation practices, initial respiratory support, nutritional management, and prevention of infections. Application of systematic QI methods has the potential to reduce various forms of preventable neonatal morbidity and mortality through reliable and consistent application of existing high-level evidence, without depending on new medications, technology, or innovations to be developed. Such efforts are described below.

> **EDITORIAL COMMENT:** A mantra of quality improvement is to "borrow shamelessly," and indeed, healthcare quality improvement efforts have looked to other high-reliability industries such as aviation, nuclear power plants, naval aircraft carriers, and other industries that operate in complex, high-risk environments. Crew resource management, for example, which has been used in the aviation industry for years to improve communication, has been incorporated relatively recently in neonatal resuscitation as a way to improve teamwork.

IMPROVING THE QUALITY OF CARE

QI is now an established movement in health care. QI in health care has developed in the past three decades by using principles, tools, and techniques from other industries about improving product quality to meet their customers' needs and expectations. The basic premise of QI in health care is that improvement in patient care and outcomes can be achieved by making intentional and systematic efforts using a defined set of scientific methods and by constantly reflecting on and learning from the results of attempts to improve care. QI is based on systems thinking and therefore emphasizes the organization and systems of care. Although there are multiple QI models and frameworks—IMPROVE, Model for Improvement, Lean or Lean Six Sigma (define, measure, analyze, improve, and control; DMAIC), the Toyota Production System, Rapid Cycle Improvement, four key habits (VON), Advanced Training Program of Intermountain Healthcare, and the Microsystems approach—they are all broadly similar in their approaches. The Model for Improvement (Fig. 1.2), which was formalized by Langley, Nolan, and colleagues, is a simple and effective approach that can be used to improve the quality of care.[21] The use of this model and Plan-Do-Study-Act (PDSA) cycles to achieve improvement is discussed below.

Assessment of the neonatal unit as a clinical microsystem is the start of the improvement journey.[9,10] Using a framework known as the "Five Ps," various aspects of the microsystem—its **p**urpose, the **p**atients cared for, the **p**rofessionals that provide care, the **p**rocesses of care, and **p**atterns (culture, history, and interpersonal dynamics)—can be understood and defined. Such an analysis provides a rich and deep understanding of the context of improvement that subsequently helps with change management and strategic planning.

The Improvement Team

At the start of a QI project, it is important to obtain support and resources from the department's leaders. This will allow for time, personnel, and resource allocation for improvement. An early step in a QI project is the creation of a QI team that consists of personnel from multiple disciplines. QI teams usually are comprised of physicians, nurses, respiratory therapists, and other stakeholders who are directly or indirectly involved in aspects of the topic that is targeted for improvement. The more disciplines represented, the better the QI efforts will be. However, time and resources are limited and have to be used efficiently and effectively. The members of the QI team have to become skilled in several techniques, such as how to have productive meetings, how to work together as a team, how to bring about change in a unit, how to deal with barriers to improvement, and how to collect, analyze, and display data. A key responsibility for the QI team is to increase buy-in among the staff of the neonatal unit and heighten awareness of the problem being addressed, thereby creating a Hawthorne effect, which facilitates improvement.

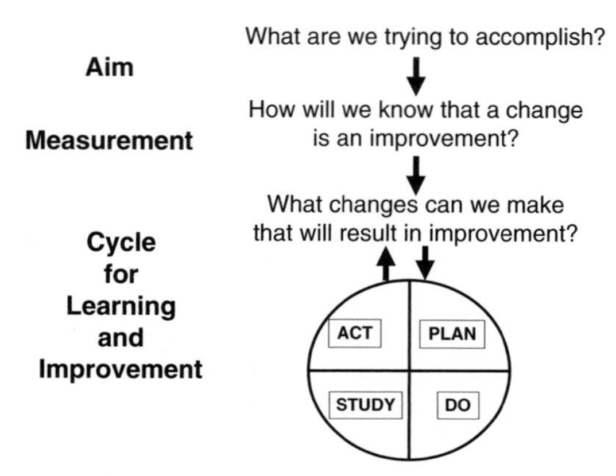
Aim
What are we trying to accomplish?
Measurement
How will we know that a change is an improvement?
Cycle for Learning and Improvement
What changes can we make that will result in improvement?
ACT
PLAN
STUDY
DO

Fig. 1.2 The Model for Improvement.

Cooperation and Collaboration

Improvement in patient care is impossible without cooperation—working together to produce mutual benefit or attain a common purpose. Collaboration and cooperation have to occur within each unit. Collaboration is a powerful force in motivating people toward improvement and in sustaining the momentum for change in each unit. Often, individual team members will need to be excused from their clinical duties when they participate in a QI project, with these clinical duties assigned to other unit personnel. The improvement team has to ensure "buy-in" from other members in their unit and get them to participate in the improvement effort. Such buy-in of all the professionals will decrease resistance to change as improvement interventions are implemented. Collaboration and cooperation among different units that can work together, share ideas, and help each other can also help improve care. Clemmer and colleagues[22] suggest five methods to foster cooperation: (1) develop a shared purpose; (2) create an open, safe environment; (3) include all those who share the common purpose and encourage diverse viewpoints; (4) learn how to negotiate agreement; and (5) insist on fairness and equity in applying rules.

Aim: What Are We Trying to Accomplish?

Any improvement project should start with a clear aim of what needs to be accomplished, or the global aim. This should next be narrowed down to a specific aim statement (Fig. 1.3). This can be done in three stages. First, a list of problems faced by the unit or opportunities for change is made in two to three sentences followed by why the current system or process needs improvement. This should include baseline data and relevant benchmarks from the published literature or other sources. The existence of quality indicators as described above will assist the compilation of such a list. Second, the problems or opportunities for change that are listed are then prioritized using criteria such as the resources available, the probability of achieving change, emotional appeal, the importance to stakeholders (including patients and their families), and practicality. Third, one item is finally selected from this list as the aim for improvement. The aim statement defines a goal, a population, and a time period. For those unfamiliar with QI, it is best to choose for the initial project a small and well-focused topic on which data are easy to obtain and that will generate interest among clinicians and nurses. VLBW neonates have been the obvious target for QI in many QI initiatives. VLBW neonates contribute significantly to the mortality and morbidity burden in the neonatal units, consume the largest proportion of resources, are easily identified, and develop potentially preventable outcomes like nosocomial infections, intraventricular hemorrhage, BPD, and ROP. When an aim is selected, it should be specified as a SMART aim, i.e., it should be specific, measurable, achievable, realistic, and time-bound. Fig. 1.3 provides a template for a SMART aim.

Measurement: How Will We Know That a Change Is an Improvement?

Measurement is key to knowing whether a change is an improvement or not. Without objective measurement, clinicians will be left guessing or relying on subjective impressions. Objective measurement of structures, processes, and outcomes provides strong motivation for a unit to embark on an improvement project. Measurement serves three purposes: (1) it indicates the current status of the unit or practice. This is called assessing "current reality"; (2) it informs QI teams whether or not they are actually making an improvement, without having to rely on subjective impressions or opinions (which can be misleading); and (3) measuring quality helps teams learn from attempts to make improvements and learn from successes as well as failures.

What Changes Can We Make That Will Result in an Improvement?

Prior to understanding what changes one can make, it is important to understand the "forces that are holding the unchanged present in place before selecting changes." For every problem, the QI team needs to understand the potential causes, the facilitators, and the barriers to change. There are many steps one can take to understand the current situation and the changes one can make that will result in an improvement. These include:

1. A detailed analysis and mapping of the process by which care is provided (process mapping). An overview of the process can be obtained using a flowchart. A flowchart helps understand the systematic flow of information in the system. The basic element of a flowchart is a simple action. It is a map of what follows what, with arrows between sequential action boxes and symbols for start and end steps in the sequence. Other symbols are used in flowcharts to represent different kinds of steps, e.g., process, decision, start, delay, cloud;
2. A review of published literature and using the principles of evidence-based medicine;
3. Benchmarking, i.e., learning from superior performers in the area chosen for improvement;
4. Advice from experts or others who have attempted improvement in similar topics;
5. Brainstorming, critical thinking, and hunches about the current system of care, especially involving individuals who are at the front line for delivering the care and intimately involved in a process. An Ishikawa/Fishbone diagram offers a useful outline for brainstorming and to identify potential factors causing an overall effect. Each cause is a source of variation. Causes are usually grouped into major categories to identify and classify these sources of variation;
6. Use of "change concepts," a set of principles of redesign of process or work flow (such as "change the sequence of steps" or "eliminate unnecessary steps")[21]; and
7. In analyzing medical errors and adverse events, a detailed systems analysis[23] is recommended. Such an analysis (the most extensive form of which is a root cause analysis [RCA][24]) attempts to identify workplace-related, human-re lated, and organizational factors[25] that contributed to the occurrence and propagation of the event. An RCA reveals key relationships among various variables, and the possible causes provide additional insight into process behavior. Box 1.2 details the steps involved in the RCA process. The leader of the RCA should be well versed in RCA methodology and also be focused on identifying system-related challenges rather than assignment of individual blame. The well-known Swiss cheese model[26] (Fig. 1.4) depicts how an error reaches a patient in spite of a series of existing safety mechanisms because the "holes in the Swiss cheese line up" (multiple safety

SPECIFIC AIM TEMPLATE

We aim to ______________________________

(increase/decrease/improve, etc.)

The ______________________________

(number, %, scores, time taken, etc.)

Of ______________________________

(name the exact thing you want to improve)

By/from ______________________________

(exact amount of improvement, e.g., from 50% to 90%)

By ______________________________

(enter month/year)

Fig. 1.3 Template for Aim Statement

BOX 1.2 Steps of a Root Cause Analysis

Step 1: Identify a sentinel event.
Step 2: Assemble a multidisciplinary team including executive and operational leadership, QI coaches, and providers who come in contact with the system.
Step 3: Verify facts surrounding the event and collect associated data.
Step 4: Chart causal factors using process maps, brainstorming, pareto charts, fishbone diagrams, etc.
Step 5: Identify root causes by asking "why" five times for each issue to get to the bottom of the cause.
Step 6: Develop strategies and make recommendations for process change.
Step 7: Present results to all stakeholders.
Step 8: Perform "tests of change."

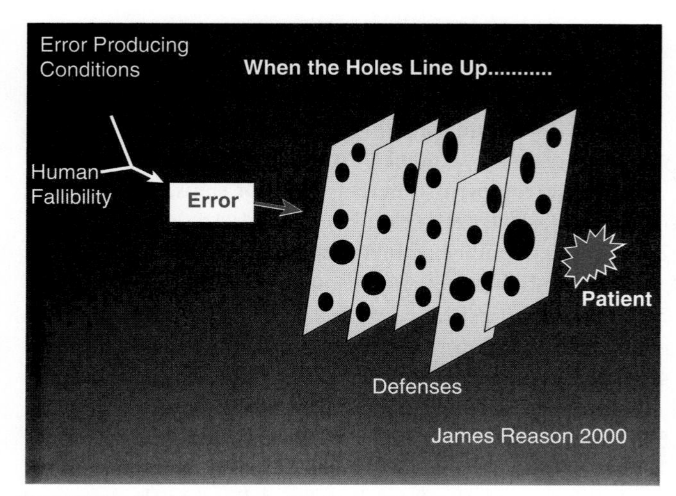

Fig. 1.4 Swiss-Cheese Model. (From Reason J. Human error: models and management. *BMJ*. 2000;320(7237):768–770.)

mechanisms fail concurrently or serially and allow propagation of the error). A key principle of improving patient safety and reducing medical errors is to focus not on individual healthcare providers as the cause of errors (the "person approach"), but more broadly on the system of care (in which the provider is embedded) as the desired locus of prevention (the "system approach"). Ensuring patient safety involves the establishment of operational systems and processes that minimize the likelihood of errors and maximize the likelihood of intercepting them when they occur.[5] Optimal design of equipment, tasks, and the work environment can enhance error-free human performance, and the use of principles of human factors engineering as well as principles of cognitive psychology can successfully guide such optimal design.

Using one or a combination of these approaches, one or more interventions are identified that, if implemented, have the potential to result in improvements in patient care and outcomes. These interventions are variously known as "change concepts," "potentially better practices,"[27] "key clinical activities,"[28] or, for patient safety events, "safety practices." They are sometimes grouped into a set of synergistic or complementary interventions that are known as "bundles."

After the changes or potentially better practices or safety practices are selected, it is not sufficient to implement them and assume that patient outcomes will improve. The next step in the improvement process is to carry out a series of PDSA cycles.

Plan-Do-Study-Act Cycles

In 1924, Walter Shewhart showed that the constant evaluation of management policy and procedures leads to continuous improvement. The Shewhart cycle, or Shewhart learning and improvement cycle, combines management thinking with statistical analysis. This cycle has also been called the Deming cycle, the Plan-Do-Check-Act cycle, or the PDSA cycle. The QI team, using the aforementioned steps, will have to decide what change concept to test. No matter what the sources of ideas for improvement are, there is no guarantee that these changes, if tried, will make things better. The results of the implementation of these changes have to be studied, using the measures that have previously been set up when answering the question, "How will we know that a change is an improvement?" In other words, the change has to be tested. This process also allows process-related obstacles to be identified and resolved. This process of testing a change is called a PDSA cycle. This is a critical step in the process of QI, since it allows troubleshooting prior to widespread implementation. Each PDSA cycle includes planning an intervention (e.g., steps to enhance adherence to hand hygiene), carrying out the intervention, studying its effect (e.g., hand hygiene compliance rate, hospital-acquired infection rate), and finally, implementing the intervention in day-to-day practice. Common questions the QI team should ask itself are: Why did we succeed? Why did we fail? What further changes do we now need to make in order to succeed? By doing a series of PDSA cycles and thus learning from each effort at improvement, the team can achieve lasting improvements in the way they provide patient care and in patient outcomes. The apparent simplicity of the PDSA cycle is deceptive. The cycle is a sophisticated, demanding way to achieve learning and change in complex systems.[29]

Ensuring Success of Quality Improvement Projects

QI projects often are not completed as intended, unsuccessful in achieving the desired results, or unable to achieve sustained results. The following ten tips can contribute to successful completion and sustained results:

1. Gain a deep understanding of the problem first using systems thinking[30] ("formulate the mess") before trying to implement solutions and resist quick "off-the-shelf" solutions.
2. Avoid solely using a research mentality, especially with measurement. Successful QI requires a combination of rigorous scientific thinking and pragmatism. Particularly with measurement, seek usefulness, not perfection.[31]
3. Focus on sustainability from the beginning, and not just on short-term wins.
4. Develop a consensus-based approach to decision-making when the evidence for interventions is sparse, incomplete, or flawed.
5. Manage change carefully using published expert recommendations.[32,33]
6. Learn from "failure" through multiple PDSA cycles. Understanding the reasons for failure can guide future refinements of the changes implemented, with eventual success.
7. Use the principles and methods of project management,[34] including good meeting skills.
8. Go beyond just using jargon such as "silo," "low-hanging" fruit, and "checklist."
9. Use a QI coach if possible. Coaching can enhance the success of QI teams.[35]
10. Do not feel compelled to adhere rigidly to any one model or framework for QI.

Leadership and Unit Culture

Finally, the involvement, support, and encouragement of the leaders of the organization or the clinical unit, as well as a favorable organizational culture, are crucial elements for the success of quality and safety improvement efforts. Without such support, many improvement efforts will be doomed to failure and frustration. Leaders of neonatal units must focus on the quality of care as an important part of the mission of their units and must actively work to create an organizational culture in the unit that will encourage efforts to improve the quality of care. For patient safety in particular, this involves fostering a culture where staff feel safe (i.e., not intimidated) in pointing out safety hazards, challenging authority, and stopping a work process or procedure if they feel it is unsafe ("stopping the line"[36]). One useful method to promote safety culture is "executive walk rounds,"[37] where senior organizational leaders periodically walk through the neonatal unit and talk to front-line staff about their perceptions of patient safety problems, hazards, and requirements.

EDITORIAL COMMENT: The Toyota Andon Cord was a rope on the assembly line that any employee could pull when they discovered a problem. The entire assembly line would stop, and the team could work to solve the problem and then restart production. The concept that any employee, not just management, could "stop the line" was revolutionary. Many other industries have adopted the principle of the Andon Cord; if a customer reports a problem with an item to an Amazon representative, that representative can halt distribution of the product until the issue has been resolved.

Examples of Quality and Safety Improvement in Neonatal Care

Quality Improvement Projects in Individual Units

Birenbaum et al reported a significant reduction in the rate of CLD as a result of a QI project in their unit.[38] The rate of BPD in VLBW neonates was reduced by more than half by avoidance of intubation, adoption of new pulse oximeter limits, and early use of nasal CPAP therapy.

Nowadzky et al[39] used QI methods to reduce CLD by implementing nasal bubble CPAP to reduce mechanical ventilation. Although the group was successful in implementing the use of bubble CPAP, the rate of CLD was unchanged, and a concomitant increase in ROP rate was noted.

Merkel et al[40] reduced unplanned extubations from 2.38 to 0.41 per 100 patient-intubated days by having at least two staff members participate in procedures such as retaping and securing endotracheal tubes, weighing and transferring the patient out of the bed; placement of alert cards at the bedside indicating the risk level for an unplanned extubation, the security of the endotracheal tube, and the depth of placement at the gums along with documentation of proper care of the endotracheal tube; use of a commercial product to secure the endotracheal tube, education of staff by staff experts ("champions"); use of a real-time analysis form to identify causes of unplanned extubations; use of a centrally located display of the days since last unplanned extubation; and placing mittens or socks on infants' hands for intubated patients greater than 34 weeks' postmenstrual age. They suggest that the benchmark for unplanned extubation should be a rate less than 1 per 100 patient-intubated days.

Collaborative Quality Improvement Projects

One successful approach that has been used in neonatology by the VON is that of collaborative QI in which a group of neonatal units collaborate for the purpose of improving the quality of neonatal care.[41,42] With this approach, a team of personnel from each hospital (from multiple disciplines involved in neonatal care, such as neonatologists, nurses, respiratory therapists, and others) meet periodically, with ongoing collaboration in between meetings carried on by the use of e-mail and telephone calls among these team members. The network acts as a coordinator, facilitator, and motivator of this collaborative effort and provides expert faculty members who work with individual sets of teams to facilitate their improvement efforts.

VON has implemented a number of such collaborative projects called the Neonatal Intensive Care Quality (NICQ) projects. The major components of NICQ projects included multidisciplinary collaboration within and among hospitals, feedback of information from the network database regarding clinical practice and patient outcome, training and QI methods, site visits to project NICUs, benchmarking visits to superior performers within the network, identification and implementation of potentially better practices, and evaluation of the results. In the first NICQ project, teams from the 10 hospitals worked together in cross-institutional improvement groups.[42] Six NICUs focused on reducing nosocomial infection, and four units focused on reducing CLD. The potentially best practices that were proposed were based on an evidence review and careful analysis of other practices at best-performing centers. During the period of the project, from 1994 to 1996, the rate of infection with coagulase-negative *Staphylococcus* decreased from 22.0% to 16.6% at the six project NICUs in the infection group; the rate of supplemental oxygen at 36 weeks' adjusted gestational age decreased from 43.5% to 31.5% at the four NICUs in the CLD group. Another NICQ project was implemented in 16 centers of VON during 2001–2003 to reduce the incidence of BPD among VLBW neonates.[43] BPD rates dropped significantly in 2003 compared with the baseline year. In addition, severe ROP, severe intraventricular hemorrhage, and supplemental oxygen at discharge dropped significantly. VON reported anther QI project with an objective of promoting evidence-based surfactant treatment of preterm neonates.[44] Participating centers were randomized to control or intervention arm. Hospitals in intervention arm received QI advice including audit and feedback, evidence reviews, an interactive training workshop, and ongoing faculty support via conference calls and email. Although there was no significant difference in incidence of pneumothorax or mortality, neonates born in intervention hospitals were more likely to receive surfactant in delivery room or within 2 hours of birth.

Payne et al[45] reported the results over 9 years from eight NICUs that participated in a VON collaborative to reduce lung injury (the ReLI group). This group successfully decreased delivery room intubation, conventional ventilation, and the use of postnatal steroids for BPD. They increased the use of nasal CPAP, and survival to discharge increased. Nosocomial infections decreased. However, BPD-free survival remained unchanged, and the BPD rate increased.

In a cluster randomized trial done by the Canadian Neonatal Network,[46] six NICUs were assigned to reduce nosocomial infection (infection group) and six units to reduce BPD (pulmonary group). Practice change interventions were implemented using rapid-change cycles for 2 years. The incidence of BPD decreased in the pulmonary group, and the incidence of nosocomial infections decreased significantly in both the infection and pulmonary groups.

In a cluster-randomized QI trial, 14 centers of the National Institute of Child Health and Human Development Neonatal Research Network were randomized to intervention or control clusters.[47] Intervention centers implemented practices of three best-performing centers of the network to reduce rate of BPD. Although intervention centers successfully implemented practices of best-performing centers, the rate of BPD was not reduced in intervention or control centers. Explanations given for failure to reduce the rate of BPD were choosing interventions that were not evidence based and targeting a multifactorial disease with a single-prong strategy of reducing oxygen exposure.

In the past decade, statewide collaboratives have been developed in multiple US states where some or all NICUs in the state work collaboratively on the same clinical topics using QI methods, share data, and learn from each other to make improvements in clinical outcomes and processes. Such statewide collaboratives[48–51] have reported significant decreases in central line–associated bloodstream infections, and are targeting other clinical outcomes as well. Since 1995, QI collaboratives (QICs) have proliferated as an approach to shared learning and improvement in health care. A systematic review of published results of such QICs reported significant improvements in targeted clinical processes and patient outcomes[52]; however, not all institutions participating in QICs are successful in making sustained improvements. Suggestions about how to make QICs more successful, and how to adapt interventions for local context, have been made by experts.[53,54]

CONCLUSIONS

Every neonatal unit should monitor the quality of care provided using structural, process, and outcome measures. Such monitoring should help identify priority topics for improvement, and formal QI projects should be conducted to improve these priority topics. QI projects should be conducted by multidisciplinary teams using formal systematic methods and a framework such as the Model for Improvement. After specifying the aim, indicators of improvement should be defined and measured. Using evidence-based practices adapted to local context, changes that might plausibly lead to improvement should be selected and tested serially in PDSA cycles using quality metrics of improvement. QI teams should be supported by institutional leaders and provided with adequate resources. Participation in a multicenter collaborative project may enhance local QI projects.

EDITORIAL COMMENT: "Team cohesion, engagement of families, and culture of improvement supported by measurement and institutional support from the hospital are some of the key contextual and managerial features critical to high-quality NICU care."

Dhurjati R, Wahid N, Sigurdson, et al. Never judge a book by its cover: how NICU evaluators reach conclusions about quality of care. *J Perinatol* 2018;38:751–758.

2

Antenatal and Intrapartum Care of the High-Risk Infant

Felicia L. Bahadue, Kimberly S. Gecsi

Everything ought to be done to ensure that an infant be born at term, well developed, and in a healthy condition. But in spite of every care, infants are born prematurely.

Pierre Budin, The Nursling

IDENTIFICATION OF THE PREGNANCY AT RISK

The goal of prenatal care is to ensure optimal outcomes for both baby and mother. Prenatal care involves a series of assessments over time, as well as education and counseling that help guide the interventions that may be offered. A significant part of the process involves identifying a pregnancy as high risk. Early and accurate establishment of gestational age, identification of the patient at risk for complications, anticipation of complications, and the timely implementation of screening, diagnosis, and treatment help achieve these goals. The distinction between a high-risk and a low-risk pregnancy and/or mother gives the provider the opportunity to potentially intervene prior to the advent of adverse outcomes. This chapter will discuss the identification of the high-risk pregnancy, focusing on some of the more commonly encountered fetal and maternal conditions.

Many of the principal determinants of perinatal morbidity and mortality have been delineated. Included among these are maternal age, race, socioeconomic status, nutritional status, past obstetric history, family history, associated medical illness, and current pregnancy problems. Ideally, the process of risk identification is established prior to conception because this is the time when counseling for and against certain behaviors, foods and nutritional supplements, medications, work, and environmental risks is likely to have the most beneficial outcome.[1] Preparations can be made for certain medical and obstetrical conditions long before untoward effects have occurred. Therefore any such assessment should include a detailed history that involves elements of personal and demographic information; personal and familial medical, psychiatric, and genetic histories; past obstetrical, gynecological, menstrual, and surgical histories; current pregnancy history; domestic violence history; and drug and tobacco use history. The care provider should also assess for any barriers to care and whether the patient has any social concerns that would be better evaluated and managed by someone with social services expertise.[2]

Accurate estimation of date of delivery is crucial to the timing of interventions, monitoring fetal growth, and timing of delivery, as well as to overall management. This is usually calculated from the date of the last known menstrual period and can be confirmed by ultrasound (US) if dating is uncertain due to irregular menses or if conception occurred while on hormonal contraception. The American College of Obstetricians and Gynecologists (ACOG) considers first-trimester ultrasonography to be the most accurate method to establish or confirm gestational age. Pregnancies without an ultrasonographic examination confirming or revising the estimated due date before 22 0/7 weeks of gestation should be considered suboptimally dated.[3] A standard panel of tests is ordered for all pregnant women at their first prenatal visit. This workup is modified based on the woman's risk profile. What constitutes optimal prenatal care and performed by whom and how often may still be up for debate.[4] Screening and treatment of asymptomatic bacteriuria, group B beta-hemolytic *Streptococcus* (GBS), and sexually transmitted diseases for at-risk women to prevent the consequences of horizontal and vertical transmission is indicated. Screening should also be offered for fetal structural and chromosomal abnormalities, and women who are Rh(D) negative should receive anti-(D) immune globulin to prevent alloimmunization and reduce the risk of hemolytic disease of the newborn. Screening for malpresentation of the fetus, as well as development of preeclampsia in the mother, is also likely to have a great impact on pregnancy outcomes.

In the United States, about 12% to 13% of all live births are premature, and about 2% are born at less than 32 weeks' gestation.[5] Approximately 50% of these births are the result of spontaneous preterm labor, 30% from preterm rupture of membranes, and 20% from induced delivery secondary to maternal or fetal indications. Prematurity remains a significant perinatal problem because prematurity, along with the associated low birth weight, is the most significant contributor to infant mortality. Mortality increases with both decreasing gestational age and birth weight. Additional causes of mortality include congenital anomalies and delivering in a hospital with a lower level of resources and experience in providing

TABLE 2.1 **Scoring System[a] for Risk of Preterm Delivery**

	Socioeconomic Status	Past History	Daily Habits
1	Two children at home Low socioeconomic status	One abortion <1 year since last birth	Works outside home
2	<20 years >40 years Single parent	Two abortions	>10 cigarettes/day
3	Very low socioeconomic status Height <150 cm Weight <45 kg	Three abortions	Heavy work Long, tiring trip
4	<18 years	Pyelonephritis	
5		Uterine anomaly Second-trimester abortion Diethylstilbestrol exposure	
10		Premature delivery Repeated second-trimester abortion	

[a]Score is computed by addition of number of points given any item. 0–5 = Low risk; 6–9 = medium risk; ≥10 = high risk.
Adapted from Creasy R, Gummer B, Liggins G. System for predicting spontaneous preterm birth. *Obstet Gynecol* 1980; 55:692.

such complex neonatal care. Improvements in obstetric and neonatal care, including surfactant, antenatal steroids, and maternal transport to an appropriate delivery facility capable of caring for high-risk neonates, have decreased the mortality rates except in those at the limit of viability.

The goal remains to identify at-risk women as soon as possible. Careful analysis indicates that determinants of morbidity and mortality are composed of historical factors existing before pregnancy as well as factors and events associated directly with pregnancy. Historically, an attempt was made to put these together into some type of assessment technique capable of distinguishing most of the high-risk patients from the low-risk patients before delivery (Table 2.1). Unfortunately, when these scoring systems have been applied to a large population base, they have not resulted in significant changes in the prematurity rates. Still, the grouping of risk factors may be of some use to the obstetrical provider because it allows for the identification of the woman who might need additional surveillance, counseling, referral, and resources.

Birth Defects and Congenital Disorders

Birth defects affect approximately 2% to 4% of liveborn infants. Contributing factors include genetic and environmental influences such as maternal age, illness, industrial agents, intrauterine environment, infection, and drug exposure. The frequency of the various etiologies of birth defects can be broken down as follows: unknown and multifactorial origin, about 65% to 75%; genetic origin, about 25%; and environmental exposures, about 10% (Table 2.2).

TABLE 2.2 **Leading Categories of Birth Defects**

Birth Defect	Estimated Incidence (Births)
Structural/Metabolic	
Heart and circulation	1 in 115
Muscles and skeleton	1 in 130
Genital and urinary tract	1 in 135
Nervous system and eye	1 in 235
Chromosomal syndromes	1 in 600
Club foot	1 in 735
Down syndrome (trisomy 21)	1 in 900
Respiratory tract	1 in 900
Cleft lip/palate	1 in 930
Spina bifida	1 in 2000
Metabolic disorders	1 in 3500
Anencephaly	1 in 8000
Phenylketonuria (PKU)	1 in 12,000
Congenital Infections	
Congenital syphilis	1 in 2000
Congenital HIV infection	1 in 2700
Congenital rubella syndrome	1 in 100,000
Other	
Rh disease	1 in 1400
Fetal alcohol syndrome	1 in 1000

The terminology used to describe these anomalies is based on their underlying cause: malformation, deformation, disruption, and dysplasia. Dysmorphology is the study of individuals with abnormal features, and increased scholarship in this area has led to specialists who study birth defects and establish patterns. The result has been a better understanding of many conditions, which has improved the quality of counseling for families, including possible recurrence rates in future pregnancies.

Malformations are considered major if they have medical or social implications and they require surgical repair in many cases. Defects are considered to be minor if they have only cosmetic relevance. They can arise from genetic or environmental factors. Deformations are defects in the position of body parts arising from some intrauterine mechanical force that interferes with the normal formation of the organ or structure. Such uterine forces could include oligohydramnios, uterine malformations or tumors, and fetal crowding from multiple gestations. Disruptions refer to defects that result from the destruction of or interference with normal development. These are typically single events that may involve infection, vascular compromise, or mechanical factors. Amniotic band syndrome is the most common example of a disruption, and the timing occurs from 28 days' postconception to 18 weeks' gestation. Dysplasias are defects that result from the abnormal organization of cells into tissues. There are recognizable patterns in many congenital defects. The terminology

TABLE 2.3 Common Teratogens

Type of Teratogen	Agent	Defect
Chemical	Retinoic acid	Hydrocephalus, central nervous system (CNS) migrations
	Thalidomide	Limb reduction
	Valproic acid	Neural tube defects
	Phenytoin	Heart defects, nail hypoplasia, dysmorphic features
	Lithium	Ebstein anomaly
	Angiotensin-converting enzyme (ACE) inhibitors	Renal and skull defects
	Misoprostol	Fetal death, vascular disruptions
	DES (diethylstilbestrol)	Cervical cancer in daughters, genital anomalies in males and females
Physical	Ionizing radiation	Fetal death, growth restriction, leukemia
	Hyperthermia	Microcephaly, mental retardation, seizures
Biological	Cytomegalovirus	Microcephaly, mental retardation, deafness
	Toxoplasmosis	Hydrocephalus, mental retardation, chorioretinitis
Maternal	Diabetes	Congenital heart anomalies, neural tube defects, sacral anomalies
	Phenylketonuria (PKU)	Microcephaly, mental retardation

Adapted from Reece EA, Hobbins JC, eds. Developmental toxicology, drugs and fetal teratogenesis. In: *Clinical Obstetrics: The Fetus and Mother*. 3rd ed. Malden: Blackwell; 2008:215.

TABLE 2.4 Viral-Induced Teratogenesis and Selected Fetal Infections

Agent	Observed Effects	Exposure Risk
Cytomegalovirus (CMV)	Birth defects, low birth weight, developmental disorders	Healthcare workers, childcare workers
Hepatitis B virus	Low birth weight	Healthcare workers, household members, sexual activity
Human immunodeficiency virus (HIV)	Low birth weight, childhood cancers, lifelong disease	Healthcare workers, sexual partners
Human parvovirus B19	Miscarriage, fetal heart failure	Healthcare workers, childcare workers
Rubella (German measles)	Birth defects, low birth weight	Healthcare workers, childcare workers
Toxoplasmosis	Miscarriage, birth defects, developmental disorders	Animal care workers, veterinarians
Varicella zoster virus (chicken pox)	Birth defects, low birth weight	Healthcare workers, childcare workers
Herpes simplex virus	Late transmission, skin lesions, convulsions, systemic disease	Sexual activity

Adapted from Reese EA, Hobbins JC, eds. Teratogenic infections. In: *Clinical Obstetrics: The Fetus and Mother*. 3rd ed. Malden: Blackwell; 2008:248.

to describe these patterns includes syndrome, sequence, association, and developmental field defect.

The study of congenital malformations caused by environmental or drug exposure is called teratology. An agent that causes an abnormality in the function or structure of a fetus is called a teratogen (Table 2.3). About 4% to 6% of birth defects are caused by teratogens, and include maternal illnesses, infectious agents, physical agents and drugs, and chemical agents. Timing of exposure to the agent plays a great role in the resulting malformation. Exposure during the first 10 to 14 days' postconception can result in cell death and spontaneous miscarriage. The all-or-none theory refers to the possibility that if only a few cells are damaged, then the other cells may compensate for their loss and result in no abnormality. Most effects are seen after fertilization, but exposure prior to conception can cause genetic mutations. Mechanisms of teratogenesis are varied and include cell death, altered cell growth, proliferation, migration, and interaction. The embryo is most vulnerable during the period of organogenesis, and this occurs up to the 8th week postconception, but certain organ systems, including the eye, central nervous system (CNS), genitalia, and hematopoietic systems, continue to develop through the fetal stage and remain susceptible.

Maternal illness that can present a teratogenic risk involves conditions in which a metabolite or antibody travels across the placenta and affects the fetus. Maternal illness can include pregestational diabetes, phenylketonuria, androgen-producing tumors, maternal obesity, and systemic lupus erythematosus. The mother may be infected but asymptomatic. Ultrasonic findings suggestive of fetal infection include microcephaly, cerebral and/or hepatic calcifications, intrauterine growth restriction (IUGR), hepatosplenomegaly, cardiac malformations, limb hypoplasia, hydrocephalus, and hydrops. Maternal fever or hyperthermia has also been associated with teratogenesis when it occurs in the first trimester, and may be associated with miscarriage and/or neural tube defects (NTDs) (Table 2.4).[6]

Maternal ingestion of certain drugs can cause birth defects or adverse fetal outcomes. It is important that nonpregnant women are counseled about the need for contraception when using a medication that is classified as category X by the U.S. Food and Drug Administration. Maternal exposure to numerous physical and environmental agents has also been implicated as a cause of birth defects. High plasma levels of lead, mercury, and other heavy metals have been associated with CNS damage and negative neurobehavioral effects in infants and children.[7] More controversial are the recent concerns over maternal exposure to so-called endocrine disruptors, bisphenol A phthalates, and airborne polycyclic aromatic hydrocarbons. These entities are chemicals that mimic the action of naturally occurring hormones such as estrogen. These chemicals can be found in pesticides, leaching from plastics found in water and infant bottles, medical devices, personal care products, tobacco smoke, and other materials. Exposure to them is widespread, and a large portion of the population has measurable levels.[8] The chemicals have been associated with adverse changes in behavior, the brain, male and female reproductive systems, and mammary glands.

Our knowledge of the effects of ionizing radiation on the fetus has been based on case reports and extrapolation of data from survivors of atomic bombs and nuclear reactor accidents. Radiation exposure during pregnancy is a clinical issue when diagnostic imaging in a pregnant woman is required. Possible hazards of radiation exposure include: pregnancy loss, congenital malformation, disturbances of growth and/or development, and carcinogenic effects.[9] The U.S. Nuclear Regulatory Commission recommends that occupational radiation exposure of pregnant women not exceed 5 mGy (500 mrad) to the fetus during the entire pregnancy. Diagnostic procedures typically expose the fetus to less than 0.05 Gy (5 rad), and there is no evidence of an increased risk of fetal anomalies or adverse neurologic outcome.

Diagnostic X-rays of the head, neck, chest, and limbs do not result in any measurable exposure to the embryo/fetus, but it is advised that the pregnant woman wear a shield for such studies. Fetal exposure from nonabdominal pelvic computed tomography (CT) scans is minimal, but again, the pregnant woman should have her abdomen shielded. US imaging has demonstrated no untoward biologic effects on the fetus or mother because the acoustic output does not generate harmful levels of heat. US has been used extensively since the 1980s. Magnetic resonance imaging (MRI) also has not demonstrated any negative effects.

Genetic Origins

Chromosomal abnormalities affect about 1 of 140 live births. In addition, approximately 50% of spontaneous abortions have an abnormal chromosomal pattern. More than 90% of fetuses with chromosomal abnormalities do not survive to term. In fetuses with congenital anomalies, the prevalence of chromosomal abnormalities ranges from 2% to 35%.[10] A comprehensive three-generation family history and ethnic origin assessment should be taken, whether evaluating preconceptionally or after birth. Congenital anomalies of a genetic origin can be sporadic or heritable and have a number of etiologies. They can involve nondisjunction, nonallelic homologous recombination, inversions, deletions and duplications, and translocations. Infants are also at a risk for having birth defects if their parents are carriers of genetic mutations. This single gene transmission pattern in humans follows three typical patterns: autosomal dominant, autosomal recessive, and x-linked conditions. These typically follow traditional Mendelian genetics. Non-Mendelian patterns of transmission include unstable DNA and fragile X syndrome, imprinting, mitochondrial inheritance, germline or gonadal mosaicism, and multifactorial inheritance. The most common genetic disorders for which prenatal screening may be offered are trisomy 21, trisomy 18, hemoglobinopathies (such as hemoglobin C disease, hemoglobin SC disease, sickle cell anemia, thalassemia), cystic fibrosis, fragile X syndrome, and a variety of disorders seen most commonly in the Ashkenazi Jewish population.

EDITORIAL COMMENT: Whole gene sequencing has not only provided the ability to quickly solve complex disorders but has also helped attribute underlying genetic changes to what were formerly thought of as disorders of unknown etiology.

Prenatal Genetic Testing for Trisomy 21. Caring for a child or adult with special needs has a significant impact on a couple and family. Down syndrome is the most common chromosomal abnormality causing mental disability in the United States. In addition to cognitive deficits, these children are also at risk for congenital heart disease, duodenal atresia, urinary tract malformations, epilepsy, and leukemia. Prenatal testing for chromosomal abnormalities is a matter of weighing the risks of the genetic condition in question with the ultimate risks of the tests available to identify that abnormality. This should include the risks of a false-negative result in an affected pregnancy and the false-positive result in the unaffected pregnancy and the possible riskier diagnostic tests that may follow. Since the late 2000s, the ability to more effectively and safely diagnose Down syndrome has improved.

Prenatal testing for Down syndrome has moved away from the traditional invasive diagnostic testing based on age alone. Presently, a combination of maternal blood tests and US screening provides women with choices beyond routine chorionic villus sampling (CVS) or amniocentesis. Optimally, this prenatal screening should minimize the number of women identified as screen positive while maximizing the overall detection rate. These screening tests therefore require a high sensitivity and a low false-positive rate. The improvements in testing have achieved this and ultimately reduced the number of invasive tests performed and, in turn, decreased the rate of procedure-related losses. Historically, the first screening tests used maternal age as a cutoff for risk assessment because the prevalence of trisomy 21 rises with age. Women aged 35 and

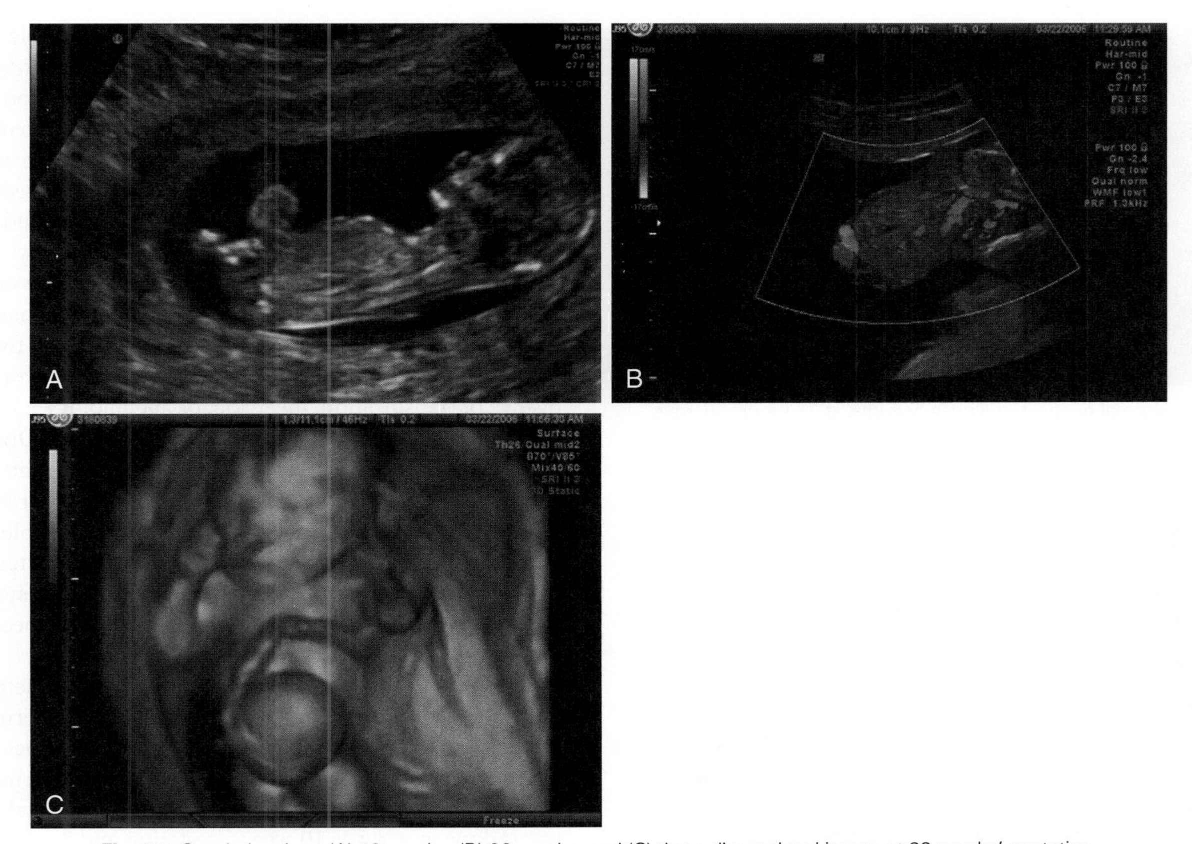

Fig. 2.1 Omphalocele at (A) 12 weeks, (B) 26 weeks, and (C) three-dimensional image at 22 weeks' gestation.

above were eligible for screening based on a cost-benefit analysis and an attempt to match the risk of an affected fetus with a procedure-related loss. Screening based on this parameter of advanced maternal age (AMA) alone had a detection rate of about 30%, with a false-positive rate of 5% when implemented in the 1970s.

From 1974 to 2002, the mean age of women giving birth in the United States increased from 24.4 to 27.4 years, and the percentage of women aged 35 years and older at birth increased from 4.7% to 13.8%. Using AMA as the main parameter became less efficacious.[11] In 1984, the association between aneuploidy and low levels of maternal serum alpha-fetoprotein (MS-AFP) was reported. In 1987, the association between high maternal serum human chorionic gonadotropin (hCG) value and a low conjugated estriol level in Down syndrome pregnancies was reported. In 1988, this information was first integrated and called the "triple screen test." Combining MS-AFP, hCG, and unconjugated estriol values with maternal age risk and performing it between 15 and 22 weeks' gestation doubled the age-related detection rate to 60% and maintained the false-positive rate at 5%. The test is considered positive when the result, stated as an estimate of risk, is above the set cutoff range. This is usually about 1:270 and based on the second-trimester age-related risk of a 35-year-old woman. In 1996, the "quad screen" was created when the level of inhibin-A was added to the triple screen. This test has a detection rate of 76% and a false-positive rate that remains at 5%.

Since the 1980s, the addition of ultrasonography to the practice of obstetrics has allowed for the detection of significant fetal abnormalities prior to delivery (Fig. 2.1). About 20% to 27% of second-trimester fetuses with Down syndrome have a major anatomic abnormality.[12] Over time, sonographic markers were identified that, when present, increase the likelihood that a chromosomal abnormality may exist. The risk increases as the number of markers increases. Sonographic markers are seen in 50% to 80% of fetuses with Down syndrome. The most common markers are cardiac defects, increased nuchal fold thickness, hyperechoic bowel, shortened extremities, and renal pyelectasis. When a second-trimester US is performed to search for these markers, it is called a "genetic sonogram." The overall sensitivity of this US is 70% to 85%.

Nuchal translucency is a standard US technique and is most accurately measured in skilled hands between 10 to 14 weeks' gestation (Figs. 2.2 and 2.3). There is a direct correlation between an increased measurement and a risk for Down syndrome, other aneuploidy, and major structural malformations.[13] In fact, a very large nuchal translucency suggests a very high risk for aneuploidy. Down syndrome, trisomy 18, and Turner syndrome are the most likely chromosomal abnormalities, and cardiac defects are the most likely malformations.

Serum genetic screening and genetic sonography evolved into a combined testing approach. With this method, the sensitivity of Down syndrome screening increased, whereas the false-positive rate decreased. The rationale involves modifying the prior maternal age risk up or down. If the pattern seen

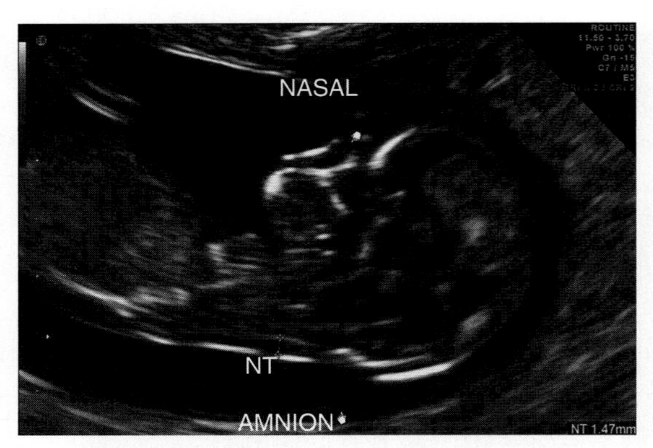

Fig. 2.2 Normal nuchal translucency width at 11 weeks, 6 days.

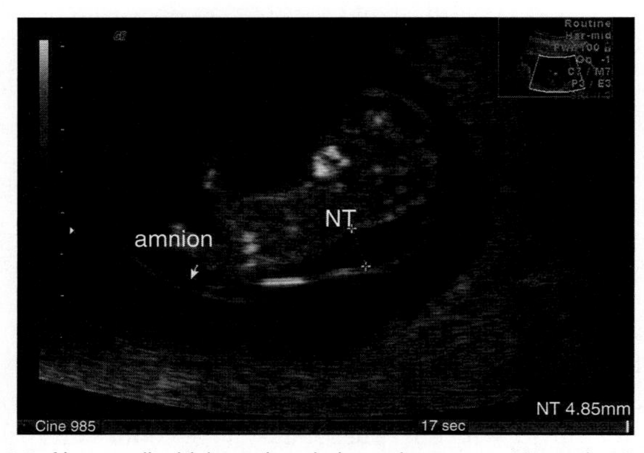

Fig. 2.3 Abnormally thickened nuchal translucency at 10 weeks, 5 days.

is similar to the pattern in a Down syndrome pregnancy, then the risk is increased; if it is the opposite, then it is decreased. The magnitude of this difference is expressed in multiples of the median (MoM), and it determines how much the risk is modified. For sonographic markers, the magnitude of these differences is measured by a likelihood ratio (LR = sensitivity/false-positive rate) that is then multiplied by the a priori risk.

This next phase of screening became the "first-trimester screening" protocol. The US component involves the sonographic measurement of the nuchal translucency. If this measurement is increased for the gestational age, it can indicate an affected fetus. This is an operator-dependent measurement, but it has demonstrated a 62% to 92% detection rate. The serum markers that are measured are maternal serum beta-hCG and maternal serum pregnancy-associated plasma protein A (PAPP-A). In the first trimester, pregnancies in which the fetus has Down syndrome have higher levels of hCG and lower levels of PAPP-A than do unaffected pregnancies. This combination of maternal age, nuchal translucency, hCG, and PAPP-A is now the standard first-trimester screening and is called the "first-trimester combined test." It has a detection rate of 85% and a false-positive rate of 5%. This is better than the quadruple screen detection rate of 80% and false-positive rate of 5%, and therefore it became the recommended screen for women who presented early in pregnancy.

It makes sense to offer Down syndrome screening as early in pregnancy as possible. Performed between 11 and 13 weeks' gestation, the first-trimester screening combined test provides for as early an evaluation and diagnosis as possible for fetal abnormalities. It also provides for maximum decision-making time and adjustment, privacy, and safer termination options if desired. One of the issues with such sophisticated screening protocols is the timing and availability of such methods. The ACOG recommends that all women be offered screening before 20 weeks' gestation, and all women should have an option of invasive testing regardless of age.[14] They also recommend that prenatal fetal karyotyping should be offered to women of any age with a history of another pregnancy with trisomy 21 or other aneuploidy, at least one major or two minor anomalies in the present pregnancy, or a personal or partner history of translocation, inversion, or aneuploidy.

The impact of prenatal screening is significant. During this age of first-trimester screening, the number of amniocentesis and CVS procedures performed has dropped. In areas where Down syndrome screening tests have been implemented, there has been an increase in the detection of affected fetuses and a drop in the number of live births with Down syndrome.

Major advances in aneuploidy screening have been made. Noninvasive prenatal screening (NIPS) evaluates cell-free DNA from maternal blood to screen for a variety of fetal conditions. The fetal component of cell-free DNA in maternal blood is mainly from apoptotic placental cells. Not only does cell-free DNA screen for aneuploidies, but it also can determine fetal sex, an Rh-positive fetus, and some genetic abnormalities. The test is done as early as 10 weeks' gestation and has the highest detection rate for Down syndrome at 98%. Advantages of NIPS are the ease and accuracy of the test. The main disadvantage is that it is still a screening test, and many women may choose to have it done over more invasive testing, leading to a delay in diagnosis and management of fetal aneuploidy.[15]

EDITORIAL COMMENT: Vanstone[a] reported that women who have had personal experience with noninvasive pregnancy testing (NIPT) have concerns and priorities that sometimes contrast dramatically with the theoretical ethics literature. NIPT raises many ethical issues. It is important to communicate effectively with patients undergoing NIPT and to address their fears and concerns. In addition to the diagnosis of fetal aneuploidy, NIPS is valuable for families with neurofibromatosis and cystic fibrosis, among many other single-gene anomalies. Clausen[b] noted that with noninvasive prenatal testing of cell-free DNA, predicting the fetal *Rh(D)* type has become highly feasible based on analysis of the fetal *Rh(D)* gene. Fetal *Rh(D)* screening can guide targeted antenatal prophylaxis, treating only women who carry an *Rh(D)*-positive fetus, thereby avoiding the unnecessary treatment of approximately 40% of the Rh(D)-negative women. Fetal *Rh(D)* screening is highly accurate, so that from gestational week 10, sensitivities are approximately 99%, and its future widespread use is expected.

[a]Vanstone M, Cernat A, Nisker J, Schwartz L. Women's perspectives on the ethical implications of non-invasive prenatal testing: a qualitative analysis to inform health policy decisions. *BMC Med Ethics.* 2018;19(1):27.

[b]Clausen FB. Lessons learned from the implementation of non-invasive fetal RhD screening. *Expert Rev Mol Diagn.* 2018;19:1-9.

Prenatal Screening for Trisomy 18. Trisomy 18 is also called Edwards syndrome and is the second most common autosomal trisomy, occurring in 1 in 8000 births. Many fetuses with trisomy 18 die in utero, and so the prevalence of this abnormality is three to five times higher in the first and second trimesters than at birth. Prenatal screening for trisomy 18 is included with screening for Down syndrome. The analyte pattern of the first-trimester test is a very low beta-hCG and a very low PAPP-A with an increased nuchal translucency.[16] Advanced maternal age increases the risk of having a pregnancy affected with trisomy 18. These fetuses have an extensive clinical spectrum disorder, and many organ systems can be affected. Fifty percent of these infants die within the first week of life, and only 5% to 10% survive the first year of life. The combined and integrated tests are especially effective at detecting these affected pregnancies. The earliest detection provides for the most comprehensive counseling and earliest intervention, if desired.

Prenatal Screening for Neural Tube Defects. The incidence of NTDs in the United States is considered to be highly variable because it depends on geographic factors and ethnic background. Typically seen in 1 in 1000 pregnancies, they are considered to be the second most prevalent congenital anomaly in the United States, with only cardiac anomalies occurring more often. It has been recommended by ACOG that screening for NTDs should be offered to all pregnant women. The American College of Medical Genetics also recommends screening using the MS-AFP and/or ultrasonography between 15 and 20 weeks' gestation.[17]

The majority of NTDs are isolated malformations caused by multiple factors such as folic acid deficiency, drug exposure, excessive vitamin A intake, maternal diabetes mellitus, maternal hyperthermia, and obesity. A genetic origin is also suggested by the fact that a high concordance rate is found in monozygotic twins. NTDs are also more common in first-degree relatives and are seen more often in females than males. Family history also supports a genetic mode of transmission. The recurrence risk for NTDs is about 2% to 4% when there is one affected sibling and as high as 10% when there are two affected siblings.[18] There is also some evidence that NTDs are associated with the genetic variance seen in the homocysteine pathways (*MTHFR* gene) and the *VANGL1* gene.[19] There is also a high prevalence of other karyotypic abnormalities, and trisomy 18 is typically the most common aneuploidy found.

In the 1970s and through the 1980s, maternal serum screening programs were instituted and combined with preconception supplementation with folic acid. In the 1990s, folic acid food fortification was implemented. During this time, screening protocols were also instituted, and initially they involved just the MS-AFP and amniocentesis for abnormal results and then went on to include sonography. Where these methods were employed, a decrease in the prevalence of NTDs was seen—largely due to the prevention of preconceptual folic acid deficiency in women.[20]

Screening for open NTDs typically involves the MS-AFP, which is most optimally drawn between 16 and 18 weeks' gestation. It is made by the fetal yolk sac, gastrointestinal tract, and liver, and is a fetal-specific globulin. It is similar to albumin and can be found in the maternal serum, amniotic fluid (from fetal urine), and fetal plasma. It is found in much lower concentrations in the maternal serum than in the amniotic fluid or fetal plasma. The primary intent is to detect open spina bifida and anencephaly, but when concentrations are abnormal, it can also suggest the presence of other nonneural abnormalities such as ventral wall defects.

For each gestational week, these results are expressed as MoM. A value above 2.0 to 2.5 MoM is considered abnormal. Some characteristics can significantly affect the interpretation of the results. A screen performed before 15 weeks and after 20 weeks' gestation will falsely raise or lower the MoM. Maternal weight affects the results because the AFP is diluted in the larger blood volume of obese women.[21] Women with diabetes mellitus have an increased risk of NTDs, and so their threshold value has to be adjusted to give a more accurate sensitivity. The presence of other fetal anomalies increases the level of the MS-AFP. The MoM level also has to be adjusted in pregnancies with multiple gestations because the MS-AFP level is proportional to the number of fetuses. Race can affect the results of the MS-AFP: African American women have a baseline level that is 10% higher than that of non–African American women. Finally, MS-AFP cannot be interpreted in the face of fetal death; therefore it cannot be used as a screening method when there is a nonviable fetus present in a multiple gestation.

US can potentially detect more NTDs than MS-AFP.[22] Detection rates depend on the type of anomaly and the trimester during which it is used. One large cohort study found that US detected 100% of NTDs and that MS-AFP was not as useful as previously believed.[23] Anencephaly and encephalocele have detection rates between 80% and 90% in the first trimester, whereas detection rates of over 90% for spina bifida are not seen until the second trimester.[24] Although the vast majority of NTDs can be seen on US and the sensitivity of the US evaluation is high, the ultimate diagnosis depends on the position of the fetus, the size and location of the defect, the maternal body habitus, and the skill of the ultrasonographer.

Women who have a screen-positive pregnancy will be counseled to undergo an US to document accurate gestational age, fetal viability, and possible presence of multiple gestation. A detailed anatomic survey of the fetus will also be performed. The use of amniocentesis may also be employed if there is some discrepancy found on US that does not explain the abnormal MS-AFP. Elevations in both amniotic fluid AFP and amniotic fluid acetylcholinesterase suggests an open NTD with almost 96% accuracy. There is some conflict today regarding the use of amniocentesis, and some experts believe that US alone should be used, given its high detection rate, absent procedure loss rate, and cost-savings advantage. ACOG now recommends a second-trimester US between 18–22 weeks' gestation to screen for anomalies, including NTDs. First-trimester US may detect some NTDs, but the rate of detection is much lower than with second-trimester ultrasonography.[25] MRI of the fetus can also be used when there is some factor that is interfering with US diagnosis of the defect.[26] This additional modality can be of great significance when planning for potential fetal or neonatal surgery, route of delivery, and overall counseling of the parents.

Fetal surgery for myelomeningocele was studied in a randomized trial comparing outcomes of in utero repair to standard postnatal repair.[27] The trial was stopped early because of the improvements seen with prenatal surgery. A composite outcome of fetal or neonatal death or the need for placement of cerebrospinal fluid shunt by the age of 12 months was seen in 98% of the postnatal surgery group versus 68% of the infants in the prenatal surgery group. Prenatal surgery, however, was associated with more preterm delivery as well as uterine dehiscence at delivery.

EDITORIAL COMMENT: Formerly, screening was largely focused on trisomy 21 and on neural tube defects. A new comprehensive paradigm that provides information on all three groups of genetic disorders, chromosomal, submicroscopic and single-gene, causing intellectual and neurodevelopmental disability has become the common approach.

In reviewing trends in birth defects in Europe between 1980 and 2012, despite efforts in prevention by means of folic acid supplementation, no decrease in neural tube defects was detected.[a]

[a]Morris JK, Springett AL, Greenlees R, et al. Trends in congenital anomalies in Europe from 1980 to 2012. *PLoS One.* 2018;13(4):e0194986.

Multiple Gestation

Multiple gestation has been increasing in the United States. In the most recent data for 2014, the twin birth rate was 33.9 per 1000 births. The rate was stable between the years 2009 and 2012 and then rose 2% from 2012 to 2013. The rate remained stable in 2014, with an observed rise of almost 80% between 1980 and 2009. The likely reasons for the increasing numbers of multiple births are the increasing maternal age at childbirth and the use of assisted reproductive technology (ART). Maternal age, ART, parity, race, geographic origin, family history, and maternal weight and height have all been associated with an increased risk of twins.

Zygosity is an important concept for multiple gestation. Twins are most commonly referred to as either di- or monozygotic. Dizygotic twins result from ovulation and fertilization of two separate oocytes. Monozygotic twins result from the ovulation and fertilization of one oocyte followed by division of the zygote. The timing of the egg division determines placentation. Diamniotic, dichorionic placentation occurs with division prior to the morula stage. Diamniotic, monochorionic placentation occurs with division between days 4 and 8 postfertilization. Monoamniotic, monochorionic placentation occurs with division between days 8 and 12 postfertilization. Division after day 12 results in conjoined twins. Placentation is typically dichorionic for dizygotic twins and can be mono- or dichorionic for monozygotic twins. Sixty-nine percent of naturally occurring twins are dizygotic, whereas 31% are monozygotic. Dizygotic twins are also more common with ART pregnancies and account for 95% of all twins conceived with ART.

Chorionicity is also an important concept because the presence of monochorionicity places those monozygotic twins at an increased risk for complications: twin-to-twin transfusion syndrome, twin anemia-polycythemia sequence, twin reversed arterial perfusion (TRAP) sequence, and selective IUGR.[28] The risk of neurologic morbidity and perinatal mortality in these twins is higher than that of dichorionic twins.

Early US assessment is a reliable way to not only diagnose multiple gestation but also to establish amnionicity and chorionicity. It provides accurate assessment of gestational age, which can be of vital importance, given the risk of preterm birth and intrauterine growth abnormalities in multiple gestation. The optimal time for this US would be in the first and early second trimester. Offering early US can also include screening for Down syndrome because each fetus is at the same risk for having a chromosomal abnormality based on maternal age and family history, and all women should be offered options for risk assessment. Maternal serum analyte interpretation can be difficult in multiple gestation because all fetuses, living or not, contribute to the concentration. Measurement of the nuchal translucency can improve the detection rate by helping identify the affected fetus. The first trimester combined test can be offered to the woman carrying multiples when CVS is available.

Although twins are not predisposed to any one type of congenital anomaly, monozygotic twins are two to three times more likely to have structural defects than singletons and dizygotic twins. Anencephaly, holoprosencephaly, bladder exstrophy, VATER association (***v***ertebral defects, imperforate ***a***nus, ***t***racheo***e***sophageal fistula, ***r***adial and ***r***enal dysplasia), sacrococcygeal teratoma, and sirenomelia are the anomalies seen with increasing frequency. Most often, the co-twin is structurally normal. The diagnosis of an anomalous twin is especially problematic if management might require early delivery or therapy that ultimately affects both twins. In the setting of conjoined twins, this process is even more complicated. The incidence is 1 in 50,000 live births, but given the high rate of stillbirth, the true incidence is 1 in 200,000 live births.[29] Additional causes for concern in monozygotic twins are monochorionic placentas that have vascular connections. The connections occur frequently and can lead to artery-to-artery shunts and, ultimately, the TRAP sequence with reversed arterial perfusion. This results in the fetal malformation, acardiac twins. Acardia is lethal in the affected twin, but also can result in a mortality rate of 50% to 75% in the donor twin. This condition occurs in about 1% of monozygotic twins.

Growth restriction and premature birth are major causes of the higher morbidity and mortality in twins compared to singletons. The growth curve of twins deviates from that of singletons after 32 weeks' gestation, and 15% to 30% of twin gestations may have growth abnormalities. This is more likely to be seen in monochorionic twins, but discordant growth can be seen in dichorionic twins depending on the placental surface area available to each. Twin growth should be monitored with serial US, and if there is evidence of discordance, then additional evaluation is needed. Starting in the second trimester, monochorionic pregnancies are followed every 2 to 3 weeks, whereas dichorionic pregnancies are followed every 4 to 6 weeks. There is no consensus on the optimal definition of discordance, because a difference of 15% to 40% has been found to be predictive of a poor outcome.[30] Presently, an estimated fetal weight (EFW) below the 10th percentile using singleton growth curves or a 20% discordance in EFW between the twins is the working definition of abnormal growth. Doppler velocimetry of the umbilical artery can be added to the US evaluation and may improve the detection rate of growth restriction.

The risk of preterm birth is higher for multiple gestations than for singletons, and represents the most serious risk to these pregnancies. When compared to singletons, the risk of preterm birth for twins and triplets was five and nine times higher, respectively. As the number of fetuses increases, the gestational age at the time of birth decreases. In 2008, the average gestational ages were 35.3, 32, 30.7, and 28.5 weeks' gestation for twins, triplets, quadruplets, and quintuplets and higher-order multiples, respectively. The rate of preterm birth for twins in the United States in 2008 was 59% before 37 weeks' gestation and 12% before 32 weeks' gestation. Additionally, 57% of these twins were of low birth weight (<2500 g), and 10% were of very low birth weight (<1500 g). Interestingly, the outcomes after delivery are similar between twins and singletons born prematurely.[31] Preterm premature rupture of membranes is also a cause of preterm birth in multiple gestations and most often occurs in the presenting sac, but can occur in the nonpresenting twin. It seems that multiple gestations have a shorter period of latency before delivery when compared to singleton gestations.

Triplet Gestation

The incidence of natural spontaneous triplet births is about 1 in 8000. Triplet pregnancy has a higher risk of maternal, fetal, and neonatal morbidity than does twin pregnancy. As the number of fetuses increases to that of the higher-order multiples, these risks increase even more significantly. Some consequences found more often in these pregnancies include growth restriction, fetal death, preterm labor, premature preterm rupture of membranes, preterm birth, neonatal neurologic impairment, pregnancy-related hypertension, eclampsia, abruption, placenta previa, and cesarean delivery.[32]

Diagnosis of a triplet or higher-order multiple gestation is done by US, and most instances are found in the first trimester because the vast majority of these pregnancies are conceived via ART. As with twin pregnancy, chorionicity identification is important. Monozygotic gestations can occur even though most of these pregnancies originate from three or more separate oocytes, especially in those that are spontaneously conceived. Spontaneous loss is common, and it occurs in 53% of triplet pregnancies. Given the inherent increased maternal and fetal risks involved with these pregnancies, historically, fetal reduction has been offered in hopes that fewer fetuses would translate into a reduced risk. Higher gestational ages at delivery, lower rates of gestational diabetes and preterm labor, and reduced hospital stay length have been the result for women electing to reduce a triplet pregnancy to twins.[33]

The risk of premature delivery or fetal death in utero of one fetus is specific to multiple gestation. The surviving fetus(es) is (are) affected by the chorionicity and the number of fetuses. There is an ethical dilemma not seen in singleton pregnancies because one must weigh the benefits for the affected fetus against the risks of the potential interventions to the remaining fetus(es). Typically, delivery before 26 weeks' gestation is not considered because the risk of mortality is significant for all fetuses. After 32 weeks' gestation, it is appropriate to move to deliver all if one is at risk because the morbidity is considered low. Between 26 and 32 weeks' gestation is a more difficult period and remains a time when parental preference is taken into great consideration after counseling has occurred. Chorionicity helps guide delivery when fetal death occurs because optimal management is unclear. As with twins, the risk is associated with monochorionicity and mortality is higher when this fetal demise occurs later in pregnancy.

A majority of triplets are born prematurely; 95% of them weigh less than 2500 g (low birth weight), and 35% are less than 1500 g (very low birth weight). The primary cause of these preterm births is premature labor. Multiple protocols have failed to reduce the risk of preterm birth, including decreased activity, bed rest hospitalization, home uterine activity monitoring, and tocolysis. Unfortunately, elective cerclage, progesterone supplementation, and sonographic cervical assessment also do not seem to have reduced the spontaneous preterm birth rate.

Although great strides have been made in the management of the neonate, the goal remains to reduce the risk and numbers of preterm birth or at least uncover a reliable method to predict women at the highest risk of developing preterm labor or premature rupture of membranes. This will be discussed in more detail in a separate section.

Antepartum Assessment of the Fetal Condition

Improved physiologic understanding and multiple technologic advancements provide the obstetrician with tools for objective evaluation of the fetus. In particular, specific information can be sought and obtained relative to maternal health and risk, fetal anatomy, growth, well-being, and functional maturity, and these data are used to provide a rational approach to clinical management of the high-risk infant before birth. It is important to emphasize that no procedure or laboratory result can supplant the data obtained from a careful history and physical examination, and these have to be interpreted in light of the true or presumed gestational age of the fetus. The initial prenatal examination and subsequent physical examinations are approached with these facts in mind to ascertain whether the uterine size and growth are consistent with the supposed length of gestation. In the era prior to routine US dating, the milestones of quickening (16 to 18 weeks' gestation) and fetal heart tone auscultation by Doppler US (12 to 14 weeks' gestation) were important and needed to be systematically recorded. Although most of this information is gathered early in pregnancy, the significance may not be appreciated until later in gestation when decisions regarding the appropriateness of fetal size and the timing of delivery are contemplated.

Ultrasonography

A clear role for antenatal US has been established in dating pregnancies, diagnosing multiple gestations, monitoring intrauterine growth, and detecting congenital malformations. It is

BOX 2.1 Uses of Ultrasound

- Confirmation of pregnancy
- Determination of:
  - Gestational age
  - Fetal number, chorionicity, presentation
  - Placental location, placentation
  - Fetal anatomy (previous malformations)
- Assessment of:
  - Size/date discrepancy
  - Fetal well-being (biophysical profile, Doppler measurements of umbilical vessels, middle cerebral artery)
  - Volume of amniotic fluid (suspected oligohydramnios or polyhydramnios)
  - Fetal arrhythmias
  - Fetal anatomy (abnormal alpha-fetoprotein)
- Assist with procedures:
  - CVS, PUBS
  - External version
  - Amniocentesis
  - Intrauterine transfusion

CVS, Chorionic villus sampling; *PUBS*, percutaneous umbilical blood sampling.

also integral to locating the placental site and documenting any pelvic organ abnormalities. US is valuable when performing CVS or amniocentesis. US may be used during labor to detect problems related to vaginal bleeding, size or date discrepancies, suspected abnormal presentation, amniotic fluid levels, loss of fetal heart tones (FHT), delivery of a twin, attempted version of a breech presentation, and diagnosis of fetal anomalies.

US is a technique by which short pulses (2 μsec) of high-frequency (approximately 2.5 MHz), low-intensity sound waves are transmitted from a piezoelectric crystal (transducer) through the maternal abdomen to the uterus and the fetus. The echo signals reflected back from tissue interfaces provide a two-dimensional picture of the uterine wall, placenta, amniotic fluid, and fetus. Some indications for US are contained in Box 2.1. In certain instances, US is performed to comply with the mother's request only.

As noted earlier, gestational age is most accurately determined the earlier it is performed during pregnancy. In the first trimester, the gestational age of the fetus is assessed by a crown-to-rump measurement, and this is the most accurate means for US dating.[34] After the 13th week of gestation, measurement of the fetal biparietal diameter (BPD) or cephalometry is the most commonly used technique. Before 20 weeks' gestation, this measurement provides a good estimation of gestational age within a range of plus or minus 10 days. After 20 weeks' gestation, the predictability of the measurement is less reliable, so an initial examination should be obtained before this time whenever possible. Such early examination also assists in interpretation of prenatal genetic screening as well as in detection of major malformations. Follow-up examinations can then be done to ascertain whether fetal growth in utero is proceeding at a normal rate.

EDITORIAL COMMENT: In countries with greater access to prenatal care, the problem of attending a delivery with uncertain gestational age occurs much less frequently.[4]

When fetal growth is restricted, however, brain sparing may result in an abnormal ratio of growth between the head and the rest of the body. Because the BPD may then be within normal limits, other measurements are needed to detect the true restriction of growth. The measurement of the ratio between the circumferences of head and abdomen is particularly valuable under these circumstances.[35]

Femur length (FL), which may be less affected by alterations in growth than the head or abdomen, is used to aid in determining gestational age and to identify the fetus with abnormal growth. Serial assessment of growth and deviations from normal, including both macrosomia and growth restriction, helps identify the fetus at risk during the perinatal period. Calculation of EFW based on various fetal biometric parameters (BPD, head circumference [HC], abdominal circumference [AC], and FL) plotted against gestational age using various sonographic nomograms is an extremely useful method for serial assessment of fetal growth. Sophisticated computer software to serially plot EFW and provide percentile ranking of a given fetus is commonly used.

Three-dimensional and four-dimensional ultrasonography have added technological advancement to the imaging possibilities. Using these modalities, the volume of the targeted anatomic area can be acquired and displayed. When the vectors have been formatted, the anatomy can be demonstrated topographically. This has been a promising technique for delineating malformations of the fetal face, neural tube, and skeletal systems, but proof of clinical advantage over two-dimensional sonography is still lacking.

Antepartum Surveillance

Early identification of any risk for neurologic injury or fetal death is the primary goal of any fetal assessment technique. The process of antenatal assessment was introduced to help pursue this underlying risk of fetal jeopardy and thereby prevent adverse outcomes. It is based on the rationale that fetal hypoxia and acidosis create the final common pathway to fetal injury and death, and that prior to their development there is a sequence of events that can be identified.

There is a general pattern of fetal response to an intrauterine challenge or chronic stress. The most widely used tests to evaluate the function and reserve of the fetoplacental unit and the well-being of the fetus before labor are maternal monitoring of fetal activity, contraction stress test (CST) and nonstress test (NST) monitoring of the fetal heart rate (FHR), fetal biophysical profile (BPP), and Doppler velocimetry.

Formal Maternal Monitoring of Fetal Activity. Fetal movement perception is routinely taught in obstetrical practice as an expression of fetal well-being in utero, and its counting is purported to be a simple method of fetal oxygenation monitoring. With a goal of decreasing the stillbirth rate near term, there has been an increased tendency to use fetal movements as an indicator of fetal well-being. It is monitored by maternal recording of perceived activity or using pressure-sensitive electromechanical devices and real-time US. A diagnosis of decreased fetal movement is a qualitative maternal perception of reduced normally perceived fetal movement. There is no consensus regarding a perfect definition, nor is there

TABLE 2.5 Criteria for Interpreting Nonstress Test and Acoustic Stimulation Test

Reactivity Terms	Criteria
Reactive nonstress test (NST)	Two fetal heart rate (FHR) accelerations of at least 15 beats per minute (bpm), lasting a total of 15 sec in 10-min period
Nonreactive NST	No 10-min window containing two acceptable (as defined by reactive NST) accelerations for maximum of 40 min
Reactive acoustic stimulation testing (AST)	Two FHR accelerations of at least 15 bpm, lasting a total of 15 sec, within 5 min after application of acoustic stimulus or one acceleration of at least 15 bpm above baseline lasting 120 sec
Nonreactive AST	After three applications of acoustic stimulation at 5-min intervals, no acceptable accelerations (as defined by reactive AST) for 5 min after third stimulus

consensus regarding the most accurate method for counting. Whereas evidence of an active or vigorous fetus is reassuring, an inactive fetus is not necessarily an ominous finding and may merely reflect fetal state (fetal activity is reduced during quiet sleep, by certain drugs including alcohol and barbiturates, and by cigarette smoking). Three commonly used methods for fetal kick counts include perception of at least 10 fetal movements during 12 hours of normal maternal activity, perception of at least 10 fetal movements over 2 hours when the mother is at rest and concentrating on counting, and perception of at least four fetal movements in 1 hour when the mother is at rest and focused on counting. Fetal movement does decrease with hypoxemia, but there are conflicting data regarding its use to prevent stillbirth.[36] Nonetheless, maternal perceived fetal inactivity requires prompt reassessment, including real-time US or electronic FHR monitoring.

EDITORIAL COMMENT: Just as pediatricians are taught to "listen to the parents," prudent obstetricians pay attention when a pregnant woman thinks something is different about the pregnancy.

Antepartum Fetal Heart Rate Monitoring. Antepartum electronic monitoring of the FHR has provided a useful approach to fetal evaluation (Table 2.5). It essentially involves the identification of two FHR patterns: nonreassuring (associated with adverse outcomes) and reassuring (associated with fetal well-being). These patterns are interpreted in the context of gestational age, maternal conditions, and fetal conditions, and compared to any prior evaluations. Electronic fetal monitors use a small Doppler US device that is placed on the maternal abdomen. It focuses a small beam on the fetal heart, and the monitor interprets these signals of the heartbeat wave and reflects its peak in a continuously recording graphic form. This pattern is then evaluated for the presence and absence of certain components that help identify fetal well-being.

BOX 2.2 Indications for Antepartum Fetal Surveillance

- Maternal antiphospholipid syndrome
- Poorly controlled hyperthyroidism
- Hemoglobinopathies
- Cyanotic heart diseases
- Systemic lupus erythematosus
- Chronic renal disease
- Type 1 diabetes mellitus
- Hypertensive disorders
- Pregnancy complications:
  - Preeclampsia
  - Decreased fetal movement
  - Oligohydramnios
  - Polyhydramnios
  - Intrauterine growth restriction
- Postterm pregnancy
- Isoimmunization
- Previous unexplained fetal demise
- Multiple gestation

Antepartum testing is performed to observe pregnancies with an increased risk of fetal death or neurologic consequences (Box 2.2). The NST is the most commonly used method. It is performed at daily or weekly intervals, but there are no high-quality data regarding the optimal interval of testing. Frequency is based on clinical judgment, and the presence of a reassuring test only indicates that there is no fetal hypoxemia at that time. It is commonly understood that a reactive NST assures fetal well-being for 7 days, but this is not proven. The management of a nonreactive NST depends on the gestational age and clinical context. The false-positive rate of an NST may be as high as 50% to 60%, so additional testing such as vibroacoustic stimulation, BPP, and possibly CST are useful adjuncts.

The oxytocin challenge test, or CST, records the responsiveness of the FHR to the stress of induced uterine contractions and thereby attempts to assess the functional reserve of the placenta. A negative CST (no FHR decelerations in response to adequate uterine contractions) gives reassurance that the fetus is not in immediate jeopardy. The CST evaluates uteroplacental function and was traditionally performed by initiating uterine contractions with oxytocin (pitocin). Because continuous supervision and an electronic pump is required for regulated oxytocin infusion and because of the invasiveness of intravenous infusion, attempts have been made to induce uterine contractions with nipple stimulation either by automanipulation or with warm compresses. Nipple stimulation has a variable success rate and, because of inability to regulate the contractions, as well as concerns raised by the observation of uterine hyperstimulation accompanied by FHR decelerations, it has not gained wide acceptance. Nonetheless, breast stimulation provides an alternative, cheap technique for initiating uterine contractions and evaluating placental reserve. Similar information may be obtained by evaluating the response of the FHR to spontaneous uterine contractions and perhaps also from the resting heart rate

TABLE 2.6 Technique of Biophysical Profile Scoring

Biophysical Variable	Normal (Score = 2)	Abnormal (Score = 0)
Fetal breathing movements	At least one episode of at least 30 sec in 30 min	Absent or no episode of ≥30 sec in 30 min
Gross body movement	At least three discrete body/limb movements in 30 min (episodes of active continuous movement considered as single movement)	Two or fewer episodes of body/limb movements in 30 min
Fetal tone	At least one episode of active extension with return to flexion of fetal limb(s) or trunk; opening and closing of hand considered normal tone	Either slow extension with return to partial flexion or movement of limb in full extension or absent fetal movement
Reactive fetal heart rate	At least two episodes of acceleration of ≥15 beats per minute (bpm) and at least 15 sec associated with fetal movement in 30 min	Less than two accelerations or accelerations <15 bpm in 30 min
Qualitative amniotic fluid volume	At least one pocket of amniotic fluid that measures at least 1 cm in two perpendicular planes	Either no amniotic fluid pockets or a pocket <1 cm in two perpendicular planes

From Manning F, Morrison I, Lange I, et al. Antepartum determination of fetal health: composite biophysical profile scoring. *Clin Perinatol* 1982;9:285.

patterns without contractions. Because the CST requires the presence of contractions and has the major drawback of a high false-positive rate, its use has diminished with the better understanding of the NST and the use of the BPP and Doppler velocimetry.

As understanding of the NST evolved, it was noted that the absence of accelerations on the FHR tracing was associated with poor fetal outcomes, and the presence of two or more accelerations on a CST was associated with a negative CST. Although the false-negative and false-positive rates are higher for an NST than a CST, it is more easily used and therefore is the initial method of choice for first-line antenatal testing.

The modified NST has become the initial testing scheme of choice. The modified NST comprises vibroacoustic stimulation, initiated if no acceleration is noted within 5 minutes during the standard NST. Because reactivity is defined by two accelerations within 10 minutes, the sound is repeated if 9 minutes have elapsed since the first acceleration. Vibroacoustic stimulation, using devices emitting sound levels of approximately 80 dB at a frequency of 80 Hz, results in FHR acceleration and reduces the rate of falsely worrisome NSTs. Thus, the specificity of the NST may be improved by adding sound stimulation.

Amniotic Fluid Volume. The amniotic fluid volume (AFV) is measured via US using the value of the amniotic fluid index (AFI). This is the sum of the measured vertical amniotic fluid pockets in each quadrant of the uterus that does not contain the umbilical cord. The value can be associated with a number of potential complications depending on whether it is too high (polyhydramnios) or too low (oligohydramnios), although set recommendations for monitoring are not established.[37] When found, alterations in AFV can suggest the presence of premature rupture of membranes, fetal congenital and chromosomal anomalies, fetal growth restriction, and the potential for adverse perinatal outcomes such as intrauterine fetal demise. Pregnancies that are at risk for AFV abnormalities where surveillance may be indicated include those with such conditions as preterm premature rupture of membranes (PPROM), hypertension, certain fetal congenital abnormalities, maternal infection conditions, diabetes, IUGR, and post-term pregnancies.

Fetal Biophysical Profile. Five components—the NST, fetal movements of flexion and extension, fetal breathing movements, fetal tone, and AFV—constitute the fetal BPP (Table 2.6). It is performed over a 30-minute period, and the presence of each component is assigned a score of 2 points for a maximum of 10 of 10. A normal score is considered to be 8 of 10 with a nonreactive NST or 8 of 8 without the NST. Equivocal is 6 of 10, and abnormal is ≤4 of 10. This test assesses the presence of acute hypoxia (changes in the NST, fetal breathing, body movements) and chronic hypoxia (decreased AFV). A modified BPP refers to an NST and an AFI. The risk of developing fetal asphyxia within the next 7 days is about 1 in 1000 with a score of 8 to 10 of 10 (when the AFI is normal). The false-negative rate is 0.4 to 0.6 per 1000. A normal fetal BPP appears to indicate intact CNS mechanisms, whereas factors depressing the fetal CNS reduce or abolish fetal activities. Thus, hypoxemia decreases fetal breathing and, with acidemia, reduces body movements. The BPP offers a broader approach to fetal well-being than does the NST but still allows for a noninvasive, easily learned and performed method for predicting fetal jeopardy. Guidelines for implementation parallel that for other antenatal fetal assessment techniques, and so the BPP is usually initiated at 32 to 34 weeks' gestation for most pregnancies at risk for stillbirth.

Doppler Velocimetry. Doppler velocimetry has been used to assess the fetoplacental circulation since 1978, but still has a limited role in fetal evaluation. Because the placental bed is characterized by low resistance and high flow, the umbilical artery maintains flow throughout diastole. Diastolic flow steadily increases from 16 weeks' gestation to term. A decrease in diastolic flow, indicated by an elevated systolic-to-diastolic ratio, reflects an increase in downstream placental resistance. A normal waveform is considered reassuring and presumes normal fetal oxygenation. Elevated systolic-to-diastolic ratios are best interpreted in conjunction with NSTs and the fetal

BPP. The information gathered from the study of Doppler waveform patterns depends on the vessel being studied. Measurement of these velocities in the maternal and fetal vessels suggests information about blood flow through the placenta and the fetal response to any negative changes, and so any challenge to the fetoplacental circulation can ultimately result over time in a compromise of the vascular tree. These indices in the umbilical artery will rise when 60% to 70% of the vascular tree has been altered. The ultimate development of absent or reversed diastolic flow (defined as the absence or reversal of end-diastolic frequencies before the next systolic upstroke) in the umbilical artery is regarded as an ominous finding and is associated with fetal hypoxia and fetal acidosis with subsequent adverse perinatal outcome.[38] Umbilical artery Doppler evaluation is most useful in monitoring the pregnancy that is associated with maternal disease (hypertension or diabetes), uteroplacental insufficiency, and fetal IUGR, and it is not supported in the routine surveillance in other settings.

When a fetus is compromised, the systemic blood flow is redistributed to the brain.[39] Doppler assessment of the fetal middle cerebral artery is presently the best tool for evaluating for the presence of fetal anemia in the at-risk pregnancy. It has all but replaced the use of percutaneous fetal umbilical blood sampling (cordocentesis or percutaneous umbilical cord blood sampling [PUBS]) in the evaluation of pregnancies involving Rh isoimmunization and other causes of severe fetal anemia, such as parvovirus-induced hydrops fetalis or hemolytic anemia.

Fetal Blood Sampling. In the past, fetal blood sampling was indicated for rapid karyotyping and diagnosis of the heritable disorders of the fetus, diagnosis of fetal infection, and determination and treatment of fetal Rh(D) disease and severe anemia. Historically, PUBS, or cordocentesis, provided direct access to the fetal circulation for both diagnostic and therapeutic purposes. Presently, the procedures of CVS and amniocentesis allow for the acquisition of the same information at an earlier time and with lower risk to the fetus. Fetal diagnostic tests for karyotype can be performed on the amniocytes or chorionic villi. Fetal involvement in maternal infections, such as parvovirus B19, can also be determined through identification of infection in amniotic fluid, fetal ascites, or pleural fluid, and Doppler of the middle cerebral artery is used to evaluate and follow subsequent fetal anemia. Inherited coagulopathies, hemoglobinopathies, and platelet disorders can also be identified through CVS and amniocentesis, but the immunologic platelet disorders such as idiopathic thrombocytopenia purpura and alloimmune thrombocytopenia may benefit from fetal blood sampling with antepartum PUBS and during labor through fetal scalp sampling. Preparations for and ability to transfuse must be available. Suspected fetal thyroid dysfunction remains an area where fetal blood sampling by PUBS may be necessary and plays a critical role in the diagnosis and management of the disease.[40]

Chorionic Villus Sampling and Amniocentesis. CVS is a method of prenatal diagnosis of genetic abnormalities that can be used during the first trimester of pregnancy. Small samples of placenta are obtained for genetic analysis. It can be performed either transcervically or transabdominally. The major indication for CVS is an increased risk for fetal aneuploidies owing to AMA, family history, and abnormal first-trimester screening for Down syndrome. It can also be used to detect hemoglobinopathies. Amniocentesis is a transabdominal technique by which amniotic fluid is withdrawn so it may be assessed. The most common indications include prenatal genetic analysis and assessment for intrauterine infection and fetal lung maturity. It may also be used to evaluate for other fetal conditions associated with hemoglobinopathies, blood and platelet disorders, NTDs, twin-to-twin transfusion, and polyhydramnios. It is usually performed under US guidance and has a low rate of direct fetal injury from placement of the needle.

Procedure-related loss rates for CVS have been identified as 0.2% in a recent metaanalysis. The pregnancy loss rate associated with amniocentesis has been reported to be from 1 in 300 to 1 in 750.[41] Although the safety and efficacy of both procedures has been established, CVS is considered to be the method of choice for first-trimester evaluation because it has a lower risk of pregnancy-related loss than does amniocentesis before 15 weeks' gestation. Second-trimester amniocentesis is associated with the lowest risk of pregnancy loss.

Assessing Fetal Maturity. Because respiratory distress syndrome (RDS) is a frequent consequence of premature birth, both spontaneous and iatrogenic, and is also a major component of neonatal morbidity and mortality in many high-risk situations, it is critical that an antenatal assessment of pulmonary status be performed when indicated. The main value of fetal lung maturity testing is predicting the absence of RDS. It is not typically performed prior to 32 weeks' gestation because physiologically the fetus is likely to have not yet matured. Fetal pulmonary maturity should be confirmed in pregnancies scheduled for delivery before 39 weeks' gestation unless the following criteria can be satisfied: US measurement at less than 20 weeks of gestation that supports gestational age of 39 weeks or greater, FHT by Doppler ultrasonography have been present for 30 weeks, or it has been 36 weeks since a positive serum or urine pregnancy test. If any of these confirm a gestational age of 39 weeks, amniocentesis can be waived for delivery. Lung maturity does not need to be performed when delivery is mandated for fetal or maternal indications.

Historically, the introduction of amniocentesis for study of amniotic fluid and Rh-immunized women paved the way for development of the battery of tests currently available to assess fetal maturity. The initial methods developed were based on amniotic fluid levels of creatinine, bilirubin, and fetal fat cells, and these provided a good correlation with fetal size and gestational age. They were, however, inadequate predictors of fetal pulmonary maturity.

Amniocentesis to assess fetal pulmonary maturity is the currently accepted technique. Fetal lung secretions can be found in amniotic fluid. Evaluation of the amniotic fluid tests either for the components of the fetal pulmonary surfactant (biochemical tests) or for the surface-active effects of these phospholipids (biophysical tests). The lecithin-to-sphingomyelin ratio (L:S) and the presence of phosphatidylglycerol are biochemical tests, whereas the fluorescence polarization or the surfactant-to-albumin ratio (TDx-FLM II) is a biophysical test. Lamellar body counts can also be used. No test has been shown to be more superior to the other at predicting RDS, and each has its own defined level of risk. The predictive values of RDS vary with gestational age and with the population.[42]

The risk of RDS is least when the L:S ratio is greater than 2.0. However, this does not preclude the development of RDS in certain circumstances (e.g., infant of a diabetic mother or erythroblastosis). Given the physiology of fetal lung maturity, the presence of phosphatidylglycerol is a good indication of advanced maturity and therefore a correlated lessened risk of RDS with fewer false-negative results. Phosphatidylglycerol can be measured by rapid tests, is not influenced by blood or vaginal secretion, and can be sampled from a vaginal pool of fluid. The surfactant-to-albumin ratio is a true direct measurement of surfactant concentration. Levels greater than 55 mg of surfactant per gram of albumin correlate well with maturity, whereas those less than 40 mg are considered immature. Lamellar body count, with a size similar to platelets, is a direct measurement of surfactant production by type I pneumocytes. Given their size, a standard hematology counter can be used for their measurement; values of greater than 50,000/μL indicate maturity.[43] The negative predictive value of these tests is high so that when one result is positive, the development of RDS is unlikely.

EDITORIAL COMMENT: To mature the lungs if the indices are immature, corticosteroids are recommended. Treatment with a single course of antenatal corticosteroids (compared with placebo or no treatment) is associated with a reduction in the most serious adverse outcomes related to prematurity, including: perinatal death, moderate/severe respiratory distress syndrome, intraventricular hemorrhage, necrotizing enterocolitis, systemic infections, and need for mechanical ventilation in the first 48 hours of life.

A single course of antenatal corticosteroids could be considered routine for preterm delivery. It is important to note that most of the evidence comes from high-income countries and hospital settings; therefore the results may not be applicable to low-resource settings with high rates of infections. There is very little data available from low-income and low-resource settings. Surprisingly, we have still not established beyond reasonable doubt the optimal dose-to-delivery interval and the optimal corticosteroid to use.

Intrapartum Fetal Surveillance

The ultimate goal of FHR monitoring is to identify the fetus that may suffer neurologic injury or death, and to intervene prior to the development of these events. The rationale behind this goal is that FHR patterns reflect states of hypoxemia and subsequent acidosis. It is the relationship between the condition of the mother, fetus, placenta, and labor course that can result in a poor neonatal outcome. Although one can identify risk factors such as maternal hypertension and diabetes, fetal growth restriction, and preterm birth, these conditions account for only a small number of the neonates with asphyxia at birth.[44]

The two most common approaches are intermittent auscultation and continuous electronic FHR monitoring. There are no studies comparing the efficacy of electronic fetal monitoring (EFM) to no fetal monitoring to decrease complications such as neonatal seizures, cerebral palsy (CP), or intrapartum fetal death.[45] A metaanalysis comparing intermittent auscultation to continuous EFM found as follows: the use of EFM increased the risk of both operative vaginal delivery and cesarean delivery, did not reduce CP or perinatal mortality, and did not change Apgar scores or neonatal unit admission rates, although it did reduce the risk of neonatal seizures. The reason for this is unknown, although it is suspected that 70% of cases of CP occur before the onset of labor.[46] Also, the use of EFM instead of intermittent auscultation has not resulted in a decrease of the overall risk of perinatal death. Given these findings, the ACOG stated that high-risk pregnancies should be monitored continuously during labor and that either EFM or intermittent auscultation is acceptable in uncomplicated patients.

At present, continuous EFM is the preferred method of identifying the FHR pattern. This is typically performed externally through a Doppler US device belted to the maternal abdomen. The device plots the continuous FHR while another pressure transducer attached to the maternal abdomen simultaneously plots the frequency and duration of uterine contractions. These patterns can also be obtained from internal measurement of the FHR and uterine tone by a fetal scalp electrode and intrauterine pressure catheter (IUPC). The scalp electrode yields a fetal electrocardiogram and calculates the FHR based on the interval between the R waves. External monitoring is usually as reliable as internal and is the preferred method as long as it remains interpretable. A fetal scalp pH can be measured when the FHR record is difficult to interpret or in the presence of decelerations.[47] Complications of fetal scalp blood sampling and fetal scalp electrode monitoring may include significant fetal blood loss and infections in the newborn, although these occur rarely. Fetal scalp pH sampling has largely been abandoned due to its problematic collection and poor sensitivity and positive predictive value. An alternative to fetal scalp pH determination is digital stimulation of the fetal scalp in the absence of uterine contractions and when the FHR is at the baseline. A positive test (i.e., an acceleration [15 beats per minute {bpm} for 15 seconds] response to such stimulation) is considered fairly reliable evidence of the absence of fetal acidosis and a pH of 7.2 or greater, and clinical investigation supports its use.

Principles Related to FHR Monitoring

Despite the frequency of its use, the EFM has poor inter- and intraobserver reproducibility and a high false-positive rate.[48] Almost 99% of nonreassuring FHR abnormalities are not associated with the development of CP. For this reason, in 2008, the National Institutes of Child Health and Human

TABLE 2.7 **2008 Electronic Fetal Monitoring Definitions**

Pattern	Definition
Baseline	Bradycardia = below 100 beats per minute (bpm) Normal = 110 to 160 bpm Tachycardia = over 160 bpm The baseline must be for a minimum of 2 min in any 10-min period or the baseline for that time is indeterminate. May refer to prior 10-min segment to exclude periodic changes, areas of marked variability.
Variability	Fluctuations in the baseline that are irregular in amplitude and frequency Absent = amplitude undetectable Minimal = amplitude is 0–5 bpm Moderate = amplitude is 6–25 bpm Marked = amplitude greater than 25 bpm Measured in a 10-min window, peak to trough. There is no longer a distinction between short- and long-term variability.
Acceleration	A visually abrupt increase in the fetal heart rate (FHR) (onset to peak is less than 20 sec) Before 32 weeks, 10 beats above the baseline for 10 sec. After 32 weeks, 15 beats above the baseline for 15 sec. A prolonged acceleration lasts 2 min or more, but less than 10 min. If it lasts longer than 10 min, then it is a baseline change.
Early deceleration	A gradual, usually symmetrical decrease from the baseline of the FHR with a contraction. The nadir occurs at the same time as the peak of the contraction.
Late deceleration	A gradual, usually symmetrical decrease from the baseline of the FHR with a uterine contraction. The deceleration is delayed in timing, with the nadir occurring after the peak of the contraction.
Variable deceleration	An abrupt decrease in the FHR below the baseline. The decrease is ≥15 bpm, lasting ≥15 sec and <2 min from the onset to return to baseline. The onset, depth, and duration of the variable commonly vary with successive contractions.
Prolonged deceleration	A decrease in FHR below the baseline of more than 15 bpm lasting at least 2 min but <10 min from the onset to return to baseline. A prolonged deceleration of 10 min or more is considered a change in baseline.

Adapted from Macones GA, Hankins GD, Spong CY, et al. The 2008 National Institute of Child Health and Human Development workshop report on electronic fetal monitoring: update on definitions, interpretation, and research guidelines. *Obstet Gynecol* 2008;112:661.

Development convened a workshop with experts from the ACOG and the Society for Maternal-Fetal Medicine to try to reach a consensus on the definitions of FHR patterns. This is a standard that has been adopted and endorsed by ACOG (Table 2.7). Two major assumptions that have been made are that these definitions are primarily for visual interpretation of FHR patterns and that they should be applied to intrapartum patterns but are applicable to antepartum testing as well.

Terminology used to describe uterine activity has been revised to include[49] the following:

Normal: five contractions or less in 10 minutes averaged over a 30-minute period.

Tachysystole: more than five contractions in 10 minutes, averaged over a 20-minute window.

The terms *hyperstimulation* and *hypercontractility* are not defined and should be abandoned.

Tachysystole should always be qualified as to the presence or absence of associated FHR decelerations. The term *tachysystole* applies to both spontaneous and stimulated labor.

The FHR pattern is usually identified as either reassuring or nonreassuring in order to guide clinical management.

The presence of a reassuring tracing suggests that there is no fetal acidemia at that point in time. To be considered reassuring, a tracing must have the following components: a baseline FHR of 110 to 160 bpm, absence of late or variable FHR decelerations, moderate FHR variability, and age-appropriate FHR accelerations (two accelerations in 20 minutes of 15 beats above the baseline for 15 seconds for 32 weeks' gestation and above, and two accelerations of 10 beats above the baseline for 10 seconds for less than 32 weeks' gestation).

Nonreassuring tracings are associated with an altered fetal acid-base status and require immediate attention and intervention. In addition to the new definitions, a three-tiered interpretation system was established to help facilitate management (Box 2.3).

A category I tracing represents a normal FHR pattern, category II represents an indeterminate tracing, and category III represents an abnormal tracing.

Serial evaluation of the tracing is necessary because the FHR pattern represents only a risk of acidosis at that point in time and does not predict future status, because the pattern can change in response to labor and maternal and fetal predisposing conditions. Transient tachycardia with heart rates of more than 160 bpm (Fig. 2.4A) may be an isolated finding. It frequently precedes a variable deceleration pattern as a brief episode (Figs. 2.4B,C), which may reflect umbilical cord venous compression.

BOX 2.3 Three-Tiered Fetal Heart Rate Interpretation System

Category I

All of the following criteria must be present and, when present, are predictive of normal acid-base status at that time:

- Baseline rate: 110–160 beats per minute (bpm)
- Moderate variability
- Absent late or variable decelerations
- Present or absent early decelerations
- Present or absent accelerations

Category II

Includes all fetal heart rates (FHRs) that are neither Category I nor Category III. They are considered indeterminate.

Category III

These tracings are predictive of abnormal fetal acid–base status at the time of observation and need to be promptly evaluated.

FHR tracings include either:

- Absent baseline FHR variability *and* any of the following:
  Recurrent late decelerations
  Recurrent variable decelerations
  Bradycardia
  Sinusoidal pattern

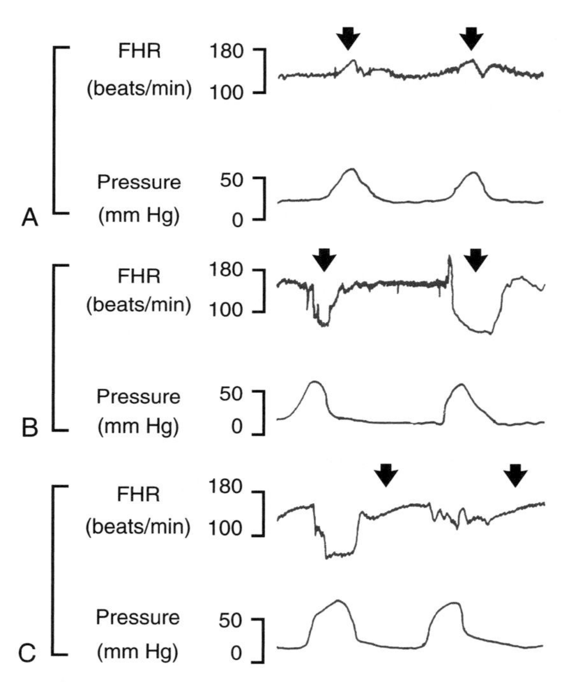

Fig. 2.4 Changes in fetal heart rate *(FHR)* during uterine contractions as a reflection of fetal distress. Arrows indicate (A) transient tachycardia, (B) variable deceleration, and (C) variable deceleration with slow recovery after uterine relaxation. Pressure is uterine pressure. (See text for explanation.)

A late deceleration pattern (Fig. 2.5) is commonly associated with uteroplacental insufficiency. Either of these patterns may be compatible with fetal stress (Box 2.4).

Some additional principles include[44,49] the following:

- The presence of FHR accelerations with moderate variability almost always indicates a fetus that is not acidotic.

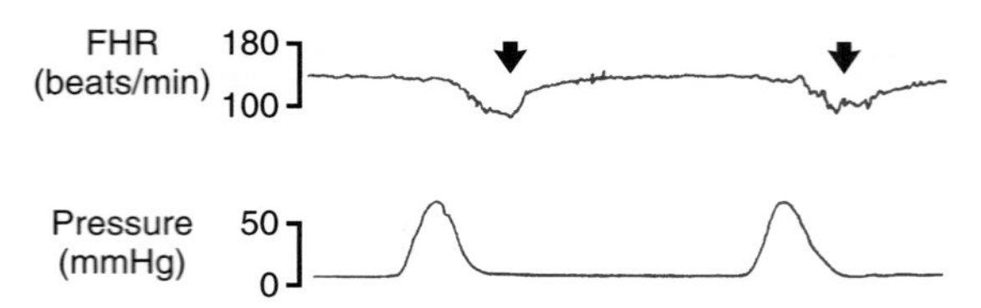

Fig. 2.5 Changes in fetal heart rate *(FHR)* during uterine relaxation as reflection of fetal distress. *Arrows* indicate late deceleration pattern with slow recovery after uterine relaxation. Pressure is uterine pressure. (See text for explanation.)

BOX 2.4 Fetal Heart Rate Patterns and Underlying Mechanisms

Reflecting fetal reserve

- Normal baseline heart rate and fetal heart rate (FHR)
- Tachycardia (>160 beats per minute [bpm])
- Diminished variability (<6 bpm variation)
- Bradycardia (<120 bpm)
- Sinusoidal pattern

Reflecting acute environmental change

- Early deceleration
- Variable deceleration
- Late deceleration
- Acceleration
- Head compression
- Cord compression
- Acute hemorrhage
- Contraction-induced hypoxia
- Intact autonomic response to intrinsic or extrinsic stimuli

Underlying mechanisms

- Intact autonomic cardiovascular reflexes, "sleep cycle," normal variant
- Prematurity
- Maternal fever, hypothermia, drug effects
- Congenital heart block, cardiac anomaly, congenital anomaly
- Fetal anemia
- Fetal acidosis and hypoxia

- In the presence of normal FHR variability, a fetus without accelerations is unlikely to be acidotic because moderate variability is strongly associated with an umbilical cord pH of greater than 7.15. An attempt can be made via vibroacoustic stimulation or scalp stimulation to elicit an acceleration.
- Neither baseline bradycardia nor tachycardia alone is predictive of acidosis.
- Baseline tachycardia may be due to early asphyxia but is more frequently the result of maternal fever, fetal infection, maternal drugs, or prematurity.
- Persistent fetal bradycardia with good variability is generally not associated with acidosis. It is more likely to be the result of drugs (medications) or fetal arrhythmias. However, persistent bradycardia below 100, even with variability present, is nonreassuring because this level of FHR may not be able to perfuse tissue adequately.
- Variability is a measure of fetal reserve. Absent or minimal variability is suggestive of fetal acidosis, especially when combined with recurrent late decelerations. Normal

baseline variability and accelerations occurring spontaneously or after stimulation indicate intact fetal reserves.

- Recurrent variable decelerations may be relieved with intrauterine amnioinfusion of saline to relieve cord compression.
- A sinusoidal pattern is no longer considered a preterminal condition in all cases and may not be due to acidosis. An attempt should be made to identify the cause. Fetal scalp stimulation may provide some reassurance.
- With any FHR tracing, if there is an increase in FHR at the time of digital stimulation of the fetal scalp, then the pH is likely to be greater than 7.15.
- Transient episodes of hypoxemia due to contraction or temporary cord occlusion are generally well tolerated, but prolonged or repeated episodes, especially if severe and/or associated with decreased variability, can lead to acidosis.

Treatment of the Category II and III Tracings

Most category II and III tracings require expeditious intervention. Administration of a high concentration of oxygen to the mother of a fetus under stress is one of the few methods of treating acute fetal hypoxemia. Maternal position changes are made to displace the gravid uterus or an occult cord prolapse. Treatment of maternal hypotension with intravenous crystalloid fluid bolus or ephedrine is given if hypotension is related to neuraxial anesthesia. Medications such as pitocin are discontinued if tachysystole is present. Beta-adrenergics such as terbutaline can be used for tachysystole that is unrelenting; these agents contribute to intrauterine resuscitation. These are just a few of the measures that can be taken to correct the nonreassuring FHR pattern changes. If the FHR tracing continues to indicate fetal compromise and it remains unresolved by interventions, a prompt delivery may be indicated. The method of delivery, operative vaginal or cesarean section, will depend on cervical dilation, station, position of the fetal head, maternal obstetrical history, and the urgency of the situation.

Adequate preparation is desirable for prompt effective resuscitation of the newborn. The pediatrician should be alerted when a decision is being made to intervene operatively for a fetus in distress (Box 2.5). A nonreassuring FHR tracing may or may not be associated with birth asphyxia, because only 30% to 40% of newborns who have low Apgar scores at birth (depressed) are actually acidotic as well. Historically, low 1- and 5-minute Apgar scores were used to define birth asphyxia. In our modern understanding of the development of CP and neurologic impairment, this is considered a misuse of the Apgar score. In general, because measurement of the process that leads to birth asphyxia is almost impossible in the fetus, asphyxia is described as the presence of hypoxia and metabolic acidosis that is severe enough to result in hypoxic encephalopathy.[50]

Neonatal encephalopathy is the present preferred terminology to describe CNS abnormalities during the newborn period of a neonate who was born after 36 weeks' gestation.[51] Birth asphyxia, now called hypoxic-ischemic (anoxic) encephalopathy, is a subset of neonatal encephalopathy. The underlying cause of brain injury in the neonate is oftentimes poorly understood, so the criteria for diagnosing HIE have not been completely established. The task force that was convened by ACOG and the American Academy of Pediatrics determined that four criteria must be met in order to define an intrapartum event as the cause of neonatal encephalopathy that would lead to CP[52]: profound metabolic acidosis (pH <7.0 and base deficit >12 mmol/L) on umbilical cord

BOX 2.5 Planning Care of the High-Risk Infant

Fetal disorders (suspected or confirmed)
- Size for dates discrepancy
- Abnormal karyotype
- Polyhydramnios or oligohydramnios
- Hydrops fetalis
- Fetal anomalies
- Abnormal alpha-fetoprotein
- Abnormal stress or nonstress contraction test
- Reduced biophysical profile score
- Reduced fetal movement
- Immature lecithin-to-sphingomyelin ratio (L:S) ratio
- Cardiac dysrhythmias

Maternal problems
- Pregnancy-associated hypertension
- Diabetes
- Previous stillbirth or neonatal death
- Maternal age <18 or >34 years
- Anemia or abnormal hemoglobin
- Rh sensitization
- Maternal infection
- Prematurity or postmaturity
- Malnutrition or poor weight gain
- Premature rupture of membranes
- Antepartum hemorrhage
- Collagen vascular disorders
- Drug therapy
- Maternal drug or alcohol abuse
- Multiple gestation

Intrapartum factors associated with maternal/fetal compromise
- Extreme prematurity or postmaturity
- Placenta previa or abruptio placentae
- Abnormal presentation
- Prolapsed cord
- Prolonged rupture of membranes >24 hours
- Maternal fever or chorioamnionitis
- Abnormal labor pattern
- Prolonged labor >24 hours
- Prolonged second stage of labor >2 hours
- Persistent fetal tachycardia
- Persistent abnormal fetal heart rate (FHR) pattern
- Loss of beat-to-beat variability in FHR
- Meconium-stained amniotic fluid
- Fetal acidosis
- General anesthesia
- Narcotic administered to mother within 4 hours of delivery
- Cesarean delivery
- Difficult delivery

arterial sample, early onset of severe or moderate neonatal encephalopathy in infants past 34 weeks' gestation, CP of the spastic quadriplegic or dyskinetic type, and exclusion of other identifiable etiologies. Additional supportive findings of an intrapartum origin that are discussed also include a sentinel hypoxic event in labor, electronic FHR abnormalities, Apgar score of 0 to 5 after 5 minutes, onset of multiorgan involvement within 72 hours, and early neuroimaging studies that show evidence of an acute nonfocal abnormality.

There are a number of antenatal risk factors that are associated with neonatal encephalopathy and CP, and it is not surprising that they include maternal medical conditions, placental abnormalities, postterm gestation, preeclampsia, prematurity, maternal fever and infection, and IUGR. Further discussion of the etiologies, diagnostic options, and management strategies of this condition will be discussed in subsequent chapters.

EDITORIAL COMMENT: *Cerebral palsy* (CP) is an umbrella term encompassing disorders of movement and posture, attributed to nonprogressive disturbances occurring in the developing fetal or infant brain.

There was a 30% reduction in CP in children born to women at risk of preterm birth who received magnesium sulfate for neuroprotection of the fetus compared with placebo. However, there was nearly a twofold increase in CP in children born to mothers in preterm labor with intact membranes who received any prophylactic antibiotics versus no antibiotics.

Shepherd E. Antenatal and intrapartum interventions for preventing cerebral palsy: an overview of Cochrane systematic reviews. *Cochrane Database Syst Rev.* 2017;8:CD012077.

BOX 2.6 An Overview of Fetal Therapy

Prevention of birth defects
- Folic acid
- Periconceptual glucose control in diabetes

Hormonal therapy
- Thyroid hormone
- Antenatal corticosteroids for acceleration of pulmonary maturation
- Corticosteroids for congenital adrenal hyperplasia

Prevention and treatment of anemia/jaundice
- Anti-D globulin (Rhogam) at 28 weeks' gestation to prevent erythroblastosis
- Direct transfusions for severe anemia/hydrops

Treatment and prevention of infection
- Spiramycin for toxoplasmosis
- Zidovudine or other agents for human immunodeficiency virus
- Antibiotics for premature rupture of membranes
- Intrapartum penicillin for group B streptococcal disease

Treatment of cardiac arrhythmias
- Agents administered to mother, injected into amniotic fluid or directly into the fetus

Fetal surgery: highly selected cases
- Usually with hydrops fetalis or gross alterations in amniotic fluid volume
- Congenital diaphragmatic hernia
- Congenital cystic adenomatoid malformation
- Fetal hydrothorax
- Sacrococcygeal teratoma
- Obstructive uropathy
- Fetal airway obstruction due to giant neck masses
- Neural tube defects

Fetal Treatment

A combination of medical and surgical therapies is available for the prevention and treatment of fetal disorders. As noted in Box 2.6, these range from simple dietary supplements (which prevent birth defects) to complex surgical procedures, usually mandated by severe fetal compromise with hydrops fetalis or gross disturbances in the volume of amniotic fluid. The development of invasive fetal therapy can be attributed to advances in prenatal ultrasonography. Ultrasonography has been critical in following the natural history of many of the birth defects and disorders. It has also permitted early identification of structural anomalies and served as a guide for the minimally invasive prenatal therapy as well as intraoperative monitoring during open fetal surgery. MRI can now be used when US is limited or its evaluation is incomplete.

Direct or indirect treatment of the fetus continues to evolve slowly. These treatments include short-term oxygen therapy for IUGR, blood transfusions for fetal anemia, antibiotics and antiretrovirals for toxoplasmosis and HIV, steroid replacement for congenital adrenal hyperplasia, stem cell therapy for immune deficiency disorders, therapy for fetal arrhythmias, and thyroxine instillation for severe hypothyroidism.

The field of fetal surgery has continued to grow, and even diaphragmatic hernias, cystadenomatous malformations of the lung, NTDs, hydrocephalus, and hydronephrosis are conditions that may be managed with in utero interventions and surgery.

EDITORIAL COMMENT: Close monitoring of fetuses with malformations has diminished the need for invasive therapies. It is only when the situation is dire and the chances of losing the extremely immature fetus are great that it becomes necessary to intervene rather than deliver the infant prematurely. Any major intervention is inevitably followed by premature delivery.

SELECTED DISORDERS OF THE MATERNAL–FETAL INTERFACE

Pregnancy-Related Hypertension

Hypertensive disorders in pregnancy can be grouped into four main classes: chronic hypertension, preeclampsia and eclampsia, preeclampsia superimposed on chronic

BOX 2.7 Criteria for the Diagnosis of Severe Preeclampsia

- Blood pressure of 160 mm Hg systolic or higher or 110 mm Hg diastolic or higher on two occasions at least 6 hours apart while the patient is on bed rest
- Oliguria of less than 500 mL in 24 hours
- Cerebral or visual disturbances
- Pulmonary edema or cyanosis
- Epigastric or right upper quadrant pain
- Impaired liver function
- Thrombocytopenia

hypertension, and gestational hypertension. This system was prepared by the National Institutes of Health (NIH) Working Group on Hypertension in Pregnancy.[53] Chronic hypertension is defined as persistent blood pressure greater than 140/90 mm Hg observed prior to pregnancy or in the first 20 weeks of gestation. Hypertension that is diagnosed after the 20th week of gestation and accompanied by proteinuria (>300 mg in 24-hour specimen) is defined as preeclampsia. Preeclampsia can be further divided on the basis of the presence or absence of severe features based on the criteria in Box 2.7. The degree of proteinuria no longer is a determining factor for differentiating between milder and more severe forms of the disease. In addition, IUGR is no longer criterion for preeclampsia. The Task Force on Hypertension in Pregnancy eliminated the term "mild preeclampsia" and instead now use "preeclampsia with or without severe features."[54] When seizure activity is present, the diagnosis of eclampsia is made. Preeclampsia superimposed on chronic hypertension can have a worse prognosis for mother and fetus than either condition alone. The diagnosis of superimposed preeclampsia can be difficult and should be suspected when worsening hypertension and new onset or worsening proteinuria is noted. A woman who is noted to have new-onset hypertension without proteinuria after 20 weeks' gestation can be classified as having gestational hypertension. Many of these women will go on to develop preeclampsia or be diagnosed postpregnancy with chronic hypertension.

Preeclampsia occurs in about 4% of pregnancies, and two-thirds of cases occur in nulliparous women.[55] Other risk factors include AMA, chronic hypertension, chronic renal insufficiency, obesity, diabetes, systemic lupus erythematosus, and multiple gestation. Numerous tests have been proposed for the prediction or early detection of preeclampsia. At present, there is no single screening test that is considered reliable and cost-effective for predicting preeclampsia.[57] Concurrently, numerous trials have described the use of various interventions to reduce the rate or severity of preeclampsia, including use of magnesium, zinc, vitamin C, vitamin E, fish oil, and calcium. Many of these studies show minimal to no benefit or conflicting results, and at present, none are recommended. Recently, the Maternal Fetal Medicine Units Network found promising new data in low-dose aspirin therapy. It was found that aspirin reduced the risk for late-onset preeclampsia by 29% when initiated before 17 weeks' gestation, supporting the practice of early initiation of aspirin in high-risk women.[57]

Maternal and neonatal outcomes in preeclampsia depend on the severity of the disease and the gestational age affected, as well as presence of other comorbidities. In a study that examined 10,614,679 singleton pregnancies in the United States from 1995 to 1997 after 24 weeks' gestation, the relative risk (RR) for fetal death was 1.4 for any hypertensive disorder and 2.7 for those born to women with chronic hypertensive disorders compared to low-risk controls.[58] Causes of perinatal death in preeclampsia include abruption, placental insufficiency, and prematurity. The perinatal mortality rate is greatest for women with preeclampsia superimposed on preexisting vascular disease. Maternal morbidity and mortality is also increased with preeclampsia. Seizures, pulmonary edema, acute renal or liver failure, liver hemorrhage, disseminated intravascular coagulopathy, and stroke can be seen in severe preeclampsia and are more common in women who develop the disease before 32 weeks' gestation or in those with preexisting medical conditions.[59] The currently used combination of magnesium sulfate and antihypertensive drugs, followed by timely delivery, has reduced the maternal mortality rate to almost zero.

Given the progressive deteriorating course of severe preeclampsia and the increased risk of maternal and neonatal morbidity and mortality, prompt delivery after 34 weeks' gestation is recommended. However, in women with severe persistent symptoms, eclampsia, multiorgan dysfunction, severe fetal growth restriction, abruptio placentae, or nonreassuring fetal testing, the recommendation is to undergo prompt delivery regardless of gestational age.[60] There is disagreement about the treatment of severe preeclampsia before 34 weeks' gestation in which the maternal condition is stable and fetal status is reassuring. Although delivery is always appropriate for the mother, it may not be optimal for the premature fetus. Several studies have shown that with close monitoring, pregnancies with severe preeclampsia can be expectantly managed with good maternal and neonatal outcomes. Continuing a pregnancy long enough to administer corticosteroids has been shown to be beneficial for infants born before 34 weeks' gestation in the setting of severe preeclampsia to reduce the rate of RDS, neonatal intraventricular hemorrhage (IVH), neonatal infection, and neonatal death.

Preeclampsia without severe features can be expectantly managed until 37 weeks' gestation, when delivery is recommended. At gestational ages less than 37 weeks, inpatient or outpatient management is acceptable depending on patient compliance with home blood pressure and symptom monitoring, resources available to return to the hospital if needed, and ability to maintain modified bed rest. These women need to have twice-weekly testing including NST and US evaluation. Women with gestational hypertension should be considered for induction of labor at 37 weeks' gestation.[61]

Intrapartum management of preeclampsia centers on prevention of seizures, detection of FHR abnormalities, and detection and treatment of worsening maternal disease. Magnesium sulfate is the drug of choice to prevent seizures

TABLE 2.8 Normal Weight and Obesity According to Body Mass Index

Weight	Body mass index (BMI)
Normal	18.5–24.9
Overweight	25–29.9
Obesity class I	30–34.9
Obesity class II	35–39.9
Obesity class III	≥ 40

Adapted from World Health Organization. Obesity: preventing and managing a global epidemic. *World Health Organ Tech Rep Ser* 2000;894:1.

in women with preeclampsia with severe features. The efficacy of magnesium for seizure prevention in severe disease is well established; however, the benefit for women with mild disease remains unclear.[62] The Task Force on Hypertension in Pregnancy now recommends against magnesium sulfate for preeclampsia without severe features. Control of severe hypertension is imperative to prevent cardiovascular and cerebrovascular complications. Recommended agents include hydralazine, labetalol, and nifedipine. The mode of delivery is based on obstetric considerations, and a vaginal delivery should be attempted in most women. Continuous FHR monitoring and evaluation for vaginal bleeding is essential during the labor process. Monitoring for signs of worsening disease with laboratory evaluation is also recommended for some patients. Women with HELLP syndrome—intravascular ***h***emolysis, ***e***levated ***l***iver function test results, and ***l***ow ***p***latelets (thrombocytopenia)—require more intense monitoring and evaluation.

Obesity in Pregnancy

Obesity is an epidemic in the United States and worldwide. The NIH and the World Health Organization define normal weight and obesity according to body mass index (BMI) as shown in Table 2.8. The Centers for Disease Control and Prevention reports that in women of reproductive age in the United States, the prevalence of obesity was 30.2%, and the prevalence of overweight was 56.7%. Obesity is a risk factor for a number of pregnancy complications. Therefore, as recommended by ACOG in Committee Opinion No. 315, obese women should be encouraged to decrease weight before considering pregnancy.[63] Given the high number of unplanned pregnancies, this goal is often not achieved. In 2009, the Institute of Medicine revised the recommendations for weight gain in pregnancy to account for the increasing prevalence of obesity and the resultant complications.[64]

Miscarriage and recurrent miscarriage are increased in obese women compared to normal-weight controls. Fetal malformations, specifically NTDs, heart defects, and omphalocele are increased in obesity. Obese gravidas have an increased incidence of gestational diabetes above that in the general obstetrical population (6% to 12% versus 2% to 4%), and the magnitude of this risk is positively correlated with increases in maternal weight. An association between obesity and hypertensive disorders during pregnancy also exists. A review of 13 cohort studies comprising nearly 1.4 million women found that the risk of preeclampsia doubled with each 5 to 7 kg/m^2 increase in prepregnancy BMI. Because of the underlying medical issues and pregnancy complications present in morbidly obese women, an increased risk of preterm delivery (odds ratio [OR]: 1.5; 95% confidence interval [CI]: 1.1–2.1) is observed compared to normal-weight controls.[65]

Obesity is also associated with an increased risk of unexplained stillbirth. Data from the Danish National Birth Cohort noted an increased hazard rate of stillbirth in obese women from 37 to 39 weeks' gestation of 3.5 (95% CI: 1.9–6.4) and at 40 weeks of 4.6 (95% CI: 1.6–13.4).[66] Furthermore, a Canadian study revealed that the factor most strongly associated with unexplained fetal death was increased prepregnancy weight. Fetal macrosomia, defined as weight greater than 4000 g, is increased in the obese population from 8.3% in nonobese women to 13.3% in the obese, and 14.6% in the morbidly obese. Although the risk of macrosomia is greater in women with gestational diabetes (OR 4.4 versus 1.6), the high prevalence of obesity correlates to a fourfold higher number of large-for-gestational-age and macrosomic infants than is seen as a result of diabetes. Being born macrosomic or large for gestational age correlates with an increased risk of obesity in the adolescent and adult years.[67] Macrosomia also contributes to the increased risk for cesarean section in obese gravidas and decreased success when attempting vaginal birth after cesarean section. Increased difficulties with regional and general anesthesia are also concerns and should prompt consideration for antepartum anesthesia consultation.

Diabetic Pregnancy

Major advances in the knowledge of carbohydrate metabolism provide the opportunity for improved screening and identification of the gestational diabetic woman.[68] Physiologic studies currently offer a better rationale for management of the chemical and the overt diabetic pregnant woman and her fetus. The increased risks for stillbirth, prematurity, and neonatal morbidity associated with diabetes pose a direct challenge to the efficacy of antenatal surveillance and neonatal intensive care.

Pregnancy increases the risks of adverse outcomes for mother and infant in women with type 1 diabetes. Reducing the risk of adverse outcomes in diabetic pregnancies to the level of risk in nondiabetic pregnancies is a major goal in diabetes care. Tight glycemic control before and during pregnancy is crucial. Preconception care is effective with an approximately threefold reduction in the risk of malformations. Supplementation with folic acid may also reduce the risk of malformations.[69,70] Insulin is now considered the gold standard for treatment of pregnancies affected by diabetes. It is imperative to minimize episodes of severe hypoglycemia during pregnancy to optimize outcomes. Screening for diabetic retinopathy, diabetic nephropathy, and thyroid dysfunction is important, and indications for antihypertensive treatment and treatment of thyroid dysfunction need to be in focus before and during pregnancy. Pregnancy in women with pregestational diabetes is associated with high perinatal morbidity and mortality. Stillbirth accounts for the majority of cases of perinatal death. Maternal smoking, hypertension (preeclampsia), and substandard utilization of antenatal care are significantly associated with stillbirths in diabetic women. IUGR, fetal hypoxia, and congenital malformations may be additional contributing factors, but more than 50% of stillbirths remain unexplained. The majority of stillbirths are characterized by suboptimal glycemic control during pregnancy. Better glycemic control together with regularly scheduled antenatal surveillance tests, including US examinations of the fetal growth rate, kick counting, and nonstress testing of fetal cardiac function, are necessary but do not ensure a favorable outcome. In summary, all known diabetic women should plan their pregnancies and optimize glycemic control preconceptually and throughout pregnancy to reduce the frequency of congenital abnormalities, obstetric complications, and perinatal mortality.

Because of the increasing incidence of type 1 diabetes, the recent emergence of type 2 diabetes as a condition that can begin during childhood, and the increasing prevalence of gestational diabetes mellitus (GDM), the number of women who have some form of diabetes during their pregnancies is increasing. Together, diabetes and obesity are the most common and important metabolic disorders. These women and their babies are at increased risk of morbidity, not just during pregnancy and birth, but for the long term as well. Between 1989 and 2004, the prevalence of GDM in the United States increased by 122%. Glycosylated hemoglobin, as measured by hemoglobin A1C (A1C), can potentially identify pregnant women at high risk for adverse outcomes associated with GDM, including macrosomia and postpartum glucose intolerance. An elevated A1C at GDM diagnosis was positively associated with postpartum abnormal glucose tolerance. A 1% increase in A1C at GDM diagnosis was associated with 2.36 times higher odds of postpartum abnormal glucose 6 weeks after delivery.[71] Women with pregnancies complicated by preeclampsia or GDM had an increased risk of later diabetes, especially those having GDM.

Leary and associates wrote, "The impact of gestational diabetes on maternal and fetal health has been increasingly recognized."[72] However, universal consensus on the diagnostic methods and thresholds has long been lacking. Published guidelines from major societies differ considerably from one another, ranging in recommendations from aggressive screening to no routine screening at all. As a result, real-world practice is equally varied. The Hyperglycemia and Adverse Pregnancy Outcomes (HAPO) study[73] and two randomized controlled trials evaluating treatment of mild maternal hyperglycemia have confirmed the findings of smaller, nonrandomized studies solidifying the link between maternal hyperglycemia and adverse perinatal outcomes. Two-step screening is commonly used by obstetricians in the United States. It is based on first screening with a 50-g oral glucose load followed by a venous glucose level 1 hour after ingestion. Women whose glucose levels are above that of an institution's specified threshold will then complete a 100-g 3-hour oral glucose tolerance test. Two values elevated above set criteria would diagnose gestational diabetes. The International Association of Diabetes and Pregnancy Study Groups (IADPSG) have formulated guidelines for screening and diagnosis of diabetes in pregnancy. Key components of the IADPSG guidelines include the recommendation to screen high-risk women at the first encounter for pregestational diabetes, to screen universally at 24 to 28 weeks' gestation, and to screen with the 75-g oral glucose tolerance test interpreting abnormal fasting, with 1-hour and 2-hour plasma glucose concentrations as individually sufficient for the diagnosis of gestational diabetes. The diagnosis of gestational diabetes is made when any of the following three 75-g, 2-hour oral glucose tolerance test thresholds are met or exceeded:

- Fasting—92 mg/dL
- 1 hour—180 mg/dL
- 2 hours—153 mg/dL

Increases in each of the three values on the 75-g, 2-hour oral glucose tolerance test are associated with graded increases in the likelihood of pregnancy outcomes such as large for gestational age, cesarean section, fetal insulin levels, and neonatal fat content. Furthermore, to translate the continuous association between maternal glucose and adverse outcomes demonstrated in the HAPO cohort, they recommend thresholds for positive screening tests at which the odds of elevated birth weight, cord blood C-peptide, and fetal body fat percent are 1.75 relative to odds of those outcomes at mean glucose values.[73]

In 2015, a Cochrane review concluded that there was no optimal universal screening test. The American College of Obstetricians and Gynecologists supports the two-step approach over the IADPSG guidelines. Providers may choose the 2-g oral glucose tolerance test if appropriate, depending on patient population.

Despite insulin therapy, the perinatal mortality rate among offspring of diabetic mothers remains higher than the general population. Note that the infant survival rate at the Joslin Clinic from 1922 to 1938 was only 54%. From 1938 to 1958, the survival rate improved to 86%, and from 1958 to 1974, a 90% survival was achieved. Thus, the combined toll from stillbirth and neonatal death may persist at five times the rate of nondiabetic women, even at major medical centers. Where care is less intensive, perinatal mortality rate for women with diabetes of 20% to 30% still exists. Congenital malformations are responsible for 30% to 50% of perinatal deaths in diabetics compared with 20% to 30% in nondiabetics.

Based on the increased risk of stillbirth during the last month of pregnancy, preterm delivery at 36 to 37 weeks' gestation was the generally accepted recommendation for many years. Möller was one of the first to strive for an avoidance of premature deliveries.[74] In 1970, she reported from Sweden a series of diabetic women carried closer to term when blood sugar regulation comparable to the nondiabetic pregnancy had been achieved and when evidence of fetal jeopardy or pregnancy complications such as toxemia did not appear. The perinatal mortality rate in her series of 47 patients was 2.1% as compared with a 21% mortality rate in a prior series from the same obstetric unit.

Similar favorable results have been reported from other institutions in Europe and in the United States.[75–77] Gyves and coworkers described a reduction in perinatal mortality rate from 13.5% to 4.1% in a group of 96 diabetic patients in whom the modern technology was applied and preterm delivery was not routinely employed.[75] These statistics continue to improve.

EDITORIAL COMMENT: On the basis of a literature review, Syed and colleagues concluded that optimal control of serum blood glucose versus suboptimal control was associated with a significant reduction in the risk of perinatal mortality but not stillbirths.[78] Preconception care of diabetes (information about need for optimization of glycemic control before pregnancy, assessment of diabetes complications, review of dietary habits, intensification of capillary blood glucose self-monitoring, and optimization of insulin therapy) versus none was associated with a reduction in perinatal mortality. They estimate that the stillbirth rate can be reduced by 10%.

For many years, good control of maternal blood sugar concentration has been considered important for the well-being of the fetus of the diabetic mother. However, wide differences of opinion exist as to what constitutes good control. The fasting plasma glucose concentration in pregnancy, in normal and diabetic mothers, has been shown to be lower than in women in the nongravid state. The continuous siphoning of glucose by the fetus profoundly affects maternal carbohydrate metabolism, and as a result, fasting glucose levels are 15 to 20 mg/dL lower during pregnancy than postpartum. Physiologic studies describing diurnal profiles for blood glucose concentrations in normal pregnancies have shown a remarkable constancy of these concentrations throughout the day. The fetus is thus, under normal circumstances, provided with a constant glucose environment.

These physiologic principles have provided a rational basis for the care of pregnant diabetic women, and the importance of rigid blood glucose control has been illustrated by several clinical studies. The marked improvement in perinatal mortality rates and morbidity obtained by Möller and Gyves and colleagues was with a mean preprandial blood glucose concentration kept close to 100 mg/dL, particularly during the third trimester.[74,75] The latter series also described a significant reduction in macrosomia among the infants of such well-controlled diabetic mothers. Karlsson and Kjellmer reported that their perinatal mortality rate could be directly correlated with maternal mean blood glucose concentrations.[79] When mean concentrations were greater than 150 mg/dL, the mortality rate was 23.6%. At concentrations between 100 and 150 mg/dL, the rate declined to 15.3%, and at less than 100 mg/dL, mortality of 3.8% was achieved. The King's College group in London reported on deliveries of 100 diabetic pregnant women in whom the mean preprandial blood glucose concentrations were maintained at approximately 100 mg/dL. There was no perinatal loss in this series.

TABLE 2.9 Clinical Status of Diabetes: Timing of Assessments

ASSESSMENT CONSIDERATIONS IN DIABETIC PREGNANCIES	
Maternal	**Fetal**
History and physical examination	Viability scan/nuchal translucency
Ophthalmology referral/evaluation	Anatomy scan
Electrocardiogram	Growth ultrasounds at 28, 32, and 36 weeks
Prenatal screen and bacteriuria screen	Fetal movement
Glycosylated proteins	Nonstress tests (NSTs)
Thyroid panel screen	
Creatinine clearance	
Urine protein	
Urine dipstick	
Lipid profile	

Adapted from *Guidelines for Care: California Diabetes and Pregnancy Program*. Maternal and Child Health Branch, Department of Health Services, Sacramento, CA; 1986.

Because improvements in obstetric and neonatal management have evolved over the same time span as these studies of intensive blood sugar control, it is difficult to attribute marked improvements in outcome to only one variable. Nevertheless, it seems prudent that the therapeutic objective in pregnant diabetic patients be an effort at normalization of plasma glucose throughout the day. This approach should apply to the woman with gestational diabetes as well as to the woman who was diabetic before pregnancy.[80]

EDITORIAL COMMENT: Newer technologies, such as the ability to continuously monitor the blood glucose, facilitate better control of diabetic pregnancy. Nonetheless, it remains a daunting task to further improve outcomes.

Principles of Management of Diabetes in Pregnancy

1. Metabolic derangements are the major abnormality affecting individuals with diabetes mellitus.
2. Pregnant women with diabetes should be managed by suitably trained individuals and teams who comprehensively monitor mother and fetus throughout pregnancy (Table 2.9).
3. Optimal care of women with diabetes must begin before conception because it has been demonstrated that careful preconception control of diabetes reduces the incidence of major anomalies.
4. All pregnancies should be screened so that women with gestational diabetes can be identified and appropriately managed.

Management of Diabetic Women Before Conception. The rationale of the preconception program for diabetic women is to optimize the pregnancy outcome for the woman and her offspring. Optimal care of gravidas with prepregnancy diabetes must begin before conception. A well-disciplined, well-coordinated, and well-organized multidisciplinary team and a compliant patient are the prime ingredients for a successful pregnancy outcome. The team comprises internists, perinatologists, and selected other medical subspecialists; a nutritionist, a social worker, and other perinatal nurse specialists who coordinate the dietary needs; and specialists in ongoing education, exercise, and blood glucose regulation. The goal is to achieve a mean fasting glucose of less than 95 mg/dL and a 1-hour postprandial level less than 140 mg/dL. Glycosylated hemoglobin should be maintained within the normal range. The objective is to achieve glycemic control before conception and throughout embryogenesis and then continue throughout gestation. In this way, major abnormalities may be averted. In addition, prophylactic folate supplementation is advocated during the periconceptual period to reduce the risk of NTDs. Strict glucose control may also diminish other perinatal complications including intrauterine demise, macrosomia, and neonatal disorders such as hypoglycemia and polycythemia in addition to a cardiomyopathy. Ongoing surveillance, continued education, and careful monitoring throughout the pregnancy are necessary to achieve optimal maternal and perinatal outcome.

Outpatient management of the diabetic pregnancy has replaced the obligatory period of hospitalization. However, in the face of deteriorating glycemic control, maternal complications including hypertensive disorders, infection, preterm labor, or evidence of fetal compromise, hospitalization is mandated.

A critical determinant of the outcome of diabetic pregnancy is the timing of delivery. The risk of intrauterine death increases as term approaches. Alternatively, the infant delivered preterm is exposed to the risks of prematurity, particularly that of respiratory distress, which may result in neonatal loss. The risk of RDS is higher in diabetic pregnancies compared with nondiabetic pregnancies. Over the past 35 years, the feasibility of extending the gestational period and of individualizing delivery timing for the diabetic mother has been enhanced by the availability of objective tests for fetal surveillance.

Because the major consequence of premature birth is respiratory distress, fetal pulmonary functional maturity is the most critical objective of current care. Biochemical estimations of this maturity can be obtained from the amniotic fluid with either the L:S ratio, the foam stability test, or the measurement of phosphatidylglycerol, indicating mature surfactant.[81,82] These determinations provide an important dimension in the management of the pregnant diabetic woman, particularly when maternal blood sugar control has been good and a normal physiologic milieu has been approximated.

> **EDITORIAL COMMENT:** Despite technological advances in the field, testing for fetal lung maturity at a more advanced gestational age (>36 weeks) is neither reliable nor cost-effective. Data mandate reconsideration of our current recommendation of amniocentesis to confirm fetal lung maturity prior to elective delivery at 36 to 39 weeks' gestation in well-dated pregnancies.

Congenital malformations have assumed a major role in diabetic pregnancies. In a prospective study, Simpson et al.[83] documented a 6.6% incidence of major anomalies among offspring of diabetic mothers as compared with a 2.4% incidence in control mothers. (Other centers report even higher rates.) Because the anomaly rate in those patients whose diabetes was aggressively managed was similar to that observed by others in patients whose diabetes was less vigorously managed, the researchers hypothesized that abnormal development had occurred before the patients entered the study. There is a major emphasis on carefully managing diabetes before conception and even in the first trimester to reduce the high anomaly rate associated with diabetic pregnancies.

Patients with high hemoglobin (HbA_{1C}) (variably defined as greater than 7.99 or greater than 9.0) have extremely high (22.5% to 40%) risk of congenital malformation compared with women whose HbA_{1C} is less than that level (5%). This is supported by data generated by Ylinen et al.,[84] who measured maternal HbA_{1C} as an indication of maternal hyperglycemia during pregnancy to determine its relationship to fetal malformations. Maternal HbA_{1C} was measured at least once before the end of the 15th week of gestation in 139 insulin-dependent patients who delivered after 24 weeks' gestation. The mean initial HbA_{1C} was 9.5% of the total hemoglobin concentration in the 17 pregnancies complicated by malformations, which was significantly higher than in pregnancies without malformations (8.0%). Fetal anomalies occurred in 6 of 17 cases (35%) with values initially of 8% to 9.9%, and only 3 of 63 (5%) anomalies occurred in babies of patients who had an initial level less than 8%. These data support the notion that there is an increased risk of malformation associated with poor glucose control. Unplanned pregnancies should be avoided in diabetic women, and determination of HbA_{1C} before conception may assist in planning the optimal time for conception.

> **EDITORIAL COMMENT:** Many studies confirm the extensive work of Fuhrman et al. that strict diabetic control before conception significantly reduces the incidence of congenital malformations.[85] To have a meaningful effect, this information must be widely disseminated. It is unfortunate that these results have not been achieved because appropriate preconceptional control was not attempted. The reasons for this remain undefined but are probably shared. Examples are (1) unplanned nature of pregnancies (i.e., lack of planned, or recommendation for, contraception by internist); (2) noncompliance by the patient; and (3) lack of effort by healthcare provider (generally internist) to attempt to achieve good control because of lack of consideration of the possibility of pregnancy.

The application of current technology provides the clinical team with the means of minimizing both fetal death in utero and preventable neonatal morbidity and mortality from the hazards of prematurity. Together with intensive control of maternal blood glucose, the technology of fetal surveillance offers the possibility of normalizing perinatal outcomes in large numbers of diabetic pregnancies.

EDITORIAL COMMENT: Infants of diabetic mothers are at risk for many physiologic, metabolic, and congenital complications that include, but are not limited to, malformations, macrosomia, asphyxia, birth injury, respiratory distress, hypoglycemia, hypocalcemia, hyperbilirubinemia, polycythemia and hyperviscosity, cardiomegaly, cardiomyopathy, and CNS disruption. Interestingly, macrosomia is common, but serious perinatal complications specifically associated with gestational diabetes are rare. Maternal obesity is an additional risk factor for complications, regardless of diabetes status.

The definition of macrosomia may be a birth weight more than 4000 or 4500 or 5000 g or, if you are a stickler for taking gender and gestational age into consideration, a birth weight above the 90th percentile for gestation, or, if you are a statistical purist, above the 97.75th percentile of a reference population corrected for gestational age and sex have been proposed. Whatever you select, these are large babies with considerable risk for morbidity before, during, and after birth. Because the number of adverse outcomes increases substantially above 4500 g, this is widely accepted. Macrosomia is associated with a higher risk of emergency cesarean section, longer maternal hospital stay of more than 3 days, and a four times higher risk of shoulder dystocia, together with a greater need for neonatal resuscitation and intensive care admission of the babies.

Preterm Labor and Preterm Delivery

Preterm birth, defined as birth before 37 weeks' gestation, remains an unsolved problem of paramount importance in perinatal medicine. The rate of preterm delivery in the United States has increased over 33% in the past 25 years from 9.4% in 1981 to approximately 12.8% in 2006 (one in eight births).[86] Although advances in neonatal intensive care have improved outcomes for preterm infants, the complications of prematurity remain the most common underlying cause of perinatal and infant morbidity and mortality. Approximately 75% of preterm births occur between 34 and 36 weeks' gestation, and although these infants experience morbidity, the majority of perinatal mortality and serious morbidity occurs among the 15% of preterm infants who are born before 32 weeks' gestation.

Preterm birth may fall into two broad categories: spontaneous preterm birth or indicated preterm birth. Spontaneous preterm birth includes preterm labor with intact membranes, preterm PPROM prior to the onset of labor, and cervical insufficiency. Indicated preterm births are those that occur secondary to an underlying fetal or maternal medical conditions or compromise. Seventy-five percent of all preterm births are spontaneous, whereas the remaining 25% are indicated. Although a distinction between indicated and spontaneous preterm birth may not always be clear or clinically evident, the distinction provides a conceptual framework for evaluating etiologies and trends of preterm birth. Notably, the overall rise in preterm birth rate in the United States is largely attributed to indicated preterm birth. This rise in preterm birth has been accompanied by an overall decline in fetal mortality, which suggests that this rise may reflect improved perinatal care (Fig. 2.6).

Spontaneous preterm birth represents a multifactorial disorder in which multiple modifiable and nonmodifiable risk factors interact, predispose, and cause disease. Maternal characteristics and behavior, maternal reproductive history, and characteristics of the index pregnancy all affect the risk of preterm delivery (Box 2.8). Although risk factors may identify patients at risk for preterm birth, many preterm deliveries occur in women without risk factors.

The diagnosis and treatment of preterm labor remains a challenging, inexact process for a multitude of reasons: the signs and symptoms of early preterm labor are often noted in normal pregnancy (menstrual-like cramping, low back or abdominal pain, nausea), the progression from subclinical to overt preterm labor may be gradual and unpredictable, and no threshold of contraction frequency has been shown to correlate with the risk of preterm delivery. Traditional diagnostic criteria—persistent uterine contractions accompanied by dilation and/or effacement of the cervix—demonstrate reasonable accuracy if contraction frequency is greater than six per hour and cervical dilation is greater than or equal to 3 cm and effacement is 80% or greater. However, many symptomatic women present with lower thresholds of cervical dilation or progression, and therefore overdiagnosis remains prevalent. Initial evaluation includes a detailed obstetric and medical history, physical examination, establishment of gestational age, evaluation of fetal status (monitoring or US), a consideration of other etiologies (PPROM, cervical insufficiency, abruption), and an evaluation for underlying infection. Transvaginal US and/or fetal fibronectin (fFN) testing in cervicovaginal fluid may improve diagnostic accuracy and decrease false-positive diagnoses. Women with a cervical length of 30 mm by transvaginal US are at a very low risk for preterm delivery.[87] These women may be discharged home after a period of observation with confirmation of fetal well-being, lack of cervical change, and exclusion of a precipitating event. Fetal fibronectin, a glycoprotein thought to promote cellular adhesion at the fetal–maternal interface, is released into cervicovaginal secretions when the chorionic/decidual interface is disrupted. Although this is a likely candidate to predict preterm labor and preterm delivery if present, numerous studies have demonstrated that the principal utility of fFN testing rests in the very high negative predictive value (>99% for prediction of preterm labor and preterm delivery in the next 14 days). The positive predictive value (less than 30% in most populations) limits the utility of a positive test.[88] Therefore negative tests remain highly useful in the initial triage of patients presenting with symptoms of preterm labor because patients with negative tests may reliably be discharged home.

After diagnosis of acute preterm labor and prior to the initiation of treatment, contraindications must be excluded, and gestational age must be established. Contraindications to tocolysis include placental abruption, chorioamnionitis, fetal demise, and acute fetal or maternal compromise, among

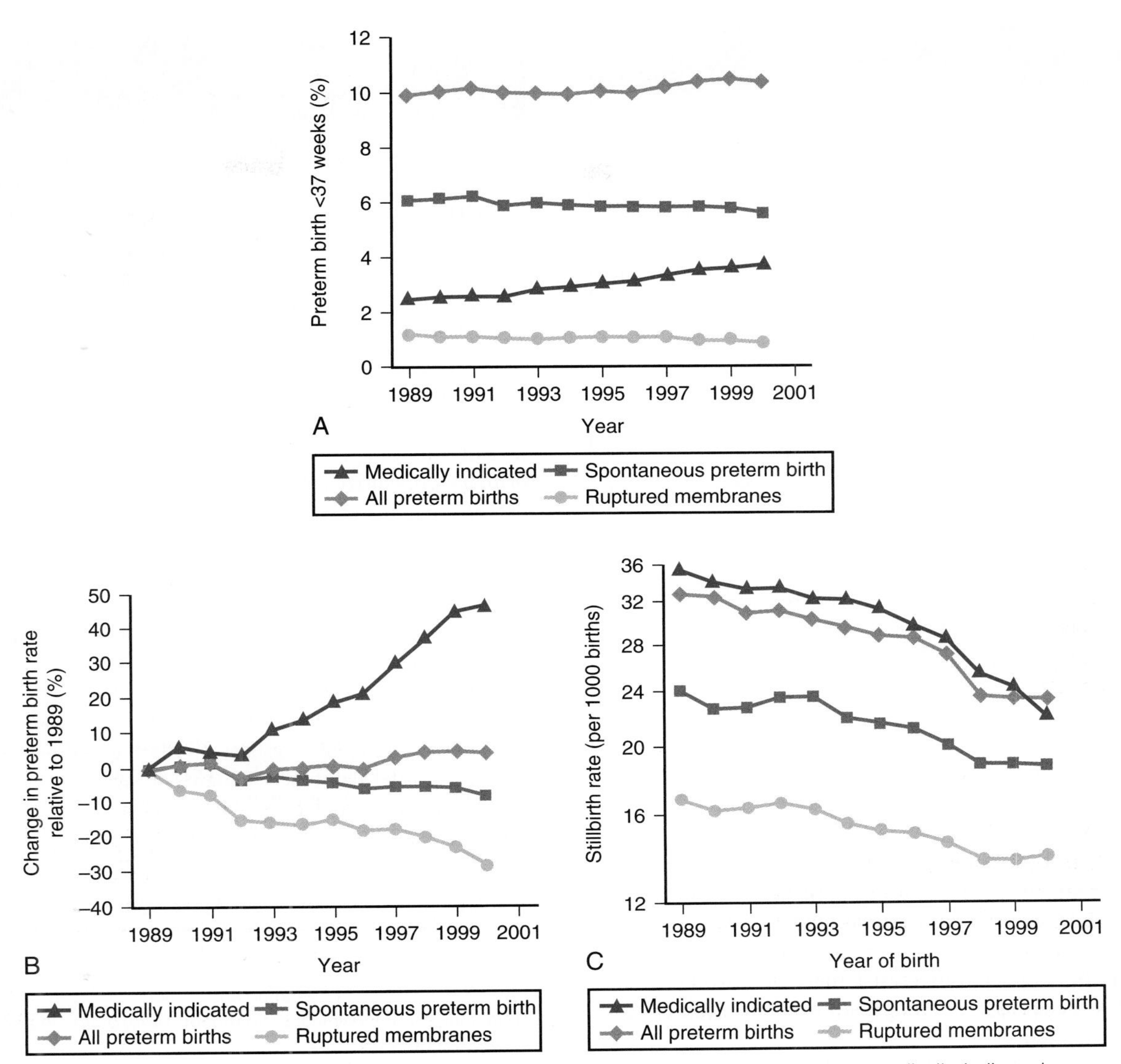

Fig. 2.6 Temporal change in singleton preterm births <37 weeks' gestation: overall, medically indicated, from spontaneous preterm labor, from ruptured membranes, and from stillbirth. (A) Rates in each group by year. (B) Change (%) in rates relative to 1989. (C) Trend of stillbirth by year. (Adapted from Ananth CVP, Joseph KSM, Oyelese YM, et al. Trends in preterm birth and perinatal mortality among singletons: United States, 1989 through 2000. *Obstet Gynecol.* 2005;105:1084.)

others. Regarding gestational age, the lower limit at which therapy should be offered is controversial, and no definitive data from randomized trials exist to support a recommendation. However, greater consensus regarding an upper gestational age limit exists. At 34 weeks' gestation, the perinatal morbidity and mortality are too low to justify the potential maternal and fetal complications or cost associated with inhibition of labor. Treatment of preterm labor consists of administration of GBS prophylaxis, magnesium sulfate for neuroprotection, if appropriate (see later discussion), and the administration of tocolytic therapy to inhibit uterine contractions and antenatal corticosteroids.

The goal of tocolysis is to reduce neonatal morbidity and mortality long enough to allow for the administration of antenatal corticosteroids and maternal transport to an appropriately equipped hospital. Metaanalyses have demonstrated the utility of tocolytic therapy for preterm labor in that all agents were more effective than no therapy or placebo at delaying delivery for 48 hours to 7 days. However, this prolongation was not associated with a statistically significant decrease in respiratory distress or neonatal death.[89] Tocolytic therapy includes many classes of drugs: calcium channel blockers, cyclooxygenase inhibitors, magnesium sulfate, oxytocin antagonists, nitric oxide donors, and betamimetics. However, no tocolytic drug is currently FDA approved for the indication of arresting labor. Selection of appropriate tocolytic therapy requires consideration of the maternal and fetal risk, efficacy, and side effects. A detailed discussion of

BOX 2.8 Danger Factors That Increase Risk of Spontaneous Preterm Delivery

Nonmodifiable
- Familial risk
- Low socioeconomic status
- Low education status
- Low or high maternal age (<18 or >40 years)
- African American race
- Uterine anomalies
- Prior spontaneous PTD
- Multiple gestation
- ART (singleton or multiple gestation)
- Uterine volume
- Cervical length ("short cervix")

Modifiable
- Maternal smoking
- Substance abuse
- Nutritional status (low BMI)
- Genital tract infection/colonization
- Prior pelvic surgery
- Antenatal stress or depression

ART, Assisted reproductive technology; *BMI,* body mass index; *PTD,* preterm delivery.

the numerous trials comparing tocolytic agents is beyond the scope of this discussion. However, recent evidence shows the following:[90]

- Nifedipine and indomethacin are suggested first-line agents, with some authorities suggesting indomethacin as the first-line agent in patients less than 32 weeks' gestation who are also receiving magnesium sulfate for neuroprotection (potential for increased maternal adverse events with simultaneous use of magnesium sulfate and a calcium channel blocker).
- Magnesium sulfate should be used with caution as a primary tocolytic, given that data support less efficacy and increased side effects or adverse events.
- The use of multiple tocolytic agents ("double tocolysis") should be performed with caution because the propensity for adverse events increases and no evidence supports increased efficacy.
- Data from poorly designed studies do not support maintenance or repeat tocolysis after initial inhibition of preterm labor.

Although the identification and inhibition of acute preterm labor remains an important strategy aimed at reducing neonatal morbidity and mortality, primary prevention strategies have remained slow to develop owing to the multifactorial, complex pathophysiology of preterm labor and delivery. However, over the past 10 years, secondary prevention has made a marked impact on recurrent preterm delivery. Meis et al. published a landmark trial in 2003 demonstrating a decrease in recurrent[91] spontaneous preterm delivery for women receiving weekly intramuscular (IM) injections of 17α-hydroxyprogesterone caproate (17-OHP) from 16 to 36 weeks' gestation (Table 2.10). Notably, the risk reduction

TABLE 2.10 Impact of 17α-Hydroxyprogesterone Caproate (17-OHP) on Spontaneous Preterm Delivery

	*N**	<37 wk (%)	<35 wk (%)	<32 wk (%)
Placebo	153	54.9	30.7	19.6
17-OHP	306	36.3	20.6	11.4

Abbreviations: *17-OHP,* 17α-Hydroxyprogesterone caproate.
Adapted from Meis PJ, Klebanoff M, Thom E, et al. Prevention of recurrent preterm delivery by 17α-hydroxyprogesterone caproate, *N Engl J Med* 2003;348:2379.

increased with earlier gestational age of the index preterm delivery. Subsequent studies confirmed that supplementation in multiple gestation does not provide any benefit. With primary preventive strategies still in development, secondary prevention with 17-OHP has been estimated to save in excess of $2 billion annually in the United States alone.[92]

EDITORIAL COMMENT: Administration of vaginal progesterone to asymptomatic women with a twin gestation and a sonographic short cervix in the midtrimester reduces the risk of preterm birth occurring at <30 to <35 gestational weeks, neonatal mortality, and some measures of neonatal morbidity, without any demonstrable deleterious effects on childhood neurodevelopment.[a] However, progestogen administration does not prolong pregnancy in singleton gestations with preterm prelabor rupture of membranes.[b] Vaginal progesterone and 17α-hydroxyprogesterone were comparable for the prevention of recurrent spontaneous preterm delivery in singleton pregnancies; vaginal progesterone could be superior.[c]

[a]Romero R, Conde-Agudelo A, El-Refaie W, et al. Vaginal progesterone decreases preterm birth and neonatal morbidity and mortality in women with a twin gestation and a short cervix: an updated meta-analysis of individual patient data. *Ultrasound Obstet Gynecol.* 2017;49(3):303-314.
[b]Quist-Nelson J, Parker P, Mokhtari N, et al. Progestogens in singleton gestations with preterm prelabor rupture of membranes: a systematic review and metaanalysis of randomized controlled trials. *Am J Obstet Gynecol.* 2018;219(4):346-355.
[c]Oler E, Eke AC, Hesson A. Meta-analysis of randomized controlled trials comparing 17α-hydroxyprogesterone caproate and vaginal progesterone for the prevention of recurrent spontaneous preterm delivery. *Int J Gynaecol Obstet.* 2017;138(1):12–16.

Preterm Premature Rupture of the Membranes

PPROM, defined as spontaneous membrane rupture before labor *and* before 37 weeks' gestational age, occurs in approximately 3% of pregnancies and affects more than 120,000 pregnancies annually in the United States. PPROM is responsible for more than one-third of all preterm births and remains an important cause of maternal, fetal, and neonatal morbidity and mortality. The etiology of PPROM is multifactorial, and many patients will have multiple risk and etiologic factors (Box 2.9). Many of these factors are involved with pathways that result in accelerated membrane weakening such as increased stretch or degradation from local inflammation or ascending infection. A history of early preterm birth (23–27

BOX 2.9 Factors and Etiologies of Preterm Premature Rupture of Membranes

- Amniocentesis
- Cerclage
- Cervical insufficiency
- Cigarette smoking
- Collagen defect or degradation
- Low socioeconomic status
- History of cervical conization
- History of preterm delivery
- History of preterm premature rupture of membranes (PPROM)
- Sexually transmitted infection
- Other choriodecidual infection or inflammation
- Uterine overdistention (polyhydramnios, multifetal gestation)
- Vaginal bleeding in pregnancy (subchorionic hemorrhage, abruption, abnormal placentation)

weeks' gestation) after PPROM is the strongest risk factor for PPROM, which carries a threefold increase in risk of recurrence. In the majority of cases, an exact etiology of PPROM remains unknown after diagnosis.

The frequency and severity of neonatal complications after PPROM vary with gestational age at which membrane rupture and delivery occur. Additional factors that increase perinatal morbidity and mortality are perinatal infection, placental abruption, and umbilical cord compression. The most notable morbidities include RDS, necrotizing enterocolitis, IVH, and sepsis, which are common with early preterm birth. However, the risk of sepsis is twofold higher in the context of PPROM relative to preterm labor without PPROM. With conservative management after PPROM, the risk of intrauterine fetal demise is approximately 1% to 2%. Additionally, with expectant or conservative management of PPROM in the early midtrimester, the risk of pulmonary hypoplasia increases with estimated risks of 0% to 26% of births after PPROM at 16 to 26 weeks' gestation and approximately 50% when PPROM occurs before 20 weeks' gestation.

In the majority of cases, PPROM can be diagnosed clinically by a combination of clinical suspicion, patient history, and physical examination. Notably, patient history has 90% accuracy for diagnosis of PPROM. Physical examination should include a sterile speculum investigation with collection of fluid from the posterior vaginal fornix to evaluate by the nitrazine and ferning tests. Both of these tests are highly sensitive and specific for the diagnosis of PPROM, with nitrazine being more susceptible to contamination. In rare cases where history and examination remain equivocal, a dye test by amniocentesis (intrauterine injection of indigo carmine followed by observation for passage of blue fluid onto a perineal pad) may be performed to confirm PPROM. Notably, digital cervical examination should be avoided because multiple trials have demonstrated decreased latency periods with one to two cervical examinations in patients with PPROM.

Given that gestational age at membrane rupture and delivery substantially affects the risk of perinatal morbidity and mortality, a gestational age–based model guides management in the context of PPROM. This model balances the risks of fetal and neonatal complications with immediate delivery compared with the potential risks and benefits of conservative management to prolong pregnancy. Although practice variation exists, a few general principles and trials deserve attention:

- Gestational age must be established based on clinical history and ultrasound evaluation.
- Ultrasound should be performed to evaluate fetal growth, position, amniotic fluid volume, and anatomy.
- Women with PPROM must undergo clinical evaluation for preterm labor, chorioamnionitis, placental abruption, or fetal distress, which are indications for delivery independent of gestational age.
- A patient must be admitted to a facility that is appropriately equipped to provide emergent obstetric services as well as neonatal intensive care, and therefore transfer may be appropriate.

A large National Institute of Child Health and Human Development Maternal-Fetal Medicine Units Network study demonstrated the safety and efficacy of intravenous erythromycin and ampicillin followed by oral therapy to complete a 1-week course. In this trial, antibiotics improved neonatal outcomes by reducing the risk of death, RDS, early neonatal sepsis, severe IVH, severe necrotizing enterocolitis, patent ductus arteriosus, and bronchopulmonary dysplasia (from 53% to 44%; $p < 0.05$). A decrease in amnionitis and increase in latency of at least 1 week was also demonstrated.[93]

Several studies have evaluated other antibiotic regimens. The use of oral amoxicillin–clavulanic acid has been associated with an increased risk of necrotizing enterocolitis and should be avoided. The algorithm in Fig. 2.7 outlines the management of PPROM by gestational age.

Cervical Insufficiency

Cervical insufficiency describes a presumed physical or structural weakness that causes or contributes to the loss of an otherwise healthy pregnancy. Classically, cervical insufficiency manifests in the midtrimester with painless cervical dilation. Although anatomic, biochemical, and clinical evidence support structural weakness as an underlying cause of midtrimester birth, cervical integrity or competence represents only one variable of a multifactorial problem. Other factors such as uterine overdistention, hemorrhage, decidual infection, or inflammation may trigger the parturition process leading to changes that ripen, shorten, or weaken the cervix. When this occurs, the clinical presentation may be indistinguishable from so-called "weakness"-mediated cervical insufficiency. Therefore in the absence of definitive tests to discriminate between underlying etiologies or mechanisms, cervical insufficiency may be defined when other variables (labor, intrauterine infection, hemorrhage, etc.) that may precipitate midtrimester loss are not clinically evident.

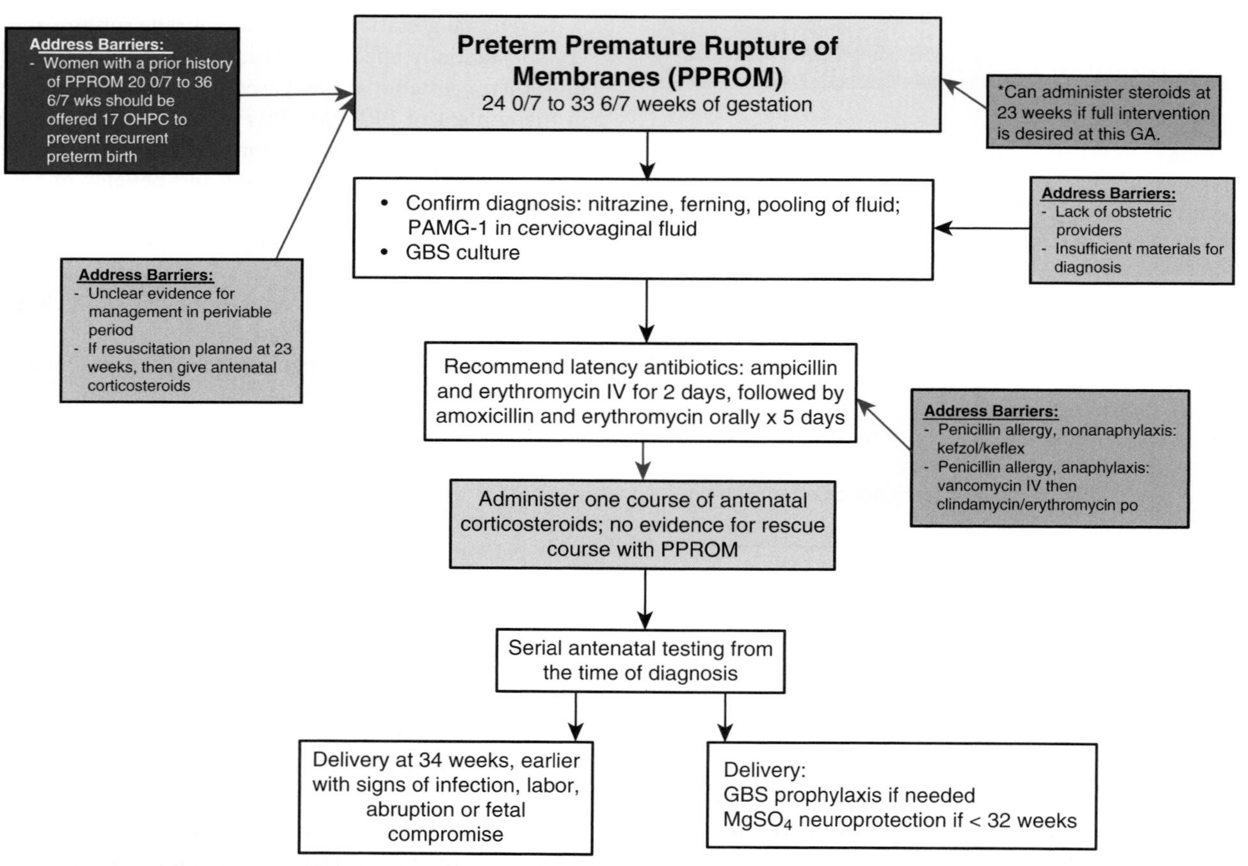

Preterm Premature Rupture of Membranes (PPROM)
24 0/7 to 33 6/7 weeks of gestation
Address Barriers:
- Women with a prior history of PPROM 20 0/7 to 36 6/7 wks should be offered 17 OHPC to prevent recurrent preterm birth
*Can administer steroids at 23 weeks if full intervention is desired at this GA.
• Confirm diagnosis: nitrazine, ferning, pooling of fluid; PAMG-1 in cervicovaginal fluid
• GBS culture
Address Barriers:
- Lack of obstetric providers
- Insufficient materials for diagnosis
Address Barriers:
- Unclear evidence for management in periviable period
- If resuscitation planned at 23 weeks, then give antenatal corticosteroids
Recommend latency antibiotics: ampicillin and erythromycin IV for 2 days, followed by amoxicillin and erythromycin orally x 5 days
Address Barriers:
- Penicillin allergy, nonanaphylaxis: kefzol/keflex
- Penicillin allergy, anaphylaxis: vancomycin IV then clindamycin/erythromycin po
Administer one course of antenatal corticosteroids; no evidence for rescue course with PPROM
Serial antenatal testing from the time of diagnosis
Delivery at 34 weeks, earlier with signs of infection, labor, abruption or fetal compromise
Delivery:
GBS prophylaxis if needed
$MgSO_4$ neuroprotection if < 32 weeks

Fig. 2.7 An algorithm for evaluation and management of preterm premature rupture of the membranes (PPROM). *GA*, gestational age; *GBS*, group B beta-hemolytic *Streptococcus*; *IV*, intravenously; *$MgSO_4$*, magnesium suphate; *OHPC*, alpha hydroxyprogesterone caproate; PAMG-1, placental alpha microglobulin-1; *po*, orally. (From Mercer BM. Treatment of preterm premature rupture of the membranes. *Obstet Gynecol.* 2003;101(1):178.)

Many patients who present with cervical insufficiency do not have underlying risk factors. However, some patients may have congenital or acquired forms of cervical insufficiency that include those with a history of collagen disorders (e.g., Ehlers-Danlos syndrome), uterine anomalies, diethylstilbestrol exposure, prior cervical trauma, or surgery. Notably, the cervix is a dynamic organ, and it undergoes various biological changes during normal pregnancy, parturition, and postpartum, which include softening, ripening, dilation, and repair.[94] In normal pregnancies, the cervix begins to efface at 32 to 34 weeks' gestation in preparation for term birth. Over the past 15 years, cervical length (measured by transvaginal US) has emerged as a notable risk factor for preterm delivery. A landmark study by Iams and coworkers, published in 1996, demonstrated a few important principles: (1) cervical length is normally distributed in the population (Fig. 2.8); and (2) the risk of spontaneous preterm birth before 35 weeks' gestation increases as cervical length shortens, particularly for those in the lowest quartile of the distribution. Although US may identify women at risk for preterm delivery due to a "short" cervix, US cannot distinguish the diagnosis of cervical insufficiency compared with other causes of premature cervical effacement. Attempts to characterize the cervix with percentile cervical length alone or in combination with other sonographic characteristics to predict cervical insufficiency have been unsuccessful.

Therefore cervical insufficiency remains a clinical diagnosis informed by history, physical examination, and US evaluation. Notable historical factors include the following: history of cervical trauma; repeat midtrimester pregnancy loss; absence of painful contractions, bleeding, or infection; advanced cervical dilation or effacement on presentation; and US findings of a cervical length less than the 10th percentile before 24 weeks' gestation. Notable elements of a physical exam include a speculum evaluation for prolapsing or "hourglassing" membranes, which are always abnormal, and a sterile vaginal exam to evaluate for advanced dilation or effacement. A comprehensive physical evaluation for symptoms of intrauterine infection (tachycardia, uterine tenderness) should also be completed. Laboratory evaluation includes a white blood cell count to exclude leukocytosis. Some authorities recommend amniocentesis to exclude intrauterine infection (glucose >20 mg/dL) prior to offering treatment with an emergent cerclage. The treatment of cervical insufficiency may vary based on gestational age at presentation and on the history and clinical scenario.

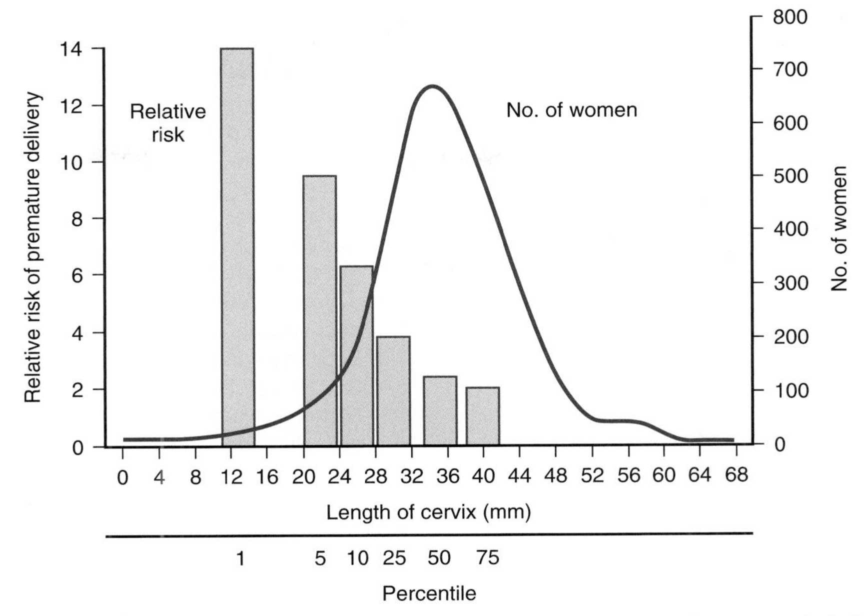

Fig. 2.8 Distribution of subjects among percentiles for cervical length measured by transvaginal ultrasonography at 24 weeks of gestation *(solid line)* and relative risk of spontaneous preterm delivery before 35 weeks of gestation according to percentiles for cervical length *(bars)*. (From Creasy RK, Resnik R. Preterm labor and delivery. In: Creasy RK, Resnik R, eds. *Maternal-fetal medicine.* 4th ed. Philadelphia, PA: WB Saunders; 1999.)

Presentation With Unanticipated Advanced Cervical Dilation or Effacement

Management of cervical insufficiency in the emergent setting (when advanced dilation or effacement is discovered before 24 weeks' gestation in the absence of infection, hemorrhage, or labor) remains controversial. Very limited data exist to guide management; however, data from one small randomized trial and a larger observational trial suggest that increased gestational time can be gained by placement of an emergent cerclage compared with expectant management.[95] The benefits of this increased latency remain unclear because many patients deliver children at the threshold of viability who suffer from the complications and sequelae of extreme prematurity. A retrospective study of 116 patients with emergent cerclage placement concluded that nulliparity, the presence of prolapsing membranes beyond the external cervical os, and gestational age less than 22 weeks at the time of cerclage placement are associated with a decreased likelihood of delivery at or after 28 weeks' gestation.[96] Additionally, the risks of cerclage placement, particularly membrane rupture, increase with the degree of cervical dilation and effacement as well as the gestational age at the time of placement. These factors should inform counseling regarding emergent cerclage, and the decision should be individualized to the clinical scenario at hand.

Documented History of Cervical Insufficiency

Patients with a history of cervical insufficiency in a previous pregnancy may be followed by either serial US surveillance of cervical length or with prophylactic cerclage, which is generally placed between 12 to 15 weeks' gestation. Recommendations may include history-indicated prophylactic cerclage over US surveillance when history is confirmed. Prophylactic cerclage is an accepted treatment in this subset of patients, with success rates reported to be as high as 75% to 90%.

Incidental Observation of Short Cervix by Ultrasound

This increasingly common scenario has no evidence-based recommendation for management. Many of these women are asymptomatic, and a short cervix is discovered incidentally by a midtrimester US to assess fetal anatomy. Women with singleton pregnancies with cervical shortening and normal obstetric histories do not benefit from cerclage.[97] Several randomized controlled trials have been done to suggest the use of vaginal progesterone in the setting of an incidentally found short cervix and no prior history of preterm birth will be beneficial to the current pregnancy in asymptomatic women.[98,100] In 2012, a multicenter randomized control trial found that 17-OHP in nulliparous women with incidentally discovered short cervix did not reduce the risk of preterm birth.[99]

Women With a History of Spontaneous Preterm Delivery

Data from a recent randomized controlled trial supports a role for cerclage placement for women with a history of preterm birth (defined between 16 and 34 weeks' gestation). As a part of this trial, 301 women with a history of preterm birth were screened with serial cervical length assessment beginning at 16 weeks' gestation, and those with a cervical length below 25 mm were randomly assigned to cerclage or no cerclage. Cerclage did not result in a significant reduction in the primary outcome of preterm birth before 35 weeks' gestation for

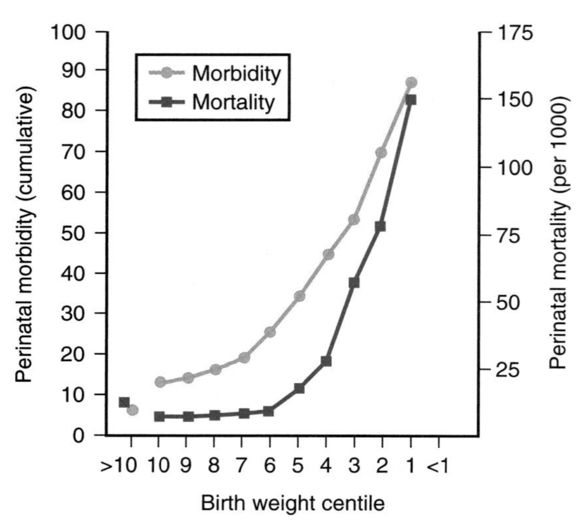

Fig. 2.9 Relationship between birth weight percentiles and adverse perinatal outcomes in infants with intrauterine growth restriction. (From Creasy RK, Resnik R: Intrauterine growth restriction. In: Creasy RK, Resnik R, eds. *Maternal-fetal medicine.* 4th ed. Philadelphia, PA: WB Saunders; 1999.)

the study cohort (OR: 0.67; 95% CI: 0.42–1.07), except in the women with cervical length less than 15 mm (OR: 0.23; 95% CI: 0.08–0.66). Additionally, the cerclage group was noted to have improvement in the following secondary outcomes: perinatal death (8.8% versus 16%), birth before 24 weeks' gestation (6.1% versus 14%), and birth before 37 weeks' gestation (45% versus 60%).[101] This benefit was also reaffirmed by an individual, patient-level metaanalysis that demonstrated a reduction in composite perinatal morbidity and mortality as well as preterm birth at less than 24, 28, 32, and 37 weeks' gestation.[102]

Intrauterine Growth Restriction

Identifying a fetus at risk for or with growth restriction remains a major focus of prenatal care. The classification of newborns by birth weight percentile cannot be understated because there is an inverse relationship between birth weight and adverse perinatal outcomes: newborns in the lowest percentiles are at increased risk of immediate perinatal morbidity and mortality (Fig. 2.9) as well as subsequent adult cardiovascular disease (hypertension, hyperlipidemia, coronary artery disease, diabetes mellitus) as described in the Barker hypothesis. In the 1960s, Lubchenco and colleagues published a series of classic papers with detailed graphs depicting birth weight as a function of gestational age and adverse outcomes. Since that time, various classification schemes and terminology have been adapted to describe infants that fail to reach their growth potential, such as "premature," "low birth weight," "small for gestational age," "small for dates," or "growth restricted." The evolution of these differing terms highlights the complexity of this problem as well as the difficulty of establishing uniform diagnostic criteria. The most common definition for IUGR today is an EFW less than the 10th percentile for gestational age by US evaluation. However, this criterion remains controversial given that it relies on a population-based reference standard and does not provide a means to distinguish fetuses that are constitutionally small, growth restricted and small, and growth restricted but not small. Studies evaluating customized, individual fetal growth curves have been published in Spain, France, and New Zealand and demonstrate improved accuracy in detecting fetuses at risk for adverse outcome, but are not currently employed in the United States.[103,104]

BOX 2.10 Factors and Disorders Associated With Intrauterine Growth Rate

Maternal factors
- Hypertensive disease, chronic or preeclampsia
- Renal disease
- Diabetes mellitus
- Antiphospholipid syndrome
- Hemoglobinopathy
- Collagen vascular disease
- Severe nutrition deficiency (inflammatory bowel disease, poor weight gain)
- Body mass index (BMI)
- Smoking and substance abuse
- Maternal hypoxia (cyanotic heart disease, lung disease, high altitude)
- Medications

Fetal factors
- Multiple gestation
- Placental abnormalities
- Infection (viral, protozoal)
- Congenital anomalies
- Chromosomal abnormalities

Numerous maternal and fetal factors have been associated with IUGR, and these etiologies are listed in Box 2.10. Often, the underlying etiology is clinically apparent, and in such cases a diagnosis and management plan can be established. In other cases, the underlying cause may be more elusive. Importantly, an attempt should be made to determine the cause antenatally to provide appropriate counseling and management plans. Additionally, the underlying etiology may have implications for future pregnancies. Therefore when IUGR is identified, additional testing such as a detailed anatomic US evaluation, karyotype, or evaluation for viral infections may be warranted—depending on the clinical scenario.

Typically, the fundal height measurement in centimeters should approximate the weeks of gestational age. Therefore a fundal height measurement significantly less than the estimated gestational age may suggest an IUGR fetus. However, clinical diagnosis of IUGR is inaccurate. In fact, studies demonstrate that with the use of physical exam alone, IUGR remains undetected or is incorrectly diagnosed in about 50% of cases. Currently, US is the preferred modality for the diagnosis of IUGR. Therefore one essential principle of the antenatal recognition of IUGR is identification of the maternal and fetal risk factors that may prompt US surveillance.

US measurements of the BPD, HC, AC, and FL are four standard measurements used to estimate fetal weight and allow for the determination of the pattern of growth aberration. Symmetrical IUGR, which accounts for approximately 20% to 30% of cases, occurs after an insult early in pregnancy (infection, drug or environmental exposure, chromosomal abnormality) affects fetal growth equally at all morphologic parameters. Conversely, asymmetrical IUGR occurs more frequently and results from placental insufficiency later in pregnancy. In asymmetrical IUGR, the FL and HC are preserved, but the AC is decreased secondary to the redistribution of blood flow to vital organs (heart, brain, placenta) at the expense of less vital organs (lungs, abdominal viscera, skin). Notably, the finding of a normal AC reliably excludes IUGR with a false-negative rate of less than 10%.

An optimal or standard management of pregnancies complicated by IUGR has not been established. The cornerstones of management for a fetus with IUGR include antenatal testing with serial NSTs or BPPs; serial US surveillance of fetal growth, AFV, and umbilical artery Doppler velocimetry; and the administration of antenatal corticosteroids if preterm delivery is anticipated. Notably, the weekly monitoring of umbilical artery Doppler velocimetry is the recommended primary surveillance tool for the fetus with IUGR. Numerous studies and metaanalyses have demonstrated a reduction in perinatal mortality and iatrogenic prematurity (premature or unnecessary induction of labor) for a preterm infant with IUGR when umbilical artery Doppler is utilized in decisions regarding timing of delivery. Normal or decreased umbilical artery flow is rarely associated with significant morbidity, whereas absence or reversal of end-diastolic flow suggests poor fetal condition.

The optimal timing of delivery for the IUGR fetus remains controversial and without consensus. However, although opinions vary, experts generally agree that the growth-restricted infants should be delivered close to term, assuming that growth continues and antenatal testing remains reassuring. The Growth Restriction Intervention Trial highlighted the difficulty in selecting the appropriate timing of delivery. This trial randomized 548 preterm IUGR pregnancies for which both fetal compromise and uncertainty regarding delivery were identified to immediate or delayed delivery. In the delayed group, delivery occurred when the primary obstetrician felt certainty regarding delivery timing (median delay: 4.9 days). The primary finding was that delayed delivery results in more stillbirths than immediate delivery; however, the number of stillbirths was equal to the increase in neonatal deaths observed in the immediate delivery arm. The long-term outcomes failed to demonstrate any neurodevelopmental differences in either group among survivors.[107]

Therefore timing of delivery should be individualized and based on gestational age and fetal condition. The following principles may guide management of pregnancies complicated by IUGR:

- Remote from term, conservative management to prolong pregnancy may be performed safely with serial antepartum surveillance as described earlier to achieve further fetal maturity.
- The term or late preterm (>34 weeks) IUGR fetus should be delivered when there is evidence of maternal hypertension, poor interval growth (over 2- to 4-week intervals), nonreassuring antenatal testing (NST, BPP), and/or umbilical artery Doppler testing to demonstrate absence or reversal of flow.
- When growth restriction is mild, no complicating maternal or fetal factors are present, and the umbilical artery Doppler and fetal testing are reassuring, delivery can be delayed until at least 37 weeks' gestation to minimize the risks of prematurity.
- Each specific clinical scenario requires close consideration and an individualization of management plans.

Magnesium for Neuroprotection

CP comprises a heterogeneous group of chronic, nonprogressive disabilities of the CNS, primarily of movement and/or posture. CP represents the most common cause of childhood motor disability, and the prevalence has remained stable over time at approximately 1–2 per 1000 live births. Prematurity is one of the most powerful risk factors for CP, and in one study, the prevalence of CP rose from 0.1% in term infants to 0.7% at 32 to 36 weeks' gestation, 6% at 28 to 31 weeks' gestation, and to 14% at 22 to 27 weeks' gestation.[108] Observational studies, primarily secondary analyses of trials involving very-low-birth-weight infants whose mothers received magnesium sulfate either for tocolysis or eclampsia prophylaxis, emerged in the 1980s–1990s, describing an association between magnesium sulfate exposure and neurologic outcomes. Many of these studies noted that exposure conferred a protective effect against the development of CP. Importantly, animal models have supported the biological plausibility for a neuroprotective effect, which may involve the inhibition of *N*-methyl-D-aspartate excitotoxic neuronal damage, promotion of cerebral vasodilation, scavenging of free radicals, or reduction of inflammatory cytokines.

Subsequently, multiple randomized controlled trials were conducted to evaluate the efficacy of magnesium sulfate specifically for neuroprotection in women at risk for preterm delivery.[110] Notably, all trials demonstrated a decrease in the risk of moderate or severe CP in the magnesium-exposed trial arms. In the largest trial, the Benefits of Antenatal Magnesium by Rouse and associates,[111] magnesium reduced the risk of moderate to severe CP from 7.3% to 4.2% ($p < 0.004$). Although there was no statistically significant difference noted in the primary composite outcome (death or CP) in the larger two trials, the published analysis included data demonstrating that there was no impact of magnesium on the risk of death, thereby eliminating the possibility that the lower rate of CP in the treatment arm was caused by increased death with magnesium. No increase in serious maternal adverse events was reported in any trial. Additionally, multiple metaanalyses have been performed that confirm the findings of the individual trials (reduction in moderate to severe CP, no impact on death alone) and also demonstrate a statistically significant reduction in the primary outcome of death or CP (summary RR: 0.85; 95% CI: 0.74–0.98).[112]

Therefore the weight of the available evidence supports the use of magnesium for neuroprotection, and ACOG published a Committee Opinion in March 2010 supporting its use.[113] Notably, the number of women who must be treated to prevent one case of CP decreases with decreasing gestational age: at less than 32 weeks' gestation, 63 women must receive magnesium to prevent one case of moderate to severe CP; at less than 28 weeks' gestation, 29 women must be treated. If magnesium sulfate were administered uniformly to women at risk of preterm delivery before 32 weeks' gestation in the United States, more than 1000 cases of handicapping CP would be prevented yearly. Institutions adopting the use of magnesium sulfate for neuroprotection should develop specific treatment protocols, guidelines, and inclusion criteria in accordance with trials that have demonstrated benefit.

Antenatal Corticosteroids

In a landmark paper published in 1972, Liggins and Howie demonstrated a decrease in RDS and neonatal mortality in the offspring of women treated with antenatal corticosteroids. Subsequently, the efficacy of antenatal glucocorticoid therapy has been confirmed by more than 12 randomized controlled trials and multiple metaanalyses. In 1994, the NIH held a consensus conference to address antenatal corticosteroids use, which resulted in the recommendation for the administration of a single course of corticosteroids to all pregnant women between 24 and 34 weeks' gestation at risk for preterm delivery within 7 days, including patients with PPROM prior to 32 weeks' gestational age. A 2017 update of the ACOG committee opinion recommends steroid administration for pregnant women with an increased risk of preterm birth in the next 7 days including those with PPROM and multiple gestations. The update also suggests that a single course of betamethasone may be considered in pregnant women who are between 34 weeks' gestation and 36 weeks and 6 days' gestation who are at risk for preterm birth in the next 7 days, and who have not received a course of antenatal steroids.[114] See Fig. 2.7, recommendations for steroids in the context of PPROM.

Corticosteroid therapy is thought to improve neonatal lung function through multiple mechanisms: accelerating the morphologic development and maturation of both type I and type II alveolar pneumocytes, stimulating surfactant production from type II pneumocytes, and increasing the synthesis of surfactant-binding proteins and lung antioxidant enzymes. The cumulative effect is a maturation of the lung architecture and the biochemical pathways that improve the mechanical function of the lungs and gas exchange. Regarding clinical respiratory morbidity and mortality outcomes, a Cochrane systematic review concluded that treatment with antenatal corticosteroids was associated with an overall reduction in RDS as well as severe RDS (RR reduction of approximately 40% to 50%), thereby decreasing requirements for respiratory support. Importantly, numerous studies and systematic reviews have demonstrated that antenatal corticosteroid administration decreases the risk of other severe morbidities related to prematurity. The aforementioned Cochrane review also concluded that corticosteroid treatment decreases the risk of IVH (RR: 0.54; 95% CI: 0.43–0.69), necrotizing enterocolitis (RR: 0.46; 95% CI: 0.29–0.74), neonatal mortality (RR: 0.69; 95% CI: 0.58–0.81), and systemic infection within the first 48 hours of life (RR: 0.56, 95% CI: 0.38–0.85).

Betamethasone and dexamethasone are the preferred corticosteroids for antenatal treatment and have been the most widely studied agents. Both drugs cross the placenta in their active form and have similar biological activity. Although comparative trials between betamethasone and dexamethasone exist, results have been inconsistent and conflicting, and there is insufficient evidence to recommend one steroid over the other. The most commonly used regimens that constitute a single course include the following:

- *Betamethasone*—12 mg IM every 24 hours for two doses
- *Dexamethasone*—6 mg IM every 12 hours for four doses

There is no evidence to support the efficacy or safety of increasing the quantity of the dose or accelerating a dosing regimen should prompt delivery be expected.

The initial data of Liggins and Howie suggested that the benefits of antenatal corticosteroid administration decreased beyond 7 days after administration, which was also evident in the aforementioned Cochrane analysis. However, other retrospective studies have challenged this view, and, subsequently, various trials have examined the role for repeat courses of corticosteroids.[115,117] In 2000, the NIH reconvened another consensus panel to update the 1994 recommendations with regard to repeat courses of antenatal corticosteroids. The panel concluded that although existing evidence suggested a possible benefit in respiratory outcomes, animal and human studies demonstrated evidence of adverse fetal effects on fetal growth (HC), lung growth and organization, retinal development, insulin resistance, renal glomerular number, and maturation and myelination of the CNS. Two studies with long-term follow-up of children exposed to multiple courses of steroids to 2 years of age did not demonstrate any significant difference in neurocognitive outcomes.[109,116] However, a large randomized controlled trial demonstrated a trend, albeit statistically insignificant, toward an increased incidence of CP with repeat courses of corticosteroids.[117] Both the NIH and ACOG do not recommend repeat courses of corticosteroids.[114]

However, a single rescue course of antenatal corticosteroids may significantly improve short-term neonatal respiratory morbidity. A multicenter randomized control trial of a single rescue course was conducted in 437 patients without PPROM who had completed a course of antenatal corticosteroids before 30 weeks of gestation. Other inclusion criteria included completion of a course of corticosteroids more than 14 days before randomization and a recurring threat of preterm delivery before 33 weeks' gestation. The study demonstrated a significant reduction in RDS, surfactant use, and composite morbidity in those delivering before 34 weeks' gestation and for the overall cohort without any increase in other fetal, neonatal, or maternal outcomes.[117] Long-term data have not yet been published. Since publication of this trial, ACOG has released a committee opinion stating that in the appropriate candidates, a single rescue course of steroids "may be considered."[114]

Little evidence supports the use of antenatal corticosteroids for the previable fetus. Administration prior to 24 weeks' gestation will unlikely have a significant impact on the improvement of lung function, given that lungs are still in the canalicular phase of development with few primitive alveoli available on which steroids can exert an effect. Few studies regarding neonatal outcomes after steroid administration prior to 24 weeks' gestation have been conducted, and the available data are limited to case series and observational studies. The largest study conducted to date evaluated 181 neonates born between 23 0/7 and 23 6/7 weeks' gestation and noted that neonates exposed to a complete course of corticosteroids had a decreased mortality risk (OR: 0.18; 95% CI: 0.06–0.54). However, exposure to corticosteroids had no impact on the risk of severe IVH or necrotizing enterocolitis.[118] Although a detailed discussion of the management of the periviable fetus is beyond the scope of this chapter, the authors believe that the administration of antenatal corticosteroids prior to 24 weeks' gestation may be considered in select circumstances. This decision should be individualized after a careful consideration of the clinical scenario, prognostic factors (weight, fetal gender, presence of intraamniotic infection, etc.), and parental wishes regarding neonatal resuscitation.

EDITORIAL COMMENT: There has been a change in practice in many units so that antenatal corticosteroids are administered routinely at 22 weeks' gestation.

Normal and Abnormal Labor

Labor and delivery is dependent on the complex interaction of three variables: the powers, the passenger, and the passage. The powers refer to the forces generated by the uterus. Uterine activity is characterized by the intensity, frequency, and duration of contractions. The passenger is the fetus: the absolute size, lie, position, presentation, attitude, and number. The passage refers to the pelvis and its ability to allow for delivery of the fetus. The bony limits of the pelvis can be assessed using clinical pelvimetry or, rarely, radiography and CT.

Labor occurs in three distinct stages. The first stage is the interval between the onset of labor and full cervical dilation. This stage has been further subdivided into three phases: latent, active, and deceleration. The second stage is the interval between full cervical dilation and delivery of the infant. The mother assists in this stage with active pushing, although this is not a requirement. The third stage is the interval between delivery of the infant and delivery of the placenta and fetal membranes. Each of these stages has an expected length, although recent research has questioned this older data.[119] Abnormalities of the labor process can occur at any of these stages.

Intrapartum management depends on assessment of risk and evaluation for current or pending complications. Complications can arise rapidly during labor. Approximately 20% to 25% of all perinatal morbidity and mortality occurs in pregnancies with no underlying risk factors.[120] The presence of medical comorbidities such as diabetes, hypertension, asthma, HIV, and obesity will affect management. Labor will also be affected by complications of pregnancy: preeclampsia, macrosomia, chorioamnionitis, PPROM preterm labor, and fetal anomalies. When possible, the assessment and management of these complications and comorbidities antenatally is essential for the proper care of the patient during her labor course.

During labor, all pregnant women require surveillance of vital signs and FHR. The value of routine continuous EFM during labor is controversial. The U.S. Preventive Services Task Force states that "routine electronic fetal monitoring for low-risk women in labor is not mandatory and there is insufficient evidence to recommend for or against intrapartum EFM for high-risk pregnant women." Regardless, some form of FHR monitoring has become a standard of care for all women in the United States, either by continuous electronic or manual auscultation.

Assessment of contractions and cervical change are also done at regular intervals to follow the progress of labor and guide the need for intervention. There is no standard interval for cervical assessment, and many practitioners weigh the risk of chorioamnionitis with frequent cervical examinations versus the prolongation of labor due to lack of progress.

EDITORIAL COMMENT: The association between maternal chorioamnionitis and early-onset sepsis in the newborn has long been recognized. Established guidelines recommended treating all exposed infants with broad-spectrum antibiotics until infection was ruled out. A management strategy consisting of close observation of well-appearing term and late preterm infants exposed to suspected intrauterine infection will reduce exposure to empiric antimicrobial therapy.[a] A panel has recommended replacement of the term *chorioamnionitis* with a more general, descriptive term: *intrauterine inflammation or infection or both,* abbreviated as *Triple I*.[b]

Among patients with preterm clinical chorioamnionitis, 24% had no evidence of either intraamniotic infection or intraamniotic inflammation, and 66% had negative amniotic fluid cultures, using standard microbiologic techniques. These observations call for a reexamination of the criteria used to diagnose preterm clinical chorioamnionitis and support the restricted use of empiric antibiotic therapy.[c]

[a]Randis TM, Polin RA, Saade G. Chorioamnionitis: time for a new approach. *Curr Opin Pediatr.* 2017;29(2):159-164.

[b]Higgins RD, Saade G, Polin RA, et al. Chorioamnionitis Workshop Participants. Evaluation and management of women and newborns with a maternal diagnosis of chorioamnionitis: summary of a workshop. *Obstet Gynecol.* 2016;127(3):426-436.

[c]Oh KJ, Kim SM, Hong JS, et al. Twenty-four percent of patients with clinical chorioamnionitis in preterm gestations have no evidence of either culture-proven intraamniotic infection or intraamniotic inflammation. *Am J Obstet Gynecol.* 2017;216(6):604.e1-604.e11.

Contraction frequency and duration can be monitored using simple observation and palpation of the fundus or with internal or external tocodynamometry. However, only internal tocodynamometry with an IUPC can measure the strength of contractions. Contractions or cervical change that is not deemed adequate for labor, a lack of powers, can be augmented using oxytocin. The use of oxytocin in most institutions is given under a standard protocol to ensure safe administration and low incidence of hyperstimulation that can lead to FHR abnormalities and acidemia.

In otherwise uncomplicated patients without maternal of fetal indications for induction of labor, timing of delivery recommendations vary widely among providers. The general consensus is to recommend delivery by 42 weeks' gestation. Postterm deliveries were also more likely to be associated with macrosomia, shoulder dystocia, low Apgar scores, and oligohydramnios. More importantly, postterm pregnancies carry an increased risk of intrauterine fetal demise and intrapartum death.[121] A recently completed multicenter trial on labor induction reported that elective induction of labor for women at 39 weeks' gestation improves neonatal and maternal outcomes without increasing rates of cesarean section.[122] Abnormalities in labor progression that lead to arrest or protraction disorders can occur in the first or second stages. Typically, first-stage arrest that is not amenable to oxytocin administration is treated with cesarean delivery. Second-stage arrest can also be treated by cesarean delivery if an operative vaginal delivery cannot be safely completed. In the United States, 4.5% of births are completed by operative vaginal delivery, and the success rate is high.[123] Choice of instrument is determined by level of training with either forceps or vacuum. Other considerations include the degree of maternal anesthesia, gestational age of the fetus, and anticipated difficulty of the procedure. Maternal and fetal complications rates depend on a number of factors and may be more related to abnormal labor than to the devices themselves. A metaanalysis of 10 trials comparing vacuum with forceps delivery found vacuum deliveries were associated with less maternal soft tissue trauma and required less anesthesia, but were less likely to result in successful vaginal delivery. Neonates delivered by vacuum extraction had more cephalohematoma and retinal hemorrhages than those delivered by forceps. Sequential attempts at operative vaginal delivery using different instruments should be avoided due to an increased risk of fetal injury.

Reducing infectious complications in the mother and the neonate are important in the management of labor. In the United States, a universal screening program for group B-hemolytic *Streptococcus* (GBS) has been implemented. This screening program, combined with the chemoprophylaxis of screen-positive patients, has dramatically reduced the incidence of early onset GBS infections in neonates.[124] The diagnosis of chorioamnionitis can contribute to significant morbidity for the mother and infant. Risk factors for intrauterine infection include nulliparity, spontaneous labor, prolonged rupture of membranes (>18 hours), multiple digital vaginal examinations, meconium-stained fluid, internal fetal or uterine monitoring, and the presence of genital tract pathogens. Maternal fever and two of the following symptoms contribute to the diagnosis: maternal or fetal tachycardia, uterine fundal tenderness, foul-smelling amniotic fluid, or elevated maternal white blood cell count. Prompt treatment with broad-spectrum intravenous antibiotics is recommended to improve maternal and neonatal outcomes. Typically, ampicillin, gentamycin, and clindamycin or metronidazole is used. Alternative regimens include ampicillin-sulbactam or cefoxitin.

Labor is a painful process, and women use different methods to relieve this discomfort. While some prefer nonpharmacologic methods, ACOG supports the concept that maternal request alone is a sufficient medical indication for labor analgesia. Pharmacologic approaches can be classified as systemic, regional, or local. Systemic methods involve intravenous or IM administration of typically opioid agents or opioid agonist-antagonists. These agents provide only minimal relief unless high dosages are used. When used in higher dosages, opioid analgesics can cause respiratory depression and an increased risk of aspiration in the mother, as well as neonatal respiratory depression. Regional techniques include epidurals, spinals, and combined spinal-epidurals. The methods typically use a mixture of a local anesthetic and opioid agent. Neuraxial anesthesia is very widely used in the United States, with approximately 70% of patients receiving this type of labor pain relief.[125] Maternal risks of neuraxial anesthesia are rare, including systemic toxicity, high spinal, hypotension resulting in fetal bradycardia, postdural puncture headache, infection, hematoma, and urinary retention. The effects on the neonate have been studied and show either no difference or improvement in neonatal neurobehavior after epidural compared to systemic opioid analgesia or no medication. The effect of neuraxial analgesia in labor on breast feeding is controversial, and studies to date are inconclusive. ACOG concluded that breast feeding is not affected by choice of anesthetic; thus anesthetic choice should be based on other considerations. Local injections of anesthesia in the area of the pudendal nerve (pudendal block) can be used in the second or third stage of labor without any effect on the neonate.

Human Immunodeficiency Virus

Pregnant women with HIV require comprehensive medical care to achieve good maternal outcomes and low rates of perinatal HIV transmission. Antiretroviral therapy is recommended to reduce perinatal transmission. Transmission can occur during pregnancy, labor and delivery, or the breast-feeding period. The risk has been reduced to less than 2% in the United States with the administration of antiretroviral prophylaxis and viral suppression.[126] The first study in 1994 showed the benefit of administering a single agent, zidovudine, intrapartum and to the infant after delivery. It was effective in significantly decreasing transmission, from 25% to 8%. Since that time, other studies have shown benefit of multiple agents and administration earlier in pregnancy.[127] The current recommendation is to start antiretroviral therapy immediately if the patient requires it for her own health, or otherwise after the first trimester. Delaying treatment until after 28 weeks' gestation may result in an increased risk of transmission. Treatment regimens for pregnant patients with HIV are the topic of guidelines produced and regularly updated by the U.S. Department of Health and Human Services.[128]

In addition to standard screening, pregnant women with HIV should be screened for other infectious diseases including hepatitis B and C, toxoplasmosis, tuberculosis, and cytomegalovirus. For women with CD4 counts lower than 200 cells/mm^3, pneumocystis pneumonia prophylaxis is recommended. Counseling on sexually transmitted disease prevention and reduction of other risk factors should be performed. Women should be informed that in resource-rich areas, such as the United States, breast feeding is not recommended because of the increased risk of transmission to the infant.

QUESTION

True or False

Insulin is the first line of treatment for gestational diabetics with elevated glucose levels.

While oral antidiabetic agents were almost universally endorsed as first-line drugs in the treatment of intrauterine growth restriction (gestational diabetes mellitus) in the past, recent evidence suggest insulin is considered the preferred pharmacologic treatment of gestational diabetes mellitus. Oral hypoglycemic agents such as metformin and glyburide are reasonable choices for women who cannot administer or cannot afford insulin, though oral hypoglycemic agents are not approved by the U.S. Food and Drug Administration, cross the placenta, and lack long-term neonatal safety data, making insulin superior to oral antidiabetic medication.[129] Therefore the answer is true.

The reference list for this chapter can be found online at www.expertconsult.com.

3

Resuscitation and Initial Stabilization

Amy E. Heiderich, Tina A. Leone

The transition from fetal to neonatal life is a dramatic and complex process involving extensive physiologic changes that are most obvious at the time of birth. Individuals who care for newly born infants during these first few minutes of neonatal life must monitor the progress of the transition and be prepared to intervene when necessary. In the majority of births, this transition occurs without a requirement for any significant assistance. However, when the need for intervention arises, the presence of providers who are skilled in neonatal resuscitation can be life saving. Each year approximately 4 million children are born in the United States, and more than 30 times as many are born worldwide.[1,2] It is estimated that approximately 5% to 10% of all births will require some form of resuscitation beyond basic care, thereby making neonatal resuscitation the most frequently practiced form of resuscitation in medical care. Throughout the world, approximately 1 million newborn deaths are associated with birth asphyxia. Although it cannot be expected that neonatal resuscitation will eliminate all early neonatal mortality, it has the potential for helping save many lives and for significantly reducing associated morbidities.

Attempts at reviving nonbreathing infants immediately after birth have occurred throughout recorded time, with references in literature, religion, and early medicine. Although the organization and sophistication has changed, the basic principle and goal of initiating breathing has remained constant throughout time. It has only been since the late 20th century that the process of neonatal resuscitation has been more officially regimented. Resuscitation programs in other areas of medicine were initiated in the 1970s in an effort to improve knowledge about effective resuscitation and provide an action plan for early responders. The first of such programs was focused on adult cardiopulmonary resuscitation.[3] These programs then began increasing in complexity and becoming more specific to different types of resuscitation needs. With the collaboration of the American Heart Association and the American Academy of Pediatrics, the Neonatal Resuscitation Program (NRP) was initiated in 1987 and was designed to address the specific needs of the newly born infant. Since the origination of the NRP, ongoing evaluation of the program has resulted in changes when new evidence becomes available. The most recent edition of the NRP textbook, published in 2016, made several revisions, including the use of monitoring in the delivery room and management of infants born through meconium-stained amniotic fluid.[4] Various groups throughout the world also provide resuscitation recommendations that may be more specific to the practices in certain regions. An international group of scientists, the International Liaison Committee on Resuscitation, completes a thorough review of the literature about each of the relevant questions of resuscitation, which is published and utilized by the different groups that provide recommendations for practice.[5]

The overall goal of the NRP is similar to other resuscitation programs in that it intends to teach large groups of individuals of varying backgrounds the principles of resuscitation and to provide an action plan for providers. Similarly, a satisfactory end result of resuscitation would be common to all forms of resuscitation, namely to provide adequate tissue oxygenation to prevent tissue injury and restore spontaneous cardiopulmonary function. When comparing neonatal resuscitation with other forms of resuscitation, several distinctions can be noted. First, the birth of an infant is a more predictable occurrence than most other events that require resuscitation. Although not every birth will require "resuscitation," it is more reasonable to expect that skilled individuals can be present when the need for neonatal resuscitation arises. It is possible to anticipate with some accuracy which neonates will more likely require resuscitation based on perinatal factors and thus allow time for preparation. The second distinction of neonatal resuscitation compared with other forms of resuscitation involves the unique physiology involved in the normal fetal transition to neonatal life. The fetus exists in the protected environment of the uterus where temperature is closely controlled, continuous fetal breathing is not essential to provide gas exchange, the lungs are filled with fluid, and gas exchange occurs in the placenta. The transition that occurs at birth requires the neonate to increase heat production, initiate continuous breathing, replace the lung fluid with air, and significantly increase pulmonary blood flow so that gas exchange can occur in the lungs. The expectations for this transitional process and knowledge of how to effectively assist the process help guide the current practice of neonatal resuscitation.

FETAL TRANSITION TO EXTRAUTERINE LIFE

The key elements necessary for a successful transition to extrauterine life involve changes in thermoregulation, respiration, and circulation. In utero, the fetal core temperature is approximately 0.5° C greater than the mother's temperature.[6] Heat is produced by metabolic processes and is lost over this small temperature gradient through the placenta and skin.[7] After birth, the temperature gradient between the infant and the environment becomes much greater, and heat is lost through the skin by radiation, convection, conduction, and evaporation. The newly born infant must begin producing heat through other mechanisms such as lipolysis of brown adipose tissue.[8] If heat is lost at a pace greater than it is produced, the infant will become hypothermic. Preterm infants are at particular risk because of increased heat loss through immature skin, a greater surface area–to–body weight ratio, and decreased brown adipose tissue stores. Preterm hypothermic infants who are admitted to the nursery have decreased chances of survival.[9] Routine measures during neonatal resuscitation, such as the use of radiant warmers and drying the infant, are aimed at preventing heat loss. For the preterm infant, special measures for temperature management, such as the use of plastic wrap as a barrier to evaporative heat loss, are necessary to ensure adequate thermoregulation.

The fetus lives in a fluid-filled environment and, as lung development occurs, the developing alveolar spaces are filled with lung fluid. Lung fluid production decreases in the days prior to delivery, and the remainder of lung fluid is resorbed into the pulmonary interstitial spaces after delivery.[10,11] As the infant takes the first breaths after birth, a negative intrathoracic pressure of approximately 50 cm H_2O is generated to help fill the lung with air replacing the lung fluid.[12,13] The alveoli become filled with air, and with the help of pulmonary surfactant, the lungs retain a small amount of air at the end of exhalation, known as the functional residual capacity (FRC). Although the fetus makes breathing movements in utero, these efforts are intermittent and are not required for gas exchange. Continuous spontaneous breathing is maintained after birth by several mechanisms including the activation of chemoreceptors, the decrease in placental hormones, which inhibit respirations, and the presence of natural environmental stimulation. Spontaneous breathing can be suppressed at birth for several reasons, most critical of which is the presence of acidosis secondary to compromised fetal circulation. The natural history of the physiologic responses to acidosis has been described by researchers creating such conditions in animal models. Dawes described the breathing response to acidosis in different animal species.[14] He noted that when pH was decreased, animals typically have a relatively short period of apnea followed by gasping. The gasping pattern then increases in rate until breathing ceases again for a second period of apnea. Dawes also noted that the first period of apnea or primary apnea could be reversed with stimulation, whereas the second period of apnea, secondary or terminal apnea, required assisted ventilation to establish spontaneous breathing. In the clinical situation, the exact timing of onset of acidosis is generally unknown, and therefore any observed apnea may be either primary or secondary. This is the basis of the resuscitation recommendation that stimulation may be attempted in the presence of apnea, but if not quickly successful, assisted ventilation should be initiated promptly. Without the presence of acidosis, a newborn may also develop apnea because of recent exposure to respiratory-suppressing medications such as narcotics, anesthetics, and magnesium. These medications, when given to the mother, cross the placenta and, depending on the time of administration and dose, may act on the newborn.

Fetal circulation is unique because gas exchange takes place in the placenta. In the fetal heart, oxygenated blood returning via the umbilical vein is mixed with deoxygenated blood from the superior and inferior vena cava and is differentially distributed throughout the body. The most oxygenated blood is directed toward the brain, while the most deoxygenated blood is directed toward the placenta. Thus, blood returning from the placenta to the right atrium is preferentially streamed via the foramen ovale to the left atrium and ventricle, and then to the ascending aorta, providing the brain with the most oxygenated blood. Fetal channels, including the ductus arteriosus and foramen ovale, allow blood flow to mostly bypass the lungs with their intrinsically high vascular resistance, which will receive only approximately 10%–30% of the total cardiac output.[15] Thus, the fetal circulation is unique in that the pulmonary and systemic circulations are not equal as occurs after these channels close. In the mature postnatal circulation, the lungs must receive 100% of the cardiac output. When the low-resistance placental circulation is removed after birth, the infant's systemic vascular resistance increases while the pulmonary vascular resistance begins to fall as a result of pulmonary inflation, increased arterial oxygen tension, and local vasodilators. These changes result in a dramatic increase in pulmonary blood flow. Near the end of gestation the placenta contains about 30%–50% of the feto-placental blood volume.[16] When the umbilical cord remains patent following birth, some of the placental blood volume is transferred into the newborn, leading to higher newborn hematocrit levels and a more stable hemodynamic transition. It has also recently been shown in animal models that when newly born lambs are ventilated prior to cord clamping, hemodynamic parameters such as blood pressure and cerebral blood flow remain more stable after birth.[17] The average fetal oxyhemoglobin saturation as measured in fetal lambs is approximately 50%,[18] but ranges in different sites within the fetal circulation between values of 20% to 80%.[19] The oxyhemoglobin saturation rises gradually over the first 5 to 15 minutes of life to 90% or greater as the air spaces are cleared of fluid.[20] In the face of poor transition secondary to asphyxia, meconium aspiration, pneumonia, or extreme prematurity, the lungs may not be able to provide efficient gas exchange, and the oxygen saturation may not increase as expected. In addition, in some situations, the normal reduction in pulmonary vascular resistance may not fully occur, resulting in persisting pulmonary hypertension and decreased effective pulmonary blood flow with continued right-to-left shunting through the aforementioned fetal channels. Although the complete transition from fetal to extrauterine life is complex and much more intricate than can be discussed in these few short paragraphs, a basic knowledge of these processes will contribute to the understanding of the rationale for resuscitation practices.

Preparation

The environment in which the infant is born should facilitate the transition to neonatal life as much as possible and should readily accommodate the needs of a resuscitation team when necessary. Hospitals may vary in the approach to the details of how to prepare for resuscitation. For example, some hospitals may have a separate room designated for resuscitation where the infant will be taken after birth, others bring all the necessary equipment into the delivery room when resuscitation is expected, and some have every delivery room already equipped for any resuscitation. Wherever the resuscitation will take place, a few key elements should be ensured. The room should be warm enough to prevent excessive newborn heat loss, bright enough to assess the infant's clinical status, and large enough to accommodate the necessary personnel and equipment to care for the baby.

When no added risks to the newborn are identified, the term birth frequently may occur without the attendance of a specific neonatal resuscitation team. However, it is frequently recommended that one individual be present who is only responsible for the infant and can quickly alert a neonatal resuscitation team if necessary. Even the best neonatal resuscitation triage systems will not anticipate the need for resuscitation in all cases. Using a retrospective risk assessment scoring system, Smith and colleagues found that 6% of newborns requiring resuscitation would not be identified based on risk factors.[21] Antenatal determination of neonatal risk allows the neonatal resuscitation team to be present for the delivery and to be more thoroughly prepared for the situation. Preterm infants require resuscitation more frequently than term infants and therefore require the presence of a prepared neonatal resuscitation team at the delivery. Any situation in which the infant's respirations may be suppressed or the fetus is showing signs of distress should signal the need for a neonatal resuscitation team. A list of factors that may be associated with an increased risk of need for resuscitation can be found in Box 3.1. Hospitals may vary to some extent about which conditions require presence of the neonatal resuscitation team at delivery.

The composition of the neonatal resuscitation team will also vary tremendously among institutions. Probably the most important factor in how well a team functions is how well the group has prepared for the delivery. When there is a high index of suspicion that the newborn infant will be born in a compromised state, the minimum requirements for an effective team includes at least three members, one of whom has significant previous experience leading neonatal resuscitations. Preparation involves both the immediate tasks of readying equipment and personnel, as well as the broader institutional preparation of training team members and providing appropriate space and equipment. Teams that regularly work together and divide tasks in a routine manner will have a better chance of functioning smoothly during a critical situation. Although much attention has been raised in the literature regarding teamwork and team and leadership training, minimal evidence is available to recommend a specific team composition or training approach. Regular simulation and debriefing experiences have been useful in helping keep teams prepared for emergency situations. The use of video debriefing during simulation and real-life resuscitation can help identify areas for quality improvement.[22,23]

BOX 3.1 Risk Factors Related to Resuscitation at Birth

Maternal factors	Fetal factors	Placental factors
Diabetes mellitus	Preterm birth	Placenta previa
Preeclampsia	Known fetal anomalies	Placenta accreta
Chronic illness	Multiple gestation	Vasa previa
Poor prenatal care	Hydrops fetalis	Placental abruption
Substance abuse	Oligohydramnios	Premature rupture of membranes
Uterine rupture	Polyhydramnios	
General anesthesia	Intrauterine growth restriction	
Chorioamnionitis	Signs of fetal distress	
	Decreased fetal movement	

EDITORIAL COMMENT: Quality improvement by means of simulation has been implemented in many units with great success. Furthermore, quality improvement aimed at preventing low temperatures on admission to the neonatal intensive care unit have substantially reduced the prevalence of moderate hypothermia (temperature below 36°C) on admission. This may alter mortality and morbidity.

Cord Management

After the infant is delivered, the umbilical cord must be clamped and cut. The recommended timing for clamping the umbilical cord has changed over recent years. The obstetric practice had been to immediately clamp the cord after delivery in an effort to prevent maternal hemorrhage. However, a number of randomized controlled trials have shown that "delayed cord clamping" of at least 60 seconds after birth has benefits for the newborn infant without having adverse effects for the mother. In preterm infants, several studies have shown decreases in the rates of intraventricular hemorrhage, necrotizing enterocolitis, and need for blood transfusion. The most recent metaanalysis of studies comparing delayed cord clamping with immediate cord clamping showed a decrease in mortality in the infants treated with at least 60 seconds of delayed cord clamping.[24] In term infants, delayed cord clamping increases hemoglobin levels and iron stores in the first few months of life.[25] Delayed cord clamping is now recommended by the American College of Obstetrics and Gynecology[26] as well as the NRP.[4] In infants who are depressed at birth, the suggested management is less clear. Some investigators have studied and suggested performing milking of the umbilical cord to increase the transfer of blood from the placenta to the infant.[27] This practice has been equivalent to delayed cord clamping in small studies, but is not currently recommended by any guidelines. Ongoing studies are evaluating the practice of beginning resuscitation with the cord intact for infants who are depressed at birth. There is not sufficient evidence to recommend this practice outside of research protocols.

EDITORIAL COMMENT: Delayed or optimal clamping of the cord has been readily accepted and is becoming standard care. Longer-term follow-up is needed, but the data so far are encouraging, and the limited reports demonstrate improved motor function, especially in boys. As noted, questions remain around whether delayed cord clamping in nonvigorous infants is beneficial. Additionally, research is ongoing using a specially designed resuscitation bed that allows neonatal resuscitation simultaneously with delayed cord clamping.

Assessment

Immediately after birth, the infant's condition is evaluated by general observation as well as measurement of specific parameters to ensure the transition to neonatal life proceeds appropriately. Typically, after birth, a healthy newborn will cry vigorously and maintain adequate respirations. The color will transition from blue to pink over the first 2 to 5 minutes, the heart rate (HR) will remain in the 140s to 160s, and the infant will demonstrate adequate muscle tone with some flexion of the extremities. The assessment of an infant who is having difficulty with the transition to extrauterine life will often reveal apnea, bradycardia, cyanosis, and hypotonia. Resuscitation interventions are based mainly on the evaluation of spontaneous respiratory effort and HR. These parameters need to be accurately and continually assessed throughout the resuscitation to determine the need for further intervention. HR can be monitored by auscultation or by palpation of the cord pulsations, with auscultation being a more reliable method; however, both methods have been shown to be imprecise and often underestimate the HR.[28] In many situations, the use of a device for more extensive and more accurate monitoring such as a pulse oximeter or electrocardiogram (ECG) monitor can be helpful during resuscitation.[29] A pulse oximeter or ECG monitor can provide the resuscitation team with a continuous audible and visual indication of the newborn's HR throughout the various steps of resuscitation while freeing a team member to perform other tasks. Studies demonstrated that ECG monitors allow for faster and more accurate HR detection than do pulse oximeters in the delivery room.[29–32] In addition to measuring HR, the pulse oximeter can be used as a more accurate measure of oxygenation than the evaluation of color alone and can be used to guide the titration of supplemental oxygen. It has been well established that color alone is an unreliable measure to accurately assess the infant's oxygen saturation, especially where the room lighting is suboptimal. The NRP guidelines currently recommend that whenever an infant requires mask positive pressure ventilation (PPV), a pulse oximeter should be used for additional monitoring of the infant. Additionally, whenever the infant requires prolonged mask PPV, intubation, and certainly chest compressions, ECG leads should be applied to allow reliable, continuous HR monitoring in addition to pulse oximetry.

The overall assessment of a newborn was quantified by Virginia Apgar in the 1950s with the Apgar score.[33] The score describes the infant's condition at the time it is assigned, and consists of a 10-point scale with a maximum of 2 points assigned for each of the following categories: respirations, HR, color, tone, and reflex irritability. The score was initially intended to provide a uniform, objective assessment of the infant's condition and was used as a tool to compare different practices, especially obstetrical anesthetic practices. Despite the intent of objectivity, there is often disagreement in score assignment among various practitioners.[34,35] Low scores have been consistently associated with increased risk of neonatal mortality,[36,37] but have not been predictive of neurodevelopmental outcome.[38] Interpreting the score when interventions are being provided may be difficult, and current recommendations suggest that clinicians should document the utilized interventions at the time the score is assigned.[39]

Initial Steps: Stimulation and Maintaining the Airway

In the first few seconds after birth, all infants are evaluated for signs of life, and a determination of the need for further assistance is made. The initial screen for neonatal well-being includes checking for spontaneous breathing and tone. As recommended by NRP, an infant who is term, has good tone, and is breathing can continue transitioning with his/her mother, whereas all other infants should be brought to a radiant warmer for further assessment and treatment. When placing the infant on the warmer, the first step is to position the baby in an optimal manner. Appropriate positioning includes placing the infant supine on the warmer with the baby's head toward the open end of the warmer to allow care providers to have easy access to the infant. In addition, the head should be in a neutral or "sniffing" position to facilitate maintenance of an open airway. Providers may provide gentle stimulation, usually performed simultaneously with drying the infant, to encourage spontaneous breathing; however, this should not delay other interventions if the infant does not respond with a strong cry and spontaneous breathing quickly. The oropharynx may be suctioned if there is excess fluid causing airway obstruction. Care should be taken to avoid excessive suctioning, and the provider must be conscious of the possibility of causing vagal-induced bradycardia while suctioning. A metaanalysis on the benefits of oropharyngeal suctioning demonstrated that in term babies, the available evidence is inconclusive regarding the benefits and harms of routine oronasopharyngeal suction.[40]

An infant born through meconium-stained amniotic fluid is at risk for aspirating meconium and developing significant pulmonary disease known as meconium aspiration syndrome (MAS), which may also be accompanied by persistent pulmonary hypertension. For many years, routine management of all infants with meconium-stained amniotic fluid included endotracheal intubation and tracheal suctioning in an attempt to remove any meconium from the trachea and prevent the development of MAS. Recognizing that intubation may not be necessary for all infants and that the procedure may be associated with complications, a more selective approach was followed for approximately 15 years where only those infants who were nonvigorous (HR <100, apneic, poor tone) at birth were intubated and underwent tracheal suctioning.[41–43] More recent, small, randomized trials have evaluated whether tracheal suctioning is beneficial in reducing severe MAS or death in nonvigorous infants. These small trials have demonstrated no difference in the incidence of MAS or death between nonvigorous infants who received tracheal suctioning and those who did not receive routine tracheal suctioning.[44,45] Acknowledging the lack of evidence for benefit of routine intubation and suctioning and the potential for harm associated with delayed initiation of ventilation and potential complications of intubation, the most recent NRP guidelines do not recommend routine tracheal intubation and suctioning of nonvigorous infants born through meconium-stained fluid. Additional future studies may help clarify this issue further.

Temperature Management

The provision of warmth is crucial for all infants but is particularly important for the extremely preterm infant. Preterm infants are commonly admitted to the neonatal intensive care unit (NICU) hypothermic, with core temperatures well below 37°C. In a population-based analysis of all infants less than 26 weeks' gestation, greater than one-third of these preterm infants had admission temperatures less than 35°C. More disturbing is the fact that infants with such admission temperatures survived less often than those with admission temperatures greater than 35°C.[9,46] Admission temperature is considered a strong predictor of morbidity and mortality at all gestations, and all attempts should be made to maintain the temperature in the normothermic range. The recommended temperature on admission is between 36.5°C and 37.5°C. Routine documentation of the admission temperature should be standardized in each neonatal unit to ensure ongoing quality of care.

In order to assist infants in maintaining adequate thermoregulation, on arrival to the warmer, all infants should have any wet towels removed and a warmed hat placed on their head to prevent heat loss. Vohra and colleagues have shown that admission temperatures may be improved in infants less than 28 weeks' gestation by immediately covering the infant's body with polyethylene wrap prior to drying the infant.[47,48] With this approach, the infant's head is left out of the wrap and is dried, but the body is not dried prior to wrap application. The plastic blocks evaporation and minimizes heat loss from convection. A recent meta-analysis examined 18 studies and concluded that the use of plastic wrap or a plastic bag led to increased NICU admission temperatures and fewer infants outside of the normothermic range.[49] Other measures for maintaining infant temperatures include performing resuscitation in a room that is kept at an ambient temperature of approximately 23°C to 25°C (73°F to 77°F), using radiant warmers with servo-controlled temperature probes placed on the infant within minutes of delivery, and the use of prewarmed thermal mattress/heating pads for the tiniest of infants. A meta-analysis has shown that the use of thermal mattresses for infants less than 1500 g is associated with warmer infants and reduced hypothermia on admission to the NICU[49]; however, one must be careful to avoid hyperthermia when using these mattresses in combination with other strategies to prevent hypothermia.[50] It is important to note that as a required safety feature, radiant warmers will substantially decrease their power output after 15 minutes of continuous operation in full-power mode. If this decrease in power is unrecognized, the infant will be exposed to a much cooler radiant temperature. By applying the temperature probe and using the warmer in servo mode, the temperature output will adjust as needed and the power will not automatically decrease; however, it is also important to apply the temperature probe to the infant promptly to avoid overheating the newborn.

Assisting Ventilation

As the newborn infant begins breathing and replaces the lung fluid with air, the lung becomes inflated, and an FRC is developed and maintained. With inadequate development of FRC, the infant will not adequately oxygenate, and if prolonged, the infant will develop bradycardia. The steps involved in performing resuscitation include providing assisted PPV when the infant shows signs of inadequate lung inflation. The indications for provision of PPV include apnea or inadequate respiratory effort and HR less than 100 beats per minute (bpm). PPV can be delivered noninvasively with a pressure delivery device and a face mask or invasively with the same pressure delivery device and an endotracheal tube. Pressure delivery devices can include self-inflating bags, flow-inflating or anesthesia bags, and T-piece resuscitators, each with its own advantages and disadvantages. A self-inflating bag requires a reservoir to provide nearly 100% oxygen and allows the operator to change pressure delivered easily, but may deliver very high pressure if not used carefully and even with a positive end-expiratory pressure (PEEP) valve does not deliver reliable PEEP. These devices have pressure release valves, but these valves do not always open at the target release pressures.[51] The self-inflating bag is easy to use for inexperienced personnel and will work in the absence of a gas source. An anesthesia bag or flow-inflating bag requires a gas source for use and allows the operator to "instinctively" vary delivery pressures, but requires significant practice to develop expertise with use. A T-piece resuscitator is easy to use, requires a gas source for use, and delivers the most consistent levels of pressure, but requires intentional effort to vary pressure levels.[52,53] The flow-inflating bag and T-piece resuscitator allow the operator to deliver continuous positive airway pressure (CPAP) or PEEP relatively easily.[53,54]

A level of experience is required to perform assisted ventilation using a face mask and resuscitation device, especially for an extremely low-birth-weight infant. It is important to maintain a patent airway for the air to reach the lungs. The procedure of obtaining and maintaining a patent airway includes, at minimum, clearing of fluid with a suction device, holding the head in a neutral position, and sometimes lifting the jaw slightly anteriorly. The face mask must make an adequate seal with the face for air to pass to the lungs effectively. No device will adequately inflate the lungs if there is a large leak between the mask and the face. The face mask must cover the mouth and nose while avoiding the eyes. Masks for infants of all sizes are available, including the smallest of infants. Studies have demonstrated that mask leak and airway obstruction are common challenges encountered, and their recognition is often delayed while providing face mask ventilation.[55,56] Signs that the airway is patent and air is being delivered to the lungs include visual inspection of chest rise with each breath and improvement in the clinical condition, including HR and color. The use of a colorimetric carbon dioxide detector during mask ventilation will allow confirmation that gas exchange is occurring by the observed color change of the device or alerting the operator of an obstructed airway with lack of such color change.[57] It is important to remember that these devices will not change color in the absence of pulmonary blood flow, as occurs with inadequate cardiac output. At times, multiple maneuvers are required to achieve a patent airway, such as readjusting the head and mask positions, choosing a mask of more appropriate size, and further suctioning of the pharynx. Alternate methods of providing a patent airway include the use of a nasopharyngeal tube,[58] a laryngeal mask airway (LMA) device,[59] or an endotracheal tube. These interventions for improving ventilation are summarized in NRP by the pneumonic MR. SOPA (***M***ask readjustment, ***R***epositioning, ***S***uction, ***O***pen the mouth, ***P***ressure increase, and ***A***lternate Airway).

The amount of pressure provided with each breath during assisted ventilation is critical to the establishment of lung inflation, FRC and therefore adequate oxygenation. Although it is important to provide adequate pressure for ventilation, excessive pressure can contribute to lung injury. Achieving the correct balance of these goals is not simple and is an area of resuscitation that requires more study. A specific level of inspiratory pressure will never be appropriate for every baby. During the transition to neonatal life, there are vast changes in compliance and resistance of the lungs, and therefore pressure used to provide the same tidal volume is likely dynamic throughout the resuscitation. A manometer in the circuit during assisted ventilation provides the clinician with an indication of the actual administered pressure, allowing better awareness of the pressures being supplied, although if the airway is blocked, this pressure is not delivered to the lungs. The current NRP textbook recommends initial pressures of 20 to 25 mm Hg for preterm infants. The first few breaths may require increased pressure if lung fluid has not been cleared, as occurs when the infant does not initiate spontaneous breathing. It has been shown that using enough pressure to produce visible chest rise may be associated with hypocarbia on blood gas evaluation, and excessive pressure may decrease the effectiveness of surfactant therapy.[60,61] Visible inspection of chest rise can be somewhat subjective, and while it is a good indicator of a patent airway, it is not an accurate gauge of the delivered tidal volume.[62] Choosing the actual initial inspiratory pressure is less important than continuously assessing the progress of the intervention. It has been shown in both manikin and human studies that T-piece resuscitators deliver more consistent peak inspiratory pressure (PIP) and less often deliver inflations of excessive pressure compared to the self-inflating bag.[53] Despite these findings, there is felt to be insufficient evidence to recommend against the self-inflating bag, as clinical outcomes have not been shown to be different between the two devices.[63,64] Additionally, since the self-inflating bag does not require a gas source, it may be necessary to use in areas with limited resources.

It may be possible to establish FRC without increasing peak inspiratory pressures by providing a sustained inflation.[65] Multiple animal and human studies have assessed sustained inflations of varying pressures (ranging from 20–30 cm H_2O) and durations (ranging from 10–20 seconds). A recent metaanalysis showed that the use of sustained inflation may be associated with a decreased duration of mechanical ventilation compared with conventional breaths.[66] However, safety of this approach has not been established, and there may, in fact, be considerable harm caused by the practice of providing sustained inflation. Therefore this practice is not recommended.

The most critical component of continued assessment is evaluation of the infant's response to the intervention. If, after initiating ventilation, the condition of the infant does not improve (specifically, improved HR, breathing, and color), then the ventilation is most likely inadequate. The two most common reasons for inadequate ventilation are a blocked airway or insufficient inspiratory pressure. The blocked airway frequently can be corrected with changes in position or suctioning, whereas inadequate pressure is corrected by adjusting the ventilating device.

In addition to consideration of inspiratory pressure, use of continuous pressure throughout the breathing cycle seems to be beneficial for the establishment of FRC and improvement in surfactant function.[67,68] This is accomplished during assisted ventilation with the use of PEEP or CPAP when additional inspiratory pressure is not needed. In the absence of PEEP, a lung that has been inflated with assisted inspiratory pressure will lose, on expiration, most of the volume that had been delivered on inspiration. This pattern of repeated inflation and deflation is frequently thought to be associated with lung injury. In preterm infants, a general approach of using CPAP as a primary mode of respiratory support in NICUs has been associated with a low incidence of chronic lung disease.[69] A recent metaanalysis assessed studies comparing early CPAP with early assisted ventilation with or without surfactant and found that early CPAP was associated with a "small, but clinically significant" reduction in the incidence of bronchopulmonary dysplasia (BPD), death or BPD, and the need for mechanical ventilation as well as surfactant.[70] It is therefore reasonable to begin CPAP for all spontaneously breathing preterm infants soon after birth.

If the infant is not breathing and assisted ventilation is necessary for a prolonged period of time or if other resuscitative measures have been unsuccessful, ventilation should be provided via an endotracheal tube. The NRP recommends placing an endotracheal tube and providing 30 seconds of high-quality ventilation prior to initiating chest compressions in a depressed infant.

The intubation procedure, although potentially critical for successful resuscitation, requires a significant amount of skill and experience to perform reliably and may be associated with serious complications. The procedure entails using a laryngoscope to visualize the vocal cords and passing the endotracheal tube between the vocal cords. The placement of the laryngoscope in the pharynx often produces vagal nerve stimulation, which leads to bradycardia. Assisted ventilation must be paused for the procedure, which, if prolonged, will lead to hypoxemia and bradycardia. Intubation has been shown to increase blood pressure and intracranial pressure.[71] Trauma to the mouth, pharynx, vocal cords, and trachea are all possible complications of intubation. Performing the intubation procedure when the infant already has bradycardia and is hypoxic can lead to further decline in HR and oxygenation.[72] Therefore it is most appropriate to make an attempt to stabilize the infant with noninvasive ventilation prior to performing the procedure, limit each attempt to 30 seconds or less, and stabilize the infant between attempts. If misplacement of the endotracheal tube into the esophagus goes unrecognized, the infant may experience further clinical deterioration. Clinical signs that the endotracheal tube has been correctly placed in the trachea include the following: auscultation of breath sounds over the anterolateral aspects of the lungs (near the axilla), mist visible on the endotracheal tube, chest rise, and clinical improvement in HR and color or oxygen saturation. The use of a colorimetric carbon dioxide detector to confirm intubation decreases the amount of time necessary to determine correct placement of the endotracheal tube[73] and is recommended by the NRP as one of the primary methods of determining endotracheal tube placement.

Given the significant skill required to place an endotracheal tube, another device, the LMA, was developed as an alternative airway that is particularly useful for infants with small chins, cleft lip/palate, or other upper-airway anomalies. The LMA is a small oval mask with an inflatable cuff that sits over the laryngeal opening. The cuff fits on the hypopharynx and occludes the opening to the esophagus, allowing ventilation directed to the larynx. It can be used to provide PPV in apneic infants or for airway control in spontaneously breathing patients. Development of a size 1 LMA allowed for its introduction to neonatal resuscitation in the 1990s and to the NRP guidelines in 2000. Studies have evaluated its use compared to a face mask as a primary ventilation device for PPV in newborns over 34 weeks' gestation and have shown that it is at least as effective as the face mask for achieving stable vital signs and avoiding the need for intubation.[74–76] Three small studies have compared the LMA with endotracheal intubation for newborns who have not responded to face mask PPV in the delivery room, and demonstrated similar rates of successful resuscitation between the two devices.[77–79] Although more studies of the LMA are needed, currently the NRP guidelines suggest the use of the LMA as an alternative to intubation in newborns over 34 weeks' gestation if face mask ventilation fails, and recommends the LMA when intubation is not feasible.

EDITORIAL COMMENT: The laryngeal mask airway (LMA) can achieve effective ventilation during neonatal resuscitation in a time frame consistent with current neonatal resuscitation guidelines. Compared to bag and mask ventilation (BMV), the LMA is more effective in terms of shorter resuscitation and ventilation times and less need for endotracheal intubation; however, there is lack of evidence to support LMA in more premature infants. LMA may be successful when BMV fails and intubation can be avoided. This is a relatively new skill for the neonatal community and requires training and preparation.

The difficulty of intubation and the need for training is highlighted by O'Connell's study in which 55 physicians and nurses performed four intubations in succession on a high-fidelity extremely low-birth-weight manikin with size 0 Miller and size 00 Miller blades from two different manufacturers. There was no difference in total laryngoscopy time (median 23.7 versus 20.6 seconds) or first-attempt success in <30 seconds (67.3% versus 69.1%) between the size 0 and size 00 blades. With inexperienced operators, the success rate is lower and time to intubation longer.

O'Connell J, Weiner G. Intubating extremely premature newborns: a randomised crossover simulation study. *BMJ Paediatr Open.* 2017;1(1):e000157.

Oxygen Use

In the past, the use of 100% oxygen for assisted ventilation was routine when neonates required assisted ventilation, as was done in all other types of resuscitation without any specific evidence. Over time, however, the potential toxicity of oxygen, especially through the creation of free radicals, led investigators to study this well-accepted practice. For term or near-term infants, many trials have compared using 100% oxygen to using room air (21%) for neonatal resuscitation. Overall, these trials found that room air was as successful as 100% oxygen in achieving resuscitation, and demonstrated less oxidative stress.[80–83] Subsequent metaanalyses of up to 10 trials showed that infants resuscitated with room air had less risk of mortality than those resuscitated with 100% oxygen, and also demonstrated a trend toward less risk of severe hypoxic-ischemic encephalopathy (HIE).[84–86] NRP guidelines currently recommend initiating resuscitation of term and near-term infants (>35 weeks' gestation) with room air and using a pulse oximeter to allow titration of the oxygen

TABLE 3.1 Target Oxygen Saturation According to Time After Birth

Time After Birth (min)	Target SpO_2 (%)
1	60–65
2	65–70
3	70–75
4	75–80
5	80–85
10	85–95

delivered based on target oxygen saturations. These target oxygen saturations can be found in Table 3.1 and were derived from a study of healthy mostly term infants who did not require resuscitation in the delivery room.[20] The values demonstrate that the transition from fetal life normally starts at a relatively low oxygen saturation around 50%–60% and gradually increases to over 90%. For the vast majority of newborns who require respiratory support for stabilization, targeting oxygen levels to mimic healthy transitioning infants is logical. However, for those who are severely depressed and require significant resuscitation, the evidence is less clear. In fact, in some of the initial trials comparing 21% versus 100% oxygen, if infants did not respond to ventilation with 21% oxygen, the amount of oxygen delivered was increased to 100%. It is therefore unknown whether providing less than pure oxygen during times of severely diminished cardiac output is safe. It is recommended that if the infant has significant bradycardia (HR <60 bpm) requiring chest compressions, 100% oxygen be used to ventilate the baby.

The best concentration with which to initiate resuscitation for preterm infants is not the same as for term infants. Preterm infants have decreased antioxidant enzyme capacity and may therefore be more susceptible to harmful effects of excessive oxygen exposure. Multiple studies have evaluated starting resuscitation of preterm infants with low oxygen concentrations (≤30%) compared with high initial oxygen concentrations (≥60%). These trials consistently found that infants in the lower oxygen group needed more than 21% oxygen to achieve resuscitation targets.[87–92] In the largest of these trials in which preterm infants were initially resuscitated with either 21% or 100% oxygen, a subgroup analysis of babies less than 28 weeks' gestation revealed increased mortality in the infants initially treated with room air.[90] A metaanalysis of studies evaluating infants less than 28 weeks' gestation demonstrated no difference in overall mortality prior to discharge, BPD, retinopathy of prematurity, intraventricular hemorrhage, or necrotizing enterocolitis between infants resuscitated with an initial low (≤30%) versus high (≥60%) concentration of oxygen.[93] Current NRP guidelines recommend initiating resuscitation of infants less than 35 weeks' gestation with a low oxygen concentration of 21%–30% and against starting resuscitation with high oxygen (>65%). As with term infants, oxygen delivered should be titrated based on the HR and preductal oxygen saturations obtained using a pulse oximetry probe.

Assisting Circulation

In newly born infants, the need for resuscitative measures beyond assisted ventilation is extremely rare. Additional circulatory assistance can include chest compressions, administration of epinephrine, and volume infusion. In a large urban delivery center with a resuscitation registry, 0.12% of all infants delivered received chest compressions and/or epinephrine from 1991 to 1993, and 0.06% of all infants delivered received epinephrine from 1999 to 2004.[94,95]

The importance of chest compressions in resuscitation is currently being emphasized in adult and pediatric resuscitation programs. However, because of the unique characteristics of the transitioning newborn infant as discussed previously, ventilation remains the most critical priority in neonatal resuscitation. Chest compressions can be necessary when prolonged cardiorespiratory insufficiency has been present. They are indicated when the HR remains below 60 bpm despite adequate ventilation for 30 seconds. The preferred method of chest compressions is the two-thumb method, which involves encircling the chest with both hands and placing the thumbs on the sternum. The chest is then compressed in a 3:1 ratio coordinated with ventilation breaths to provide 90 compressions to 30 breaths per minute. Chest compressions can be provided from the head of the bed, allowing another team member access to the umbilical cord for venous catheter placement.

Further circulatory support may be necessary if adequate chest compressions do not result in an increase in HR after 60 seconds. Epinephrine is then indicated as a vasoactive substance, which increases blood pressure by alpha-receptor agonist effects, improves coronary perfusion pressure, and increases HR by beta-receptor agonist effects. The strongly recommended method of epinephrine administration is intravenous in a dose of 0.01 to 0.03 mg/kg (0.1 to 0.3 mL/kg of a 1:10,000 solution). Therefore early placement of an umbilical venous catheter during a difficult resuscitation is important for both volume and epinephrine administration. If there is any prenatal indication that substantial resuscitation will be required, the necessary equipment for umbilical venous catheter placement should be prepared before delivery as completely as possible. It is probably advisable to initiate the process of umbilical venous catheter placement when the need for chest compressions arises. Epinephrine may be given by endotracheal tube, but the drug delivery is not as certain, and therefore an increased dose of 0.05-0.1 mg/kg (0.5-1 mL/kg of a 1:10,000 solution) is currently recommended. Epinephrine doses may be repeated every 3 minutes if HR does not increase. Excessive epinephrine administration may result in hypertension, which, in preterm infants, may be a factor in the development of intraventricular hemorrhage. However, the risks are balanced by the benefit of successful resuscitation in an infant who might not otherwise survive.

If the infant has not responded to all of the prior measures, a trial of increasing intravascular volume should be considered by the administration of crystalloid or blood. Situations associated with fetal blood loss are also frequently associated with the need for resuscitation. These include placental abruption, cord prolapse, and fetal-maternal transfusion. Some of these clinical circumstances will have an obvious history associated with blood loss, whereas others may not be readily evident at the time of birth. Signs of hypovolemia in the newly born infant are nonspecific but include pallor and weak pulses. Volume replacement requires intravenous access for which emergent placement of an umbilical venous catheter is essential. Any infant who has signs of hypovolemia and has not responded to other resuscitative measures should have an umbilical venous line placed and a volume infusion administered. The most common volume replacement (and currently recommended fluid) is isotonic saline. A trial volume of 10 mL/kg is given initially and repeated if necessary. If a substantial blood loss has occurred, the infant may require infusion of red blood cells to provide adequate oxygen-carrying capacity. Because not all blood loss is obvious and resuscitation algorithms usually discuss volume replacement as a last resort of a difficult resuscitation, the clinician needs to keep an index of suspicion for significant hypovolemia so that action may be taken to correct the problem as promptly as possible. Therefore in situations where the possibility for hypovolemia is known prior to birth, it would be wise to prepare an umbilical catheter and an initial syringe of isotonic saline, and prepare for the possibility that uncross-matched blood may be required.

Specific Problems Encountered During Resuscitation

Neonatal Response to Maternal Anesthesia/Analgesia. Medications administered to the mother during labor can affect the fetus by transfer across the placenta and directly affecting the fetus or by adversely affecting the mother's condition, thereby altering uteroplacental circulation and placental oxygen delivery. One of the possible complications of intrapartum medication exposure is perinatal respiratory depression after maternal opiate administration. Because opiates can cross the placenta, the fetus may develop respiratory depression from the direct effect of the drug. Naloxone has been used in the past during neonatal resuscitation as an opiate receptor antagonist to reverse the effects of fetal opiate exposure. However, due to a lack of evidence of beneficial effect and possible adverse effects, naloxone hydrochloride is no longer recommended for use in neonatal resuscitation.

Conditions Complicating Resuscitation. When resuscitation has proceeded through the described steps without improvement in the infant's clinical condition, other problems should be considered. Some of these problems may be modifiable with interventions that could improve the course of the resuscitation. For example, an unrecognized pneumothorax could prevent adequate pulmonary inflation and, if under tension, could impair cardiac function. If the pneumothorax is recognized and drained, both gas exchange and circulation can be improved. Some congenital anomalies that were not diagnosed antenatally make resuscitation more difficult. Congenital diaphragmatic hernia is one such anomaly that is difficult to recognize on initial inspection of the infant but can cause significant problems with resuscitation. The abdominal organs are displaced into one hemithorax, and the lungs are unable to develop normally, causing ventilation to be quite difficult. If the intestines are displaced into the thorax and mask ventilation is provided, the intestines will become inflated, making ventilation even more difficult. Therefore when the congenital diaphragmatic hernia is known before delivery or a presumptive diagnosis is made in the delivery room, the baby should be intubated early to prevent intestinal inflation. A large (10 French) orogastric suction tube should also be placed to decompress the inflated intestines. Many other congenital anomalies that can lead to a difficult resuscitation will be more visibly obvious when the baby is born. For example, hydrops fetalis occurring for any reason can be associated with very difficult resuscitation. Frequently, peritoneal and/or pleural fluid will need to be drained to achieve adequate ventilation.

A situation that may create a particularly difficult resuscitation is an airway obstruction, especially if not diagnosed prior to delivery. If a significant airway obstruction is diagnosed antenatally, an EXIT procedure (***ex***-utero ***i***ntrapartum ***t***reatment) can be planned. This allows for establishment of a stable airway prior to clamping of the umbilical cord, which maintains placental function until the airway is secure. The therapy will vary depending on the cause of obstruction. An alternate airway (oral or nasopharyngeal) can be helpful if endotracheal intubation is not possible, as can occur with micrognathia. Tracheal suctioning can be attempted if a tracheal plug is suspected. In extreme situations of airway obstruction, an emergency cricothyroidotomy may be attempted.

After Resuscitation. In infants born without a HR or any respiratory effort, if resuscitation is performed to the full extent without any response, discontinuation may be appropriate after 10 minutes. This recommendation is based on the high incidence of mortality and morbidity among infants born without any signs of life and poor response to resuscitation.[96,97] The decision of when to discontinue resuscitation must be individualized depending on the condition of the infant and response to resuscitation.

Infants who do survive a significant resuscitation may require special attention in the hours to days that follow. Frequent complications immediately following resuscitation include hypoglycemia, hypotension, and persistent metabolic acidosis. In addition, infants with evidence of HIE may benefit from mild therapeutic hypothermia.[98] This therapy is most beneficial when initiated as quickly as possible after an insult and is not available at every center. Institutions that do not provide this therapy should coordinate in advance with centers that do to ensure that treatment is started in a timely manner.

CASE STUDY 3.1

A woman presents to the labor and delivery unit in active labor after having had no prenatal care. She precipitously delivers the baby, and you are called urgently to the room. Who will go with you to the delivery room?
Each institution must decide the composition of their delivery resuscitation team. The individuals intended to participate on any given day should be identified prior to the start of the day. A team that has worked well together consistently would be expected to work well together in difficult situations.

The baby is handed to you; you place the baby on a radiant warmer and begin to evaluate the baby. You suction the mouth and remove the wet linens. The baby is making intermittent respiratory effort, and the heart rate is over 100 bpm.

As you are drying the baby, you are stimulating him, and his breathing becomes more regular by 1 minute of life. His heart rate always remains greater than 100 bpm; his color transitions from blue to pink centrally by 2 minutes of life. You note that his extremities are flexed, and he cries when you examine him.

What Apgar score do you assign him at 5 minutes of life?
By 5 minutes of life, the baby has a heart rate greater than 100 bpm (2 points), adequate regular spontaneous respirations (2 points), good tone (2 points), good reflex irritability (2 points), and is centrally pink (1 point). Therefore the Apgar score at 5 minutes of life is 9.

Once the initial stabilization has been completed, what do you look for in this infant whose mother had no prenatal care?
Among the most important observations to make is an approximation of gestational age. In addition to evaluating the size of the baby, a quick physical examination with attention to physical maturity findings will indicate an approximate gestational age, which will be important in determining the further care necessary for this newborn. A brief physical examination will also be important as a preliminary screen for congenital anomalies. Further evaluation and observation will be necessary because of the lack of prenatal screening. Some of these routine prenatal screens may be completed by testing the mother at the time of admission. The pediatrician needs to be aware of these screens to treat the baby properly. Urgent considerations for the baby include rapid HIV testing, hepatitis B screening, syphilis screening, blood type assessment, and a sepsis risk assessment, as group B *Streptococcus* carrier status is unknown. An urgent or early therapy for each of these conditions can be life altering. Further evaluation may also be indicated but is not necessarily as urgent.

CASE STUDY 3.2

A woman with a twin gestation at 25 weeks is admitted to the labor and delivery unit with preterm labor. Fetal monitoring is initiated, a dose of betamethasone is administered, and a course of antibiotics is begun. You have a chance to talk with the parents; in addition to discussing general issues of prematurity at 25 weeks, what do you tell them to expect in the delivery room?
To begin the discussion, it would be helpful to inform the parents who will be caring for the babies at the delivery and where they will be cared for immediately after delivery. When multiples are delivered, it is best to have a separate resuscitation team planned for each infant. This may take extra preparation to ensure that enough resources are available at the time of delivery. It would be appropriate to inform the parents that preterm babies at 25 weeks have a higher chance of requiring resuscitation, including the need for intubation.

Later that evening, her labor is progressing, and late decelerations (a category II tracing) develop on fetal heart rate monitoring. Your team is called to the delivery, and a cesarean section is performed. The first baby is handed to you and does not have any apparent respiratory effort. Describe what you expect to occur in the first 1 minute of life.
The infant will be brought to a radiant warmer, and wet linens will be removed. On the warmer, there will be a plastic wrap/bag waiting, which will cover the infant's body as soon as the wet linens are removed. While one team member places electrocardiogram (ECG) leads and then assesses the heart rate by auscultation providing a visual display for the entire team until the ECG is functioning, a second team member will bulb suction the infant's mouth and position the baby on the bed in a straight fashion with the neck neutral. After suctioning the mouth, the second team member will place a face mask and initiate assisted ventilation. The third person will place a pulse oximeter and adjust the delivered oxygen concentration to meet the saturation targets recommended by the Neonatal Resuscitation Program (NRP) (Table 3.1).

You begin positive pressure ventilation (PPV) because the baby's spontaneous respiratory effort was inadequate. The nurse auscultates the heart rate and finds it to be approximately 80 beats per minute (bpm) and not yet increasing. How do you proceed?
Because you are already giving PPV, you need to assess whether the breaths are being delivered adequately—in other words, whether the airway is open. Observe the chest for movement with inflations, although this is sometimes difficult to see in very small babies. An additional indication of an open airway is detection of carbon dioxide on a disposable device placed in line with the face mask and breathing device. If there is not adequate chest rise or there is no color change on the CO_2 detector, the first step would be to readjust the head position, ensuring that there is a good seal with the face mask and the neck is neutral. It can be helpful to gently hold upward pressure on the corners of the mandible while stabilizing the face mask. If there remains no chest rise or measured end-tidal CO_2, the pharynx should be suctioned and the mouth opened. If the

Continued

CASE STUDY 3.2—cont'd

heart rate does not improve with these initial measures, the positive inspiratory pressure of the delivered breaths should be increased (done differently depending on the device used) or the inspiratory time of each breath could be increased. These measures frequently lead to improvement but should not be prolonged and delay more definitive therapy.

At this point (it is now approximately 1.5 minutes of life), the baby has a functioning pulse oximeter on the right hand, which displays a heart rate of 85 bpm and an oxygen saturation of 30%. The baby has made some attempts at breathing but does not have sustained spontaneous respirations. Why do you think the baby is not making further improvements, and what is your next step?

The most likely cause of the continued bradycardia is lack of development of an adequate functional residual capacity (FRC). Because attempts to stabilize the baby with noninvasive ventilation have failed, it is necessary to intubate the baby to provide a more direct and secure method of providing positive pressure. The equipment necessary for intubation had been prepared and inspected prior to delivery and is waiting at the bedside. An appropriately sized endotracheal tube is available. The designated operator performs the procedure with the assistance of a second team member. Because the pulse oximeter is functioning, the baby will be monitored throughout the procedure. An additional team member will track the time and notify the operator if 30 seconds has elapsed prior to passing the endotracheal tube. If the attempt is unsuccessful, the laryngoscope will be removed from the baby's mouth, and the PPV will be reinstituted to allow the baby to recover prior to another attempt. Once the endotracheal tube is positioned, a carbon dioxide detector will be used to ensure placement in the trachea. Breath sounds will be auscultated, and the depth of the tube will be adjusted as necessary.

When the endotracheal tube is inserted and positive pressure is restarted, the heart rate increases to 150 bpm, and the baby becomes pink with an oxygen saturation that increases to 95%. How would you care for the baby until transport to the neonatal intensive care unit (NICU)?

Attention will be paid to the infant's temperature, breathing, and heart rate throughout the entire time in the delivery room and through transport to the NICU. A temperature probe will be placed and the radiant warmer switched to servo mode. The pulse oximeter will be kept in place throughout the time in the delivery room and transport to the NICU. The delivered oxygen concentration will be adjusted to maintain the oxygen saturation appropriate for the time of life. Continued PPV with end-expiratory pressure will be provided with delivered pressures adjusted as needed for the infant. In this case, the pressure was increased prior to intubation. If a T-piece resuscitator is being used for ventilation, the pressure will need to be manually adjusted to obtain desired levels and should be decreased once the intubation is performed and the heart rate and oxygen saturation have improved. The most consistent methods of providing continued ventilation with consistent levels of pressure would be either with a T-piece resuscitator or a ventilator. The use of either the self-inflating bag or flow-inflating bag for prolonged periods of time will likely lead to inconsistent pressure delivery with the potential for delivery of excess peak inspiratory pressure or inadequate positive end-expiratory pressure levels, both of which may contribute to lung injury. Some institutions determine the level of pressure provided by measuring the tidal volume delivered, targeting an exhaled volume of 5 to 6 mL/kg. Additional care for an infant of this gestational age who has required intubation and mechanical ventilation would be administration of exogenous surfactant once appropriate endotracheal tube position has been confirmed.

CASE STUDY 3.3

A 27-year-old gravida 2, para 0 woman presents to labor and delivery at 30 weeks' gestation with rupture of membranes. She is admitted to the hospital, betamethasone is administered, and fetal monitoring is initiated. After she has been hospitalized for 4 days, the fetal heart rate is noted to increase to the 170s. On examination, it is noted that the umbilical cord is palpable in the vagina. The mother is rushed to the operating room, and an emergency cesarean section is performed. The pediatric team is called to the delivery room and is handed the baby, who is limp and pale and has no respiratory effort. How do you proceed?

The baby is positioned on a radiant warmer and quickly dried, wet linens are removed, and the mouth is bulb suctioned. If these simple measures, which also act to stimulate the baby, do not cause the infant to begin breathing spontaneously, then assisted ventilation must be initiated without delay. The face mask and ventilating device are then immediately applied, and positive pressure ventilation (PPV) is initiated. At the same time, a second team member is evaluating the heart rate and a third team member is placing a pulse oximeter.

The heart rate is not appreciable by auscultation or palpation. What is your next step?

The effectiveness of ventilation is evaluated, looking for evidence of a patent airway. The mask and head position are adjusted. The pharynx is suctioned, the mouth is opened, and the level of positive pressure delivered is increased. If these actions have made no difference in heart rate, then an alternate airway should be placed to provide effective ventilation. Ideally, this means an endotracheal tube is placed. After intubation is confirmed and PPV is given for 30 seconds with 100% oxygen, chest compressions are initiated if the heart rate remains less than 60 beats per minute (bpm). One team member should place electrocardiogram (ECG) leads, if not already done. Chest compressions and breaths are coordinated in a three-compressions-to-one breath rhythm, with the team member performing chest compressions counting the actions

CASE STUDY 3.3—cont'd

out loud. The pace will be such that in 1 minute there will be approximately 90 compressions and 30 breaths. Depending on the number of individuals present at the resuscitation, more help should be called at this point, if necessary.

The heart rate is reevaluated after 30 seconds of assisted ventilation and chest compressions and continues to be undetectable. What do you do now?
Because the baby is intubated with a low (absent) heart rate and is already intubated and receiving chest compressions, it will most likely be necessary to give epinephrine. Therefore one team member should prepare and place an umbilical venous line. An additional (fourth) individual could be preparing the epinephrine dose. A fifth team member can be recording all of the events of the resuscitation in real time to accurately document the interventions and response. This individual can also serve as a timekeeper and prompter for key resuscitation events.

Can you do anything else to help the baby at this point?
A dose of intravenous epinephrine should be given as soon as the umbilical venous catheter (UVC) is placed. If the time to place the UVC is prolonged and an endotracheal tube is in place, a dose of epinephrine may be given via endotracheal tube while IV access is obtained. Because the baby appeared pale from the start and there was a history of cord prolapse, it may be helpful to provide intravenous fluid volume. A bolus of 10 mL/kg of normal saline can be given initially and repeated if necessary. If suspicion of blood loss is high, a transfusion of emergency blood may be provided. In addition, repeat doses of epinephrine can be administered every 3 minutes. An evaluation for other causes of cardiopulmonary insufficiency should be done. A pneumothorax may cause circulatory compromise and may be evaluated by auscultation of breath sounds and transillumination of the chest. A brief survey for congenital anomalies might disclose a cause for difficulty with resuscitation.

After you have given one dose of intravenous epinephrine and one bolus of normal saline, the baby's heart rate becomes detectable and steadily increases to greater than 100 bpm. How long would you have continued resuscitation if there had been no improvement?
In a situation where there are no signs of life (no heart rate or respiratory effort), and full resuscitative efforts are continued for 10 minutes with no effect, it is considered appropriate to stop the resuscitation. Each team may vary the time frame based on when resuscitative efforts were felt to be truly adequate and whether there is any clinical evidence of signs of life.

CASE STUDY 3.4

A 32-year-old gravida 1, para 1 woman presents to labor and delivery at 28 weeks' gestation with severe preeclampsia. She is given betamethasone on admission and 24 hours later. Forty-eight hours from admission, her symptoms worsen despite medications, and the decision is made to perform a cesarean section and deliver her baby. The baby is born through clear fluids, she has a spontaneous cry at birth, and delayed cord clamping is provided for 60 seconds. She is handed to the pediatrician. What are the initial steps when you bring the baby to the warmer?
The baby is placed in plastic wrap and a hat is placed on her head. She is positioned supine with her head in a neutral position. She is assessed for continued spontaneous respirations, heart rate (HR) by auscultation, color, and tone. Gentle suction is provided to clear secretions from her mouth. A pulse oximeter is placed on the right wrist, and electrocardiogram (ECG) leads placed for continued HR monitoring reveal an HR of 100 beats per minute. You notice that she has stopped breathing, however, and the HR falls to 80 beats per minute. What is your next action?

Given the infant is apneic, you begin positive pressure ventilation (PPV) via face mask with a T-piece resuscitator set to 25/5 cm H_2O with 30% oxygen. After 30 seconds of PPV, her HR improves, and she has spontaneous respirations. You notice that the baby is making a grunting sound and has significant retractions. Her oxygen saturation is 45% at 2.5 minutes of life. What do you do next?
Since the baby has signs of respiratory distress and inadequate oxygenation but is breathing spontaneously, you start the baby on continuous positive airway pressure (CPAP) 5 cm H_2O with 30% supplemental oxygen. Her oxygen saturation improves, and by 4 minutes she is meeting the target saturations on 40% oxygen by 4 minutes of life. Her grunting persists but is slightly quieter. You decide to transition to nasal-prong CPAP and continue monitoring the oxygen requirement.

CASE STUDY 3.5

A 30-year-old gravida 2, para 1 woman presents to labor and delivery at 35 weeks' gestation with spontaneous rupture of membranes and early labor. She develops a fever and is started on antibiotics for presumed chorioamnionitis. Labor is progressing slowly, but ultimately a cesarean section is performed. You are called to the cesarean section, and your team of three individuals attends the delivery. The baby is handed to you, and you place her on the radiant warmer. She is dried, and the wet blankets are removed. You suction her mouth and note that she is not breathing. How do you proceed?

Continued

CASE STUDY 3.5—cont'd

The drying and suctioning that you previously performed would be adequate to stimulate breathing if breathing could have been stimulated. It is therefore necessary to initiate positive pressure ventilation (PPV). You do this while a second team member auscultates the heart rate (HR) and taps out the beats. You ensure that the assisted breaths that you are providing are being adequately delivered to the lungs by looking for chest rise and continuously monitoring the HR to determine the occurrence and direction of change. Throughout these initial steps, the third team member is placing a pulse oximeter.

The HR prior to starting ventilation was 70 beats per minute (bpm), and it has increased slightly to 90 bpm when ventilation was initiated. You note that there appears to be chest rise, and you have used a carbon dioxide detector between the mask and ventilating device, which is changing color, indicating that you have an open airway. The baby continues to be apneic, and the HR remains at approximately 90 bpm. What would you do next?

Ventilation was somewhat effective but did not improve the HR to normal, and spontaneous respirations have not yet begun. An increase in the amount of positive pressure may help to develop the functional residual capacity (FRC) and improve the HR. After increasing the pressure for several breaths, if there is no further improvement, the next step would be to intubate the baby.

You now have a functioning pulse oximeter, which indicates that the HR is 95 bpm and the oxygen saturation on the right hand is 35%. The baby is now 2 minutes old, and you proceed with the intubation. Describe the procedure.

The baby is positioned on the bed with the body straight, neck in the neutral position, and back flat against the bed. You obtain the correctly sized endotracheal tube (a 3.5 mm for this infant of 35 weeks' gestational age), and you insert a stylet into the endotracheal tube to the appropriate depth above the side hole if so desired. You ensure that the pharynx is suctioned, and you quickly test the function of the light bulb before inserting the laryngoscope into the mouth. Because the pulse oximeter is functioning, you are comfortable that the baby is being monitored while you are performing the procedure, and you ask another team member to watch the time while you are performing the procedure. You move the laryngoscope blade to the locked and functioning position. You open the baby's mouth with your right hand, insert the laryngoscope blade into the mouth with your left hand, and advance it toward the base of the tongue. The laryngoscope handle should be along the baby's midline, making approximately a 45-degree angle with the baby's chin. You then lift the tongue with the laryngoscope blade, maintaining the same angle of the laryngoscope handle with the chin. The tendency when lifting the tongue is to make a rocking motion with the laryngoscope handle, which will increase the angle that the laryngoscope handle makes with the chin and will obscure the view of the larynx. After you have inserted the blade and have lifted the tongue, you identify the normal airway landmarks, including the epiglottis and vocal cords. When you see the vocal cords, a second team member places the endotracheal tube in your right hand, and you pass it through the glottis. You then remove the laryngoscope while holding the endotracheal tube with your right hand, and a second team member helps remove the stylet and attach a carbon dioxide detector and ventilating device. You look for cyclical color change on the carbon dioxide detector and mist on the tube. You listen for breath sounds bilaterally. You can also palpate the tip of the tube in the suprasternal notch to ensure that the tube is not placed too far distally, which could potentially result in a right main stem bronchus intubation. When you have confirmed tube placement, you tape the tube in place.

After you successfully intubate the baby, the HR increases to approximately 100 to 110 bpm, the baby begins to make gasping respirations, and the oxygen saturation is 40%. Despite continued assisted ventilation, the HR and oxygen saturation do not increase beyond these levels. How do you proceed at this point?

This baby has not followed the usual pattern of improvement after provision of what seems to be adequate ventilation. It is therefore necessary to evaluate for other problems that might be hindering resuscitation. You have a second team member providing ventilation, and the third team member is ensuring adequate temperature control. You do a quick survey of the baby for any obvious anomalies. You note that the face appears normally formed; there is no evidence of compression deformations, which would be associated with long-standing oligohydramnios and could lead to pulmonary hypoplasia. There is no obvious edema to suggest hydrops fetalis or ascites, which could lead to compression of the thoracic cavity and respiratory compromise. You auscultate the chest on both sides and hear breath sounds louder on the right, and note that the abdomen appears scaphoid. Transillumination of the chest is unremarkable. You therefore suspect a congenital diaphragmatic hernia on the left and insert an orogastric tube. You aspirate the syringe and obtain 10 mL of air. The HR slowly increases, and the oxygen saturation has increased slowly to 55%. You now consider administering surfactant and move the infant to the NICU for further management.

QUESTIONS

True or False

The majority of extremely preterm infants are apneic at birth.

O'Donnell et al. reviewed the videos of 61 extremely preterm infants taken immediately after birth. The majority cried (69%) and breathed (80%) without intervention. Most preterm infants are not apneic at birth. Therefore the answer is false.

O'Donnell CP, Kamlin CO, Davis PG, et al. Crying and breathing by extremely preterm infants immediately after birth, *J Pediatr.* 2010;156:846.

True or False

Some neonatologists state that at the delivery of extremely premature infants they rely on "how the baby looks" when deciding whether to initiate resuscitation. This is a reliable and precise method to determine whether to initiate resuscitation.

Previous studies have reported poor correlation between early clinical signs and prognosis. To determine if neonatologists can accurately predict survival to discharge of extremely premature infants on the basis of observations in the first minutes after birth, Manley et al. showed videos of the resuscitation of 10 extremely premature infants (<26 weeks' gestation) to 17 attending neonatologists and 17 fellows from the three major perinatal centers in Melbourne, Australia. Antenatal information was available to the observers. A monitor visible in each video displayed the heart rate and oxygen saturation of the infant. Observers were asked to estimate the likelihood of survival to discharge for each infant at three time points: 20 seconds, 2 minutes, and 5 minutes after birth. Observers' ability to predict survival was poor and not influenced by their level of experience.

Neonatologists' reliance on initial appearance and early response to resuscitation in predicting survival for extremely premature infants is misplaced. Therefore the answer is false.

Manley BJ, Dawson JA, Kamlin CO, et al. Clinical assessment of extremely premature infants in the delivery room is a poor predictor of survival, *Pediatrics.* 2010;125:e559.

The reference list for this chapter can be found online at www.expertconsult.com.

4

Physical Growth

Physical Examination of the Newborn Infant and the Physical Environment

Avroy A. Fanaroff, Tom Lissauer, Jonathan M. Fanaroff

There are tiny, puny infants with great vitality. Their movements are untiring and their crying lusty, for their organs are quite capable of performing their allotted functions. These infants will live, for although their weight is inferior ... their sojourn in the womb was longer.

Pierre Budin, The Nursling

An infant's problems and prognosis are in large part determined by birth weight and gestational age. The designations low birth weight (LBW), very low birth weight (VLBW), and extremely low birth weight (ELBW) have been applied to all infants weighing less than 2500 g, 1500 g, and 1000 g at birth, respectively, regardless of the duration of gestation. Infants are further classified by gestational age into the designations of preterm, early term, term, and postterm, if they have completed less than 37, 37–38, 39–41, and more than 41 weeks of pregnancy, respectively. Formerly referred to as *near-term* infants, *late preterm* infants, who have completed more than 34 and less than 37 weeks' gestation, account for almost three-quarters of preterm births. Therefore prevention of late preterm delivery would make the biggest impact in reducing the overall rate of premature birth. Late preterm infants have significant in-hospital morbidity and a threefold higher mortality rate when compared with term infants. Late preterm infants are also at higher risk of neurodevelopmental impairment when compared with age-matched infants born at term.

An infant's size at birth is dependent on two factors: gestational age and intrauterine growth velocity. The proportion of LBW infants who are preterm as opposed to those with abnormal intrauterine growth varies among countries. In developed countries, the majority of LBW infants are premature, whereas in developing countries, intrauterine growth restriction (IUGR) is the major contributing factor. However, as the standard of living improves in developing countries, the proportion of LBW infants who are premature rises in comparison to those who have been growth restricted, suggesting a relationship between socioeconomic status and appropriate intrauterine growth.

Infants are classified as appropriate for gestational age (AGA) if their birth weight falls between the 10th and 90th percentiles, small for gestational age (SGA) if their birth weight is below the 10th percentile, and large for gestational age (LGA) if their birth weight is above the 90th percentile (Fig. 4.1)[1,2]

DETERMINANTS OF FETAL GROWTH

Normal fetal growth requires contributions from the mother, the placenta, and the fetus. Numerous maternal metabolic adjustments are made during pregnancy to provide an uninterrupted supply of nutrients to the developing fetus. Foremost among these are adjustments in carbohydrate metabolism. During a normal pregnancy, a mother will experience mild fasting hypoglycemia and postprandial hyperglycemia, associated with an increased basal insulin level and relative insulin resistance. Maternal glucose use is attenuated, whereas ketones and free fatty acids increasingly serve as substrate for maternal tissues. These alterations in maternal metabolism allow for a continuous supply of glucose to the developing fetus from the mother, which is the primary substrate used for fetal oxidative metabolism, even during periods of maternal fasting. However, during relatively extended periods of maternal fasting, the fetus is also able to use ketones to serve its energy and synthetic needs. Maternal serum levels of lipids increase during gestation. In midpregnancy, fat is stored for fetal use during late pregnancy, when demands increase. Maternal metabolic adaptions to pregnancy are so effective in supplying the fetus with required nutrients that only severe maternal malnutrition (e.g., wartime famine) during the third trimester may cause a reduction in birth weight. Starvation during the first trimester results in placental growth to compensate for the reduced energy supply to the fetus. If nutrition is then restored in the second and third trimester, birth weight is actually increased above what it would have been in the absence of early malnutrition.

The human placenta is a highly active endocrine organ, and produces hormones with direct effect on growth, including growth factors and human placental lactogen (HPL), also known as chorionic somatomammotropin. HPL is produced by the syncytiotrophoblast cells. Its growth-promoting effects are mediated by the stimulation of fetal insulin-like growth factors (IGF) production and increasing nutrient availability. Elevation of maternal serum lipids plays a role here as

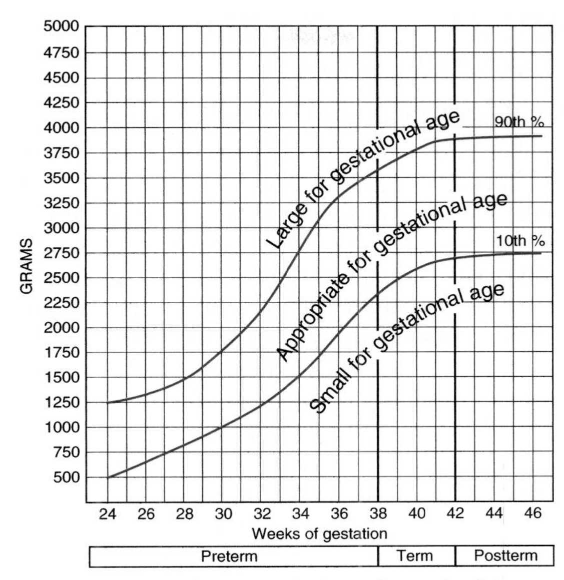

Fig. 4.1 Birth weights of liveborn singleton Caucasian infants at gestational ages from 24 to 42 weeks. (From Battaglia F, Lubchenco L. A practical classification of newborn infants by weight and gestational age. *J Pediatr.* 1967;7:159.)

well. The expression of the HPL gene is regulated, in part, by apoprotein A1, the major protein component of high-density lipoprotein. The fetus plays a role in its own growth by producing a variety of polypeptide IGF molecules and modulating binding proteins. These substances are produced by a variety of fetal tissues, with site, timing, and control of expression varying with each IGF.

INTRAUTERINE GROWTH RESTRICTION

The growth trajectory of a fetus results from the combined effects of genetic programming and the growth support it receives from its mother. A fetus' genetic growth potential is determined by contributions from the mother and the father, but these contributions are not necessarily of equal influence. For example, genomic imprinting causes approximately 30 genes to be active or inactive, depending on the individual parent from whom they are inherited. Paternal imprinting tends to encourage fetal growth, whereas maternal imprinting tends to restrict fetal growth. Although maternal and paternal genes have an approximately equal contribution to adult height and weight, the height and weight of the mother contribute more than 90% of the influence on birth weight.

IUGR is often defined as failure of the fetus to reach its genetic growth potential, but this definition is not comprehensive, as genetic potential can be modified according to nutrient supply. In addition, some babies' genetic growth potential is inherently abnormal because of genetic diseases such as aneuploidy. For example, a high proportion of babies with trisomy 21 fail to reach their expected "genetic growth potential" based solely on parental size.

Ideally, the classification of fetuses as growth restricted should rely on functional measures,[3] the most obvious of which is the risk of intrauterine or neonatal demise. Other typical indicators of inadequate growth status include an inability to cope with the hypoxia of labor resulting in fetal acidosis and neonatal depression, the passage of meconium during labor, and neonatal dysfunction such as hypoglycemia and hypothermia. In the longer term, catch-up growth may be either incomplete (resulting in reduced adult size) or excessive (leading to adult obesity, hypertension, and insulin resistance with an increased risk of diabetes). The concept of IUGR leading to long-term sequelae has led to the "fetal origins of adult disease or metabolic syndrome" hypothesis proposed by Barker and his colleagues.[4,5]

IUGR does not relate directly to percentile birth weight. Although babies who are SGA are at increased risk of the dysfunction typical of IUGR, many will be small but healthy babies. There is no clear threshold of percentile birth weight below which the risk of dysfunction increases; rather, the risk rises steadily as the percentile birth weight falls.[6] One approach that could improve the correlation between percentile birth weight and neonatal health is that of using "customized birth weight percentiles" in which the percentile birth weight of a particular baby is adjusted to take into account the mother's height, weight, racial origin, and other relevant factors.[7] However, some factors known to influence birth weight are pathologic. For example, severely underweight or overweight mothers are more likely to have babies who are born preterm or become macrosomic, and it would be inappropriate to correct percentiles to this extent.[8] Mothers from some racial groups are twice as likely to deliver stillborn infants if the pregnancy is complicated by fetal growth restriction,[9] and again, correction for this would clearly be inappropriate. It has been argued that using percentile charts based on estimated fetal weights of fetuses growing normally, instead of percentiles based on actual birth weights, may give a better indication of the incidence and role of fetal growth restriction on neonatal disease; however, this approach is limited by the inherent difficulty of obtaining accurate fetal measurements.[10,11]

Perhaps the most appropriate way of defining IUGR is using serial ultrasound measurements of fetal size. Measurements from 22 weeks' gestation onward can be used to establish the "normal" growth velocity for an individual fetus, and a subsequent decline in this growth trajectory fulfills the requirements for the definition of growth restriction. Prospective studies have shown that such measurements are at least as good a predictor of intrapartum dysfunction as percentile birth weight.[12] It is possible for a fetus who was initially growing on the 90th percentile to experience slowing of growth typical of IUGR and sustain associated perinatal problems despite having a birth weight within the "normal" range. This phenomenon demonstrates that it is possible to have IUGR without being born SGA.

PATTERN OF FETAL GROWTH

With the use of anthropometric measurements, including fetal weight, length, and head circumference, fetal growth standards have been determined for different reference populations from various locations.[13–15] From these data, it is apparent that there are variations in "normal" weight at any given gestational age from one environment to another. This variation is related to a number of factors including sex, race, socioeconomic status, and even altitude. But this brings into question what is meant by "normal". For example, babies born at high altitude are, on average, smaller than those born at sea level. Thus, when growth charts for babies born at altitude are constructed, the 10th percentile, commonly used as the boundary between AGA and SGA, will be at a lower birth weight than that for babies born at sea level. (For example, babies that are on the 11th percentile for altitude might be on the 8th percentile for sea level and would be categorized as AGA for altitude but as SGA for sea level.) However, infants born at altitude are at higher risk for intrauterine or intrapartum demise. This begs the question: Should it be regarded as "normal" if more babies are stillborn? The purpose of customized percentiles is to correct for variations in birth weight because of physiologic variations in the mother and her environment, not to correct for conditions that may be pathologic or that are associated with a worse outcome.

The Colorado data, presented by Lubchenco et al in the 1960s,[14] summarized standards of intrauterine growth for Caucasian (55%), African American (15%), and Hispanic (30%) newborns born between 1948 and 1961 in Denver. The graphic display of this relationship provides a useful and simple method for determining the birth weight percentiles with respect to gestational age and the local population. What such standards cannot do, however, is indicate whether the population as a whole (e.g., Hispanics compared with Caucasians) is disadvantaged. Equivalent designations of weight for gestational age between two different populations should be based on equivalent risk of poor outcome, rather than simply on the population distribution of birth weight.

Ten years after the Colorado data were published, Brenner et al published fetal weight curves based on more than 30,000 pregnancies (including live born, electively terminated, or spontaneous intrauterine demise).[16] These curves, which were adjusted for parity, race, and sex, demonstrated nearly linear growth between 20 and 38 weeks of gestation, with slowing thereafter. Using such nomograms, fetal growth may be longitudinally plotted throughout pregnancy, and a decline in growth velocity may be detected, which would indicate IUGR. A decline in fetal growth velocity is indicative of risk of poor fetal or neonatal outcome, regardless of the absolute weight percentile at the time of delivery. For example, a fetus that had been growing along the 80th percentile but experiences a decline in growth velocity and is born with a weight at the 40th percentile for gestational age (IUGR but AGA) can be as clinically significant as a fetus that is growing along the 10th percentile and declines in growth velocity to eventually be born at the fifth percentile for gestational age (IUGR and SGA). Thus, many clinicians consider that the best descriptor of IUGR is "a decline in fetal growth velocity," rather than being on, or falling below, a particular percentile.

ANTENATAL ASSESSMENT OF INTRAUTERINE GROWTH

Clinical Assessment of Gestational Age

Optimal management of the pregnant woman and her fetus is highly dependent on an accurate knowledge of the gestational age of the fetus. Gestational age is important for interpretation of common tests (e.g., nuchal translucency screening for trisomy 21), scheduling invasive procedures (e.g., amniocentesis), planning the delivery of high-risk fetuses (e.g., assessing the risk of respiratory distress syndrome [RDS]), and assessing fetal growth and size. Determination of the expected date of delivery (due date) can be made with varying degrees of certainty by history of menstrual cycles, physical examination of the pregnant woman, and a variety of clinical obstetrical milestones. Serial ultrasound examination of the developing fetus is the most accurate predictor of gestational age, except in cases where the date of conception is precisely known (as with pregnancies conceived by in vitro fertilization).

In Caucasian women, the average duration of pregnancy is 280 days, counting from the first day of the last menstrual period. However, because conception occurs, on average, on day 14 of the menstrual cycle, the true duration of gestation is 266 days. There is now good evidence that gestational age varies among racial groups, being 5 to 7 days shorter, for example, in South Asians and black Africans.[17] Between 22 and 34 weeks' gestation, in an appropriately growing singleton fetus, there is a reasonable correlation between the age of the fetus in weeks and the height of the uterine fundus in centimeters when measured as the distance over the abdominal wall from the superior border of the symphysis pubis to the top of the fundus. This measurement is frequently used for screening, but it is very unreliable in obese individuals, who account for 30% or more of Western populations. Obesity also makes ultrasound measurements more difficult and less reliable. For these reasons, the efficiency of screening for growth restriction is particularly poor in obese women. The size of the uterus changes more slowly in late pregnancy because as the fetus grows, the relative proportion of amniotic fluid decreases. Although physical examination estimates of gestational age have a standard deviation of plus or minus 2 weeks in the first trimester, this extends to 4 weeks in the second trimester and 6 weeks in the third trimester.

Assessment of Gestational Age

Forty percent of pregnant women have an uncertain last menstrual period, making accurate estimation of gestational age by history alone challenging. Since the 1970s, antenatal determination of gestational age using serial ultrasound studies of the fetus has become universal in developed countries. The type of ultrasound, the parameters measured, and the accuracy of the study vary with the progression of pregnancy.

It is possible to visualize the gestational sac by ultrasound as early as 5 weeks' gestation. The optimal time to determine gestational age by ultrasound is between 7 and 9 weeks' gestation using a high-resolution transvaginal ultrasound probe to measure crown-rump length. Routine ultrasound screens for dating, however, are usually performed between 11 and 14 weeks' gestation, the optimal time to evaluate the nuchal translucency thickness, which is used as a marker for risk of Down syndrome. Another scan at 20 to 22 weeks' gestational age is usually done for comprehensive fetal anomaly screening. Measurements at this stage of pregnancy are less reliable for assessing gestational age because to estimate gestational age from the size of the fetus, one must assume that the fetus is growing appropriately. By definition, 10% of babies will be SGA, and another 10% will be LGA. When the fetus is growing rapidly during the first trimester, the change in size from week to week is substantial; therefore the standard deviation of likely gestational age is small. Typically, 2 standard deviations are only 3 to 4 days different from the mean. Thus, it can be assumed that the fetus is likely to be of the average gestational age for a particular size, plus or minus 3 to 4 days. During the first trimester, fetuses smaller than 2 standard deviations below the mean for gestational age are at high risk for demise. However, the normal range of size increases as gestation advances, and accuracy of dating in the second trimester is generally no better than plus or minus 7 days. Ultrasound measures size and not gestational age. The most commonly used ultrasound measurements for determining estimated gestational age during the second trimester are head circumference, biparietal diameter, abdominal circumference, and femur length. Each of these measurements decreases in accuracy with increasing gestational age, particularly after 20 weeks, because of increasing normal variation with advancing gestation. A composite fetal size based on the average of these four measurements is used to enhance the accuracy of the assessment. Fetal abdominal circumference provides the most accurate estimate of fetal weight and growth velocity.

Intrauterine Growth Restriction

IUGR can result from a multitude of pathologic and nonpathologic processes (see later discussion). The terms IUGR and SGA are often used interchangeably but actually describe two different phenomena that may occur concurrently, but each may also exist without the other. IUGR describes a decrease in fetal growth velocity independent of absolute weight, whereas SGA describes an infant with a birth weight less than the 10th percentile for gestational age, independent of fetal growth velocity. Approximately 70% of babies who have IUGR will also be SGA. However, most babies who are born SGA were not growth restricted as fetuses and thus will not have the risk of physiologic dysfunction associated with IUGR. If the 3rd percentile were used as the cutoff (approximately 2 standard deviations below the mean), a much higher proportion of babies would actually show dysfunction secondary to growth restriction.

EPIDEMIOLOGY AND ETIOLOGY OF FETAL GROWTH RESTRICTION

Normal fetal growth is dependent on contributions of the mother, the placenta, and the fetus, and aberrant growth may result from disturbances in any of these contributors.

Race

Almost without exception, studies in the United States have demonstrated a significantly higher rate of IUGR, preterm birth, and LBW in African Americans when compared with their Caucasian contemporaries. European studies have shown that black African mothers have an average gestational length that is about 5 days shorter than that of Caucasian mothers.[17] This is compensated for by accelerated maturity in black Africans.[18] A study conducted in South Carolina over a 20-year period showed that between 1975 and 1979,[19] African American babies born at less than 37 weeks of gestation consistently had a lower perinatal mortality for gestational age than did Caucasian babies. However, this relationship reversed at term, with African American babies born at greater than 37 weeks' gestation having a higher rate of perinatal mortality as compared with Caucasian babies, and they were more likely to suffer from obstructed labor and meconium aspiration syndrome.

Analysis of data between 1990 and 1994 showed that although gestation-specific perinatal mortality had reduced in both groups, the same pattern of lower mortality before 37 weeks and higher mortality after 37 weeks in black infants persisted. More recently, 22 million infants born between 1989 and 1991 in the United States were studied, and the results were similar.[20]

European studies have shown that babies of South Asian origin have increased perinatal mortality at all gestational ages when compared with Caucasian babies.[9] This is likely because of the fact that South Asian babies have a lower birth weight across the gestational age range when compared with Caucasian infants. Babies born in India are, on average, approximately 600 g lighter than those born in Europe. Studies of South Asian babies born in developed countries show that the deficit persists but on average is reduced to 300 g. It may be conjectured that infants of South Asian descent have a lower average birth weight when compared to gestational age–matched Caucasian infants as an adaptation to smaller average maternal size of South Asian women, thus minimizing perinatal death as a result of obstructed labor.[21] However, South Asian individuals born in Europe have a very high incidence of diabetes and cardiovascular disease.[22–24] This highlights one of the pitfalls of customized fetal growth nomograms. Although South Asian infants born in Europe may, on average, be larger than babies born in India, correcting for this difference may actually be correcting for a pathologic process with serious long-term sequela.

Prior Obstetric and Family History

Women who are younger than 15 years of age, older than 45 years of age, have a history of miscarriages or unexplained stillbirths after 20 weeks' gestation, or have prior preterm deliveries are at increased risk for delivering a growth-restricted baby.[25] Familial factors also appear to play a role in the birth weight of babies. Mothers of one LBW infant were frequently LBW infants themselves and are more likely to deliver subsequent LBW babies than other age-matched mothers, and their siblings are more likely to parent LBW infants than other age-matched parents.[26,27]

Altitude

Infants born at altitude are, on average, smaller than infants born at sea level. When comparing growth curves, most authors note that Lubchenco's data were generated in Denver, the "mile-high city," and that the 10th percentile on these nomograms is lower than the 10th percentile of data collected from centers closer to sea level. Yip was able to demonstrate a "dose-dependent" effect of altitude on the LBW rate,[28] with a two- to threefold greater rate of LBW seen at altitudes greater than 2000 meters than at sea level.

Maternal Factors Contributing to Intrauterine Growth Restriction

In developed countries, factors that are known to contribute to IUGR include race, prior obstetric history, maternal nutritional status (prepregnancy weight and weight gain during pregnancy), maternal short stature, smoking, preeclampsia, chronic hypertension, multiple gestation, and female sex of the fetus. In developing nations, malaria is also a significant factor.

Maternal Nutritional Status

Although prepregnancy weight and weight gain during pregnancy are both indicators of maternal nutritional status, they affect fetal growth and birth weight independently of one another. It remains controversial as to whether preconception nutritional intervention in women who are poorly nourished may be beneficial to future pregnancy outcomes.[29] However, it does not confer additional benefit to pregnancy outcomes to provide preconception nutritional supplementation to women who are already well nourished. An obese mother, without other comorbid risk factors such as hypertension, is unlikely to deliver a growth-restricted baby, even if she gains relatively little weight during the pregnancy.

Smoking

Cigarette smoking has consistently been identified as a dose-dependent contributor to abruptio placentae, late intrauterine fetal demise, LBW, and IUGR. Women who smoke during pregnancy are 3 to 4.5 times more likely to have a fetus affected by IUGR, with average birth weights decreasing by 70 g to 400 g, and these effects are particularly pronounced in babies born to mothers of advanced maternal age. Multiple mechanisms may contribute to the detrimental effect of smoking on fetal growth and overall pregnancy outcomes. Nicotine and subsequent catecholamine release, along with reduced synthesis of prostacycline, result in placental vasoconstriction and elevated vascular resistance. This causes decreased delivery of nutrients and oxygen from mother to fetus across the placenta. Fetal carboxyhemoglobin levels also increase, which further interferes with delivery of oxygen to the developing fetal tissues. It has also been suggested that smoking causes indirect effects on fetal growth by causing suboptimal nutritional status both before and during pregnancy. The mechanism for this is thought to be an increased metabolic rate in woman who smoke, rather than decreased maternal caloric intake. In contrast, smoking mothers actually may consume more calories than their nonsmoking counterparts, and supplementing the diet of smoking mothers is ineffective in offsetting the detrimental effects on the fetus. However, if a pregnant woman successfully ceases to smoke before the third trimester, her infant's birth weight will be indistinguishable from those babies whose mothers did not smoke during pregnancy at all.

A variety of other drug exposures, including alcohol, marijuana, cocaine, and amphetamines, have been associated with adverse fetal effects. With the exception of alcohol, the effects of these agents are not as well established or as pervasive as is tobacco. Certain prescription drugs, particularly antiepileptic drugs, can result in fetal growth restriction and specific malformation syndromes.

TABLE 4.1 Effect of Chronic Hypertension on the Risk of Small for Gestational Age by Maternal Age

	SMALL FOR GESTATIONAL AGE BIRTHS (%)	
Maternal Age	Normotensive	Chronic Hypertension
<26 years	10	6
26–30 years	7	14
>30 years	5	18

Preeclampsia/Hypertension

Maternal chronic hypertension is an independent risk factor for IUGR and subsequent SGA infants. Advanced maternal age further increases the risk of SGA in infants born to mothers with chronic hypertension (Table 4.1). Superimposed preeclampsia on chronic hypertension poses the greatest risk of severe IUGR and subsequent adverse perinatal outcomes to infants of hypertensive mothers. Chronic hypertension and preeclampsia are both vascular problems in nature and are likely to have a common pathophysiologic effect on the placenta. Potential medical therapies aimed at preventing fetal growth restriction by improving placentation and placental blood flow is an area of active research.[30]

Multiple Gestations

The presence of more than one fetus in the uterus often results in SGA offspring. The presence and time of onset of fetal growth restriction is determined by the number of fetuses: the more fetuses, the more likely there is to be growth restriction, and the earlier it is likely to be observed.

Other

Finally, a variety of chronic maternal medical conditions are likely to have a negative effect on fetal growth. Gastrointestinal conditions that jeopardize maternal overall nutrition, or the mother's ability to absorb certain nutrients, such as inflammatory bowel disease or short gut syndrome, may have a negative effect on fetal growth or availability of certain nutrients to the developing fetus. Diseases that affect the oxygen content of the mother's blood, such as hemoglobinopathies, severe maternal anemia, or cyanotic heart disease, may all

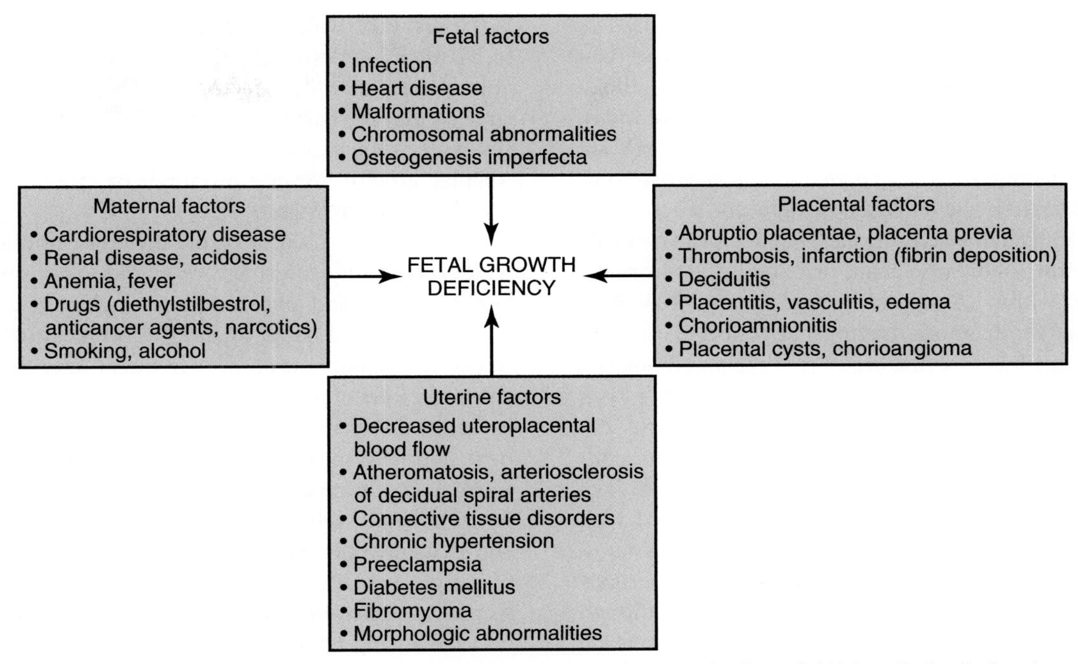

Fig. 4.2 Causes of growth restriction by compartment. (From James D, Steer P, Weiner C, Gonik B, eds. *High Risk Pregnancy*. 4th ed. Philadelphia, PA: Saunders; 2010.)

affect availability of oxygen to the fetus, thus having a negative effect on fetal growth. Maternal vasculopathies, such as can be seen with advanced diabetes mellitus, can result in IUGR. The potential role of psychosocial stressors in IUGR is unclear.[31,32] A summary of the relative contributions of the various factors with direct causal impact is provided in Fig. 4.2.

PLACENTAL CONTRIBUTIONS

The placenta is comprised of fetal tissue. It follows that circumstances that ultimately result in abnormal fetal growth often similarly affect placental growth. There is a known significant correlation between infant birth weight and both placental weight and villus surface area. Likewise, there are placental pathologic correlates of known causes of IUGR (intrauterine infections, chromosomal anomalies, hypertensive disorders, multiple gestations) and gross placental and cord abnormalities (chronic abruptio placentae, choriohemangioma, extensive infarction, and abnormal cord insertions), which are likely to result in restricted fetal growth. However, the majority of cases of IUGR are idiopathic, with the epidemiologic risk factors discussed earlier (e.g., previous fetal losses, extremes of maternal age, previous preterm or SGA infant, substance abuse) as the only clue. The cause of growth failure in these infants is presumed to be the result of the ill-defined uteroplacental insufficiency. Human and animal in vivo studies, Doppler ultrasound investigations, and pathologic evaluations have identified an array of placental abnormalities that may well shed a unifying light on these apparently disparate groups of mother–infant dyads[25,33] (Box 4.1). As a result of these investigations, the central role of the placenta in the development of the growth-restricted baby is coming to the forefront.

BOX 4.1 Findings in the Placenta in Fetal Growth Restriction

Uteroplacental Blood Flow
- Diminished blood flow
- Increased vascular resistance
- Absent spiral artery remodeling
- Atherosis of vessels of parietal decidua

Fetoplacental Blood Flow
- Increased irregularity of luminal size
- Abnormal umbilical Doppler flow studies
- Decreased number of placental arterial vessels
- Decreased size of placental vessels
- Decreased artery to villus ratio

Interface of Maternal and Fetal Circulations
- Cytotrophoblastic hyperplasia
- Thickened basement membrane
- Chronic villitis

DIMINISHED POTENTIAL: FETAL CONTRIBUTIONS

Genetic potential for fetal growth is inherited from both parents. Although this is the major determinant of early fetal growth, fetal growth is subsequently modulated by a multitude of environmental factors. IUGR can result from a variety of conditions (e.g., congenital infections) in which a genetically normal fetus is prohibited from growing appropriately, or as a result of a genetic aberration that precludes the fetus from growing appropriately.

Congenital Infections

During the rubella pandemic of 1962 to 1964, IUGR was found to be the most consistent characteristic of congenitally infected infants, with 60% of affected infants weighing less than the 10th percentile at birth and 90% weighing less than the 50th percentile.[34] Cytomegalovirus (CMV) is the infectious organism most commonly associated with IUGR today, although 90% of infants congenitally infected with CMV are asymptomatic. Symptomatic congenial CMV is most commonly characterized by hepatosplenomegaly and microcephaly with paraventricular calcifications. Diagnosis can be made reliably with viral polymerase chain reaction (PCR) from the urine obtained within 14 days of birth. Salivary CMV PCR may also be used for diagnosis, but must be collected immediately following birth before first breast feeding, and if positive should be confirmed with urine, as false positives have been derived from saliva.[35] Human immunodeficiency virus has also been associated with IUGR, even when adjusted for confounding variables, which can be difficult to separate.[36] Zika virus infection during pregnancy has been associated with an array of adverse clinical outcomes in the developing fetus, including intrauterine demise, IUGR, and central nervous system abnormalities with marked microcephaly.[37] Although numerous other bacterial, protozoal, and viral pathogens are known to invade the developing fetus, most of these infants develop appropriately.

Genetic Factors

About 8% of all SGA infants have a major congenital anomaly.[38] Conversely, the incidence of growth restriction in infants with significant congenital anomalies is 22%, nearly three times that of the general population, and a correlation exists between the number of malformations and frequency of IUGR.[39] A wide array of chromosomal aberrations (aneuploidy, deletions, translocations) are associated with IUGR. The likelihood of finding a chromosomal disorder in an SGA infant with a congenital anomaly is approximately 6%.[40] Uniparental disomy, a chromosomal disorder wherein a pair of homologous chromosomes are inherited from the same parent, has been associated with IUGR. Single-gene disorders and inborn errors of metabolism (such as maternal and fetal phenylketonuria) are likewise represented in this population. In addition, there are well over 100 syndromes without identified chromosomal abnormalities that are associated with IUGR.

IDENTIFICATION AND MANAGEMENT OF GROWTH RESTRICTION

A major problem is knowing which babies are at risk of growth restriction and should therefore have their growth monitored. Using classic risk factors and uterine fundal height measurements, at best, two-thirds of babies with growth restriction can be detected antenatally. In routine clinical practice, the proportion is actually often much lower, with typically about 30% detected in antenatal screening. Attempts have been made to detect intrauterine growth restriction in low-risk populations using a single assessment at 32 to 34 weeks' gestation. However, a single measurement cannot indicate growth trajectory as opposed to size; therefore it could be used to determine that a fetus is SGA but not whether this is the result of IUGR. Conversely, a fetus that is AGA at 32 to 34 weeks' gestational age has not necessarily followed an appropriate growth trajectory. Indeed, a Cochrane review showed that the harm from false-positive ultrasound diagnoses exceeds the benefit when screening is done in this way.[41] Regular growth velocity profiling for every baby would be prohibitively expensive.

Currently, usual obstetric practice is to monitor the fetuses with risk factors for growth restriction from maternal (e.g., hypertension) and epidemiologic factors (e.g., a previous growth-restricted baby) by ultrasound measurement every 2 weeks. Measurements at more frequent intervals are not reliable indicators of poor growth because the change in fetal size is within the error of the measurement. If growth slows, the next step is to measure umbilical artery blood flow velocity waveforms.[42] A raised pulsatility index (ratio of systolic velocity to diastolic velocity), or even worse, absent or reversed end-diastolic flow, indicates increased resistance to perfusion of the placenta, putting the fetus at risk for hypoxia. If these factors are identified, fetal medicine specialists can move on to assessing fetal vascular redistribution as a response to early hypoxia. This redistribution can be detected by Doppler studies of key fetal organs, including the brain (by study of the middle cerebral artery), to detect the maintenance of the oxygen supply to them, thereby protecting their vital functions. At the same time, flow to less vital organs is reduced. Impaired cardiac function in the fetus can be demonstrated using venous Doppler examination of the precordial veins (ductus venosus, inferior vena cava, or superior vena cava), hepatic veins, and head and neck veins. Combining the umbilical artery, middle cerebral artery, and venous Doppler examinations provides information about the degree of placental insufficiency, the level of blood flow redistribution, and the degree of cardiac compromise, respectively.

There is no currently known effective treatment to improve the growth pattern of a fetus. If it is likely that delivery will be indicated because of IUGR at less than 35 weeks' gestation, antenatal steroids should be given to improve lung maturity before delivery. Recent data suggests that there may be benefit to the infant if antenatal steroids are administered before delivery at less than 37 weeks' gestational age, as long as there are no comorbidities affecting the pregnancy that are potential contraindications to antenatal steroids (such as gestational diabetes or chorioamnionitis).[43] Antenatal steroids will help abate RDS, one of the most common and potentially severe morbidities related to prematurity.

Prenatal management of IUGR fetus is aimed at determining the best time and mode of delivery. Gestational age is a critical factor in this decision. Deciding on the appropriate time of delivery is particularly difficult before 30 weeks' gestation, when the risks of prematurity to the neonate are substantial. Early delivery of growth-restricted fetuses with an abnormal umbilical artery waveform results in a high live born rate but at the cost of rates of high neonatal mortality and morbidity. Alternatively, delaying delivery until the fetal heart rate pattern is abnormal has been reported to result in a nearly five-fold increase in fetal demise. However, neonatal deaths before discharge fall by more than one-third when delayed until there is a nonreassuring fetal heart rate tracing, and overall the total mortality is unchanged. Further, there is some evidence that long-term outcome may be improved by delaying delivery until there is a nonreassuring fetal heart rate tracing.[44]

SMALL-FOR-GESTATIONAL-AGE INFANTS

Lubchenco et al defined SGA as having a birth weight less than the 10th percentile. By definition then, 10% of all newborns in a given population are too small. Others have proposed other cutoff percentiles (e.g., the 25th, 15th, 5th, or 3rd), or 2 standard deviations from the mean, which would correspond to approximately 2.5% of the population. However, as previously noted, being SGA does not necessarily mean an infant was growth restricted. This distinction is made between the growth trajectory throughout fetal development (IUGR) and the absolute weight of a fetus or infant at a given time (percentile weight for gestational age).

Excluding SGA infants who have significant congenital anomalies and infections, there is a group of SGA infants with a relatively characteristic physical appearance: head disproportionately large as compared to the trunk, thin extremities, long nails, large anterior fontanelle, wide or overlapping cranial sutures, thin umbilical cord with little Wharton jelly, scaphoid abdomen, diminished subcutaneous fat, and loose skin on the arms, legs, back, abdomen, and buttocks, which may be dry and flaky with little vernix caseosa. The facial appearance has been likened to that of a "wizened old man."

Measuring the weight, length, and head circumference allows for further classification of the SGA infant as either symmetrically SGA (those infants with decreased length and head circumference) or asymmetrically SGA (relatively normal length with relative "head sparing"). The distinction between symmetric and asymmetric SGA is often used as both a diagnostic tool and a prognostic indicator. The symmetrically SGA newborn, historically representing approximately 20% of all SGA infants, is thought to result from an injury or process (congenital infection, genetic disorders) that occurred or began in the early stages of the pregnancy, during the phase of growth primarily characterized by cellular hyperplasia. The prognosis for eventual growth and development of these infants is somewhat guarded, in large part because of the underlying etiology. The asymmetrical ("wasted") SGA baby, on the other hand, has been proposed to result from a third-trimester insult interfering with delivery of oxygen and nutrients (the effect of maternal hypertensive disorders, maternal starvation, advanced diabetes) during the cellular hypertrophy phase of fetal growth. This latter group has a much better prognosis than the symmetric SGA.

Body proportionality is often measured as weight/length, with the three most common being weight for length (weight/length), body mass index (weight/length), and ponderal index (weight/length), and all of these indices have been used to attempt to further differentiate between the subgroups of symmetric and asymmetric SGA.[46] Similarly, a normal frequency distribution of head-to-abdominal circumference ratio is seen in antenatal ultrasound assessments of growth-restricted fetuses, with increased severity of growth restriction being associated with increased asymmetry.[47]

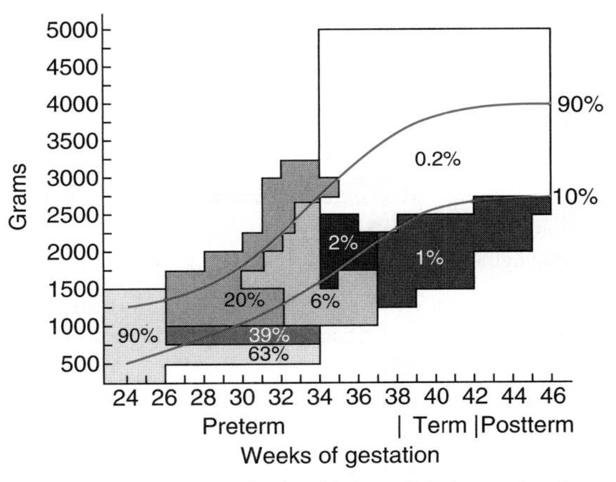

Fig. 4.3 Mortality risk according to birth weight/gestational age relationship. Based on 14,413 live births at University of Colorado Health Sciences Center (1974 to 1980). (From Koops B, Morgan LJ, Battaglia FC. Neonatal mortality risk in relation to birth weight and gestational age: update. *J Pediatr.* 1982;101:969.)

However, the clinical significance of symmetry of SGA has come into question. In some populations, symmetrical SGA infants are found more frequently than asymmetrical infants.[48] Salafia[33] found that IUGR preterm infants born to mothers suffering from preeclampsia were far more likely to be symmetrical than asymmetrical, and David[47] found an equal distribution of a small number of chromosomal abnormalities between the symmetrical and asymmetrical populations. These data suggest that although body proportionality helps characterize an SGA infant, they are certainly not the only factors guiding diagnosis and prognosis.

CLINICAL PROBLEMS

Perinatal and Neonatal Morbidity and Mortality

The growth-restricted fetus and newborn have a higher rate of perinatal mortality as compared to those of normal fetal growth trajectory, whether preterm, term, or postterm (Fig. 4.3). They are also at risk for many other adverse outcomes as a result of the intrauterine condition that resulted in IUGR (either inherent to the fetus, such as with a chromosomal abnormality, or related to the environment, such as with maternal hypertensive disorders). Overall, the rate of perinatal mortality among growth-restricted infants is 8 to 10 times that of infants who have grown normally, and the risk of perinatal morbidity and mortality increases markedly with the severity of IUGR (Fig. 4.4).[49]

Acute Neonatal Problems

Asphyxia

Perinatal asphyxia is the most significant risk for the growth-restricted fetus and newborn, who is often marginally oxygenated and who has limited carbohydrate reserves. With the stresses associated with labor and delivery, the IUGR fetus is at risk of fetal demise or hypoxic-ischemic encephalopathy.

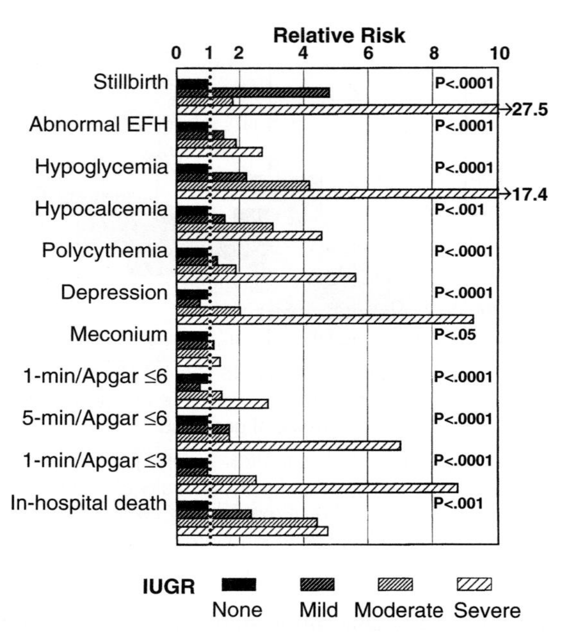

Fig. 4.4 Morbidity and mortality varies with degree of growth restriction. *EFH,* Electronic fetal heart pattern; *IUGR,* intrauterine growth restriction. (From Kramer MS, Olivier M, McLean FH, et al. Impact of intrauterine growth retardation and body proportionality on fetal and neonatal outcome. *Pediatrics* 1990;86:707.)

Respiratory Difficulties

Relative intolerance of the IUGR infant to the stresses of labor and delivery increases the risk of intrauterine passage and aspiration of meconium. Because of risk of intrauterine fetal demise, growth-restricted infants are more likely to be electively delivered prematurely, which places the infant at risk for all of the morbidities associated with prematurity, including RDS.

Hypoglycemia and Hypocalcemia

SGA infants are at risk of hypoglycemia, which usually resolves after the first 48 to 72 hours of life but may sometimes be severe and prolonged. Blood glucose homeostasis in SGA infants requires frequent monitoring and, in some cases, treatment, as severe hypoglycemia is a risk factor for long-term neurodevelopmental morbidity. Hypoglycemia can result from inadequate glycogen stores, diminished gluconeogenesis, relatively reduced alternative energy substrates (e.g., free fatty acids), hyperinsulinemia, and/or increased sensitivity to insulin, asphyxia, polycythemia, or hypothermia. Hypocalcemia is seen less frequently than hypoglycemia in SGA infants but must also be considered and monitored for as a possible complication in these infants (see Chapter 12).

Thermoregulation

SGA babies often have difficulty with maintaining body temperature in the normal range, and easily become hypothermic. This may stem from a diminished supply of glucose, diminished insulating subcutaneous fat, and impaired lipid metabolism. Brown adipose tissue stores are depleted in some SGA infants, which may diminish the infants' ability to adequately respond to hypothermia. The range of thermoneutral environmental temperatures for SGA infants is narrowed when contrasted with AGA infants of the same gestational age.

Hematologic Issues

Polycythemia, defined as a central venous hematocrit greater than 65%, occurs in as many as 40% of term or near-term IUGR infants. The etiology is thought to be poor placental function with resultant relative fetal hypoxia leading to elevated levels of fetal erythropoietin production. Elevated circulating nucleated red blood cells have also been observed in IUGR newborns. Polycythemia has been associated with cardiopulmonary, metabolic, and neurologic complications. It is important to closely monitor the cardiorespiratory status and blood glucose concentration of polycythemic infants. If an infant is asymptomatic and has normal or increased intravascular volume and the hematocrit is 65% to 75%, this monitoring may be sufficient. If an infant has a hematocrit greater than 65% and is symptomatic, partial exchange transfusion with normal saline is indicated to reduce blood viscosity, improve blood flow, and improve tissue perfusion. If the central venous hematocrit remains greater than 75% despite normal intravascular blood volume, partial exchange transfusion with normal saline may also be indicated.[50]

Polycythemia is not the only hematologic problem seen commonly in IUGR infants; white blood cells and platelets may be compromised. Serum immunoglobin G concentrations are depressed in term SGA infants when compared with their AGA peers, neutropenia is common in infants who had IUGR, and in some instances there are deficiencies in lymphocyte function, which all contribute to potential immunologic dysfunction. Growth-restricted infants may also exhibit thrombocytopenia. Infants with congenital infections and infants delivered to mothers with preeclampsia are particularly at risk for these issues.

THE PRETERM GROWTH-RESTRICTED INFANT

There have been animal and clinical research data that have both suggested that growth-restricted preterm infants may have a more favorable respiratory prognosis than equally premature infants with normal fetal growth. It has been postulated that this effect is as a result of a stress-induced acceleration of fetal lung maturation. However, other studies have demonstrated the opposite effect (Table 4.2). A study of a very large number of VLBW infants born between 25 and 30 weeks' gestation, free of major congenital anomalies, showed increased risk of neonatal death (odds ratio 2.77), necrotizing enterocolitis (odds ratio [OR] 1.27), and RDS (OR 1.19) in the SGA infants, as opposed to gestational age–matched AGA infants.[51]

GROWTH AND LONG-TERM OUTCOME

Growth

Many SGA infants show some degree of catch-up growth in the first year of life. In a large cohort study in the Netherlands evaluating catch-up growth of infants who were born AGA at less than 32 weeks' gestation, SGA at less than 32 weeks' gestation, and SGA at 32 weeks' (or higher) gestation, AGA infants born less than 32 weeks' gestational age showed no

TABLE 4.2 Incidence of Respiratory Distress in Small-for-Gestational-Age and Appropriate-for-Gestational-Age Infants According to Gestational Age

	INFANTS WITH RDS (%)	
Gestation (wk)	**SGA**	**AGA**
27–28	50	37
29–30	43	23
31–32	39	13
33–34	16	2.5
35–36	6	0
37–38	1.5	0.1

AGA, Appropriate for gestational age; *RDS,* respiratory distress syndrome; *SGA,* small for gestational age.

growth stunting by age 10 years, but SGA infants, both less than 32 weeks and 32 weeks (or higher), were likely to have continued stunting of growth at age 10 years, and this difference is most significant in infants who were born both SGA and less than 32 weeks. Early weight gain seems to be an important factor in predicting overall catch-up growth by age 10 years.[52] Infants with poor prenatal and postnatal head growth are at most risk of growth stunting and poor neurodevelopmental outcomes. The presence or absence of symmetry does not reliably indicate adequacy of growth in early childhood.[53]

Neurodevelopmental Outcome

Fetal growth restriction has been associated with an increased incidence of cognitive deficits (reduced IQ, impaired executive function, poor memory), motor deficits (impaired fine and gross motor skills, reduced visuomotor skills, clumsiness, cerebral palsy), and behavioral issues (attention deficits, hyperactivity, irritability, mood disorders, anxiety).[54-56] Poor prenatal head growth is associated with worse cognitive outcome, but impaired cognitive development has also been observed in growth-restricted infants with appropriate head growth. The severity of overall neurodevelopmental consequence of fetal growth restriction is complicated by a number of factors, including the severity of IUGR, the timing of onset of fetal growth restriction (early versus late), and the gestational age at delivery.[56]

LARGE FOR GESTATIONAL AGE

Babies whose birth weight is greater than the 90th percentile for gestational age are considered to be LGA. Much like infants born SGA, by definition, this category will characterize 10% of the population. Because the delivery of an LGA baby is potentially associated with significant perinatal morbidity and mortality, efforts are made to predict and confirm the presence of fetal macrosomia in an affected pregnancy before labor to facilitate appropriate management of the mother and infant. The LGA infants are especially at risk of birth trauma (shoulder dystocia, clavicular or humeral fractures, brachial plexus injuries, etc.), and there is an increased likelihood of instrumental vaginal delivery or cesarean delivery.[57]

There are a number of risk factors for fetal macrosomia, including maternal multiparity, maternal obesity, postterm pregnancy, gestational diabetes, and maternal history of a previous macrosomic infant and fetal Beckwith-Wiedemann syndrome.

Fetal macrosomia is commonly associated with pregnancies complicated by maternal diabetes. Even in expert centers, the rates of fetal macrosomia are between 20% and 40% for offspring of women with insulin-dependent diabetes, non-insulin-dependent diabetes, and gestational diabetes.[58] Being an infant of a diabetic mother is also associated with RDS, perinatal asphyxia, hypoglycemia, hypocalcemia, polycythemia, and, less frequently, hypertrophic cardiomyopathy or structural congenital heart disease.[59,60]

PHYSICAL EXAMINATION OF THE NEWBORN INFANT

Preparation

Before embarking on the physical examination of the infant, the clinician must review the mother's medical and pregnancy history to help focus the examination and to ensure that no pertinent findings are overlooked. For example, a history of maternal insulin-dependent diabetes should alert the examiner to the risk of a variety of congenital anomalies as well as aberrant growth. A history of polyhydramnios raises the suspicion of a proximal gastrointestinal obstruction or an underlying neurologic problem. A history of oligohydramnios may raise the question of structural renal anomalies. A mother reporting weak fetal movements would raise suspicion of a neuromuscular disorder. Knowing that a fetus presented in breech position should lead the examiner to focus on examination of the hips. As noted in the previous sections of this chapter, the presence of IUGR should alert the examiner to search for the stigmata of intrauterine infections and various syndromes.

Transfer of pathogenic microbes from the examiner to the baby must be prevented by thorough hand hygiene, and the stethoscope or any other instruments used should be cleaned thoroughly with an antiseptic. For all newborns, but in particular the premature or sick neonate, the thermal environment must be appropriate. Attention must also be given to the lighting and noise in the examination area. Lighting needs to be adequate but avoid very bright light. A thorough examination of the newborn should take no more than 5 to 10 minutes.

Varying Purpose of the Examination

The extent and focus of the examination varies with circumstances. There are typically three distinct periods during which the infant is examined: (1) a brief examination immediately after birth; (2) a complete examination in the newborn nursery or mother's room within 24 hours after birth; and (3) a focused examination within 24 hours before discharge.

The purpose of the initial examination, immediately following delivery, is twofold: (1) to ensure that there is no evidence of significant cardiopulmonary instability that requires intervention; and (2) to identify significant congenital anomalies. For the high-risk neonate, it may be advantageous to use this setting to perform a complete examination, to forgo a subsequent examination, and thereby avoid an unnecessary disturbance of the baby in the intensive care nursery.

The assessment of cardiopulmonary adaptation to extrauterine life begins as soon as the infant is delivered, and this initial evaluation is, in part, quantified by the Apgar score. Assessment of the presence, regularity, and effectiveness of respiratory effort is the first step in evaluating any newborn. Apnea or signs of respiratory distress must be noted to determine the need for intervention. It is not unusual for a healthy newborn to require a few minutes to establish a regular respiratory pattern, and unlabored respiratory rates of 60 to 80 breaths per minute may be seen for the first 1 to 2 hours in some normal infants during transition. If the respiratory rate persists to be above 60 breaths per minute, or if there are signs of distress such as grunting, flaring of the nostrils, or intercostal retractions, a detailed evaluation including pulse oximetry, chest x-ray, blood gas, hematocrit, and sepsis evaluation is warranted (see also Chapter 9).

Cardiovascular adaptation is simultaneously assessed with the pulmonary adjustment to extrauterine life. The normal heart rate of newborn infant is 100–160 beats per minute, although it may exceed 160 beats per minute for brief periods. Sustained tachycardia is not a normal finding and may indicate hypovolemia, inadequate oxygen delivery to the tissues, sepsis, anemia, or, rarely, an arrhythmia.

To assess oxygenation and circulation in the delivery room, it is important to assess color of the infant centrally (gums, inner lips, tongue), because acrocyanosis (blue discoloration of the hands and feet) is often present in the normal infant during the first 24 hours of life. Pallor and poor perfusion require further evaluation. Circulation may also be evaluated by assessing capillary refill time. Normal capillary refill time is less than 2 seconds. Capillary refill time is measured by pressing gently on the sternum for five seconds until the skin blanches beneath the practitioner's finger, and then releasing. Capillary refill time is time for the color to return once the pressure is released.

Evaluation of responsiveness and muscle tone are the next steps in evaluation of the success of transition. Normal tone varies considerably with gestational age, but flaccidity, hypertonicity, and asymmetry of tone are never normal.

Following the initial assessment for physiologic stability, an efficient physical examination, specifically looking for major congenital anomalies, should be conducted. This should include survey of the face, mouth, abdomen, back, extremities, genitalia, and perineum. This should be done while the mother and infant are still in the delivery room, so that the presence, significance, and preliminary plans for the evaluation of any anomalies discovered can be discussed with the family. Even relatively minor anomalies can precipitate strong reactions from anxious parents.

After medical assessment of the infant, assuming the conditions of the baby and mother permit, the parents should be provided with some private time with their new baby. The baby is usually in a state of quiet alertness, which facilitates initial parent–infant bonding. This state of quiet alertness will also allow the mother to attempt to latch the infant onto the breast for the first time, and early latching increases the likelihood of future breast-feeding success. The infant should be assessed at least once every 30 minutes until there has been continued stability for 2 hours of life.[45]

Transition Period

During the first 15 to 30 minutes of life, the first period of reactivity, the infant is in a state of sympathetic discharge. During this period, the normal newborn is alert and responsive and exhibits spontaneous startle reactions (Moro reflex), bursts of crying, side-to-side movements of the head, smacking of the lips, and tremors of the extremities. As the infant begins to exhibit parasympathetic discharge, bowel sounds, passage of meconium, and saliva production become evident. Preterm infants and term infants who are ill or under perinatal stress may have a prolonged period of initial reactivity.

During the first hour of life, the infant spends up to 40 minutes in a quiet alert state. This is often the longest period of quiet alert behavior during the first 4 days of life. After this period of alertness, the baby passes into a 1- to 2-hour period of decreased activity and sleep. A second period of reactivity occurs between 2 and 6 hours of age, with many of the same motor and autonomic manifestations previously described for the first period of reactivity; however, gagging and vomiting are also often observed during this time. The duration of this phase is variable, lasting from 10 minutes to several hours. For more information on the transition period, see Chapter 3.

Postnatal Assessment of Gestational Age

Ultrasound assessment during early pregnancy is the most accurate method of assessing gestational age and is the standard of care in high-income countries.[61] A variety of assessment tools have been developed to estimate the gestational age of a newborn infant. Currently, the most widely used assessment tool for the postnatal estimation of gestational age in the United States is the New Ballard Score (NBS), which estimates gestational age based on a combination of physical examination and neurological examination characteristics (Box 4.2 and Fig. 4.5).[62,63] The advantage of the NBS is the relative ease with which it can be carried out, even in the newborn requiring mechanical ventilation. However, even in the most experienced hands, the NBS demonstrates up to a 2-week variance in the postnatal assessment of gestational age from well-established antenatal ultrasound-based dating.

EDITORIAL COMMENT: Donovan et al. determined the accuracy of the New Ballard Score (NBS) for infants less than 28 weeks' gestational age (GA) by accurate menstrual history. They reported that for each week from 22 to 28 weeks' GA by accurate menstrual history, NBS estimates exceeded GA by dates by 1.3 to 3.3 weeks, and estimates varied widely. NBS did not contribute significantly to regression models of death, poor outcome, or duration of hospital stay. Therefore the most accurate estimates of GA are obtained before delivery.

(Donovan EF, Tyson JE, Ehrenkranz RA, et al. Inaccuracy of Ballard scores before 28 weeks' gestation. National Institute of Child Health and Human Development Neonatal Research Network. *J Pediatr.* 1999;135(2 Pt 1):147-152.)

BOX 4.2 Technique for New Ballard Score

Neuromuscular Maturity

There is a general replacement of extensor tone by flexor tone in a cephalocaudal progression with advancing gestational age.

Posture: Observe the unrestrained infant in the supine position.

Square window: Flex the wrist and measure the minimal angle between the ventral surface of the forearm and the palm.

Arm recoil: With the infant supine and the head midline, hold the forearm against the arm for 5 seconds, then fully extend and release the arm. Note the time it takes the infant to resume a flexed posture.

Popliteal angle: Flex the hips with the thighs on the abdomen. Then, without lifting the hips from the bed surface, extend the knee as far as possible until resistance is met. (One may overestimate the extent of extension if one attempts to continue extending the knee beyond the point where resistance is first met.)

Scarf sign: Keeping the head in the midline, pull the hand across the chest to encircle the neck as a scarf and note the position of the elbow relative to the midline.

Heel to ear: With the infant supine and the pelvis kept on the examining surface, the feet are brought back as far as possible toward the head, allowing the knees to be positioned alongside the abdomen.

Physical Maturity

Skin: With maturation, the skin becomes thicker, less translucent, and, eventually, dry and peeling.

Lanugo: This fine, nonpigmented hair is evenly distributed over the body and is most prominent at 27 to 28 weeks' gestation, then it gradually disappears, usually first from the lower back. Although present over the entire body, the lanugo over the back is used for gestational age assessment.

Plantar surface: As with the hands, the presence of creases in the foot is a reflection of intrauterine activity as well as maturation. The absence of creases may indicate an underlying neurologic problem as well as immaturity. Accelerated crease development is observed when oligohydramnios was present. An addition in the New Ballard Score (NBS) is the requirement for measuring the plantar surface.

Breast: The areola development is not dependent on adequacy of intrauterine nutrition. There is no difference in male or female infants.

Ear cartilage: With maturation, the ear cartilage becomes increasingly stiff, and the auricle thickens. Fold the top of the ear and assess the recoil.

Eyelid opening: Used (incorrectly) by some as a sign of nonviability. Dr. Ballard included the degree of fusion of the lids as a new assessment tool. She defined tightly fused as both lids being inseparable by gentle traction, and loosely fused as either lid being able to be partly separated by gentle traction. Tightly fused lids were observed in 20% of infants born at 26 weeks' gestation and only 5% of babies delivered at 27 weeks. The presence of fused eyelids alone should never be used as a sign of nonviability.

External genitalia, male: Palpate for level of testicular descent, and observe the degree of rugation.

External genitalia, female: The labia minora and clitoris are prominent in the immature newborn, at times leading the inexperienced examiner to suspect clitoromegaly. With maturation, the labia majora becomes fat filled and therefore prominent. The undernourished fetus may have relatively thin labia majora.

The Complete Examination

The complete examination of the healthy newborn can be carried out either in the newborn nursery or in the mother's room. When the infant is examined at the mother's bedside, the infant's family is more easily able to express any concerns about the baby, and the physician is better able to observe parent–infant interactions.

The purpose of the complete examination is to

- detect any congenital anomalies that may not have been anticipated based on prenatal care (a significant congenital anomaly is present in 10 to 20 per 1000 live births);
- confirm any abnormalities detected prenatally and consider postnatal evaluation and care;
- consider potential problems related to maternal pregnancy history or family history;
- allow the parents to ask any questions and raise any concerns about their baby;
- determine whether there is concern by caregivers about the ability of the parents to care for the baby following discharge;
- provide anticipatory guidance; and
- ensure appropriate follow-up care has been arranged.

The clinician needs to find a method that will allow for a comprehensive examination while minimizing the disturbance of the baby. General observation (hands and stethoscope off) is combined with a head-to-toe physical examination. Sometimes it is necessary to be opportunistic in the approach of the newborn, for example, checking red reflexes when the infant has his eyes open, or listening to the heart, lungs, and abdomen with a stethoscope at a moment when the infant is not crying, but it is important to ensure that all aspects of the examination are eventually covered.

Body Measurements and Gestational Age Assessment

Note the birth weight, length, and head circumference and plot them on a growth chart with respect to gestational age. The gestational age is usually based on the maternal estimated date of delivery (EDD), which is derived from prenatal ultrasound evaluation and date of last menstrual period. Gestational age can also be assessed by physical examination of the infant, using the New Ballard score, which is helpful in cases where infant maturity and maternal EDD appear to be discordant, or when pregnancy dating is uncertain before delivery.

Vital Signs

The respiratory rate and heart rate of the normal newborn vary considerably in the first few hours of life. During the

Neuromuscular maturity

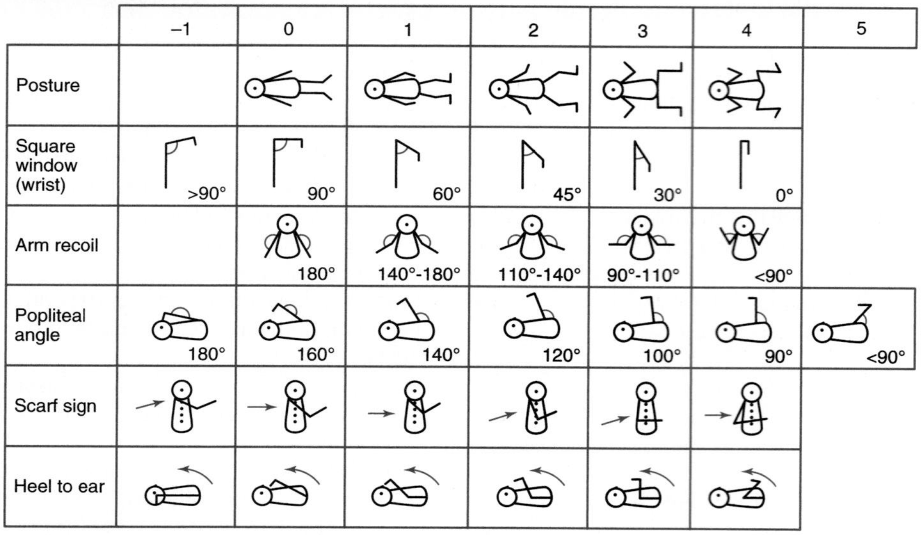

	−1	0	1	2	3	4	5
Posture							
Square window (wrist)	>90°	90°	60°	45°	30°	0°	
Arm recoil		180°	140°-180°	110°-140°	90°-110°	<90°	
Popliteal angle	180°	160°	140°	120°	100°	90°	<90°
Scarf sign							
Heel to ear							

Physical maturity

Skin	Sticky, friable, transparent	Gelatinous, red, translucent	Smooth, pink, visible veins	Superficial peeling &/or rash, few veins	Cracking pale areas, rare veins	Parchment, deep cracking, no vessels	Leathery, cracked, wrinkled
Lanugo	None	Sparse	Abundant	Thinning	Bald areas	Mostly bald	
Plantar surface	Heel-toe 40-50 mm: −1 <40 mm: −2	>50 mm no crease	Faint red marks	Anterior transverse crease only	Creases anterior 2/3	Creases over entire sole	
Breast	Imperceptible	Barely perceptible	Flat areola, no bud	Stippled areola 1-2 mm bud	Raised areola 3-4 mm bud	Full areola 5-10 mm bud	
Eye/ear	Lids fused Loosely:−1 Tightly:−2	Lids open, pinna flat, stays folded	slightly curved pinna; soft; slow recoil	Well-curved pinna; soft but ready recoil	Formed & firm, instant recoil	Thick cartilage, ear stiff	
Genitals, male	Scrotum flat, smooth	Scrotum empty, faint rugae	Testes in upper canal, rare rugae	Testes descending, few rugae	Testes down, good rugae	Testes pendulous, deep rugae	
Genitals, female	Clitoris prominent, labia flat	Prominent clitoris, small labia minora	Prominent clitoris, enlarging minora	Majora & minora equally prominent	Majora large, minora small	Majora covers clitoris & minora	

Maturity Rating

Score	Weeks
−10	20
−5	22
0	24
5	26
10	28
15	30
20	32
25	34
30	36
35	38
40	40
45	42
50	44

Fig. 4.5 New Ballard Score. (From Ballard J, Wednig K, Wang L, et al. New Ballard Score, expanded to include extremely premature infants. *J Pediatr.* 1991;119:417.)

remainder of the first day of life, most newborns have a respiratory rate of 40 to 60 breaths per minute and a heart rate of 120 to 160 beats per minute. The temperature is also evaluated in the delivery room, and a normal newborn's axillary temperature should be between 35.5°C and 37.5°C. An elevated temperature may represent a fever but is more commonly the result of environmental factors, such as heat applied to the infant from the radiant warmer or overbundling.

OBSERVATION

Initially, examiners uses only their eyes and unaided ears to evaluate the baby (hands and stethoscope off). This is usually best done in stages, observing one exposed part of the baby at a time.

Respiratory Effort

The respiratory effort of the newborn varies with activity level of the infant at the time of observation. During deep sleep, the infant usually has a regular breathing pattern, whereas during awake states, bursts of more rapid breathing are often observed. Because of the newborn's compliant chest wall and almost exclusive diaphragmatic breathing, it is not unusual to observe mild subcostal and intercostal retractions, as well as paradoxical movement during inspiration, with the thorax being drawn inward accompanied by outward abdominal excursion. Even though this "seesaw" pattern is often seen in neonates with respiratory distress, in the absence of further evidence of respiratory difficulties, this movement should not cause alarm. However, suprasternal and supraclavicular retractions are not normal findings. Likewise, asymmetrical chest wall movement is abnormal and may indicate unilateral lesions of the diaphragm (diaphragmatic hernia or diaphragmatic paralysis associated with a difficult delivery) or pleural space (effusion or pneumothorax). The normal newborn thorax has a relatively narrow anteroposterior diameter. A barrel chest appearance suggests cardiomegaly or air trapping, as may be seen with meconium aspiration syndrome or a pneumothorax. Audible grunting results from the infant expiring against a partially closed glottis in an effort to maintain a functional residual capacity in the face of atelectasis. This finding should be assumed to indicate a potentially significant cardiopulmonary disorder until proven otherwise.

Color and Perfusion

The normal newborn is pink, and they may have acrocyanosis (blue discoloration of the hands, feet, and perioral area) on the first day of life. Central cyanosis (involving the tongue and mucous membranes of the mouth) persisting beyond the first few minutes of life is always abnormal and may indicate significant cardiopulmonary disease. Occasionally, infants with polycythemia appear cyanotic despite adequate oxygenation because they have a relatively high concentration of reduced hemoglobin. As noted previously, polycythemia is more likely to present in postdates, LGA, and IUGR infants, and in infants of mothers with diabetes.

> **EDITORIAL COMMENT:** Despite the now common practice of delaying clamping of the cord at birth, polycythemia has become relatively uncommon, which is in large part a result of prevention of postterm delivery and better management of gestational diabetes. Polycythemia is now seen predominantly in the "recipient" twin in monochorionic-diamniotic twin pregnancies affected by twin-to-twin transfusion syndrome (see Chapter 16).

The presenting fetal parts may be bruised during delivery, resulting in a localized bluish-purple discoloration. This can be particularly striking in a facial presentation, and petechiae may accompany the ecchymosis. Bruising may be easily differentiated from cyanosis by applying gentle pressure to the affected area. A bruise will remain unchanged with pressure, whereas an area of cyanosis will blanch. A similar discoloration of the face may occur in an infant delivered with a nuchal cord as the result of transient obstruction of venous drainage of blood from the head.

A vigorous infant may turn nearly purple during a Valsalva maneuver, which often occurs before crying or during stooling. Occasionally, an infant may exhibit Harlequin color change, wherein there is a striking division into pale and red halves in an infant, with a sharp line of demarcation along the midline from head to foot. Although striking in appearance, this finding is of no clinical significance and will resolve without intervention.

Although jaundice develops in 80% of newborns, this finding in the first 24 hours of life is abnormal and requires investigation. If jaundice is suspected within the first 24 hours of life, a transcutaneous or serum measurement should be performed and plotted on a nomogram. The clinician should not rely on visual inspection of the jaundiced infant to estimate serum bilirubin concentration, as this is highly unreliable. Rarely, direct hyperbilirubinemia is seen in the first hours of life, which typically provides a green cast to the infant's skin. Greenish staining of the skin and nails is much more commonly observed when an infant has passed meconium in utero.

Mottling may be observed in well preterm infants or term infants, especially when hypothermic. However, mottling can also be a sign of significant systemic illness. Pallor, however, is never normal and may result from poor cardiac output, subcutaneous edema, asphyxia, or anemia. Finally, a grayish hue may be associated with significant metabolic acidosis.

Position and Movement

Observation of an infant's position at rest (an indicator of underlying tone) and spontaneous movement provides a great deal of information about his or her neurologic status. Gestational age, illness, maternal medications, and sleep state influence tone and spontaneous movements and must be considered during the evaluation. Muscle tone generally increases in a caudocephalad direction with advancing gestational age. In the infant of 28 weeks' gestation, there is little tone in either upper or lower extremities, and the infant generally remains in the position in which he is placed. By 32 weeks, the infant should have developed tone in the lower extremities, resulting in flexion at the hips and knees. At 36 weeks, strong flexor tone is present in the lower extremities, and the arms begin to display some flexion. At term, an infant in the supine position holds all four extremities in moderate flexion. When placed prone, the term infant should be able to briefly lift his head above the plane of the body, and often elevates the pelvis above the flexed hips and knees. Most of the time the term infant will hold his hands fisted with the thumb adducted and folded (cortical thumbs), although he will intermittently open them.

The character of normal spontaneous movements varies with gestational age. Before 32 weeks, infants demonstrate random, slow writhing movements with interspersed myoclonic jerks of the extremities. This writhing quality often persists through 44 weeks' gestational age. By 32 weeks, flexor movements of the lower extremities begin to predominate and typically occur in unison. A month later, these movements alternate, a pattern seen more frequently in the term infant. This progression of findings is entirely dependent on gestational, not postnatal, age.

Normal babies of all gestational ages have symmetrical tone and movements. Finding more than mild asymmetry in position and range of spontaneous movement may indicate the presence of local birth trauma (brachial plexus injury or fractures of the clavicle, humerus, or femur) or, rarely, a central nervous system insult, lesion, or anomaly. Asymmetry of position may also reflect in utero positioning, which should improve with time. The finding of extremes of flexion or extension requires a more in-depth neurologic evaluation.

Face and Crying

A normal infant should display symmetry of the mouth and eyes, both at rest and with crying. An asymmetric mouth (the abnormal side does not "droop" with crying) with an ipsilateral eye that does not close and a forehead that does not wrinkle usually indicates an injury to the peripheral facial nerve (cranial nerve VII), as may occur with a forceps-assisted vaginal delivery. This situation must be differentiated from a congenital degeneration or maldevelopment of the cranial nerves VI and VII nuclei (Möbius sequence), which is typically manifested by bilateral palsy. A palsy confined to the lower portion of the face (central facial palsy) may indicate an intracranial hemorrhage or infarct. This latter finding should be distinguished from congenital absence of the depressor anguli oris muscle (asymmetrical crying facies), which is a benign condition but one that may be associated with congenital cardiac anomalies.

A healthy newborn should have a strong, lusty cry. A weak or whining cry may indicate illness, developing respiratory distress, depression from maternal medication exposure before delivery (such as magnesium or opioids), or central nervous system disturbance. Central nervous system abnormalities may also result in persistent high-pitched crying. Hoarseness can be caused by laryngeal edema resulting from airway manipulation in the delivery room, hypocalcemia, unilateral vocal cord paresis, or airway anomalies. Conditions resulting in either internal obstruction or external compression of the airway often cause stridor, which is exacerbated by crying, and must always be considered a potentially serious finding.

Congenital Anomalies

A quick head-to-toe survey for dysmorphic features must be undertaken for each newborn infant.

Skin

In the extremely premature infant (<29 weeks' gestation), the skin is translucent with little subcutaneous fat and easily visualized superficial veins. Because the stratum corneum is thin, the skin of the extremely premature infant is easily injured by seemingly innocuous procedures or manipulation, which may result in denudation of the stratum corneum and a raw, weeping surface. Insensible losses of water through this immature integument can be considerable and may result in marked fluid and electrolyte imbalances. This effect may be attenuated by raising humidity in the incubator. The stratum corneum of even the extremely premature infant quickly matures so that by 1 to 2 weeks of postnatal age, the insensible water losses are reduced to levels seen in the mature infant. By term, skin is relatively opaque with considerable subcutaneous fat.

At 35 to 36 weeks' gestational age, the infant is covered with greasy vernix caseosa, which then thins by term and is usually absent in the postterm infant. The postmature infant has parchment-like skin with deep cracks on the trunk and extremities, long fingernails, and peeling of the distal extremities.

A variety of benign, transient skin conditions are found in the newborn. Erythema toxicum neonatorum is a rash seen generally in term infants beginning on the second or third day of life. It is characterized by 1- to 2-mm white papules (which may become vesicular) on an erythematous base of varying diameter. The lesions appear and disappear on different parts of the body, although they are infrequently seen on the face and are never found on the palms or soles. On microscopic evaluation of the papule or vesicle, eosinophils will be present.

Milia are 1- to 2-mm whitish papules and are frequently found on the face of newborns. Miliaria is a result of eccrine sweat duct obstruction, and it manifests as glistening vesiculopapular lesions over the forehead and on the scalp and skinfolds. Miliaria appears during the first day and disappears within the first week of life.

Transient neonatal pustular melanosis, which is seen predominantly in African American infants, is a benign generalized eruption of superficial pustules overlying hyperpigmented macules. The pustules, which can be found on any area of the skin, including the palms and soles, may be removed when vernix is being wiped off or during the first bath, so that the physician may see only macules surrounded by a fine, scaly collarette. Caucasian infants may also have transient pustular melanosis but often do not exhibit the hyperpigmentation. On microscopic evaluations, the pustules contain an occasional polymorphonuclear leukocyte and cellular debris.

Cerulean spots are macular areas of slate-blue hyperpigmentation seen predominantly over the buttocks or trunk. They are seen most commonly in African American, Native American, and Asian infants.

A large number of skin, nail, and hair abnormalities may be found in the newborn. Some of these are important clues in the identification of an underlying syndrome or generalized disease process. Examination of the newborn's skin should be made to identify any congenital nevi, hemangiomas, areas of abnormal pigmentation, tags, pits, scaling, blistering, abnormal laxity, or dysplasia. The color, distribution, and texture of hair is noted. Nail hypoplasia, dysplasia, aplasia, or hypertrophy should be further investigated. A large hemangioma on the face or neck can potentially cause airway obstruction. Port wine stains are capillary malformations that present as pink macular lesions that become purple with time. They are usually on the face, but can be anywhere on the body. When the port wine stain involves the distribution of the trigeminal nerve, it may be associated with an underlying vascular malformation of the meninges and cerebral cortex, and may cause seizures and developmental delay (Sturge-Weber syndrome). If the port wine stain involves the distribution of the first and second divisions of the trigeminal nerve, congenital glaucoma may also be present, and the infant should undergo ophthalmologic evaluation.

Head

There are several potential findings on the scalp, face, and head that may result from the delivery process. Small lacerations or puncture wounds may be present on the scalp if the infant was monitored during labor using a fetal scalp electrode. Use of forceps can result in superficial marks, edema, or bruising of the skin on the sides of the skull and face, whereas the vacuum extractor can leave a circumferential area of edema, bruising, and occasionally blisters. Use of either forceps or vacuum extractor is associated with an increased likelihood of injuries to the extracranial structures.

Caput succedaneum is a boggy area of edema located at the presenting part of the often-molded head; it is present at birth, crosses suture lines, and disappears within a few days. In contrast, cephalohematomas, present in 1% to 2% of all newborns, are subperiosteal collections of blood that do not cross suture lines. They are often bilateral, and they usually increase in size after birth. Depending on the amount of blood present, cephalohematomas may be fluctuant or tense. Cephalohematomas may take weeks to months to resolve. Subgaleal hemorrhages are the least common of the extracranial injuries but are the most dangerous. Newborns can lose tremendous amounts of blood from this injury, and they must be monitored carefully for shock when the diagnosis is suspected. Subgaleal hemorrhages are fluctuant, can cross suture lines, and may expand rapidly following delivery. It is possible for a subgaleal hemorrhage to cover the entire scalp, push the ears anteriorly, and even extend into the neck.

Unusual configuration of the scalp hair, such as double or anterior whorls or prominent cowlicks, may be associated with abnormalities of the skull or brain, particularly if there are associated unusual facies. A low-set posterior hairline may indicate a short or webbed neck, as in Turner syndrome. Cutis aplasia, a condition in which a 2- to 5-cm-diameter portion of the scalp appears to be totally absent, may be an isolated problem, but it is also a common finding in trisomy 13.

Accurate measurement of the head circumference is an important aspect of the physical examination. Macro- or microcephaly may indicate significant underlying neuropathology. The true circumference of the skull may be difficult to ascertain immediately after birth because of the molding that occurs during the birth process, and some time may be required before one can be sure of the presence or absence of an abnormality.

Babies delivered by cesarean section without a trial of labor typically have little to no molding, whereas vaginal delivery usually results in an enhanced occipitomental dimension with a relatively narrow biparietal diameter. Infants who were in breech presentation characteristically have an accentuation of the occipitofrontal measurement with a resultant occipital shelf and apparent frontal bossing. The effects of intrauterine positioning and birth are transient and should recede within days. If molding appears to persist beyond the first few days, underlying abnormalities should be considered. A head with a short occipitofrontal dimension (brachycephaly) is characteristic of trisomy 21. Palpation of the skull should reveal bones with mobile edges along the sagittal, coronal, and lambdoidal suture lines. Initial overlapping of the sutures is normal. A palpable ridge along suture lines should always be considered abnormal, possibly indicating premature closure of the sutures (craniosynostosis). The impact of craniosynostosis on the final configuration of the skull depends on the suture involved. The most commonly involved is the sagittal suture, with resultant dolichocephaly. Even though most instances of craniosynostosis are isolated events, it is also characteristic of some syndromes, such as Apert and Crouzon. The normal width of the various sutures of the skull is quite variable. African American infants tend to have wider metopic and sagittal sutures. Wide lambdoidal and squamosal sutures in term infants may be a sign of raised intracranial pressure. Craniotabes, soft pliable parietal bone along the sagittal suture, is a common finding in preterm infants as well as in the term infant whose head had been resting on the pelvic brim for the last few weeks of pregnancy. As its name implies, craniotabes can be seen in congenital syphilis, but this is much less common.

Palpation of the anterior and posterior fontanelles should take place when the infant is relatively quiet. The normal anterior fontanelle has slight pulsations accompanying the heart beat and should be flat or slightly sunken. There is a wide range of normal for fontanelle size, and thus routine measurement of fontanelles is not particularly useful and not recommended. There are differences in normal fontanelle size among different racial populations; for example, African American babies have statistically larger fontanelles than do Caucasian infants. If an infant has an audible bruit when the fontanelle is auscultated with a stethoscope, this may signify an intracranial arteriovenous malformation.

Eyes

Salmon-colored patches on the eyelids, midforehead, and nape of the neck are common. Those on the face fade by 1 year of age, whereas those on the nape are more persistent, and may be present into adulthood, but are often hidden by hair. Dysmorphologies of the eye and ocular region are the most frequently cited findings in malformation syndromes. Abnormal eyes may also indicate inborn errors of metabolism, central nervous system defects, or congenital infections. Although careful evaluation of the eyes is clearly important, it is potentially one of the most difficult aspects of the examination. Most infants will open their eyes at some point during the course of the examination. Dimming the ambient light and gently holding the infant upright and rocking backward and forward often prompts the baby to open his eyes.

The size, orientation, and position of the eyes should be noted. The diameters of the cornea and eye at term are approximately 10 mm and 17 mm, respectively. Microphthalmia is seen in a number of malformation syndromes, including trisomy 13, whereas an enlarged or cloudy cornea should suggest congenital glaucoma. Trisomy 21 is characterized by palpebral fissures that slant upward from the inner canthus, whereas Treacher Collins, Apert, and DiGeorge syndromes are all characterized in part by downward-slanting palpebral fissures. A large number of syndromes, including Alpert syndrome and trisomy 13, are associated with hypertelorism (a wide interpupillary distance), whereas hypotelorism is less common but can be seen in holoprosencephaly and trisomy 13.

Newborns often demonstrate random and, at times, disconjugate movements of the eyes. Persistent strabismus should be further evaluated. Subconjunctival hemorrhages can occur during the birthing process, but they are benign and resolve spontaneously. The iris is blue in nearly all newborns, although some more heavily pigmented infants have dark irises at birth. Reaction of the pupil to light begins to appear by 30 weeks' gestation, but reaction may not be consistently seen for another 2 to 5 weeks. Detailed visualization of the retina is unnecessary in most infants. The goal of routine funduscopic examinations is to ensure the absence of intraocular pathology and opacities of the cornea and lens by establishing the presence of a normal light reflex (red reflex). Whereas the normal light reflex is red in Caucasian infants, more darkly pigmented infants may have a pearly gray reflex. The finding of a white pupillary reflex (leukocoria) can suggest the presence of a variety of ocular pathologies (cataracts, trauma, persistent hyperplastic primary vitreous, tumor, retinopathy of prematurity) and requires urgent evaluation by an ophthalmologist.

EDITORIAL COMMENT: Callaway reported that fundus hemorrhages (FHs) are common and detectable by retinal photographs in 20% of term newborns. They often involve multiple areas and layers of the retina. Some 95% of FHs involved the periphery, 83% involved the macula, and 71% involved multiple layers of the retina. Vaginal delivery was associated with a significantly increased risk of FH, whereas self-identified Hispanic or Latino ethnicity was protective against FH in this study. Birth trauma from forceps delivery and asphyxia have also been identified as risk factors for FH. The long-term consequences of FH on visual development remain unknown, but close follow-up is recommended, especially if the macula is involved.

Retinal hemorrhages occur in less than 10% of LBW neonates (i.e., a prevalence one-half that observed in term neonates). The hemorrhages tend to resolve without sequelae in the first 10 days of life and occur more commonly in infants born to women with uterine infection. Retinal hemorrhages in very premature neonates are not predictive of intraventricular hemorrhage–related brain damage.

Callaway NF, Judwig CA, Blumenkranz MS, et al. Retinal and optic nerve hemorrhages in the newborn infant: one-year results of the Newborn Eye Screen Test Study. *Ophthalmology.* 2016;123:1043-1052.

Ears

The appearance of the normal external ear can vary widely. Many syndromes include malformed auricles or low-set ears as part of their spectrum, but the findings are not pathognomonic. The patency of the external ear canals should be ensured. All infants should have hearing screening performed before discharge from their newborn hospitalization. If there is an ear anomaly, including preauricular skin tags or pits, some centers perform ultrasound evaluation of the kidneys because there is a slight increase in associated incidence of renal abnormalities.

Nose

The nose may appear misshapen because of in utero positioning, and it usually self-corrects in a few days. Conversely, nasal asymmetry may be the result of septal displacement, which requires evaluation by an otolaryngologist. Several syndromes and teratogens have nasal manifestations including small (fetal alcohol syndrome) to large (trisomy 13) noses and low (achondroplasia) to prominent (Seckel syndrome) nasal bridges. Nasal obstruction may be caused by mucus, or it may represent true anatomic obstruction caused by tumors, encephalocele, or choanal atresia. Choanal atresia may be unilateral or bilateral, and may require the use of an oral airway or endotracheal intubation to maintain a patent airway. Choanal atresia may be isolated, or found as part of the CHARGE association (*c*oloboma, *h*eart disease, *a*tresia choanae, *r*estricted growth and development and/or central nervous system [CNS] anomalies, *g*enital anomalies and/or hypogonadism, and *e*ar anomalies and/or deafness).

Mouth

Micrognathia is a component of many malformation syndromes. The interior of the mouth should be evaluated with a light and tongue blade as well as a gloved finger. The frenulum labialis superior is a band of tissue that connects the central portion of the upper lip to the alveolar ridge of the maxilla. It may be prominent and be associated with a notch in the maxillary ridge where it originates. Likewise, the frenulum linguae is a band of tissue that connects the floor of the mouth to the tongue. This may extend to the tip of the tongue (tongue-tie). Natal (present at birth) and neonatal (present in the first month of life) teeth are usually found in the mandibular central incisor region, and are bilateral approximately half of the time. They may be removed to avoid the risk of aspiration. White epithelial cysts on the palate known as Epstein pearls are present in many babies, and similar lesions may be seen along the gums. Clefts of the palate may be obvious to the eye or only found by palpation (submucosal cleft). This latter abnormality may be accompanied by a bifid uvula.

Face

One should be careful during the examination not to focus too much on specific problems, but to consider the overall picture. Take a moment, step back, and just observe the baby to ensure that, as the saying goes, you don't "miss the forest for the trees." Is there anything that just looks unusual?

Neck, Lymph Nodes, and Clavicles

The neck of the newborn is relatively short. Redundant skin along the posterolateral line (webbing) is seen in approximately one-half of girls with Turner syndrome (karyotype 45 X,0), whereas the neck of the infant with trisomy 21 is notable for excess skin concentrated at the base of the neck posteriorly. A variety of branchial cleft remnants are manifested by pits, tags, and cysts. The most common neck mass is a lymphangioma (cystic hygroma), which is a multiloculated cyst composed of dilated lymphatics. Occasionally containing a hemangiomatous component, these are usually posterior to the sternocleidomastoid muscle with potential extension into the scapulae and thoracic and axillary compartments. The anterior neck should be evaluated for a midline trachea, thyromegaly, and thyroglossal duct cysts. Lymph nodes are sometimes palpable in the cervical area in healthy newborns, but congenital infections can also result in lymphadenopathy. Palpable supraclavicular lymph nodes are never normal. The clavicles are palpated for their presence or absence (cleidocranial dysostosis) and the presence of fractures, which typically manifest as asymmetrical arm movements, tenderness, and crepitus.

Respiratory System and Chest

The most important part of the respiratory system examination is performed while simply observing the infant breathe. If the infant has respiratory distress, the stethoscope is used to assess the quality and equality of breath sounds. Alveolar pathology (atelectasis, pneumonia) may be suggested by the presence of inspiratory crackles, whereas crepitant sounds heard both in inspiration and expiration are usually the result of airway secretions. Asymmetric breath sounds, with much more air entry on one side of the chest as opposed to the other, may suggest a pneumothorax. Bowel sounds may be heard in the chest if the infant has a congenital diaphragmatic hernia.

The chest is evaluated for size, symmetry, bony structure, musculature, and position of the nipples. The thorax may be malformed or small in a variety of neuromuscular disorders, osteochondrodysplasias, and processes associated with pulmonary hypoplasia. The presence of pectus excavatum (funnel chest) and carinatum (pigeon breast) can be of considerable concern to the family, and both can be associated with Marfan, Noonan, and other syndromes. Palpable pectoralis major muscle tissue in the axillae assures the presence of the muscle, the absence of which is suggestive of Poland syndrome. Supernumerary nipples, found inferomedial to the true breasts, are seen in approximately 1% of the general population, with a higher incidence in African Americans. Breast hypertrophy, at times asymmetrical, can be seen in both male and female infants in response to maternal hormones and may be accompanied by the secretion of a thin, white, milky fluid for a few days to weeks. Erythema and tenderness of the breasts warrant further evaluation.

Cardiac System

The goal of the cardiac examination generally falls into one of two categories: (1) assess the rate, rhythm, and heart sounds in an asymptomatic neonate; or (2) to evaluate the heart in an unwell infant as the possible source of illness.

The normal resting heart rate of the term newborn is between 100 and 160 beats per minute, with occasional brief fluctuations above and below these values. The premature infant's baseline heart rate tends to be slightly higher. Persistent bradycardia or tachycardia can be an indication of primary cardiac or, more commonly, other systemic processes.

Examination of the cardiovascular system begins with an assessment of general appearance, color, perfusion, and respiratory status. The presence of congenital anomalies increases the likelihood of associated congenital heart defects. Central cyanosis accompanied by a comfortable respiratory effort is suggestive of a structural heart defect with diminished pulmonary blood flow (such as pulmonary atresia). Because of relative hypertrophy of the right ventricle, the point of maximal impulse (PMI) of the newborn is found just to the left of the lower sternal border. In the term newborn, the precordial impulse is visible during the first few hours of life but generally disappears by 6 hours of age. Because of the lack of subcutaneous tissue in the preterm and growth-restricted newborn, the PMI may be visible for a somewhat longer time. Abnormal persistence of the visible or easily palpated PMI is seen in transposition of the great vessels and structural defects characterized by right-sided volume overload. The femoral pulses should be evaluated by palpation. The femoral pulses are diminished in coarctation of the aorta, but may initially be palpable if blood flow is maintained by right-to-left shunting across the ductus arteriosus.

Auscultation should begin with a warmed stethoscope. Identifying abnormal heart sounds is made difficult by the rapid heart rate in the neonatal period. The first heart sound is typically single and is accentuated at birth and in conditions in which there is increased flow across an atrioventricular valve. The second heart sound is best heard at the upper left sternal border. In most infants, the second heart sound (S_2) is split, although this can be difficult to appreciate because of the high heart rate. The presence of a normally split S_2 is an important physical finding. The absence of a split S_2 can indicate the presence of a single ventricular valve (aortic atresia, pulmonary atresia, and truncus arteriosus) and transposition of the great vessels (as a result of the orientation of the valves). Widely split S_2 is seldom indicative of increased pulmonary blood flow (atrial septal defect) in neonates, but it can be heard in total anomalous venous return and lesions characterized by an abnormal pulmonary valve. A narrowly split, accentuated S_2 is characteristic of persistent pulmonary hypertension of the newborn.

The absence of a heart murmur does not eliminate the possibility of important structural heart defects, and classic murmurs ascribed to specific lesions in older children may not be present in the neonate. Even though some infants may have a heart murmur noted during their first week of life, most of these murmurs are related to ongoing circulatory adaptation to an extrauterine environment, and they are transient and inconsequential. Innocent murmurs are soft, systolic, and at the left sternal edge or pulmonary area, and the infant is well and examination is otherwise normal. The murmur of pulmonary artery branch stenosis is best heard in the pulmonary area, is a systolic flow murmur best heard in the pulmonary area, and radiates to the axilla and back, and it resolves in a few weeks. The most concerning murmurs are those that arise from congenital heart disease, especially ductal-dependent lesions that may result in circulatory failure or cyanosis when the ductus arteriosus closes. Harsh grade 2 or 3 murmurs in the first hours of life (ventricular outflow tract obstruction), pansystolic (atrioventricular valve insufficiency), and continuous (absent pulmonary valve, valvular regurgitation) murmurs require more extensive evaluation with echocardiography. Finally, the disappearance of a previously noted murmur in a baby who is clinically deteriorating should make one suspect the closure of the ductus arteriosus with a ductal-dependent lesion (coarctation of the aorta, tricuspid atresia, or pulmonary atresia).

If a murmur is heard, the cardiac system is carefully evaluated. A chest x-ray and electrocardiogram may provide clues to the diagnosis, but the definitive diagnosis is by echocardiography. Pulse oximetry should be done to assess arterial oxygenation. If there are features of an innocent flow murmur, the infant should be assessed within a few days to check that the murmur has disappeared. The parents should be informed of the clinical signs of heart failure (sweating or cyanosis with feeds, slow-feeding tachypnea at rest or with feeds) for which they should seek medical attention. If the murmur persists or has pathologic features, or if the infant becomes unwell, referral to a pediatric cardiologist and echocardiography are indicated.

EDITORIAL COMMENT: Routine pulse oximetry screening for the detection of critical cyanotic congenital heart disease has been very successful, not only in the earlier detection of these cardiac anomalies but also for identifying respiratory disorders. The net effect has been to reduce mortality from these disorders by earlier recognition and intervention (see Chapter 14).

Blood pressure is not measured routinely, but it is performed in infants who are unwell or preterm and require admission to a neonatal unit. If the femoral pulses are diminished and coarctation of the aorta is suspected, blood pressure is measured in the arms and legs. Blood pressure in the legs is normally the same or slightly higher than that found in the arms, but is markedly reduced if coarctation of the aorta is present. Normal systemic blood pressure varies with postnatal and gestational age (see Appendix C for tables of normal blood pressure).

Abdomen

Patience and warm hands are the keys to a successful abdominal examination. In most infants, inspection reveals a rounded abdomen. A flat or scaphoid abdomen may be observed in the presence of a congenital diaphragmatic hernia. A full upper abdomen in the presence of a flattened lower abdomen suggests a proximal bowel obstruction. Distention is usually apparent at birth when there are massive ascites, meconium ileus or peritonitis, or intrauterine midgut volvulus. Clearly visible intestinal loops are not normal in the term infant, but the thin abdominal wall of the extremely premature baby may result in easily observed loops and peristalsis. Abdominal wall defects (omphalocele and gastroschisis) are usually readily apparent, and these require urgent surgical evaluation and intervention. Bowel sounds are nearly always present, and their absence is a concerning finding.

Palpation of the abdomen is facilitated by having the infant's legs in a flexed position. Palpation should begin in the lower abdomen, with the hand allowed to rest there until the infant relaxes. The kidneys are normally palpable bilaterally if the infant is very relaxed. Enlargement of the kidneys caused by hydronephrosis or cystic kidney disease is the most common abdominal mass found in the newborn. The liver is usually palpable 1 to 3 cm below the right costal margin, and the left lobe extends across the midline. The liver should be smooth, and its edge should be soft and thin. It may be enlarged in cases of cardiac failure, congenital infections, extramedullary hematopoiesis, tumors, and a variety of inborn errors of metabolism. The spleen is less frequently palpable than the liver and should be considered abnormally large if palpable more than 1 cm below the left costal margin.

The umbilical cord normally has two umbilical arteries and one umbilical vein. A single umbilical artery is a soft marker for chromosomal abnormalities, but in an otherwise normal newborn, a single umbilical artery is associated with an increased risk of renal malformation.[64] Infants with limited fetal activity as a result of congenital neuromuscular disorders, including trisomy 21, often have relatively short umbilical cords, which the obstetrician may note at the delivery.

Genitalia

The appearance of the genitalia is certainly one of the first, if not the first, areas of interest to the parents. If there is a disorder of sexual differentiation, assignment of the infant's gender should never be made until a detailed assessment has been performed by an experienced multidisciplinary team, including, but not limited to, neonatology, genetics, endocrinology, and urology, and a karyotype should be done urgently.

Male. The penile size, position of the meatus, appearance of the scrotum, and position of the testes must all be assessed. The penis of a term infant stretched along its length until resistance is met should be at least 2.5 cm long. It is not necessary, and potentially painful and damaging, to retract the foreskin over the glans penis to determine the placement of the meatus. Hypospadias, a meatal opening on the ventral surface of the penis, is relatively common and is readily apparent on inspection. Far less common is an epispadias, in which the meatus is present on the dorsal surface of the penis. This is usually not an isolated defect, more often being associated with exstrophy of the bladder. If an infant has hypospadias or epispadias, an infant should not have a routine circumcision in the newborn period, and merits an evaluation by a urologist. At the tip of the foreskin may be found a 1-mm-diameter pearly white sebaceous cyst, which is of no clinical significance. The testes should be palpable in the scrotum of the term infant. In approximately 2% to 4% of term infants, either one or both testes have not descended, but in three-fourths of these infants, the testes have descended at 3 months of age. Premature infants are far more likely to have an undescended testis at birth than the term infant. A hydrocele can usually be distinguished from a hernia by a combination of palpation and transillumination.

Female. The external female genitalia changes in appearance with advancing gestational age. The premature female infant has a prominent clitoris and labia minora, whereas in the term infant the labia majora completely covers these structures. The prominence of the clitoris in the premature infant is a result of this structure being fully developed by 27 weeks' gestation but there being very little adipose tissue in the labia majora until later in gestation. In the term female, outpouching of the vaginal mucosa (vaginal skin tags) is often seen at the posterior aspect of vaginal opening. Vaginal skin tags are inconsequential and regress within a few weeks. A newborn female infant may have a small amount of vaginal discharge, which may be mucous or even bloody, and occurs in response to maternal hormones. The passage of large amounts of blood, or clots, is not normal. The hymen has some opening in the majority of females. A completely imperforate hymen may result in the development of hydrometrocolpos. This is usually characterized by the bulging hymen, which is particularly prominent with crying. Virilization of the female infant consists of varying degrees of clitoral hypertrophy and labioscrotal fusion. A mass in the labia or groin may be a hernia, but consideration must be given to the possibility of an ectopic gonad, which may be either an ovary or a testis.

Anus

The presence, patency, and location of the anus should be noted. An imperforate anus will require surgery, but should also bring to mind the possibility of other associated anomalies, in particular VACTERL association—*v*ertebral defects, *a*nal defects, *c*ardiac defects, *t*racheoesophageal atresia, *r*enal defects, *l*imbs defects.

Hips

Examination of the hips of the neonate is performed on all infants to detect developmental dysplasia of the hip. This disorder is more common in females, if there is a family history, infants with underlying neurologic abnormalities, and those presenting in the breech position. The infant must be relaxed, because crying or kicking results in tightening of the muscles around the hip. There may be asymmetry of skinfolds around the hip and shortening of the affected leg. It should be possible to abduct both hips; full abduction may not be possible if the hip is dislocated. The Barlow maneuver is performed to check if the hip is dislocatable posteriorly by adducting a flexed hip with gentle posterior force to push the femoral head posteriorly out of the acetabulum. The Ortolani maneuver checks if a dislocated hip can be relocated into the acetabulum by abducting a flexed hip with gentle anterior leverage of the femur. If the examination is abnormal, a hip ultrasound and orthopedic consultation should be arranged. The American Academy of Pediatrics does not recommend routine ultrasound screening of all infants, but only for female infants born in the breech position and optional hip ultrasound for boys born in the breech position or girls with a positive family history.[65] Although screening leads to earlier identification, 60% to 80% of the hips identified as abnormal by physical examination and more than 90% of those identified by ultrasound resolve spontaneously. Avascular necrosis of the hip is reported in up to 60% of treated children, and no screening method has been shown to reduce the need for operation for the disorder.[66]

The Extremities

Careful inspection of the extremities alone usually determines whether the extremities are well formed. Joint contractures, asymmetries, or dislocations should be noted. Erb palsy, which may result from brachial plexus injury during the delivery process, is manifested by an arm that is extended alongside the body with internal rotation and demonstrates limited movement. The humerus and femur are the second and third most commonly fractured bones at delivery. Abnormalities of the digits (shortening, tapering, syndactyly, polydactyly), single palmar creases, and nail hypoplasia can be important clues to dysmorphic syndromes. Variations caused by intrauterine positioning are seen and need to be differentiated from true equinovarus deformities. Positional deformities of the foot can usually be distinguished by the presence of a normal range of motion and ability to establish a normal position and appearance of the foot with gentle pressure, as opposed to club foot, which cannot easily be straightened by applying gentle pressure.

The Back

The back is examined for the presence of abnormal curvatures and evidence of an abnormality overlying the spine. The presence of a tuft of hair, a subcutaneous lipoma, sinus, hemangioma, dimples separate from the gluteal crease, aplasia cutis, or skin tag should raise suspicion regarding the possibility of an underlying occult spinal dysraphism. If these abnormalities are found, an ultrasound examination of the involved area of the spine should be undertaken. A structural aberration of the spine requires neurosurgical evaluation, and possibly intervention.

Concluding the Physical Examination

After completion of the examination, any abnormalities or potential problems should be explained to the parents. Parents should be provided with the opportunity to inquire about any concerns they have about their baby. This time also provides an opportunity to inquire about difficulties with feeding, provide anticipatory guidance, and ensure appropriate pediatric care has been established. It is also a good time to discuss immunization, universal neonatal biochemical screening, hearing screening, and advice about safe sleep practices.

CASE 4.1

A male infant is born at 40 weeks' gestation with a birth weight of 2200 g, length of 46 cm, and head circumference of 32 cm. The physical examination is remarkable for short palpebral fissures, a small jaw, a smooth philtrum, and thin upper lip.

What is this combination of features most consistent with?

A. Trisomy 21.
B. Fetal alcohol syndrome (FAS).
C. Congenital cytomegalovirus infection.
D. Beckwith-Wiedemann syndrome.

This constellation of findings is most suggestive of (B), FAS. Trisomy 21, FAS, and congenital cytomegalovirus (CMV) infection may be associated with growth restriction, which is often "symmetrical." Beckwith-Wiedemann syndrome, in contrast, is typically associated with macrosomia. Other physical findings suggestive of FAS include ptosis of the eyelids, short nose, small distal phalanges, and small fifth fingernails. Long-term prognosis for these children is somewhat guarded, with the majority being developmentally delayed, often to a severe degree.

CASE 4.2

You are called to attend the delivery of male infant at an uncertain gestational age, who is to be delivered by emergency cesarean section because of nonreassuring fetal heart rate tracing, with fetal heart rate decelerations occurring following the peak of uterine contractions. The fetal membranes are intact. The estimated fetal weight (determined by ultrasound during labor) is 2 kg. The mother is a 15-year-old primigravid woman whose pregnancy was notable for smoking, a weight gain of 12 pounds, and infrequent visits to the clinic for prenatal care. She was admitted to the labor and delivery service in active labor, at which time she was found to have a blood pressure of 160/110 and proteinuria. She was subsequently given magnesium sulfate for preeclampsia for several hours before the delivery.

What problems do you anticipate that you will need to address in the delivery room, and what measures will you take to be prepared?

This is a complicated but not uncommon scenario. With a lack of regular obstetrical care, the gestational age of the baby is uncertain. The baby may be preterm or term. In either case, the infant care center must be warm, and towels for drying the baby must be available. If the infant is at term, he appears to be growth restricted and has shown evidence of not tolerating the stress of labor. The necessary supplies for airway management and suctioning must be present in the area. If the infant is preterm, meconium passage and aspiration are less likely, but respiratory distress related to prematurity remains a possibility.

At delivery, there was no meconium, and the baby needed only towel drying, clearing of the airway, and a brief period of supplemental oxygen for resuscitation. In the delivery room, the following are noted: bilaterally descended testes, stiff ear cartilage, scant vernix caseosa, well-developed areolae but poor breast tissue development, and decreased muscle tone. The baby's weight is 1800 g, length is 48 cm, and head circumference is 32 cm. There are no obvious anomalies on the initial examination, and the examination of the abdomen, heart, and lungs is normal.

What is your assessment of his gestational age and his classification?

This baby is likely a term, small-for-gestational age (SGA) infant. The findings of the descended testes, stiff ear cartilage, lack of vernix, and well-developed areolae support this contention. The decreased muscle tone may be related to exposure to magnesium. A complete New Ballard examination should be carried out during the first 24 hours to confirm the gestational age.

What problems will you anticipate for this infant in the next 24 to 48 hours?

As a term infant who is SGA, he is at risk for thermoregulation difficulties, hypoglycemia, polycythemia, and possibly hypocalcemia.

Why is this baby so small?

This infant had several risk factors for IUGR/SGA: teenage mother, poor maternal weight gain during pregnancy, smoking, and preeclampsia. How far to pursue further evaluation for other etiologies (chromosomal abnormalities, congenital infections) will vary among clinicians, but in the absence of other clinical abnormalities, the yield from further investigations is very low.

CASE 4.3

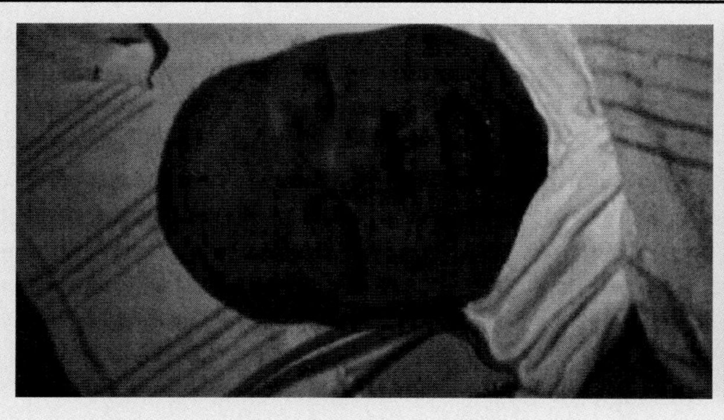

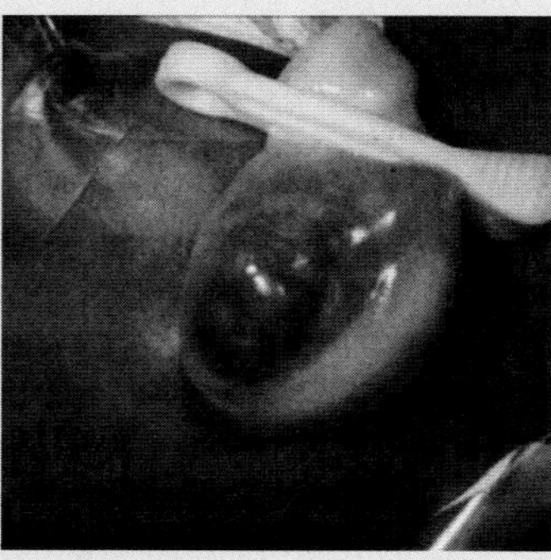

This is a large-for-gestational-age infant with a protuberant tongue and omphalocele. The infant is jittery. What is the most likely cause of the jitteriness, what is the mechanism for that, and what is the genetic abnormality in infants with this syndrome?

This infant has Beckwith–Wiedemann syndrome. The main features of Beckwith–Wiedemann syndrome are:

- macroglossia (large tongue)
- macrosomia (above average birth weight and length)
- sometimes hemihypertrophy
- microcephaly
- midline abdominal wall defects (omphalocele/exomphalos, umbilical hernia, diastasis recti)
- ear creases or ear pits
- neonatal hypoglycemia
- hepatoblastoma

The most likely etiology for jitteriness in an infant with Beckwith-Wiedemann syndrome is hypoglycemia.

1. What are the ear anomalies in Beckwith–Wiedemann syndrome?
2. What is the pathogenesis of the hypoglycemia in these infants?
3. What chromosomal anomaly is found in 20% of affected infants?

Beckwith–Wiedemann syndrome is an overgrowth disorder usually present at birth, characterized by an increased risk of childhood cancer (especially hepatoblastoma and Wilm tumor) and certain congenital physical features.

CASE STUDY 4.3—cont'd

What are the ear anomalies in Beckwith–Wiedemann syndrome? Pits and clefts

What is the pathogenesis of the hypoglycemia in these infants? Hyperinsulinism

What chromosomal anomaly is found in 20% of affected infants? Uniparental disomy (UPD) 11P15.5

Uniparental Disomy

UPD occurs when an individual receives two copies of a chromosome, or part of a chromosome, from one parent and no copies from the other parent. Examples include:

- Prader Willi syndrome
- Angelman syndrome—chromosome 15
- Beckwith–Wiedemann syndrome—chromosome 14
- neonatal diabetes—chromosome 9

5

Nutrition and Selected Disorders of the Gastrointestinal Tract

PART 1: NUTRITION FOR THE HIGH-RISK INFANT

David H. Adamkin, Paula G. Radmacher

KEY POINTS

1. Begin intravenous amino acids in the first hours of life.
2. Consider using lipid emulsions early with long-chain polyunsaturated fatty acids (LCPUFA) (especially docosahexaenoic acid [DHA], arachidonic acid [ARA], and eicosapentaenoic acid [EPA]) to prevent omega 3 deficiencies.
3. Prioritize the use of human milk. If mother's own milk is unavailable, use donor milk.
4. Human milk should be fortified early so that protein intake is not compromised during the transition from parenteral to enteral nutrition.
5. Early malnutrition may have serious long-term consequences.

INTRODUCTION

The goal of nutritional support for the high-risk infant is to provide sufficient nutrients postnatally to ensure continuation of growth at rates similar to those observed in utero. The preterm infant presents a particular challenge in that the nutritional intake must be sufficient to both replenish tissue losses and permit tissue accretion. However, during the early days after birth, acute illnesses such as respiratory distress and patent ductus arteriosus with fluid restriction preclude maximal nutritional support. Functional immaturity of the renal, gastrointestinal (GI), and metabolic systems limits optimal nutrient delivery. Substrate intolerances are common, limiting the nutrients available for tissue maintenance and growth.

During the last trimester of pregnancy, nutrient stores are established in preparation for birth at 40 weeks' gestation. Fat and glycogen are stored to provide ready energy during times of caloric deficit. Iron reserves accumulate to prevent iron-deficiency anemia during the first 4 to 6 months of life. Calcium and phosphorus are deposited in the soft bones to begin mineralization, which continues through early adult life. However, the infants who are delivered before term have minimal nutrient stores and higher nutrient requirements per kilogram than their term-born counterparts.

Infants weighing less than 1.5 kg have a body composition of approximately 85% to 95% water, 9% to 10% protein, and 0.1% to 5% fat. The fat is primarily structural with only negligible amounts of subcutaneous fat; hepatic glycogen stores are virtually nonexistent. The growth of these infants lags considerably after birth.[1] Such infants, especially those less than 1000 g birth weight (extremely low birth weight [ELBW]), historically did not regain birth weight until 2 to 3 weeks of age. The growth of most less than 1500 g (very low-birth-weight [VLBW]) infants proceeds at a slower rate than in utero, often by a large margin.[1] Although many of the smallest VLBW infants are also born small for gestational age (less than the 10th percentile [SGA]), both appropriate for gestational age (AGA), VLBW, and SGA infants develop extrauterine growth restriction (EUGR). Fig. 5.1 from the National Institute of Child Health and Human Development (NICHD) Neonatal Research Network demonstrates the differences between normal intrauterine growth and the observed rates of postnatal growth in the NICHD study.[1] These postnatal growth curves are shifted to the right of the reference curve in each gestational age category. This "growth faltering" is common in ELBW infants. It has been over 20 years since the publication of this data and, despite newer strategies, EUGR or postnatal growth failure (PGF) persists. Epidemiologic data from across the United States demonstrate that in 2013, over half of VLBW infants left the neonatal intensive care unit with a weight below the 10th percentile for gestational age.[2]

In 1998, the American Academy of Pediatrics (AAP) Committee on the Fetus and Newborn stated that the goal of nutrition of these VLBW infants is to achieve a postnatal growth rate approximating that of the normal fetus of the same gestational age. Although reaffirmed by the AAP and other neonatal and pediatric organizations worldwide, this goal continues to be elusive. Many questions remain: Is this the best approach? If it is the best approach, how can it be safely achieved? And how can it be supported by measurable outcomes?

Nutrient intakes received by VLBW infants are much lower than what the fetus receives in utero—an intake deficit that persists throughout much of the infants' stay in the hospital and even after discharge.[2] Although nonnutritional factors (comorbidities) contribute to the slower growth of VLBW infants, suboptimal nutrient intakes are critical in explaining their poor growth outcomes. Considerable evidence exists that early growth deficits, which reflect inadequate

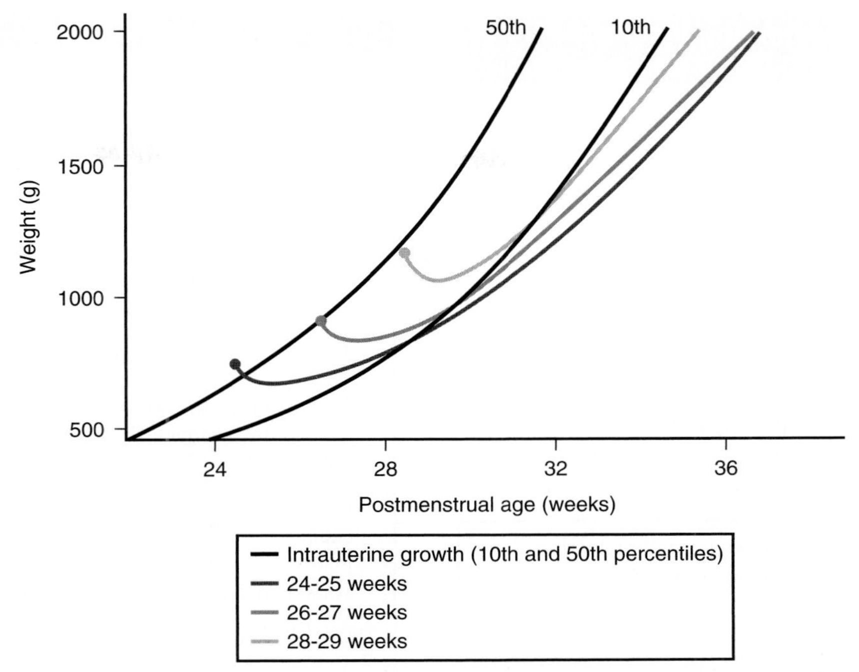

Fig. 5.1 Postnatal shifts in weight percentiles (10th and 50th) compared with in utero growth curves.[1]

nutrition, have long-lasting effects, including short stature and poor neurodevelopmental outcomes. Therefore another frequently occurring morbidity seen in VLBW infants is neurodevelopmental impairment. These infants demonstrate difficulties across a wide range of domains, including cognitive, motor, language, and behavioral functioning.[3,4] Links between neurodevelopmental impairment and early nutrition are well established[5] and are explained by the sensitivity of the developing brain to nutrition.[6]

In a 2016 commentary on growth failure, Hay and Ziegler state, "The significance of growth failure is that it puts all these infants at risk for neurodevelopmental impairment. Growth failure is, however, preventable and so is neurodevelopmental impairment, as both are attributed to inadequate nutrition."[7] Undernutrition is, by definition, nonphysiologic and undesirable. Any measure that diminishes it is inherently good, providing safety is not compromised. Avoiding inadequate nutrition must be a priority. This chapter will provide guidance on steps to prevent growth failure and thereby reduce the risk of developmental impairment. For growth failure to occur, nutrient intakes must be inadequate for more than just a few days. The nutrient that is virtually always limiting for growth is protein, whereas energy tends to be provided in amounts that cover at least basic needs, but often to excess.[7–9] First, we will review the fluid and electrolyte challenges in managing these VLBW infants and then specifically address nutritional support.

FLUID

In the fetus at 24 weeks' gestation, the total body water (TBW) represents more than 90% of the total body weight, with approximately 65% in the extracellular compartment, 25% in the intracellular compartment, and 1% in fat stores. The TBW and extracellular fluid volumes decrease as gestational age increases. By term, the infant's TBW represents 75% of total body weight, with extracellular and intracellular compartments comprising 40% and 35%, respectively.

Compared with the full-term infant, the preterm infant is in a state of relative extracellular fluid volume expansion with an excess of TBW. The dilute urine and negative sodium balance observed during the first few days after birth in the preterm infant may constitute an appropriate adaptive response to extrauterine life. Therefore the initial diuresis should be regarded as physiologic, reflecting changes in interstitial fluid volume. This should be included in the calculation of daily fluid needs. As a result, a gradual weight loss of 10% to 15% in a VLBW infant and 5% to 10% in a larger baby during the first week of life is to be expected without adversely affecting urine output, urine osmolality, or clinical status. Provision of large volumes of fluid (160–180 mL/kg/day) to prevent this weight loss appears to increase the risk of the development of patent ductus arteriosus, cerebral intraventricular hemorrhage, bronchopulmonary dysplasia (BPD), and necrotizing enterocolitis (NEC). Therefore a careful approach to fluid management is currently appropriate. It appears that the preterm infant can adjust water excretion within a relatively broad range of fluid intake (65–70 mL/kg/day to 140 mL/kg/day) without disturbing renal concentrating abilities or electrolyte balance.

Estimation of daily fluid requirements includes insensible water losses (IWL) from the respiratory tract and skin, GI losses (emesis, ostomy output, and diarrhea), urinary losses, and losses from drainage catheters (chest tubes). IWL is a passive process and is not regulated by the infant. However, the environmental conditions in which the infant is nursed should be controlled to minimize losses (Box 5.1).

The transepithelial losses are dependent on gestational age, the thickness of the skin and stratum corneum, and blood flow to the skin. The preterm infant has a high body surface

BOX 5.1 Factors Affecting Insensible Water Loss in Preterm Neonates

- Severe prematurity
- Open warmer bed
- Forced convection
- Phototherapy
- Hyperthermia
- Tachypnea

area-to-body weight ratio, with thinner, more permeable skin that is highly vascularized. These factors increase heat and fluid losses. In addition, the use of open bed platforms with radiant warmers as well as phototherapy lights may increase the IWL by more than 50%. This excessive IWL may be reduced with the use of humidified incubators to care for the infant.[10]

EDITORIAL COMMENT: Although phototherapy has long been included in the causes of increased insensible water loss, with the use of LED phototherapy units, it is unlikely that this is still a significant factor.

The measurement of urine specific gravity is commonly used to predict urine osmolality. Although this is a reliable means of predicting hyperosmolality (urine osmolality >290 mOsm/kg water with a urine specific gravity ≥1.012), its reliability in predicting hypo-osmolality (urine osmolality <270 mOsm/kg water with a urine specific gravity ≤1.008) is variable, ranging from 71% to 95% accuracy. Accuracy is even lower in predicting iso-osmolality (urine osmolality of 270–290 mOsm/kg water with a urine specific gravity of 1.008–1.012). In addition, glucose and protein in the urine may increase the urine specific gravity, giving a falsely high estimate of urine osmolality. Therefore urine specific gravity should be checked only to rule out hyperosmolar urine. A test for sugars and proteins in the urine should be conducted at the same time. The maximal concentrating capabilities in the neonate are limited compared with those in adults. Thus an infant with a urine osmolality of approximately 700 mOsm/kg water (urine specific gravity of 1.019) may be dehydrated. One can estimate the urine osmolality by determining the potential renal solute load of the infant's feeding and the fluid intake (Box 5.2). The infants at risk for high urine osmolality are those who are receiving a concentrated formula and those whose fluid intake is restricted.

Water balance may be maintained with careful attention to input and output. Infants should be weighed nude and at approximately the same time of day. During the first week of life, VLBW infants should be weighed daily; ELBW infants should be weighed twice daily. Meticulous records of fluid intake (with the use of accurate infusion pumps and careful measurement of enteral feedings) and output (by weighing diapers and collecting urine, ostomy output, and drainage from any indwelling catheters) are necessary to compute fluid requirements. Serum glucose, electrolytes, blood urea nitrogen (BUN), and creatinine may be monitored two times per day during the first 2 days in critically ill ELBW infants and then daily or as needed thereafter. Urine glucose is routinely tested, and urine specific gravity is measured as necessary.

BOX 5.2 Renal Solute Load Calculation

Potential renal solute load (PRSL):
4 × (g protein/L) + mEq sodium/L + mEq potassium/L + mEq chloride/L = PRSL (mOsm/L)

Example:
Preterm formula$_{24}$ (PT_{24}) contains:

22 g protein/L × 4	= 88.0
15.2 mEq sodium/L × 1	= 15.2
26.9 mEq potassium/L × 1	= 26.9
18.6 mEq chloride/L × 1	= 18.6
	PRSL = 148.7 mOsm/L

Baby A is a 2-week-old former 32 week AGA infant weighing 1400 g now receiving 150 mL/kg/d of PT_{24}

Estimated fluid losses are:

Stool	10 mL/kg/d
Insensible water loss	70 mL/kg/d
Total fluid loss	80 mL/kg/d

150 mL/kg/d intake – 80 mL/kg/d output = 70 mL/kg/d available for urine output

The PRSL of PT_{24} is 148.7 mOsm/L:

$$\frac{148.7\text{ mOsm}}{1000\text{ mL}} \times \frac{X\text{ mOsm}}{150\text{ mL}}$$

X = 22.3 mOsm/L

This infant has 70 mL/kg/d to excrete 22.3 mOsm of PRSL.

$$\frac{22.3\text{ mOsm}}{70\text{ mL}} \times 1000 = X\text{ mOsm/L}$$

X = 318.6 mOsm/L

Therefore, the estimated osmolality of the urine is 319 mOsm/L.

AGA, Appropriate for gestational age.

Senterre and Rigo showed that optimizing nutritional support based on nutritional recommendations profoundly affected postnatal weight loss, limiting that loss to day 3 in the majority and dramatically reducing PGF.[11] This was a prospective, nonrandomized, observational study in 120 consecutive infants less than 1250 g over 2 years. First-day nutritional intake was 38 ± 6 kcal/kg/day with 2.4 g/kg/day of protein. Mean intake during the first week of life was 80 ± 14 kcal/kg/day with 3.2 g/kg/day of protein.[11] On average from birth to discharge, 122 ± 10 kcal/kg/day and 3.7 g/kg/day of protein were administered. Postnatal weight loss was limited to the first 3 days of life, and birth weight was regained after a mean of 7 days. Catch-up growth occurred after the second week in all groups of VLBW infants.[11] This study confirmed that the first week of life is a critical period to promote growth and that early nutrition from the first day of life is essential. Postnatal weight loss may be limited, and subsequent growth may be optimized with a dramatic reduction in PGF.[11]

ELECTROLYTES

Sodium is required in quantities sufficient to maintain normal extracellular fluid volume expansion, which accompanies tissue growth. In animal studies, if insufficient amounts are provided, the extracellular fluid volume expansion is suppressed, and there are subsequent alterations in quantitative and qualitative somatic growth.

Catheter flushes (using isotonic saline solution) may contribute significant quantities of electrolytes, including chloride, to the infant's total intake. Hyperchloremic metabolic acidosis in LBW infants has been associated with chloride loads greater than 6 mEq/kg/day. The intake can easily be decreased by substituting acetate or phosphate for chloride in the intravenous (IV) solution.

Hypochloremia has also been associated with poor growth. Supplementation with chloride to normalize serum chloride concentrations in infants with BPD resulted in improved growth. Hypochloremia has been noted in infants with BPD who did not survive. However, whether this is a predictor of poor outcome or a symptom of severe illness remains to be resolved.

EDITORIAL COMMENT: Sodium may be considered a growth hormone in preterm infants. In infants who are not thriving, paying careful attention to their serum sodium and supplementation may be in order.

Isemann et al tested the hypothesis that sodium supplementation in early preterm infants prevents late-onset hyponatremia and improves growth without increasing common morbidities during birth hospitalization. They performed a randomized controlled trial of 4 mEq/kg/d of sodium (intervention) versus sterile water (placebo) from days-of-life 7 to 35 in infants born at less than 32 weeks' corrected gestational age. The primary outcome was weight gain in the first 6 weeks of life.

Infants receiving the intervention had greater velocity of weight gain and fewer reports of serum sodium concentrations less than 135 mmol/L. The supplemented infants more closely followed and maintained fetal reference birth percentile for body weight compared with infants receiving placebo. There were no increases in comorbidities.

(Isemann B, Mueller EW, Narendran V, Akinbi H. Impact of early sodium supplementation on hyponatremia and growth in premature infants: a randomized controlled trial. *J Parenter Enteral Nutr.* 2016;40:342-349.)

Potassium chloride (2 mEq/kg/day) is added to the IV fluid within the first days of life as soon as urinary output is established and hyperkalemia is not present. The potassium dose may be adjusted depending on urine output and use of diuretics. However, it is often difficult to obtain accurate determinations of serum potassium, especially when the blood samples are from heel-sticks, which may lead to excessive red blood cell hemolysis and spuriously high serum potassium levels. If an elevated potassium concentration is obtained, a second blood sample from venipuncture should be obtained for confirmation of the level. If infused via a peripheral vein, concentrations of potassium chloride up to 40 mEq/L are usually tolerated and do not cause localized pain. However, if higher concentrations are needed because of fluid restriction, a central vein should be used. See Table 5.1 for characteristics of various intravenous fluids.

EDITORIAL COMMENT: The immature kidney has a diminished ability to reabsorb water and respond to mineralocorticoids, in addition to a high excretion of filtered sodium. Their renal function may be compromised by perinatal complications and the use of medications such as diuretics, indomethacin, and amphotericin B, which affects tubular function. All these factors contribute to sodium and potassium imbalances.

Although hyperkalemia is defined as a potassium greater than 6 mmol/L, treatment is unnecessary in preterm infants unless potassium is above 6.5 mmol/L. This is unusual.

Total Parenteral Nutrition

The early postnatal period for the preterm infant represents a critical developmental stage with significant nutritional needs. In fact, it can be viewed as a nutritional emergency.[12] Because these VLBW infants are unable to receive adequate nutrition enterally because of GI immaturity and critical illness, parenteral nutrition serves as a bridge. Over the past decade, clinicians have come to recognize the safety of and need for immediate provision of amino acids with the appropriate amount of energy to promote positive nitrogen balance and to minimize the protein deficit that would accumulate without it.[13,14] Consideration of the correct timing to add lipids as well as the best dose are less well understood. Inadequate nutritional support, especially over the first days to weeks of life, may set the stage for postnatal growth faltering, which may have implications for long-term neurodevelopmental outcomes.

Amino Acids

The fetus receives a continuous supply of amino acids via active transport by the placenta. Animal studies have shown that fetal amino acid uptake is higher than that needed solely for protein accretion.[15,16] When that supply of amino acids ends with preterm delivery, the infant immediately experiences a reduction in protein accretion that, unless addressed, will result in a significant deficit of protein by hospital discharge.[14] Early institution of parenteral nutrition with sufficient amino acid content to meet fetal growth requirements (2.0–4.0 g/kg/day)[7] is important to minimize such deficits, improve glucose tolerance,[17] avoid metabolic shock,[18] and prevent negative nitrogen balance.[19,20] Even the administration of as little as 1 g/kg/day of amino acids has been shown to eliminate negative nitrogen balance, whereas 3 g/kg/day leads to protein accretion.[21]

Numerous studies have shown the benefits of early amino acid administration in the VLBW infant.[17,22–25] In addition to preventing the catabolism of body protein, the provision of amino acids in the first administered fluids smooths the metabolic transition to extrauterine life. Early amino acids may stimulate insulin secretion and improve glucose tolerance. A study from Rivera et al[17] of early amino acid infusion in preterm infants showed that VLBW infants receiving early amino acids with glucose were able to receive more glucose (and consequently more energy) than infants receiving

TABLE 5.1 **Characteristics of Intravenous Fluids**

	CATIONS			ANIONS		
Type of fluid	**Na (mEq/L)**	**K (mEq/L)**	**Ca (mEq/L)**	**Cl (mEq/L)**	**HCO_3[a] (mEq/L)**	**Osmolarity (mOsm/L)[b]**
Dextrose in water						
D_5W						253
$D_{7.5}W$						378
$D_{10}W$						505
$D_{12.5}W$						939
$D_{15}W$						757
$D_{20}W$						1009
$D_{25}W$						1261
Dextrose in saline						
D_5W and 0.225% NaCl (¼ NS)	38.5			38.5		329
D_5W and 0.45% NaCl	77			77		406
D_5W and 0.9% NaCl	154			154		559
D_{10} and 0.225% NaCl	38.5			38.5		582
D_{10} and 0.45% NaCl	77			77		659
$D_{10}W$ and 0.9% NaCl	154			154		812
Saline solutions						
¼ NS (0.225% NaCl)	38.5			38.5		77
½ NS (0.45% NaCl)	77			77		154
NS (0.9% NaCl)	154			154		308
3% NaCl	513			513		1026
Multiple electrolyte solutions						
Ringer's solution	147	4	5	155		309
Lactated Ringer's solution	130	4	3	109	28	273
D_5W in Lactated Ringer's	130	4	3	109	28	524
Lipid emulsions						
20% only						258–315

For example:

$D_{10}W$ and 0.45% NaCl (½ NS)

$D_{10}W$ = (10 x 51)	= 510 mOsm/L
0.45% NaCl = (0.45 x 340)	= 153 mOsm/L
TOTAL	663 mOsm/L

$D_{10}W$ and 4% amino acids (no calcium or heparin)

$D_{10}W$ = (10 x 51)	= 510 mOsm/L
4% AA = (4 x 87.5)	= 350 mOsm/L
TOTAL	860 mOsm/L

An easy way to approximate the osmolarity of an intravenous fluid is to consider that for each 1% dextrose there are 51 mOsm/L; for each 1% amino acids there are 87.5 mOsm/L; and for each 1% NaCl there are 340 mOsm/L.

[a]Or its equivalent in lactate, acetate, or citrate.

[b]Osmolarity of the blood is 285–295 mOsm/L.

Modified from Wolf BM, Yamahata WI. Fluid, electrolyte, and acid-base balance. In Zeman FJ, ed. *Clinical Nutrition and Dietetics*. New York, NY: MacMillan; 1991:40-41.

glucose alone. Mahaveer et al[26] compared data from a clinical nutrition practice change (early initiation of amino acids at a higher dose) to historical experiences with glucose tolerance in infants less than 29 weeks. Cumulative protein intake (mean ± standard error of the mean) over the first 7 days was statistically higher in the change group (15.3 ± 0.4 g/kg vs. 11.8 ± 0.4). The proportion of infants that required insulin in the change group was half that of the historical group (26% vs. 53%). The mechanism for this finding is that hypoaminoacidemia leads to decreased insulin secretion and down-regulation of glucose transporters at the cell membrane, leading to a decrease in Na^+, K^+ ATPase activity, and intracellular energy failure.[27] Data from Radmacher et al[28] showed that in the first 5 days of life, ELBW infants receiving earlier and higher doses of amino acids (~3 g/kg/day) had lower glucose levels than those initiating amino acids at a lower dose. Glucose tolerance was enhanced with a higher dose of amino acids.

The predicted daily rate of protein accretion in a fetus at 70% of gestation (~28 weeks) is around 2 g/kg. Studies have shown that infusions of glucose alone without amino acids will actually lead to a loss of body protein that is inversely proportional to gestational age.[29–31] Fig. 5.2 compares the degree of protein loss in infants at gestational ages of 26 weeks, 32 weeks, and term when infused with glucose alone.[32] How this protein loss is manifest in the 26-week 1-kg infant is shown in Fig. 5.3. With body protein stores of around 88 g at birth and losses of around 1.5% each day

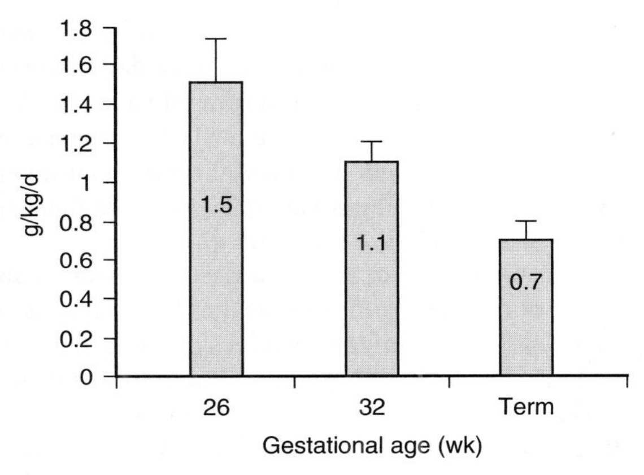

Fig. 5.2 Protein losses measured in three groups of infants receiving glucose alone at 2 to 3 days of age. Protein losses are calculated from measured rates of phenylalanine catabolism. (Modifed from Denne SC. Protein and energy requirements in preterm infants. *Semin Neonatal.* 2001;6:377.)

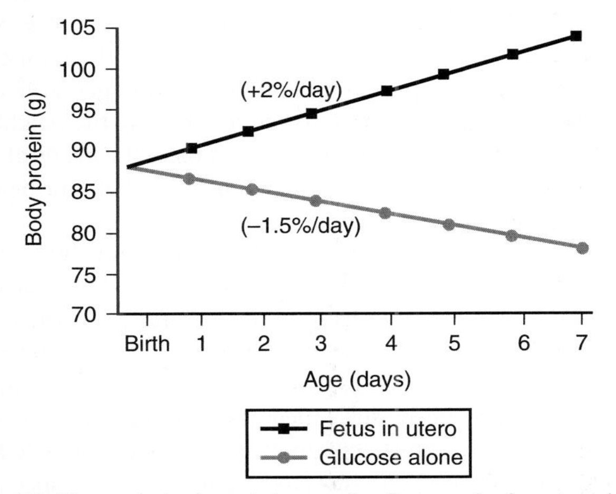

Fig. 5.3 Change in body protein over the first week of postnatal life for a theoretical 1000-g, 26 weeks' gestation infants provided with glucose alone versus protein accretion of the fetus in utero at the same gestational age. (Modifed from Denne SC. Protein and energy requirements in preterm infants. *Semin Neonatal.* 2001;6:377.)

without exogenous amino acids, this infant's body protein pool shrinks by more than 10% in the first week of life. The comparable fetus in utero would be increasing body protein by around 2% each day or up to 15% for the week. The provision of amino acids at a dose as little as 1 to 1.5 g/kg/day can meet losses, but higher doses are necessary for protein accretion.

Studies have shown that early amino acid administration in VLBW infants can improve protein balance, minimize protein deficits, and improve growth.[23,25,33] Initiating amino acids at doses of 2 to 3.5 g/kg/day within hours of birth has been shown to be safe.[17,24,34–36] In short-term toxicity studies, acid–base status in VLBW infants receiving early amino acids has not been negatively affected.[17,23–25,34,36] Studies have reported no rise in ammonia levels in infants receiving amino acids compared with those receiving glucose alone.[17]

Many clinicians follow BUN levels as an indicator of amino acid tolerance. Multiple investigators have reported that BUN concentrations do not correlate with the dose of intravenous amino acids.[28,37] Modest increases in BUN with no change in serum creatinine or other indicators of metabolic disturbance have been seen with early amino acid administration.[33] BUN reflects not only intake but also acuity of illness, renal function, hepatic synthesis, and hydration status. Thus a comprehensive evaluation of the infant, not a single blood test, is necessary to determine a need to reduce amino acid intake in an infant with an "elevated" BUN.[28,37]

Most amino acids formulations have not changed in over 25 years, and the optimal intake of individual parenteral amino acids for premature infants remains unknown. Pediatric amino acid solutions are more appropriate for the preterm infant than those designed for adults. However, the original safety data were compiled in the 1990s and may need to be revisited, as amino acid dosing was much lower, was usually initiated later, and did not include the higher doses being used today. Conditionally essential amino acids such as tyrosine, glutamine, and cysteine are unstable in current products and have been shown to be in low plasma concentrations in parenterally nourished infants.

Morgan et al[38] conducted a single-center randomized controlled trial to compare a standard neonatal parenteral nutrition plan to one with enhanced macronutrient content. The protocol was followed for up to the first 28 days of life as long as parenteral nutrition was required. Clinical care (fluid management, enteral nutrition introduction, and biochemical monitoring) for both groups was by unit protocol. Parenteral nutrition was discontinued when enteral intake exceeded 75%. Plasma profiles were analyzed for 20 specific amino acids. Among the conditionally essential amino acids, there was little difference between groups, despite the higher total amino acid intake in the enhanced group. The median plasma levels of glutamine, arginine, and cysteine were all below reference values.

Lipids

Preterm birth leads to early termination of placental delivery of fatty acids. This coincides with a period of rapid brain growth and significant lipid accretion in VLBW infants. Coupled with scarce amounts of adipose tissue, these infants are fully dependent on postnatal nutritional strategies to meet their needs during this period because they are not able to form sufficient quantities of needed long-chain polyunsaturated fatty acids (LCPUFA) from precursor fatty acids (Fig. 5.4). Intravenous lipid infusions serve as a source of LCPUFA, including the n-3 (linolenic LNA, 18:3n-3) and n-6 (linoleic LA, 18:2n-6) fatty acids, to prevent essential fatty acid deficiency (EFAD)[39] and be a source of energy as a partial replacement for glucose. However, soybean oil–based emulsions are devoid of other important LCPUFAs, such as docosahexaenoic acid (DHA, 22:6n-3), eicosapentaenoic acid (EPA, 20:n-5), and arachidonic acid (ARA, 20:4n-6). The proper balance of lipid classes is critical, especially for the developing brain and retina, where these fatty acids serve as structural components of lipid-based cell structures.[40,41] Soybean oil–based products, originally designed for use in adults, have been the most commonly used products in the United States, even in preterm infants. Recent research has shown the importance of providing a broader mix of LCPUFA to meet the needs of infants at critical windows of development.

Martin et al[42] have shown the rapid decrease in DHA and ARA levels in preterm infants in the first postnatal week. This rapid loss of structural lipids cannot be corrected with soybean oil–based products. Research from multiple groups in both animals and humans has shown that deficiencies in LCPUFAs may have roles to play in the development of such neonatal complications as chronic lung disease,[42] NEC,[43,44] and retinopathy of prematurity (ROP).[45]

When to start intravenous lipids is not universally agreed among clinicians, especially in critically ill VLBW infants with respiratory disease. Concerns related to potential adverse effects on gas exchange and bilirubin displacement from albumin because of increases in free fatty acids (FFA) have been raised. A number of studies have shown that with

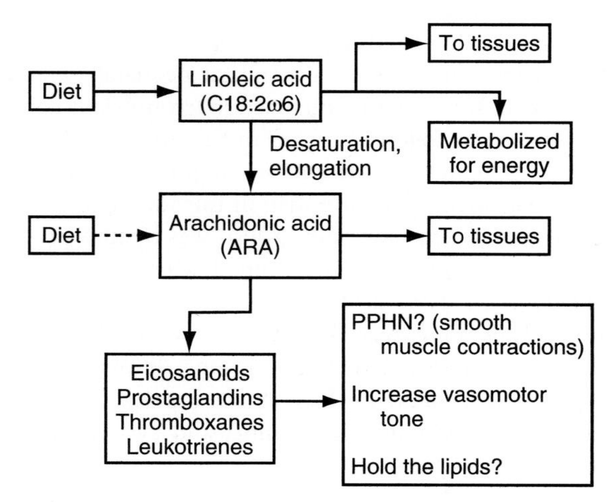

Fig. 5.4 Metabolic derivatives of linoleic acid and arachidonic acid. *ARA,* Arachidonic acid; *PPHN,* persistent pulmonary hypertension. (Modifed from Adamkin DH. Nutrition in very very low birth weight infants. *Clin Perinatol.* 1986;13(2):419-443.)

slow infusion rates over longer periods of time (up to 24 hours) and with careful monitoring of triglycerides, modest amounts of lipids can be infused in most infants, even in the first days of life, without adverse effects.[46–49] In vitro, the displacement of bilirubin from binding sites on serum albumin by the increased FFA depends on the relative concentrations of all three compounds and may occur even with adequate metabolism of infused lipid. Andrew et al[48] found no free bilirubin (B_f) generated in vivo if the molar FFA/albumin remained less than 6. Adamkin et al[47] also found acceptable FFA/albumin (<3) when lipids were infused over long periods (18–24 hours).

Amin et al conducted a prospective, nested study of bilirubin binding during intravenous lipid infusions in infants 24 to 33 weeks' gestational age.[50] Infants were stratified into two cohorts based on gestational age less than or equal to 28 or greater than 28 weeks. Intralipid 20% (IL; Fresenius Kabi, Uppsala, Sweden) was infused over 16 to 20 hours at a rate less than 0.15 g/kg/hour in increasing doses (0.5–3 g/kg/day) over the first 10 days of life. Triglycerides were monitored, and IL was held less than or equal to 2 g/kg/day in the presence of hyperbilirubinemia. Total serum bilirubin (TSB) and B_f were analyzed with each increase in IL; albumin was analyzed by the third postnatal day. The bilirubin/albumin equilibrium association binding constant (*K*) was calculated at IL intakes of 1.5, 2.0, 2.5, and 3.0 g/kg/day.

For infants greater than 28 weeks' gestational age, TSB, *K*, and B_f did not change significantly as the IL dose increased to 2.5 or 3.0 g/kg/day. For infants 28 weeks or lower, the median differences in B_f and *K* at 1 gm/kg/day were not statistically significant compared with that in the more mature infants. However, as the dose increased above 1.5 g/kg/day, *K* was significantly lower ($P < .01$), and B_f was significantly higher ($P < .05$) in the more immature infants. Although there are no data that define the intake of lipid at which clinically significant bilirubin displacement occurs, these results suggest there may be a maturational effect.

Concerns about adverse effects of intravenous lipid on pulmonary function have been raised but have not generally been found to be an issue. For infants with significant respiratory disease, providing lipid at low dosages sufficient to prevent EFAD may be more prudent during the height of pulmonary disease, although it will not meet the needs of the preterm infant. It should only be a short period of time before lipids can be advanced.

The most commonly used lipid emulsions in the United States are Intralipid 20% (Fresenius Kabi USA, Lake Zurich, IL) and Liposyn III 20% (Hospira, Lake Forest, IL). These are 100% soybean oil and provide alpha-linolenic and linoleic acids, but no DHA, EPA, or ARA. Alternative lipid source emulsions have been developed, as evidence increasingly suggests that excessive polyunsaturated fatty acid (PUFA) and linoleic acid content may have harmful effects, especially regarding the inflammatory response and oxidative stress.[51] Few large randomized trials are available to evaluate these newer products. Table 5.2 lists commercial products both in and outside the United States. Smoflipid, a mixed-oil product

TABLE 5.2 **Commercially Available Intravenous Fat Emulsion Products in the United States and Elsewhere**

Product	Manufacturer or Distributor	Lipid Source	CONCENTRATIONS OF SELECTED FA (% BY WEIGHT)				n-6/n-3 RATIO	Alpha-Tocopherol (mg/L)
			Linoleic	Alpha-Linolenic	EPA	DHA		
Available in the United States								
Intralipid	Fresenius Kabi/ Baxter	100% soybean oil	44–62	4–11	0	0	7:1	38
Liposyn III	Hospira	100% soybean oil	54.5	8.3	0	0	7:1	NA
Available outside the United States								
Intralipid	Fresenius Kabi	100% soybean oil	44–62	4–11	0	0	7:1	38
Ivelip	Baxter Teva	100% soybean oil	52	8.5	0	0	7:1	NA
Lipovenoes	Fresenius Kabi	100% soybean oil	54	8	0	0	7:1	NA
Lipovenoes 10% PLR	Fresenius Kabi	100% soybean oil	54	8	0	0	7:1	NA
Intralipos 10%	Mitsubishi Pharma Guangzhou/ Tempo Green Cross Otsuka Pharmaceutical Group	100% soybean oil	53	5	0	0	7:1	NA
Lipofundin-N	B. Braun	100% soybean oil	50	7	0	0	7:1	180 ± 40
Soyacal	Grifols Alpha Therapeutics	100% soybean oil	46.4	8.8	0	0	7:1	NA
Intrafat	Nihon	100% soybean oil	NA	NA	0	0	7:1	NA
Structolipid 20%[a]	Fresenius Kabi	64% soybean oil; 36% MCT oil	35	5	0	0	7:1	6.9
Lipofundin MCT/LCT	B. Braun	50% soybean oil; 50% MCT oil	27	4	0	0	7:1	85 ± 20
Lipovenoes MCT	Fresenius Kabi	50% soybean oil; 50% MCT oil	25.9	3.9	0	0	7:1	NA
ClinOleic 20%	Baxter	20% soybean oil; 80% olive oil	18.5	2	0	0	9:1	32
Lipoplus	B. Braun	40% soybean oil; 50% MCT oil; 10% fish oil	25.7	3.4	3.7	2.5	2.7:1	190 ± 30
SMOFlipid	Fresenius Kabi	30% soybean oil; 30% MCT; 25% olive oil; 15% fish oil	21.4	2.5	3.0	2.0	2.5:1	200
Omegaven	Fresenius Kabi	100% fish oil	4.4	1.8	19.2	12.1	1:8	150–296

[a]Fat source uses structured lipids

EPA, Eicosapentaenoic acid; *FA*, fatty acid; *MCT*, medium-chain triglyceride; *n-6/n-3 ratio*, ratio of ω-6 fatty acids to ω-3 fatty acids; *NA*, not available.

From Vanek VW, Seidner DL, Allen P, et al. ASPEN position paper: clinical role for alternative intravenous fat emulsions. *Nutr Clin Pract.* 2012; 27:157. With permission.

(soybean, medium-chain triglycerides [MCT], olive, and fish; Fresenius Kabi, Bad Homburg, Germany) was approved for use in adults by the U.S. Food and Drug Administration (FDA) in 2016. However, it comes with a warning regarding use in preterm infants. Two studies with Smoflipid have been published from Europe.

Tomsits et al[52] randomized 60 premature infants to Intralipid or Smoflipid and stratified them into three birth weight groups. The primary safety parameter was serum triglyceride concentrations. Some 51 infants completed the study with mean durations of 11 and 10 days (study vs. control, respectively).

Triglyceride values were similar between groups at the beginning and end of the study period, showing a slight rise with lipid infusion but remaining within expected limits. No significant differences between groups were noted for vital signs, growth, occurrence of adverse events, and hematological and clinical chemistry lab results, with the exception of gamma-glutamyl transferase, which remained relatively constant in both groups through study day 8 but was significantly increased in the control group ($P < .05$) at the end of treatment. Alpha-tocopherol levels were significantly increased in the study group compared with the control group ($P < .05$). Red blood cell phospholipid fatty acid patterns were similar at baseline, but significant differences were seen at study termination for linoleic, alpha-linolenic, and EPA fatty acids that reflected the differences in lipid profile of the two emulsions: a significant increase in EPA and smaller decrease in DHA in the study group. Linoleic and alpha-linolenic acids significantly increased in the control group. Overall, Smoflipid was well tolerated.

Rayyan et al[53] conducted a randomized trial of Smoflipid and Intralipid in 53 preterm infants less than 34 weeks' gestation and stratified into three weight groups. Lipid solutions were infused 1 g/kg/day for 3 days and then increased to 2, 3, and 3.5 g/kg/day from day 6 on. The maximum infusion rate was 0.17 g/kg over 18 hours/day. Routine labs were collected as well as blood for fatty acid analysis (plasma and red blood cells). The primary safety parameter was change in serum triglycerides from baseline to study day 8.

There were no significant differences in nutrient intake or occurrence of adverse/serious events between groups. The rise in triglycerides was similar between groups (baseline to day 8). With the exception of total and LDL cholesterol, lipid parameters were similar between groups. Cholesterol values were higher in the study group but remained within expected ranges. In the control group, the direct bilirubin increased significantly from baseline to final observation ($P = .036$). Plasma phospholipids were significantly different between groups at the end of the study period: total n-6 PUFA (control > study, $P < .001$), total n-3 PUFA (study > control $P < .001$), n-6/n-3 ratio (control > study, $P < .001$).

Omegaven (Fresenius Kabi, Bad Homburg, Germany) is 100% fish oil, approved for use in Germany, but only in expanded access protocols in the United States. Fish oil is rich in n-3 fatty acids, especial EPA and DHA. Gura et al[54] showed that using a fish oil–based emulsion helped reverse cholestasis that developed in infants with short bowel syndrome after receiving a soybean-based emulsion for a prolonged period of time. The investigators noted the absence of EFAD, hypertriglyceridemia, coagulopathy, infections, or growth delay in these infants. Other investigators[55–58] have noted a role for alternative lipid emulsions in preventing/ameliorating liver compromise related to use of soybean oil products.

Carnitine is an essential cofactor required for the transport of long-chain fatty acids (LCFA) across the mitochondrial membrane for beta-oxidation. Because of the limited carnitine reserves and low plasma carnitine levels in preterm infants, some investigators have recommended supplementing parenteral nutrition.[59,60] A secondary analysis of metabolic profile data by Clark et al[61] showed that supplementation with L-carnitine during parenteral nutrition significantly increased plasma free carnitine concentrations within the first week compared with infants not supplemented. During the transition to enteral nutrition, free carnitine content decreased but remained higher in the most immature infants who received supplementation. Thus carnitine supplementation is recommended only for VLBW infants who require prolonged parenteral nutrition (2–3 weeks). Dosage at 8 to 10 mg/kg/day has been used without observable side effects.[62]

EDITORIAL COMMENT: Premature birth occurs at a critical time when the fetus is undergoing rapid intrauterine brain and body growth. It is challenging yet most important to maintain this growth trajectory postnatally. Despite adoption of a more aggressive approach with amino acid infusions, there is still some hesitation to use early intravenous lipids because of concerns that lipid infusions may cause or exacerbate lung disease, displace bilirubin from albumin, aggravate sepsis, lower platelets, and cause central nervous system injury. The case for using intravenous lipids is strongly summarized above. Further well-designed and adequately powered studies are necessary to determine the optimal product and dose of lipid infusion and the long-term effects on morbidity, growth, and neurodevelopment. The fish oil–based products appear to be gaining momentum.

Parenteral Vitamins

Adequate supplies of vitamins are essential for normal growth and development. The optimal requirement for vitamins in neonates has not been determined, and little additional information has been developed in the past 20 years. Current recommendations are generally based on expert opinion. With commercially available products, dosing is generally done by adding one-third, two-thirds, or a full vial to total parenteral nutrition (TPN) based on weight groups (<1 kg or 1–3 kg) (see Table 5.3).

Parenteral vitamin preparations are exposed to light, oxygen, and the lipophilic surfaces of tubing materials

TABLE 5.3 **Vitamins for Total Parenteral Nutrition Solutions**

	MVI Pediatric[b]	INFUVITE PEDIATRIC[c]	
Vitamin	**5 mL**	**Vial 1 (4 mL)**	**Vial 2 (1 mL)**
Vitamin C (ascorbic acid)	80 mg	80 mg	
Vitamin A[a]	0.7 mg (retinol)	2300 IU (0.7 mg) (retinyl palmitate)	
Vitamin D[a]	10 mcg (ergocalciferol)	400 IU (10 mcg) (cholecalciferol)	
Thiamine (Vitamin B_1) (as the hydrochloride)	1.2 mg	1.2 mg	
Riboflavin (Vitamin B_2) (as riboflavin-5-phosphate sodium)	1.4 mg	1.4 mg	
Pyridoxine (Vitamin B_6) (as the hydrochloride)	1.0 mg	1.0 mg	
Niacinamide	17 mg	17 mg	
Dexpanthenol (d-pantothenyl alcohol)	5 mg	5 mg	
Vitamin E (dl-alpha-tocopheryl acetate)[a]	7 mg	7 IU (7 mg)	
Biotin	20 mcg		20 mcg
Folic acid	140 mcg		140 mcg
Vitamin B_{12} (cyanocobalamin)	1 mcg		1 mcg
Vitamin K_1 (phytonadione)[a]	200 mcg	0.2 mg	

[a]Vitamins A, D, E, and K_1 water solubilized with polysorbate 80.
[b]Hospira, Inc., Lake Forest, IL
[c]Baxter Healthcare Corp., Deerfield, IL

during administration, which may reduce the amounts delivered to VLBW infants. For these reasons, vitamins are usually added to TPN shortly before infusing. Some nurseries cover the TPN bags and tubing with foil or opaque materials. Others choose to add vitamin preparations to the lipid emulsion. See Table 5.4 for recommended parenteral and enteral intakes.

Trace Minerals

As with vitamins, precise requirements for individual trace minerals remain unknown, especially in the low-birth-weight (LBW) infant who has inadequate stores and rapid growth demands. Parenteral preparations are designed to provide sufficient amounts to prevent deficiencies and to match in utero accretion rates. Contaminants such as aluminum and chromium require monitoring in cases of long-term parenteral nutrition. Copper levels may need to be monitored in infants with cholestasis to avoid toxicity. See Table 5.5 for parenteral and enteral recommended intakes.

Calcium and Phosphorus

Preterm infants require increased intakes of calcium and phosphorus for optimal bone mineralization. The fetus accretes calcium at a rate of around 104 to 125 mg/kg/day at 26 weeks' gestation; phosphorus uptake is around 63 to 86 mg/kg/day.[63,64] It is difficult to deliver adequate amounts of these mineral in conventional TPN solutions because of Ca/P precipitation. The addition of cysteine hydrochloride lowers the pH of the solution and improves solubility. Suggested parenteral intake of calcium is 60 to 80 mg/kg/day and phosphorus 45 to 60 mg/kg/day. See Table 5.5 and chapter on glucose calcium and magnesium.

Carbohydrates

In the fetus, glucose is the main carbohydrate used for fuel and is provided by the placenta at a rate of around 7 g/day in the last trimester of pregnancy. In the early postnatal period, carbohydrates continue to serve as the primary energy substrate for the preterm infant receiving parenteral nutrition, supplying metabolic fuel for all major organs, especially the brain.

The glucose infusion rate should maintain euglycemia. Depending on the degree of immaturity, 5% or 10% glucose is commonly used; higher concentrations may require a central line for infusion. Glucose intolerance, defined as an inability maintain euglycemia at glucose administration rates of less than 6 mg/kg/minute, is a frequent problem with VLBW infants, especially those less than 1000 g birth weight, and must be avoided. Endogenous glucose production is elevated in VLBW infants (8 mg/kg/minute) compared with term infants and adults.[65] Additionally, high glucose production rates are found in VLBW infants who receive only glucose compared with those receiving glucose plus amino acids and/or lipids.[65] Clinical experience with glucose intolerance suggests that glucose alone does not always suppress glucose production in these infants. Although not all of the contributing factors to hyperglycemia are entirely clear, it appears likely that persistent glucose production is the main cause, fueled by ongoing proteolysis that is not suppressed by physiologic

TABLE 5.4 Comparison of Parenteral and Enteral Macronutrient and Vitamin Intake Recommendations for Stable, Growing Preterm Infants

	RECOMMENDATIONS (UNIT/KG/DAY UNLESS NOTED)	
Component, units	**Parenteral**	**Enteral**
Water/fluids, mL	120–160	135–190
Energy, kcal	90–100	110–130
Protein, g	3.2–3.8	3.4–4.2
Carbohydrate, g	9.7–15	7–17
Fat, g	3–4	5.3–7.2
Linoleic acid, mg	340–800	600–1440
Vitamins: fat soluble		
Vitamin A, IU	700–1500	700–1500
Vitamin D, IU	40–160	150–400
Vitamin E, IU	2.8–3.5	6–12
Vitamin K,[a] mcg	10	8–10
Vitamins: water soluble		
Ascorbate, mg	15–25	15–25
Thiamine (vitamin B1), mcg	200–350	200–350
Riboflavin (Vitamin B2), mcg	150–200	250–360
Pyridoxine (Vitamin B6), mcg	150–200	150–210
Niacin, mg	4–6.8	3.6–4.8
Biotin, mcg	5–8	5–8
Folic acid, mcg	56	25–50
Vitamin B_{12}, mcg	0.3	0.3

Conversion factors:
Vitamin A: 1 mcg retinol = 3.33 IU Vitamin A = 6 mcg beta-carotene = 1.83 mcg retinyl palmitate = 1 retinol equivalent (RE)
Vitamin E: 1 mg α-tocopherol = 1 IU Vitamin E
Vitamin D: 1 mcg Vitamin D (cholecalciferol) = 40 IU Vitamin D (cholecalciferol)
Niacin: 1 mg niacin = 1 niacin equivalent (NE) = 60 mg tryptophan

[a]Vitamin K: 0.5 to 1 mg given at birth
From Schanler RJ, Anderson D. The low birth-weight infant: inpatient care. In: Duggan C, Watkins JB, Walker WA, eds. *Nutrition in Pediatrics*. 4th ed. Hamilton, Ontario, Canada: BC Decker Inc; 2008. With permission.

TABLE 5.5 Comparison of Parenteral and Enteral Electrolyte and Mineral Intakes for Stable, Growing Preterm Infants

	RECOMMENDATIONS (UNIT/KG/DAY UNLESS NOTED)	
Component, units	**Parenteral**	**Enteral**
Electrolytes		
Sodium, mg	69–115	69–115
Potassium, mg	78–117	78–117
Chloride, mg	107–249	107–249
Minerals		
Calcium, mg	60–80	100–220
Phosphorus, mg	45–60	60–140
Magnesium, mg	4.3–7.2	7.9–15
Trace elements		
Iron, mg	100–200	2000–4000
Zinc, mcg	400	1000–3000
Copper, mcg	20	120–150
Chromium, mcg	0.05–0.3	0.1–2.25
Manganese, mcg	1	0.7–7.5
Selenium, mcg	1.5–4.5	1.3–4.5
Other		
Carnitine, mg	~3	~3

Conversion factors:
Calcium: 40 mg = 1 mmol = 2 mEq
Phosphorus: 31 mg = 1 mmol
Magnesium: 24 mg = 1 mmol = 2 mEq
Sodium: 23 mg = 1 mmol = 1 mEq
Potassium: 39 mg = 1 mmol = 1 mEq
Chloride: 35 = mg 1 mmol = 1 mEq

From Schanler RJ, Anderson D. The low birth-weight infant: inpatient care. In: Duggan C, Watkins JB, Walker WA, eds. *Nutrition in Pediatrics*. 4th ed. Hamilton, Ontario, Canada: BC Decker Inc; 2008. With permission.

concentrations of insulin. Hyperglycemia can also occur in the presence of nonoliguric hyperkalemia.[66]

Strategies to treat early hyperglycemia include:

1. decreasing the glucose infusion rate until the hyperglycemia resolves;
2. administering parenteral amino acids, which results in lowering glucose concentrations, presumably by enhancing endogenous insulin secretion;
3. initiation of exogenous insulin at rates to control hyperglycemia[67,68]; and
4. infusion of insulin as a nutritional adjuvant (to control hyperglycemia and to increase nutrient uptake).[69]

The first and third options limit the amount of energy available to the infant, and the last approach has been shown to lead to lactic acidemia. The second strategy is preferred because it more closely mimics the fetal circumstance and has been shown to work.[17,26,28] The decline of specific amino acids at the time of birth may trigger the starvation response, which includes an increase in endogenous glucose production. By smoothing the metabolic transition to extrauterine life with early amino acid infusion, one may forestall the starvation response and improve glucose tolerance. With the current practice of earlier initiation of parenteral amino acids, the frequency of early hyperglycemia can be reduced.[28]

TABLE 5.6 Estimation of the Energy Requirement of the Infant With Low Birth Weight

	Average Estimation, kcal/kg/day
Energy expended	40–60
Resting metabolic rate	40–50[a]
Activity	0–5[a]
Thermoregulation	0–5[a]
Synthesis	15[b]
Energy stored	20–30[b]
Energy excreted	15
Energy intake	90–120

[a]Energy for maintenance
[b]Energy cost of growth
Modified from the Committee on Nutrition of the Preterm Infant, European Society of Paediatric Gastroenterology and Nutrition, Bremer HJ, Wharton BA. Nutrition and feeding of preterm infants, Oxford, 1987; Kleinman RE, ed. *Pediatric Nutrition Handbook*. 6th ed. Elk Grove Village, IL: American Academy of Pediatrics; 2009:83.

Excessive glucose infusion may result in increased energy expenditure, oxygen consumption, serum osmolality, osmotic diuresis, and fat deposition.[8] A study by Poindexter et al[31] examined the effect of insulin using a hyperinsulinemic-euglycemic clamp in normoglycemic ELBW infants receiving only glucose. They reported significant increases in plasma lactate concentrations and metabolic acidosis. A study by Beardsall et al[70] showed in a randomized trial in VLBW infants that 20% glucose coupled with insulin in the first 7 days of life led to increased episodes of hypoglycemia and increased mortality at 28 days compared with standard practice. Thus routine use of insulin is not recommended.

(For further details on glucose management, see Chapter 11.)

Energy

Energy needs are dependent on age, weight, rate of growth, thermal environment, activity, hormonal activity, nature of feedings, and organ size and maturation (Table 5.6). Measurement of a true basal metabolic rate requires a prolonged fast and cannot ethically be determined in VLBW infants. Therefore resting metabolic rate (RMR) is used to estimate energy needs, dietary-induced thermogenesis, minimum energy expended in activity, and the metabolic cost of growth. The metabolic rate increases during the first weeks of life from an RMR of 40 to 41 kcal/kg/day during the first week to 62 to 64 kcal/kg/day by the third week of life. The extra energy expenditure is primarily as a result of the energy cost of growth related to various synthetic processes. The metabolic rate of the nongrowing infant is approximately 51 kcal/kg/day, which includes 47 kcal/kg/day for basal metabolism and 4 kcal/kg/day for activity. Excessive energy intake may result in hyperglycemia, increased fat deposition, fatty liver, and other complications.[12]

The contribution of activity to overall energy expenditure seems to be small, between 3 and 5 kcal/kg/day. Because of the large amount of time spent in the sleep state, energy expenditure in muscular activity in immature infants is relatively small in comparison to their resting metabolism. As infants mature, they become more active; therefore energy expenditure from activity increases.

The exposure of infants to a cold environment affects energy expenditure with small alterations in the thermal environment, making a significant contribution to energy expenditure. Infants nursed in an environment just below thermal neutrality increase energy expenditure by 7 to 8 kcal/kg/day; any handling adds to this energy loss. A daily increase of 10 kcal/kg/day should be allowed to cover incidental cold stress in the preterm infant. Infants who are intrauterine growth restricted, particularly the asymmetrical type, have a higher RMR on a per-kilogram body weight basis because of their relatively high proportion of metabolically active mass. Other factors that may increase metabolic rate include the effects of fever, sepsis, and surgery. The degree to which the infant's energy requirements are increased is uncertain.

Caloric intake above maintenance contributes to growth. On average, for each 1-g increment in weight, approximately 4.5 kcals above maintenance energy needs are required. Therefore to attain the equivalent of the third-trimester intrauterine weight gain (10–15 g/kg/day), a metabolizable energy intake of approximately 45 to 70 kcal/kg/day above the 51 kcal/kg/day required for maintenance must be provided, or approximately 100 to 120 kcal/kg/day. Increasing metabolizable energy intakes beyond 120 kcal/kg/day with energy supplementation alone does not result in proportionate increases in weight gain. However, when energy, protein, vitamins, and minerals are all increased, weight gain with increases in rates of protein and fat accretion can be realized. The higher the caloric intake, the more energy that is expended through excretion, dietary-induced thermogenesis, and tissue synthesis. The energy cost of weight gain at 130 kcal/kg/day has been shown to be 3.0 kcal per gram of weight gain. However, at an intake of 149 kcal/kg/day and 181 kcal/kg/day, the energy cost of weight gain has been estimated to be 4.9 and 5.7 kcal/g of weight gain, respectively. In summary, to increase lean body mass accretion and limit fat mass deposition, an increase in protein-to-energy ratio in enteral diets is necessary.

The energy needs of the parenterally nourished infant differ from the enterally fed infant in that there is no fecal loss of nutrients. Preterm infants who are appropriately grown for gestational age are able to maintain positive nitrogen balance when receiving 50 nonprotein calories (NPCs)/kg/day and 2.5 g protein/kg/day. At an NPC intake of greater than 70 NPC/kg/day and a protein intake of 2.7 to 3.5 g/kg/day, preterm infants exhibit nitrogen accretion and growth rates similar to in utero levels. In the ELBW infant with minimal respiratory disease but requiring mechanical ventilation, energy expenditure may be as high as 85 kcal/kg/day in early postnatal life.[71] There are few data that describe energy expenditure in these infants, as a result of technical difficulties and methodologic limitations affecting the interpretation of data.

The primary sources of energy for parenteral nutrition in infants are either glucose or lipid or a combination of the two. Although both glucose and fat provide equivalent nitrogen-sparing effects in the neonate, studies have demonstrated that a nutrient mixture using IV glucose and lipid as the nonprotein energy source is more physiologic than supplying glucose alone.[9] The amount of glucose required to meet the total energy needs approximates 7 mg/kg/min (10 g/kg/day). Excess glucose is converted to fat or triglycerides. When lipids supply 60% to 63% of the NPCs given to LBW infants, nitrogen retention is decreased, and temperature control is adversely affected.[72] A moderate IV fat intake, comprising approximately 35% of the NPCs, is preferred.

Practical hints for fluid and TPN management in the first few days of life:

- Provide sufficient fluid to result in a urine output of 1–3 mL/kg/hour, a urine specific gravity of 1.008 to 1.012, check for sugar and protein.
- Target a weight loss of 5% or less in full term or 15% or less in VLBW infants.
- Weigh infants twice daily in the first 2 days, then daily.
- Use birth weight to calculate intake until birth weight is regained.
- Record fluid intake, output, and weight.
- Use only 20% lipid emulsions. Infuse lipids slowly, not to exceed 0.17 g/kg/hour. If the infant is hyperbilirubinemic, limit lipids to 0.5 to 1.0 g/kg/day. The maximum lipid dose should be 3 to 4 gm/kg/day while maintaining serum triglyceride less than 200 mg/dL. Check before starting lipids, when lipids are advanced, and weekly thereafter;
- Aim to provide a parenteral energy intake of 90 to 100 kcal/kg/day and an amino acid dose up to 3.5 gm/kg/day. The NPC:N ratio should be 150 to 250.
- (Lipid calories + dextrose calories) ÷ (protein [grams] * 0.16) = NPC/N (grams)

ENTERAL NUTRITION

When parenteral nutrition is used exclusively for the provision of nutrients, morphologic and functional changes occur in the gut with a significant decrease in intestinal mass, a decrease in mucosal enzyme activity, and an increase in gut permeability. The changes are due primarily to the lack of luminal nutrients rather than the TPN. The timing of the initial feedings for the VLBW infant should be within the first days of life, with many clinicians now initiating gut priming as soon as day 1. This strategy of early feeding replaces the one in which feedings were held during the first days of life because of concerns about NEC with early feedings. Physicians chose to use parenteral nutrition alone in the sick, ventilated, preterm infant. Total parenteral nutrition was thought to be a logical continuation of the transplacental nutrition the infants would have received in utero.

However, this view discounts any role that swallowed amniotic fluid plays in nutrition and in the development of the GI tract. In fact, by the end of the third trimester, amniotic fluid provides the fetus with the same enteral volume intake and approximately 25% of the enteral protein intake as that of a term, breast-fed infant. Parenteral nutrition does little to support the function of the GI tract. Enteral feedings have direct trophic effects and indirect effects secondary to the release of intestinal hormones, for example, significant rises in plasma concentrations of enteroglucagon.[73]

Regardless of feeding strategy, the advancement of feedings has been based on the absence of significant pregavage residuals or greenish aspirates. These gastric residuals are very frequent in the early neonatal period, are virtually always benign when not accompanied by other signs of GI abnormalities, and not associated with NEC.[74,75] One study demonstrated that in ELBW infants, excessive gastric residual volume either determined by percent of the previous feed or an absolute volume (>2 mL or >3 mL) did not necessarily affect feeding success as determined by the volume of total feeding on day 14.[76] Similarly, the color of the gastric residual volume (green, milky, clear) did not predict feeding intolerance. Nonetheless, the volume of feeding on day 14 did correlate with a higher proportion of episodes of zero gastric residual volumes and with predominantly milky gastric residuals. Thus isolated findings related to gastric emptying alone should not be the sole criterion in initiating or advancing feeds. Stooling pattern, abdominal distention, and the nature of the stools should also be considered.[74] Some units have now abandoned checking gastric residuals at all, and randomized trials support such an approach.

The etiology and pathophysiology of NEC remain unclear. Because NEC rarely occurs in infants who are not being fed, feedings have come to be seen as a cause of NEC. However, intestinal immaturity, abnormal microbial colonization, and a highly immunoreactive intestinal mucosa appear to be leading elements of a multifactorial cause. The association between feedings and NEC is likely explained by the fact that feedings can act as vehicles for the introduction of bacterial or viral pathogens or toxins. They are more likely to survive the gastric barrier because of low acidity, against which the immature gut is poorly able to defend itself. Efforts aimed at minimizing the risk of NEC have focused on the time of introduction of feedings, on feeding volumes, and on the rate of feeding volume increments. One by one, the strategies that had been developed with the aim of reducing the risk of NEC were shown to be ineffective. Therefore, as discussed above, feedings should not be reduced in volume or held altogether because of minor GI irregularities, such as gastric emptying defined by residuals. If PGF is to be avoided, the neonatologist must pay close attention to nutrition from the minute the infant is born.[7]

Finally, the withholding of feeding for prolonged periods of time to prevent NEC eventually came under scrutiny and was compared in a number of controlled trials with early introduction of feedings. A systematic review of the results of these trials concluded that early introduction of feedings shortens the time to full feeds, as well as the length of hospitalization, and does not lead to an increase in the incidence of NEC.[77] A controlled study involving 100 VLBW infants confirmed these findings and found a significant reduction in serious infections when feedings were introduced early.[78]

Another strategy aimed at preventing NEC has been to keep the rate increments low. Unnecessarily slowing advancement of nutrition will adversely affect growth. The strategy was based on the findings of Anderson and Kliegman,[79] who conducted a retrospective analysis of 19 cases of NEC with two matched controls per case of NEC. They found that in infants who went on to develop NEC, feedings were advanced more rapidly than in control infants without NEC. Based on these findings, they recommended that feedings not be advanced by more than 20 mL/kg each day. In this study, some of the feeding advancements were much beyond current practices and bear no resemblance to how infants are fed today. However, the recommendation has found wide acceptance, although its validity has not been confirmed in randomized controlled trials.

In a prospective randomized trial, Rayyis et al[80] compared increments of 15 mL/kg/day with increments of 35 mL/kg/day. They found that with fast advancement, return to birth weight occurred earlier, full intakes were achieved sooner, weight gain set in earlier, and there was no difference in the incidence of NEC. A Cochrane review found 10 randomized controlled trials (RCTs) with a total of 3753 infants (2804 participated in one large trial) to compare feeding advancement.[81] Although most participants were stable AGA, very preterm infants, about one-third were ELBW and 20% were SGA, or compromised in utero, as indicated by absent or reversed-end diastolic flow velocity in the fetal umbilical artery. Trials typically defined slow advancement as daily increments of 15 to 20 mL/kg and faster advancement as daily increments of 30 to 40 mL/kg/day. Meta-analyses did not show effects on risk of NEC or all-cause mortality.[81] Subgroup analyses of extremely preterm or of SGA or growth restricted/growth compromised infants showed no evidence of an effect on risk of NEC or death. Slow feed advancement delayed establishment of full enteral nutrition by between 1 and 5 days. Meta-analyses showed a borderline increased risk of invasive infection. Therefore advancing feeds at a slow rate results in several days of delay in establishing of full enteral feedings and may be associated with metabolic and infectious morbidities secondary to prolonged exposure to parenteral nutrition.

When initiating early enteral feedings, infants may still have umbilical artery catheters (UACs) in place, and safety is often a concern. The presence of a UAC has led to delay of feedings until catheters are removed. This may make early gut priming and day 1 feeding more difficult. However, few data from controlled studies support this policy of delaying feeds because of the UAC. Davey et al[82] examined feeding tolerance in 47 infants weighing less than 2000 g at birth who had respiratory distress and UACs in place. Infants were assigned randomly to begin feedings as soon as they met the predefined criterion of stability or to delay feeding until their UACs were removed for 24 hours. Infants who were fed with catheters in place started feeding significantly sooner and required half the number of days of parenteral nutrition. The incidence of NEC was comparable for infants fed with catheters in place and those whose catheters were removed before initiation of feedings. In addition, large epidemiologic surveys have not shown a cause-and-effect relationship between low-lying UACs and NEC.[74,75]

The decision when to start these early enteral or trophic feeds may be influenced by what milk is available to feed the infant. Donor milk (DM) is widely used when own mother's milk (OMM) is unavailable.[83] Both older and more recent studies suggest that DM is as efficacious as OMM in preventing NEC in preterm infants.[84–86] A recent meta-analysis of data from six trials found a statistically significantly increased incidence of NEC (twice the risk) and feeding intolerance in the formula-fed group compared with the human milk fed groups. It has been estimated that one extra case of NEC will occur in every 25 preterm infants who receive formula.[87] (See also Section 3 of this chapter on NEC.)

Feedings with human milk for the VLBW infant may have to include DM to be able to start within the first days of life. A frequently encountered problem is that own mother's breast milk takes at least 2 days to come in and often does not come in for 3, 4, or 5 days. During that time, only small amounts of colostrum are available, which is very beneficial to the infant and must be fed, but will not provide enough volume. Gastric residuals should not interfere with feeding. Initial feeding volumes should be kept low (1–2 mL/feed) and provided at 3-hour intervals. Incremental advances should be about 20 mL/kg/day when a decision is made to advance feedings.

EDITORIAL COMMENT: The old wives' tale was that all babies regurgitated human milk, including through their nose, so that the upper respiratory tract would be lined and protected by secretory immunoglobulin A and other factors from the milk.

Indeed, cytokines applied to the oropharynx may stimulate the lymphoid tissue, enhancing the immune system. Colostrum is rich in cytokines and other immune agents that provide bacteriostatic, bactericidal, antiviral, antiinflammatory, and immunomodulatory protection against infection. Oropharyngeal administration of colostrum may decrease clinical sepsis, inhibit secretion of proinflammatory cytokines, and increase levels of circulating immune protective factors in extremely premature infants. Placing the colostrum with a small syringe into the cheek pouch has become commonplace. even if they are on the ventilator.

For ELBW infants on life support with invasive monitoring, trophic feedings may be introduced with 1 mL/feed every 8 hours for a period of a few days and then proceed as above. Each nursery should establish criteria for feeding readiness; standardization of feeding protocols leads to better results. These may include normal blood pressure and pH, PaO_2 greater than 55, at least 12 hours from last surfactant or indomethacin dose, normal GI examination, heme-negative stools, and fewer than two desaturation episodes (SaO_2 <80%) per hour. Collectively, these signs are a surrogate for establishing "physiologic" stability before feeding initiation.

EDITORIAL COMMENT: Standardization of feeding protocols reduces time to full feeds, enhances growth, and reduces necrotizing enterocolitis.

Carbohydrate

Carbohydrate provides 41% to 44% of the calories in human milk and most infant formulas. In human milk and standard infant formulas, it is present as lactose, which has been shown to enhance calcium absorption. Once the infant's condition stabilizes, the requirement for carbohydrate is estimated at 40% to 50% of calories, or approximately 10 to 14 g/kg/day. In soy and other lactose-free formulas, the carbohydrate is in the form of sucrose, maltodextrins, and glucose polymers (corn syrup solids or modified starches). The three major disaccharidases responsible for the digestion of disaccharides are lactase, maltase, and sucrase-isomaltase. Maltase and sucrase-isomaltase first appear at 10 weeks' gestation, reaching approximately 70% of newborn levels at 28 weeks. However, by 28 to 34 weeks' gestation, lactase has only 30% of the activity found in the term infant.[88] However, in clinical settings, lactose intolerance is rarely a problem. Human milk is usually well tolerated, possibly because preterm infants acquire a relatively efficient capacity to hydrolyze lactose in the small intestine at an earlier developmental stage that do infants in utero.[89]

When lactose is not hydrolyzed in the small intestine, bacterial fermentation of the undigested portion occurs in the colon, producing short-chain fatty acids, which enhance mineral and water absorption and may stimulate growth and cell replication in the gut lumen. Thus colonic salvage is apparently important in disposal of unabsorbed lactose; however, its exact quantitative contribution remains unknown. Colonic bacterial fermentation of unabsorbed lactose to absorbable organic acids enables the infant to reclaim this carbohydrate energy and appears to prevent clinical symptoms of diarrhea.

Although pancreatic alpha-amylase, the major enzyme in starch hydrolysis, is either absent or in very low concentrations in the first 6 months of life, newborns are capable of tolerating small amounts of starch without side effects, and preterm infants are able to hydrolyze glucose polymers. Several enzymes may compensate for the physiologic pancreatic amylase deficiency in infancy. Glucoamylase, an enzyme found in the brush border of the small intestine, is present in the neonate in concentrations similar to those in adults. Also, salivary and human milk amylases may provide additional pathways for glucose polymer digestion in infancy.

Because lactase is found only at the tip of the villus, it is very sensitive to mucosal injury. Lactose intolerance may develop in infants with diarrhea, those suffering from undernutrition, or those recovering from NEC, necessitating temporary use of a lactose-free formula. In contrast, glucoamylase is able to survive partial intestinal atrophy because it is located at the base of the villi, thus enabling glucose polymers to be an alternative carbohydrate source when enteritis is present and lactase may be in low concentrations.

In premature infant formulas, lactose has been partially replaced by glucose polymers, polysaccharides with chains of 5 to 10 glucose residues joined linearly by 1, 4-alpha linkages to decrease the osmolality of the formula and to decrease the lactose load in the diet. Glucose polymers are well tolerated by preterm infants with glucose and insulin responses similar to those of a lactose feeding. Because glucose polymers add fewer osmotic particles to the formula per unit weight than does lactose, they permit the use of a high-carbohydrate formula with an osmolality less than 300 mOsm/kg of water. Special formulas for preterm infants contain approximately 40% to 50% lactose and 50% to 60% glucose polymers, a ratio that does not impair mineral absorption.[90]

Protein

The protein requirement of the preterm infant is estimated to be 3.2 to 4.2 g/kg/day for VLBW infants and 3.5 to 4.4 g/kg/day for ELBW infants.[7] One study suggests that in VLBW infants, a formula with higher protein content (3.6 g/100 kcal) versus 3.0 g/100 kcal in standard formula results in increased protein accretion and weight gain without evidence of metabolic stress.[91] The quality and quantity of protein that the infant receives are important. Although weight gain and growth of VLBW infants fed protein intakes of 2.2 to 4.5 g/kg/day of either a casein- or whey-predominant formula have been shown to be no different from those receiving pooled human milk, the metabolic responses can be significantly different. Serum BUN, ammonia, albumin, and plasma methionine and cysteine concentrations were higher in the infants receiving high-protein formulas. Elevated levels of phenylalanine and tyrosine were seen in infants fed the casein-predominant, high-protein formula, and lower concentrations of taurine were noted in infants fed casein-predominant formulas regardless of quantity. Preterm infants fed soy protein formula supplemented with methionine exhibit slower weight gain and lower serum protein and albumin concentrations than infants fed a whey-predominant formula. Thus premature infant formulas are whey predominant with a 60 to 40 whey-to-casein ratio; soy protein-based formulas are not recommended for the preterm infant.[92]

Human milk is considered to have the ideal amino acid distribution for the human infant. Preterm infants fed their OMM have more rapid growth than infants fed pooled, banked human milk with accretion of protein and fat similar to that of the fetus.[93] Human milk is lower in mineral content, especially magnesium, calcium, phosphorus, sodium, chloride, and iron. To attain intrauterine growth rates in

TABLE 5.7 Comparison of Enteral Electrolyte and Mineral Intake Recommendations for Stable, Growing Preterm Infants

	RECOMMENDATIONS (UNITS/KG/DAY UNLESS NOTED)	
Components, units	**≤1000 g**	**1001–1500 g**
Electrolytes		
Sodium, mg	69–115	69–115
Potassium, mg	78–117	78–117
Chloride, mg	107–249	107–249
Minerals		
Calcium, mg	100–220	100–220
Phosphorus, mg	60–140	60–140
Magnesium, mg	7.9–15	7.9–15
Iron, mg	2–4	2–4
Zinc, mcg	1000–3000	1000–3000
Copper, mcg	120–150	120–150
Selenium, mcg	1.3–4.5	1.3–4.5
Chromium, mcg	0.1–2.25	0.1–2.25
Manganese, mcg	0.7–7.75	0.7–7.75
Molybdenum, mcg	0.3	0.3
Other		
Iodine, mcg	10–60	10–60
Taurine, mg	4.5–9.0	4.5–9.0
Carnitine, mg	~2.9	~2.9

From Tsang RC, Uauy R, Koletzko B, Zlotkin SH. eds. *Nutrition of the Preterm Infant: Scientific Basis and Practical Guidelines.* Cincinnati, OH: Digital Educational Publishing Inc; 2005:417-418. With permission; Kleinman RE, ed. *Pediatric Nutrition Handbook.* 6th ed. Elk Grove Village, IL: American Academy of Pediatrics; 2009:80.

larger preterms, large volumes (180–200 mL/kg/day) of human milk must be fed. Fortification of human milk is discussed below.

The recommended dietary allowances for infants and children to age 12 months are listed in Table 5.7.

Lipids

Fat is a major source of energy for the infant, with approximately 50% of the calories in human milk derived from fat. In commercial formulas, fat provides 40% to 50% of the energy. These feedings provide 5 to 7 g of fat per kg per day. The saturated fat of human milk is well absorbed by the preterm infant, in part because of the distribution pattern of fatty acids on the triglyceride molecule. Palmitic acid is present in the beta position in human milk fat and more easily absorbed than palmitic acid in the alpha position, which occurs in cow milk.

Human milk contains a bile salt–activated lipase that enhances lipid digestion in the duodenum. The special formulas for preterm infants contain a mixture of medium-chain triglycerides and vegetable oils rich in polyunsaturated long-chain triglycerides (LCTs), both of which are well absorbed by preterm infants.[94,95]

MCTs are oils with an 8 to 12 carbon chain length. Unlike LCTs, MCTs do not require bile for emulsification. MCTs are rapidly hydrolyzed in the gut and pass directly to the liver through the portal circulation, whereas LCFAs must be re-esterified once absorbed and are transported via the lymph system into the blood circulation, where they are hydrolyzed by lipoprotein lipase. Medium-chain fatty acid (MCFA) metabolism differs from that of LCFA in that it does not require carnitine for transport into the mitochondria and is not regulated by cytosolic acyl-CoA synthetase. MCFAs enter the mitochondria directly and are rapidly oxidized. Formulas with MCTs have been shown to improve nitrogen, calcium, and magnesium absorption. Preterm infant formulas have been developed with approximately half the fat as MCTs.

Vitamins

Vitamin A

Vitamin A is a fat-soluble vitamin that promotes normal growth and differentiation of epithelial tissues. At birth, preterm infants less than 36 weeks' gestational age have been reported to have lower plasma retinol concentrations as compared with full-term infants, although the measured levels are quite variable. There is a further decrease in the plasma retinol and retinol-binding protein levels during the first 2 weeks after birth, particularly when sufficient amounts of vitamin A are not provided. A number of reasons, including impaired absorption and low concentrations of intestinal carrier proteins for retinol, place the preterm infant at risk of vitamin A deficiency. The measured hepatic levels of retinol expressed as μmol/g in preterm infants are reported to be the same as in infants born at term gestation but lower than those in older children and adults. The preterm infant's vitamin A status may affect the maintenance and development of pulmonary epithelial tissue. Recommendations for vitamin A intake range from 700 to 1500 IU/kg/day.[96]

Retinol has been shown to be essential for the growth and differentiation of epithelial cells and has been suggested to have a role in prevention and repair of lung injury. Vitamin A deficiency is associated with histopathologic changes in the lung similar to those seen in BPD. For these reasons, the impact of vitamin A supplementation on BPD in VLBW infants has been examined.[96,97] In a multicenter, blinded, randomized trial, the use of vitamin A 5000 IU (1.5 mg) administered intramuscularly three times per week for 4 weeks improved the biochemical vitamin A status and resulted in a modest advantage in relation to prevention of chronic lung disease.[96] Vitamin A in such large doses was shown to have no clinically measurable toxic effects. In a meta-analysis of seven randomized trials, supplementation with vitamin A resulted in reduction of death or oxygen requirement at 1 month of age and oxygen requirement at 36 weeks' postmenstrual age (chronic lung disease) as well as trends toward a reduction in oxygen requirement in survivors at 1 month of age.[98] Clinicians must weigh the modest benefits against necessity for repeated intramuscular injections.

Vitamin E

Vitamin E, or alpha-tocopherol, serves as an antioxidant to protect double bonds of cellular lipids. Vitamin E requirements are increased with increasing PUFA intake and in the presence of oxidant stress, such as high iron intake. Vitamin E deficiency is rarely seen in infants because infant formulas are supplemented with vitamin E in proportion to the PUFA content. However, infants who are breast-fed and receiving supplemental iron should be given additional vitamin E. Preterm infants have low serum vitamin E levels and may be at increased risk for oxidative damage to cell membranes. Studies to investigate the effectiveness of pharmaceutical doses of vitamin E on ROP and BPD have not demonstrated benefits of this therapy. The VLBW infant should receive 6 to 12 IU/kg of vitamin E per day enterally. The formulas for preterm infants supply 4 to 6 IU/100 kcal per day.

Vitamin K

Vitamin K, an important cofactor in the activation of intracellular precursor proteins to blood clotting proteins, is synthesized endogenously by bacterial flora. Hemorrhagic disease of the newborn infant, most commonly seen in exclusively breastfed infants, results from vitamin K deficiency.[99]

As a preventive measure, an intramuscular injection of vitamin K is routinely provided after birth. In preterm infants weighing more than 1 kg at birth, the standard prophylactic dose of 1 mg of phylloquinone is appropriate. For those infants weighing less than 1 kg, a dose of 0.3 mg/kg of phylloquinone is recommended.

Calcium, Phosphorus, Magnesium, and Vitamin D

The amount of enteral calcium, phosphorus, and magnesium intake required to match intrauterine accretion rates is high: calcium 185 to 200 mg/kg/day, phosphorus 100 to 113 mg/kg/day, and magnesium 5.3 to 6.1 mg/kg/day. VLBW infants with minimal illness may require lower intakes.[100] The AAP recommends calcium intakes of 185 to 210 mg/kg/day, phosphorus 123 to 140 mg/kg/day, and magnesium 8.5 to 10 mg/kg/day. However, magnesium intake at this level with such high calcium and phosphorus intake results in negative magnesium balance. Therefore a higher intake of magnesium, approximately 20 mg/kg/day, may be needed.[101]

The recommendation for vitamin D, which is required for normal metabolism of calcium, phosphorus, and magnesium, has ranged from 200 to 2000 IU per day for the preterm infant. VLBW infants can maintain normal vitamin D status with 400 IU/day; high-dose vitamin D supplementation does not decrease the incidence of rickets in VLBW infants.

Human milk has concentrations of calcium and phosphorus that are appropriate for full-term infants but not for the VLBW infant. Breast milk should be supplemented with additional calcium, phosphorus, and vitamin D, which can easily be done with human milk fortifiers. Fortification yields better mineral accretion than breast milk alone, similar to that of VLBW infants fed a premature infant formula.[93]

Inadequate intakes of calcium, phosphorus, and vitamin D result in metabolic bone disease of prematurity, also called rickets of prematurity. This disease is characterized by reduced bone mineralization and, in severe cases, frank radiologic evidence of rickets and spontaneous fractures. The biochemical findings, although not highly sensitive, include an elevated alkaline phosphatase (>500 IU/L), decreased serum phosphorus (<4 mg/dL), and normal serum calcium. The 25-hydroxycholecalciferol (25-OH vitamin D) level is usually normal, but 1,25 dihydroxycholecalciferol (1,25-OH vitamin D) levels may be elevated as a result of increased parathyroid hormone levels and low serum phosphorus levels. The incidence of rickets was higher before institution of the current practices of higher calcium and phosphorus levels in parenteral nutrition solutions and early enteral feedings. The etiology of rickets remains unclear but is thought to be primarily because of an insufficient intake of calcium and phosphorus. Risk factors for rickets are listed in Box 5.3. Confirming the diagnosis requires radiologic evidence of osteopenia.

EDITORIAL COMMENT: Osteopenia of prematurity, also called metabolic bone disease of prematurity or rickets of prematurity, is characterized by a reduction in bone mineral content usually manifest between the 6th to 12th weeks of corrected gestational age. It occurs in over 50% of infants born with weight less than 1000 g and 25% of infants weighing less than 1500 g.

High levels of alkaline phosphatase can be considered a reliable biomarker to predict the status of bone mineralization and the need for radiological evaluation in premature infants.

Dual-energy x-ray absorptiometry and quantitative ultrasonogram are important diagnostic tools. Standard x-ray only detects osteopenia when there is about 20% loss of bone mineralization. The focus on prevention has largely centered on providing adequate intake of phosphorus and calcium.

Exercise consisting of passive range of motion exercise with gentle compression of both the upper and lower extremities lasting 5 to 10 minutes each day may improve biochemical and imaging parameters.

BOX 5.3 Risk Factors for Metabolic Bone Disease of Prematurity

- Extremely low birth weight (ELBW, ≤1000 g)
- Prolonged parenteral nutrition
- Unfortified human milk
- Use of elemental and/or soy formulas
- Chronic diuretic therapy (especially furosemide)
- Chronic problems such as necrotizing enterocolitis, bronchopulmonary dysplasia, cholestasis, and acidosis

Fortified human milk or premature infant formula is the preferred feeding for VLBW infants. The use of soy formulas is not recommended for infants with birth weights less than 1800 g. If continuous infusion feeding of human milk is necessary, the syringe and the pump should be placed upright to prevent loss of calcium, phosphorus, and milk fat by separation and adherence to the tubing.

Vitamin B_{12} and Folate

Vitamin B_{12} requires intrinsic factor for its absorption in the distal ileum. Therefore particular attention to this vitamin is necessary in infants who have had gastric resection or resection of the terminal ileum (e.g., NEC surgery). The potential neurologic complications of vitamin B_{12} deficiency are irreversible.

Serum folate levels may be low in the preterm infant. Folate is supplemented in the pediatric IV multivitamin preparation and in infant formulas. It is not available in the infant multivitamin drops because of its instability in the liquid form. Folate plays an important role in DNA synthesis. Deficiency of this vitamin may result in megaloblastic anemia, neutropenia, thrombocytopenia, and growth failure. Requirements for fat- and water-soluble vitamins in VLBW and ELBW infants are shown in Table 5.7. Advisable intakes for infants 0 to 12 months are shown in Table 5.8.

Iron

There has been increased interest in iron deficiency, with data suggesting that mental and developmental test scores are lower in infants with iron deficiency anemia and that iron therapy sufficient to correct the anemia is insufficient to reverse the behavioral and developmental disorders in many infants.[102,103] This indicates that certain ill effects are persistent depending on the timing, severity, and/or degree of iron deficiency anemia during infancy.

Iron stores in the preterm infant are lower than in the term baby because iron stores are relatively proportional to body weight.[104] Iron depletion occurs around the time the baby doubles her/his birth weight, and thus iron therapy should begin by 4 weeks of life in the preterm infant when enteral feedings are tolerated. Smaller preterm infants may need as much as 4 to 6 mg/kg/day, with about 2 mg/kg/day provided by iron-fortified formula and the remainder as iron supplementation at 2 to 4 mg/kg/day. A higher dose is also necessary for infants being given erythropoietin. Oral iron supplementation can interfere with vitamin E metabolism in the VLBW infant,[102] thereby further increasing the need for vitamin E in an infant who is at risk for low serum tocopherol levels. Although premature infant formulas, both with and without iron fortification, are manufactured with ample amounts of vitamin E and a PUFA-to-E ratio of 6 or greater, premature infants on human milk and receiving supplemental iron can be also supplemented with 4 to 5 mg (6–8 IU) of vitamin E per day. This can be readily accomplished by use of an oral multivitamin with iron.

The impression that low-iron formulas are associated with fewer GI disturbances is not supported by controlled studies.

TABLE 5.8 Dietary Reference Intakes: Recommended Daily Intakes for Infants

Nutrient	0–6 Months	7–12 Months
Protein, g/kg	**1.52**	1.05
Carbohydrate, g	**60**[a]	95[a]
Fat, g	**31**[a]	30 [a]
N–6 PUFA (linoleic acid) g	**4.4**[a]	4.6[a]
N–3 PUFA (alpha-linolenic acid), g		
Sodium, g	**0.12**[a]	0.37[a]
Potassium, g	**0.4**[a]	0.7[a]
Chloride, g	**0.18**[a]	0.57[a]
Calcium, mg	**210**[a]	270[a]
Phosphorus, mg	**100**[a]	275[a]
Magnesium, mg	**30**[a]	75[a]
Iron, mg	**0.27**[a]	**11**
Zinc, mg	**2**[a]	**3**
Copper, mcg	**200**[a]	220[a]
Selenium, mcg	**15**[a]	20[a]
Vitamin A, mcg	**400**[a]	500[a]
Vitamin C, mg	**40**[a]	50[a]
Vitamin D, mcg	**5**[a]	5[a]
Vitamin E, mg	**4**[a]	5[a]
Vitamin K, mcg	**2**[a]	2.5[a]
Thiamin, mg	**0.2**[a]	0.3[a]
Riboflavin, mg	**0.3**[a]	0.4[a]
Niacin, mg	**2**[a]	4[a]
Vitamin B_6, mg	**0.1**[a]	0.3[a]
Folate, mcg	**65**[a]	80[a]
Vitamin B_{12}, mg	**0.4**	0.5
Pantothenic acid, mg	**1.7**[a]	1.8[a]
Biotin, mcg	**5**[a]	6[a]

[a]Adequate intakes (AI) represent the mean intake for healthy, breast-fed infants.

Bold type: Recommended dietary allowances (RDA) are set to meet the needs of 97%–98% of individuals in a group. *PUFA,* Polyunsaturated fatty acid.

From DRI Reports. http://www.iom.edu/CMS/3788/21370.aspx and Kleinman RE, ed. *Pediatric Nutrition Handbook.* 6th ed. Elk Grove Village, IL: American Academy of Pediatrics; 2009:1294-1296.

Because the bioavailability of iron from iron-fortified infant cereals is somewhat low, it is recommended that iron-fortified formulas or daily iron supplements be continued through the first year of life.[102]

Among term infants, breast feeding usually provides adequate iron intake during the first 4 to 6 months of life, and supplementation during this time is not necessary. Although the iron content of human milk is low, averaging 0.8 mg iron/L, the bioavailability is high, with term infants absorbing about 49% of the iron content compared with 10% to 12% from iron-fortified cow milk formula. Infants who are exclusively breast fed can maintain normal hemoglobin and ferritin levels, and do not need iron supplementation until 4 to 6 months. See Table 5.5.

The late Frank Oski, MD, a brilliant pediatrician and hematologist, claimed that he never saw evidence of iron deficiency in breast-fed infants. He maintained that although the iron content of human milk was extremely low, it was well absorbed.

There is overwhelming evidence that iron deficiency impairs intelligence. Optimal cord clamping may therefore be a critical means of providing extra hemoglobin and iron and may have a global impact on intelligence.

TABLE 5.9 Dietary Reference Intake for Fluoride

Age Group	Adequate Intake (mg/day)	Tolerable Upper Intake (mg/day)
Infants		
0–6 months	0.01	0.7
7–12 months	0.5	0.9
Children		
1–3 yr	0.7	1.3
4–8 yr	1	2.2
9–13	2	10
Boys 14–18 yr	2	10
Girls 14–18 yr	3	10
Males 19 yr and older	4	10
Females 19 yr and older	3	10

From Kleinman RE, ed. *Pediatric Nutrition Handbook*. 6th ed. Elk Grove Village, IL: American Academy of Pediatrics; 2009:1050. With permission.

Fluoride

Because of reports of dental fluorosis in infants and toddlers, fluoride supplementation is no longer recommended in the infant younger than 6 months of age. The supplementation schedule (Table 5.9) recommended by the AAP and the American Dental Association should be followed according to the fluoride content of the local water supply.[105]

GROWTH IN THE NEONATAL INTENSIVE CARE UNIT INFLUENCES NEURODEVELOPMENTAL AND GROWTH OUTCOMES

A multicenter cohort study from the NICHD included 600 infants with birth weights from 501 to 1000 g. These infants were stratified by 100 g–birth weight increments and divided into quartiles based on in-hospital growth velocity rates.[106] As the rate of weight gain increased between quartile 1 and quartile 4 (from 12–21.2 g/kg/day), the incidence of cerebral palsy, Bayley II Mental Developmental Index (MDI) and/or Psychomotor Developmental Index (PDI) scores of less than 70, abnormal neurologic examination findings, neurodevelopmental impairment, and need for rehospitalization fell significantly at 18 to 22 months' corrected age. Similar findings were observed as the rate of head circumference (HC) growth increased from 0.67 to 1.12 cm/week. Higher in-hospital growth rates were associated with a decreased likelihood of anthropometric measurements below the 10th percentile at 18 months' corrected age. The influence of growth velocity remained after controlling for variables known at birth or identified during the infants' neonatal intensive care unit hospitalizations that affect outcome, including comorbid conditions such as NEC or BPD. This study emphasizes the importance of closely monitoring the rate of in-hospital growth once birth weight has been regained. Goals for growth, including HC gain of more than 0.9 cm/week and weight gain of 18 g/kg/day from return to birth weight through discharge, were associated with better neurodevelopmental and growth outcomes. If growth rates falter, the infants' diets should be reviewed to ensure adequate nutritional support, including protein/energy ratios of feeds and the use of calorically dense milks (>24 kcal/ounce).

METHOD OF FEEDING

The method of feeding for each infant should be chosen on the basis of gestational age, birth weight, clinical condition, and experience of the hospital personnel. An important consideration in feeding the newborn is the development of sucking, swallowing, gastric motility, and emptying. Swallowing is first detected at 11 weeks' gestation, and the sucking reflex is first observed at 24 weeks' gestation. However, a coordinated suck-swallow is not present until 32 to 34 weeks' gestation, and even then, it is immature. The maturation of the swallowing reflex is related to postnatal age. Swallowing must be coordinated with respiration in that the two processes share the common channels of the nasopharynx and laryngopharynx. The inability of the infant to coordinate this action results in choking, aspiration of feedings, and vomiting. To evaluate the suck-swallow reflex, one should observe the number of swallows per second. An infant with a good suck-swallow reflex swallows approximately once per second. If greater than two per second are observed, the infant is probably not able to coordinate the swallowing. With a good suck, the temporal muscle will bulge.

When starting to introduce the nipple, a rule of thumb is to bottle-feed for 20 minutes, then gavage the remainder. At first, the infant may be offered nipple feeding once in a 24-hour period; the number of feedings is then increased as the infant becomes more able to nurse. Because of the additional work of sucking, the energy expenditure increases; therefore an increased caloric intake may be required to maintain an adequate rate of growth. Weight gain during the start of nipple feeding should be closely monitored. It is not necessary for an infant to be able to bottle-feed before attempting to breast feed. Infants who will be breast feeding may actually be able to nurse from the breast sooner than they will be able to coordinate bottle-feeding. If an infant's respiratory rate is 70 to 80 breaths per minute or more, he or she should be tube fed because of the increased risk of aspiration.

If an infant is unable to nipple feed, he or she needs to be fed through an orogastric or nasogastric tube or, rarely, transpylorically. Intragastric tube feedings are preferable in that they allow for normal digestive processes and hormonal responses. The acid content of the stomach may impart bactericidal effects. Other benefits of intragastric tube feeding include ease of insertion of tube, tolerance of greater osmotic loads with less cramping, distention, diarrhea, and less risk of developing dumping syndrome. Continuous transpyloric feeding is rarely used in infants who cannot tolerate feedings because of impaired gastric emptying or a high risk of aspiration. However, this route of infusion has a higher risk of perforation of the gut, may not enable delivery of a large volume of feedings, and may result in inefficient nutrient assimilation because bypassing the gastric phase of digestion limits the exposure of food to acid hydrolysis and the lipolytic effects of lingual and gastric lipases.

If using tube feedings, the decision to feed intermittently or continuously must be made. There are differences seen in the endocrine milieu between infants fed continuously compared with those fed intermittently. The significance of these differences is unclear, and it is not possible to state with certainty which method is best for the prematurely born neonate. It has been suggested that the cyclic changes in circulating hormones and metabolites, as seen in intermittent bolus feeding, may have quite different effects on cell metabolism,[107] gallbladder emptying, and gut development. Continuous infusion of human milk is not recommended because there is a loss of fat and, consequently, calories in the tubing of the pump. Additionally, at the end of the infusion, a large bolus of fat is delivered to the infant, owing to the separation of the fat during the infusion period.

Gastrostomy feedings are chosen when it becomes apparent that there will be long-term tube feeding (e.g., for a neurologically impaired infant), when there is persistent gastroesophageal reflux that is unresponsive to medical treatment, or when esophageal anomalies prevent the use of an orogastric or nasogastric tube.

Positioning of the infant during feeding is important for more efficient stomach emptying. Infants with respiratory distress fed in the supine position have delayed gastric emptying. The stomach empties more rapidly in the prone or right lateral positions; thus these positions are preferred, especially in infants with respiratory distress and in those infants who have the potential for feeding intolerance.

The evaluation of an infant's feeding tolerance is an ongoing process to determine the appropriate feeding method, type of formula to feed, and increment of feeding advancement. Vomiting, abdominal distention, significant gastric residuals, abnormal stooling patterns, and presence of reducing substances or frank or occult blood in the stool are indicators of intolerance. Sepsis and NEC may first manifest with one or more of these signs of feeding intolerance. Vomiting or spitting in the high-risk infant increases the risk of aspiration.

Another consideration in promoting feeding tolerance is the use of compressed, intermittent feedings. In a study of duodenal motility patterns, the same volume of full-strength formula produced a normal duodenal motility administered with "slow bolus" technique (i.e., intermittent feedings lasting from 30 minutes to 2 hours) and may be the best tolerated feeding method versus the 15-minute bolus.[108]

HUMAN MILK

Human milk is recommended as the first choice for feeding the VLBW infant.[83,109] The AAP supports the feeding of human milk for all infants, term and preterm. Human milk has both nutritional and antiinfective properties, which are especially important for infants at risk for sepsis and NEC. When OMM is not available or the amount produced is not sufficient to meet daily needs, donor human milk may (should) be used in its place. However, DM is generally term milk in quality and likely has insufficient protein to promote appropriate growth. Whether donor or OMM is provided, fortification of human milk is necessary to meet nutrient requirements for growth and development for these VLBW infants who are at high risk for growth faltering during the hospital stay. DM and OMM intended for her preterm infant have inadequate amounts of several nutrients, especially protein, vitamin D, calcium, phosphorus, and sodium. When the protein content is suboptimal, especially for VLBW infants weighing less than 1500 g, it results in lower serum albumin and transthyretin (prealbumin) levels, which are reliable indicators of protein nutriture in preterm infants.[110] Poor growth will be the ultimate outcome with inadequate protein. The calcium and phosphorus content is low in unsupplemented human milk in comparison to that required to achieve intrauterine accretion rates, resulting in poor bone mineralization in VLBW infants. In addition, the sodium content of human milk results in less sodium retention than intrauterine estimates and may result in hyponatremia.

The benefits of human milk over formula feeding include nutritional, immunologic, developmental, psychological, social, and economic. Breast milk influences major short-term outcomes in VLBW. These include a reduction in three widely occurring morbidities: NEC, BPD, and ROP.[111–115] The prevention of BPD has been less clear until recently, when a multicenter cohort study from the German Neonatal Network compared almost 500 VLBW infants who received formula only with exclusive human milk feeding.[114] They found an increased risk of BPD with an odds ratio of 2.6 with exclusive formula feeding. They also found increased odds ratios for ROP and NEC of 1.8 and 12.6, respectively, for those fed only formula versus exclusively fed human milk.[114]

There are also unique long-term beneficial effects of human milk for ELBW infant cognitive outcomes. Data from the Eunice Kennedy Shriver National Institute of Child Health and Developmental Neonatal Research Network, including nutritional data on 773 ELBW infants, showed positive effects related to human milk intake for developmental outcomes at 18 months of age.[116] Studied again at 30 months of age, these infants with higher volumes of human milk received during their neonatal hospitalization, continued to have higher Bayley Mental Developmental Index (MDI) and Bayley behavior score percentiles for emotional regulation, and had fewer rehospitalizations between discharge and 30 months. Incredibly, every 10 mL/kg/day of human milk received increased the MDI by 0.59 points.

The German Neonatal Network study[114] and a recent study of our own,[117] showing short-term benefits in preventing BPD and NEC, both found that with disease prevention comes a reduction in growth in those VLBW infants receiving exclusive human milk feedings. Thus the conundrum: to prevent disease with exclusive human milk feeding, clinicians increase the risk for growth failure, which is itself associated with increased risk of adverse neurologic and developmental outcomes.[118,119] As seen in the previous section on growth in the neonatal intensive care unit (NICU), poor growth during the neonatal hospitalization was associated with an increased risk of cerebral palsy, lower MDI and PDI scores less than 70, as well as an increased risk of blindness and deafness at 18- to 22-month follow-up.[106]

Because the composition of preterm milk varies greatly from one mother to another and the concentration of nutrients in preterm milk changes over time, it is difficult to determine the actual macronutrient intake of an infant. However, new technology (infrared spectrophotometry) in human milk analyzers (HMA) allows accurate bedside analysis of the macronutrients in human milk. To confer the potential nonnutritional advantages yet provide optimal nutrient intake, human milk should be fortified with protein, calcium, phosphorus, vitamin D, and sodium.

There are a few strategies when it comes to fortification of human milk for the VLBW. Standard fortification adds a fixed amount of fortifier as recommended by the manufacturer and is the most widely used method. It does not take into account the variability of the macronutrient contents of the native milk and often fails to meet the nutritional needs of preterm infants.[120]

Two new fortification strategies (adjustable and individualized) have been suggested to improve nutritional intakes and growth outcomes in VLBW infants. Arslanoglu and Ziegler adjusted fortification (by increasing or decreasing fortifier packets) according to the values of BUN, considered a marker of metabolic response for protein adequacy for these VLBW infants.[121] The BUN method is easy to apply and does not require HMA daily milk analyses. However, it has been shown that BUN is not correlated with protein intakes during the first weeks of life but rather reflects renal immaturity of VLBW infants. Therefore the use of BUN as a threshold did not allow the provision of adequate nutrition and growth during the first weeks of life.[121]

Targeted fortification uses data from HMA, which permits the clinician to tailor macronutrient content based on real-time analysis of the native human milk sample. It aims to "standardize" the composition of breast milk and provide VLBW infants with a constant and defined intake. Much of the work with the HMAs have been in research protocols, but the hope is that in the near future, they become available for routine clinical use when they are approved by the FDA.

It is difficult for the mothers of ELBW infants to provide sufficient volumes of milk to meet their infants' needs over the entire hospitalization. Therefore pasteurized human milk from DM banks and now industry is available as a potential proxy for the mother's own milk.[122] Studies showing a lower rate of NEC with DM were conducted before the use of human milk fortifiers. Many of these infants suffered growth failure and osteopenia of prematurity secondary to inadequate protein, calcium, and phosphorous in DM.

A randomized controlled multicenter trial to evaluate an exclusively human milk diet in extreme premature infants (500–1250 g birth weight) was done and was the first to use a human milk–based fortifier.[115] Three study groups received, on average, 70% of their feeds as mother's own milk. One group of infants received mother's milk fortified with powdered bovine fortifier. This group actually received 89% of their diet with their OMM. When mother's milk was unavailable, these infants received preterm formula. The other two groups were fed pasteurized DM when the OMM was not available and were fortified with human milk–derived fortifier at two different intake volumes. The rates of NEC (medical and surgical) were lower in the exclusively human milk–fed infants. There was a 50% reduction in medical NEC and almost a 90% reduction in surgical NEC for the infants fed an exclusive human milk diet compared with a diet containing bovine milk–based products.

Editorials and commentaries concerning this study point out that the study was powered to look at days of TPN between the groups (not NEC), but the prospective randomized trial had 16% NEC in the bovine cohort, a much higher rate of NEC than that seen in many units. In fact, de Halleux et al reported that in units from the Belgium Network using only preterm formula or bovine-based fortifier, the rate of NEC was 4.4%.[123] Was the effect caused by the novel fortifier or the benefit of giving human milk? Concerns remain about the study being underpowered and not having a bovine-based fortifier for comparison.[124]

To be able to select the proper formula for feeding a sick infant, a clear understanding of the differences between formulas and unique qualities of a given formula is necessary (Table 5.10).

PREMATURE INFANT FORMULAS

Providing optimal nutrition to a preterm infant is complicated by a lack of a natural standard. For the healthy full-term infant, human milk is considered the ideal food; therefore it is used as the reference standard for the development of commercial infant formulas. Although early milk of mothers who deliver their infants prematurely is higher in nitrogen (early in lactation), fatty acid content, sodium, chloride, magnesium, and iron, it is still inadequate in other nutrients, especially calcium and phosphorus. It therefore cannot be used as a standard for the development of premature infant formula. Modifications in the composition of the preterm formulas

	Mature preterm human milk (unfortified)	Enfamil Premature[a]	Enfamil Premature 24 Cal High Protein[a]	Similac Special Care with Iron[b]	Similac Special Care 24 High Protein[b]	Gerber Good Start Premature[c]	Gerber Good Start Premature 24 High Protein[c]
Nutrient density (kcal/oz)	19–21	24	24	24	24	24	24
Energy (kcal)	100	100	100	100	100	100	100
Protein (g)	2.2 ± 0.2	3.3	3.6	3	3.3	3	3.6
% Total calories	8	13	14	12	13	12	14
Source	Human milk	Whey protein concentrate, nonfat milk	Whey protein concentrate, nonfat milk	Whey protein concentrate, nonfat milk	Whey protein concentrate, nonfat milk	Whey partially hydrolyzed	Whey partially hydrolyzed
Fat (g)	5.4 ± 0.9	5	5	5.43	5.43	5.2	5.2
% Total calories	44–52	44	44	47	47	40	47
Source	Triglycerides	MCT oil, soy oil, high oleic vegetable oil, single-cell oil products (DHA and ARA)	MCT oil, soy oil, high oleic vegetable oil, single-cell oil products (DHA and ARA)	MCT oil, soy oil, coconut oil, single-cell oil products (DHA and ARA)	MCT oil, soy oil, coconut oil, single-cell oil products (DHA and ARA)	MCT oil, high oleic vegetable oil, soy oil, single-cell oil products (DHA and ARA)	MCT oil, high oleic vegetable oil, soy oil, single-cell oil products (DHA and ARA)
Oil ratio (approximate)	99	40:30.5:27:2.5	40:30:27:2:1	50:30:18.3:0.25:0.4	50:30:18.3:0.25:0.4	40:29:29:2	40:29:29:2
Linoleic acid (mg)	440–1500	810	810	700	700	990	990
Carbohydrate (g)	10 ± 0.6	10.8	10.5	10.3	10	10.5	9.7
% Total calories	40–44	43	42	41	40	42	39
Source	Lactose, glucose	Corn syrup solids, lactose	Corn syrup solids, lactose	Corn syrup solids, lactose	Corn syrup solids, lactose	Lactose, maltodextrin	Lactose, maltodextrin
Minerals							
Calcium (mg)	37–44	165	165	180	180	164	164
Phosphorus (mg)	19–21	90	90	100	100	85	85
Ca:P	1.9–2.2:1	2:1	1.8:1	1.8:1	1.8:1	1:9	1:9
Sodium (mg)	30–37	70	70	43	43	55	55
Potassium (mg)	78–85	98	98	129	129	120	120
Chloride (mg)	63–82	106	106	81	81	85	85
Iron (mg)	0.2	1.8	1.8	1.8	1.8	1.8	1.8
Zinc (mg)	0.5	1.5	1.5	1.5	1.5	1.3	1.3
Magnesium (mg)	4.4–4.9	9	9	12	12	10	10
Other							
Nucleotides (mg)	7.6–9.1	4.25	4.25	9	9	4.6	4.6
Osmolality (mOsm/kg H_2O)	290	320	300	280	280	275	299

[a]Mead Johnson Nutritionals, Evansville, IN, USA
[b]Abbott Nutrition, Columbus, OH, USA
[c]Nestlé S.A., Vevey, Switzerland
ARA, Arachidonic acid; *DHA*, docosahexaenoic acid; *MCT*, medium-chain triglyceride.
Modified from Hay WW and Hendrickson KC. Preterm formula use in the preterm very low birth weight infants. *Semin Fetal Neonatal Med*. 2017;22(1):15-22.

followed review of a number of studies that provided more rational evidence of the nutritional requirements that were specific to VLBW and ELBW infants. The special premature infant formulas have been developed from knowledge of the accretion rates of various nutrients relative to the reference fetus, from studies of the development of the GI tract that have defined absorptive efficiency and function, and from metabolic studies.

Premature infant formulas have a lower lactose concentration, with approximately 50% of the carbohydrate as lactose to reduce the lactose load because of relative lactase deficiency. The remainder of the carbohydrate is provided as glucose polymers, which are readily hydrolyzed by glucoamylase and result in a product with low osmolality. Nevertheless, lactose remains important for normal nutrition and especially for prevention of NEC, perhaps in part by lowering distal intestinal pH, which suppresses growth of opportunistic bacteria and promotes growth of *Lactobacillus* and *Bifidobacterium* organisms.

The premature infant formulas are whey predominant, which has been shown to result in less metabolic acidosis in VLBW infants. The risk of lactobezoar formation is reduced when a whey-predominant formula is used. In addition, the concentration of protein per liter is approximately 50% greater than that of standard infant formula and can provide 3.6 to 4.2 g protein/kg/day. The newer 60% whey and 40% casein ratio produces more rapid gastric emptying, digestion, and amino acid absorption, and less metabolic acidosis. The whey-predominant preterm formulas also produce free amino acid concentrations that are more similar to those produced by human milk than the casein formulas.[125] The protein content of many standard preterm formulas (2.2–2.4 g/100 cal) does not meet the protein requirements for growth of the VLBW. Newer generations of high-protein preterm formulas containing 2.7 to 2.9 g/100 mL or 3.3 to 3.6 g/100 kcal and providing up to 4.5 g/kg/day of protein are indicated for ELBW and VLBW infants who have experienced a large cumulative protein deficit, have inadequate growth in length and/or HC, or who are volume restricted.[126]

The fat source in the newer preterm formulas is a blend of vegetable oils, but also contains between 10% and 50% MCTs. The necessity of MCTs is controversial. However, the MCTs are potentially better for energy production than longer-chain fatty acids and do not contribute to fat storage.

The vitamin concentration is higher because the volume of formula consumed is significantly less in the tiny baby. The calcium and phosphorus content is greater than standard formula, with variation between formula manufacturers. The calcium-to-phosphorus ratio generally is 2:1 as compared with 1.4:1 to 1.5:1 with standard infant formulas. Too much calcium and phosphorus may result in intestinal milk bolus obstruction. As with all formulas, it is important to shake the formula before use because precipitation may occur, and the precipitate, containing high amounts of calcium and phosphorus, may remain in the bottom of the container.

Premature infant formulas have always been low in iron content (3 mg elemental iron/L) because these infants were often receiving transfusions and because the use of iron would increase the requirement for vitamin E. However, because some infants are receiving this type of formula for greater than 2 months and because the advantages of continuing a baby on premature infant formula after hospital discharge have been recognized, premature infant formulas have been available with low iron content (3 mg elemental iron/L) and with iron fortification (15 mg elemental iron/L).

The sodium content of premature infant formula is greater than human milk or standard infant formula. Because sodium requirements vary considerably between infants and are influenced by receipt of diuretics, this amount may be inadequate to maintain normal serum levels. Supplementation with 3% sodium chloride (0.5 mEq sodium and chloride/mL) may be necessary. Because this is a highly osmolar solution (see Table 5.1), the dose should be divided and administered several times throughout the day. One distinct advantage of premature infant formula is that, despite the high concentration of nutrients, the 24-calorie/oz. premature infant formula is iso-osmolar, with osmolalities ranging from 280 to 300 mOsm/kg H_2O.

Preterm infants fed human milk have advanced neurodevelopmental outcome as compared with formula-fed infants, measured by electroretinograms, visual evoked potentials, and psychometric tests.[106,127,128] The better performance, in part, has been related to dietary DHA and ARA acids because plasma and erythrocyte phospholipid concentrations of ARA and DHA are higher in breast-fed infants than in infants fed formulas lacking these fatty acids. Inadequate LCFA in the diet may be related to performances on tests of cognitive function.[128] The inability to synthesize enough DHA and ARA from their precursors and the lack of preformed DHA may be the cause of lower content of these fatty acids in formula-fed infants. The addition of these fatty acids to formulas in the United States has led to renewed interest and debate about the effects of LCFA on later neurodevelopmental outcome and has been reviewed elsewhere.[129]

STANDARD INFANT FORMULAS

The carbohydrate in standard infant formula is 100% lactose, and the fat is all LCTs of vegetable origin, usually soy and coconut oils. Most standard formulas are whey predominant, with 60% of the protein whey and 40% casein. Standard formulas are available in iron-fortified and non–iron-fortified (or "low iron") forms. Iron-fortified formula contains elemental iron of 12 mg/L or approximately 2 mg/kg/day for an infant receiving approximately 108 kcal/kg/day. Low-iron formula contains elemental iron 1.5 mg/L or 0.2 mg/kg/day.

Most standard infant formulas are available as ready to feed, liquid concentrate, and powder. The concentrate and the powder provide the option of concentrating the formula to a higher caloric density. Concentrations above 1 calorie per milliliter or 30 calories per ounce are not recommended because of the high renal solute load that results from the decrease in free water intake. As the formula is concentrated, the osmolality increases to approximately the same degree as the concentration. Thus for a 20 kcal/oz. formula with an osmolality of 300 mOsm/kg H_2O, if concentrated 135%, or to 27 kcal/oz. formula, the osmolality increases to approximately 405 mOsm/kg H_2O. If formula is to be concentrated, a written recipe should be given to the caregiver because overconcentration may be hazardous to small preterm infants.

Caloric density of a formula may also be increased by the addition of glucose polymers, which increases the osmolality of the formula, or by adding fat (e.g., vegetable oil, MCT oil). However, when an infant formula is supplemented with calories only, the intake of nutrients must be calculated and compared with recommended guidelines (see Tables 5.4, 5.5, and 5.8) to ensure adequacy of intake. The distribution of calories will be affected using this method of increasing calories; therefore the percent of calories from carbohydrate, protein, and fat should be determined. Approximately 35% to 65% of the total calories should be derived from carbohydrate, 30% to 55% from fat, and 8% to 16% from protein. LBW infants fed a formula contributing 7.8% of calories as protein grew at a significantly slower rate than infants fed formulas with either 9.4% or 12.5% of the calories from protein.

SOY FORMULA

Soybean-based formulas with soy protein isolate or soybean solids with added methionine as the protein source are lactose free and, therefore are recommended for infants with galactosemia with primary lactase deficiency, or recovering from secondary lactose intolerance. The carbohydrate is provided as sucrose or corn syrup solids or as a combination of the two. The fat is provided as a vegetable oil (LCTs), usually soy and coconut oils. All soy formulas are iron fortified. Although soy formulas have been used when cow milk protein allergy is suspected, the AAP cautions that infants allergic to cow's milk may also develop an allergy to soy-based milk.[92] A protein hydrolysate formula should be the initial formula of choice. Infants with a family history of allergy who have not shown clinical manifestations may benefit from soy protein formula; however, such infants should be closely monitored for soy protein allergy. Soy protein formulas are appropriate for infants of vegetarian families who eat no animal products.

The use of soy protein formulas for VLBW infants is not recommended because of the low calcium and phosphorus content of these formulas. Preterm infants fed soy protein formulas have significantly lower serum phosphorus, higher serum alkaline phosphatase levels, and an increased risk of development of osteopenia. Even when supplemented with additional calcium, phosphorus, and vitamin D, VLBW infants fed these formulas exhibit slower weight gain and lower serum protein and albumin concentrations than infants receiving a whey-predominant premature infant formula.

PROTEIN HYDROLYSATE FORMULA

Protein hydrolysate formulas are designed for infants who are allergic to cow milk or soy proteins. Some protein hydrolysate formulas are also elemental, with the carbohydrate in easily absorbable forms, such as glucose polymers or monosaccharides, and the fat as both MCTs and LCTs. These are sometimes used in the management of infants with intestinal resection or intractable diarrhea.

FOLLOW-UP FORMULA

Although considerable attention has been directed toward improving the nutrition of hospitalized VLBW infants with nutrient-enriched formulas and multinutrient fortifiers for human milk, only recently has attention been paid to nutrition support of such infants after hospital discharge. The first postnatal year may provide an important opportunity for human somatic and brain growth to compensate for earlier deprivation. A key question is whether VLBW infants have special nutrient requirements in the postdischarge period. In more biological terms, it is reasonable to ask whether this period is also critical for later health and development because it is common for human milk fortifiers to be stopped or term formulas to be substituted at hospital discharge. Available data suggest that preterm infants are in a state of suboptimal nutrition at the time of discharge from the hospital and beyond. Improving this situation would be beneficial in the short term and potentially for longer-term health and development.

Nutrient-enriched formulas for preterm infants after hospital discharge (postdischarge formulas) are generally intermediate in composition between preterm and term formulas. Compared with term formula, preterm formula contains an increased amount of protein with sufficient additional energy to permit utilization. Postdischarge formula contains extra calcium, phosphorus, and zinc, all of which are necessary to promote linear growth. Additional vitamins and trace elements are included to support the projected increased growth. A pilot study of 32 preterm infants was the first to show that infants randomized to receive the postdischarge formula up to 9 months postterm showed significantly greater weight and length gains and had higher bone mineral content in the distal radius than infants who received a standard term formula.[130] Studies have provided additional insight into the role for postdischarge formula, suggesting that benefits may be related to birth weight,[131] gender,[132–134] and a "window of opportunity" (a critical growth epoch) when supplemental nutrients can promote catch-up and subsequent growth, even after discontinuation of postdischarge formula. The reports also raise the possibility that postdischarge nutrition may benefit long-term development.[132,134]

Lucas et al reported results of a study with 284 preterm infants who received either term formula or postdischarge formula for the first 9 months postterm.[134] At 9 months postterm, postdischarge formula–fed infants were significantly heavier (mean difference, 370 g) and longer (1.1 cm) than term formula-fed infants, and the length difference persisted to 18 months postterm or 9 months after postdischarge formula was discontinued. Differences between diet groups were significantly greater in boys, who had a length advantage of 1.5 cm at 18 months if they received postdischarge formula. There was no evidence that the postdischarge formula had made infants fat. Their mean weight percentile was still below the 50th percentile, and skinfold thickness was not increased. HC and developmental outcomes at 9 or 18 months did not differ significantly between groups, although postdischarge formula–fed infants had a 2.8 ± 0.25-point advantage in the Bayley MDI Score.[134] In another study, Carver found improved growth in preterm infants who were fed a postdischarge formula after discharge up to 12 months corrected age, with the significant differences in weight, length, or HC.[131] This was more pronounced for smaller infants (birth weight <1250 g) and male infants. The differences in growth produced by postdischarge formula occurred early (critical growth epoch) but did not increase appreciably over time, suggesting that the benefit of postdischarge formula with respect to catch-up occurred soon after discharge. The benefits persisted throughout the period of observation, and, for infants whose birth weights were less than 1250 g, growth in HC was the most beneficial effect.

Another study examined the use of preterm formula after discharge in 129 preterm infants randomly assigned to one of three dietary regimens until 6 months postterm: term formula, preterm formula, or preterm formula until term followed by term formula to 6 months.[132] Males fed preterm formula after discharge showed significantly greater weight and length gain and larger HC by 6 months postterm than those fed term formula throughout the study period. Infants fed preterm formula consumed an average of 180 mL/kg/day, resulting in a protein intake of approximately 4 g/kg/day. Those fed term formula took more milk and increased consumption to about 220 mL/kg/day, but their protein intake still did not match that of the preterm formula group. At 18 months postterm, boys previously fed preterm formula were on average 1 kg heavier, 1 cm longer, and had 1 cm greater HC than those fed term formula. Body composition measurement using dual-energy x-ray absorptiometry suggested that the additional weight gain was composed predominantly of lean tissue rather than fat.[133] There were no significant differences in neurodevelopment measured using Bayley Scales of Infant Development at 18 months.

Randomized studies demonstrate that the use of either preterm formula or postdischarge formula after discharge in preterm infants results in improved growth, with differences in weight and length persisting beyond the period of intervention in two studies. Such findings raise the hypothesis that nutrition during the postdischarge period may have longer-term effects on growth trajectory. Evidence from three randomized trials suggests that the effect of a nutrient-enriched postdischarge diet is greatest in boys, possibly reflecting their higher growth rates and protein requirements. Whether the observed growth effects persist or have consequences for other aspects of health or development requires further investigation.

PRACTICAL HINTS FOR ENTERAL NUTRITION

Start minimal enteral nutrition as soon as possible—preferably day 1.

Feed colostrum to ELBW infants as per protocol discussed above.

Start small breast milk or formula feedings (10–20 mL/kg/day) as soon as possible. It is unnecessary to start with 5% glucose water.

Assess the infant's ability to nipple feed. Infants younger than 32 weeks' gestational age and infants with respiratory rates between 60 and 80 breaths per minute need to be tube fed.

Use premature infant formula or fortified breast milk for infants weighing less than 1800 g. Encourage the mother to provide her milk. If breast milk is to be used, start feedings with unfortified breast milk until tolerance is established, then add fortifier.

Intermittent gavage feedings are preferred; continuous feedings or "compressed" feedings over an hour or so may be helpful for infants with feeding intolerance.

Monitor feeding tolerance. Vomiting, a sudden increase in abdominal girth, and frank or occult blood in the stool with large gastric residuals may be signs of infection or NEC. The feedings should be stopped, the stomach should be aspirated, and a #8 Fr nasogastric tube should be inserted for gastric decompression.

Record fluid intake, output, weight, type of feeding given, and feeding tolerance.

Reduce parenteral feedings proportionate to the increase of enteral feedings to prevent excess fluid intake.

Increase feedings at a rate of 20 mL/kg/day and monitor tolerance to previous volume before increasing rate. Feed the infant in a prone position to facilitate gastric emptying and maintain better oxygenation. Once the infant is receiving 90 to 100 mL/kg/day enterally, the TPN should be discontinued; if greater fluid volume is required, provide it as an IV glucose-electrolyte solution.

Aim for a goal of 110 to 130 kcal/kg/day and 3.5 to 4 g protein/kg/day with a weight gain of approximately 15 to 18 g/kg/day.

Offer a pacifier to the infant, especially while being gavage fed.

Encourage the parents to feed the infant after the infant is feeding well. It may be very frustrating for the parents to attempt feeding when the infant is resistant.

NUTRITIONAL ASSESSMENT

An in-depth nutritional assessment requires anthropometric, biochemical, dietary, and clinical data. However, interpreting anthropometric and biochemical measurements is difficult; therefore nutritional assessment in neonates receiving intensive care treatment is often confined to detecting fluctuations in weight gain and in caloric intake. Nonetheless, it is necessary for the clinician to be able to assess the neonate's nutritional status because of the potentially serious sequelae of malnutrition on multiple organ systems and the importance of growth (especially brain growth) on developmental outcome.

In nutritional assessment, one must consider the length of gestation and adequacy of intrauterine growth and nutrient tolerance. There should be a static assessment (current balance between intake and output) as well as a dynamic assessment (evaluation of infant's growth over time or growth velocity) of each infant. Also, the nonnutritional factors such as disease state, medication, and stress (e.g., infection and surgery) must be considered.

Weight gain is the most frequently used anthropometric measure. It is important to use the same scale, obtain weight measurements at the same time each day to avoid diurnal changes, and indicate any equipment being weighed (especially arm boards and dressings); if equipment is not recorded, changes in weight may be spurious. In preterm infants, weight gain should be expressed on a gram per kilogram per day basis. Table 5.11 contains suggested postterm weight gain goals.

When assessing weight, there are several problems to consider. In the first week of life, all newborns lose weight as a result of the loss of free water and low intake; however, most preterm infants are also calorie and fluid restricted during that period as a result of illness, so that it may be difficult to separate changes in growth measurements caused by diuresis from those caused by poor protein-calorie intake. Weight gain does not necessarily reflect growth, which is a deposition of new tissue of normal composition; weight increase may reflect excessive fat deposition or water retention, neither of which is truly growth.

Length measurements are the most inaccurate anthropometric measurement. Accurate technique is important in performing length measurements to detect small changes. Two trained individuals are needed to measure the infant on a measuring board containing a stationary head board, movable foot board, and a built-in tape measure. Skeletal growth is often spared relative to weight in mildly malnourished infants; therefore initially, linear growth is often slow or stops. Serial length measures obtained weekly are helpful in assessing nutritional status when plotted over time; length measures are especially useful in infants, such as those with BPD, whose weight fluctuates greatly. A gain in length of 1 cm per week is expected.

An increase in HC, the measurement of the largest occipitofrontal circumference, correlates well with cellular growth of the brain in normal infants. During acute illness, the velocity of head growth for the sick preterm infant is less than that of the normal fetus. During recovery, head growth parallels that of normal fetal growth, and subsequently, rapid "catch-up" growth in HC may occur. Normal growth does not occur until the acute illness has resolved, despite high energy intake. Preterm infants who were calorically deprived for the longest periods showed slower growth rates and longer duration of catch-up growth. In this respect, the longer these infants remain with suboptimal head size, the greater is their developmental risk.

HC is usually measured once a week using a paper tape; a new tape should be used for each infant. A goal of about 0.9 cm per week is to be expected. If hydrocephalus is of concern, more frequent measuring is warranted. The initial HC may differ from subsequent measurements because of molding of the head. Measuring HC may be difficult because of interfering equipment such as IV lines on the scalp. Serial weight, length, and HC measurements should be plotted on an appropriate growth chart.[135] The Fenton growth curve is commonly used in the NICU.

TABLE 5.11 Growth Velocity of Preterm Infants From Term to 18 Months

Age from Term (month)	Weight (g/day)	Length (cm/month)	Head Circumference (cm/month)
1	26–40	3.0–4.5	1.6–2.5
4	15–25	2.3–3.6	0.8–1.4
8	12–17	1.0–2.0	0.3–0.8
12	9–12	0.8–1.5	0.2–0.4
18	4–10	0.7–1.3	0.1–0.4

From Theriot L. Routine nutrition care during follow-up. In: Groh-Wargo S, Thompson M, Cox JH, eds. *Nutrition Care for High Risk Newborns*, Chicago, IL: Precept Press; 2000:570. With permission.

Skinfold measures of several sites have been used to estimate body fat stores and the percent of body fat in children and adults. These determinations are made by using a variety of formulas that are based on the assumption that the percent of TBW and fat distribution remains constant. In the neonate, these assumptions are not valid because the percentage of body water decreases with increasing gestational age and postnatal age, and fat increases with increasing gestational age.

The biochemical assessment of nutritional status may be more specific than anthropometric measures and may be useful in combination with anthropometric indices for nutritional assessment of the sick neonate. Many routine tests may signal nutrition-related problems. For example, an elevated alkaline phosphatase level (>500 IU) and a low serum phosphorus level (<4 mg/dL) may occur during the active phase of rickets. This combination of biochemical findings indicates the need to obtain diagnostic x-ray studies. However, abnormal alkaline phosphatase levels may occur because of hepatic dysfunction; therefore heat fractionation of the isoenzyme is suggested to determine its origin. As rickets begins to heal, the serum phosphorus levels normalize, whereas the alkaline phosphatase continues to be elevated during the radiographic picture of healing. Elevated alkaline phosphatase levels generally precede radiologic changes by 2 to 4 weeks.

Albumin is a serum protein commonly measured in routine laboratory tests. Although it has limited value for nutritional assessment, it may serve as an indicator of inadequate energy and protein intake. The average serum albumin concentration in infants younger than 37 weeks' gestation ranges from 2 to 2.7 mg/dL. This relative hypoalbuminemia of the preterm infant appears to be a result of a more rapid turnover of a small plasma pool versus a decreased rate of albumin synthesis; the half-life of albumin is approximately 7.5 days in the preterm infant versus 14.8 days in adults. Despite the relatively rapid turnover, serum albumin concentration changes slowly in response to nutrition rehabilitation.

To quickly assess response to nutrition support, a serum protein with a shorter half-life is necessary. Transthyretin (prealbumin), with a half-life of approximately 2 days in adults, has been shown to be a suitable marker for evaluation of nutritional status in VLBW infants.[79] Because transthyretin increases with gestational age as well as with protein and energy intake, the direction of change in serial tests may be more useful than striving for absolute values.

Because of the various metabolic, renal, respiratory, and GI abnormalities to which VLBW infants are subjected, close monitoring of blood gases, serum electrolytes, calcium, phosphorus, glucose, BUN, and creatinine is necessary. Ongoing nutritional assessment includes careful calculation of dietary intake relative to estimated requirements, determination of fluid balance and hydration status, and tolerance to feeding method. In combination with anthropometric, clinical, and biochemical data, adjustments in intake or method of nutrient delivery can be made to achieve effective nutritional support.

CASE 5.1

A 26 4/7-week preterm infant was just born weighing 900 g, head circumference 23.5 cm, and length 35 cm.

What can be said about growth?

This infant is considered ELBW (extremely low birth weight) with a birth weight less than 1000 g. If the gestational age and anthropometric measurements are considered accurate, size for gestational age can be determined. This infant plots AGA (appropriate for gestational age) on the Olsen (2010) or Fenton (2013) charts. If calculators are available in the electronic health record or accessed online, *z*-scores can also be documented.

What is an appropriate nutrition plan?

Fluid needs for a preterm infant are 80 to 100 mL/kg. A stock solution containing dextrose and amino acids is commonly available for infants born weighing less than 1500 g. D10% at 80 mL/kg = 0.10 g dextrose/mL x 80 mL/kg x 3.4 kcal/g dextrose = 27.2 kcal/kg. A 4% amino acid solution at 80 mL/kg = 0.04 g dextrose/mL x 80 mL/kg = 3.2 g/kg protein x 4 kcal/g protein = 12.8 kcal/kg. Calcium and heparin would be added. This solution would run at 80 mL/kg/day x 0.9 kg x 1 day/24 hours = 3mL/hr and would provide 40 kcal/kg and 3.2 g/kg protein. Full total parenteral nutrition (TPN) with lipids would be ordered the next day. The infant could receive oral therapy with swabs of mother's expressed colostrum until trophic feedings could be started.

On day of life #3, the weight is 830 g. and the infant is on D10% AA 3.5 g/kg at 3.8 mL/hr (at 100 mL/kg) and lipids 2 g/kg at 0.38 mL/hr at 10 mL/kg). Labs show a glucose of 76, blood urea nitrogen (BUN) of 29, and triglyceride of 137. Trophic feedings of mother's breast milk or donor breast milk 1 mL every 3 hours are started.

What can be said about growth?

The infant is down 70 g total from a birth weight of 900 g, so this is 7.8% (70 g/900 g) and is appropriate. Goal is approximately 3% per day until nadir of around 10% is reached.

What is an appropriate nutrition plan?

The infant is getting 110 mL/kg from TPN/lipids and less than 10 mL/kg trophic feedings. The TPN and lipids provide 66 kcal/kg and 3.5 g/kg protein. Based on the glucose level, the dextrose-based energy could be advanced by increasing the dextrose concentration, the dextrose rate, or both to provide more calories. Based on the triglyceride level, the lipids could be advanced to provide more calories. Enteral feedings would be advanced in volume and then fortified to provide more calories, protein, and nutrients. As enteral feedings increase, the TPN could be weaned down, especially when fortification is started. Osmolarity limits may require weaning of TPN components earlier than anticipated.

On day of life #10, the infant has returned to birth weight of 900 g. The infant is on D11% AA 3.5 g/kg at 2.4 mL/hr (65 mL/kg) and lipids 3 g/kg at 0.56 mL/hr (15 mL/kg). Enteral feedings of mother's breast milk or donor milk will stay at 9 mL q 3 hours (80 mL/kg) but will be fortified to 24 kcal/oz (2.4 g/dL protein).

What can be said about growth?

The infant returned to birth weight by day of life 10, which is appropriate.

What is an appropriate nutrition plan?

The TPN/lipids provides 80 mL/kg, 65 kcal/kg, and 3.5 g/kg protein. The plain breast milk provides 53 kcal/kg (assuming 20 kcal/30 mL × 80 mL/kg) and 0.7 to 1.2 g/kg protein (assuming 0.9 g/dL in term donor milk and 1.5 g/dL in mom's preterm milk). The current nutrition provides 160 mL/kg, 118 kcal/kg, and 4.2 to 4.7 g/kg protein. When the breast milk is fortified, it will provide 64 kcal/kg and 1.9 g/kg protein. If the TPN/lipids are not adjusted, the infant will get 129 kcal/kg and 5.4 g/kg protein. The TPN/lipids can start to be weaned when enteral fortification begins. Fortification can be adjusted based on total fluid goals to meet estimated energy and protein needs. Vitamin D and iron will likely need to be supplemented, depending on the breast milk fortifier that is used.

On day of life #20, the infant's weight is up 140 g to 1040 g, and is still AGA on the growth chart. Labs show Na 139, K 4.1, Cl 105, BUN 3, Cr 0.4, and glucose 82. The infant is being fed breast milk fortified to 24 kcal/oz (2.4 g/dL protein) at 19 mL q 3 hours with appropriate vitamin D and iron supplementation.

What can be said about growth?

The growth velocity is less than 15 to 20 g/kg, so a nutrition intervention is needed. Growth velocity will falter before the overall trend on the growth chart is impacted. The practitioner should act now.

What is an appropriate nutrition plan?

The infant is receiving 146 mL/kg, 117 kcal/kg, and 3.5 g/kg protein. Additional calories and protein can be provided by increasing the total feeding volume to 160 mL/kg and weight adjusting frequently every 2 to 3 days for optimal intake. If volume cannot be increased, the team could consider adding a liquid protein modular to increase protein intake or increasing fortification to increase calorie and protein intake. The impact on

Continued

CASE 5.1—cont'd

the volume of breast milk should be considered, as increasing fortification most often decreases the volume of breast milk.

On day of life #45, the infant's weight is up to 1650 g and is still AGA on the growth chart. Labs show Na 138, K 4.2, Cl 104, BUN 10, Cr 0.3, glucose 77, Alk Phos 330, and phosphorus 6.1. According to unit policy, the infant is 33 weeks and appropriate to transition off donor milk to feedings of mother's milk as available or formula. Recent growth has been 19 g/kg. The infant is rooting in skin to skin but is otherwise sleepy.

What can be said about growth?

Growth is appropriate. The practitioner should also be following for head circumference and linear growth measurements. The bone labs show low risk for osteopenia.

What is an appropriate nutrition plan?

Mother's milk would still be provided as available. If quantities are sufficient for fortification and waste would be minimal, fortification could be continued. As the infant cues, he could transition to breast feeding. Donor milk could be changed to a preterm formula to provide the most calories, protein, and micronutrients to this former ELBW infant who still has increased needs for catch-up growth. Vitamin D and iron supplements could be adjusted as needed to account for additional amounts in formula. As breast feeding is established and the infant shows feeding cues, the infant could work on bottle-feeding. Depending on growth at discharge, this infant could be sent home on a variety of feeding options including plain human milk with a few supplements of fortified human milk, preterm formula, or preterm discharge formula. Special considerations should be made to optimize breast feeding success and minimize risk with powder infant formulas, which are not sterile.

PART 2: SELECTED DISORDERS OF THE GASTROINTESTINAL TRACT

Michael Dingeldein

Anomalies of the GI tract may involve any part of the primitive tube from the hypopharynx to the anal dimple. The most common are atresias, stenoses, duplications, and functional obstructions. Vascular occlusions, sometimes resulting from rotational anomalies and intussusceptions, may be in utero factors in atresias and stenoses. Findings can include the following:

- History of hydramnios
- Increased salivation, cyanosis, and choking with feedings
- Large gastric aspirate (>25 mL) in delivery room
- Vomiting, especially bile stained
- Abdominal distention with or without visible peristalsis
- Failure to pass a stool or delayed passage of stool

Definitions

Atresia is complete luminal discontinuity of the GI tract, ranging from the shortest segment web to complete loss of a major segment of bowel and mesentery. Multiple atresias may occur throughout the intestinal tract, especially in the jejunoileal segments.

Stenosis is a narrowing that may involve the entire thickness of the bowel wall or may be merely a partial web.

Duplications may vary from simple cyst like projections into the mesentery to complete replication of any length of the GI tube, with or without luminal continuity with the in-line segment. They may occur anywhere along the GI tract and manifest as obstructions, as perforations, or a palpable mass.

Functional obstructions are those that are not associated with anatomic malformation. They include achalasia, pyloric stenosis, and aganglionic megacolon, all of which have some component of myoneural dyscoordination in their etiologies. Meconium ileus and meconium plug syndrome caused by abnormalities of intraluminal contents represent another type of functional obstruction.

Imaging

The role of imaging varies from helping establish a diagnosis to evaluating associated abnormalities and planning surgical solutions. Imaging may serve as a therapy for conditions such as meconium ileus and meconium plug syndrome. Plain radiographs and bowel contrast examinations serve as primary imaging modalities. Ultrasound, computed tomography (CT) scan, and magnetic resonance imaging (MRI) play roles in more complex cases.

Ultrasound can help correctly identify meconium ileus and meconium peritonitis, and is useful in the diagnosis of enteric duplication cysts and intussusception. CT and MRI can provide superb anatomic detail and added diagnostic specificity in malrotation and anorectal anomalies. Intestinal duplications manifest as an abdominal mass at radiography, contrast enema examination, or ultrasound. On CT scan, most duplications manifest as smoothly rounded, fluid-filled cysts or tubular structures with thin, slightly enhancing walls. On MRI scan, the intracystic fluid has heterogeneous signal density on T1-weighted images and homogeneous high signal intensity on T2-weighted images. Familiarity with these GI abnormalities is essential for correct diagnosis and appropriate management.

CASE 5.2

A pregnancy is complicated by polyhydramnios. A full-term male infant presents with increased salivation and choking with feedings. Vomitus is never bile stained. Subsequently, respiratory distress develops. On physical examination, the infant is noted to be blue when crying and salivating excessively. The abdomen is distended. No obvious external malformation is noted. The x-ray film from the referring hospital is reported to demonstrate aspiration pneumonia.

Discussion: With a history of polyhydramnios and increased salivation, a likely diagnosis is esophageal atresia. The presence of abdominal distention suggests that atresia is associated with a fistula between the esophagus and trachea. The absence of bile staining of the vomitus indicates obstruction proximal to the entry of the common duct into the duodenum, that is, the esophagus.

A baby with esophageal atresia plus or minus tracheoesophageal fistula classically manifests with respiratory distress, choking, feeding difficulties, and frothing in the first few hours after birth. Neonates are unable to swallow, which accounts for the overflow of saliva, and they are vulnerable to aspirate into their lungs. A nasogastric tube will stop in the upper pouch.

The diagnosis may be suspected antenatally because of polyhydramnios and an absent fetal stomach bubble detected on ultrasound. In the absence of other anomalies, the prenatal detection rate approaches 50%. A karyotype should be obtained because of potential association with trisomy 18. Mortality is significantly higher in prenatally diagnosed infants and in infants with additional congenital anomalies and prematurity. Isolated esophageal atresia is associated with good outcome.[136]

Diagnostic Maneuver

Pass a radiopaque nasogastric tube until it stops, and obtain an x-ray film, including neck, chest, and upper abdomen. When passing a nasogastric tube for a diagnostic maneuver in suspected esophageal atresia, use as large a tube as will pass the nares. A small tube may enter the larynx and pass down the trachea, through the fistula to the esophagus, and into the stomach, giving the false impression of esophageal continuity. A large tube will not be tolerated in the larynx. If the tube passes through the esophagus to the stomach, esophageal atresia is ruled out.

X-Ray Findings in Esophageal Atresia With Tracheoesophageal Fistula

- There is a wide, air-filled pouch in the neck or upper mediastinum.
- The nasogastric tube is seen to stop in the upper mediastinum at about T3.
- Aspiration pneumonia may be noted, usually in the right upper lobe.
- Parts of the abdomen show air in the intestines (often as an excess amount). With atresia and no fistula, there is a gasless abdomen.
- Often, skeletal anomalies are present (vertebrae/ribs).
- The VATER association is a nonrandom association of vertebral defects, imperforate anus, tracheoesophageal fistula, and radial and renal dysplasia. The association may be broadened by the inclusion of cardiac defects and limb abnormalities (VACTERL).

Management Considerations in Esophageal Atresia[136–141]

More than 90% of all patients with esophageal atresia have the common variety of blind upper esophagus with the lower segment entering into the membranous posterior portion of the trachea above the carina as a fistula. This connects the acid-filled stomach to the tracheobronchial tree. A small percentage of cases have esophageal atresia without tracheoesophageal fistula, in which case the abdomen is airless. From the first suspicion that a fistula exists until complete separation of the esophagus from the trachea is achieved, proper management is essential to prevent the fatal complication of aspiration pneumonia. Aspiration from the proximal pouch into the larynx is prevented by withholding all feedings and continuously aspirating the pouch with a sump tube. Reflux of gastric juice into the fistula is more damaging and more difficult to prevent but can be offset by attention to optimal positioning and by early surgical intervention. The child should be maintained in the prone, head-elevated position, which allows the stomach to fall anteriorly away from the esophagus and provides an inclined esophagus as a retardant to reflux of gastric juice.

Fistula ligation and primary repair of the tracheoesophageal fistula should be done early in the hospitalization to prevent respiratory deterioration. Preoperative chest x-ray and echocardiogram are key to evaluate for other anomalies and help determine the aortic arch position. The surgical repair can be done open or thoracoscopically, depending on the comfort of the surgeon.

In patients who have respiratory instability, or extreme prematurity, it may only be possible to initially control the fistula. Once the fistula is ligated, either transthoracic or transabdominal, and the respiratory status stabilizes, then a staged operation can be done to establish esophageal continuity.

In unstable patients or patients with long-gap esophageal atresias, primary esophageal repair may not be possible. Mouth-to-stomach continuity can then be restored either by a staged repair such as a Foker procedure or by esophageal replacement using the stomach or colon. The goal, if possible, is to always use native esophagus. Cervical esophagostomy in esophageal atresia when initial repair cannot be made makes sham feeding necessary. This teaches the child the mechanics of swallowing and supports the oral gratification so essential in this period for later motor development.

Choudhury and colleagues have confirmed excellent results even in infants with birth weights less than 1500 g.[141] Death is associated with complex cardiac and chromosomal anomalies.

Overall survival now exceeds 90% in dedicated centers. Associated congenital heart defects and LBW can affect survival. Early mortality is usually attributed to cardiac and chromosomal abnormalities. Late mortality is usually attributed to respiratory complications.

DUODENAL OBSTRUCTION

Sonographic findings suggestive of duodenal atresia include a dilated fluid-filled stomach adjacent to a dilated proximal intestinal segment, showing the classic fetal "double bubble" sign. The diagnosis can be made in the early second trimester but more commonly is made in the third trimester when the duodenum becomes more dilated. Polyhydramnios develops in up to 50% of cases.

Fetal dilated or echogenic bowel is a marker for a variety of conditions, including bowel obstruction, chromosomal and congenital infectious disorders, and cystic fibrosis. Jackson reported on 35 fetuses with echogenic bowel, of whom 12 babies underwent surgery for intestinal atresia,[142] meconium ileus, and duplication cysts. Postoperative courses and outcomes were good. They concluded that echogenic bowel on antenatal ultrasound is a nonspecific marker for a variety of disorders, including intestinal atresia. Although associated with higher rates of fetal loss, the majority of neonates are normal at delivery. Obstruction of the duodenum may be complete or partial and caused by extrinsic (malrotation, annular pancreas) or intrinsic lesions (duodenal atresia, duodenal stenosis). Malrotation is the most common extrinsic lesion obstructing the duodenum and, because of the potential for vascular compromise to the bowel, it constitutes a true emergency in the neonate. Vomiting is the predominant manifesting symptom and, if the obstruction is below the second part of the duodenum, it will be bile stained. Duodenal atresia is commonly associated with trisomy 21.

X-Ray Findings in Duodenal Obstruction

- Plain x-ray film of the abdomen revealing a "double bubble," that is, the air- and fluid-filled stomach and duodenum.
- The presence of air bubbles beyond the second part of the duodenum suggests incomplete obstruction.

Management Considerations in Duodenal Obstruction

Killbride warned that infants with congenital duodenal obstruction,[143] particularly if breast fed, may not present with classic findings of upper GI obstruction in the first days of life. Careful in-hospital evaluation of infants with persistent regurgitation, even low volume, is recommended to avoid missing this diagnosis. There are other diagnoses that warrant emergent surgery that may be confused with duodenal obstruction. An upper GI series is indicated if malrotation is suspected. It is also important to rule out midgut volvulus, either by foregut contrast study or directly by diagnostic laparoscopy.

St. Peter reported on 408 patients with duodenal atresia.[144] There was a 28% incidence of trisomy 21. Only two patients (0.5%) were identified as having a second intestinal atresia. In this, the largest series of duodenal atresia patients compiled to date, the rate of a concomitant jejunoileal atresia is less than 1%. This low incidence is not high enough to mandate extensive inspection of the entire bowel in these patients, and a second atresia should not be a concern during laparoscopic repair of duodenal atresia. Duodenoduodenostomy is the procedure of choice to correct duodenal atresia and may be done open or laparoscopically.

JEJUNOILEAL ANOMALIES

Atresia is more common than stenosis, with ileal lesions being more common than jejunal lesions.[145] It has been postulated that these lesions arise from intrauterine bowel ischemia. Anomalies that produce obstruction of the small intestine may manifest with bilious vomiting, abdominal distention, and obstipation. The combination of bilious vomiting and passage of blood by rectum signifies vascular compromise of the intestine, necessitating immediate operative intervention. Atresias and stenoses must be differentiated from meconium ileus and meconium peritonitis, as described later.

X-Ray and Other Imaging Findings in Jejunoileal Anomalies

- Plain radiographic studies may show nonspecific bowel dilation. It is extremely difficult to distinguish small bowel from colon in the neonatal period.
- Contrast enemas may show a microcolon together with one or more focal small bowel stenoses.

Dalla Vecchia et al encountered 277 neonates with intestinal atresia and stenosis between 1972 and 1997.[146] The level of obstruction was duodenal in 138 infants, jejunoileal in 128, and colonic in 21. Of the 277 neonates, 10 had obstruction in more than one site. Duodenal atresia was associated with prematurity (46%), maternal polyhydramnios (33%), Down syndrome (24%), annular pancreas (33%), and malrotation (28%). Jejunoileal atresia was associated with intrauterine volvulus (27%), gastroschisis (16%), and meconium ileus (11.7%). Operative mortality for neonates with duodenal atresia was 4%; with jejunoileal atresia, 0.8%; and with colonic atresia, 0%. Cardiac anomalies (with duodenal atresia) and ultrashort bowel syndrome (<40 cm) requiring long-term total parenteral nutrition, which can be complicated by liver disease (with jejunoileal atresia), are the major causes of morbidity and mortality. The long-term survival rate for children with duodenal atresia was 86%; with jejunoileal atresia, 84%; and with colon atresia, 100%.

Management Considerations for Jejunal Abnormalities

The majority of patients with intestinal atresia have a single lesion and normal length of bowel, making the primary repair relatively straightforward, although they can take a prolonged time postoperatively to achieve all of their caloric needs enterally. The atretic bowel did not develop normally, with the distal part small and proximal part grossly distended, leading to motility issues, especially early in the course. Patients with complex atretic bowel, such as type IIIB lesions, can be particularly challenging to manage. Associated congenital anomalies adversely affect outcomes in jejunoileal atresia.[147]

There are several surgical approaches, but all with the same objective: to restore intestinal continuity. They may be managed with laparoscopic or open procedures.

MALROTATION/VOLVULUS

Incomplete rotation and fixation of the embryonic intestine as it returns to the fetal abdominal cavity from its embryonic extracoelomic position is referred to as malrotation.[148] The normal alignment of the gut has the distal duodenum crossing to the left of the vertebral column to join the jejunum at a normally positioned ligament of Treitz with the cecum in the right lower quadrant. With malrotation, the cecum is undescended and situated in the right hypochondrium, abnormally fixed by bands crossing the second part of the duodenum.

Fetal bowel obstruction has a prevalence of 1 in 3000 to 5000 live births. Ultrasonographic diagnosis is made by demonstrating distended loops of bowel, fetal ascites, or echogenic bowel. Echogenic bowel, defined as small bowel more echogenic than liver or bone, in addition to bowel obstruction, has also been associated with congenital infections, cystic fibrosis, and chromosomal abnormalities.

Malrotation may be associated with other GI lesions, including duodenal atresia, small intestinal atresia, gastroschisis, omphalocele, and congenital diaphragmatic hernia as well as cardiac, renal, and other major anomalies. Malrotation may manifest with bile-stained vomiting and abdominal distention. The obstruction may be intermittent, causing a mild presentation. Alternatively, there may be a dramatic manifestation with bile-stained vomiting, abdominal distention, possibly an abdominal mass, shock, pallor, and bloody stools. This manifestation signifies a volvulus (i.e., occlusion of blood flow to the gut), which mandates emergent exploration.

X-Ray and Other Imaging Findings for Malrotation/Volvulus

- Plain films of the abdomen may reveal a distended proximal bowel and stomach, with air patterns visible beyond the duodenum.
- Malrotation or volvulus is standardly diagnosed with upper GI contrast studies. The major purpose of the study is to establish the anatomic relationships with the duodenum crossing the midline.
- A sharp cutoff with curved narrowing of the distal duodenum is characteristic of an obstruction secondary to a volvulus.

If there is any doubt concerning the diagnosis, an exploratory laparoscopy or laparotomy is mandatory because the integrity of the bowel may be rapidly compromised by vascular occlusion.

Management Considerations

Volvulus of the bowel can be a fulminant and fatal condition. Rapid diagnosis and prompt surgical intervention are mandatory. The traditional approach to a suspected volvulus was a barium enema examination; however, this only provided indirect evidence of a volvulus if the cecum was not in the right lower quadrant. Volvulus of the small bowel may occur with a normal rotation and position of the colon. Therefore an upper GI approach has been adopted to establish the diagnosis. Both the site of obstruction and often the cause can be identified in this manner.

Intestinal malrotation in neonates or infants requires urgent surgical treatment, especially when volvulus and vascular compromise of the midgut are suspected. Hagendoorn wished to determine whether laparoscopy for the treatment of malrotation has a success rate equal to that of open surgery.[149] Successful laparoscopic treatment of intestinal malrotation could be performed in 75% of the cases ($n = 28$), and conversion to an open procedure was necessary in 25% of the cases ($n = 9$). Postoperative clinical relapse because of recurrence of malrotation, volvulus, or both occurred in 19% of the laparoscopically treated patients ($n = 7$). They concluded that "diagnostic laparoscopy is the procedure of choice when intestinal malrotation is suspected." If present, malrotation can be treated adequately with laparoscopic surgery in the majority of cases. Nevertheless, to prevent recurrence of malrotation or volvulus, a low threshold for conversion to an open procedure is mandated."

MECONIUM ILEUS

Meconium ileus is a luminal obstruction of the distal small intestine by abnormal meconium, in contrast to meconium plug syndrome, which is a colonic obstruction. Meconium ileus is seen predominantly in patients with cystic fibrosis. The infants present with bile-stained vomiting and abdominal distention, and the meconium-filled loops have a doughy feel. The sonographic findings associated with meconium peritonitis in utero include polyhydramnios, ascites, dilatation of the bowel, hyperechoic bowel, and the telltale sign of intraabdominal calcification, which is pathognomonic of meconium ileus.

Imaging Findings of Meconium Ileus

- Obstruction with a characteristic soap bubble appearance produced by the air trapped in the thick meconium. Intrauterine perforation (meconium peritonitis) with the passage of sterile meconium into the peritoneal cavity may be reflected by calcification and predisposes to intestinal obstruction from adhesive bands.
- The diagnosis may be confirmed with a water-soluble diatrizoate enema, which may also be therapeutic because it facilitates passage of the tenacious meconium. The study is contraindicated if signs of peritonitis or pneumoperitoneum are present.

Management Considerations of Meconium Ileus

The preferred treatment for simple meconium ileus is a gastrografin enema. Complicated meconium ileus and those who fail nonoperative management will need to undergo a bowel resection with temporary enterostomy or resection with primary anastomosis. The prognosis for these patients is very promising, with recent studies showing 1-year survival rates as high as 100%.

MECKEL DIVERTICULUM

The omphalomesenteric duct usually obliterates spontaneously during embryonic development. Umbilical anomalies arise from fetal structures such as the omphalomesenteric duct or urachus, or from failure of closure of the umbilical fascial ring. Persistence of the omphalomesenteric duct may lead to several anomalies including umbilical sinus, umbilical cyst, Meckel diverticulum, or patent omphalomesenteric duct.[150] A patent omphalomesenteric duct is usually associated with the ileum; rarely, it may be associated with the cecum or appendix. If the duct remains patent at the umbilicus, the umbilicus is constantly moist from intestinal secretions, whereas persistence of a blind duct produces a "strawberry" tumor at the umbilicus. Persistence at the ileal end is noted in 2% of the population and results in Meckel diverticulum, which often also contains ectopic gastric and pancreatic tissue. Meckel diverticulum may be asymptomatic, or it may manifest with painless rectal bleeding (the result of ulceration caused by gastric secretions) or obstruction. The diverticulum may also serve as the point for an intussusception. Meckel diverticulum can be diagnosed with a Meckel scan if suspected. If the diverticulum is symptomatic or found incidentally, it can be removed by diverticulectomy. If the base of the Meckel diverticulum is so wide that simple transection would narrow the adjacent ileal lumen, a sleeve resection of the ilium should be performed to preserve patency of ilium.

COLONIC LESIONS

Meconium Plug Syndrome

Meconium plug syndrome is part of the spectrum of colonic hypomotility and is seen predominantly in preterm infants and infants of diabetic mothers. Infants with meconium plug syndrome fail to pass meconium in the first 24 hours of life and present with clinical and radiologic features of intestinal obstruction. Rectal examination may prompt passage of meconium with a characteristic white plug; otherwise, a radiographic contrast enema is indicated. This may serve the dual function of diagnosis and therapy. Inspissated meconium may be documented in the distal colon with dilation above. The contrast examination may precipitate passage of the meconium plug and relieve the symptoms. It is important to recognize that a meconium plug may be associated with cystic fibrosis and Hirschsprung disease. Hence if the symptoms persist or recur, the infant should have a sweat chloride test and rectal mucosal biopsy.

Krasna reported a series of 20 babies with birth weights between 480 and 1500 g who appeared to have an unusual type of "meconium plug syndrome,"[151] which required a contrast enema or Gastrografin upper GI series to evacuate the plugs and relieve the obstruction. Many of the mothers were on magnesium sulfate or had eclampsia. The plugs were diagnosed late rather than shortly after birth, and the plugs were significant, extending to the right colon.

Greenholz identified 13 patients who underwent treatment for intestinal obstruction secondary to inspissated meconium.[152] The average birth weight was 760 g. Prenatal and postnatal risk factors included intrauterine growth restriction, maternal hypertension, prolonged administration of tocolytic agents, patent ductus arteriosus, respiratory distress syndrome, and intraventricular hemorrhage. Stooling was absent or infrequent during the first 2 weeks of life. The infants had abdominal distention or perforation between days 2 and 17 of life. Twelve patients required operative intervention. Findings invariably included one or more obstructing meconium plugs with proximal distention, and the dilated segments were frequently necrotic. None of the patients had cystic fibrosis. The markedly premature infant is at risk for obstruction and eventual perforation secondary to meconium plugs, presumably formed in conjunction with intestinal dysmotility. This entity must be distinguished from spontaneous intestinal perforation (IP), which occurs in the absence of plugs (see later text). Prompt diagnosis and timely intervention require a high index of suspicion, including close attention to stooling patterns, careful abdominal examinations, and screening radiographs when indicated. Patients with this disorder should be evaluated for cystic fibrosis and may need to undergo a rectal biopsy to rule out Hirschsprung disease.

Neonatal Small Left Colon

Small left colon is a rare entity encountered predominantly among infants of diabetic mothers. The presenting features characteristically include delayed passage of meconium. Radiographic evidence includes dilation of the proximal colon, a clearly delineated transition zone, usually the splenic flexure, and narrowing of the distal colon. Resolution of the problem may be anticipated in the first month of life. Management is expectant, and the need for surgical intervention is rare.

Congenital Aganglionic Megacolon (Hirschsprung Disease)

Congenital aganglionic megacolon occurs in approximately 1 in 5000 births and is the most common cause of large-bowel obstruction in the newborn. It can be life-threatening and should be considered in any neonate with intestinal obstruction. It is more common in males, infants with trisomy 21, and siblings of children with the disorder. Hirschsprung disease is thought to result from defective migration of neural crest cells to the distal colon, leaving a segment of bowel aganglionic and dysfunctional.

Only 10% to 20% of patients with this disorder are first seen in the newborn period. In the infant, symptoms may manifest as acute obstruction, abdominal distention, vomiting, and delay in passing or failure to pass meconium (95% of normal term newborns pass meconium in the first 24 hours of life). Constipation is a prominent feature. Irritability, poor feeding, and failure to thrive are other presenting features. Rectal examination or rectal stimulation, such as with a rectal thermometer, may produce an explosive gush of gas, and meconium may obscure the diagnosis; however, in the absence of rectal stimulation, no stools are passed.

Radiographic Findings of Hirschsprung Disease

- Nonspecific obstructive features, such as dilated loops of bowel and multiple fluid levels with the absence of air in the rectum.
- Barium studies should be performed without prior cleansing enemas. The findings include proximal dilation and distal narrowing in the aganglionic segment. Note, however, that the transition zone may not be clearly defined in the neonate, and the barium may be retained for more than 24 hours.

The diagnosis is established by biopsy, which must be of adequate depth to confirm the absence of ganglia in the nerve plexus.

Management Considerations for Hirschsprung Disease

The most important aspect of early Hirschsprung disease management is the decompression of the colon and decrease of intestinal bacterial load using colonic irrigations. Hirschsprung enterocolitis can cause significant morbidity and mortality. Hirschsprung disease can be successfully treated in the neonatal period with a one-stage endorectal pull-through resecting the aganglionic portion of the colon. Occasionally, because of patient size, stability, or other congenital anomalies, a leveling colostomy is done as a first-stage procedure.

ABDOMINAL WALL DEFECTS

Omphalocele and gastroschisis are major defects of the abdominal wall, resulting in parts of the GI tract remaining outside the abdominal cavity. An omphalocele is covered by peritoneum and is frequently associated with other anomalies (congenital heart disease, trisomy 13 or 18, urinary tract anomalies), and Beckwith-Wiedemann syndrome, which includes macrosomia, macroglossia, omphalocele, and hypoglycemia (see Chapter 11). Omphalocele and gastroschisis patients have malrotation. The pentalogy of Cantrell refers to an omphalocele accompanied by defects in the diaphragm, sternum, heart, and pericardium.

Gastroschisis is a full-thickness opening in the abdominal wall to the right of the umbilicus. The extruded loops of bowel are thickened and covered by a fibrinous peel that develops in the latter part of the third trimester. Atresias, strictures, adhesions, and stenoses of the bowel accompany gastroschisis, but other malformation syndromes are unusual. The atretic areas are secondary to vascular insults.

Both lesions may be identified relatively early in gestation through alpha-fetoprotein screening (see Chapter 2), and the lesions can be accurately delineated with antenatal ultrasound. Delivery should take place at a tertiary center because these cases represent complex management problems. The mode of delivery is determined by obstetric factors; vaginal delivery has not been proven to increase morbidity, mortality risk, or length of stay. Thermal regulation, fluid and electrolyte management, nutritional support, and measures to prevent infection are needed to complement the surgical team.

Gastroschisis and omphalocele are usually considered together because both are congenital abdominal wall defects, yet their anatomy, embryogenesis, clinical presentation, and associated problems are quite different. For gastroschisis, evidence points to environmental teratogens as the cause with little evidence for a genetic cause,[153] whereas for omphalocele, substantial data support genetic or familial factors as a cause, with little evidence for environmental factors. Gastroschisis is rarely associated with other anomalies, although about 15% have intestinal atresias. Some 25% of patients with omphalocele have other serious congenital anomalies, with cardiac lesions being the most common. Definitive treatment for both is a reduction and surgical closure.

INGUINAL HERNIA

Inguinal hernias occur in 1% to 3% of all children, more often in premature infants, in boys more frequently than girls, and more often on the right side than left, but can also occur on both sides. Hernias occur more often in children with a parent or sibling who had a hernia as an infant, cystic fibrosis, developmental dysplasia of the hip, or undescended testes or urethral abnormalities. The prevalence of incarceration of the hernia in infants discharged home is very low. Inguinal hernia repair is one of the most common surgical procedures performed on premature infants. Improved survival rates in the NICU have led to an increase in the incidence of premature infants with inguinal hernias.

CASE 5.3

An infant takes initial feedings and then vomits bile-stained material. He is otherwise asymptomatic. Examination reveals abdominal distention. The anus is patent, and meconium is passed.

Discussion: Any GI obstruction distal to the entry of the common duct into the duodenum can lead to bile-stained vomiting. As a general rule (but not an infallible one), the earlier the onset of bile-stained vomiting, the higher the level of obstruction. Lower-level obstructions usually manifest initially with distention and failure to pass meconium with bile-stained vomiting occurring hours to days later.

X-ray findings vary with the level and type of obstruction. They may be clearly diagnostic, as is the case with complete obstruction of the duodenum (double bubble; duodenal atresia, annular pancreas, occasionally malrotation), or they may be equivocal, as in meconium ileus or Hirschsprung disease.

Eventual diagnosis is forthcoming in every case, given enough time and persistence. In the interim, effective nasogastric decompression and parenteral fluid, electrolyte, and nutritional support by vein sustain most of these infants, even if significant time lapses before diagnosis and definitive therapy. Only those lesions that may lead to catastrophe require urgent diagnosis and treatment, so attention should be directed to recognizing these disorders rapidly. These disorders include malrotation, volvulus, bowel perforations, and aganglionic megacolon.

CASE 5.4

Bilious vomiting, usually with some abdominal distention, occurs in a baby who passed normal meconium and has an open anus. X-ray films may show duodenal obstruction and usually show some gas throughout the abdomen.

Discussion: Malrotation is the most malevolent lesion of infancy because of its propensity toward volvulus with resultant strangulation of the superior mesenteric artery. This catastrophe can lead to total destruction of the digestive-absorptive segment of the intestinal tract—the jejunoileum. Furthermore, compared with any other single anomaly, this lesion is quite common. It must therefore always be in the differential diagnostic forefront to be rapidly ruled in or out. The most direct method for doing so is by upper GI contrast study, which demonstrates obstruction of the duodenum. If obstruction is incomplete, the study reveals that the duodenal C loop fails to complete its normal course to a position in the left upper quadrant behind the stomach—the ligament of Treitz.

Contrast enemas, frequently recommended for diagnosis of malrotation in the past, may be confusing. The high-riding cecum with malpositioned appendix is diagnostic if clearly present, but often the cecal position is equivocal and difficult to locate clearly. Reflux of dye into the ileum may mask the position of the cecum. Therapeutic delay is intolerable here. One should quickly intervene operatively in any duodenal obstruction not clearly caused by an entity other than malrotation.

Intestinal malrotation is a common cause of upper GI obstruction and manifests with duodenal obstruction caused by volvulus of the midgut loop. Patients are at risk of catastrophic midgut infarction, and malrotation is a more frequent cause of duodenal obstruction in infants than duodenal atresia. Bilious vomiting and bloody stools are the two most common clinical presentations in neonates. Rectal bleeding is an ominous sign. Most patients manifesting such bleeding have a gangrenous bowel. Urgent upper contrast studies are necessary. Ultrasound studies may also be helpful as a characteristic pattern of echogenic ascites, thickened bowel wall; dilated, fluid-filled bowel lumen, and lack of peristalsis may be seen in children with gangrenous bowel.

BLOOD IN STOOL

Blood in the stool[154] is a frequent problem confronting the neonatal team. Whether gross blood is present, streaks of blood are on the outside of an otherwise normal-appearing stool, or only occult blood is present, a prompt and diligent search for the cause is mandatory. In many instances, no cause will be found; however, major pathologic disorders accounting for the blood in the stool must be ruled out.

Disorders causing frank blood in the stool range from swallowed maternal blood, an inconsequential problem, to life-threatening disorders, including NEC, malrotation with volvulus, disturbances of coagulation, ulcerative disorders, and infections. Blood-streaked stools are most commonly seen with an anal fissure or following trauma to the rectum with temperature probes and thermometers. Occult blood may signify blood swallowed during breast feeding, upper GI disorders, milk intolerance, hemorrhagic disorders, or NEC.

GI bleeding in the newborn must be differentiated from swallowed maternal blood caused by antepartum hemorrhage, the episiotomy, or cracked, bleeding nipples. The Apt test distinguishes maternal from fetal red blood cells in that the fetal cells are resistant to alkali denaturation (addition of sodium hydroxide). Hence a solution containing maternal blood changes from pink to brown. Other laboratory tests include a complete blood count with a differential and smear; platelet count; coagulation studies such as partial thromboplastin time, prothrombin time, and fibrinogen level; blood culture; and a plain film of the abdomen. These tests should point to the cause of the bleeding, which can then be managed appropriately.

SPONTANEOUS INTESTINAL PERFORATION

Another disorder has emerged among the premature infants. It has been designated spontaneous IP and may be indistinguishable from NEC. Spontaneous perforation, however, occurs much less frequently than NEC in preterm infants. The infants may have dramatic abdominal distention often associated with blue discoloration of the abdominal wall. Obvious clinical signs of bowel perforation are infrequent with spontaneous IP.

Infants with spontaneous perforation are smaller and born more prematurely when compared with infants who had NEC.[155,156] The onset of illness was earlier and was associated with antecedent hypotension, leukocytosis, and a gasless appearance on abdominal radiograph. Infants with spontaneous perforations are more likely to have received postnatal steroids or to have systemic candidiasis. Conditions associated with fetal or neonatal hypoxia are important antecedents for this emerging distinct clinical entity. Other factors implicated in the etiology include indomethacin therapy, patent ductus arteriosus, and intraventricular hemorrhage. Peritoneal drainage alone may be considered definitive therapy for IP in the majority of extremely immature infants. The prognosis for spontaneous IP is better than for NEC (see later).

SUMMARY

Understanding of the basic entities and familiarity with some of the common presentations can help differentiate the conditions. The following are key points when considering neonatal and infant bowel problems:

- Intestinal obstruction may be anticipated in 1 of every 1000 births. Multiple anomalies occur frequently.
- Lesions producing obstruction of the upper GI tract may be associated with maternal polyhydramnios and large gastric aspirates at birth.
- Green (bilious) vomitus is considered an indication of midgut volvulus until proven otherwise.
- Clinical features of intestinal obstruction include vomiting, abdominal distention, visible peristalsis, and delayed passage of meconium. With upper GI obstruction, meconium may be passed, but no transitional stool is seen.
- GI obstruction between the pylorus and the ligament of Treitz is considered malrotation until proven otherwise.
- When the continuity of the GI tract is clearly demonstrated postnatally by the passage of transitional stools, air, or contrast medium, congenital atresia can be excluded as the cause of the obstruction. Meconium may be passed from the bowel distal to a complete obstruction, so passage of meconium does not exclude obstruction.
- Colonic obstruction may manifest with the same constellation of symptoms as upper GI obstruction. Particular note is taken of delayed passage of meconium (Hirschsprung disease, meconium plug syndrome).
- In patients younger than 2 years, it is hazardous to attempt to differentiate large from small bowel on the basis of plain abdominal radiographs, particularly because the frequent errors in this evaluation may lead to delay in diagnosis and therapy for an obstructive bowel lesion.
- An entity that can obstruct the bowel may also lead to perforation and the resulting signs and symptoms of peritonitis. Thus when peritonitis is the presenting symptom, an obstructing lesion must be sought and corrected.

TABLE 5.12 **Modified Bell's Staging Criteria for Neonatal Necrotizing Enterocolitis**

Stage	Systemic Signs	Intestinal Signs	Radiologic Signs	Treatment
IA—Suspected NEC	Temperature instability, apnea, bradycardia, lethargy	Elevated pregavage residuals, mild abdominal distention, emesis, guaiac-positive stool	Normal or intestinal dilation, mild ileus	Nothing by mouth, antibiotics for 3 days pending cultures
IB—Suspected NEC	Same as above	Bright red blood from rectum	Same as above	Same as above
IIA—Definite NEC: mildly ill	Same as above	Same as above, *plus* diminished or absent bowel sounds with or without abdominal tenderness	Intestinal dilation, ileus, pneumatosis intestinalis	Nothing by mouth, antibiotics for 7–10 days if examination is normal in 24–48 hr
IIB—Definite NEC: moderately ill	Same as above *plus* mild metabolic acidosis and mild thrombocytopenia	Same as above *plus* definite abdominal tenderness, with or without abdominal cellulitis or right lower quadrant mass, absent bowel sounds	Same as stage IIA with or without portal vein gas, with or without ascites	Nothing by mouth, antibiotics for 14 days, $NaHCO_3$ for acidosis
IIIA—Advanced NEC: severely ill, bowel intact	Same as IIB *plus* hypotension, bradycardia, severe apneas, combined respiratory and metabolic acidosis, disseminated intravascular coagulation, neutropenia, anuria	Same as above *plus* signs of generalized peritonitis, marked tenderness, distention of abdomen, and abdominal wall erythema	Same as stage IIB, definite ascites	Same as above *plus* 200 mL/kg/day fluids, fresh frozen plasma, inotropic agents; intubation, ventilation therapy; paracentesis; surgical intervention if patient fails to improve with medical management within 24–48 hr
IIIB—Advanced NEC: severely ill, bowel perforation	Same as stage IIIA	Same as stage IIIA	Same as stage IIB *plus* pneumoperitoneum	Same as above *plus* surgical intervention

PART 3: NECROTIZING ENTEROCOLITIS

Michael Caplan

NEC remains the major GI cause of morbidity and mortality among the neonatal intensive care population. The incidence varies among countries and among units. Uauy et al,[157] reporting on behalf of the National Institute of Child Health and Development Neonatal Multicenter Research Network, noted that 10% of 2681 infants with birth weights between 501 and 1500 g had proven NEC (Bell stage II and beyond) (Table 5.12). Approximately 7% of all babies with birth weights below 1500 g will develop NEC. Most infants with NEC have a low birth weight, are immature, and develop the disease between 28 to 32 weeks postconceptional age.[158–160]

The age of onset for NEC varies inversely with gestational age. In approximately half of the term infants with NEC, symptoms manifest in the first day of life. Specific risk factors for NEC among term infants include cyanotic heart disease, polycythemia, birth asphyxia, and twin gestation. Whereas sporadic cases of endemic NEC occur throughout the year, temporal and geographic epidemic clusters are associated with a variety of pathogens, including *Staphylococcus Aureus*, *Clostridia*, and other organisms.

An altered intestinal microbiome coupled with an unbalanced proinflammatory response in a high-risk premature infant may lead to the final common pathway of intestinal necrosis. Many studies have identified an abnormal microbiome in preterm infants (as compared with full-term infants), and furthermore, there is a different microflora in preterm infants who develop NEC compared with those whose intestinal tracts remain healthy. The inflammatory response in preterm infants is weighted toward proinflammatory signaling; these patients have impaired antiinflammatory capacity to down-regulate an activated response. Studies have identified several potential factors that contribute to this exaggerated proinflammatory signaling, including excessive nuclear factor kappa beta and interleukin 8, and decreased platelet activating factor acetylhydrolase and single immunoglobulin interleukin-1 related receptor function, and these factors may have genetic underpinnings.

Clinical classifications and the pathogenesis of the disease are outlined in Tables 5.13 and Figs. 5.5. In addition to the abnormal intestinal microbiome and dysregulated inflammatory responses, inciting events for NEC may include hypoxemia, sepsis, low cardiac output, and factors within the bowel such as hypertonic and high-volume feeding. Although feeding precedes the onset of symptoms in most cases, delayed feeding has not been shown to clearly reduce the risk for NEC, and therefore early hypocaloric feedings are recommended to

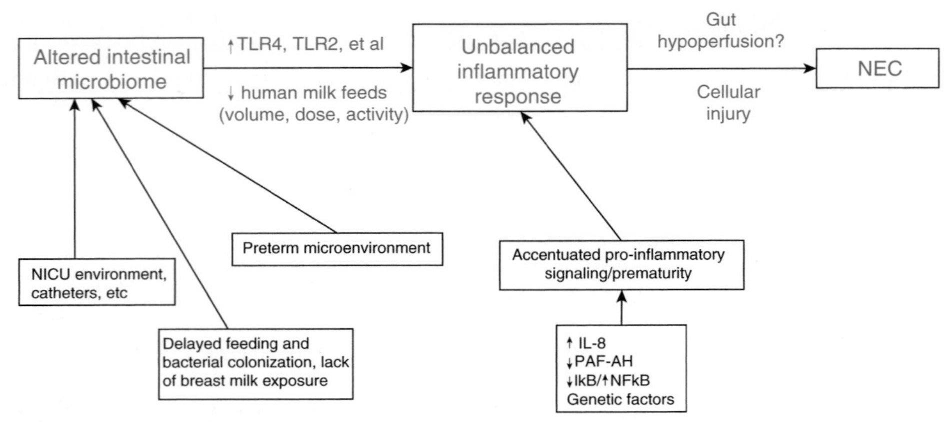

Fig. 5.5 Proposed pathophysiology of necrotizing enterocolitis *(NEC)*. *NICU*, neonatal intensive care unit.

prevent hyperbilirubinemia, mucosal atrophy, and feeding intolerance.[161]

Gut ischemia is a potential risk factor for NEC. Intrauterine growth-restricted infants with aberrant fetal Doppler blood flow velocity waveforms and infants born to cocaine-abusing mothers show increased rates of NEC.[162–164] In addition, cocaine-exposed infants with NEC are more likely to require surgical intervention, have massive gangrene, or die.[162]

EDITORIAL COMMENT: The search for predictive markers of NEC has been inconsistent, although some might have clinical utility, including C-reactive protein, hydrogen breath test, interleukin-8 (IL-8), platelet-activating factor, stool calcitonin, and, most recently, complement 5a, cytosolic beta-glucosidase, serum amyloid A, and salivary H secretor phenotype.[165–167] In these studies, most markers were measured at the time of NEC diagnosis, and unfortunately, patients will only benefit if a marker is discovered that predicts NEC before the diagnosis is made. Chabaan has identified interalpha inhibitor protein (Ialp) as a potential marker of NEC.[168] Ialps are serine protease inhibitors that modulate endogenous protease activity and improve survival in adult models of sepsis. The beneficial effects of Ialp appear to be via suppression of proinflammatory cytokines such as tumor necrosis factor alpha rather than augmentation of IL-10. The impact of Ialp may be significantly greater than that of a just as reliable predictive marker for NEC—Ialp may be useful in the treatment of this dreaded disease. It has been shown that serine proteases initiate a cell death pathway in epithelial cells, and this mechanism may contribute to the pathogenesis of NEC.[169] If so, low Ialp levels because of consumption or immaturity would lead to prolonged serine protease exposure and may contribute to increased epithelial cell death. It seems plausible that exogenous Ialp could reduce serine protease effects, and in animals, Ialp treatment has reduced the risk of death in a neonatal sepsis model.[170] Additional studies are needed to explore the possible role of Ialp in the diagnosis and treatment of neonatal NEC.

In summary, NEC is a multifactorial disorder with a delicate balance between nutritional exposures, bowel perfusion, intestinal microflora, and host inflammatory responses. In small studies completed many years ago, the disorder was reduced by prenatal and/or postnatal administration of steroids,[171] and by the postnatal administration of immunoglobulin A.[172] Breast milk is also protective, as shown by Lucas and Cole in a multicenter study addressing the role of diet in NEC.[61] Furthermore, pasteurizing the milk did not reduce its effectiveness, and the combination of breast milk and formula was less likely to be associated with NEC than formula alone. Breast milk contains a myriad of bioactive factors that modulate bacterial adherence and pathogenicity, increase probiotic colonization, and reduce proinflammatory signaling. For many reasons, human milk should be the standard-of-care feeding regimen for all premature infants.

Late-onset sepsis and NEC may result from bacterial translocation. Lactoferrin (LF) is a multifunctional protein and has antimicrobial, antiinflammatory, immunoregulatory, and growth-promoting properties. All of these contribute to the prevention of bacterial translocation in VLBW infants. Manzoni et al observed a significant reduction in late-onset sepsis among VLBW infants fed bovine LF (BLF).[86] Incidence of late-onset sepsis was significantly lower in the BLF and BLF plus *Lactobacillus rhamnosus* GG groups (5.9% and 4.6%, respectively), compared with the control group receiving placebo (17.3%). The decrease occurred for both bacterial and fungal sepsis. No adverse effects or intolerances to treatment occurred. When BLF and *L. rhamnosus* GG were given enterally to the infants, NEC was significantly decreased compared with controls.

Aceti et al included 6600 premature infants in a meta-analysis of prospective, randomized trials, and demonstrated significant reduction in NEC for those supplemented with probiotics compared with placebo (2.6% vs. 5.7%, $P < .05$, risk ratio 0.47) without any significant side effects.[173] Although probiotics are used as standard of care in several countries, they are currently not approved by the FDA for use in the

United States to prevent NEC in premature infants, as efficacy with specific product formulations, adequate quality control, and safety considerations have not been completed.

CLINICAL FEATURES

The clinical features of NEC are variable, and the signs and symptoms may not be specific.[174] Most often, temperature instability, lethargy, abdominal distention, and retention of feedings develop. Occult blood is present in the stools, which may sometimes reveal frank blood. Reducing substances are often detected before the onset of NEC. Apnea may be a prominent feature as well as bilious vomiting, increased abdominal distention, acidosis, and disseminated intravascular coagulation. The characteristic x-ray features are pneumatosis intestinalis, with bubbles or layers of gas in the wall of the bowel as well as portal venous gas. Free air within the peritoneum is associated with perforation of a viscus. Engel et al demonstrated that about 30% of the gas in the wall of the bowel is hydrogen,[175] the product of bacterial fermentation of carbohydrate substrate.

Medical management includes nasogastric suction, IV fluids, and broad-spectrum systemic antibiotics (Appendix A-2). Frequent abdominal examinations as well as determination of abdominal girth and cross-table lateral x-ray films are important to detect free air. Infants should be maintained on a regimen of nothing per os for 7 to 14 days while they receive all nutritional support intravenously. The main indication for surgery is perforation, which is demonstrated by free air in the peritoneum. However, surgery may also be considered for infants with worsening clinical status, refractory disseminated intravascular coagulation, or acidosis. The discovery of an abdominal mass and gas in the portal venous system is not necessarily an indication for surgery. Some infants may require surgery at a later stage because of the development of strictures. With present vigorous medical and surgical management as outlined earlier, 75% of infants with birth weights above 1 kg should survive.

Perforated NEC is a major cause of morbidity and mortality in premature infants, and the optimal treatment is uncertain. Blakely documented that survival to hospital discharge after operation for NEC or isolated IP in ELBW (<1 kg) neonates was only 51%. Among the 156 enrolled infants, 80 underwent initial peritoneal drainage, and 76 had initial laparotomy.[176,177] Patients with a preoperative diagnosis of NEC have a relative risk for death of 1.4 compared with those with a preoperative diagnosis of isolated IP. They could distinguish on the basis of radiologic findings and age at surgery preoperatively between NEC and isolated IP. The overall incidence of postoperative intestinal stricture was 10.3%, wound dehiscence 4.4%, and intraabdominal abscess 5.8%, and did not significantly differ between groups undergoing initial laparotomy versus initial drainage. By 18 to 22 months, 78 (50%) had died; 112 (72%) had died or were shown to be impaired. Outcome was worse in the subgroup with NEC.

Subsequently, Moss reported from a multicenter randomized trial that compared outcomes of primary peritoneal drainage with laparotomy and bowel resection in preterm infants with perforated NEC.[178] At 90 days postoperatively, 19 of 55 infants assigned to primary peritoneal drainage had died (34.5%), as compared with 22 of 62 infants assigned to laparotomy (35.5%, $P = .92$). They concluded that the type of operation performed for perforated NEC does not influence survival or other clinically important early outcomes in preterm infants.[178] Among ELBW infants, surgical NEC, which is likely to be associated with a greater severity of disease, is associated with significant growth delay and adverse neurodevelopmental outcomes at 18 to 22 months' corrected age compared with infants who did not have NEC.[179] Medically treated NEC does not seem to confer additional risk, and the outcomes are similar to VLBW babies without NEC.

The incidence of surgical short bowel syndrome in a cohort of 12,316 VLBW infants (<1.5 kg) was 0.7%.[180] NEC was the most common diagnosis associated with surgical short bowel syndrome. More VLBW infants with short bowel syndrome (20%) died during initial hospitalization than those without NEC or short bowel syndrome (12%), but fewer than the infants with surgical NEC without short bowel syndrome (53%). Among 5657 ELBW infants (<1 kg birth weight), the incidence of surgical short bowel syndrome was 1.1%. At 18 to 22 months, ELBW infants with short bowel syndrome were more likely to still require tube feeding (33%) and to have been rehospitalized (79%). Moreover, these infants had growth delay with shorter lengths and smaller HCs than infants without NEC or short bowel.

CASE 5.5

C. K. weighs 1300 g at 32 weeks' gestation. His Apgar scores were 4 at 1 minute and 6 at 5 minutes. Respiratory distress syndrome (RDS) develops on the first day of life, an arterial catheter is placed at the level of T10, and 60% oxygen but no assisted ventilation is used. The RDS resolves by 48 hours of life, and the catheter is removed. Standard formula is first fed on the third day of life. On the eighth day, abdominal tenderness and distention are observed, and the nurses reported guaiac-positive stools, 5 mL residual from the last feeding, and a higher incubator temperature required to maintain body temperature.

What is the most likely preliminary diagnosis?

1. Meconium plug syndrome.
2. Necrotizing enterocolitis.
3. Septicemia.
4. Malrotation.
5. Hirschsprung disease.

Any neonate with a triad of abdominal distention, Hematest or guaiac-positive stools, and retention of gastric formula should be suspected of having NEC and should be immediately evaluated for it. The initial manifestation of NEC may be indistinguishable from septicemia, and a positive blood culture is obtained from 30% of infants with NEC. The answer is 2, necrotizing enterocolitis.

Initially, how should this patient be evaluated?

1. Culture of blood, urine, cerebrospinal fluid, and stool.
2. Complete blood count and clotting profile.
3. Barium swallow.
4. Gastrografin enema.
5. Anteroposterior and lateral film of abdomen.
6. Blood gases and serum electrolytes.

1. Because sepsis is present in many of these, blood, urine, and stool cultures should be obtained. In those with positive blood cultures, cerebrospinal fluid collection is warranted.
2. A complete blood count, blood smear, and clotting profile should be ordered and the type and cross-match sent to the blood bank. Take specific note of fragmented red blood cells (disseminated intravascular coagulation), neutropenia (margination of white blood cells), and thrombocytopenia.
3. Barium swallow is not indicated immediately. If there is evidence of obstruction without pneumatosis intestinalis on the flat film, then a barium swallow may be necessary to exclude malrotation.
4. Gastrografin enema may be curative if there is a meconium plug but is contraindicated in this case because the hyperosmolar contrast medium may produce further damage to already compromised bowel and result in perforation.
5. Abdominal x-ray films, both KUB (kidney, ureter, and bladder) and cross-table lateral, should be obtained to detect the presence of pneumatosis intestinalis, hepatic portal gas, or free intraabdominal gas, indicating a perforated viscus. If no free air is seen initially but there is pneumatosis intestinalis present, the cross-table lateral x-ray film should be repeated every 4 to 6 hours or sooner if there is clinical deterioration.
6. Evaluate acid–base status and serum electrolytes in infants with suspected GI disturbances. Correction of these metabolic derangements is crucial before submitting these precarious infants to major surgery.

The x-ray films reveal pneumatosis intestinalis with no air in the liver or free intraperitoneal air. The blood pressure is 55/35; blood gases pH 7.32, PaO2 65, and Pco_2 40; bicarbonate 20; serum sodium 132; potassium 4.8; chloride 105; BUN 10; hematocrit 38%; white blood cell count 14,900 with 70% segmented cells; platelets adequate and clotting profile normal. Pediatric surgeons were consulted and, together with the nursery staff, they managed the case.

The following treatments should be instituted (True or False):

1. Nasogastric suction, IV fluids, and nothing per os (NPO).
2. Systemic and orogastric antibiotics.
3. Laparotomy.
4. Exchange transfusion.
5. Placement of central hyperalimentation line.

1. True. It is imperative to decompress the abdomen with a large oral or nasogastric tube. Carefully record all intake and output, weigh the baby twice daily, and measure abdominal girth frequently. IV fluid therapy must take into consideration significant third-space losses, and significant volume resuscitation is typically required. Patients with documented NEC should be managed with NPO for at least 7 to 10 days.
2. True. The patient was started on appropriate doses of IV ampicillin and an aminoglycoside. False. Antibiotics via nasogastric tube are not efficacious for this condition.
3. False. There is no clear-cut indication for laparotomy at this stage. Whereas surgery is clearly indicated for IP, some centers operate when medical management fails to correct the shock-acidosis, if there is persistent cellulitis of the anterior abdominal wall, or if, radiologically, a single dilated loop of bowel persists.
4. False. Exchange transfusion has not been shown to influence the outcome of NEC.
5. False. TPN is going to be necessary for this infant. However, with septicemia possible, it is advisable to wait until the sepsis has been controlled and the general condition is stabilized before placing a central line for IV nutrition. Some centers provide all nutritive support with peripheral lines using glucose-amino acid mixtures supplemented with IV lipid.

Four hours later, the blood pressure drops from 55/35 to 40/0. The urine output decreases to less than 1 mL/hour, and the abdomen is more distended, edematous, and tender. On physical examination, the infant is pink with a wide pulse pressure, tachycardia, and warm extremities. Repeat complete blood count reveals white blood cell count of 3.1, with 10% segmented cells and 10% bands.

These data should be interpreted as (True or False):

1. Septic shock.
2. Perforated abdominal viscus.
3. Patent ductus arteriosus with congestive heart failure.
4. Pneumothorax.
5. Third-space loss.

1. 1 and 5, True. The patient as described—pink with wide pulse pressure, tachycardia, and warm extremities—has the classic features of warm shock. When such cases are untreated, the blood pressure decreases further, and vasoconstriction predominates, transforming the "warm" shock to "cold" shock. A major factor contributing to shock in patients with

CASE 5.5—cont'd

NEC is the massive third space that develops in the abdomen, which results from the inflammatory response and bowel necrosis. These large fluid and protein losses result in hypovolemia and require urgent therapy. The mainstay of treatment is to elevate the blood pressure by supporting the intravascular space with sufficient blood, plasma, or crystalloid to maintain the blood pressure and urine output. Whole blood is preferred because it remains in the intravascular space, whereas other fluids leak through the damaged capillaries and contribute to intestinal edema. Large volumes of crystalloid may be required. Neutropenia may be documented in NEC without bacteremia. Margination of neutrophils is assumed because marrow reserves are not depleted.

2. False. Although the sudden deterioration is suggestive of perforation and evaluation by transillumination and an x-ray film is certainly indicated, no perforation was present at the time. The wide pulse pressure is not usually detected at the time of perforation.
3. False. Tachycardia, edema, and wide pulse pressure are present with patent ductus arteriosus and congestive heart failure. However, the striking abdominal findings, together with the diminished blood pressure, suggest that this is not the primary problem. Patent ductus arteriosus, however, is found frequently in infants with NEC.
4. False. This is unlikely, given the complete picture, particularly with a pink baby and wide pulse pressure.

Two hours later, x-ray films show increased distention and no evidence of free air but the appearance of bowel "floating" in the abdomen.

What is the significance of this finding?

Bowel floating in the abdomen in a patient with sepsis and a distended tender abdomen indicates ascites caused by peritonitis. Because many cases of "intraabdominal sepsis" are caused by anaerobic bacteria, anaerobic antimicrobial coverage should be started following paracentesis. (Clindamycin is instituted for infants with suspected NEC and perforation.)

On surgically introducing a drain into the left lower quadrant, 10 mL of purulent fluid is removed. The cell count shows 90,000 white blood cells with 75% polymorphonuclear leukocytes. Gram stain shows both gram-positive and gram-negative rods.

The patient is noted to have blood oozing from venipuncture sites, with petechiae and a falling hematocrit despite multiple blood transfusions.

Laboratory Data

CBC: Hct 28; platelets 5000; smear shows fragmented red blood cells and burr cells
Prothrombin time: patient, 50 seconds; control, 10 seconds
Partial thromboplastin time: patient, 180 seconds; control, 30 seconds
Fibrinogen: 50 mg/dL (normal 200 mg/dL)
International normalized ratio (INR): 3.0

Disseminated intravascular coagulation has complicated the picture, and therefore treatment with platelets and fresh frozen plasma is provided.

Blood pressure, urine output, and activity are normal for 3 days. The abdomen is softer, but there is still some edema of the abdominal wall. Repeated x-ray films fail to reveal free intraabdominal air. After 5 days of relative stability, the patient becomes acutely distended with signs of respiratory embarrassment.

Which of the following management options is appropriate?

1. Repeat clotting profile and exchange transfusion.
2. Percuss abdomen and then transilluminate while awaiting x-ray film.
3. Repeat blood cultures and change antibiotics.
4. Measure blood gas and increase environmental oxygen.

1. This acute episode following a period of stability cannot entirely be attributed to disseminated intravascular coagulation.
2. This acute change is probably as a result of IP. Abdominal percussion used to demonstrate the absence of hepatic dullness and positive transillumination may confirm suspicions before the cross-table lateral x-ray film has been developed. The film in this instance demonstrated free air.
3. Blood culture should be repeated, but there is no reason to change antibiotics at this time.
4. This is only symptomatic management. The basic cause for the abdominal distention and respiratory embarrassment must be determined. The blood gas will indicate the need for ventilatory support.

The child is brought to the operating room where the perforated area of ileum is resected and an ileostomy and colostomy are performed. Two days postoperatively, a central line is placed in the NICU operating room, and TPN is administered via this route for 21 days. After 14 days of being NPO, he was started on breast milk and did well.

CASE 5.6

M. P. is born at 34 weeks' gestation, weighing 1200 g. His perinatal course is complicated by intrauterine growth restriction, hyperbilirubinemia, and polycythemia, requiring a single volume exchange transfusion done through an umbilical venous catheter. At 8 days of age, abdominal distention, hematochezia, acidosis, and hypotension develop. NEC is diagnosed and is treated with medical management. He recovers and begins enteral feedings 14 days after the onset of acute NEC.

M. P. is discharged home at 6 weeks of age, having tolerated full-volume enteral feedings for 2 weeks. Three weeks after discharge, he has acute abdominal distention, vomiting, and hematochezia. Abdominal examination reveals guarding and tenderness.

What is the most likely diagnosis?

1. Clostridium difficile infection.
2. Intestinal stricture.
3. Anal fissure.
4. Milk protein allergy.

Strictures are one of the most common complications of NEC, occurring in 10% to 35% of all survivors.[181,182] They result from healing and cicatricial scarring of an ischemic area

Continued

CASE 5.6—cont'd

of bowel.[183] Signs include hematochezia, vomiting, abdominal distention, and sudden bowel obstruction. Strictures usually manifest in the first 2 months following acute NEC, but may occur as late as years later.

Which of the following management options is appropriate?

1. Perform stool culture and start oral antibiotics.
2. Change infant to soy formula feedings.
3. Obtain abdominal x-ray, do barium enema, and consult pediatric surgery.
4. Reassure the mother that rectal bleeding is common; send child home with office follow-up in 1 to 2 days.

1, 2, and 4. False. Any neonate with history of NEC followed by the onset of hematochezia and vomiting should undergo evaluation to rule out strictures. Recent reports have suggested that clinical observation alone is associated with significant morbidity in this population. Failure to rapidly detect and manage stricture complications has resulted in IP and life-threatening sepsis.[184]

3. True. Proper management includes abdominal x-rays, barium enema, and pediatric surgical evaluation.

Abdominal x-rays reveal acute intestinal obstruction. Barium enema demonstrates multiple strictures of the ileum, transverse and descending colon, and rectosigmoid region, as well as perforation with intraperitoneal contrast extravasation.

Emergency ileostomy is performed. Postoperatively, M. P. has a rocky course, complicated by multiple episodes of sepsis and feeding intolerance. He is given several courses of antibiotics and nearly 3 weeks of total parenteral nutrition.

Approximately 1 month after surgery, M. P. is noted to have direct hyperbilirubinemia, poor growth, hepatomegaly, and elevated liver function tests. Work-up includes a negative hepatitis panel, normal hepatic and gallbladder ultrasound, negative sepsis, TORCH (*to*xoplasmosis, *r*ubella, *c*ytomegalovirus, and *h*erpes simplex) work-ups, and a normal newborn screen.

What is the most likely diagnosis?

1. Biliary atresia.
2. TPN cholestasis.
3. Alpha-1 antitrypsin deficiency.
4. Cystic fibrosis.

Although all of the above are possible, the most likely diagnosis is TPN cholestasis. It typically develops after 2 or more weeks of enteral fasting with TPN providing the sole nutritional support. With initiation of trophic feeding to enhance bile flow, TPN cholestasis gradually resolves over 1 to 3 months. Some studies have suggested that the exclusive saturated fatty acids with no PUFAs in the United States. TPN preparations contribute to this condition. If symptoms persist despite enteral feeding, a full diagnostic work-up is indicated.

By 6 weeks after operation, M. P. has advanced to full-volume enteral feedings with slow resolution of the TPN cholestasis. However, he continues to demonstrate poor growth and develops increasing stool output through the ileostomy. He undergoes a second surgery to reanastomose the bowel. Following reanastomosis, M. P.'s nutritional status improves, and he is discharged to home. At 10 months of age, he is tolerating a normal diet, although he remains at the third percentile for all growth parameters.

6

Genetics, Inborn Errors of Metabolism, and Newborn Screening

Shawn E. McCandless, Kimberly A. Kripps

The Human Genome Project and the technological and information advances that it enabled mark the shift in clinical genetics from an observational and descriptive field to one of precise molecular diagnosis with a growing repertoire of meaningful therapeutic interventions. In the lifetime of most practicing senior neonatologists, that means going from a few recognizable syndromes, chromosome anomalies, and multifactorial birth defects to the more than 6000 phenotypes listed at the Online Mendelian Inheritance in Man (OMIM) website that have a "known" molecular basis. Using the search term "congenital" in OMIM identifies nearly 3600 listings.

Regardless of one's experience, the volume of genetic information now available can be overwhelming. New tests and new testing methods seem to appear daily. New (and staggeringly expensive, in some cases) treatments for rare diseases emerge regularly. The reality is that the essential elements of good patient care have not changed, but more than ever, the practicing clinician needs a framework around which to organize their thinking about genetic problems. This chapter aims to accomplish that goal using an approach based on presentation in the NICU. It addresses birth defects, inborn errors of metabolism (IEM), newborn screening (NBS), and congenital neurologic abnormalities, providing an overall approach to diagnosis, critical elements of the initial evaluation and management, and when and how to involve other specialists. Finally, there is a brief discussion of newer methods of genetic testing that are revolutionizing care of the ill neonate.

EDITORIAL COMMENT: Regarding the newer methods of genetic testing, "The rapid advancement of next-generation sequencing (NGS) technology and the decrease in costs for whole-exome sequencing (WES) and whole-genome sequencing (WGS), has prompted its clinical application in several fields of medicine. Currently, there are no specific guidelines for the use of NGS in the field of neonatal medicine and in the diagnosis of genetic diseases in critically ill newborn infants. As a consequence, NGS may be underused with reduced diagnostic success rate, or overused, with increased costs for the healthcare system."[a] Van Diemen[b] prospectively studied the speed and yield of rapid targeted genomic diagnostics in 23 critically ill children younger than 12 months where a quick diagnosis could not be made after routine clinical evaluation and diagnostics. Targeted analysis of 3426 known disease genes was performed by using WGS data. They measured diagnostic yield, turnaround times, and clinical consequences. A genetic diagnosis was obtained in 7 patients (30%), with a median turnaround time of 12 days (ranging from 5–23 days), including the identification of a new microdeletion in a child with a cardiomyopathy. They concluded that rapid targeted genomics combined with copy number variant detection adds important value in the neonatal and pediatric intensive care setting. We concur.

([a]Borghesi A, Mencarelli MA, Memo L, et al. Intersociety policy statement on the use of whole-exome sequencing in the critically ill newborn infant. *Ital J Pediatr.* 2017;43:100;
[b]van Diemen CC, Kerstjens-Frederikse WS, Bergman KA, et al. Rapid targeted genomics in critically ill newborns. *Pediatrics.* 2017;140(4). e20162854.)

HISTORY AND PHYSICAL EXAMINATION

Most of the information needed for genetic assessment is standard in the evaluation of the ill neonate. Pregnancy history, including careful documentation of exposures to medications and potential environmental toxins, is important, as is information about maternal illness that may impact embryonic development (e.g., diabetes mellitus, thyroid disease, or autoimmune disorders). Special attention should be paid to the history of pregnancy loss in the parents or family, other infants and children with health problems, and potential consanguinity (often associated with parents from a social structure with limited diversity or cultural norms that encourage marriage between cousins).

Physical examination is not different from standard approaches in the neonatal intensive care unit (NICU), although special attention should be paid to some aspects that may be overlooked during the initial assessment. Examples include evaluation of the umbilical cord looking for the typical three vessels; evaluation of the placenta for abnormalities or diagnostic clues; careful evaluation of the palate and uvula, looking for evidence of subtle manifestations of clefting (palpable defects of the hard palate with a submucosal cleft or bifid uvula), especially if the infant is to be intubated; evidence of skeletal malformation of extremities or chest, or even evaluating number and appearance of digits before tape is applied during intravenous (IV) placement; hypogonadism in females may be indicated by lack of the typical clitoral enlargement present in the newborn; skin pigmentation defects can be easily overlooked in the ill neonate, and should be specifically looked for as surrounding equipment and coverings are applied; and absence of typical posturing in the newborn as an indicator of subtle hypotonia.

Historically, there has been a perception that certain "dysmorphic" findings are critical. This can sometimes be misleading. "Low-set ears," fifth finger clinodactyly, unilateral single transverse palmar crease, and increased "sandal gap" between the first and second toes are all examples of findings that may have some diagnostic significance but should not by themselves be drivers of further investigation. An infant with low muscle tone and "low-set ears" requires a careful genetic evaluation for the hypotonia, regardless of the facial appearance. It is rare that subtle "dysmorphic" findings in the absence of other more significant medical issues will lead to a diagnosis that changes patient management. There are certain findings that are critical in that they may indicate underlying defects not apparent superficially. Examples include very closely spaced eyes that can be associated with holoprosencephaly, abnormal chest shape or disproportion of extremities that may indicate an underlying skeletal abnormality, or patchy skin hyper- or hypopigmentation that may indicate a variety of genetic disorders.

Common laboratory tests performed in ill neonates may also carry clues to genetic abnormalities, particularly persistent abnormal findings that are not explained by other known diagnoses. Examples include persistent metabolic acidosis that may indicate a defect in metabolism of a specific organic acid (high anion gap) or underlying kidney disease (normal anion gap, hyperchloremic acidosis), persistent increases alanine aminotransferase and aspartate transaminase, which may indicate underlying liver or muscle disease, unexplained abnormal blood clotting parameters that could indicate liver disease or inherited coagulation defects, or persistent diffuse abnormalities of urine analytes that are reported normalized to urine creatinine that could indicate an underlying defect of creatine (and creatinine) synthesis.

Other clinical signs that suggest the possibility of an underlying genetic disorder are the involvement of multiple organ systems that are not easily explained by hypoxia or other findings. Any organ malformation, especially the brain, should raise the question of a genetic abnormality. Premature delivery or fetal distress during delivery that are not clearly related to recognizable causes should also raise the level of suspicion for an underlying genetic disorder. It is worth remembering that problems in labor and delivery with abnormal neurological status in the first days of life are common in infants eventually determined to have underlying genetic disorders; thus, difficulty in labor and delivery may be the first indication of an underlying genetic disorder, rather than the cause of later neurological findings.

BIRTH DEFECTS AND MULTIPLE CONGENITAL ANOMALIES

Major structural birth defects are discovered in 1 of every 33 births.[1] Birth defects may occur as a result of maternal exposures or an abnormal uterine environment; however, the vast majority have an underlying genetic cause.

The first steps in the workup of any infant found to have a birth defect are a thorough physical examination to look for any other abnormalities that may be associated with the original finding and to define the phenotype through ancillary tests and imaging (Box 6.1). Imaging studies to look for internal defects of the heart and kidneys should be performed and an ophthalmologist consulted to do a formal eye examination. Depending on the malformations present, further imaging and laboratory evaluation may be warranted.

BOX 6.1 Recommendations Following the Discovery of any Major Birth Defect

Physical Examination

- Examine the head for shape and size, patency of the fontanelles, ridging of the sutures, presence of cutis aplasia or other scalp defects.
- Examine the sclera of the eyes, assess for colobomas.
- Examine palate (palpate with finger and also be sure to visualize the uvula—an abnormally shaped uvula may be indicative of a subtle soft palate defect).
- Assess the extremities paying attention to limb lengths, bowing or abnormal alignment of the limbs, range of motion of the joints, number and shape of the digits, presence of syndactyly.
- Examine the abdomen for the presence of large hernias, other abdominal wall defects, and hepatosplenomegaly.
- Assess the genitalia for development of the external sex organs, ensure anal position and patency.
- Examine the spine, looking for hair tufts or dimples indicative of a vertebral defect or cord tethering.
- Examine the skin for appropriate pigmentation, hypo- or hyperpigmented lesions, bullae, abnormal scaling, abnormal hair growth.

Imaging/Procedures

- Echocardiogram
- Renal ultrasound
- Hearing examination

Consultations

- Ophthalmology for eye examination
- As indicated by findings

Aneuploidies

Multiple, severe congenital anomalies in conjunction with or without an underlying heart defect should always raise suspicion for a chromosomal abnormality (Table 6.1). Chromosomal microarray (CMA) is now the preferred method of assessing for gains and losses of genetic material (also referred to as copy number variants, or CNV). In the case that an aneuploidy is highly likely, evaluation by karyotype or fluorescence in situ hybridization may be sufficient to confirm the diagnosis. If CMA is performed, a karyotype can still be valuable and can be performed at the same time or in series to rule out a complex rearrangement or balanced translocation disrupting an important gene or genomic region.

FISH (fluorescence in situ hybridization) testing utilizes fluorescent probes that are designed to hybridize to specific regions of interest on the chromosomes. It can generally yield a result within 24 to 72 hours and is one of the fastest genetic

TABLE 6.1 **Cardiac Findings Frequently Associated With Specific Genetic Disorders**

Syndrome	Associated Heart Defects (Most Common)	Gene(s)	Other Physical Findings
Turner syndrome (monosomy X)	Coarctation of the aorta Bicuspid aortic valve	*NA*	Short stature Low-set ears Short neck (webbed neck, low posterior hairline) Broad chest, widely spaced nipples Lymphedema Kidney malformations
Down syndrome (trisomy 21)	Endocardial cushion defects	*NA*	Epicanthal folds Upturned palpebral fissures Flat facial profile, flattened nasal bridge Small mouth, large tongue Hypotonia Single palmar creases, clinodactyly Space between first and second toes (sandal gap toes)
22q11 deletion syndrome	Conotruncal heart defects	*NA*	Low-set ears Tubular nose (hypoplastic ala nasi) Cleft palate, submucosal cleft, bifid uvula Laryngotracheoesophageal abnormalities Kidney anomalies Hypocalcemia Thymus aplasia
Williams syndrome (deletion 7q11.23)	Supravalvular aortic stenosis Peripheral pulmonic stenosis	*NA*	Broad forehead Stellate pattern of the iris Wide mouth with full lips Small chin Hypercalcemia
CHARGE syndrome	Conotruncal defects AV canal defects Aortic arch defects ASD/VSD/PDA	*CHD7*	Colobomas Choanal atresia/stenosis Cranial nerve defects Hearing loss Abnormal external ears Cryptorchidism/hypogonadotropic hypogonadism Growth deficiency Cleft lip/palate Tracheoesophageal fistula
Noonan syndrome	Pulmonary valve stenosis ASD Hypertrophic cardiomyopathy	*PTPN11* *SOS1* *RAF1* *RIT1* *KRAS* *NRAS* *BRAF* *MAP2K1*	Low set ears Hypertelorism Down-slanting palpebral fissures Ptosis Broad/webbed neck Pectus Widely spaced nipples Cryptorchidism
Holt-Oram syndrome	ASD VSD Cardiac conduction defect	*TBX5*	Upper limb malformation (involving the carpal, redial, and thenar bones)
Alagille syndrome	Peripheral pulmonary artery stenosis Tetralogy of Fallot VSD ASD Aortic stenosis Coarctation of the aorta	*JAG1* *NOTCH2*	Liver dysfunction Cholestasis Bile duct paucity Posterior embryotoxon Butterfly vertebrae Kidney abnormalities Pancreatic insufficiency Facial features: prominent forehead, pointed chin, deep-set eyes, hypertelorism, saddle or straight nose

continued

TABLE 6.1 Cardiac Findings Frequently Associated With Specific Genetic Disorders—cont'd

Syndrome	Associated Heart Defects (Most Common)	Gene(s)	Other Physical Findings
Kabuki syndrome	Left-sided obstructive lesions Septal defects	*KMT2D* *KDM6A*	Elongated palpebral fissures with eversion of lateral lower eyelid Arched/broad eyebrows Short columella Large cupped ears Ear pits Cleft lip/palpate Blue sclerae Strabismus Ptosis Anorectal abnormalities Genitourinary abnormalities

ASD, Atrial septal defect; *NA,* not applicable; *PDA,* patent ductus arteriosus; *VSD,* ventricular septal defect.

testing modalities available. FISH can rule in or out a chromosomal aneuploidy with a high level of confidence. However, FISH testing will only reveal the presence or absence of the specific chromosome anomaly that is being assessed and will not yield additional findings of chromosomal duplications or deletions outside of those indicated in the test order. If a specific defect is likely, for example, trisomy 21, FISH is currently the fastest and most cost-effective test.

A karyotype will also determine the presence of aneuploidy with high confidence and would additionally provide information regarding the presence of large chromosomal duplications or deletions, as well as whether the aneuploidy resulted from a balanced translocation in the parent. Karyotypes generally take a longer time to result compared with FISH, which should be considered if making a diagnosis is time sensitive.

Microdeletions and Microduplications

22q11.2 Deletion Syndrome

The 22q11.2 deletion syndrome, previously referred to as DiGeorge syndrome or velo-cardio-facial syndrome before a common genetic etiology was identified, has a prevalence around 1 in 6000 births. The phenotypic spectrum of 22q11.2 deletions is quite variable, and occasionally a previously unrecognized parent will be discovered to carry the deletion after their child is born with a serious cyanotic heart lesion. Thus, any infant born with a conotruncal heart defect should be evaluated for the 22q11.2 deletion, even in the absence of other features of the syndrome, which include palatal or laryngotracheoesophageal abnormalities, low-set ears, hypoplastic alae nasae (nostrils), kidney anomalies, hypocalcemia, or an immune defect. Given the potential for serious adverse symptoms of hypocalcemia, if 22q11.2 deletion is suspected, calcium levels should be monitored while awaiting the genetic testing results.

Williams Syndrome

A diagnosis of Williams syndrome (7q11.23 deletion syndrome) may be difficult to make in the neonatal period based on physical features alone, as the unique facial appearance and personality typical of Williams syndrome may not become clearly apparent until later in childhood. The finding of supravalvular aortic stenosis or peripheral pulmonic stenosis should raise suspicion for the condition and lead to genetic testing. Additional findings of a broad forehead, stellate pattern of the iris, wide mouth with full lips, small chin, or hypercalcemia on laboratory testing would further support testing for Williams syndrome.

Testing for Microdeletions and Microduplications

Targeted FISH testing can be used for the evaluation of common microdeletion syndromes such as 22q11.2 and Williams syndrome (7q11.23 deletion). As with aneuploidy testing, FISH for a specified microdeletion can yield a result in 24 to 72 hours.

For isolated cardiac defects, or when multiple congenital anomalies are present but do not necessarily fit with a classically described syndrome, CMA is the recommended first-tier test. CMA offers a platform for broader testing for small chromosome microdeletions and duplications across the genome. A CMA can be used to test for both 22q11.2 deletion syndrome and Williams syndrome, and also identifies other aneuploidies and CNVs. The turnaround time for a CMA result is generally longer than FISH, ranging from 1 to 2 weeks. Thus, FISH testing offers a faster means to make a diagnosis when a particular chromosomal abnormality is suspected.

Given the large amount of normal variation in the genome across the population, there is always potential for a CMA to reveal a copy number variant of uncertain significance. These variants may represent pathogenic changes, or they could represent benign, normal variation. Testing of asymptomatic parents can usually help to clarify the significance of these changes, although this adds another step to the diagnostic workup. As these variants of uncertain significance can cloud and confuse the diagnostic picture, generally, if there is high suspicion for a particular condition such as 22q11.2 deletion syndrome, targeted testing through FISH is preferred over broader based testing, as this excludes the possibility for unclear variants to be discovered.

Congenital Heart Disease

Congenital heart malformations are a frequent finding in newborns, with an incidence of about 1% in the United States.[2] Of these, about 25% have major structural defects leading to cyanotic disease that often requires early surgical or medical intervention.[2] Any significant heart defect should raise the physician's suspicion for a possible genetic abnormality and prompt a careful investigation to look for other clues that may point to a recognizable underlying syndrome. Associated findings of a cleft lip or palate, eye abnormalities, limb anomalies, kidney and genital defects, or a family history of cardiac malformations can help further guide the genetic evaluation by narrowing the differential diagnosis. A genetic etiology for isolated heart defects is often difficult to identify, given the broad differential diagnosis it encompasses. Many experts, although certainly not all, consider any major cardiac malformation, even in the absence of other syndromic features, as an indication for a basic genetic evaluation, specifically chromosome analysis.

The differential diagnosis for genetic causes of congenital heart disease is extensive, including both chromosomal abnormalities and single-gene defects. Among the chromosomal abnormalities, aneuploidy syndromes such as trisomy 21, trisomy 13, trisomy 18, and monosomy X often have major structural heart malformations. Microdeletion syndromes, including both the 22q11.2 deletion (velocardiofacial and DiGeorge syndrome) and 7q11.23 deletion (Williams syndrome), are also commonly associated with heart defects. Single-gene disorders to consider include CHARGE, Noonan, Holt-Oram, Alagille, and Kabuki syndromes. Heart malformations may also stem from nongenetic causes such as exposure to teratogens. The VACTERL spectrum featuring vertebral anomalies, anogenital defects, cardiac malformations, tracheoesophageal fistula, renal anomalies, and limb defects is not uncommon but should not be considered as a final diagnosis; rather, it is a phenotypic description. Children with VACTERL spectrum defects have been shown to occasionally have CNVs on CMA testing,[3] and recently, overlap with defects of nicotinamide adenine dinucleotide (NAD+) synthesis was identified by genomic sequencing.[4]

Establishing the genetic basis of a cardiac defect in the neonatal time period may not be practical in all circumstances. The diagnostic process may be prolonged, but ruling out the common genetic conditions early on is important, as a confirmed diagnosis will have significant implications for future care. For example, identifying a 22q11.2 deletion would prompt careful monitoring of calcium levels and investigation for an underlying immunodeficiency, both critical elements for management and for counseling the family before taking the child home. Identification of a patient with Alagille syndrome has major implications for monitoring and management of hepatic manifestations. Given the associated morbidity and shortened life expectancy seen with trisomies 13 and 18, diagnosis of either of these conditions may impact decisions to pursue major corrective heart surgery or how aggressive to be with medical therapies.

Evaluation: Many genetic syndromes have characteristic heart lesions, and the finding of a particular lesion should certainly lead to the inclusion of the associated syndrome in the differential diagnosis. The physician should always keep in mind that with most genetic conditions, a wide phenotypic spectrum of disease exists. Thus, the absence of the classic cardiac malformation does not exclude a syndrome from the differential. Table 6.1 lists some of the more common associations.

Following characterization of the underlying heart defect, further evaluation of a neonate with congenital heart disease should focus on identifying any other abnormalities that may help focus the genetic evaluation. These include:

- ophthalmologic examination
- thorough examination of the palate
- renal ultrasound
- examination of the genitalia and determination of patency of the anus
- careful examination of the limbs and digits
- X-rays of the spine

Single-Gene Disorders

There are numerous single-gene disorders that are associated with cardiac defects. As mentioned previously, some of the more commonly described single-gene syndromes shown in Table 6.1 include CHARGE syndrome, Noonan syndrome, Holt-Oram, Alagille syndrome, and Kabuki syndrome. Testing for these conditions involves sequencing of the genes in question. Consultation with a clinical geneticist who is familiar with ordering these tests is recommended when one of these conditions is being considered.

Orofacial Clefts

Orofacial clefts affect approximately 1 in 700 neonates.[5] Cleft lip and/or palate (CLP) is a common feature of many syndromes; thus, once a cleft has been identified, as with other major birth defects, a thorough evaluation for other anomalies needs to take place.

Any child identified with a cleft palate should be evaluated for the Pierre Robin sequence. The Pierre Robin sequence is characterized by a U-shaped palatal cleft accompanied by micrognathia and backward displacement of the tongue (glossoptosis). This can have significant consequences for the airway and may even necessitate intubation or placement of a tracheostomy to ensure airway patency.

Syndromic Cleft Lip and/or Palate

Syndromic causes of CLP include (but are not limited to) Stickler, 22q11.2 deletion (discussed earlier), Treacher Collins, CHARGE, and Smith-Lemli-Opitz (SLO) syndromes.

Stickler Syndrome

Stickler syndrome is an important cause of cleft palate, often in the setting of the Pierre Robin sequence. Apart from morbidity associated with the airway, individuals with Stickler syndrome have high myopia with a significant risk for retinal detachment. Thus, evaluation and long-term follow-up by an ophthalmologist is critical, as is prompt treatment by ophthalmology should any change in vision occur. Stickler syndrome should be suspected in infants with significant myopia in the neonatal period, when hyperopia is the norm. Stickler syndrome is also associated with hearing loss, and thus, audiometry should be performed in the NICU and followed routinely. Stickler syndrome is a clinical diagnosis, but the genetic basis for Stickler syndrome has been established in recent years and includes mutations in one of six collagen genes. Molecular panel testing for these genes should be performed when Stickler syndrome is suspected.

Treacher Collins Syndrome

Treacher Collins syndrome (TCS) is a recognizable autosomal dominant condition caused by mutations in one of three genes: *TCOF1*, *POLR1C*, or *POLR1D*. TCS is characterized by underdevelopment of the facial bones (namely the zygomatic arch and mandible) leading to midface hypoplasia and retrognathia. Choanal atresia and the Pierre Robin sequence can lead to significant airway issues necessitating a tracheostomy. External ear anomalies, hearing loss, colobomas of the lower eyelid, and other refractive errors of the eyes are also common. Cognition in TCS individuals is generally normal, and other organ systems, apart from the facial abnormalities, are usually unaffected.

CHARGE Syndrome

CHARGE syndrome features **C**oloboma, **H**eart defects, **C**hoanal atresia, **R**estricted growth and development, **G**enital anomalies, and **E**ar anomalies. Orofacial clefts are seen in approximately 15% to 20% of patients with CHARGE. Tracheoesophageal fistulas can sometimes be seen, as well as cranial nerve dysfunction, hearing loss, and swallowing problems. The only known gene associated with CHARGE is *CHD7*, which is inherited in an autosomal dominant manner, usually attributed to a de novo mutation in the affected child. One-third of patients with a clinical diagnosis of CHARGE have no diagnostic genetic change in *CHD7*, however, and the diagnosis is made clinically based on the presence of enough features of the condition to meet diagnostic criteria.

Smith-Lemli Opitz

Smith-Lemli Opitz (SLO) syndrome is a congenital disorder resulting from a defect in cholesterol biosynthesis (7-dehydrocholesterol reductase deficiency). A high-arched or cleft palate is a common feature of this disorder. Patients present with a variable degree of other features, which can include microcephaly, facial dysmorphisms (short nose with anteverted nares, broad nasal bridge, long philtrum, micro/retrognathia, blepharoptosis, low-set ears), 2-3 toe syndactyly (a hallmark sign of the condition), genital abnormalities, congenital heart defects, and abnormalities of the kidneys, adrenal glands, lungs, and intestinal tract. Patients may also present with a disorder of sex development (see later). Cholestatic jaundice and neonatal ascites can be observed, likely as a result of liver injury caused by accumulations of upstream products of the cholesterol pathway. Poor growth, intellectual disability, and behavior problems become apparent as the child grows older. Screening for SLO is accomplished by measuring serum 7,8-dehydrocholesterol levels. Significant elevations are indicative of disease. Low cholesterol levels are often observed as well, and there is a correlation with disease severity, magnitude of elevation in 7,8-dehydrocholesterol, and the degree of cholesterol deficiency.[6]

Isolated Cleft Lip and/or Palate

It is not uncommon for CLP to be found as an isolated defect. Numerous studies have been performed in recent years to try and identify the etiology of isolated CLP, and mutations in numerous genes have been revealed. The most common genetic etiology for isolated CLP is Van der Woude syndrome, resulting from mutations in the gene *IRF6*. However, it has become clear that most of the implicated genes, including *IRF6*, have reduced penetrance, and there is a great deal of influence from environmental factors, as well as background genetics, in CLP. As the various genetic causes of isolated CLP have not been found to be associated with the development of any other major medical issues, identifying a genetic basis is typically not pursued, although, in light of the variable penetrance of mutations, a clinically unaffected parent could have an increased recurrence risk identified by molecular testing. It is likely that molecular testing will become more common with increasing knowledge of causative genetic defects and reduction in the cost of testing. Referral to a center experienced in multidisciplinary care of orofacial clefts will allow up-to-date counseling for the family.

The most important information to provide families of a newborn with isolated CLP is the risk for recurrence in future offspring. Generally, regardless of the genetic mutation, a 4% risk for recurrence of CLP can be quoted for any future sibling or offspring of the affected individual. In the case of a unilateral cleft lip without a cleft palate, or a cleft palate without a cleft lip, the recurrence risk to siblings or offspring falls to 2%. In the case of a bilateral cleft lip and palate, the recurrence risk is 6%. The risk further increases in when another affected sibling or offspring is born.[7]

Disorders of Sex Development (Ambiguous Genitalia)

Disorders of sex development (DSD) often present with ambiguous genitalia, but can sometimes not manifest until the neonate displays signs of hypoglycemia, hyponatremia, or shock without appreciable abnormal physical signs. Other DSDs may not be apparent until later in life, such as when a phenotypic female fails to undergo menstruation and is found to have male internal anatomy. The etiologies of the different disorders are numerous and stem from defects in hormonal pathways, chromosomal disorders, as well as defects in genes involved in male patterning during development. Thus, workup for DSD warrants consultation with both endocrinology and genetics.

Ambiguous genitalia can lead to significant parental anxiety and strife. It is important not to label the infant with any particular gender until a genetic sex and etiology of the disordered sex development is determined. Providing the family with resources for psychosocial support in dealing with the uncertainty may be necessary. Furthermore, consultation with urology and surgery may also be warranted for surgical correction of the genitalia once a decision has been made as to which sex the baby will be raised.

For any infant presenting with ambiguous genitalia, the priority is to ensure that they are medically stable with normal blood pressure, heart rate, serum sodium concentrations, and glucose levels. Any abnormalities of these parameters should prompt medical intervention. Once the neonate is appropriately stabilized, the next step is to determine the genetic sex of the baby. This involves sending a karyotype or FISH testing for the sex chromosomes. Knowing the genetic sex of the baby allows the physician to determine if the baby is over- or undervirilized and thus guide further workup. Roughly 80% of all neonates with ambiguous genitalia have an XY karyotype, with 10% to 15% carrying an XX genotype and the rest demonstrating sex chromosome abnormalities.[8]

Abnormalities in blood pressure, hyponatremia, or hypoglycemia, especially in the setting of ambiguous genitalia, should raise concern for adrenal insufficiency. Testing considerations include a serum cortisol, 17-hydroxyprogesterone, testosterone, and growth hormone. Further recommendations may be added by endocrinology. In all cases of ambiguous genitalia, testosterone levels should be measured, even in the absence of blood pressure or chemistry abnormalities. Abnormalities in hormone levels should be addressed by an endocrinologist and treated appropriately. Further investigation as to the etiology of these abnormalities may be warranted as addressed later.

Careful examination of the genitalia should be performed, paying attention to presence of palpable testes, scrotal/labial fusion, phallic/clitoral size, and presence of a urogenital slit/hypospadias. Furthermore, imaging of the internal anatomy to characterize the reproductive organs should be performed. Attention should also be paid to other minor anomalies on physical exam that may indicate a specific disorder of sex development. Hypotonia and feeding issues, in conjunction with hypoplasia of the genitalia in a male, may indicate Prader-Willi syndrome (PWS). Dysmorphic facies, 2-3 toe syndactyly, and undervirilized male genitalia would be suspicious for SLO syndrome. Testicular tissue in a female should be removed to reduce risk of later malignancy.

Congenital Adrenal Hyperplasia

The most common cause of congenital adrenal hyperplasia is 21-hydroxylase deficiency. In this disorder, there is a block in the pathway for aldosterone and cortisol synthesis. Thus, the infant presents with adrenal insufficiency that can manifest with shock-like symptoms of hypotension, hyponatremia, and hypoglycemia. In addition to lack of cortisol and mineralocorticoids, metabolites before the enzymatic block accumulate and are shunted toward the sex-steroid pathway with a consequent increase in androgen production. Increased androgens lead to virilization in females. Genotypic males may not have any apparent genital anomalies but will present similar to females with adrenal insufficiency and salt wasting. Cortisol levels will be low in these patients, and elevations in 17-hydroxyprogesterone are observed.

Other defects in the adrenal-steroid hormone synthesis pathway that can lead to disordered sex development include 11-beta-hydroxylase deficiency, 17-alpha-hydroxylase deficiency, and 3-beta-hydroxysteroid dehydrogenase deficiency. In 11-beta-hydroxylase deficiency, the enzymatic block is distal to that of 21-hydroxylase, and although aldosterone and cortisol production is impaired, there is enough activity in the metabolites before the block to prevent adrenal crisis. However, as the regulatory axis is impaired, the precursors of 11-beta-hydroxylase deficiency accumulate and can be shunted toward androgen synthesis and cause female virilization as well as salt retention and consequent hypertension from the accumulation of mineralocorticoids. 17-alpha-hydroxylase deficiency results in a block in sex hormone synthesis and leads to ambiguous genitalia in XY individuals and failure of pubertal development in all affected individuals. 3-beta-hydroxysteroid dehydrogenase deficiency causes a block in the synthesis of cortisol, aldosterone, and sex-steroid hormones and thus will lead to adrenal crisis in addition to undervirilization in males, with lack of puberty in both sexes. As cholesterol is the precursor for all steroid hormone synthesis, defects affecting cholesterol synthesis and transport can also lead to adrenal insufficiency and virilization issues.

In all cases of congenital adrenal hyperplasia, a definitive diagnosis with molecular testing of the suspected genetic defect should be pursued.

5-Alpha-Reductase Deficiency

Individuals with 5-alpha-reductase deficiency lack the enzyme needed to convert testosterone to dihydrotestosterone (DHT). DHT is a potent androgen for signaling the formation of the external male genitalia, and as a result, males with 5-alpha-reductase deficiency are born with ambiguous or female-appearing external genitalia. As testosterone is still produced, the internal anatomy remains male, and these individuals will still develop and display secondary sex characteristics (although often to a lesser degree than their male peers). Basal levels of serum testosterone and DHT are not reliable for the diagnosis of 5-alpha-reductase deficiency, and stimulation testing with human chorionic gonadotropin is needed to clearly assess whether the levels are abnormal. Molecular testing of the *SRD5A2* gene is generally the best initial test if 5-alpha-reductase deficiency is suspected.

Androgen Insensitivity

Androgen insensitivity syndrome, an X-linked disorder, manifests as a result of complete or partial dysfunction of the androgen receptor. Without normal androgen receptor activity, androgen hormones are unable to exert an effect (or have only a partial effect) on development of the male external genitalia. Thus, males are born with female external genitalia. Imaging studies will reveal an absent uterus and the presence of testes. The vagina often ends in a blind pouch. Unless a karyotype is performed, the diagnosis is often missed, and the baby will be considered a normal female. Other clues in the newborn period for this diagnosis are palpable testes in the inguinal area or an inguinal hernia. Many patients will not be diagnosed until the teenage years when they present for evaluation of primary amenorrhea. In the neonatal period, the diagnosis is generally made through molecular testing of the *AR* gene.

Exogenous Testosterone

A careful history should be taken for any baby born with ambiguous genitalia, but especially in any genotypic females presenting with virilization. Exogenous testosterone use by the father (or mother) during the pregnancy, which may have come in contact with the mother's skin and been absorbed into her circulation, can lead to virilization in the female neonate in the absence of any underlying genetic defect.

Non-endocrine Causes of Disordered Sex Development

When no steroid/hormonal or other phenotypic anomalies are consistent with a specific diagnosis, the next step in the workup of the infant with ambiguous genitalia is to look for genetic changes that may have affected sex differentiation in utero. The first place to start is with chromosome evaluation. The CMA will be able to identify any duplications or deletions of the chromosomes in regions containing genes known to be involved in sex differentiation. These genes include those in the SRY region on the Y chromosome, the *DMRT1* on 9p, and several others. If no chromosomal changes are evident, further investigation with molecular testing, under the guidance of a clinical geneticist or another team experienced in genetic evaluation of DSD, is warranted.

There are multiple chromosomal and single-gene causes of ambiguous genitalia. Discussed are a few of the more common diagnoses to consider, although this list is by no means exhaustive.

WAGR: WAGR syndrome (Wilms tumor, aniridia, genital anomalies, and mental retardation) is a contiguous gene deletion syndrome occurring on chromosome 11p13. The genes in the region include *WT1* predisposing to Wilms tumor and *PAX6* leading to the aniridia. The other features of the syndrome are believed to be secondary to other affected genes in the region. Genital abnormalities can include cryptorchidism (most common), hypospadias, as well uterine and ovarian abnormalities. Ambiguous genitalia can be seen.

SLO: SLO syndrome is a congenital disorder resulting from a defect in cholesterol biosynthesis described previously.

Abdominal Wall Defects

The most common abdominal wall defect identified in the neonate is an umbilical hernia. Most umbilical hernias are small, freely reducible, and do not require any intervention. General guidelines are to repair the defect only if it has not spontaneously closed by 5 years of age. Earlier repair may be required if there are concerns that the hernia is growing in size, is larger than 1.5 cm, or if there are concerns for strangulation of the intestine. In the absence of other findings, genetic workup for an umbilical hernia is not necessary. However, large umbilical hernias can, in some cases, represent an attenuated form of an omphalocele. Thus, if a large umbilical hernia is found in conjunction with other birth anomalies, genetic evaluation (similar to that of an omphalocele, discussed later) should be pursued.

The two most common major abdominal wall defects encountered in the NICU include gastroschisis and omphalocele. The largest distinction between the two is the presence of a peritoneal sac enclosing the abdominal organs extruding through the umbilical ring in an omphalocele, whereas in gastroschisis, the abdominal organs spill out of the abdominal defect without a covering membrane, typically beside the umbilical ring.

Gastroschisis is believed to stem from a vascular insult to the abdominal wall as it is forming. This insult results in failure of the abdomen to fully close, and the opening allows the abdominal organs to extrude from the abdomen during development. The defect is most often to the right of the umbilicus. The finding of gastroschisis (usually identified on prenatal ultrasound) requires careful planning in terms of delivery. It is important that the bowels are wrapped and protected in a plastic covering as soon as the baby is born to protect from water loss and thermal instability. Prompt evaluation and management by a pediatric surgeon is required.

At this time, an identifiable genetic cause for gastroschisis has not been found. The majority (~85%) of these infants do not present with other birth defects, and their prognosis is good in terms of developmental and neurologic outcomes, pending appropriate surgical correction of the abdominal defect without significant complications. Syndromic causes are identified in approximately 15%, typically with other findings or malformations. Genetic testing, specifically CMA, should be considered in most cases, and certainly if there is any other malformation.

Omphaloceles are much more commonly associated with genetic changes; thus, genetic evaluation is always warranted. These babies, too, need prompt surgical attention following birth; however, given that they already have a sac covering their abdominal contents, the risks for infection and water loss are somewhat less. The abdominal contents protrude through the umbilicus with omphaloceles.

Beckwith-Wiedemann Syndrome

Beckwith-Wiedemann syndrome (BWS) should be considered in any baby born with an omphalocele. These babies are generally large for age, can have omphalocele or large umbilical hernia, visceromegaly, large tongue, hemihypertrophy, and they are at risk for hypoglycemia in the newborn period. Given the associated risks for seizures and other morbidities associated with hypoglycemia, careful monitoring of blood sugars is warranted in the newborn period for any baby with an omphalocele or other findings concerning for BWS. BWS results from methylation defects at chromosome 11p15. Therefore, testing for BWS requires targeted methylation studies. Less commonly, maternally inherited mutations in the gene *CDKN1C* can cause BWS. If there is strong suspicion for BWS and methylation testing returns normal, sequencing of *CDKN1C* would be the next step in evaluation.

Aneuploidy

Trisomy 13 also is frequently associated with an inguinal or umbilical hernia or omphalocele. Findings of an omphalocele in conjunction with cutis aplasia, cleft lip, holoprosencephaly, heart defects, polydactyly, or other major malformations warrants an evaluation with FISH for aneuploidies or karyotyping to evaluate for trisomy 13 as well as trisomy 18, which can also be associated with omphalocele, although less commonly.

Other Single-Gene Disorders

Other considerations for a patient with an omphalocele include Donnai-Barrow syndrome, which features craniofacial dysmorphisms, eye abnormalities, hearing loss, and intellectual disability. Donnai-Barrow syndrome is caused by mutations in *LRP2* gene. Fibrochondrogenesis is a severe short-limbed skeletal dysplasia and also often features an omphalocele. Fibrochondrogenesis is caused by biallelic mutations in the *COL11A1* gene. Manitoba oculotrichoanal syndrome is caused by biallelic *FREM1* mutations and is notable for dysmorphic craniofacial features of the hairline, eyes, and nose, and imperforate anus in addition to omphalocele or large umbilical hernia. In the absence of a recognizable syndrome, CMA testing, looking for small chromosomal deletions or duplications, should be performed.

Exstrophy of the Cloaca

A more severe abdominal wall defect is cloacal exstrophy in which there is extrusion of the bladder and rectum along with the abdominal contents of an omphalocele. In individuals with omphalocele and cloacal exstrophy, imperforate anus and spinal defects are also common (sometimes referred to as OEIS complex). The genetic basis of cloacal exstrophy is not well understood, although family studies have demonstrated an increased recurrence risk. Cloacal exstrophy should be evaluated similarly to an omphalocele. Trisomy 18, as well as a few microdeletion syndromes, have been described with cloacal exstrophy; thus, any baby born with these features should have a CMA performed. Isolated bladder exstrophy can also occur. Again, the genetics for isolated bladder exstrophy are not clear, but these babies should at the very least be evaluated with a CMA.

Pentalogy of Cantrell is another complex abdominal wall defect extending rostrally and including the diaphragm and sternum, thus exposing the heart and intestines, usually occurring sporadically. CMA is indicated but typically unrevealing. Like many localized defects, this may represent mosaicism for mutation in a gene whose product is critical for embryonic development.

Diaphragmatic Hernia

As many as 15% of cases of diaphragmatic hernia may be found to have a recognized genetic basis as a result of chromosomal rearrangements and copy number variants (CNV). The most common syndromic association is Fryns syndrome, associated with facial dysmorphism, heart defects, limb anomalies, genitourinary defects, and many other associated birth defects. Death in the neonatal period is typical, and survivors typically have severe neurodevelopmental defects. For isolated cases, the degree of pulmonary underdevelopment determines the outcome, and neurologic and intellectual development can be good. The genetic basis of Fryns syndrome is yet to be identified.

Malformation of Extremities and Skeletal Dysplasia

The differential diagnosis for findings of abnormal limb defects or evidence of a skeletal dysplasia is quite large, and often requires the expertise of an experienced pediatric radiologist and medical geneticist to identify the precise diagnosis. Certain abnormal limb and skeletal findings should trigger the neonatologist to look for some of the more recognizable syndromes. In all cases, abnormal skeletal findings should initiate a workup so that further information is available to the geneticist upon consultation.

Digital Defects

Polydactyly is one of the most common digital anomalies that is encountered in the newborn period. Usually, the polydactyly is postaxial in nature, with the extra digit positioned lateral to the fifth digit. As with any other malformation, a thorough physical evaluation is warranted. In many cases of isolated postaxial polydactyly, a family history will reveal other affected family members with no other significant medical issues. Thus, although there is clearly a genetic component to the polydactyly, workup of the genetic cause is unnecessary, as it is unlikely to contribute to future care of the infant.

Preaxial polydactyly, and especially the much rarer insertional polydactyly, are more commonly associated with genetic syndromes and definitely require further evaluation for associated anomalies. Similarly, syndactyly, in which there is a failure of the involution of the skin between the fingers, can be found as a part of many syndromes. Workup will be determined by the other findings encountered.

Thumb abnormalities are particularly important to pay attention to and should never be dismissed (Table 6.2). Absent thumbs, hypoplastic thumbs, or dangling thumbs can be seen commonly in Fanconi anemia, which requires testing with a chromosomal breakage study or molecular testing. Homozygous mutations in *BRCA2*, *BRCA1*, *PALB2*, and other cancer risk variants are among the causes of Fanconi anemia and are associated with increased of cancer in the carrier parents. Absent or hypoplastic thumbs are also seen in such conditions as Holt-Oram, Duane-Radial Ray, and Yunis-Varon syndromes, all of which feature other congenital anomalies that may require management in the newborn period. Thumb abnormalities are also commonly seen in VACTERL spectrum, but as stated previously, known genetic syndromes should be ruled out before a diagnosis of VACTERL is made.

Shortened hypoplastic digits or transverse limb defects, especially when seen in conjunction with cutis aplasia, should bring to mind Adams-Oliver syndrome, which can be evaluated through molecular testing of six different genes found to be associated with the condition.

Ectrodactyly, known also as split-hand deformity or lobster claw deformity, can be associated with clefting, tooth anomalies (hypodontia, microdontia), and long bone defects. Thus, when ectrodactyly is identified, the oropharynx and long bones should be carefully examined.

Limb Defects

The limb defects that can be encountered range from short limbs, absent limbs or bones, misshapen bones, fused joints, contractures of the joints, fractures, and abnormal mineralization of the joints. When any of these findings is present, the best initial step in workup is to x-ray the affected limb, as well as a full skeletal survey, so as to better characterize the bony abnormalities.

Short Limbs

There are many different types of skeletal dysplasia that can present with foreshortened limbs. The initial evaluation should distinguish the location of the shortening (proximal or distal extremity, or both). Achondroplasia is the most recognized and should not be missed in the newborn period. The characteristic facial features seen in achondroplasia, including macrocephaly, frontal bossing, and depressed nasal bridge, are not as prominent in an infant,

TABLE 6.2 **Examples of More Common Genetic Syndromes Associated With Thumb Abnormalities**

Syndrome	Thumb Abnormality	Gene(s)	Associated Findings
Fanconi Anemia	Absent Hypoplastic Dangling Bifid Duplicated Triphalangeal Long Proximally placed	Autosomal dominant *RAD51* *FANCB* Autosomal recessive >19 genes	Pancytopenia Abnormal pigmentation Deformities of the upper limbs Microcephaly Genitourinary abnormalities Ophthalmic anomalies Congenital heart defects Gastrointestinal abnormalities
Holt-Oram	Absent Triphalangeal Anomalous thenar bones Abnormal opposition of the thumbs Abnormal carpal bone	*TBX5*	Septal defects (atrial septal defect/ventricular septal defect) Cardiac conduction defect Aplasia/hypoplasia of the radius
Duane-Radial Ray	Hypoplastic/aplastic Duplication Triphalangeal	*SALL4*	Limitation in eye abduction (Duane anomaly) Hypoplasia/aplasia/shortening of the radius Ocular anomalies Renal anomalies
Yunis-Varon	Hypoplastic/aplastic thumbs (as well as fingers)	*FIG4*	Microcephaly Micrognathia Cleidocranial dysplasia Facial dysmorphisms Hypotonia Brain malformations Congenital heart disease Absent nipples
Thrombocytopenia-Absent Radii	Thumbs are present	*RBM8A*	Thrombocytopenia Bilateral absent radii

but the limbs will be shortened in comparison to the torso, and the fingers will notably have a trident-like appearance. Respiratory status should be carefully assessed in all infants with achondroplasia, as they are at risk for upper airway obstruction, as well as central apnea as a result of a high prevalence of increased intracranial pressure, hydrocephalus, and/or Chiari malformations, which may lead to compression of the brain stem. Thus, imaging of the head and craniocervical junction should be performed to assess for these conditions in case neurosurgical intervention is required. Polysomnography to assess for apnea and a hearing screen should also be performed in the neonatal period. Achondroplasia is always caused by a mutation at position 1138 of the *FGFR3* gene. When achondroplasia is suspected, targeted testing for this mutation should be performed.

Missing Limbs/Bones

Absence of the bilateral radii should always raise suspicion for thrombocytopenia absent radius syndrome (TAR). Absent radii can also be seen in other conditions such as Fanconi anemia, but TAR is distinguished from these by the presence of both thumbs. Biallelic defects in *RBM8A*, one of which is a null allele (does not make a protein), are responsible for TAR syndrome. Close monitoring of platelet counts while confirming the diagnosis is warranted, as transfusion is often necessary. Continued monitoring of platelets is needed if a diagnosis if TAR is confirmed.

Amelia or phocomelia is classically associated with thalidomide exposure during pregnancy, although since the association was discovered and thalidomide discontinued as a treatment for morning sickness, teratogenicity from thalidomide is no longer a common consideration for these findings. Some genetic causes for phocomelia include Roberts syndrome, which usually presents with other severe congenital malformations, and Holt-Oram syndrome, which can sometimes present with unilateral or bilateral phocomelia and is associated with heart defects. Hypomelia can be associated with vascular insults such as that seen with the Poland sequence, which is proposed to be caused by a defect in the development of the subclavian artery, leading to absence of the pectoralis muscle in addition to hypoplasia of the ipsilateral limb. Amniotic bands can also lead to restricted perfusion to the limb and result in hypoplasia or aplasia of the extremity.

Fractures

The presence of fractures of long bones in the neonate is never normal (with possible exception of clavicular fracture) and should always prompt an investigation for osteogenesis imperfecta (OI).

OI usually results from changes in one of two collagen genes, *COL1A1* and *COL1A2*. The spectrum of disease in OI is quite variable and ranges from a perinatal lethal form to milder forms with increased fractures in childhood and hearing loss later in life. Severe perinatal lethal OI often results in loss of the pregnancy in utero, although some of these infants do survive to birth. Classic findings include dark blue sclera, short and bowed extremities, a disproportionately large head, skin and joint laxity, and multiple fractures or evidence of callouses from in utero fractures. Death usually occurs in the first day to week as a result of pulmonary insufficiency from a small rib cage with or without flail-chest symptoms from multiple rib fractures. More attenuated forms of OI can be seen in the neonatal period as well, with the infant appearing normal but developing fractures with simple cares, or simply having skeletal findings of femoral bowing. Presence of blue sclera is typical in most forms of OI during infancy and should raise consideration for OI if observed. Blue sclera can be seen in other connective tissue disorders, although a diagnosis specifically of OI cannot be made on that finding alone. A definitive diagnosis is achieved through molecular testing of the involved genes.

When OI is suspected, careful handling of the baby is necessary to minimize further fractures. Hearing should be evaluated in the NICU with continued monitoring through life. Treatment with bisphosphonates is common now, although data are still accumulating as to the magnitude of the benefit. When a neonate is diagnosed with OI, an investigation into whether or not the infant would meet criteria or benefit from bisphosphonate therapy should be performed.

Misshapen Bones

The differential for abnormally shaped bones is quite broad and includes many different forms of skeletal dysplasia. Obtaining a skeletal survey is key in these circumstances, as a trained pediatric radiologist is likely to assist in narrowing the differential diagnosis. Conditions to consider include collagen and other connective tissue disorders, lysosomal storage disorders, and mineralization defects such as hypophosphatasia.

Alkaline phosphatase should be measured to rule out hypophosphatasia caused by biallelic mutations in the *ALPL* gene as the cause of a skeletal dysplasia, as enzyme replacement therapy (ERT) is now available to treat this condition. In hypophosphatasia, the serum alkaline phosphatase is very low.

Furthermore, radiographic features of dysostosis multiplex (thoracolumbar kyphosis, platyspondyly, odontoid hypoplasia, paddle-shaped ribs, dysplastic femoral heads) should prompt testing for a mucopolysaccharidosis (MPS) or mucolipidosis disorders with urine mucopolysaccharide and oligosaccharide screening or enzyme testing. The skeletal features of MPS disorders can be subtle in the newborn period but should definitely be evaluated for when a skeletal dysplasia is suspected, especially in an infant with apparent (although likely subtle) coarse features, airway issues, and hepatomegaly. Early intervention with ERT therapies and/or hematopoietic stem cell transplant can significantly improve long term outcomes in some MPS disorders.

Small for Gestational Age

There are many reasons for a baby to be born small. Maternal factors leading to small size include placental insufficiency, maternal diabetes (which can lead to small babies as well as large babies), inaccurate dating, or constitutional small size. When maternal factors are not the case, a genetic etiology is likely. Common genetic causes of small for gestational age (SGA) include Turner syndrome, Russell-Silver syndrome, and other chromosomal abnormalities.

If there are signs of Turner syndrome such as a webbed neck, coarctation of the aorta, kidney abnormality, or lymphedema, FISH for aneuploidy or karyotype can be sent. In other circumstances, the best initial test is CMA. If Russell-Silver is a concern as a result of a limb-length discrepancy (hemihypotrophy), triangular facies, and clinodactyly of the fifth digit, methylation studies of chromosome 11p and testing for uniparental disomy of chromosome 7 may be diagnostic in more than half.

Extreme short stature with birth weight less than 1500 g in a term infant raises concern for a primordial dwarfism syndrome, especially when postnatal catch-up growth is not observed. There are many different types of primordial dwarfism. They can be distinguished based on the presence of certain facial features, head size in proportion to body size, and presence of other congenital malformations. However, after a CMA has been performed to rule out CNV, molecular diagnosis, performed through a large sequencing panel of the associated primordial dwarfism genes, is the best, and most definitive, method to characterize the condition.

Defects of the Intestinal Tract

Defects of the intestinal tract may be identified on prenatal ultrasound or may not be apparent until the infant demonstrates intolerance of feeding or failure to pass stool. Intestinal defects including duodenal atresia, Hirschsprung disease, meconium ileus, and small left colon syndrome are often genetic in nature, but can also stem from maternal factors.

Duodenal Atresia

Duodenal atresia, classically identified with a "double bubble" sign on ultrasound or X-ray imaging, is most commonly associated with trisomy 21. Thus, a karyotype or specific FISH test should be sent in any case of duodenal atresia. If testing for trisomy 21 is normal, CMA should be sent to look for smaller chromosomal anomalies, especially when there are other associated defects.

Meconium Ileus

Meconium ileus represents a diagnosis of cystic fibrosis (CF) until proven otherwise. Close follow-up of the NBS is warranted, as many NBS programs reflex to molecular testing of common CF mutations when there is an elevation of immunoreactive trypsinogen (IRT) on the initial screen. In the case that the NBS is low risk, a sweat test should be performed, and full sequencing of the *CFTR* gene should be sent to look for some of the less common mutations that lead to CF.

Hirschsprung Disease

Hirschsprung disease results from failed migration of neural crest cells during intestinal development leading to aganglionosis of all or part of the intestines or colon. Definitive diagnosis requires a suction biopsy with pathologic confirmation of absence of ganglion cells.

Genetically, Hirschsprung disease can be syndromic or isolated. Trisomy 21 is the most notable of the syndromic conditions. Any baby identified with trisomy 21 who fails to pass stool in the first 24 to 48 hours should be evaluated for Hirschsprung disease. Other syndromic conditions to consider include Mowat-Wilson, Waardenburg, and Goldberg-Shprintzen syndromes. Isolated Hirschsprung disease can also arise from single-gene defects.

When other features on examination and evaluation point to a specific syndrome, genetic testing to confirm that condition should be pursued. In the absence of an identifiable diagnosis, especially in the presence of other phenotypic abnormalities, CMA would be an appropriate initial step in the evaluation to look for small duplications or deletions that encompass the genes known to be associated with Hirschsprung disease. If the CMA is normal, molecular testing through a panel of known genes associated with Hirschsprung would be the next step. Consultation with a geneticist familiar with ordering the testing is advised.

Genetic diagnosis once Hirschsprung disease is identified is important, as it may have significant implications to the family regarding risk for future pregnancies. As with most genetic disease, there is a wide phenotypic spectrum of the condition; thus, a parent may carry a mutation and be unaffected or perhaps have had short-segment Hirschsprung disease, but their child may manifest with complete colonic Hirschsprung or intestinal aganglionosis, which has significantly more impact on their health and morbidity. Furthermore, with a syndromic etiology, a genetic diagnosis may prompt careful investigation or screening for other associated issues. Sensorineural hearing loss is very common with Waardenburg syndrome, and certain mutations in the gene *RET* can lead to Hirschsprung disease as well as multiple endocrine neoplasia syndrome type 2 with a high risk for malignancies in the future.

Renal Malformations

Renal malformations are often found in the context of other syndromic features and should always prompt a thorough examination to look for other abnormalities. It should be kept in mind that decreased kidney function in utero can result in the disruption of normal development; thus, associated findings may not actually be part of a syndrome (having a common underlying cause to the renal disease), but rather a sequence of morphological changes with an isolated kidney defect as the root cause. The most common example of this is when embryonic kidney failure with oligo/anuria leads to oligohydramnios with resultant lung hypoplasia and findings of Potter sequence. Similarly, disruption of urine outflow can lead to massive enlargement of structures proximal to the obstruction including the kidneys, ureters, and bladder. The girth of these structures in the abdomen can disrupt the development of the abdominal musculature, leading to Eagle-Barrett syndrome (prune belly sequence). Potter sequence is often found in association with prune belly sequence.

The finding of bilateral cystic kidneys always warrants evaluation for autosomal recessive polycystic kidney disease (ARPKD); however, other isolated kidney defects may be more difficult to characterize genetically.

Polycystic Kidney Disease

ARPKD presents with bilateral enlarged cystic kidneys. Often, the cystic kidneys are identified on prenatal ultrasound. At birth, the kidneys may be palpable on exam. In severe forms, when the cystic kidneys lead to renal failure in utero and the baby has Potter sequence, outcomes are poor as a result of lung hypoplasia and pulmonary insufficiency. In the absence of pulmonary issues, significant renal insufficiency and hypertension may present in the neonatal period and warrant management by an experienced pediatric nephrologist. With milder disease, kidney failure may not develop until later in life; however, these individuals require close monitoring by a nephrologist. ARPKD may also manifest with hepatic cysts, and thus, the liver should be evaluated with an ultrasound at birth and routinely afterward.

Rare renal cysts may also be found in infants with autosomal dominant PKD alleles, and may be part of a chromosomal deletion that includes the *TSC2* gene associated with tuberous sclerosis.

Dysplastic or Ectopic Kidneys

There are many conditions associated with dysplastic kidneys. Dysplastic kidneys alone are a nonspecific finding, and thus, reliance on other physical anomalies is key to discerning the underlying genetic diagnosis. *PAX2*-related disorders can be associated with isolated renal disease and renal dysplasia, although eye abnormalities often accompany the renal findings. Autosomal recessive defects in the genes involved in the renin-angiotensin system can also lead to isolated bilateral renal malformations. Renal anomalies can also be seen in various chromosomal and microdeletion disorders including Turner syndrome, 22q11.2 deletion syndrome, and 17q12 deletion syndrome.

Unless key features of a single-gene disorder are present, CMA is the initial test of choice in evaluating kidney dysplasia. If the microarray is normal, in the case of isolated bilateral renal disease, the next step would be to send panel testing for known single-gene causes of renal defects. This is best performed under the guidance of a clinical geneticist.

Unilateral Renal Defects

In the case of an isolated unilateral renal defect such as an absent kidney or unilateral multicystic dysplastic kidney, a genetic etiology may be elusive. Unilateral kidney malformations can occur secondary to stenosis of a single ureter, leading to backup of urine into the corresponding kidney with resultant malformation and sometimes involution. The etiology of the stenosis could possibly be genetic, but may also be related to a vascular insult or other idiopathic insult to the ureter during development. If no other anomalies are noted on exam, CMA may be considered to rule out a microdeletion syndrome, but further genetic investigation following a normal microarray is unlikely to be rewarding.

Many other types of birth defects and congenital anomalies can present in a neonate. The general principles described previously will allow the neonatal provider to begin the evaluation with confidence.

METABOLIC ISSUES

Acidosis

Acidosis is a common finding in the neonatal unit, most often resulting from respiratory insufficiency, which is clearly indicated in the blood gas measurements. Occasionally, a metabolic acidosis is present, which can be characterized as high or normal anion gap metabolic acidosis. The anion gap (= sodium-chloride-bicarbonate) represents unmeasured anions in the blood using a measured bicarb from serum electrolyte analysis, as opposed to using a calculated bicarbonate from a blood gas. Potassium is primarily an intracellular cation; thus, most metabolic experts do not include it in the calculation of the anion gap because fluctuations in serum values because of hemolysis can complicate interpretation. An excess anion gap (>15 mmol/L) in the setting of low serum bicarbonate and low pH represents an increased concentration of unmeasured organic acids in the blood and should be further investigated. Lactic acid is the most common unmeasured anion, and can be increased in a variety of settings, most typically hypoxia or hypoperfusion. If the excess of the anion gap (the difference between the measured anion gap and the upper limit of normal) is entirely explained by the measured lactate, then treatment of hypoxia and potential perfusion abnormalities are the priority.

Lactic Acidemia

Persistent lactic acidemia after correction of oxygen delivery to tissues may be an indicator of a defect in glycogen metabolism (in the setting of hypoglycemia), an organic acidemia (with secondary inhibition of pyruvate metabolism), a primary defect in pyruvate metabolism, or a primary defect of the mitochondrial respiratory chain. The first two types of defects are typically apparent from the clinical setting. The latter two defects require additional thought.

The ratio of lactate to pyruvate measured in plasma from simultaneous samples can be helpful in distinguishing primary defects of pyruvate metabolism from respiratory chain insufficiency. In the latter case, reduced nicotinamide adenine dinucleotide (NADH), which cannot be oxidized by the respiratory chain, accumulates in the cell with a matching relative deficiency of its redox partner, NAD+. NAD+ is a required substrate for lactate dehydrogenase, which transfers an electron from lactate to NAD+ to form NADH and pyruvate. If the respiratory chain is insufficient, NADH accumulates with reduction in NAD+ concentration, and as a result, lactate accumulates faster than pyruvate. Thus, the ratio of lactate:pyruvate is elevated to greater than 20. If the lactate is accumulating because of a primary defect in the oxidation of pyruvate with a normal respiratory chain, the ratio will be normal, 10 to 20. It is important to remember that the most common cause of respiratory chain insufficiency, by far, is inadequate delivery of oxygen to the tissues. Primary mitochondrial diseases should only be considered when all questions of oxygenation and perfusion are resolved.

The primary source of lactate and pyruvate is from the breakdown of glucose in the initial anaerobic step of glycolysis, or in the setting of a defect in gluconeogenesis, the production of pyruvate from the carbon backbone of gluconeogenic amino acids. If the defect is in the gluconeogenic pathway (e.g., pyruvate carboxylase deficiency), lactate and pyruvate increase with fasting, and plasma concentrations of lactate should go down with the addition of intravenous or enteral glucose. If the defect is in the oxidation of pyruvate for energy, whether because of pyruvate dehydrogenase complex deficiency or a respiratory chain defect (including hypoxia), adding more glucose will create even more lactate accumulation. Therefore, when treating a patient with lactic acidosis of unknown etiology, close monitoring of plasma lactate should accompany the initiation of IV glucose therapy or enteral carbohydrate administration. Rising lactate may indicate a defect in pyruvate oxidation requiring reduction of IV glucose to the minimum level required to maintain normal blood sugar.

In general, delivery of IV glucose is the first line of treatment for IEM because it will suppress catabolism of endogenous fat and protein. Defects of pyruvate oxidation or the respiratory chain are the exception to this rule, and sustained delivery of high concentrations of IV glucose in that setting can actually make the problem worse. In the setting of lactic acidemia of unknown cause, the response to glucose infusion, carefully monitored over the first few hours, can provide important diagnostic information and in many cases is therapeutic.

The diagnostic evaluation for primary lactic acidemia, as noted earlier, begins with meticulous attention to delivery of oxygen to tissues. When that issue is clarified, and lactic acidemia persists, response to feeding and IV glucose helps to distinguish defects of pyruvate oxidation (more common) from gluconeogenic defects (less common). An important association in the neonatal period is the combined presence of lactic acidemia, hypoglycemia, and hyperammonemia caused by severe defects of pyruvate carboxylase deficiency, the first committed step in gluconeogenesis. Unfortunately, this combination can also occur with organic acidemias and sometimes with fatty acid oxidation (FAO) defects, all of which must also be ruled out (see later). For this reason, the metabolic evaluation of high anion gap metabolic acidosis typically begins with broad-based screening tests.

Organic Acidemias and Fatty Acid Oxidation Defects

High anion gap metabolic acidosis with an excess of unmeasured anions other than lactate usually represents an inborn error of small molecule metabolism in an infant, or consumption of an anionic toxin. The latter is uncommon in neonates. The IEM of most concern in this setting are the FAO defects and the organic acidemias, including branched-chain acyl-CoA dehydrogenase deficiency, or maple syrup urine disease

(MSUD), an organic acidemia that leads to accumulation of several amino acids and is often considered an amino acidopathy. Many reviews of these disorders are available,[9] but a detailed discussion is beyond the scope of this chapter. Rather, it is critical to describe the approach to the evaluation and the initial treatment of suspected small-molecule disorders.

When high anion gap metabolic acidosis (using a measured bicarbonate) is recognized, without a rise in plasma lactic acid large enough to explain the excess gap, a critical blood sample should be obtained as therapy is beginning. Testing should include measurement of:

- blood sugar
- blood lactate
- ammonia
- plasma amino acids
- plasma carnitine and acylcarnitine
- blood or urine ketones
- plasma homocysteine
- liver function tests
- urine for organic acid analysis (obtained as soon as possible)

The laboratory should be contacted to expedite the amino acids, acylcarnitine, and organic acid analyses if there is a high suspicion of an IEM (anion gap >22–25, typically). Ammonia should be collected from free-flowing blood if possible, or with minimal tourniquet time. Rarely, a capillary sample can be used if:

1. perfusion is excellent;
2. the extremity well warmed; and
3. blood flows freely (this is also true for lactic acid measurement).

In the absence of any of these three criteria, a venous or arterial sample should be obtained. Drawing from an indwelling catheter, arterial or venous, is always best. Most laboratories can perform these tests on a surprisingly small amount of serum and plasma, so it is good to contact the lab to enquire about absolute minimum volumes.

The rationale for these tests is apparent, except for homocysteine. Several defects in the metabolic pathway of cobalamin (vitamin B12) can present with acidosis caused by accumulation of methylmalonic acid (MMA) because methylmalonyl CoA mutase requires activated cobalamin (adenosylcobalamin) as a cofactor. Homocysteine, which can be performed rapidly in most laboratories, may be increased as a result of reduced activity of methionine synthetase, another cobalamin-requiring enzyme. It can point toward one of these forms of cobalamin defect and allow initiation of therapy with a therapeutic trial of hydroxocobalamin (1 mg) given intramuscularly or subcutaneously. For short-term use, cyanocobalamin can be substituted if hydroxocobalamin is not available (although most hospitals have the hydroxy form available for treatment of cyanide poisoning).

Ammonia should always be a first-line blood test in evaluating an ill neonate, as hyperammonemia can mimic sepsis, and ammonia can be elevated in both organic acidemias and FAO defects. Ammonia can be artificially elevated if the sample is not spun down and run immediately because glutaminase in red blood cells continuously degrades glutamine to glutamate and ammonia. Plasma ammonia in the first 7 to 10 days of life may be normally up to 100 μmol/L, and most metabolic experts are unlikely to be overly concerned by values even as high as 140 μmol/L. Sample handling defects can rarely cause values higher than this, but artifacts are generally easily identified and do not interfere with diagnosis; therefore, providers should not hesitate to measure ammonia. Organic acidemias, and occasionally severe FAO disorders, can often present with ammonias of 200 to 500 μmol/L, and occasionally over 1000. In the setting of high anion gap metabolic acidosis not fully explained by lactic acidemia, the hyperammonemia is more likely attributed to an organic acidemia or FAO than a urea cycle defect (see later).

Plasma amino acids can be rapidly obtained (typically by the next day) in many institutions. The presence of alloisoleucine with marked elevation of all three branched-chain amino acids, leucine, isoleucine and valine, is pathognomonic of branched-chain 2-ketoacyl-CoA dehydrogenase deficiency, more commonly known as maple syrup urine disease (MSUD). Marked elevations of glycine are characteristic of many of the organic acidemias because the organic acids inhibit the glycine cleavage pathway. Alanine is the transamination product of pyruvate (the enzyme responsible is ALT [alanine transaminase]); thus, it can be markedly elevated in the setting of persistent lactic acidemia when the substrate, pyruvate, accumulates. Alanine can also accumulate when another substrate, ammonia, accumulates. Elevated glutamine is also a marker for hyperammonemia. High glutamine in the setting of low citrulline can be a marker for a defect in the early part of the urea cycle, most often ornithine transcarbamylase (OTC) deficiency. Some other abnormal amino acids are discussed subsequently under the "Abnormal Newborn Screen" heading.

Massive ketosis is rare in a neonate and is strongly suggestive of an organic acidemia, and argues against FAO disorders. The presence of moderate ketosis, on the other hand, should not be misinterpreted as ruling out FAO disorders. Remember that many metabolic defects are partial, and there may be compensatory mechanisms that produce unexpected metabolites.

The indirect markers of organic acidemias, namely ketosis, lactic acidosis, and hyperglycinemia, are often the only clues available in the first several days of management of the ill neonate until the results of more specific tests are available. The NICU should always contact the NBS laboratory in this situation to determine if testing is complete or can be expedited. This is particularly true if the NBS result is normal because the NBS lab will likely prioritize the reporting of abnormal values, so a low-risk result may not be reported as quickly.

Aggressive management of the acidosis, and hyperammonemia if present, are critical to optimizing the clinical and neurological outcome of IEM. The mainstay of treatment is to minimize exposure to the offending substrate, whether it is the amino acid precursor to an organic acid or a fatty acid. This is accomplished by providing safe nutrition to suppress catabolism. Safe nutrition means not giving the substrate that can't be effectively metabolized. Because the offending compound is not apparent early in the evaluation, the safest approach is to give large amounts of IV glucose. This leads to insulin release that stops the endogenous release of fatty acids and drives storage of energy in the form of fat and protein synthesis. If blood sugars are elevated to the point of spilling glucose in the urine, an intravenous insulin infusion should be considered. When the acylcarnitine results return and are not concerning for a defect of fat metabolism, IV intralipid can be added to give more nutrition. IV protein should be withheld for the first 24 hours, but prolonged avoidance can lead to protein catabolism because of inadequate circulating amino acids, which can actually make an organic acidemia (or a urea cycle defect) worse. If enteral feeding is possible, giving a modest amount of protein enterally appears to be the safest way to avoid protein catabolism.

It is worth noting that during the acute phase of treatment of acidosis or hyperammonemia caused by IEM, some anticonvulsants have been suggested to have neuroprotective function in the setting of metabolic and neurometabolic disorders. Consideration should be given to early evaluation for subclinical seizures and preemptive treatment in consultation with the pediatric neurologist.

Some providers give supplemental L-carnitine if an organic acidemia is suspected, although there are few, if any, data supporting the approach. The reasoning is that excess carnitine can help excrete the accumulating organic acid and help to reduce the sequestration of CoA in the mitochondria in the form of acyl-CoAs, which could limit the availability of free CoA needed for the tricarboxylic acid cycle, gluconeogenesis, and other critical pathways. One important caveat to giving L-carnitine is that one should be confident that there is not a long-chain FAO present because the rapid infusion of L-carnitine could, hypothetically, lead to a rapid increase in the arrhythmogenic long-chain acylcarnitines.

FAO defects that present in the neonatal period are typically quite severe variants. They may present with hypoketotic hypoglycemia, or with high anion gap metabolic acidosis, or even with cardiomyopathy. Hyperammonemia may be present. Muscles, especially cardiac muscle, prefer fat as the substrate for energy production; thus, reduced ability to utilize fat for energy production can lead to significant myopathic effects. Diagnosis is typically made by plasma acylcarnitine analysis. Carnitine can cross the mitochondrial membrane with fatty acids covalently bound. The physiological reaction is to carry long-chain fats into the mitochondria, but if there is a defect of FAO in the mitochondria, carnitine can also shuttle partially oxidized fatty acids out of the mitochondria as acylcarnitines, which can be measured in plasma. Excess long-chain acylcarnitine species are suspected to be dysrhythmogenic; therefore, if an FAO defect is suspected, treatment with L-carnitine should be held until the plasma acylcarnitine analysis is complete and is not suggestive of an FAO.

The acute treatment for decompensation in all FAO disorders is to provide glucose, both as a source of energy and to drive insulin release, which inhibits lipolysis and drives fatty acid synthesis and storage, thus alleviating the accumulation of fatty acids in the mitochondria. Treatment with a low-fat diet may be helpful in long-chain FAO defects, and supplementation with medium-chain triglycerides that bypass the block may be helpful. It is important to note that infants with long-chain FAO defects who present with cardiomyopathy have severe forms of the disease that are rarely responsive to diet or other therapy.

Once a specific diagnosis is made, dietary therapy can be initiated, usually in collaboration with a physician and dietician experienced in management of these defects. Some forms of methylmalonic acidemia are partially responsive to hydroxocobalamin, which should be given as a therapeutic trial when MMA is increased. Long-chain FAO disorders can be treated with medium-chain triglyceride oil that bypasses the defect. Supplemental carnitine is recommended by some practitioners as described earlier. Additional specific therapies may be available for other rare defects.

One specific long-chain FAO, long-chain hydroxyacyl-CoA dehydrogenase (LCHAD) deficiency is of special interest in the neonatal unit because heterozygous mothers are at high risk of developing acute fatty liver of pregnancy or HELLP syndrome (hemolysis-elevated liver enzymes-low platelets) during pregnancy with a fetus affected with LCHAD. Infants born to mothers with these conditions should be closely monitored until it is clear that the baby is not affected, either by plasma acylcarnitine analysis or by normal NBS for FAO.

Hyperammonemia

Generally speaking, plasma ammonia concentration in neonates can be higher than in older children and adults. Most metabolic experts consider ammonia values below around100 µmol/L essentially normal in a neonate; values above 150 µmol/L deserve additional evaluation.

> **EDITORIAL COMMENT:** Urea cycle disorders are inborn errors of ammonia detoxification/arginine synthesis, with an estimated incidence of 1:8000. Many patients present with hyperammonemia shortly after birth with the introduction of feeds or later, at any age, leading to death or to severe neurological handicap in survivors. The levels of ammonia will rise until effective dietary intervention is begun, and the patients will become progressively lethargic and eventually deeply comatose. Effective therapy includes alternative pathway therapy and liver transplantation. The nutritional management of patients with urea cycle disorders involves restriction of dietary protein along with provision of adequate protein-free energy, essential amino acid supplements, and vitamins and minerals in combination with nitrogen-scavenging drugs.

However, outcomes remain poor. This may be related to underrecognition and delayed diagnosis as a result of the nonspecific clinical presentation and insufficient awareness of healthcare professionals because of disease rarity. Evidence of hyperventilation and metabolic alkalosis may be a clue to measure a plasma ammonia concentration.

Markedly increased ammonia, typically 400 µmol/L or higher, requires immediate initiation of a plan to provide hemodialysis. The preparation for this should occur in parallel with other treatment maneuvers to try to minimize the total exposure of the brain to high ammonia. Giving IV 10% dextrose with appropriate crystalloid (usually normal or half-normal saline) at 1.5 times the maintenance dose is the starting point and is the highest concentration and delivery that can typically be tolerated by a peripheral vein infusion. If central access is available, more glucose can be given with insulin infusion, if needed. In most cases of organic acidemia or FAO defect, the ammonia will begin to decline with this therapy alone.

Continued rising ammonia should be treated more aggressively, either by beginning dialysis, or, if dialysis is not yet available, loading with IV nitrogen scavengers (sodium benzoate and sodium phenylacetate) as well as with IV arginine. These compounds are expensive and can have serious side effects if administered incorrectly, so involvement of a provider experienced in their use should be sought, if possible. Defects of the urea cycle presenting in the newborn period with altered mental status and ammonia greater than 400 to 500 μmol/L are unlikely to be corrected solely with scavenger therapy, so this treatment should not delay the initiation of dialysis.

Urea Cycle Defects

The amino acid analysis typically contains enough information to narrow down the diagnosis in urea cycle defects. Glutamine is typically increased, as is alanine, and potentially other amino acids that can be synthesized from transaminases. In the proximal pathway defects, with OTC deficiency the most common defect, citrulline concentrations are low. Other, rarer proximal urea cycle defects include carbamoyl phosphate synthetase (CPS) deficiency and N-acetylglutamate synthetase (NAGS) deficiency. Massive elevations of citrulline usually indicate argininosuccinic acid synthase deficiency, also known as citrullinemia type I. Moderate elevation of citrulline with the accumulation of argininosuccinic acid in the blood is diagnostic of argininosuccinic acid lyase deficiency. Arginine is typically normal or somewhat low in all of the urea cycle defects, except for argininemia as a result of arginase deficiency, where it is markedly increased. Arginase deficiency does not typically present in the newborn period with hyperammonemia.

Definitive diagnosis is usually confirmed by DNA testing, but occasionally enzyme testing is needed. OTC deficiency, in particular, may not have an identifiable mutation in 15% to 20% of cases. The proximal enzymes in the urea cycle (NAGS, CPS, and OTC) are only expressed in liver, so liver biopsy may be needed if molecular testing is not diagnostic. OTC deficiency leads to accumulation of carbamoyl phosphate in the liver, which can be shunted to pyrimidine synthesis via orotic acid that can be increased in blood and urine. Orotic acid is not elevated in CPS or NAGS, distinguishing OTC from the other proximal defects.

A specific therapy is available for NAGS deficiency. N-carbamylglutamate (Carbaglu) replaces the missing N-acetylglutamate (the product of NAGS) to activate CPS. If molecular DNA testing is not readily available, and the metabolite findings are suggestive (low orotic acid and low citrulline in the setting of hyperammonemia), one might consider a therapeutic trial of N-carbamylglutamate. In most cases of NAGS deficiency, the hyperammonemia will resolve rapidly, and other treatment can be safely withdrawn. Unfortunately, because it is most easily treated, NAGS deficiency is the rarest urea cycle defect.

Typically, it is best to avoid excessive restriction of protein intake for more than 24 to 48 hours because the resulting deficiency of plasma amino acids leads to endogenous protein breakdown and increased ammonia production. When possible, giving protein enterally is the best and most physiological approach. Most infants with urea cycle defects of organic acidemias require at least 1.5 to 1.7 g/kg/day of protein, which is often given as a mix of intact protein from breast milk or regular formula and special elemental formulas depleted in specific offending amino acids and enriched with essential amino acids. If the infant is unable to take enteral feeds, IV forms of protein can be used. IV protein should be administered as a separate infusion, rather than as part of a total parenteral nutrition formulation, as frequent adjustments in the protein infusion may be needed. If not already obtained, consultation with a physician experienced in the management of infants with hyperammonemia is valuable when ammonia has stabilized at an acceptable concentration and transition to chronic therapy is needed.

ABNORMAL NEWBORN SCREEN

The widespread implementation of population-based NBS has been a major public health success since the mid-1960s; however, in the population of premature and low-birth-weight (LBW) infants, screening is complicated. Physiological differences in these infants, and the lack of understanding of how these differences affect the appropriate cutoff values for NBS, mean that false-positive results are much more common in LBW infants than in infants with normal birth weight. Further, the treatments given in the NICU may increase the risk of uninterpretable results (i.e., blood product transfusion or IV total parenteral nutrition supplementation).

Amino Acids

One of the more common reasons to need a repeat sample for the NBS is to have multiple amino acids above the cutoff values. This has been more prominent since the recognition of improved outcomes of LBW infants started on high concentrations of amino acids in parenteral nutrition on the first day of life. This common problem can be avoided by stopping the protein component of the TPN for 2 to 3 hours before drawing the NBS sample, replacing the dextrose component of the TPN with a similar dextrose concentration in an appropriate saline solution.[10]

Single amino acids flagging as high risk should be investigated promptly, although the amino acid defects are typically not associated with decompensation and acute illness (except for elevated leucine in MSUD). Except for leucine elevations, evaluation of NBS amino acid notifications are not required emergently, but they should be completed in a timely manner.

Elevated leucine, along with the other branched-chain amino acids, isoleucine and valine, suggest branched-chain 2-ketoacyl-CoA dehydrogenase deficiency, commonly referred to as MSUD as a result of the characteristic odor apparent during episodes of metabolic decompensation. The diagnosis is confirmed by the appearance of the pathognomonic metabolite alloisoleucine in the serum amino acid analysis, along with markedly elevated leucine and the other branched-chain amino acids. Plasma ammonia concentrations may be increased during periods of metabolic decompensation. Significantly elevated leucine concentrations are toxic and can lead to encephalopathy and cerebral edema; thus, findings of elevated leucine and branched-chain amino acids on NBS requires prompt evaluation and follow-up of the infant. Initial treatment requires complete exclusion of leucine and the other branched-chain amino acids, although isoleucine and valine need to be added back promptly when their respective blood concentrations reach two to three times the upper limit of normal. This will ensure the adequacy of these essential amino acids for protein synthesis, which is the only mechanism for clearing amino acids that cannot be normally degraded because of the underlying enzyme defect.

Tyrosine

Tyrosine is a frequent abnormality of NBS in the NICU, and the vast majority of cases are either TPN related or because of transient hypertyrosinemia of the newborn, a condition that resolves spontaneously by 4 to 6 weeks of age in most cases. The cause of this is thought to be hepatic immaturity, but the specific factor has not been elucidated. No treatment is required, and demonstration of normal plasma tyrosine at 6 weeks rules out the rare case of a more significant tyrosinemia type II or III. Persistent increase in tyrosine concentrations, indicating one of these latter defects, is treated with a tyrosine-restricted diet, but there does not appear to be a compelling need to begin treatment for several months, so waiting to rule out transient hypertyrosinemia is reasonable.

Tyrosinemia type I is not reliably identified by elevated tyrosine, but many NBS programs now test for the highly sensitive marker succinylacetone. In states where succinylacetone is not measured, even modest increases in tyrosine indicate the need for measuring the succinylacetone in urine or blood, particularly in the setting of liver or renal disease. Because NBS tyrosine is often normal in newborns with tyrosinemia type I, clinicians in areas where NBS labs do not measure succinylacetone must retain a high level of suspicion in the clinical setting of unexplained kidney and/or liver disease because this condition is treatable with a drug, nitisinone. The treatment prevents the accumulation of toxic intermediates by creating a block earlier in the pathway, which also causes accumulation of tyrosine that is treated with dietary restriction.

Phenylalanine

Phenylalanine (phe) is a marker for the hyperphenylalaninemias, including classical phenylketonuria (PKU), milder variants of phenylalanine hydroxylase (PAH) deficiency, and several defects of synthesis and recycling of a cofactor of the enzyme, tetrahydrobiopterin. Tetrahydrobiopterin is also a cofactor for several enzymes involved in the synthesis of the neurotransmitters dopamine and serotonin. Therefore, deficiency in those genes may cause hyperphenylalaninemia (~1%–2% of cases of elevated phe), but also causes central nervous system (CNS) effects that are not corrected by dietary treatment of the hyperphenylalaninemia. Treatment of those disorders requires additional therapy with sepiapterin (Kuvan), a biopterin analogue, and neurotransmitter precursors. A recently described defect in a gene called *DNAJC12* appears to also cause deficiencies of neurotransmitters in addition to hyperphe, and is currently treated with neurotransmitter precursors.[11]

Elevated phe on NBS should be confirmed by measurement of plasma phenylalanine. If significantly elevated, in either the range of mild hyperphenylalaninemia (typically <500–600 μmol/L) to classic PKU values (>1200 μmol/L), defects of biopterin and *DNAJC12* should be ruled out. DNA panels are available to simultaneously sequence all of the known causative genes, or one can sequence *PAH* alone to demonstrate two mutant alleles. Absence of mutations in *PAH* indicates a need to look for other defects of tetrahydrobiopterin synthesis and recycling. Metabolite and enzyme testing can also be used to identify the majority of biopterin defects, but will miss *DNAJC12*, so they likely should no longer be the first line of testing.

Dietary treatment of high phenylalanine should begin as soon as possible and not later than 4 weeks after birth. A low-phe diet, with supplementation with tyrosine, the product of the deficient enzyme that is low in PKU patients, is the current mainstay of therapy. Specially designed formulas for this treatment are widely available and effective. Several pharmacological therapies are also approved, including sepiapterin, although diet treatment should be the first line for the majority of patients. Somewhere between 30 and 50% of PKU and hyperphe patients will have a moderate or better response to sepiapterin. High phe because of biopterin defects responds to normal or near normal soon after beginning therapy, although other clinical aspects for the biopterin defects may not respond as well.

Methionine

Increased methionine is a marker for some forms of homocystinuria (specifically cystathionine beta synthase), which can be easily and quickly ruled out by measurement of plasma total homocysteine. Therapy for affected patients should begin when they are stable enough to tolerate enteral pyridoxine therapy. Some individuals have a significant response and may need no other therapy. Others will not have a significant response and will require therapy with other cofactors for the remethylation pathway (methionine synthesis), including vitamin B12 and folic acid and use of a scavenger drug, betaine (Cystadane). Betaine donates a methyl group directly to homocysteine by way of an enzyme-mediated transferase, betaine-homocysteine methyltransferase, converting homocysteine directly to methionine. Dosing is limited by the capacity of the individual to perform this conjugation reaction.

Isolated hypermethioninemia is extremely rare because of variants in both alleles of one of three different genes involved in synthesis or degradation of S-adenosylmethionine (SAM). SAM is a critical source of methyl groups for a variety of critical cellular processes, including DNA synthesis, histone modification, and protein posttranslational modification.

Treatment is primarily with dietary restriction of methionine, although supplementation with SAM may have benefit.

Organic and Fatty Acids

Screening for organic acidemias and FAO defects by acylcarnitine analysis appears to work reasonably well in LBW infants, although they do appear to have modestly higher rates of abnormal NBS for most metabolites. Abnormalities of the acylcarnitine profile should be investigated by appropriate urine and blood tests as for any child. Repeating the NBS is typically not recommended as the follow-up test for these abnormalities because the cutoff values used to distinguish high-risk individuals are specific to infants in the first few days of life and thus are not applicable to older infants.

Enzyme Assays

Several of the longest-standing NBS conditions, galactosemia and biotinidase deficiencies, are screened by direct assay of enzyme activity in the dried blood spots. Enzymes in dried blood spots can be inactivated by excessive heat or improper sample handling. The screening test is considered high risk when the measured enzyme activity is below the cutoff value.

Galactosemia

Galactosemia is caused by a deficiency of the enzyme galactose-1-phosphate uridyl transferase (GALT) required for conversion of galactose (one of the component sugars in the disaccharide lactose) into glucose, which can be further oxidized. Classical (severe) galactosemia is associated with severe hyperbilirubinemia and possible kernicterus in the newborn, *Escherichia coli* sepsis (although other organisms may less commonly cause the sepsis), rarely, hepatic failure, and, later in life, intellectual disability and premature ovarian failure. Prompt treatment with a galactose-free diet prevents the acute symptoms and helps reduce, but does not completely ameliorate, the long-term neurodevelopmental consequences. The safest course upon receiving an abnormal NBS result is to stop breastfeeding and initiate treatment with a galactose-free formula immediately, pending results of confirmatory testing. Consultation with an expert in galactosemia treatment can be helpful when suspicion for a false-positive result is considered. In a well-appearing child who can be closely monitored in whom the NBS result suggests the possibility of a mild variant, such as Duarte variant galactosemia, it may be possible to continue breastfeeding while confirmatory testing is pending, understanding that any deterioration in clinical status, including increases in liver function tests, must immediately lead to treatment.

Confirmatory testing involves measurement of enzyme activity and measurement of an important metabolite in blood, glucose-1-phosphate. Reflex testing to a panel of common mutations or to full gene sequencing is available in some laboratories. Partially reduced activity of the GALT enzyme is sometimes identified by NBS programs, most commonly because of compound heterozygosity (different mutations on each copy of the gene) for a classical galactosemia allele and a common variant called the Duarte allele (in reference to where it was first described). The long-term outcomes of the variant forms of galactosemia appears to be good without need for dietary treatment. Generally, these infants have approximately 25% of the mean control activity of the enzyme. For infants with lower activity, and certainly when less than 10% of the mean control activity, treatment can be initiated. A therapeutic trial of galactose can be given at a year of age to children with variant galactosemia with measurement of galactose-1-phosphate after a week of exposure to functionally interrogate the adequacy of the enzyme activity.

Biotinidase

Biotinidase is an enzyme that recycles the vitamin cofactor biotin into a protein complex used by several critical carboxylase enzymes. Deficiency of the enzyme leads to deficiency of multiple carboxylases, similar to deficiency of the holocarboxylase synthetase that incorporates biotin into the complex. The later defect is not identified by the biotinidase screen, as biotinidase activity is normal in holocarboxylase synthetase deficiency. Long-term complications of untreated biotinidase deficiency include poor growth, neurodevelopmental defects, skin rash, alopecia, and gastrointestinal symptoms. Confirmatory testing is widely available using a serum biotinidase assay, but safe and simple treatment with 10 mg of biotin should begin while waiting for confirmatory results (using a crushed tablet because solutions are prone to bacterial contamination).

Lysosomal Storage Diseases

An increasing number of regions are now screening for a variety of lysosomal storage diseases (LSD) and other complex diseases, including Pompe disease, MPS-I (or Hurler disease), Krabbe disease, and X-linked adrenoleukodystrophy. These tests typically involve use of an artificial substrate to measure enzyme activity in the dried blood spot (the enzymes are released from lysed white blood cells); thus, leukopenia may increase risk of false-positive results. These conditions rarely cause symptoms in newborns, so there is generally time to consult with an expert in the evaluation of them. Best practices for follow-up are still being evaluated and vary by disorder, but repeating the NBS test is not appropriate. DNA testing is often required for confirmation.

The experience with enzymopathies thus far suggests that low birth weight (LBW) infants may not have a significantly increased false-positive rate compared with term infants.

Pompe disease is treated with enzyme replacement therapy (ERT) and should be evaluated immediately, as experience to date suggests that the earlier treatment begins the better the short- and medium-term outcome (see later). MPS-I can be treated with enzyme replacement, which is often followed by hematopoietic stem cell transplantation (HSCT) when the child is somewhat older. There are no data available demonstrating a need to begin treatment in the first month or two in a child with LBW, so the workup may be somewhat less urgent when there are more pressing medical issues. Krabbe disease is complicated, with the recommendation that infants affected with the severe early infantile form undergo HSCT by the end of the first month of life. This is clearly not possible in an LBW infant, and the high rate of milder phenotypes and false positives identified makes the decision-making complex. Involvement of a knowledgeable expert is highly recommended.

Blood transfusion may interfere with the screening of some disorders that rely on red blood cell enzymes (galactosemia). White blood cell enzymes and DNA are less affected, but most programs require repeat testing for these assays as well several weeks posttransfusion. Most NBS programs strongly encourage collection of the initial sample at 24 hours of age. If a transfusion is needed before then, an initial sample should be sent before 24 hours, with a repeat sent soon after per the recommendations of the specific NBS program.

Other Newborn Screening Tests

Congenital Adrenal Hyperplasia

Congenital adrenal hyperplasia (CAH) is discussed elsewhere, but it should be noted that LBW infants have high rates of false positives on NBS for this condition. Many state programs adjust the cutoff values used for LBW infants for this reason. Abnormal NBS for CAH should be evaluated immediately because of the risk of salt wasting and adrenal insufficiency.

Congenital Hypothyroidism

Congenital hypothyroidism is screened by blood thyroid stimulating hormone in many states, by direct thyroid hormone measurement in some, and by a combination of the two in a few states. Although this topic is discussed elsewhere, it is valuable to point out here that recent evidence suggests that repeat screening is necessary at regular intervals in LBW infants to avoid missing cases that develop in these patients in the first weeks of life.[12] Repeating the NBS test is typically not recommended unless the individual state recommends doing so because cutoff values are not optimized for this use. Further, many states are not able to assay single metabolites, so repeat testing increases the risk of a new false-positive result in another metabolite that was previously normal.

Cystic Fibrosis

NBS for CF has been shown to associate with improved weight gain and growth, which correlates in later life with improved lung function. NBS for CF most often involves first-tier testing of immunoreactive trypsinogen (IRT); those samples with the highest concentrations have second-tier testing in most states by a limited panel of relatively common mutations in the *CFTR* gene, although some NBS programs utilize a second IRT measurement at 1 to 2 weeks of age instead. Infants with two identified mutations are affected and should be referred immediately to the nearest center equipped to care for neonates with CF. Infants with a single mutation identified are screen positive, most of whom will be unaffected heterozygotes, but a few will have a second mutation that was not part of the NBS screening panel. A confirmatory sweat test should be obtained as soon as is feasible for any screen-positive infant, recognizing that in LBW infants, this may not be possible for some time. In that case, full sequencing of the *CFTR* gene may be indicated as an initial step, with sweat test to be performed when the child is older, regardless of the result of sequencing. Nutrition support, intestinal enzyme therapy, and supportive respiratory treatment for CF is most effective when initiated within the first month of life.

Spinal Muscular Atrophy

An increasing number of NBS programs are now considering screening for spinal muscular atrophy (SMA) type I, as it has recently become a treatable condition. The screening test is DNA based, so it should not be prone to false positives; however, as it only tests for the common deletion, NBS will miss approximately 5% of cases. A high index of suspicion should be maintained in neonates with significant hypotonia who screen negative. Confirmatory testing of a positive screen should be sent immediately, as outcomes appear to be strongly dependent on early initiation of treatment with cerebrospinal fluid (CSF) injection of a nucleotide therapy (details of which are beyond the scope of this discussion). Involvement of a pediatric neurologist familiar with the diagnosis and treatment is wise.

HEPATOSPLENOMEGALY AND HYDROPS FETALIS

Hepatomegaly and splenomegaly (HSM) in a neonate can have many causes, including infections, vascular occlusions and clots, cardiomyopathy, and biliary obstruction. When these are ruled out, genetic and metabolic causes predominate among the remaining potential diagnoses. A complete discussion of the genetic causes is beyond the scope of this chapter; Box 6.2 shows some of the more common, with particular attention to those that are treatable.

BOX 6.2 Metabolic Diseases That May Present With Hepatosplenomegaly

Specific Treatment Needed Promptly to Prevent Long-term Complications

- Fatty acid oxidation disorders
- Glycogen storage disease (particularly types 1a, 1b, and 3)
- Hereditary fructose intolerance
- Organic acidemias
- Pompe disease
- Urea cycle defects

Treatment May Impact Long-term Outcome or Be Less Urgent

- Congenital lactic acidemias
- Lysosomal storage diseases, including
  - Mucopolysaccharidosis
  - Niemann-Pick disease
  - Gaucher disease (especially type 2 and 3)
  - GM1 gangliosidosis
  - Galactosialidosis
  - Mucolipidoses
- Wolman disease (and the milder cholesteryl ester storage disease, both caused by deficiency of lysosomal acid lipase)
- Wilson disease

Specific Treatment Not Currently Available

- Peroxisomal biogenesis disorders (Zellweger syndrome)

The evaluation for genetic and metabolic causes of HSM begins, as always, with the context of the patient. When present at birth, HSM may indicate a severe form of one of several LSDs. Associated neurologic or renal disease could indicate a defect of peroxisomal biogenesis (Zellweger spectrum disorders), or perhaps a primary mitochondrial disease (e.g., Alpers syndrome because of biallelic mutations in the DNA polymerase *POLG*). Acidosis or hypoglycemia may suggest a defect in hepatic intermediate metabolism such as an FAO defect, organic acidemia, or a glycogen storage disease. Associated hyperammonemia may represent a defect of the urea cycle or, especially if moderate, a portovenous shunt. Associated cardiomyopathy may be seen in Pompe disease. Jaundice may indicate obstructive biliary disease outside the liver (biliary atresia) or within the liver (Alagille syndrome), or a defect in synthesis or excretion of bile acids. Hemangiomas of the skin or other organs may be associated with a hepatic hemangioma. Isolated splenomegaly is uncommon. Splenomegaly may proceed hepatomegaly with some storage diseases and rarely is the presenting finding in prolidase deficiency.

The initial evaluation of a neonate with HSM includes measurement of electrolytes, glucose, liver function markers, ammonia, lactic acid, and other typical screening tests. If acidosis is present, searching for causes described earlier is required. Pompe disease requires a specific enzyme assay, which can be performed on white blood cells or from dried blood spots. This should be requested without delay, as earlier treatment correlates with improved outcome.

Hereditary fructose intolerance because of aldolase B deficiency is uncommon before initiation of table foods, but has become increasingly recognized in newborns and infants treated with formulas that contain fructose as part of the disaccharide sucrose. These formulas are often marketed for use in perceived feeding intolerance. Immediate cessation of fructose results in rapid correction of hepatic failure, jaundice, and hypoglycemia, if caught in time. Once permanent hepatic injury and cirrhosis occurs, transplantation may be required. The diagnosis is clinical with confirmation by DNA testing.

If a structural or vascular defect is not found, and initial metabolic testing is not diagnostic, the clinician is left with the difficult decision of whether to pursue a variety of individual screening tests, for example, lysosomal enzyme screening, or to move quickly to a broad-based genetic test, either a liver disease-specific panel or whole-exome or whole-genome sequencing (see discussion later for additional information about genetic testing). At this point, it is likely that multiple specialists will be involved, and a team-based approach to decision-making should be pursued.

NEUROLOGICAL PRESENTATIONS

Encephalopathy

In the neonatal period, encephalopathy refers to a disturbance in the level of consciousness appropriate for the gestational age; it refers typically to a reduced level of consciousness and activity, but in the case of ischemic injury, it can also refer to a hyperalert state. There are many possible causes of neonatal encephalopathy, including metabolic and genetic disorders. Some of these may be responsive to specific therapy, whereas others may indicate a poor prognosis that would be a contraindication to aggressive care; thus, early and accurate diagnosis can have significant impact on the management of the patient.

Hypoxic-ischemic injury as a result of difficult labor or delivery is often the presumed cause of neonatal encephalopathy. From the perspective of the clinical geneticist, it is difficult to distinguish between a difficult labor as the first sign of fetal/infant brain dysfunction rather than the cause of the dysfunction. Recent advances in genetic testing have shown that there are many possible causes of cerebral dysfunction in the fetus and neonate that can present with difficult delivery; thus, one should not assume that just because the labor was complicated or difficult that the encephalopathy is as a result of hypoxia/ischemia. Further, even with clear clinical and imaging findings supportive of hypoxic-ischemic encephalopathy (HIE), it is impossible to know that the complicated delivery, and the resulting ischemic injury, were not caused by an underlying genetic abnormality. Although this goes against traditional thinking in the field of neonatology,[13] it is prudent to at least consider the possibility of an underlying genetic or metabolic disorder in the setting of presumed HIE.

Encephalopathy in a neonate is generally associated with hypotonia, and not infrequently with seizures; thus, the differential diagnoses and approaches to evaluation overlap significantly. A great deal of information can be obtained from routine laboratory analysis, particularly investigating acid-base status (see evaluation of metabolic acidosis), glucose concentration, and ammonia. Ammonia should always be measured promptly in an infant with altered mental status because prompt treatment of hyperammonemia is clearly associated with improved neurological outcome, regardless of the cause (see hyperammonemia earlier). Subclinical seizure activity should be actively investigated. If seizures are present, the workup will best follow the approach described for seizures.

If hypotonia is prominent, more so than the altered mental status, initially following the approach to hypotonia is logical (see hypotonia discussion subsequently). The presence of significant dysmorphism or birth defects suggests the probability of a significant defect in brain development, and imaging, generally by magnetic resonance imaging (MRI), should be considered. If MRI is obtained, MR spectroscopy is a valuable add-on to give data regarding CNS lactic acidemia, as might be seen with defects of mitochondrial metabolism. In the setting of liver disease and encephalopathy, one should consider defects of mitochondrial DNA depletion, particularly Alpers syndrome, as a result of mutations in both alleles of the DNA polymerase, POLG. Facial dysmorphism in the same setting could point to a Zellweger spectrum disease associated with defects of peroxisomal biogenesis. Defects in CNS neurotransmitter synthesis and metabolism are increasingly recognized in this setting; however, in the absence of seizure, lumbar puncture (LP) for measurement of neurotransmitters and cofactors (folate, pyridoxal-5-phosphate, pterins, etc.) is generally not a first-line test. An often-overlooked genetic cause of neonatal encephalopathy, in isolation or with a more complex phenotype including dysmorphism and/or birth defects, are the congenital disorders of glycosylation (CDGs). CDGs may manifest with multiorgan system disease secondary to defects in the posttranslational modification of proteins with carbohydrate side chains that are needed for normal protein function.

An excellent review with detailed algorithms for evaluation of neonatal encephalopathy has been published recently.[13] Recent advances in genetic testing are beginning to change the approach taken to the evaluation of neonatal encephalopathy, with or without seizures or hypotonia. Namely, early genomic testing, either whole exome or, increasingly, whole genome, is now arguably a test to do early in the course of illness when no exogenous cause or metabolic disruption is identified in the first few days of life. This is discussed later in the section on genetic testing.

Seizures

As with all neurological presentations in the neonate, there is overlap and sometimes different perspectives on problems between different specialties. In the case of seizures, the geneticist begins with the assumption that seizure activity in a neonate always represents a defect in either gross structure, microscopic structure (not visible as an MRI abnormality), or neurochemistry, and, in the absence of a clear alternative explanation (CNS infection, sepsis, blood clot, or hemorrhage), a genetic abnormality is the likely explanation. As noted previously, the presence of difficult labor with possible hypoxic-ischemic injury can now be argued to be a diagnosis of exclusion, made only after genomic testing does not identify a genetic etiology of symptoms. Further, because we do not yet have the knowledge to interpret the entire genome, genomic testing cannot definitively rule out a genetic defect. One must therefore be conservative in consideration of alternative causes of seizures in neonates.

Because the ways in which a neonate can present clinically are somewhat limited, the evaluation of possible genetic causes of seizures starts with consideration of standard laboratory tests, including the complete blood count, electrolytes and glucose, and ammonia. If there is evidence of blood loss, imaging of the brain may be needed to rule out a bleed. Severe anemia could also lead to CNS hypoperfusion. Hypoglycemia may cause seizures in a neonate, and the evaluation should proceed as described earlier in this chapter and in Chapter 11. Any of the causes of neonatal metabolic acidosis may also present with seizures, so elevated anion gap metabolic acidosis should be sought at the time of presentation and treated accordingly. Likewise, hyperammonemia as a result of defects of the urea cycle or organic or FAO defects requires specific therapy to control the seizures. As noted earlier, in the setting of acidosis or hyperammonemia, the possibility of subclinical seizures should be considered, as should the potential value of preemptive anti-epileptic therapy.

Typically, when a neonate presents with seizures, an LP will be considered to rule out infection. A valuable practice is to consider whether additional tubes of CSF may be helpful for neurometabolic testing if infection is not found. Several of the metabolites to be tested require tubes with special stabilizing agents. These tubes should be kept in the neonatal unit so that the search for tubes does not delay the LP or lead to a decision to not obtain the samples at all. Tests to be performed include lactate, amino acids (paired with serum or plasma amino acids obtained in the same time frame), neurotransmitters (dopamine, serotonin, and metabolites), folate, pyridoxal-5-phosphate, and CSF pterins (tetrahydrobiopterin is a cofactor for synthesis of both dopamine and serotonin).

Several rare metabolic disorders that present with neonatal onset of seizures deserve special mention. Pyridoxine dependent epilepsy results from a defect in the metabolism of alpha-amino adipic semialdehyde (alpha-AASA), a downstream product in the degradation of lysine. This compound is in equilibrium with 6-hydoxypiperideine-2-carboxylic acid, which also accumulates and binds the active form of pyridoxine (vitamin B6), pyridoxal-5'-phosphate (P5P). As P5P is a vital cofactor in the synthesis of multiple neurotransmitters, deficiency leads to encephalopathy and seizures. Treatment with pyridoxine is usually effective in stopping the seizure activity and improving the electroencephalogram (EEG) within a few hours or a day of giving the first dose of 100 mg of pyridoxine IV. In rare cases, for reasons that are not understood, folate or folinic acid may also reduce the seizures. A therapeutic trial of pyridoxine is often given for any infant presenting with seizures, but a lack of response is not definitive evidence against PDE, so urinary alpha-AASA measurement should be performed in all cases. Treatment with a lysine-restricted diet has been suggested to reduce the residual risk for neurodevelopmental abnormalities, even when seizures are controlled with pyridoxine. Supplementation with arginine to competitively inhibit lysine uptake into the CNS via a shared transport system may also improve outcomes. Some neurologists prefer to use P5P rather than pyridoxine because it can also treat an even more rare condition, pyridoxamine-5'-phosphate oxidase (PNPO) deficiency. Patients with PNPO deficiency often have a significant, although incomplete, response to pyridoxine. The fact that the compound is more difficult to obtain, and it can cause neuropathy, suggest that it is not an ideal alternative to pyridoxine unless the diagnosis of PNPO deficiency is confirmed.

Sulfite oxidase deficiency, which can be primary or caused by a defect in the synthesis of the molybdenum cofactor, typically presents with neonatal seizures, often resistant to anticonvulsant therapy, and can be associated with MRI changes in the brain strongly suggestive of hypoxic-ischemic injury. Molybdenum cofactor deficiency, which is also a cofactor for xanthine oxidase, appears to be the more common of the two disorders and is potentially partially treatable with an investigational therapy. Screening can include looking for low uric acid (caused by xanthine oxidase deficiency) and low plasma homocysteine (caused by sulfite oxidase deficiency). Neither is completely diagnostic, so measurement of urinary s-sulfocysteine, with or without other disulfide-containing compounds, is necessary. The sulfur-containing metabolites in these disorders can cause secondary deficiency of the alpha-AASA dehydrogenase enzyme, so s-sulfocysteine measurement should be included in the evaluation of patients with pyridoxine-dependent epilepsy.

Low CSF glucose relative to the serum glucose concentration, hypoglycorrhachia, is caused by a defect in the CNS glucose transporter, GLUT1. Treatment with a ketogenic diet significantly improves neurological and seizure outcome, so this diagnosis should not be missed. The diagnosis is suggested in the setting of low CSF glucose (<50 mg/dL) and CSF/serum ratio of less than 0.6, in the absence of a CSF infection (bacterial or viral), and is usually confirmed by DNA analysis.

A variety of other metabolic and neurometabolic disorders that specifically present with neonatal, usually intractable, seizures, for which specific treatments are not apparent include nonketotic hyperglycinemia (increased CSF and plasma glycine), mitochondrial respiratory chain defects (typically with increased CSF lactate, although plasma lactate is not always increased), peroxisomal biogenesis defects (elevated plasma very-long chain fatty acids, C:22 and C:24), defects of purine and pyrimidine metabolism, and others.

The metabolic evaluation of neonatal seizures should therefore include:

- routine metabolic tests (electrolytes, glucose, BUN);
- screening tests for IEM (plasma amino acids, plasma acylcarnitine profile, urine organic acids, biotinidase activity);
- urine AASA and pipecolic acid;
- CSF glucose, lactate, neurotransmitters, amino acids, and cofactors;
- urine s-sulfocysteine;
- plasma very-long chain fatty acid analysis; and
- urine or plasma purine and pyrimidine analysis.

In the absence of a treatable metabolic disorder, it is now standard practice to utilize newer DNA sequencing technologies to interrogate a panel of genes that are associated with infantile seizure disorders. Many of these single-gene disorders occur sporadically as a result of de novo mutations, so there is no family history. Defining the diagnosis as accurately and precisely as possible is critical to ensuring that the appropriate therapy is given, that excessive and expensive care is avoided when not helpful, that appropriate prognostic counseling is given (especially in the case of benign neonatal seizures as a result of certain mutations in the potassium channel genes *KCNQ2* and *KCNQ3*), and that future reproductive risks are identified for the family. These panels often include genes that are associated with the neurometabolic disorders so that invasive testing can be avoided in some cases, remembering that because of limitations in technology and our ability to interpret noncoding DNA changes, a negative DNA test does not definitively rule out a genetic disease. It is incumbent on the clinician to be aware of the genes tested, and those not tested, in any particular DNA panel, as well as the limitations of the assay selected.

EDITORIAL COMMENT: Among 611 consecutive newborns with seizures, 79 (13%) had epilepsy (35 epileptic encephalopathy, 32 congenital brain malformations, 11 benign familial neonatal epilepsy [BFNE], 1 benign neonatal seizures). Twenty-nine (83%) with epileptic encephalopathy had genetic testing and 24/29 (83%) had a genetic etiology. Neonatal epilepsy is often attributed to identifiable genetic causes. Thus, genetic testing is now warranted for newborns with epilepsy to guide management and inform discussions of prognosis.

Shellhaas RA, Wusthoff CJ, Tsuchida TN, et al. Neonatal Seizure Registry. Profile of neonatal epilepsies: characteristics of a prospective US cohort. *Neurology.* 2017;8:893-899.

Hypotonia

Persistent hypotonia is a common neonatal presentation that can have many causes, ranging from defects of the cerebral cortex, the brainstem and spinal cord, the anterior horn cell, and even the myocyte (Box 6.3).

(The list is not exhaustive; rather, it focuses on the more common diagnosis, those that may be less common but have effective treatment, and those that can be easily suggested or ruled out by common and inexpensive tests.)

Evaluation of a neonate with significant hypotonia involves a careful search for other major and minor malformations, careful neurological evaluation (paying particular attention to deep tendon reflexes and tongue fasciculations), evidence of more diffuse encephalopathy, subtle signs of seizures, and physical manifestations of hypogonadism. Initial diagnostic process should include immediate and rapid evaluation for the two important treatable causes (SMA type I and Pompe) and the common PWS. Initial evaluation should include:

1. DNA testing for the common deletion of the *SMN1* gene, with full sequencing if a carrier and high index of suspicion;
2. enzyme analysis for Pompe disease (alpha-glucosidase activity), which is available from a dried blood spot in some laboratories; and
3. DNA methylation analysis for PWS.

Next-tier testing should be performed in consultation with neurology, genetics, and other consultants, and may include, but is not limited to, MRI scan of the brain, testing for IEM and mitochondrial disorders (even in the setting of a normal NBS test), CMA, and EEG. Muscle biopsy is usually nondiagnostic and is rarely required for evaluation of hypotonia; it should only be considered if there is a specific clinical indication and other methods of diagnosis have been exhausted. Recent work suggests that early addition of whole-exome or whole-genome sequencing can lead to a significant reduction in other testing, reduced NICU cost, and more rapid initiation of definitive therapy. Genomic testing can be considered concurrently but should not be ordered in lieu of the three initial diagnostic maneuvers because it will delay their diagnosis (compared with standard testing) and will not identify the most common causes of SMA type I and PWS.

BOX 6.3 Important Genetic Causes of Marked Neonatal Hypotonia

- Spinal muscular atrophy (both common and with newly available treatment)
- Prader-Willi syndrome
- Chromosomal disorders
- Congenital myotonic dystrophy
- Primary myopathies
- Mitochondrial encephalomyopathies
- Inborn errors of metabolism
- Brain malformations
- Other causes of more diffuse encephalopathy (e.g., *PURA* mutations)
- Neonatal seizure disorders

Spinal Muscular Atrophy

SMA is a condition that can cause profound and progressive hypotonia and paralysis attributed to dysfunction and death of motor neuron cells. Individuals affected by severe forms of the disease eventually lose the ability to move their extremities and breathe independently. With the development of novel therapies for SMA type I (the most severe form) that appear to be more effective the earlier that they are started, it is important not to miss or delay this diagnosis. NBS as currently recommended uses DNA screening that is known to miss 5% to 7% of cases of SMA type I; thus, it is critical that clinicians maintain a high level of suspicion. This is also one of the more common genetic disorders, with incidence estimated to be 1 in 6000 to 10,000.

Typical findings of this anterior horn cell deterioration syndrome include loss of deep tendon reflexes and tongue fasciculations, both of which may not be present yet in affected neonates in the first month or two of life.

Treatment for SMA type I currently involves use of a novel antisense microRNA that leads to increased expression of the *SMN2* pseudogene that can provide some of the missing function from the lack of expression of *SMN1*. Details on the mechanism and diagnostic testing process and pitfalls, can be found elsewhere (the reader is referred to GeneReviews for regularly updated information).

Pompe Disease

Pompe disease, attributed to lysosomal alpha-glucosidase deficiency, is an important genetic/metabolic defect to consider in the setting of neonatal hypotonia. The disorder is caused by accumulation of undegraded glycogen fragments that have been transported into the lysosome, leading to cellular injury, especially in muscle. The incidence of the infantile form is not well documented but is thought to be approximately 1 in 100,000. The infantile form typically presents in the first weeks to months of life with hypotonia, weakness, and poor feeding, often leading to poor weight gain. These symptoms may precede the onset of the hypertrophic cardiomyopathy and hepatomegaly, but those findings soon follow, with death in the untreated infant occurring typically in the first 12 to 18 months of life. Treatment with recombinant alpha-glucosidase ERT can significantly alter the natural history of the disease, essentially correcting the cardiomyopathy and slowing the progressive myopathy, allowing some treated infants to live into the second decade, and perhaps beyond. Again, as with SMA type I, the earlier treatment begins, the better the expected outcome. Treatment regimens evolve rapidly, so initiation of therapy should be under the care of a physician knowledgeable in the treatment.

Both Pompe disease and SMA type 1 attributed to the common deletion of the *SMN1* gene have recently been added to the U.S. Department of Health and Human Services Recommended Uniform (Newborn) Screening Panel, but it will likely be some years before routine NBS occurs everywhere (see information on NBS previously).

Prader-Willi Syndrome

PWS is relatively common defect (incidence ~1 in 15,000–25,000) caused by the lack of expression of one or more genes in the pericentromeric region of chromosome 15. Copies of the genes on the maternally inherited chromosome 15 are epigenetically silenced by methylation. Only those genes in the region on the paternally inherited copy are expressed. The most common cause of PWS is deletion of the portion of the chromosome 15 inherited from the father (paternal deletion), although a significant minority of cases are attributed to inheritance of both copies of chromosome 15 from the mother (maternal uniparental disomy). Both causes occur sporadically and are not associated with significant recurrence risk. Identification of the specific cause is critical because 2% to 3% of cases are attributed to other types of defects that may have increased recurrence risk for future pregnancies. Details of genetic causes and the very significant later findings, including hyperphagia, short stature, behavior problems, and a wide variety of other issues, are widely available elsewhere.

PWS is typically associated with decreased fetal activity. Newborns have significant hypotonia noted in the hours immediately after delivery, with poor sucking and typically little interest in feeding. Other malformations and clinical findings are rare, although cryptorchidism is typical in males; underdevelopment of the labia and clitoris are often present, but overlooked, in the female. Although there is no specific cure, appropriate management, including appropriate nutritional support, feeding therapy, and the early initiation of growth hormone replacement therapy, can significantly improve the first years of life for the child.

Other Causes of Hypotonia

IEM may also present with hypotonia; however, it would be unusual for the hypotonia to be the only presenting finding. Additional information about the evaluation of an ill neonate for inborn errors is found earlier in this chapter. A wide variety of other neurological and myopathic disorders can present with severe neonatal hypotonia, so broad-based genomic testing is also likely to play an increasingly early part in the evaluation.

TERATOGENS

The maternal environment can have a significant impact on fetal development and at times result in consequences for the infant that very much resemble a genetic abnormality. A thorough maternal history, including maternal health issues, illness during pregnancy, medications taken during pregnancy, and substance use during pregnancy, is thus a vital aspect in the evaluation of any infant born with congenital anomalies or neurological abnormalities.

Teratogens can come in many forms. One of the most common but easily overlooked causes of fetal anomalies is uncontrolled maternal diabetes. Other maternal diseases, such as lupus or uncontrolled PKU, can result in significant consequences for the baby. Maternal infections during pregnancy, including the classic TORCH infections (toxoplasmosis, other [syphilis, varicella-zoster, parvovirus B19], rubella, cytomegalovirus, and herpes infections), can lead to sequelae for the infant, as can maternal use of drugs such as lithium, valproic acid, retinoic acid, warfarin, thalidomide, and substances such as alcohol.

Specific teratogens often manifest with characteristic fetal anomalies. Teratogens can mimic certain genetic syndromes, and in fact, the commonalities observed between certain teratogenic defects and genetic conditions, such as thalidomide and Roberts syndrome, have provided insight into the mechanisms underlying the genetic defect by means of knowing the mechanism of action of the drug, or vice versa.

Not all maternal exposures result in fetal abnormalities. Likely, the anomalies result from the exposure to the fetus in addition to the genetic background of the fetus, which may predispose more or less sensitivity to the teratogen. Timing of the exposure during pregnancy can also have a differential impact on the effect on the fetus. Therefore, if a maternal exposure is known, the physician should screen for potential consequences of that exposure, but the baby could quite probably have no abnormal findings.

If the fetal anomalies observed are consistent with the known exposure, an extensive genetic evaluation is not needed. However, if the birth defects do not fit with the known teratogen, or if there is no known history of maternal exposures, a genetic workup should be undertaken to rule out a genetic rather than teratogenic cause.

Underlying Maternal Health Conditions

Maternal Diabetes

Uncontrolled maternal diabetes is most commonly known to lead to macrosomic infants from the increased exposure to glucose during pregnancy. Macrosomia comes with risks for birth trauma such as shoulder dystocia and, in many cases, leads to requirement for cesarean section. Additionally, increased exposure to glucose in utero leads to expression of high levels of insulin in the baby, which often results in hypoglycemia following birth, as the insulin levels remain temporarily high despite the elevated glucose source being taken away.

More significant congenital anomalies are also known to result from uncontrolled maternal diabetes, although these are seen less frequently. Small left colon syndrome resulting in bowel obstruction can occur. Usually, this does not require any surgical intervention, and the infant will outgrow it; however, it may lead to a prolonged NICU stay for management of the obstruction.

Caudal regression syndrome, manifesting with varying degrees of anomalies/malformations of the caudal/sacral vertebrae, lower extremities, urogenital organs, and lower intestinal tract, can be a serious complication of maternal diabetes. The exact mechanism for how maternal diabetes contributes to caudal regression is unclear; however, a vascular insult is hypothesized.[14] There are genetic syndromes that can present with similar findings to caudal regression, and thus, even in the setting of maternal diabetes, any baby presenting with features of caudal regression should additionally be evaluated with a CMA. Examination by a clinical geneticist to rule out single-gene disorders that can present with similar features, such as Townes-Brocks Syndrome (*SALL1*), is also recommended. In the absence of genetic findings, the caudal regression syndrome features can be attributed to a teratogenic insult from the maternal diabetes.

Maternal Systemic Lupus Erythematosus

Babies born to mothers with systemic lupus erythematosus (SLE) are at risk for neonatal lupus, which is usually transient and resolves once the maternal antibodies have been cleared from their system, as well as congenital heart block. Congenital heart block can be significant and may require a lifelong cardiac pacing device. Any baby born to a mother with SLE should have an electrocardiogram (ECG) performed after birth to evaluate for heart block. Any ECG abnormalities require consultation with a cardiologist. Sometimes, a baby born with congenital heart block can be the first symptom of a mother with lupus. Thus, any mother of a baby born with congenital heart block should have testing for lupus.[15]

Maternal Phenylketonuria

PKU is a recessive condition manifesting with elevated phenylalanine levels. Because phenylalanine is concentrated by the placenta into the fetus, mothers with poorly controlled PKU may give birth to infants with problems that include microcephaly, intellectual impairment, SGA, and congenital heart defects. Unless the partner of a mother with PKU has PKU or is a carrier for PKU, the probability that the baby will have PKU is low, but the NBS result needs to be checked to confirm. Abnormal NBS is not common in these infants attributed to maternal PKU. Infants born to mothers with poorly controlled PKU should be evaluated carefully for the findings of maternal PKU. At discharge, the infant should be referred for ongoing neurodevelopmental monitoring.

Drug Exposures

Numerous drugs are known to have consequences for fetal development. Drugs are classified by the U.S. Food and Drug Administration into five categories: A, B, C, D, and X, with A being safe during pregnancy and X being absolutely contraindicated. Every drug should include its pregnancy rating in its information sheet.

Certain drugs are known to result in typical fetal anomalies, and the finding of an anomaly should prompt the physician to reevaluate and question the mother for drug exposures during pregnancy. In many cases, a mother may have taken a substance before knowing she was pregnant, or the risks of not taking the medication during pregnancy (as with some antipsychotic or seizure medications) outweighed potential risks to the fetus. Table 6.3 shows some of the more common teratogenic drugs, along with known genetic mimics.

Maternal Infections

Exposure to infectious agents in utero or at the time of birth can interfere in normal development and lead to severe neonatal complications and even death in certain circumstances, such as with neonatal herpes simplex virus (HSV). Maternal infections should always be considered when abnormal findings are seen in the baby, as many infections can be treated and lead to improved outcomes. Further descriptions of the manifestations observed with congenital infections can be found elsewhere.[16] However, a brief overview of key findings in the most significant maternal infections is provided in Table 6.4.

TABLE 6.3 Common Teratogenic Drugs and Related Abnormalities

Drug	Syndrome	Features	Genetic Mimic
Alcohol	Fetal alcohol syndrome/fetal alcohol spectrum disorder (FAS) Note: Individuals can show just the facial features of FAS without the neurologic features, or may have no facial features and only neurologic features, or they may show characteristics of both	• Typical facial features: short nose, smooth philtrum, thin upper lip, microcephaly, small palpebral fissures • Neurologic: intellectual disability/developmental delay • Hyperactivity, impulsivity • Executive functioning issues • Memory issues	
Phenytoin	Fetal hydantoin syndrome	• Facial features: wide anterior fontanelle, hypertelorism, depressed nasal bridge, short nose, bowed upper lip • Digital anomalies: stiff, tapered fingers, hypoplastic distal phalanges, fingerlike thumb • May also have rib abnormalities, hip dislocation, hernias, coarse hair, and hirsutism • Neurologic: mild to moderate intellectual disability	
Lithium		• Cardiac: Ebstein anomaly • Increased birth weight	
Warfarin	Warfarin embryopathy	• Facial features: nasal hypoplasia with depressed nasal bridge • Skeletal: stippled epiphyses, hypoplastic distal phalanges	• Vitamin K epoxide reductase deficiency (pseudo-warfarin syndrome) • X-linked recessive chondrodysplasia punctata
Valproic acid	Fetal valproate syndrome	• Facial features: high forehead, epicanthal folds, telecanthus, broad, low nasal bridge, long philtrum, small mouth and jaw • Neural tube defects • Cardiac defects • Long digits • Neurologic: developmental delays/impaired cognitive outcomes	
Methotrexate	Fetal methotrexate syndrome	• Growth deficiency • Facial features: microcephaly, hypoplastic facial bones, wide fontanelles, craniosynostosis of lambdoid and/or coronal sutures, shallow orbits, micrognathia, epicanthal folds, cleft palate occasionally seen • Skeletal: mild shortening of bones, hypodactyly, syndactyly • Neural tube defects • Can have urogenital and malformations and/or intestinal malrotation	
Angiotensin-converting enzyme (ACE) inhibitors		• Renal defects, specifically renal tubular dysgenesis, which can lead to renal insufficiency/failure in the fetus with resultant features of Potter sequence	
Retinoic acid	Retinoic acid embryopathy	• Facial features: microtia, facial asymmetry, facial nerve paralysis, micrognathia, hypertelorism, mottled teeth • Cardiac defects (mostly conotruncal) • Neurologic: hydrocephalus, microcephaly, cortical and cerebellar malformations, intellectual disability • Abnormalities of the thymus and parathyroid glands	
Thalidomide		• Limb defects (amelia, phocomelia, abnormalities of the forelimb and hands/feet)	Roberts syndrome (*ESCO2*)

TABLE 6.4 Clinical Findings in Neonates With Congenital Infections

Infectious Agent	Susceptibility Window	Neonatal Findings
Toxoplasmosis	Greater risk of transmission if mother infected later in pregnancy, but more complications in the infant if infected earlier in pregnancy	Chorioretinitis Hydrocephalus Intracranial calcifications Anemia Thrombocytopenia Hepatosplenomegaly Jaundice Seizures
Syphilis	Increased infections in mothers with active disease (RPR titer >1:4). Fetal immune system will not be able to mount a response to the infection (and thus develop signs of congenital syphilis) until after about 18 weeks' gestation.	Infant often asymptomatic at birth with development of symptoms around 1–2 months of age Skeletal lesions (diaphyseal periostitis, osteochondritis, and lucent epiphyseal bands, osteitis, dactylitis) Saddle nose deformity Snuffles Chorioretinitis, glaucoma Lymphadenopathy, anemia, leukopenia/cytosis Thrombocytopenia Hepatosplenomegaly Maculopapular rash Mucous patches Meningitis Hydrocephalus
Varicella (VZV)	Infection at <20 weeks' gestation can lead to fetal death/anomalies Infection at >20 weeks' gestation can lead to risk for typical VZV symptoms Infection around the time of birth can lead to severe neonatal illness with possible death	Ophthalmologic abnormalities Cutaneous Scarring Limb hypoplasia CNS damage Typical VZV symptoms Systemic infection
Parvovirus	Highest risk to fetus with infection at the end of the 1st trimester	Severe fetal anemia Nonimmune hydrops Thrombocytopenia
Rubella	Highest risk to fetus with maternal infection in the first trimester	SGA Sensorineural hearing loss Cataracts, microphthalmia, corneal opacity, glaucoma Cardiac defects (PDA, pulmonary artery stenosis, coarctation) Blueberry muffin rash, hepatosplenomegaly, thrombocytopenia
CMV	Higher risk to infant with primary infection in the first half of pregnancy	IUGR Sensorineural hearing loss (can present later in childhood) Microcephaly, hypotonia, seizures Optic atrophy, chorioretinitis Periventricular calcifications, cystic white matter disease Hepatosplenomegaly, elevated liver enzymes, conjugated hyperbilirubinemia
Congenital HSV[17] (neonatal HSV acquired at or shortly after birth, discussed elsewhere)	Infection acquired in utero (as opposed to intrapartum, as seen with neonatal HSV) Congenital HSV accounts for only 4%–5% of HSV infections in neonates	IUGR Preterm birth Microcephaly Hydrocephalus Encephalomalacia CNS calcifications Microphthalmia Cataracts Chorioretinitis Vesicular rash (or other rash) Bone abnormalities Visceral organ involvement (liver, adrenal glands, lungs) with organ dysfunction, necrosis, and calcification

TABLE 6.4 Clinical Findings in Neonates With Congenital Infections—cont'd

Infectious Agent	Susceptibility Window	Neonatal Findings
Congenital Zika virus[18,19]	Infection acquired in utero No recognized association with timing of maternal infections Mother may have asymptomatic infection <100% of fetuses born to affected mothers have congenital effect ~15% of affected infants have severe embryopathy	Microcephaly (not present at birth in 20% of cases) Calcifications throughout brain Enlarged ventricles/cerebral atrophy Abnormal gyration Vision and hearing defects Intellectual disability Motor disability

CMV, Cytomegalovirus; *CNS,* central nervous system; *HSV,* herpes simplex virus; *IUGR,* intrauterine growth restriction ; *RPR,* reactive plasma reagin.

GENETIC TESTING

In broad terms, genetic testing can be considered to be any test that points to a specific genetic diagnosis, for example, hemoglobin electrophoresis that diagnoses sickle cell disease, or a sweat test that diagnoses CF. Most often the term is applied specifically to tests that evaluate DNA. This includes tests of chromosomal structure and individual DNA sequencing. Advances in DNA sequencing technologies have altered the landscape in recent years to the point where traditional methods (karyotype analysis and Sanger sequencing of individual genes) have been mostly replaced by CMA technologies and next-generation (massively parallel) DNA sequencing. The cost of these methods has reached a point where single-gene testing is often no longer the most cost-effective approach, but with the large-scale sequencing approaches comes new complexity in terms of variants of unknown significance and potential to identify unrelated but clinically important variants.

Decision-making around which tests to order, and when to do them, should be made in consultation with local experts experienced in selecting and interpreting genetic tests. Particularly complex is the decision whether to order a panel of DNA tests or to take a genomic approach using whole-exome or whole-genome sequencing. Interestingly, use of genomic testing approaches has revealed that in complex phenotypes, there may be multiple genetic diagnosis present. This may occur in up to 5% of individuals with complex phenotypes.

As technologies change and improve, it seems likely that whole-genome testing will become more standard, although our ability to interpret the full genome, including all of the noncoding DNA, is likely to take many years to mature.

Although individual genetic disorders are rare, when considered together, they are among the most common problems identified in the ill newborn. Standard approaches to diagnosis, utilizing common testing and imaging results, allow the neonatal healthcare provider to rapidly narrow the differential and obtain directed testing to make a specific diagnosis.

RESOURCES

Online Mendelian Inheritance in Man, OMIM: An Online Catalog of Human Genes and Genetic Disorders website. https://omim.org/. Accessed November 12, 2018.

GeneReviews. Adam MP, Ardinger HH, Pagon RA, et al., eds. *GeneReviews.* Seattle, WA: University of Washington, Seattle; 1993-2018. https://www.ncbi.nlm.nih.gov/books/NBK1116/. Accessed November 12, 2018.

7

Care of the Parents

Kristin C. Voos, Jonathan M. Fanaroff

Unfortunately a certain number of mothers abandon the babies whose needs they have not had to meet, and in whom they have lost all interest. The life of the little one has been saved, it is true, but at the cost of the mother.[1]

Pierre Budin, The Nursling

A renewed interest in the first minutes, hours, and days of life has been stimulated by several provocative behavioral and physiologic observations in both mother and infant. These assessments and measurements have been made during labor, birth, the immediate postnatal period, and the initial breastfeedings. They provide a compelling rationale for major changes in care in the perinatal period for both mother and infant. These findings form a novel way to view the mother–infant dyad.

To understand how these observations fit together, it is necessary to appreciate that the period of labor, birth, and the ensuing several days can probably best be defined as a "sensitive period." During this time, the mother and, probably, the father, are especially open to changing their later behavior with their infant depending on the quality of their care during the sensitive period.

Winnicott also described this period.[2] He reported a special mental state of the mother in the perinatal period that involves a greatly increased sensitivity to, and focus on, the needs of her baby. He indicated that this state of "primary maternal preoccupation" starts near the end of pregnancy and continues for a few weeks after the birth of the baby. A mother needs nurturing support and a protected environment to develop and maintain this state. This special preoccupation and the openness of the mother to her baby is probably related to the bonding process. Winnicott wrote that "Only if a mother is sensitized in the way I am describing, can she feel herself into her infant's place, and so meet the infant's needs." In the state of "primary maternal preoccupation," the mother is better able to sense and provide what her new infant has signaled, which is her primary task. If she senses the needs and responds to them in a sensitive and timely manner, mother and infant will establish a pattern of synchronized and mutually rewarding interactions. It is our hypothesis that as the mother–infant pair continues this dance pattern day after day, the infant will more frequently develop a secure attachment, with the ability to be reassured by well-known caregivers and the willingness to explore and master the environment when caregivers are present.

This chapter describes studies of the process by which a parent becomes attached to the infant and the physiologic and behavioral components in the newborn, and suggests applications of these findings to the care of the parents of a normal infant, a premature or sick infant, and a stillbirth or neonatal death. Technical advances in the care of critically ill and premature infants have resulted in decreased mortality and morbidity of the high-risk infant. These developments have been accompanied by a heightened awareness of the psychologic strain and emotional stresses encountered by the family of a sick neonate and the profound effect on family functioning.[3–7] Realization of the need for a family-centered approach to perinatal care has emerged out of an enhanced understanding of individual and family functioning and the challenges in coping and adapting to stress.[8–11] It has become essential for perinatal healthcare teams to be cognizant of the overall psychological needs of families who are experiencing the painful crisis of the birth of a sick newborn.[6,12]

PREGNANCY

A mother's and father's actions and responses toward their infant are derived from a complex combination of their own genetic endowment, the way the infant responds to them, a long history of interpersonal relations with their own families and with each other, past experiences with this or previous pregnancies, the absorption of the practices and values of their cultures, and probably most importantly, how each was raised by his or her own mother and father. The parenting behavior of each woman and man, his or her ability to tolerate stresses, and his or her need for special attention differ greatly and depend on a mixture of these factors. Fig. 7.1 is a schematic diagram of the major influences on paternal and maternal behavior and the resulting disturbances that we hypothesize may arise from them.

Included under parental background are the parent's care by his or her own mother, genetics of parents, practices of their culture, relationships within the family, experiences

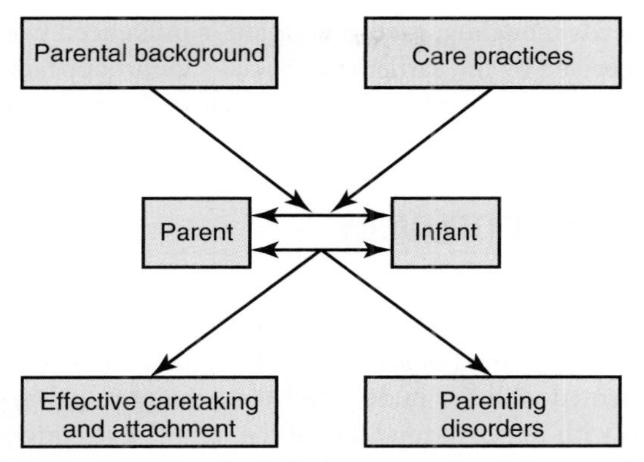

Fig. 7.1 Algorithm of major influences on parent–infant attachment and resulting outcomes.

BOX 7.1 Steps in Attachment

- Before pregnancy:
  - Planning the pregnancy
- During pregnancy:
  - Confirming the pregnancy
  - Accepting the pregnancy
  - Experiencing fetal movement
  - Beginning to accept the fetus as an individual
- Labor
- Birth
- After birth:
  - Touching and smelling
  - Seeing the baby
  - Breastfeeding
  - Caring for the baby
  - Accepting the infant as a separate individual

with previous pregnancies, and planning, course, and events during pregnancy. Strong evidence for the importance of the effect of the mother's own mothering on her caretaking comes from an elegant 35-year study by Engel et al. that documented the close correspondence between how Monica (an infant with a tracheoesophageal fistula) was fed during the first 2 years of life,[13] how she then cared for her dolls, and how as an adult she fed her own four children.

During the first hours and days of life, it is here, during this period, that studies have in part clarified some of the steps in parent–infant attachment. A diversity of observations are beginning to piece together some of the various phases and times that are helpful for this process (Box 7.1). Pregnancy for a woman has been considered a process of maturation,[14,15] with a series of adaptive tasks, each dependent on the successful completion of the preceding one.

Some mothers may be initially disturbed by feelings of grief and anger when they become pregnant because of factors ranging from economic and housing hardships to interpersonal difficulties. However, by the end of the first trimester, the majority of women who initially rejected pregnancy have accepted it. This initial stage, as outlined by Bibring, is the mother's identification of the growing fetus as an "integral part of herself."[14]

The second stage is a growing perception of the fetus as a separate individual, usually occurring with the awareness of fetal movement. After quickening, a woman generally begins to have some fantasies about what the baby may be like; she attributes some human personality characteristics and develops a sense of attachment and value toward the baby. At this time, further acceptance of the pregnancy and marked changes in attitude toward the fetus may be observed; unplanned infants can become deeply valued. Objectively, the health worker usually finds some outward evidence of the mother's preparation in such actions as the purchase of clothes or a crib, selecting a name, and arranging space for the baby.

The increased use of amniocentesis and ultrasound has appeared to affect parents' perceptions of babies in a rather unexpected fashion. Many parents have discussed the disappointment they experienced when they discovered the sex of the baby. Half of the mystery was over. Everything was possible, but once the amniocentesis was done and the sex of the baby known, the range of the unknown was considerably narrowed. However, the tests have the beneficial result of removing some of the anxiety about the possibility of the baby having an abnormality. We have noted that, following the procedure, the baby is sometimes named, and parents often carry around a picture of the very small fetus. This phenomenon requires further investigation to understand the significance of these reactions to the bonding process.

Cohen suggests the following questions to learn the special needs of each mother[16]:

- How long have you lived in this immediate area, and where does most of your family live?
- How often do you see your mother or other close relatives?
- Has anything happened to you in the past (or do you currently have any condition) that causes you to worry about the pregnancy or the baby?
- What was the father's reaction to your becoming pregnant?
- What other responsibilities do you have outside the family?

When planning to meet the needs of the mother, it is important to inquire about how the pregnant woman was mothered—did she have a neglected and deprived infancy and childhood or grow up with a warm and intact family life?

LABOR AND DELIVERY

Newton and Newton noted that those mothers who remain relaxed in labor,[17] who are supported, and who have good rapport with their attendants are more apt to be pleased with their infants at first sight.

One Cochrane review looked at the importance of continuous support for women during childbirth. Looking at 21 trials involving 15,061 mothers, the results showed that women who had continuous social support during labor and birth had labors that were significantly shorter, were more likely to have a spontaneous vaginal birth, and were less likely to have intrapartum analgesia.[18] They also were less likely to have a cesarean section or instrumented vaginal birth, regional anesthesia, or a baby with a low 5-minute Apgar score. This low-cost intervention may be a simple way to reduce the length of labor and perinatal problems for women and their infants during childbirth.

EFFECTS OF SOCIAL AND EMOTIONAL SUPPORT ON MATERNAL BEHAVIOR

Pregnancy and labor, a highly significant time in a woman's life, has been explored in depth because the care during labor appears to affect a mother's attitudes, feelings, and responses to her family, herself, and especially her new baby to a remarkable degree. In a well-conducted trial of continuous social support in South Africa, both mothers with and without doula support were interviewed immediately after delivery and 6 weeks later.[19,20] Women who had support during labor had significantly increased self-esteem, believed they had coped well with labor, and thought the labor had been easier than they had imagined. Women who received this support reported being less anxious 24 hours after birth compared with mothers without a doula. Supported mothers were significantly less depressed 6 weeks postpartum, as measured on a standard depression scale. Also, supported mothers had a significantly greater incidence of breastfeeding without supplements (52% versus 29%), and they breastfed for a longer period.

The supported mothers said it took them an average of 2.9 days to develop a relationship with their babies compared with 9.8 days for the nonsupported mothers. This feeling of attachment and readiness to fall in love with their babies made them less willing to leave their babies alone. They also reported picking up their babies more frequently when they cried than did nonsupported mothers. The supported mothers were more positive in describing the special attributes of their babies than were the nonsupported mothers. A higher percentage of supported mothers not only considered their babies beautiful, clever, healthy, and easy to manage, but also believed their infants cried less than other babies. The supported mothers believed that their babies were "better" when compared with a "standard baby," whereas the nonsupported mothers perceived their babies as "almost as good as" or "not quite as good as" a "standard baby." "Support group mothers also perceived themselves as closer to their babies, as managing better, and as communicating better with their babies than control-group mothers did," the study reported. A higher percentage of the supported mothers indicated that they were pleased to have their babies, found becoming a mother was easier than expected, and thought that they could look after their babies better than any other person could. In contrast, the nonsupported mothers perceived their adaptation to motherhood as more difficult and believed that others could care for their baby as well as they could.

A most important aspect of emotional support during childbirth may be the most unexpected internalized one—that of the calm, nurturing, accepting, and holding model provided for the parents with support during labor. Maternal care needs modeling; each generation is influenced from the care received by the earlier one. Social support appears to be an essential ingredient of childbirth that was lost when birthing moved from home to hospital.

THE DAY OF DELIVERY

Mothers after delivery appear to have common patterns of behavior when they begin to care for their babies in the first hour of life. Filmed observations reveal that when a mother is presented with her nude,[21] full-term infant in privacy, she begins with fingertip touching of the infant's extremities and within a few minutes proceeds to massaging, encompassing palm contact of the infant's trunk. Mothers of premature infants also follow this sequence, but proceed at a much slower rate. Fathers go through some of the same routines.[22]

A strong interest in eye-to-eye contact has been expressed by mothers of both full-term and premature infants. Tape recordings of the words of mothers who had been presented with their infants in privacy revealed that 73% of the statements referred to the eyes. The mothers said, "Let me see your eyes" and "Open your eyes and I'll know you love me." Robson has suggested that eye-to-eye contact appears to elicit maternal caregiving responses.[23] Mothers seem to try hard to look "en face" at their infants—that is, to keep their faces aligned with their baby's so that their eyes are in the same vertical plane of rotation as the baby's. Complementing the mother's interest in the infant's eyes is the early functional development of the infant's visual pathways. The infant is alert, active, and able to follow during the first hour of life if maternal sedation has been limited and the administration of eye drops or ointment is delayed.

Additional information about this early period was provided by Wolff,[24] who described six separate states of consciousness in the infant, ranging from deep sleep to screaming. The state in which we are most interested is state 4, the quiet, alert state. In this state, the infant's eyes are wide open, and he or she is able to respond to his or her environment. The infant may only be in this state for periods as brief as a few seconds. However, Emde et al. observed that the infant is in a wakeful state on the average for a period of 38 minutes during the first hour after birth.[25] It is currently possible to demonstrate that an infant can see, has visual preferences, has a memory for the mother's face at 4 hours of age, will turn his or her head to the spoken word, and moves in rhythm to the mother's voice in the first minutes and hours of life—a beautiful linking and synchronized dance between the mother and infant. After this, however, the infant goes into a deep sleep for 3 to 4 hours.

Therefore during the first 60 to 90 minutes of life, the infant is alert, responsive, and especially appealing. In short, the infant is ideally equipped to meet his or her parents for the first time. The infant's broad array of sensory and motor abilities evokes responses from the mother and begins the communication that may be especially helpful for attachment and the initiation of a series of reciprocal interactions. It is important to keep the mother–infant dyad together during those first critical moments whenever medically possible.

Observations by Condon and Sander reveal that newborns move in rhythm with the structure of adult speech.[26] Interestingly, synchronous movements were found at 16 hours of age with both of the two natural languages tested, English and Chinese.

Mothers also quickly become aware of their infant. Kaitz et al. demonstrated that after only 1 hour with their infants in the first hours of life,[27,28] mothers are able to discriminate their own baby from other infants. Parturient women know their infant's distinctive features after minimal exposure using olfactory and tactile cues (touching the dorsum of the hand), whereas discrimination based on sight and sound takes somewhat longer to develop. Fathers are good at quickly recognizing their newborn through visual-facial cues, although not quite as good as mothers at recognizing olfactory cues.[29]

Without attachment, there is risk for the following parenting disorders: vulnerable child syndrome,[30] child abuse,[31,32] failure to thrive,[33] and some developmental and emotional problems in high-risk infants.[34] Other determinants—such as the attitudes, statements, and practices of the nurses and physicians in the hospital, whether the mother is alone for short periods during her labor, whether there is separation from the infant in the first days of life, the nature of the infant, his or her temperament, and whether he or she is healthy, sick, or malformed—will affect parenting behavior and the parent–child relationship. Included under care practices are the behavior of physicians, nurses, and hospital personnel, care and support during labor, first days of life, separation of mother and infant, and rules of the hospital. The variables most easily remedied in this scheme are the separation of the infant from the mother and the practices in the hospital during the first hours and days of life.

CARE OF THE HEALTHY TERM INFANT AND PARENTS FOLLOWING BIRTH

After birth, the newborn should be thoroughly dried with warm towels so as not to lose heat and be observed to have good color and be active (usually within 5 minutes); ideally, this can be done on the mother. If not, the warm and dry infant should be placed between the mother's breasts or on her abdomen or, if she desires, next to her as soon as possible. The latest Neonatal Resuscitation Program guidelines emphasize that babies who do not need resuscitation should not be separated from their mothers.[35]

When newborns are kept close to their mother's body or on their mother, the transition from life in the womb to existence outside the uterus is made much easier for them. The newborn recognizes his mother's voice and smell,[36,37] and her body warms his to just the right temperature.[38] In this way, the infant can experience sensations somewhat similar to what he felt during the last several weeks of uterine life.

In the past, many caretakers believed that the newborn needs help to begin to nurse. So often, immediately after birth, the baby's lips are placed near or on the mother's nipple. In that situation, some babies do start to suckle, but most babies just lick the nipple or peer up at the mother. They appear to be much more interested in the mother's face, especially her eyes, even though the nipple is right next to their lips. They most commonly begin, when left on their own, to move toward the breast 30 to 40 minutes after birth.

THE BREAST CRAWL

One of the most exciting observations made is the discovery that the newborn has the ability to find her mother's breast all on her own and to decide for herself when to take her first feeding. In order not to remove the taste and smell of the mother's amniotic fluid, it is necessary to delay washing the baby's hands. The baby uses the taste and smell of amniotic fluid on her hands to make a connection with a certain lipid substance on the nipple related to the amniotic fluid.

The infant usually begins with a time of rest and quiet alertness, during which he rarely cries and often appears to take pleasure in looking at his mother's face. Around 30 to 40 minutes after birth, the newborn begins making mouthing movements, sometimes with lip smacking, and shortly after, saliva begins to pour down onto his chin.[39] When placed on the mother's abdomen, babies maneuver in their own ways to reach the nipple. They often use stepping motions of their legs to move ahead while horizontally moving toward the nipple, using small push-ups and lowering one arm first in the direction they wish to go. These efforts are interspersed with short rest periods. Sometimes babies change direction in the midst of their journey. These actions take effort and time. Parents find patience worth every minute if they wait and observe their infant on his first journey.

In Fig. 7.2, one newborn is seen successfully navigating his way to his mother's breast. At 10 minutes of age, he first begins to move toward the left breast, but 5 minutes later, he is back in the midline. Repeated mouthing and sucking of the hands and fingers is commonly observed. With a series of push-ups and rest periods, he makes his way to the breast completely on his own, placing his lips on the areola of the breast. He begins to suckle effectively and closely observes his mother's face.

In one group of mothers who did not receive pain medication and whose babies were not taken away during the first hours of life for a bath, vitamin K administration, or application of eye ointment, 15 of 16 babies placed on their mother's abdomen were observed to make the trip to their mother's breast, latch on their own, and begin to suckle effectively.[40]

This sequence is helpful to the mother as well, because the massage of the breast and suckling induce a large oxytocin surge into her bloodstream, which helps contract the uterus, expelling the placenta and closing off many blood vessels in the uterus, thus reducing bleeding. The stimulation and suckling also helps in the manufacture of prolactin, and the suckling enhances the closeness and new bond between mother and baby. Mother and baby appear to be carefully adapted for these first moments together.

To allow this first intimate encounter, the injection of vitamin K, application of eye ointment, washing, and any measuring of the infant's weight, height, and head circumference may be delayed for at least 1 hour. More than 90% of all

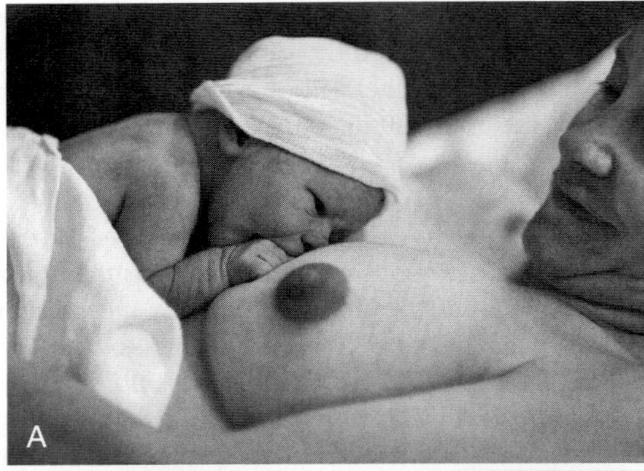

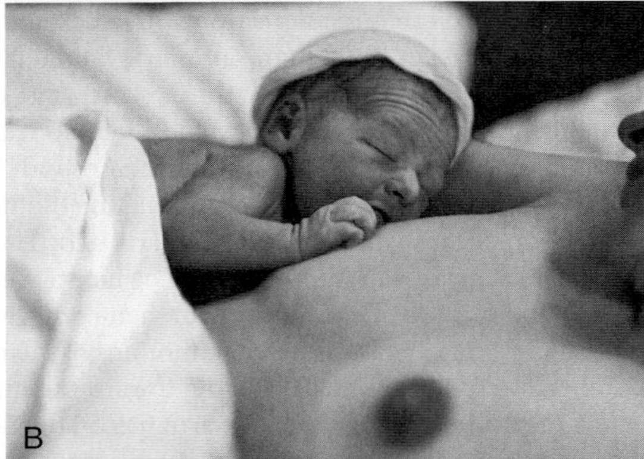

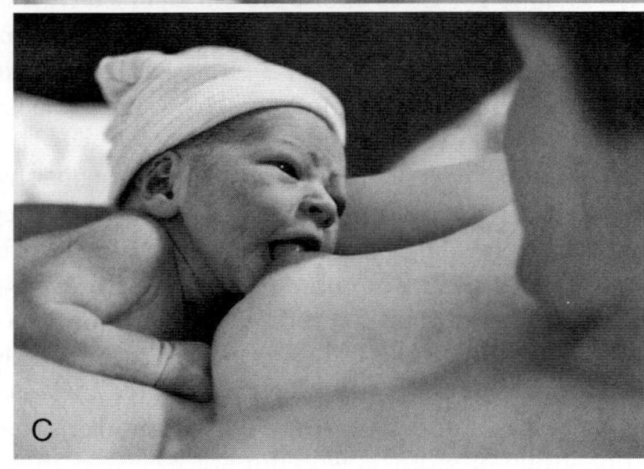

Fig. 7.2 (A) Infant about 15 minutes after birth, sucking on the unwashed hand and possibly looking at mother's left nipple. (B) An arm push-up, which helps the infant move to mother's right side. (C) At 45 minutes of age, the infant moved to the right breast without assistance and began sucking on the areola of the breast. The infant has been looking at the mother's face for 5 to 8 minutes. (Photographed by Elaine Siegel. From Klaus PH. *Your Amazing Newborn,* Cambridge: Perseus; 1998:13,16,17.)

full-term infants are normal at birth. In a few minutes, they can be easily evaluated to ensure that they are healthy.

The odor of the nipple appears to guide a newborn to the breast.[37,41] If the right breast is washed with soap and water, the infant will crawl to the left breast, and vice versa. If both breasts are washed, the infant will go to the breast that has been rubbed with the amniotic fluid of the mother. The special attraction of the newborn to the odor of *his* mother's amniotic fluid may reflect the time in utero when, as a fetus, he swallowed the liquid. Although it is not breast milk, amniotic fluid probably contains a substance that is similar to a secretion of the breast. Amniotic fluid on the infant's hands probably also explains part of the interest in sucking the hands and fingers seen in the photographs. Early hand-sucking behavior is markedly reduced when the infant is bathed before the crawl. With all these innate programs, it almost seems as if the infant comes into life carrying a small computer chip with these instructions.

At a moment such as childbirth, we come full circle to our biological origins. Many separate abilities enable a baby to do this. Stepping reflexes help the newborn push against his mother's abdomen to propel him toward the breast. Pressure of the infant's feet on the abdomen may also help in the expulsion of the placenta and in reducing uterine bleeding. The ability to move his hand in a reaching motion enables the baby to find the nipple. Taste, smell, and vision all help the newborn detect and find the breast. Muscular strength in the neck, shoulders, and arms helps newborns bob their heads and do small push-ups to inch forward and side to side. This whole scenario may take place in a matter of minutes; it usually occurs within 30 to 60 minutes, but it is within the capacity of the newborn. It appears that young humans, like other baby mammals, know how to find their mother's breast.

When the mother and infant are resting skin to skin and gazing eye to eye, they begin to learn about each other on many different levels. For the mother, the first minutes and hours after birth are a time when she is uniquely open emotionally to respond to her baby and to begin the new relationship.

A Sensitive Period?

Many studies have focused on whether additional time for close contact of the mother and infant alters the quality of attachment.[21,42,43] These studies have addressed the question of whether there is a sensitive period for parent–infant contact in the first minutes, hours, and days of life that may alter the parents' later behavior with their infant. In many biological disciplines, these moments have been called *sensitive periods.* However, in most of the examples of a sensitive period in biology, the observations are made on the young of the species rather than on the adult. Evidence for a sensitive period comes from the following series of studies. Note that in each study, increasing mother–infant time together or increased suckling improves caretaking by the mother.

In six of nine randomized trials of only early contact with suckling (during the first hour of life), both the number of women breastfeeding and the length of their lactation were significantly increased for early contact mothers compared with women in the control group.

In addition, studies of Brazelton and others have shown that if nurses spend as little as 10 minutes helping mothers discover some of their newborn infant's abilities,[44] such as turning to the mother's voice and following the mother's face, and assisting mothers with suggestions about ways to quiet their infants, the mothers become more appropriately interactive with their infants face-to-face and during feedings at 3 and 4 months of age.

O'Connor et al. carried out a randomized trial with 277 mothers in a hospital that had a high incidence of parenting disorders.[45] One group of mothers had their infants with them for 6 additional hours on the first and second day, but no early contact. The routine care group began to see their babies at the same age but only for 20-minute feedings every 4 hours, which was the custom throughout the United States at that time. In follow-up studies, 10 children in the routine care group experienced parenting disorders, including child abuse, failure to thrive, abandonment, and neglect during the first 17 months of life compared with two children in the experimental group who had 12 additional hours of mother–infant contact. A similar study in North Carolina that included 202 mothers during the first year of life did not find a statistically significant difference in the frequency of parenting disorders[33]; 10 infants failed to thrive or were neglected or abused in the control group compared with seven in the group that had extended contact. When the results of these two studies are combined in a metaanalysis ($p = 0.054$), it appears that simple techniques, such as adding additional early time for each mother and infant to be together and continuous rooming-in, may lead to a significant reduction in child abuse. A much larger study is necessary to confirm and validate these relatively small studies.

Swedish researchers have shown that the normal infant,[38] when dried and placed nude on the mother's chest and then covered with a blanket, will maintain his or her body temperature as well as when elaborate, high-tech heating devices that usually separate the mother and baby are used. The same researchers found that when the infants are skin to skin with their mothers for the first 90 minutes after birth, they cry hardly at all compared with infants who were dried, wrapped in a towel, and placed in a bassinet. It is likely that each of these features—the crawling ability of the infant, the decreased crying when close to the mother, and the warming capabilities of the mother's chest—are adaptive features that have evolved to help preserve the infant's life.

When the infant suckles from the breast, it stimulates the production of oxytocin in both the mother's and the infant's brains, and oxytocin in turn stimulates the vagal motor nucleus, releasing 19 different gastrointestinal hormones, including insulin, cholecystokinin, and gastrin. Five of the 19 hormones stimulate growth of the baby's and mother's intestinal villi and increase the surface area and the absorption of calories with each feeding.[46] Stimuli for this release are touch on the mother's nipple and the inside of the infant's mouth. The increased gut motility with each suckling may help remove meconium, with its large load of bilirubin.

These research findings may explain some of the underlying physiologic and behavioral processes and provide additional support for the importance of 2 of the 10 caregiving procedures that the United Nations International Children's Emergency Fund is promoting as part of its Baby Friendly Initiative to increase breastfeeding: (1) early mother–infant contact, with an opportunity for the baby to suckle in the first hour; and (2) mother–infant rooming-in throughout the hospital stay.

Following the introduction of the Baby Friendly Initiative in maternity units in several countries throughout the world, an unexpected observation was made. In Thailand,[47] in a hospital where a disturbing number of babies are abandoned by their mothers, the use of rooming-in and early contact with suckling significantly reduced the frequency of abandonment from 33 in 10,000 births to 1 in 10,000 births a year. Similar observations have been made in Russia, the Philippines, and Costa Rica, where early contact and rooming-in were also introduced.

These reports are additional evidence that the first hours and days of life are a sensitive period for the human mother. This may be due in part to the special interest that mothers have shortly after birth in hoping that their infant will look at them and to the infant's ability to interact in the first hour of life during the prolonged period of the quiet alert state. There is a beautiful interlocking at this early time of the mother's interest in the infant's eyes and the baby's ability to interact and to look eye to eye.

A possible key to understanding what is happening physiologically in these first minutes and hours comes from investigators who noted that if the lips of the infant touch the mother's nipple in the first hour of life, a mother will decide to keep her baby 100 minutes longer in her room every day during her hospital stay than another mother who does not have contact until later.[48] This may be partly explained by the small secretions of oxytocin (the "love hormone") that occur in both the infant's and mother's brains when breastfeeding occurs. In sheep,[49] dilation of the cervical os during birth releases oxytocin within the brain, which, acting on receptor sites, is important for the initiation of maternal behavior and for the facilitation of bonding between mother and baby. In humans, there is a blood–brain barrier for oxytocin, and only small amounts reach the brain via the bloodstream. However, multiple oxytocin receptors in the brain are supplied by de novo oxytocin synthesis in the brain. Increased levels of brain oxytocin result in slight sleepiness, euphoria, increased pain threshold, and feelings of increased love for the infant.

Measurements of plasma oxytocin levels in healthy women who had their babies skin to skin on their chests immediately after birth reveal significant elevations compared with the prepartum levels and a return to prepartum levels at 60 minutes. For most women, a significant and spontaneous peak concentration was recorded about 15 minutes after delivery, with expulsion of the placenta.[50] Most mothers had several peaks of oxytocin up to 1 hour after delivery. The vigorous oxytocin release after delivery and with breastfeeding may not only help contract uterine muscle to prevent bleeding but also enhance bonding of the mother to her infant. These findings may explain an observation made in France in the 19th century when many poor mothers were giving up their babies. Nurses recorded that mothers who breastfed for at least 8 days rarely abandoned their infants. We hypothesize that a cascade of interactions between the mother and baby occurs during this early period, locking them together and ensuring further development of attachment. The remarkable change in maternal behavior with just the touch of the infant's lips on the mother's nipple, the effects of additional time for mother–infant contact, and the reduction in abandonment with early contact, suckling, and rooming-in, as well as the elevated maternal oxytocin levels shortly after birth in conjunction with known sensory, physiologic, immunologic, and behavioral mechanisms all contribute to the attachment of the parent to the infant.

EARLY AND EXTENDED CONTACT FOR PARENTS AND THEIR INFANT

Although debate continues on the interpretation and significance of some of the research studies regarding the effects of early and extended contact for mothers and fathers on bonding with their infants, both sides agree that all parents should be offered such contact time with their infants. A Cochrane Review looked at 30 studies involving 1925 participants (mother–infant dyads) and concluded that early skin-to-skin contact for mothers and their healthy newborns reduced crying, improved mother-baby interaction, kept the baby warmer, and women breastfeed successfully.[51]

Evidence suggests that many of these early interactions also take place between the father and his newborn child. Parke has demonstrated that when fathers are given the opportunity to be alone with their newborns,[52] they spend almost exactly the same amount of time as mothers in holding, touching, and looking at them.

How strongly should physicians and nurses emphasize the importance of parent–infant contact in the first hour and extended visiting for the rest of the hospital stay? Despite a lack of early contact experienced by many parents in hospital births in the past, almost all these parents became bonded to their babies. The human is highly adaptable, and there are many fail-safe routes to attachment. Parents who miss the bonding experience can be assured that their future relationship with their infant can still develop as usual. Mothers who miss out on early and extended contact are often those at the limits of adaptability and who may benefit the most—the poor, the single, the unsupported, and the teenage mothers.

At least 60 minutes of early contact in privacy should be provided, if possible, for parents and their infant to enhance the bonding experience. If the health of the mother or infant makes this impossible, then discussion, support, and reassurance should help the parents appreciate that they can become as completely attached to their infant as if they had the usual bonding experience. If modifications are needed based on medical need, the medical team should do what they can to keep the mother and baby together while maintaining safety for both the infant and mother. The baby should remain with the mother as long as desired throughout the hospital stay so that the mother and the baby can get to know each other. This permits both mother and father more time to learn about their baby and to gradually develop a strong tie in the first weeks of life.

From these many findings are the following recommendations for changing the perinatal period for mother and for the healthy, term infant:

- Every mother should ideally have continuous physical and emotional support during the entire labor by a knowledgeable, caring woman (e.g., doula, obstetric nurse, or midwife) in addition to her partner.
- Childbirth educators and obstetric caregivers should discuss with every pregnant woman the advantages of an unmedicated labor to avoid interference with the infant's ability to interact, self-attach, and successfully breastfeed.
- Immediately after birth and a thorough drying, an infant who has good Apgar scores and appears normal should be offered to the mother for skin-to-skin contact, with warmth provided by her body and a light blanket covering the baby. The baby should not be removed for a bath, footprinting, or administration of vitamin K or eye medication until after the first hour. The baby thus can be allowed to decide when to begin his first feeding.
- The central nursery should be used infrequently. All babies should room-in with their mothers throughout the short hospital course unless this is prevented by illness of mother or infant. If rooming is not possible due to medical needs, efforts should be made for mother–infant interactions as much as possible.
- Early and continuous mother–infant contact appears to decrease the incidence of abandonment and increase the length and success of breastfeeding. All mothers should begin breastfeeding in the first hour, nurse frequently, and be encouraged to breastfeed for at least the first 2 weeks of life, even if they plan to return to work. Early, frequent breastfeeding has many advantages, including earlier removal of bilirubin from the gut as well as aiding in mother–infant attachment.

EDITORIAL COMMENT: While bonding is certainly important for multiple reasons, infant safety is equally important. New mothers are often sleep deprived, recovering from delivery and/or surgery, and possibly on a number of medications that may have a sedative effect. There have been a number of reported cases of newborns with apnea or cardiorespiratory failure related to inadvertent suffocation or entrapment. The risk of these events, referred to as sudden unexpected postnatal collapse, may be decreased with appropriate hospital skin-to-skin and safe sleep policies.

THE SICK OR PREMATURE INFANT

Parents of infants requiring neonatal intensive care often experience high levels of stress, and as a consequence, this impairs their abilities to interact optimally with their infants. For many parents, this may be the first time they have had to cope with a significant challenge in their lives. This may lead to depression, impaired recall, dysfunctional parenting patterns, and poorer child developmental outcomes.[53–56] The perinatal healthcare team is presented with a unique opportunity to practice family-centered and preventive health care.[12,57]

During this stressful time, the families' usual problem-solving mechanisms may not be adequate to cope with the events presented to them. In addition to confronting this situational crisis, the individual or family must master the normal developmental process of parenthood.

Situational factors can have an important bearing on the family's ability to cope with the crisis and thus affect the overall outcome. Uncertainty about their infant's future and separation from their infant are sources of parental stress that can dramatically affect the quality of attachment that develops.[55,58] Even when parents have close contact with their infants in the intensive care nursery, they may still experience prolonged stress.

Highly interacting mothers visit and telephone the nursery more frequently while the infants are hospitalized, and stimulate their infants more at home. Mothers who stimulate their infants very little in the nursery also visit and telephone less frequently and provide only minimal stimulation to them at home. Most perceptively, Minde et al. noted that mothers who touched their infants more in the nursery had infants who opened their eyes more often.[60] He and his associates observed the contingency between the infant's eyes being open and the mother's touching and between gross motor stretches and the mother's smiling. They could not determine to what extent the sequence of touching and eye opening was an indication of the mother's primary contribution or whether it was initiated by the infant. Thus Newman and Minde et al. predict that mothers who become involved with,[60,61] interested in, and anxious about their infants in the intensive care nursery will have an easier time when the infant is taken home.

Families are psychologically vulnerable after the birth of a sick infant. During this period of crisis, there may be a heightened receptivity to accepting help and being open and responsive to change as the family is struggling for a way to cope with the crisis. Significant potentialities exist for individual and family emotional growth and development.[4,62,63] Parental perception of support by nurses was significantly associated with maternal depressive symptoms; as the perception of nursing support decreased, there was a corresponding increase in the maternal depressive symptoms.[65] The perinatal health team has an opportunity to influence how the individual and family adapt to the crisis.[4,7,56,63,64.]

By providing appropriate supportive interventions coupled with enlightened policies and attitudes that reflect family-centered principles, the team can have a significant positive influence on the family's ability to cope. With this comes the enhanced likelihood for successful adjustment and ultimately a healthy parent–child relationship.[a]

Family-centered care principles stress that parents are the most important persons in their infant's life, that they have expertise in caring for the infant, and that their values and beliefs should be central during neonatal intensive care unit (NICU) care.[10,66] Family-centered care demands a change from task-oriented, healthcare provider–centered care to a collaborative, relationship-based model of family advocacy and empowerment.[10,63,67,68]

Family-centered care is a philosophy often strived for in the NICU, but current practice and policies can often lag behind philosophy. NICU staff verbalize acceptance of families being involved in care, but their actions do not always reflect their words.[69,70] Studies show a discrepancy between nurses' knowledge about the necessity of and their current practice of family-centered care.[71] Current practice of family-centered care scored significantly lower than scores representing necessity: NICU staff do not consistently practice what they know to be necessary. Organizational barriers to implementation include: (1) the design of the healthcare system; (2) the lack of emotional support, guidance, and direction for the staff; (3) the lack of recognition, confidence, and support for nursing autonomy and skills to perform family-centered care; and (4) beliefs that dealing with families is stressful, interferes with care of the infant, and is "not part of my job."[63,71]

EDITORIAL COMMENT: The neonatal intensive care unit, of course, is part of a much larger social system. In this regard, the United States has the shortest length of maternity leave, 12 weeks, compared to other countries. Sweden takes the prize for the longest maternity leave, at 420 days, with 80% of wages paid!

Fenwick's research reports that mothers perceive their relationship with NICU nurses as either facilitating or inhibiting their ability to mother their infants in the NICU. Actions that facilitate mothering are family centered or family integrated. Facilitative nursing actions include fostering the relationship between mother and infant by: (1) assisting mothers to gain intimate knowledge and caregiving opportunities, (2) educating parents about their infants medical condition, (3) providing ongoing positive feedback to parents, (4) acknowledging the importance of the dyadic mother–infant and father–infant relationship, (5) honoring the mother as the infant's primary caregiver, (6) enhancing mother–infant interaction opportunities, and (7) collaborating with parents and relinquishing control to parents, particularly at the bedside.[63,67]

The parents are very sensitive to the staff's attitude toward the infant, as reflected by their comments and the manner in which the staff handle the infant. If the infant is regarded with respect and treated as important, the parent is given the feeling that the infant is seen as valued and worthwhile. This is especially important for parents of an infant with a congenital anomaly; the parents could wonder if their infant is viewed as "damaged goods" by society. In describing the infant to the parent, staff present a balanced picture of both the normal and abnormal aspects of the infant. In discussing the infant with the parents, staff should refer to the infant by name, if they have named the infant; this helps personalize the infant and establish the infant's unique identity.

[a] 4,5,6,12,64,66,67

To reinforce the caregiving needs of parents, discuss with them their plans to feed their infant. Support and encouragement should be given whether the parents have decided on breastfeeding or bottle-feeding. In most situations, breastfeeding an infant even in the NICU is possible. Many mothers can pump their breasts for milk that eventually will be given to the infant. The breastfeeding or pumping experience helps the mother feel close to her infant and helps her feel that she has some control over what is happening to her infant; she can uniquely contribute to her infant's care in a way no one else can. Fathers, too, can participate in this activity by their support and interest in the actual breastfeeding or the pumping and milk collection activities. Many mothers can pump and eventually put the infant to breast, but others cannot because of emotional stresses, the condition of the infant, and the length of time until the infant can feed. Regardless of eventual success, the mother should be encouraged to try if she has an interest; then she can feel that she made an attempt to relate to her infant in this way. If a mother does not plan to breastfeed or pump or if she tries but does not continue, she should not be made to feel guilty or that she failed in her role. She is already vulnerable to these feelings.

After the delivery, when the mother is taken to her room without a healthy infant, she usually experiences a void.[16] The interventions of the staff should be flexible and sensitive to the individual needs of the family. Empathy, responsiveness, and an ability to listen to the parents are important at this time.[68]

Encouraging parents to verbalize and express their feelings and concerns (at their own pace), although difficult to do at times, is useful to the parents. Listening is as important to parents as giving them information.[72] In talking to parents, bear in mind that the parents do not remember much of what has been said; it is very difficult for them to assimilate all that has happened, both cognitively and emotionally.

Some parents are very sad, depressed, and teary, and others may be highly anxious, at times bordering on panic states; others react by having a flat affect, withdrawing, and appearing apathetic. Some parents may exhibit very angry, hostile, confrontational behavior as a way of dealing with their distress. Others may deny the situation by optimistically feeling that "everything will be OK."

Parents need permission to have their feelings. It is essential to acknowledge to parents that it is normal to be afraid of attaching to an infant who is ill. Giving permission diminishes the guilt that the parents may feel about their behavior being abnormal or about being bad parents because they are afraid. Simple statements such as "Many parents tell us they are afraid of getting close to their baby." Social workers can provide valuable emotional support to families in helping them deal with their realistic and unrealistic concerns.

Prior studies have demonstrated that when parents experience less stress, they are more able to form early attachments to their sick infants.[55] Mothers with greater stress have less positive attitudes and interactions with their infants than those with less stress.[73] This lack of parenting confidence has been associated with lower levels of child competence and poorer child developmental outcomes.[74,75] Conversely, multiple studies have shown that positive attitudes and parental confidence are associated with secure infant attachments that lead to increased child competence and better developmental outcomes.[73] Studies have found an alarmingly high rate of psychologic pathology and traumatic stress in parents of infants in the NICU. Lefkowitz et al. had 86 mothers and 41 fathers complete measures of acute stress disorder (ASD) and found that 3 to 5 days after the infant's NICU admission,[15] 35% of mothers and 24% of fathers met diagnostic criteria for ASD. Additionally, 30 days later, 15% of mothers and 8% of fathers actually met diagnostic criteria for posttraumatic stress disorder. In some units, a psychiatrist is available to regularly meet with parents who wish to speak with him/her; this is an extremely helpful and necessary program.[76] Sensitivity training for patients aimed at recognizing signs of infant stress is associated with improved cerebral white matter development in preterm infants.[77] Thus it is not surprising that supportive interventions can decrease parental stress while infants are in the NICU and thereby promote better mother–infant attachment and improved infant developmental outcomes.[78,79]

COMMUNICATING MEDICAL INFORMATION

Most of the foundational work of family-centered care rests on effective communication.[80,81] It is well established that specific healthcare provider and patient/parent communication behaviors are associated with improved patient health status, recall, treatment adherence, and satisfaction.[80,82] The role of the healthcare professionals in communicating medical information is important. Parents need a realistic assessment of the situation that is honest and direct. Acknowledge the infant's condition and possible problems, but not necessarily every potential problem that can arise.

The principles of family-centered, family-integrated neonatal care clearly promote family participation in every aspect of their infant's care. Professional attitudes that may interfere with open, honest communication include: (1) assuming that parents are too emotional to assimilate information and make a rational decision, (2) assuming that information about complications and poor outcomes may disrupt attachment to the neonate, (3) assuming that parental guilt and psychologic harm will ensue from decision-making (despite research to the contrary), and (4) cultural and language differences.[10]

Many parents desire and can handle complete, specific, honest, detailed, unbiased, and meaningful information—the same facts and interpretation of those facts as the staff—delivered in a humane and respectful manner.[10] Parents have expressed "remarkably uniform and unambiguous requests ... to receive early, honest, and detailed information in a comprehensible and sympathetic manner and to be together when given bad news."

Individuals vary in their desire to be informed and involved in decision-making. Individuals also vary in the manner in which they assimilate information. Some parents may want extensive information about their situation, whereas others may not. However, physicians have an ethical and legal obligation to give parents the facts from which to make an informed shared decision about their neonate's condition, illnesses, outcomes, and the risks and benefits of various interventions.

Poor understanding by parents may be the result of poor communication techniques, contradictory messages, poor parental health, inexperience with medical terminology, denial, language barriers, inability to ask questions, or lack of opportunity to review the information. In one study, parents claimed that a neonatologist had never spoken to them, but, in fact, the conversation did occur and had been recorded.[83] In this study, parents were given a tape recording of their initial conversation with the neonatologist and any subsequent conversations of importance. The audiotape proved useful: 96% of the mothers and 68% of the fathers listened to the tape again an average of 2.5 and 1.8 times, respectively. Eighty-five percent of parents who listened to the tape had forgotten elements of the conversation, and two mothers did not recall that the conversation had ever occurred.

Research has documented that postpartum women and parents in stressful situations have transient deficits in cognitive function, particularly in attention and memory function.[84] Because verbal communication may be poorly remembered, augmentation with written instructions is recommended.[8,84] Again, some parents may want and need this type of information, whereas others may not. All communication needs to be culturally and linguistically appropriate.

There are several other guidelines in communicating medical information to parents. As discussed, parents' perceptions of their infant's condition are extremely important, remain in parents' minds, and can affect their relationship with the infant. Parents easily misperceive information given to them. Therefore in beginning any discussion with parents, it is essential to determine and address their perceptions. A staff member might say, "Could you tell me what you understand about your baby's condition?" Starting this way will give the physician or nurse the opportunity to correct any misinformation or misconceptions and to hear about the parents' concerns. The perceived morbidity of the baby is a source of stress for both mothers and fathers. Parents' perceptions of the severity of their infant's illness are complex, change over time, and are affected by parental anxiety, infant size, amount and type of equipment and treatments, and amount and type of information received from healthcare providers. A team member might specifically ask about the parents' concerns or worries: "Could you tell me what concerns you have about your baby?" Asking this can make communication between the perinatal healthcare team and parents more meaningful and helpful; unless the team deals with the parents' anxiety, discussions become one-sided lectures and benefit only the professional. Discussions should be a dialog between parent and professional.

During the course of a discussion and again at the end, it is useful to determine parents' interpretations of what has been said and modify and clarify as needed. It is more productive to move at a pace that allows the parent to assimilate the information presented. It is important to use simple language that is understandable. For some parents, the use of statistics is helpful; for others, it is not. Statistics can be confusing because they do not apply to the individual case and can be misinterpreted easily. Finally, if a referring physician and the nursery team are both communicating with the parents, it is essential to coordinate the particular approach. It is very confusing to parents and decreases their trust level if they receive conflicting information.

The principles of family-centered neonatal care also advocate full and free access to lay and medical literature pertaining to the neonate's condition, proposed treatments, and probable outcomes.[10] Medical literature, articles, books, and videos should be available in the NICU or in the hospital library for the parents' use. Access to the internet has proven to be a source of medical information (some accurate, some inaccurate) for families, as well as professionals. When recommending the internet as a resource, professionals should make parents aware of its benefits as well as shortcomings.

Providing culturally sensitive care in a growing multicultural and diverse society is essential and needs to be a constant pursuit in providing perinatal health care to families who have an infant in the NICU. It is important for the healthcare team to understand the values, beliefs, customs, and behaviors of the particular group(s) they serve. Culture influences beliefs about what causes illness and how that illness should be treated. The perinatal healthcare team needs to address cultural, linguistic, and spiritual competencies to provide family-centered care.

If a language or educational barrier is encountered, a qualified interpreter who is bilingual and ideally bicultural should be utilized. This is especially important in obtaining informed consent. A child or children should not be used as interpreters because they may have inadequate language skills and may be embarrassed by the topics being discussed. Often information that is translated, even by a certified translator, is not understood by families if they are not literate. However, illiteracy does not mean the family is not intelligent. Many parents can comprehend complex information if explained in a relevant manner.

Pictures can augment what is being explained. Providing a list of common medical terms and educational materials in the native language of the parents is another useful tool. At times, despite numerous discussions about the infant's medical condition, the family may appear unable to comprehend what they have been told. Consider that even if the healthcare provider and family share the same language, the words may have different meanings depending on core cultural beliefs and values and the families' previous experiences.

Becoming culturally competent healthcare providers is an ongoing developmental process. One should be aware of the dimensions and complexities in caring for individuals from diverse cultural backgrounds. It is important to understand the family's core cultural dynamics, the meaning of the infant's illness, and the social context within which these life events are occurring.

INTERVENTIONS FOR FAMILIES OF PREMATURE INFANTS: FAMILY-CENTERED CARE IN THE NICU

Providing the optimal hospital environment for a critically ill newborn clearly involves a great deal of care and consideration for the needs of the family as well. Modern NICU design and planning ideally incorporate features such as healing art, family/social spaces, and respite areas for staff.[66] One randomized, controlled trial in Stockholm found that allowing parents to stay in the NICU reduced the total length of hospital stay by 5.3 days.[85] Every facility, no matter what level of resources, can take steps to improve the environment for infants and their families by developing a unit vision and philosophy that promote the principles of family-centered care. Multidisciplinary groups have created tools and lists of potentially better practices for family-centered care.[86]

Some practices that may be considered for implementing family-centered, family-integrated care include the following[87]:

- The unit vision and philosophy should clearly articulate the principles of family-centered care.
- Leaders at the center and the unit level should clearly promote the principles of family-centered care.
- Parents are not "visitors." Rather, parents should be treated as essential components of the care team. Policies should be revised to reflect this view. "Visiting policies" should be revised to address nonparent family members and friends, whereas policies related to parents should be more appropriately addressed as participants in care.
- Neonatal care is multidisciplinary and based on mutual respect among providers for their roles and expertise. Parents are integral to care and should be encouraged to participate in patient care rounds, communication with personnel at the change of shifts, and in the bedside care of their infant. Parents should have access to information in their infant's medical record, and many units have initiated parent documentation into the record.
- The physical environment should provide for the needs of parents. Parents' needs for accessing information, rest, nutrition, privacy, childcare for siblings, and support for their infants by breast milk pumping are often inadequately addressed.
- Nursery staff should receive the support they need to provide optimal family-centered care. This support includes an environment that allows staff a time to rest to meet their own needs and ongoing education and resources to support family-centered care.

Families should be incorporated at various levels as advisors. The perspective of experienced families should be integral to the unit administrative activities. These could include parents as teachers during orientation and continuing education of staff, and parent advisory committees to collaborate in planning of new policies or space and ongoing quality improvement activities.

> **EDITORIAL COMMENT:** Family-centered care has benefits for everyone involved. Unfortunately, there has been an increase in violence and disruption from a very small subset of families in hospitals as well. This includes the neonatal intensive care unit (NICU). There are a number of measures NICU leadership can implement to encourage a safe work environment, including early recognition that a problem may be developing. Additionally, the Occupational Safety and Health Administration (OSHA) has developed a number of strategies to reduce the risk of injury and harm, available at www.osha.gov.

Transporting the Mother to be Near her Small Infant

With the development of high-risk perinatal centers, an increasing number of mothers are transported to the maternity division of hospitals with a neonatal intensive care nursery just before delivery or shortly after. If there is not sufficient time to arrange for her transport before she gives birth, it is strongly recommended that the mother be moved as soon as possible.

Supporting the Relationship With the Infant

The establishment of a relationship with their infant and initiating their caregiving role is most important. Ideally, parents have been involved as partners and caretakers since their infant was admitted to the NICU. Several formalized intervention programs have been developed and tested for efficacy in assisting parents of NICU infants in relating to and parenting their vulnerable infants. An early educational-behavioral intervention program for NICU parents (Creating Opportunities for Parent Empowerment [COPE]) was developed and tested in a randomized controlled trial with 260 families.[7] Mothers in the COPE program had significantly less stress in the NICU, more positive interactions with their infants, and less depression and anxiety at 2 months corrected infant age when compared with the control mothers. Other study outcomes included: (1) stronger parental beliefs about their role, (2) parents more able to read their infant's cues and behaviors, and (3) shorter length of both NICU and hospital stays when compared with the control group.[7] Another randomized study of an early intervention program found that parents who participated had a reduction in parenting stress after birth of their infant.[88] The March of Dimes initiative to encourage family-centered care (NICU Family Support Program) has been studied at eight sites by interviewing parents, NICU staff, and administrators. Findings include: (1) culture change within the NICU resulting in increased family support; (2) enhanced overall quality of NICU care; (3) less stressed, more informed, and confident parents; and (4) increased receptivity of staff to the concept of family-centered care and its benefits.[89] Involvement in caregiving lessens the parents' feelings of helplessness and frustration and facilitates their identification with their role as parents.[6,7,12,65,67,72]

Parents can provide skincare for their infant, learn to read and respond to infant cues, help turn the infant even if a respirator is attached, diaper the infant, and feed the infant. If the parents are separated by distance, they can send family pictures that can be posted at the infant's bed; periodic pictures of the infant taken by the staff can be sent back to the family. Parents can send clothing, mobiles, simple toys, and even recordings so that the infant can hear the parents' voices. Some mothers who are pumping send frozen breast milk. All of these reminders help the nursery staff be aware of the real family that is genuinely interested. These personal attempts made by parents that help them feel they are important to their infant's development should be encouraged. Sometimes foster grandparents or volunteers can hold, feed, and talk to infants whose parents cannot visit frequently. Many units are implementing family-integrated care or intensive parenting units, involving the family in all aspects of care.[90]

Kangaroo Care

Allowing a mother to hold the infant skin to skin for prolonged periods in the hospital is known as kangaroo care, and it has salutary effects (Fig. 7.3). Several trials have noted that if the usual precautions are taken, such as hand washing, there is no increase in the infection rate or problems in oxygenation, apnea, or temperature control. A significant medical benefit appears to be a significant increase in the mother's milk supply and success at nursing.[91,92] A randomized controlled trial in Madagascar also found a significantly increased proportion of exclusive breastfeeding at 6 months of age had earlier initiated continuous kangaroo mother care.[93] Several studies noted that the mother's own confidence in her caretaking improved along with an eagerness for discharge, and many women reported feeling an increased closeness to the infant compared with a control group of mothers. At the first skin-to-skin experience, the mother is usually tense, so it is best for the nurse to stay with her to answer questions and make any necessary adjustments in position and ensure that warmth is maintained. A few mothers find that one such experience is enough. However, most mothers find repeated kangaroo care experiences especially pleasurable. Paternal attachment is also facilitated by fathers holding their infants and engaging in skin-to-skin contact.[6] A study by Sullivan[94] indicates that the earlier fathers hold their babies, the sooner they report feelings of love and warmth. The infant may become a reality to the father when he can hold his infant.[6]

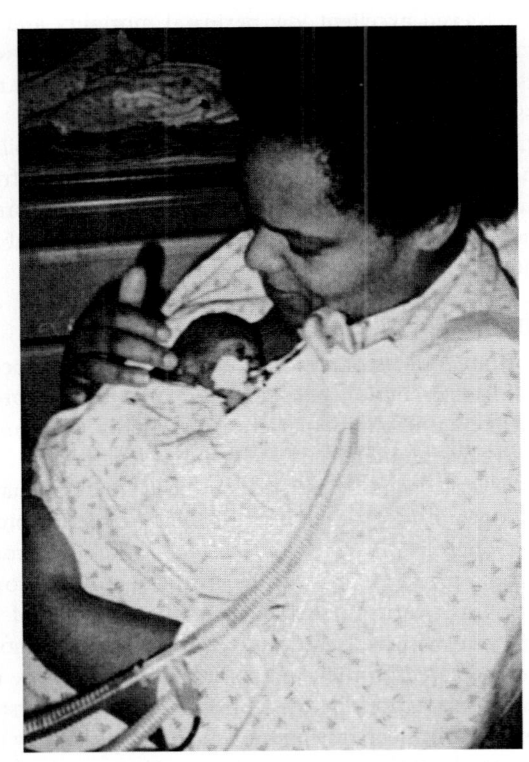

Fig. 7.3 Small immature infant (on ventilator) skin to skin with his mother.

Parent Support

A number of NICUs have formed groups of parents of premature infants who meet once each week or more often for 1- to 2-hour discussions. Documented clinical reports from these centers suggest that parents find support and considerable relief in being able to talk with each other and to express and compare their inner feelings.

Minde et al.[95] in a controlled study of a self-help group, reported that parents who participated in the group visited their infants in the hospital significantly more often than did parents in the control group. The self-help parents also touched, talked, and looked at their infants more in the en face position and rated themselves as more competent than the control group in infant care measures. The mothers in the group continued to show more involvement with their babies during feedings and were more concerned about their general development 3 months after their discharge from the nursery.

The use of "graduate parents," parents who have had an infant in the NICU and who have successfully dealt with and resolved the crisis of the birth of their infant, can be extremely valuable.[6,10] They provide support to parents by sharing common feelings, reactions, and experiences about having a hospitalized infant. Graduate parents can provide support and practical assistance for mothers interested in breastfeeding, parents who take their infant home on oxygen, or parents whose infant requires special medical care such as a gastrostomy, colostomy, or gavage feedings. Organized graduate parent groups in large tertiary settings have become a very popular means of providing support, but locating one parent or couple to talk with parents in a small community can be just as helpful. Parent classes and internet resources also can be offered on a variety of topics such as breastfeeding, infant development, sibling and family reactions, discharge, cardiopulmonary resuscitation, coping with the hospitalization, and special medical needs. These classes provide specific, didactic information combined with group discussions that are mutually supportive in nature. Social workers, nurses, and other related healthcare professionals (e.g., respiratory, occupational, and physical therapists) facilitate the group; graduate parents also participate as a resource.

Recently, telemedicine technologies have been used in the NICU to enhance medical, informational, and emotional support for families during and after hospitalization. A telemedicine program incorporates video conferencing and internet technologies to enhance interactions among families, NICU staff, and community healthcare providers. The video conferencing module enables distance learning by the family in their home during the NICU stay and remote monitoring after discharge. A survey found that families using this technology were more satisfied with the unit's physical environment and visitation policy, possibly because of the ability to facilitate visitation via teleconferencing when family members could not be present in the NICU.[96]

Support for Siblings

The inclusion of other children in the events surrounding the birth of a sick newborn is important. From a sibling's viewpoint, the anticipated birth of a new infant is a stressful time of noticeable physical and psychologic changes within the family. In preparation for the impending birth, the child is told that the mother will be going to the hospital for a few days and will return with a baby brother or sister. With the birth of a premature or sick infant, the mother may go to the hospital unexpectedly, stay a long time, and not return home with the anticipated playmate. Instead of a celebration of the expected happy event, parents are facing the current crisis of their sick infant.

Parents are often unsure about what to tell the other children and whether the children should see the infant. The siblings themselves may feel left out, rejected, or worried that they, too, may get sick. They may be disappointed and angry that they did not get the "playmate" they had wanted. Because parents are unsure about how to manage these issues, it is often helpful for the staff to introduce the topic. Most children's hospitals employ child life specialists who can consult with parents regarding siblings. Child life specialists have extensive knowledge of child development and expertise in talking with children, often using a child's own play in the process of providing support.

Infection control is the responsibility of parents and professionals. Parents must be educated about the dangers of infection and instructed on how to screen their children who may be visiting for symptoms such as fever, cough, or diarrhea. Professional staff must inquire about the health of visiting siblings, including their exposure to communicable diseases. Both parents and children must wash their hands before entering the nursery. With vigilance, no increased bacterial colonization and no increased incidence of infection occur with sibling visits.[97] Because sibling visitation may be beneficial, each NICU must evaluate the center's situation and consider instituting a sibling visitation policy.

Staff and parent response to sibling visitation has been positive in hospitals in which the policy has been implemented. Such a policy may facilitate family integrity and promote mutual support during the stressful time of hospitalization. Another advantage of visitation is that the older siblings do not endure repeated separations caused by parental visits to the hospital but are included as important and special family members. The presence of siblings in a nursery can be a rewarding experience for family and staff alike and perhaps is the ideal example of providing safe yet comprehensive family-centered care.

Preparation for Home

Rooming-in for the Parent of a Premature Infant

When Tafari and Ross in Ethiopia permitted mothers to live within their crowded premature unit 24 hours each day,[98] they were able to care for three times as many infants in their premature nursery, and at the end of 1 year, the number of surviving infants had increased 500%. Mother–infant pairs were discharged when the infants weighed an average of 1.7 kg, and most infants were breastfed. Before this, most of the infants had gone home and were bottle-fed, and usually died of intercurrent respiratory and gastrointestinal infections. When the cost of prepared milk amounts to a high proportion of the parents' weekly income, policies in support of the mother rooming-in and breastfeeding in premature nurseries have a direct impact on infant mortality. In several other countries throughout the world, including Argentina, Brazil, Estonia, and South Africa, mothers of premature infants live in a room adjoining the premature nursery, or they room in. This arrangement appears to have multiple benefits. It allows the mother to continue producing milk, permits her to take on the care of the infant more easily, greatly reduces the caregiving time required of the staff for these infants, and allows a group of mothers of premature infants to talk over their situation and gain from discussion and mutual support.

Torres,[99] in a special care unit in the slums of Santiago, Chile, achieved excellent low perinatal mortality and morbidity rates by placing special care units for low-birth-weight infants in the maternity unit, thus maintaining babies under professional observation for only as long as necessary.

Technological improvements and the resulting ability to continuously monitor sick premature infants even from a distance has allowed single-room NICUs to become a reality, and parents are encouraged to room-in with their babies in the NICU.

Nesting

In the United States, James and Wheeler first described the successful introduction of a care-by-parent unit to provide a homelike caretaking experience.[100] Parents of premature infants received nursing support before discharge.

For several years, "nesting" has been studied—namely, permitting mothers to live in with their infants before discharge. When babies reached 1.72 to 2.11 kg, each mother was given a private room with her baby where she provided all caregiving. Impressive changes in the behavior of these women were observed clinically. Even though the mothers had fed and cared for their infants in the intensive care nursery on many occasions before living-in, eight of the first nine mothers did not sleep during the first 24 hours so they could learn more about their infant's behavior. However, in the second 24-hour period, the mothers' confidence and caretaking skills improved greatly. At this time, mothers began to discuss the proposed early discharge of their infants and, often for the first time, began to make preparations at home for their arrival. Several mothers insisted on taking their babies home earlier than planned.

Early discharge, preceded by a period of isolation of the mother and infant together, may help normalize mothering behavior in the intensive care nursery. Encouraging the increasing possibilities for mother–infant interaction and total caretaking may reduce the incidence of mothering disorders among mothers of small or sick premature infants.

Parents must feel a sense of competency in relating to and caring for their infant. Discharge is an anxiety-provoking event and ushers in the "crisis" of homecoming, which parents must face and master.[6,12,64] To achieve a positive parent–child relationship after the hospitalization, provision of appropriate follow-up support through the home adjustment period is crucial.[7,12]

The perinatal healthcare team can employ many interventions to assist parents with discharge. In the hospital, adequate teaching of caregiving skills that enable the parent to develop a sense of mastery and competence is important. Parent education regarding the care and needs of their baby is a learning process that begins at admission and continues throughout the inpatient stay. In addition to tasks of care, parents should participate in planning and providing developmentally appropriate care and be able to read and respond to their infant's cues. If parents do not feel comfortable with their infant, their anxiety can cause adverse interactions. Teaching caregiving skills often can be facilitated in an environment that is less intense and crisis oriented than the NICU. Whenever possible, an infant should be transferred to a setting that is more conducive to the parents' initiation of the primary caregiving role, such as a special care or transitional nursery.

Adequate discharge planning and follow-up arrangements should include general pediatric care, home health care, nurse home visitors, referral for early intervention services if indicated, and parenting classes, especially for young or psychosocially high-risk parents.

Practical Hints for Parents of Sick or Premature Infants

- The obstetrician of a high-risk mother should consult the pediatrician early and continue to involve him or her in decisions and plans for the management of the mother and baby.
- If the baby must be moved to a hospital with an intensive care unit, it is always helpful to give the mother a chance to see and touch her infant, even if the baby has respiratory distress and is requiring respiratory support. The team should stop in the mother's room with the transport incubator and encourage her to touch her baby and look at her at close hand. A positive comment about the baby's strength and healthy features may be long remembered and appreciated.
- The father should be encouraged to come to the NICU as soon as possible so he can see what is happening with his baby. He uses his own transportation so that he can stay in the premature unit for 3 to 4 hours. This extra time allows him to get to know the nurses and physicians in the unit, to find out how the infant is being treated, and to talk with the physicians about what they expect will happen with the baby in the succeeding days. He can help by acting as a link between the NICU and his family by carrying information back to the mother. He should visit the baby in the NICU before visiting the mother so that he can let her know how the baby is doing. Taking pictures, even if the infant is on a respirator, allows him to show and describe to the baby's mother in detail how the baby is being cared for. Mothers often tell us how valuable the picture is in allowing them to maintain some contact with the infant, even while physically separated. If an institution has telemedicine or video conference technologies, including the mother remotely in these first visits promotes family-integrated care and helps the mother during the time of separation.
- Transporting both the mother and baby to the medical center that contains the intensive care nursery should be encouraged when possible for their immediate and long-term benefits.
- The intensive care nursery should be open for parental visiting 24 hours each day and should be flexible about visits from others such as grandparents, supportive relatives, and sometimes siblings. If proper precautions are taken, infection transmission will not be a problem.
- Communication is essential. The healthcare workers should communicate with the mother about her condition and about the baby's condition. This is important before, during, and after the birth of the baby, even if the information is brief and incomplete. Clinically, there may be devastating and lasting untoward effects on the mothering capacity of women who have been frightened by a physician's pessimistic outlook about the chance of survival and normal development of an infant. For example, when the newborn premature baby is doing well, but the mother is told by a physician that there is a likelihood that the baby may not survive, the mother will often show evidence of mourning (as if the baby were already dead) and reluctance to "become attached" to her baby. Such mothers may refuse to visit or will show great hesitation about any physical contact. When discussing such a situation with the physician who has spoken pessimistically with the mother, it is important to share all concerns with her so that she will be prepared in case of a bad outcome. This may be acceptable once there is a close and firm bond between the mother and infant (which may only occur after an infant has been home for several months). However, while the ties of affection are still fragile and forming, they can be easily inhibited, altered, or possibly permanently damaged. Physicians should be truthful because parents will quickly sense their true feelings, but statements must be based on the facts of the current situation, not on improbable outcomes that are causing concern for the physician. The physician should be forthright about all the medical conditions and express appropriate concern related to

these problems. Describe what the infant looks like to the medical team and how the infant will appear physically to the mother. Rather than talk about chances of survival and giving percentages, stress that most babies survive despite early and often worrisome problems. Do not emphasize problems that may occur in the future. Try to anticipate common developments (e.g., the need for phototherapy for jaundice in small premature infants).

- It is useful to talk with the mother and father together. When this is not possible, it is often wise to talk with one parent on the telephone in the presence of the other. Discuss how the child is doing with the parents; talk with them more frequently if the child is critically ill. It is essential to find out what the mother believes is going to happen or what she has read about the problem. Move at her pace during any discussion.

> **EDITORIAL COMMENT:** Although most families want and appreciate frequent communication, it should be recognized that they can vary considerably in their communication preferences. I've had multiple families actually request that I not call them every day, especially as they become "feeders and growers"—they prefer to speak with the nurses daily and the medical team when they come in for rounds. Asking families directly how they would like to handle communication can avoid misunderstandings.

- The physician should not relieve his/her anxiety by burdening the family with unnecessary concerns. For example, if there is a possibility that the child has Turner syndrome, it is not necessary to share this with the parents while the infant is still acutely ill with other problems and while affectional bonds are still weak. If the physician is worried about a slightly elevated bilirubin level that would respond promptly to phototherapy, it is not necessary to dwell on kernicterus. Once mentioned, the possibility of death or brain damage can never be completely erased. Remember, words are like a sword, and families remember forever the remarks of their caregivers. Remember, too, nonverbal communication is also important, and the demeanor of the caregivers will affect the response to information. It is important for the family to understand that they are the most important person on their baby's healthcare team. Communication is the key to providing parents with the information to have shared decision-making with the medical team. Eliciting the parents' concerns and leading them in a discussion of treatment options can help facilitate shared decision-making.
- Before the mother comes to the neonatal unit, the nurse or physician should describe in detail what the baby and the equipment will look like. When she makes her first visit, it is important to anticipate that she may become distressed when she looks at her infant. Have a chair nearby so that she can sit down, and a nurse can describe in detail the procedures being carried out, such as the monitoring of respiration and heart rate. The nurse should answer questions and give support given during the difficult period when the mother first sees her infant.
- It is important to remember that feelings of love for the baby are often elicited through contact. Therefore, if possible, try to turn off the lights and remove the eye patches from an infant under phototherapy lights so that the mother and infant can see each other.
- When the immature infant has passed the acute phase, both the father and the mother should be encouraged to touch, massage, and interact with their infant. This helps the parents get to know the baby, reduces the number of breathing pauses (if this is a problem), increases weight gain, and hastens the infant's discharge from the unit. Initially, if the infant is acutely ill, touching and fondling sometimes result in a decrease in the level of blood oxygen; therefore parents should begin this contact when the infant is stable and the nurse or physician agrees that the infant is ready. Firm massage of preterm infants 15 minutes three times a day results in markedly improved growth, less stress behavior, improved performance on the Brazelton Neonatal Behavior Assessment scale, and better performance on a developmental assessment at 8 months.[101]
- The mother and father can receive feedback from their baby in response to their caregiving. If the infant looks at their eyes, moves in response to them, quiets down, or shows any behavior in response to their efforts, the parents' feelings of attachment are encouraged. Practically speaking, this means that the mother must catch the baby's glance and be able to note that some maneuver on her part, such as picking up the baby or making soothing sounds, actually triggers a response or quiets the baby. Suggest to parents therefore that they think in terms of trying to send a message to the baby and of picking one up from them in return. Small premature infants do see and are especially interested in patterned objects, and can hear, and evidence suggests they will benefit greatly from receiving messages.
- Continue to study interventions such as rooming-in, nesting, and early discharge as well as transporting a healthy premature infant to be with his mother. It is necessary to test these various interventions in different hospital settings and to evaluate their ability to reduce the severe anxiety that many parents experience during the prolonged hospitalization and the early days following discharge.
- Nurses should support and encourage mothers during these early days and weeks.[1] The nurse's guidance in helping a mother with simple caregiving tasks can be extremely valuable in helping her overcome anxiety. In this sense, the nurse assumes a role similar to the mother's own mother and contributes much more than teaching her basic techniques of caregiving. Involving families early in the care of their infants has multiple benefits. Integrating family into care of their infants helps them identify their maternal and paternal roles, promotes attachment, decreases stress, and increases success at home. Family-integrated care and parenting units shift the model of care for neonatal units allows more effective partnership with families.

- To begin an intervention with parents early, it is necessary to identify high-risk parents who are having special difficulties in adapting. Generally, these parents visit rarely and for short periods,[23] appear frightened, and do not usually engage the medical staff in any questioning about the infant's problems. Sometimes the parents are hostile or irritable and show inappropriately low levels of anxiety, many times as a defense mechanism.
- As further understanding of the process by which normal mothers and infants interact with each other during the first months and year of life is developed, it appears that some recommendations for stimulation may be detrimental to normal development. Rather than suggesting stimulation, it may be important for a mother naturally and unconsciously to use imitation to learn about and get to know her own infant.

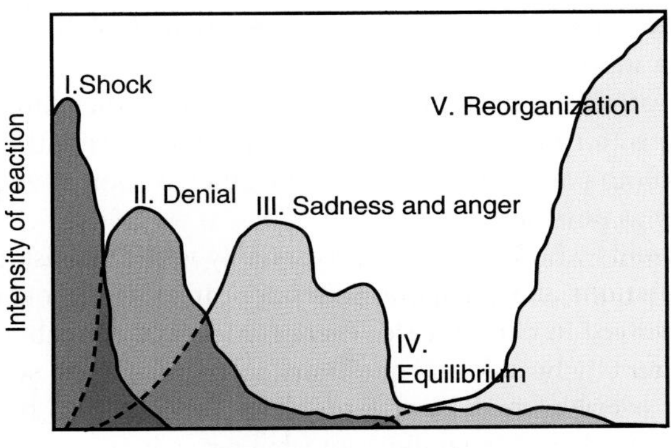

Fig. 7.4 Hypothetical model of normal sequence of parental reactions to birth of malformed infant. (Modified from Drotar D, Baskiewicz A, Irwin N, et al. The adaptation of parents to the birth of an infant with a congenital malformation: a hypothetical model. *Pediatrics* 1975;51:710. With permission of *Pediatrics*.)

CONGENITAL MALFORMATIONS

The birth of an infant with a congenital malformation presents complex challenges to the physician who will care for the affected child and his family. Although previous investigators agree that the child's birth often precipitates major family stress,[102] relatively few have described the process of family adaptation during the infant's first year of life.[102] Solnit and Stark's conceptualization of parental reactions emphasized that a significant aspect of adaptation is the mourning that parents must undergo for the loss of the normal child they had expected.[103] Observers have also noted pathologic aspects of family reactions, including the chronic sorrow that envelops the family of a child with differences.[104] Less attention has been given to the more adaptive aspects of parental attachment to children with malformations.

Parental reactions to the birth of a child with a congenital malformation appear to follow a predictable course. For most parents, initial shock, disbelief, and a period of intense emotional upset (including sadness, anger, and anxiety) are followed by a period of gradual adaptation, which is marked by a lessening of intense anxiety and emotional reaction (Fig. 7.4). This adaptation is characterized by an increased satisfaction with and ability to care for the baby. These stages in parental reactions are similar to those reported in other crises, such as those that occur with terminally ill children. The shock, disbelief, and denial reported by many parents seem to be an understandable attempt to escape the traumatic news of the baby's malformation, news so different than their expectations that it is impossible to register except gradually.

The intense emotional turmoil described by parents who have a child with a congenital malformation corresponds to a period of crisis (defined as "upset in a state of equilibrium caused by a hazardous event that creates a threat, a loss, or a challenge for the individual"). A crisis includes a period of impact, an increase in tension associated with stress, and finally a return to equilibrium. During such crisis periods, a person is at least temporarily unable to respond with his or her usual problem-solving activities to solve the crisis. Roskies notes a similar "birth crisis" in her observations of mothers of children with limb defects caused by thalidomide.[102]

With the birth of a child with a malformation, the mother must mourn the loss of her expected infant.[103] In addition, she must become attached to her actual living child. However, the sequence of parental reactions to the birth of a baby with a malformation differs from that following the death of a child in another respect. Because of the complex issues raised by the continuation of the child's life and hence the demands of his physical care, the parents' sadness, which is initially important in their relationship with the child, diminishes in most instances when they take over the physical care. Most parents reach a point at which they are able to care adequately for their child and to cope effectively with disrupting feelings of sadness and anger. The mother's initiation of the relationship with her child is a major step in the reduction of anxiety and emotional upset associated with the trauma of the birth. As with all children, the parents' initial experience with their infant seems to release positive feelings that aid the mother-child relationship following the stresses associated with the news of the child's anomaly. Lampe et al. noted a significantly greater amount of visiting if an infant with an abnormality had been at home for a short while before surgery for a cleft lip repair.[104]

Practical Suggestions for Parents of Infants With Differences

- If medically feasible, it is far better to leave the infant with the mother and father for the first 2 to 3 days or to discharge them. If the child is rushed to the hospital where special surgery will eventually be done, the mother and father will not have enough opportunity to become attached to her. Even if immediate surgery is necessary, as in the case of bowel obstruction, it is best to bring the baby to the mother first, allowing her to touch and handle her, and to point out to her how normal her baby is in all other respects.

- The parents' mental picture of the anomaly may often be far more alarming than the actual problem. Any delay greatly heightens their anxiety and causes their imaginations to run wild. Therefore it is helpful to bring the baby to both parents when they are together as soon after delivery as possible.
- Parents who are adapting reasonably well often ask many questions and indeed at times appear to be almost overinvolved in clinical care. There is more concern about the parents who ask few questions and who appear stunned or overwhelmed by the problem. Parents who become involved in trying to find out what procedures are best and who ask many questions about care often adapt best in the end.
- It's best to move at the parents' pace. It is beneficial to be a good listener and ask the parents how they view their infant and to express their concerns, which can then be addressed.
- Each parent may move through the process of shock, denial, anger, guilt, and adaptation at a different pace. If the parents are unable to talk with each other about the baby, their own relationship may be disrupted. Use the process of early crisis intervention and meet several times with the parents. During these discussions, ask the mother how she is doing, how she feels the father is doing, and how he feels about the infant. Then reverse the questions and ask the father how he is doing and how he thinks the mother is progressing. Many times a parent is surprised by the responses of his or her partner. The hope is that the parents not only will think about their own reactions, but also will begin to consider each other's. For further discussion on this subject, see Case 7.2.
- One of the major goals of postpartum discussions is to keep the family together during this early period and in subsequent years. This is best done by working hard to bring out issues early and by encouraging the parents to talk about their difficult thoughts and feelings as they arise. It is best for them to share their problems with each other. Some couples who do not seem to be close previously may move closer together as they work through the process of adaptation. As with any painful experience, the parents may be much stronger after they have gone through these reactions together. It is helpful when the father stays with his partner during the hospitalization. Sometimes the stresses of having a sick baby will ultimately disrupt the relationship of the parents.

STILLBIRTH OR DEATH OF A NEWBORN

Despite the advances in obstetrical and neonatal care, many mothers encounter a great disappointment with an early miscarriage or the perinatal loss of an infant. A mourning reaction in both parents after the death of a newborn is universal.[105] Whether the baby lives 1 hour or 2 weeks, whether the baby is a nonviable 400 g or weighs 4000 g, whether the baby was planned, and whether or not the mother has had physical contact with her baby, clearly identifiable mourning will be present. Mothers and fathers who have lost a newborn show the same mourning reactions as those reported by Lindemann,[106] who studied survivors of the Coconut Grove fire. Lindemann concludes that normal grief is a definite syndrome. It includes the following aspects:

- somatic distress with tightness of the throat, choking, shortness of breath, need for sighing, and an empty feeling in the abdomen; lack of muscular power; and an intense subjective distress described as tension or mental pain;
- preoccupation with the image of the deceased infant;
- feelings of guilt and preoccupation with one's negligence or minor omissions;
- feelings of hostility toward others; and/or
- breakdown of normal patterns of conduct.

Originally it was believed that loss of an infant was similar to the loss of a close relative; however, based on clinical studies and observations, it fits far more closely with the concepts proposed by Furman[107] and Lewis.[108] Furman eloquently notes these reactions:

- Internally, the mourning process consists of two roughly opposing mechanisms. One is the generally known process of detachment, by which each memory that ties the family to the person who is deceased has to become painfully revived and painfully loosened. This is the part of the process that involves anger, guilt, pain, and sadness. The second process is commonly called "identification." It is the means by which the deceased or parts of him are taken into the self and preserved as part of the self, thereby soothing the pain of loss. In many instances, a surviving marriage partner takes over hobbies and interests of the deceased spouse. These identifications soothe the way and make the pain of detachment balanced and bearable.
- For the surviving parents, the death of a newborn is special in several ways. Because mourning is mourning of a separate person, the process can apply only to that small part of the relationship to the newborn that was characterized by the love of a separate person, but there has not been time to build up strong ties and memories of mutual living. It is also not possible for parents—adults functioning in the adult world—to take into themselves any part of a helpless newborn and make it adaptively a part of themselves; the mechanism of identification does not work. But what about the part of the newborn that was still part of the self and that cannot be mourned? To understand this part, one has to look at the different process by which individuals cope with a loss of a part of the self (e.g., amputation or loss of function). Insofar as the newborn remains a part of the parent's self, the death has to be dealt with as would the amputation of a limb or the loss of function of the parent's body. Detachment is the mechanism with which the victim deals with such tragedies, but it

is detachment of a different kind. Acceptance that one will never ever again have that part of oneself is very different from the detachment that deals with the memories of living together with a loved one. The feelings that accompany this detachment are similar in kind and intensity: anger, guilt, fury, helplessness, and horror. In the case of the loss of a part of the self, however, they are quite unrelieved by identification.

- Next, with such a tragedy, there must be a readjustment in one's self-image. It is, however, altogether different to have to readjust to thinking of oneself as an imperfect human being, a human being that cannot walk or cannot see. That is a pain of a different kind, and the feelings that accompany it are emptiness, loss of self-esteem, and feeling low. Because the internal self never materialized in those arms and has not had a chance to be detached, it is very different from the process of mourning.
- These feelings are made particularly difficult because people around the parents are not there to help. At a conscious level, people say they simply do not understand about losing part of the self, and, indeed, they do not. Subconsciously, they understand it all too well. It fills them with fear and anxiety and makes them turn away. Parents of a dead newborn often experience this isolation. They quite often are shunned, and they may not rely on the sympathy that is usually accorded the bereaved.

This grief syndrome may appear immediately after a death or may be delayed or apparently absent. Those who have studied mourning responses have indicated that a painful period of grieving is a normal and necessary response to the loss of a loved one and the absence of a period of grieving is not a healthy sign but rather a cause for alarm.

Without any therapeutic intervention, a tragic outcome for the mother has been shown in one-third of the perinatal deaths. Cullberg found that 19 of 56 mothers studied 1 to 2 years after the deaths of their neonates had developed severe psychiatric disease (psychoses, anxiety attacks, phobias, obsessive thoughts, and deep depressions).[109] Because of the disastrous outcome in such a high proportion of mothers, it is necessary to examine in detail how to care for the family following a neonatal death.

In observations of parents who have lost newborns, the disturbance of communication between the parents has been a particularly troublesome problem. A father and mother who have communicated well before the birth of a baby often have such strong feelings after an infant's death that they are unable to share their thoughts and therefore have an unsatisfactory resolution to their grieving. In the United States, it is expected that men will be strong and not show their feelings, so a physician should encourage a father and mother to talk together about the loss and advise them not to hold back their responses—"Cry when you feel like crying." Unless told what to expect, their reactions may worry and perplex them, and this may tend further to disturb the preexisting father and mother relationship.

At the time of the baby's death, it is important to tell the parents *together* about the usual reactions to the loss of a child and the length of time these last. It is desirable to meet a second time with both parents before discharge to go over the same suggestions, which may not have been heard or may have been misunderstood under the emotional shock of the baby's death. The pediatrician or social worker should plan to meet with the parents together again 3 or 4 months after the death to check on the parents' activities and on how the mourning process is proceeding. The autopsy findings may be discussed and any further questions asked by the parents may be addressed. At this visit, the pediatrician or social worker should be alert for abnormal grief reactions, which, if present, may guide the physician to refer the parents for psychiatric assistance. It is important that these recommendations do not become an exact prescription for every parent. As noted by Leon,[110] "Such protocols can lead to a regimented assembly line approach—which impedes attempts to attune to parents individually and empathetically—the very essence of providing support."

For further discussion on this subject, see Case 7.4. Cullberg's report about severe psychiatric reactions following stillbirth or neonatal death in Swedish mothers was published in 1966 when the field of neonatology was in its infancy. Following other reports about parents' turbulent and prolonged mourning reactions, changes in the care of bereaved families were introduced. In a systematic study of 380 women following a stillbirth, Rädestad observed that mothers of stillborn infants had a diminished risk of symptoms 3 years after the death if there was a short time between diagnosis of death and initiation of the delivery,[111] if the mother was allowed to meet and say farewell to her child as long as she wished, and if there was a collection of tokens of remembrance (hand or footprints, lock of hair, and photograph). They noted that mothers living alone may have special needs for support.

Katherine Shear and Harry Shair have written about the concept of "complicated grief," which may occur with ineffective coping after the death of a loved one. They note as follows:[112]

Bereavement is a highly disruptive experience that is usually followed by a painful but time-limited period of acute grief. An unfortunate minority of individuals experience prolonged and impairing complicated grief, an identifiable syndrome that differs from usual grief, major depression, and other *DSM-IV* diagnostic entities. Underlying processes guiding symptoms are not well understood for either usual or complicated grief. We propose a provisional model of bereavement, guided by Myron Hofer's question: "What exactly is lost when a loved one dies?" We integrate insights about biobehavioral regulation from Hofer's animal studies of infant separation, research on adult human attachment, and new ideas from bereavement research. In this model, death of an attachment figure produces a state of traumatic loss and symptoms of acute grief. These symptoms usually resolve following revision of the internalized representation of the deceased to incorporate the reality of the death. Failure to accomplish this integration results in the syndrome of complicated grief.[112]

The clinical relevance of this subject can best be appreciated by the following case examples and the questions they raise. The words chosen in any discussion depend on the needs and problems of individual patients at that moment. Answers are not given as a specific formula, but to show the reader one possible approach to the parents.

CASE 7.1

Mrs. W had a normal pregnancy until 24 weeks' gestation, when she unexpectedly went into labor and delivered a 1 lb, 5 oz (600 g) female infant in a community hospital. The baby cried promptly, but then respiratory distress developed, requiring ventilator care, arterial catheterization, intubation, surfactant administration, and transfer to a tertiary level NICU at the medical center.

The following questions should be answered when caring for this mother, father, and infant.

What is the ideal method of communicating with both parents?

The best method of communicating with both parents is to have them sit down with you in a quiet, private room. You will be most effective if you can listen to the parents, let them express their worries and feelings, and then give simple, realistic explanations.

How should advice be given when discussing the situation with the parents? What should they be told about their infant and her chances for survival?

When first discussing the situation with the parents, advice should be given promptly and kept simple. As soon as possible after the birth, the mother and father can be told that the baby is small but well formed. It can be comforting to mention something positive about their baby or something their infant can do. When it is clear that the baby has respiratory distress, you can explain to the parents that the baby has a common problem of premature infants ("breathing difficulty") caused by the complex adjustments she must make from life in utero to life outside. This is called respiratory distress syndrome (RDS). In addition, it should be stated that because this condition is common, the neonatologists at the tertiary NICU in a medical center know best how to treat it, and their results with infants who are this weight can be good.

What should the mother and father be told about the ventilator?

Some of the parents' anxiety can be relieved by pointing out that the ventilator is augmenting the baby's breathing; that is, the baby is still able to breathe, but this is helping. Explaining that the baby is not able to cry audibly when an endotracheal tube is present relieves another common concern.

Can the parents see the baby before transfer?

Yes, you can explain that the mother, father, and siblings will be given time and an opportunity to see and touch the baby in the transport incubator with a nurse or neonatologist present to monitor and support the baby, siblings, and parents. Pictures of the baby will be obtained before the transfer.

Is it wise to discuss breastfeeding and the value of breast milk for a baby that will be transferred?

Yes, emphasizing the importance of pumping milk right away will increase the odds that Mrs. W will be able to provide breast milk for her baby. Discussing breastfeeding at this time when the parents are extremely anxious about their baby conveys to the parents that you expect their baby to do well. You can explain that the staff will help the mother start pumping her breasts because her breast milk will be an essential part of the treatment for her daughter, not only for her nutrition, but also to decrease the risk of infection and to improve the baby's brain development. It will also enhance the mother's bonding with her daughter, particularly when Mrs. W begins to directly breastfeed her daughter and repeatedly experiences the let-down reflex.

What other arrangements should be made before the baby is transferred?

Communication with both the referring and receiving centers and the obstetrician is necessary. Most obstetricians want to know when a baby is transferred. They can help the family by arranging for the early discharge of the mother, when medically appropriate, so she can go to her baby in the medical center. Sometimes mother and baby can both be transferred.

Baby Girl W is transported to the neonatal intensive care unit (NICU) at the medical center. She receives surfactant and gradually begins to wean off the ventilator. After 4 hours, the ventilator settings have decreased to FIO_2 27%, peak inspiratory pressure 22 mm Hg, positive end-expiratory pressure 5 mm Hg, and pulse rate 25. An arterial blood gas reveals pH 7.33, $PaCO_2$ 41 mm Hg, and PaO_2 62 mm Hg. When the mother and father arrive, the neonatologist meets with them.

The physician asks, "Would you please tell me what the doctors at the community hospital told you and what you understand about your daughter's condition?" Their answer can guide the discussion. The physician explains that the baby tolerated the transfer well and that they are beginning to decrease ventilator or breathing machine support. She agrees with the diagnosis of RDS and comments that "RDS often runs a course of increasing symptoms for a day or two and then the breathing gradually becomes easier. With RDS there is stress on the whole baby, so as the lungs improve, other organs, such as the

CASE 7.1—cont'd

intestines, may show problems. Distention or fullness of the abdomen may develop, and it may be necessary to progress slowly with feedings. Throughout the first few days, routine blood tests, ultrasound, X-rays, and other studies may be obtained repeatedly to be certain that the diagnosis and treatment are correct and to check that no other problem such as infection has developed. The overall outlook for your daughter is good."

The physician says that she will be giving their daughter routine care for a premature infant. She says, "When I have had time to complete more tests and observations, if there is any change in what I have told you, I will call you. I will keep you posted on the baby's progress. I would like you to call at other times if you have questions. I am pleased that you both came in together. In the next days, if one of you is here and I have something new to report, I will plan to talk to one of you on the telephone while the other is in the office with me. I would like you to come to the nursery as often as you can. You are the most important person on her care team. We round every morning as a medical team; you are welcomed and invited to participate in rounds. I want you to become well acquainted with your daughter and her care. Your milk will be a very important part of her treatment, and you may find your milk flows more abundantly when you are with your baby, particularly when you are skin to skin in kangaroo care."

Can the nurses help the mother adapt to the premature infant?

The nurses can aid the mother in adapting to the premature infant by standing with her and explaining the equipment being used for the baby, by welcoming the mother by name and with personalized comments at each visit and encouraging her to come back soon, by carefully considering the mother's concerns and feelings, by explaining to her that the baby will benefit from her visits, and by showing her how she assume more of the baby's care and do the mothering better than the nurses. Together, they may identify events such as loud noises and bright lights that appear to be stressful to the baby, as well as environmental changes that appear to relax her. Then they can plan modifications in positioning, feeding, and times for medications as well as environmental adjustments to increase the amount of time when the baby appears to be free of stress.

What are the normal processes that a mother goes through when she delivers a premature infant, and how can the physicians and nurses assist her?

The premature delivery often occurs before a mother is thoroughly ready to accept the idea that she is going to have an infant. Such a mother is faced with a baby who is thin, small, and very different from the ideal full-sized baby she has been picturing in her mind. She may have to grieve the loss of this anticipated ideal baby as she adjusts to the reality of the premature baby with all her problems and special needs.

All of the equipment and activities of a premature nursery are new and may be frightening to a mother. The tubes, the flashing lights, the alarms, and other instruments used in a premature nursery are disturbing. If the functions of these items are explained to the mother, her concerns may decrease. For example, "The two wires on the baby's chest and the beeping instrument tell us if the baby slows down in her respirations so we can rub her skin to remind her to keep breathing. This is frequently necessary during the first few weeks with a tiny infant." It may be helpful for the mother and infant to be together as much as possible in the early days. The mother's guilt and anxiety, and the fear that touching the infant will harm her, sometimes leads her to turn down an offer to visit the infant. No mother should be forced to visit her infant against her wishes; however, it is important for the hospital personnel to reassure her and encourage her visits, but always to move at the mother's pace. Offering and encouraging kangaroo care and early involvement can promote attachment.

What should the mother be told when she asks, "How is the baby doing?"

It is a common reflex in physicians and nurses to prepare patients for a possible poor outcome and to think in a problem-oriented manner. It is of great importance to provide encouragement to the mother so that mother–infant affectional ties develop as easily as possible, so it is desirable to approach this question in an optimistic but realistic manner. It is wise to start out by asking the mother how *she* thinks the baby is doing.

When should these parents take the baby home?

At 2 weeks, Baby Girl W developed an episode of suspected sepsis with abdominal distention that responded to nothing-by-mouth and antibiotics. The cultures were negative. At 4 weeks, Baby Girl W weighs 3 lb, 14 oz (1758 g).

The baby has been breastfeeding one or two times a day for the past 4 days and taking breast milk from the bottle. She is gaining weight and has good temperature control without an incubator. There is no infection in the home. Shortly after the baby responded to the sepsis treatment, Mrs. W called to say she was sick with the flu and would not come to the NICU. She called each day for 10 days, and her husband brought in the breast milk she had pumped. In this case, the timing of going home depended on the mother, whose visiting pattern was regular until the last week. At that time, Baby Girl W's nurse suggested that the mother spend 3 or 4 hours with her baby, give her a bath, and feed her. Mrs. W agreed, enjoyed this, and spent 6 to 8 hours caring for her baby girl over the next 3 days. Both parents take infant CPR and a class on caring for premature babies. Mrs. W has a crib and equipment to care for her daughter at home, and her husband has canceled his out-of-town trips for the next 3 weeks.

Baby Girl W went home in the winter, so the parents were advised to avoid contact with children with colds. Because she has a sibling younger than 5 years of age, Baby Girl W was given the first injection of palivizumab (Synagis) to be followed by two more injections to protect her against respiratory syncytial virus infection.

Continued

CASE 7.2

Mrs. J, a 25-year-old primiparous mother, delivered a full-term infant after a 12-hour uneventful labor. The infant was found to have a cleft lip and palate. The following questions should be answered concerning the care of this infant and mother.

Should the father be told about this before the mother has returned to her room?
Every effort should be made to tell the mother and father together about this problem; however, this is such an obvious defect that the father will notice it and the mother will at least sense that something is wrong. If this is the case, the doctor should indicate that there is a concern but that he wants to check the baby over thoroughly and will then tell both parents about the concern and what will be done about it. It is popularly believed that the father is in much better condition to learn about difficulties right after delivery than the mother, but often a woman is better able to accept news about an illness or abnormality in her baby—in an emotional sense—than the father. Any plan to give one bit of news or a different shading about the prognosis to one parent and not the other interferes with the communication between the parents. It is extremely important to support and encourage communication. The infant should be brought to the parents as soon as medically safe. The obstetrician or pediatrician should be made aware the details of the baby's health status. The appearance of a baby with an uncorrected cleft palate and lip is shocking for anyone who has not seen this before. Allow the parents time to observe, react, and ask questions. The experienced physician, advanced practitioner, or nurse will point out the underlying structures, emphasize that they are normal, and demonstrate how the surgeon will pull the skin edges of the cleft together to cover the exposed underlying tissue. Before and after pictures of surgically repaired infants are helpful and may enable parents to appreciate why the physician has been so optimistic about the baby's future appearance and normal developmental potential. It is worthwhile to repeat and emphasize the general good health and well-being of the baby.

Who should tell the mother: the obstetrician, the pediatrician, the nurse, or the father?
The obstetrician, whom the mother has known for many months, is usually the best person to tell the mother. He or she needs information from a pediatrician about the nature of the concern and the general health of the baby. Even better, the obstetrician and the pediatrician may go together to tell the parents about the medical concern. If the obstetrician can speak briefly and calmly to the mother, then the pediatrician can continue with a brief explanation about the problem. Under most circumstances, neither the nurse nor the father will be in a position to provide enough reassurance to the mother to make this first encounter progress optimally.

How should the concern be presented to the parents?
It is desirable, whenever possible, to emphasize to the parents the normal healthy features of the baby. For example, "Mr. and Mrs. Jones, you have a strong 8-pound baby boy who is kicking, screaming, and carrying out all the normal functions of a healthy baby. There is one concern present that fortunately we will be able to correct, so it will not be a continuing problem for your son. As far as I can tell, the baby is completely well otherwise."

Should the baby be present?
Yes. As shocking as a cleft palate and lip may appear to a mother, exposure to the reality of the concern is important and is usually less disturbing than the mother's imagination. Letting the mother interact, hold, have the infant skin to skin, as with all infants, can promote attachment.

CASE 7.3

At birth, the male infant of a 28-year-old mother was scrawny, with decreased subcutaneous fatty tissue and axillary and gluteal skinfolds. At 35 weeks' gestational age, the weight was 3 lb, 4.5 oz (1480 g), more than two standard deviations below the mean and 50th percentile for 31 weeks. The length was in the low normal range, and the head circumference was at the second percentile line. The baby breathed and cried promptly. The mother was upset with his thinness, saying her two previous babies were full term and "filled out." When blood was drawn and an IV line with glucose started, the infant was noted to be jittery. Glucose, calcium, electrolytes, and blood counts were normal. Examination showed no malformations.

What other causes should be considered?
The previous record of the mother was not found. When asked about prenatal care, she indicated that she had attended two prenatal visits with an obstetrician at the medical center. She said she had planned to deliver there, but when labor pains started, she had thought it best to go to the nearby community hospital. This was an unusual course of action. Obstetric patients do not often change obstetrician and hospital with onset of labor.

Shortly after delivery, a well-dressed, polite father arrived and immediately inquired which laboratory tests had been sent on his wife and son. The father remained with his wife during all postnatal care, often answering questions for her. Upon seeing his newborn son attached to an IV line, he insisted, "My child is perfectly well, just small and cold. I want both my wife and son discharged today."

Perplexed by the excessive anxiety of the family, as well as the continued jitteriness of the baby, the neonatologist sent infant urine and stool toxicology screens, which were positive for cocaine. At this point, the father picked up the baby, and with his wife, started to leave. Security personnel were called and stopped the father. He had a gun in his pocket. Emergency custody for the baby was obtained.

What other concerns should be checked when a baby is positive for cocaine?
When the mother was examined, there were large bruises on her trunk. When asked in privacy, she said her husband hit her. She agreed to go into treatment for her cocaine addiction. As an adult, she could not be kept in the hospital if she did not wish

CASE 7.3—cont'd

to stay. Photographs of the mother and her bruises were taken before she left, and she was told that these and the records of what she said would be kept if she needed them in the future. Custody of the baby was given to the maternal grandmother. Later, the mother said she came to this community hospital because she thought there would be no testing for cocaine.

Because of this incident, the hospital has installed surveillance cameras. Some hospitals have coded bracelets for the baby's arms or ankles, or umbilical tags that set off an alarm if a baby is taken. Others have a hospital public address code for a missing baby, e.g., "Baby White or Code Pink."

CASE 7.4

A 1 lb, 15-oz (880 g) infant of a 29-year-old mother with a 2-year-old and a 4.5-year-old child died suddenly at 26 hours. The pregnancy was planned. The mother had not held or touched her baby.

What are the processes this mother and father will go through?

The parents in this situation will go through intense mourning reactions. It will help the parents to see and hold the baby after the death. They may wish to bathe or undress and dress the baby. There should be no restriction on the time with their infant. The mother and father may desire to have a nurse with them or to be alone and may want relatives or friends or the two siblings to see the baby. If the parents can cry together, they themselves can best help each other. Even though the mother did not handle the infant, she and the father will be expected to show strong mourning responses, which will be intense for 1 or 2 months, and under optimal circumstances will be decreased by 6 months. In the United States, where the expression of emotion is not encouraged, the father will often force himself to hold back his emotions to provide "strong support" for the mother. This is actually harmful because a free and easy communication between the parents about their feelings is highly desirable for the resolution of mourning. On the basis of the studies that have been carried out, the stronger the mourning reaction in the early days and weeks, the more favorable the outcome.

How can the physician help them?

It is important for the physician to describe the details of the baby's death to both parents together within a few hours of the death of the baby. At that time, he should explain the type of mourning reaction they will go through. If possible, the physician should again meet with the parents 3 or 4 days later, or after the funeral, to find out how they are managing, to go over the details once more, and to indicate availability for any questions or problems. At the postpartum checkup, the obstetrician should take time to ask how the parents are managing and should evaluate the normality of their mourning and their communication. When there are other children in the family, the pediatrician should inquire about their responses. Parents are in emotional pain and are distracted with their own thoughts after a perinatal loss. It is desirable to have someone else—a grandparent or a friendly neighbor—be attentive to the surviving children and to listen to their questions and concerns. It should be explained (if appropriate) that changes in the appearance or behavior of their parents are because they feel so badly about the death. This "surrogate parent" should reassure the siblings that the baby died because of its premature birth and that nothing they thought or did caused the baby to be sick or to die.

About 3 or 4 months after the death of the baby, the physician should set aside a time to meet with both parents to present and discuss the autopsy results, review the present status of the parents and their children, and go over what has occurred since the death, their understanding of the death, and the normality of their reactions. If the mourning response is pathologic, the physician should then refer the parents for additional assistance. Using these procedures, Forrest et al. noted significantly less depression and anxiety in parents compared with control subjects.[113] Also, they noted that an early pregnancy (<6 months after the loss) was strongly associated with high depression and anxiety scores at 14 months.

This short enumeration of guidelines may incorrectly convey the impression of a mechanical quality to these discussions, which is not at all our intent. Parents appreciate evidence of human concern and reactions in a physician at times such as these, so it is appropriate for physicians to both show the sadness they feel and to "be there" for the parents.

SUMMARY

In most instances, the hospital determines the events surrounding birth and death, stripping these two most important events in life of the long-established traditions and support systems established over centuries to help families through these transitions.

Because the newborn baby completely depends on his or her parents for survival and optimal development, it is essential to understand the process of attachment. Although we are only beginning to understand this complex phenomenon, those responsible for the care of mothers and infants would be wise to reevaluate the hospital procedures that interfere with early, sustained parent-infant contact and to consider measures that promote parents' experiences with their infant, enhance communication, engage families in the care of their infant, and encourage shared decision-making.

ACKNOWLEDGMENT

The authors of this chapter gratefully acknowledge that they have built on the original chapter authored by Marshall Klaus, MD and John Kennell, MD. Both were pioneers in mother–infant bonding research and influential advocates of the principles of family-centered care. As written by Drs. Avroy Fanaroff and Richard Martin, "They paved the way to open the neonatal intensive care units for unlimited visitation and subsequently overnight visits for the parents. Their findings inspired labor wards and neonatal intensive care units to enable and encourage parents to enter the nursery to touch, hold, and care for their sick, malformed, and premature babies. They also established clinical guidance for provision of emotional support to parents, especially those dealing with the death of an infant" (*Pediatr Res.* 2018;83:6–8).

The reference list for this chapter can be found online at www.expertconsult.com.

8

Developmental Care—Understanding and Applying the Science

Sheri Ricciardi, Mary Ann Blatz

"Our doctors and nurses didn't just treat our baby. They loved her. They made us feel safe enough that we could love her, too."
***Thomas and Kelly French, parents and authors of* Juniper[1]**

INTRODUCTION

The complexity of managing the high-risk neonate and the convalescing premature infant is multifaceted. The number of surviving extremely low-birth-weight (22–25 weeks of gestation) infants has increased over the past decade, yet despite advances in lifesaving technologies, approximately 50% of these survivors are still at significant risk of morbidity or severe pulmonary and neurodevelopmental compromise.[2–4] Prematurity often thrusts these vulnerable infants on very different developmental trajectories than their term counterparts. High rates (17%–59%) of severe neurodevelopmental disabilities have been reported in short-term follow-up studies, with some improvements noted in sequential studies.[2] Long-term adverse outcomes after extreme prematurity include intellectual disability (5%–36%), cerebral palsy (9%–18%), blindness (0.7%–9%), and deafness (2%–4%).[2] Additional deficits have also been reported in cognition, behavior, sensory processing, and autism spectrum disorders.[2,5]

Striving for best patient outcomes is the goal of every neonatal intensive care unit (NICU), including minimization of neurodevelopmental issues that are onerous for families, healthcare, school systems, and the general public.[6] Immature brain development and the ability of the infant to mitigate the stressors of the extrauterine environment depend on mindful caregiving and healthy social and parental engagement.[7] Caring for a premature infant or high-risk neonate is not always instinctive in the face of significant medical complexity and can present challenges for staff and parents. This chapter will discuss theories and conceptual models of delivering developmental care in the NICU, as well as evidence-based interventions and practice applications. Although this chapter centers on the premature infant, all high-risk neonates (i.e., narcotic exposed, neonatal encephalopathy, etc.) are included in the general applications and benefits of developmental care.

DEFINING DEVELOPMENTAL CARE

Developmental care is the deliberate effort to bring all aspects of nurturing and lifesaving medical care harmoniously together by recognizing and responding to the individual needs of each and every infant. Developmental care theories and paradigms stress the importance of understanding the impact of the NICU environment on the developing infant and the benefit of adaptations to maximize short- and long-term developmental outcomes. Over the years, developmental care has evolved to include philosophical and conceptual models that enhance neurosensory and emotional development and promote parent–infant attachment opportunities. Parent engagement and education are prioritized as key aspects of developmentally supportive care. Interventions center around: decreasing stress and pain, modifying environmental stimuli (visual, auditory, tactile, and vestibular sensory input), supporting optimal positioning, protecting sleep, facilitating provision of mother's milk, and, cue-based care and feeding.[8,9] The synergistic effects of combining multiple evidence-based developmental care principles within a family-centered model of care maximize optimal outcomes for both infants and families. While researchers continue to develop practices and guidelines surrounding developmental care, most agree that pursuing an individualized, personalized approach to care should be a shared objective among neonatal clinicians.[10]

THE EVOLUTION OF NEONATAL NEURODEVELOPMENTAL CARE

In the latter part of the 19th century, a particular interest in the care of newborns emerged in Europe. In the United States, a focus on pathophysiology of the newborn arose in the early 20th century. The term *neonatology* was coined by Dr. Alexander Schaffer in 1960.[11] Since then, many advances in the clinical management of specific neonatal health conditions and improved technology have enhanced neonatal survival outcomes.[11] Pediatrician Dr. T. Barry Brazelton first studied infant development in the early 1960s.[10,12] His work was instrumental in guiding the medical community to appreciate that children have varying "temperaments" and emotional needs that impact behavior, development, and caregiver attachment. His focus on the assessment of behaviors and emotional needs of his patients created a paradigm shift in the way the medical community approached caring for children. Likewise, through years of research and dedication, his passion for promoting the bidirectional relationship between child and parent became embedded in the study of developmental pediatrics. While Dr. Brazelton and colleagues focused their research on the newborn and early child development, Dr. Heidelise Als may have been the first clinician to scrutinize early preterm development focusing on the most vulnerable newborn populations and their families.[13]

Dr. Als and her colleagues evaluated the premature infant nervous system's acceptance of sensory input and the interaction between infant behaviors and the environment. This specific approach led to the development of the conceptualized synactive theory.[14] The tenets of synactive theory and the work of Als have served as the foundation for understanding the importance of analyzing the premature infant's responses to the outside environment. Through detailed observation, they analyzed the infant's functioning across five identified subsystems: autonomic, motor, state, attentional/interactive, and self-regulation. These subsystems represent the hierarchical nature of premature infant behaviors with autonomic stability as the foundation of all systems. When stability in the autonomic subsystem is disrupted, the infant will not achieve higher levels of engagement. Each system is dynamically interdependent on one another in determining the infant's ability to interact with the world.[14] After studying thousands of infants, the Newborn Individualized Developmental Care and Assessment Program (NIDCAP) was developed. This program emphasized training clinical staff on "naturalistic observation" of infant behaviors during routine care and how to provide effective interventions.[15]

The pioneering work of Dr. Als and colleagues paved the way for a deeper appreciation of how the environment impacts brain development and the need for modifications.[16] There is now abundant evidence that preterm infants have an increased incidence and wide spectrum of altered neurodevelopmental outcomes that may be linked to perinatal factors.[2,5,17] Environmental stressors of the NICU have been shown to disrupt infant physiologic stability and impact neurodevelopmental outcomes across the life span.[5,18,19] As subsequent research emerged, neonatal units have attempted to adapt the environment to minimize stress placed on infants and their families. Clinicians gradually became aware of the importance of observing the effect of their interactions on the infant's sensory system and the need to prevent sensory overload during caregiving. Als coined this concept, "reflective caregiving."[14] She also reinforced the importance of strengthening the bidirectional relationship between the parent and infant as an important core measure of caregiving.[15]

Studies have documented significant improvements in infant outcomes and parent satisfaction utilizing the NIDCAP approach.[19,20,21] However, various metaanalyses and systematic reviews have yielded conflicting findings[22] sparking published rebuttals.[23] One explanation is that researchers have acknowledged that the strategies outlined in NIDCAP have become so integrated into the standard care in most NICUs that it is difficult to obtain a true control group. Accepting varying levels of evidence, Als' work, along with the NIDCAP Federation, has impacted the care of premature infants all over the world.[20]

"One Brain for Life......Everything Matters"

Dr. Heidelise Als [24]

BRAIN DEVELOPMENT: THE FOUNDATION OF BEHAVIOR

Behavior is an expression of brain function. From primitive reflexes to volitional movements, complex neuronal activity is responsible for these visible outward signs of the developing brain. Between 24 and 40 weeks' gestation, the brain undergoes a critically sensitive and significant period of growth.[25,26] The germinal matrix, present until 36 weeks postmenstrual age (PMA) and responsible for glial cell differentiation, is experiencing rapid proliferation and movement of neurons.[27] Excitatory and inhibitory neurons will migrate from their sites of origin on the endogenous paths outlined for them. This "neurogenic determinism" occurs in the natural maturational process; however, it is susceptible to epigenetic influences.[4] Sensory motor experiences will influence the proliferation of neurons, synaptic connections, speed of myelination, and eventual planned pruning of the unused neural pathways. It is estimated that 70% of neurons in the developing cortex will succumb to apoptosis between 28 and 40 weeks PMA if pathways are not established. [4] During this critical period of brain growth, extrauterine influences will have a significant effect on neurologic mapping and how these experiences become biophysical or biochemical pathways in the brain.[18,19]

The combination of altered endogenous and exogenous influences (epigenetics) can negatively impact developmental trajectories in terms of delayed maturation or specific injury.[26] The premature infant in this critical period is very competent in the intrauterine environment but is extremely mismatched with nature when born prematurely and thus extremely vulnerable to the outside influences of everyday life in the NICU.[28] Exposure to these clinical elements is life sustaining yet brain altering in both positive and negative ways.[29]

Extensive research in preterm birth survivors, as well as in animal models, has established a direct correlation between the degree of prematurity and loss in cortical volume with poorer neurodevelopmental outcomes.[26] The risk of cerebral palsy increases with decreasing gestation from approximately 1% at 34 weeks to 20% at 26 weeks or less of gestation.[2] Understanding the impact that prematurity, brain insult, genetic variations, and repeated stress have on the developing brain is essential in identifying and implementing strategies for mitigating negative effects and long-term sequelae. Despite the exposure to the stressors of the extrauterine world, infants may respond differently to the same experiences, which leaves researchers continuing to search for a link between epigenetics, buffering agents, genetic predisposition, and resiliency.[30]

New research is evolving to examine and understand behavioral epigenetics or experiences that impact gene expression (Fig. 8.1).[18] Extreme prematurity and prolonged medical

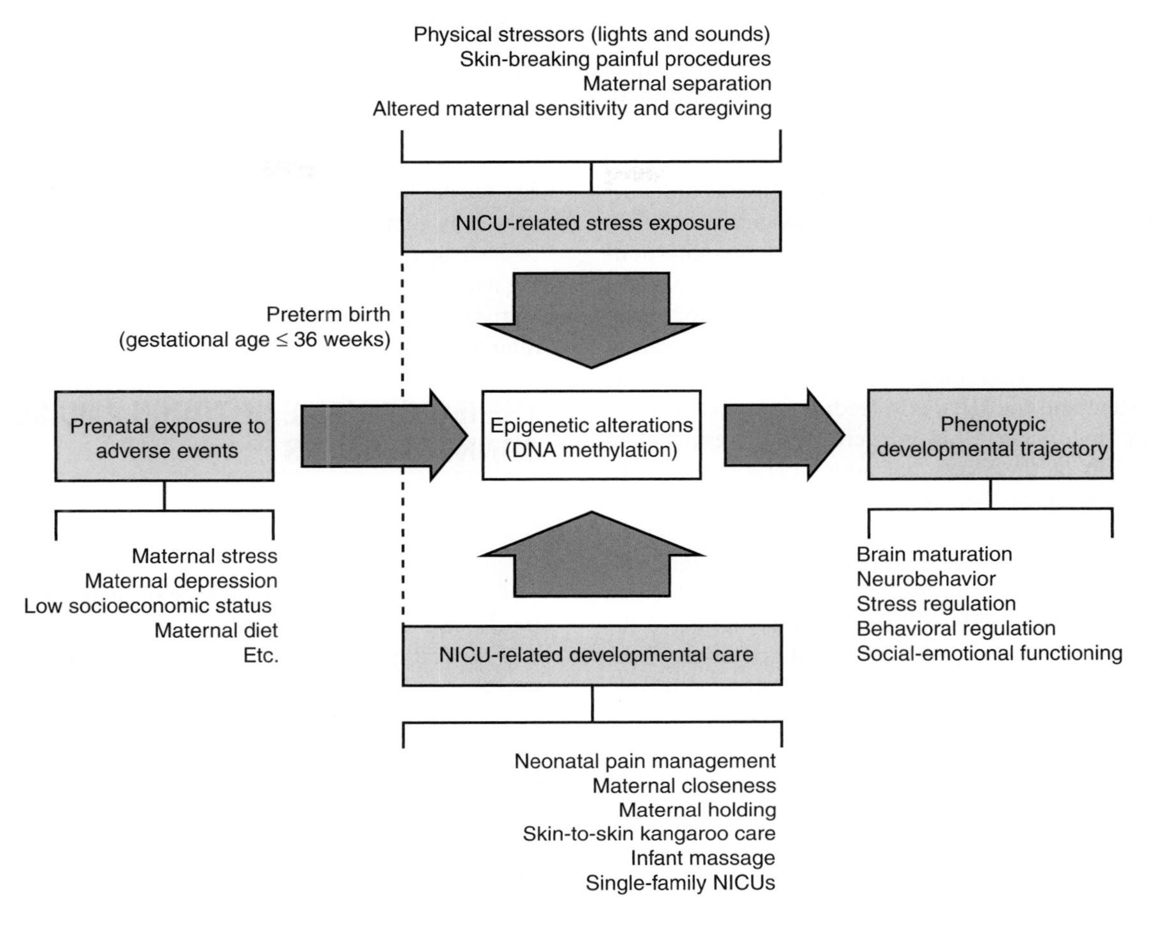

Fig. 8.1 Prospective model explaining epigenetic influences, stress factors, and developmental care strategies. (From Provenzi L, Guida E, Montirosso R. Preterm behavioral epigenetics: a systematic review. *Neurosci Biobehav Rev.* 2017;84:262-271. http://doi.org/10.1016/j.neubiorev.2017.08.020.)

stays are considered adverse life experiences despite the fact that they are also lifesaving experiences.[18] Studies examining the role of perinatal and postnatal stress in relation to dysregulation of the hypothalamic–pituitary–adrenal (HPA) system and deoxyribonucleic acid (DNA) expression may identify the genetic mechanisms behind stress.[18,31] Repeated stress on the infant is hypothesized to overactivate the HPA axis, resulting in excessive amounts of cortisol in the bloodstream. Cortisol has been implicated in the destruction of telomeres. Repeated stress results in telomere erosion, which has been correlated to chronic stress and life adversity in childhood and adult studies. Recently, the study of telomere length in very preterm infants has been investigated, with results indicating similar erosion or shortening, thus implicating the early cellular impact of repeated stress.[18]

In longitudinal studies examining telomere integrity in older children and adults, parent responsiveness has been shown to have a significant positive impact.[32,33] This has led researchers to question the role of parental, responsive caregiving, and the buffering effects this has on reducing chronic stress when applied early in the neonatal period.[18] The most investigated developmental care strategy that demonstrates epigenetic protective mechanisms is skin-to-skin care (SSC).[34] Future studies are needed to examine the impact of other stress-reducing interventions initiated early in the NICU course and the long-term impact on telomere length and adverse neurodevelopmental outcomes.[18]

PROMOTING NEUROPROTECTION

The immature brain is vulnerable and susceptible to the constant relay of sensory stimuli such as light, touch, sound, smell, temperature, and pain.[35] Every encounter with the premature infant activates sensory pathways. Implementing developmentally supportive neuroprotective interventions helps defend against neuronal injury often incurred by the cumulative effects of the NICU environment.[7] Developmental strategies to promote neuroprotection include recognition and timely responses to infant cues, protecting deep sleep, supportive containment, facilitated flexion (tucking), midline positioning, SSC, environmental modifications, positive touch, and parental engagement.[4,27] These interventions will be further discussed in detail.

THE ECO-BIO-DEVELOPMENTAL FRAMEWORK

The triad of unique early life stressors, including repetitive and cumulative stress, parental separation, and pain, have been identified as "toxic stress" and significantly disruptive to the neurodevelopmental process.[36,37] The effects of toxic stress are conceptualized in the eco-bio-developmental framework as frequent and extended activation of the infant's stress response and continual release of stress hormones.[38] The way care is delivered impacts the premature infant on many levels. Infant stress can manifest as physiological instability, motoric disorganization, irritability, hyper- or hyporesponsiveness, poor state regulation, diminished interactive and attentional abilities, and lack of self-regulation. Procedural care and undermanaged pain along with insufficient parental, or "human" nurturing contact, can overload the immature nervous system and the HPA axis, leading to an exaggerated sympathetic "fight" state. This exaggerated state results in an overproduction of the stress hormone cortisol. Ironically, heightened states of cortisol over time can eventually lead to hyporesponsivity to stress and sensory stimulation, resulting in a blunted effort on the infant's part to later attend and respond to typical and expected environmental influences such as positive touch.[37] The influence of vagal tone and the autonomic nervous system, with continual activation of the "fight-or-flight response," is known as the Polyvagal theory, and may be predictive of adverse behavioral, cognitive, and motor outcomes at 3 years of age.[39,40] Chronic repetition of stressful and painful input leads to changes in brain activity and ultimately brain architecture, resulting in long-term alterations in behavior.[38,41]

Parents of NICU infants are more likely to experience significant life stressors before their child is born. These significant life stressors, known as adverse childhood experiences, may result in diminished emotional resources and coping abilities needed to withstand the financial, situational, emotional, and mental stressors that often accompany their child's course.[37,38] It is imperative that NICUs have programs to assist families not only financially but with the emotional support needed to face the unpredictable journey that lies ahead of them.[7,46]

TRAUMA-INFORMED CARE

The trauma-informed care model attempts to explain these collective toxic stress-evoking experiences and identify interventions that NICUs should adopt to support infants and effective family coping.[7] Understanding real and perceived stressors that families experience as a result of their infant's vulnerable condition helps prevent unnecessary repetitive stress and promote feelings of "safety, security, and connectedness" between the infant and caregiver.[37] Modifications of the stress response come from deliberate and intentional efforts to provide care by buffering environmental stressors for both infant and parent, thus minimizing further adverse experiences.

Intentional caregiving, the deliberate act of thoughtful engagement in all interventions and interactions, forms the basis of trauma-informed care.[7] Mindful interventions on the part of all practitioners has been shown to reduce the effects of noxious stress, thus mitigating long-term consequences on both infant and caregiver.[42] Parents of premature infants are often not ready or able to manage the overwhelming or traumatic circumstances they encounter. Parents may feel additional emotional stress, depression, anxiety, ambiguity about their child's future, financial pressures, and posttraumatic stress than parents of term infants.[42] Family dynamics are substantially affected throughout the NICU experience as well as afterwards. Parents often leave with mental health issues triggered or intensified by their infant's experience.[43] Weaving tenets of trauma-informed care principles into the culture of care diminishes stress on caregivers as well as infants and families.[7,44,45,46]

THE IMPORTANCE OF TOUCH AND SOCIAL CONNECTEDNESS

"The first love of the human infant is for his mother"

Harry Harlow[47]

Over the years, the importance of maternal engagement, touch, and human connectedness have been shown to bolster cortical growth and synaptic connections and is a basic human need.[48,49] Classic Harlow monkey studies of the 1950s and 1960s demonstrated the importance of soft physical touch over nutrition as the rhesus monkeys sought the comfort of their soft terrycloth-simulated mothers over food. Additionally, when the monkeys were physically isolated or experienced deprivation from physical contact, they demonstrated rocking and self-stimulating behaviors as well as aggression and "autistic-like" outbursts.[50] Harlow concluded that human contact is critical for comfort and social-emotional development.[47]

Studies of Romanian orphans have yielded similar conclusions. In the 1980s and 1990s, thousands of orphans received only custodial care because of overcrowding and lack of financial resources. Many of these children suffered social isolation and lack of intimate, loving touch and attention. They were later diagnosed with "failure to thrive" and presented with diminished social, emotional, and cognitive behaviors. The impact of social deprivation was physically captured on their magnetic resonance images (MRIs), which showed 30% less cortical volume compared to their typically developing 3-year-old peers who experienced routine family interactions.[51,52] Follow-up studies found that the subgroup of children who went into highly committed and nurturing foster care along with early-intervention programming before 2 years of age showed significant improvements in their white matter and improved social and cognitive outcomes. In contrast, children who remained in the orphanages until later years had poorer outcomes. These findings suggested that neural plasticity could be achieved through promotion of high-quality caregiver–infant attachments and early-intervention programming.[53]

In the 1990s, the Humane Neonatal Care Initiative advocated that premature infants needed nurturing touch and engagement with their families not only for its medical advantages, but because it was "humane".[48] In their groundbreaking research on SSC (mother and infant in direct contact) and infant–mother bonding, Klaus and Kennell recognized that "humane touch" was essential for healing and a "right" of every infant.[48,49,54] The works of Brazelton, Kennell, Klaus, and others have significantly contributed to social bonding theories and the importance of maternal touch and engagement. Recent research has investigated the epigenetic influences of early tactile experiences and found significant effects on the biological formation of social bonds, as well as reduction of infant pain and stress regulation.[50] Early parent engagement and bonding opportunities such as SSC are now cornerstones of care in the postnatal period, including the NICU environment.

EDITORIAL COMMENT: It is hard to believe in today's world of single-room neonatal intensive care units (NICUs) and parents rooming-in, that historically the first NICUs severely restricted parental visitation, allowing visual contact only for the first 21 days in an attempt to decrease infection. It is thanks to the work of Klaus and Kennell that hospitals have become healthier and more humane places to give birth.

Skin-to-Skin Care

SSC, also known as kangaroo care, offers the most favorable extrauterine environment for the premature infant. It is the "normal environment" and the optimal venue for delivery of care.[55] The process of SSC involves the diaper-clad infant being held directly on a parent's bare chest in an upright prone position. Parental–infant SSC safeguards the premature infant from the deleterious consequences of separation, promotes optimum brain growth, encourages attachment, and fosters infant self-regulation.[55] It has been shown to be a neuroprotective intervention that diminishes infant and parental stress. Studies have shown that brain maturation and plasticity is enhanced when parent infant SSC is offered 6 hours per week for 8 weeks.[56] Parents also experience positive physiologic effects by offering SSC to their premature infants,[57] such as enhanced parent–infant attachment[58,59] and improved perceptions of parental competence.[59] Parental attachment and satisfaction are augmented with maternal–infant during SSC, while paternal depression is decreased.[60] SSC accelerates brain development, encourages healing and growth, optimizes parent–infant bonding, and decreases infections and length of hospital stay, thereby serving as the foundation for neuroprotective developmental care in the NICU.[55] SSC has become standard in most NICUs. Refer to Fig. 8.2.

***Clinical Application**: Both mothers and fathers should engage in SSC. Even though there are very few contraindications to providing SSC, infants should continue to be monitored closely and use a three-person team to assist intubated infants and families with transfer and positioning. Physicians may advise about medical appropriateness for SSC and promote the benefits to parents in daily rounds to convey the importance SSC on both medical and emotional well-being of the infant and parent. Theoretically, SSC care should rarely be limited, but there may be exceptions.*

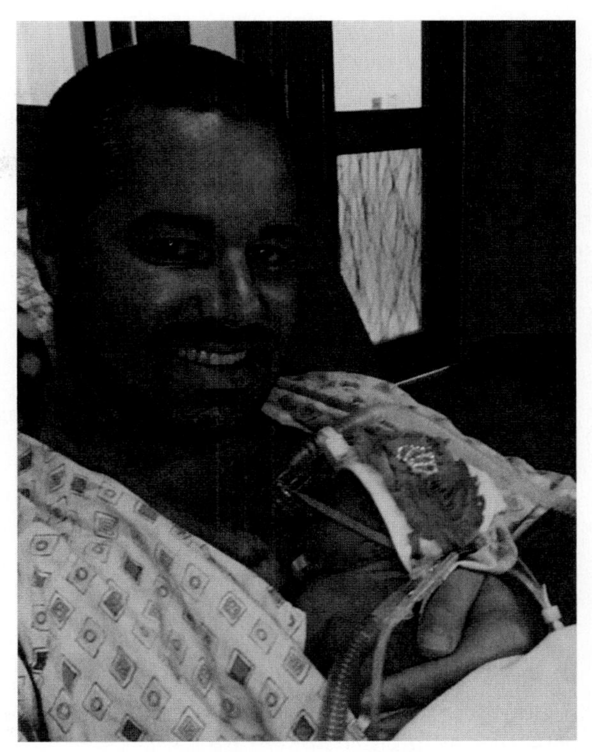

Fig. 8.2 Dad Nick and daughter Harper engaged in skin to skin. (Copyright Ricciardi SE. 2018. With permission.)

BENEFITS OF LOVING TOUCH

In addition to SSC, studies have highlighted the relationship between massage or moderate-pressure touch therapy and improved infant and mother outcomes.[61] Parental anxiety while in the NICU has been linked to compromised neurodevelopmental outcomes in very low–birth-weight infants.[62] Recent studies have revealed encouraging evidence that mothers who provided infant massage showed less psychological distress and anxiety and improved attachment.[63,64,65] Oxytocin, the neuropeptide that regulates emotions and feelings associated with love and safety, has a strong role in communicating the intention of touch.[50] Loving, nurturing touch and physical proximity have been shown to increase circulating oxytocin in term infants and improve social attachment.[66,67] Although increased circulating oxytocin has not been established in preterm infants at this time, noted improvements in behavioral responsiveness were seen when infants were socially engaged with their mothers, even at very young gestational ages (25–28 weeks).[67,68] Implications of these findings reinforce the importance of establishing social bonds and appropriate touch early in the developmental sequence.[69] Additional benefits of massage will be discussed later in this chapter. Refer to Fig. 8.3.

THE NEONATAL INTEGRATIVE MODEL OF DEVELOPMENTAL CARE

Models of developmental care have evolved over the years, leading to a currently proposed model of wide acceptance known as the Neonatal Integrative Model of Developmental

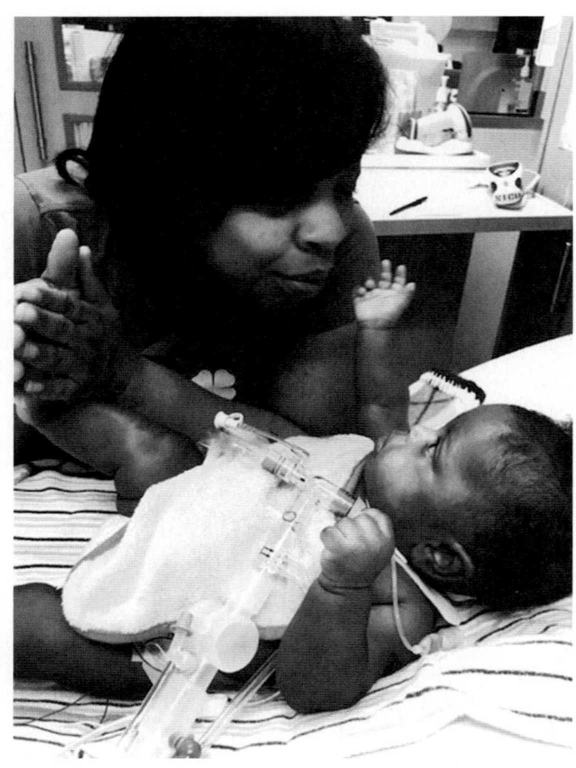

Fig. 8.3 Bonding opportunities with mom, Tere and daughter, Leah. Mutual reciprocity is promoted during massage and social engagement opportunities. (Copyright Ricciardi SE. 2018. With permission.)

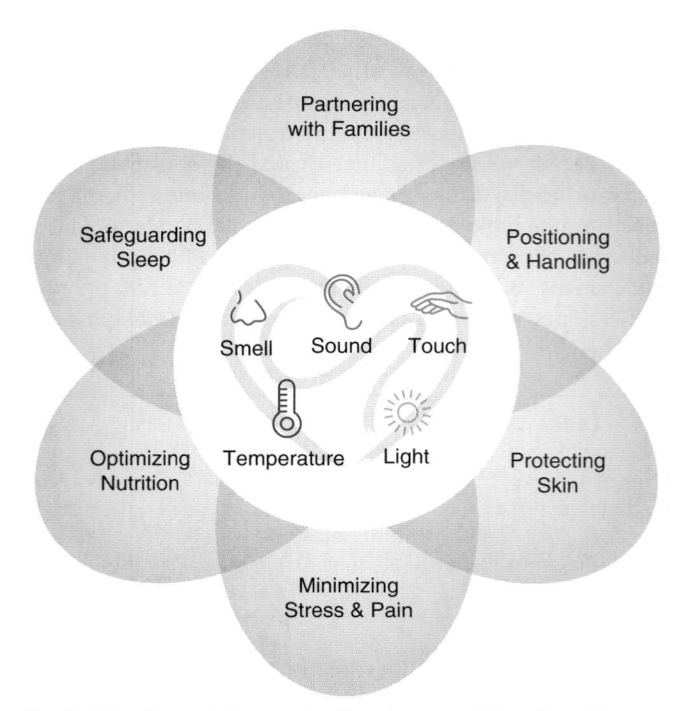

Fig. 8.4 The Neonatal Integrative Developmental Care Core Measure model. (From Altimier L, Phillips R. The Neonatal Integrative Developmental Care Model: advanced clinical applications of the seven core measures for neuroprotective family-centered developmental care. *Newborn Infant Nurs Rev*. 2016;16:230-244.)

Care. The Neonatal Integrative Model of Developmental Care[55] guides clinical practice in NICUs around the world because it suggests practical application integrating evidence and theory. The seven neuroprotective core measures of the IDC model may be envisioned as overlapping lotus petals. Refer to Fig. 8.4. The core measures are:

1. the healing environment
2. partnering with families
3. positioning and handling
4. safeguarding sleep
5. minimizing stress and pain
6. protecting skin
7. optimizing nutrition

AN INTRODUCTION TO THE SEVEN CORE MEASURES

The Neonatal Integrative Model of Developmental Care[55] weaves the seven core measures into all aspects of NICU care for vulnerable preterm infants and their families. The core measures offer clinical direction for NICU staff to provide neuroprotective family-centered developmental care to preterm infants and their families. Infants display identifiable behaviors or responses that may be considered quantifiable signs of core measure outcomes and detailed guidelines for interventions that strive to achieve the designated improvements or outcomes. Included are examples of the seven core measures along with recommendations for clinical application of important concepts of each identified area.

Core Measure #1: The Healing Environment

The physical setting of the NICU may be a healing environment that incorporates space; privacy and safety; and the sensory experiences of temperature, touch, proprioception, smell, taste, sound, and light. People, including families and healthcare professionals, and their exchanges are also significant aspects of the healing environment. When overwhelming environmental sensory stimuli are decreased by weaving neuroprotective strategies into infant care and modifying NICU design, premature infants may have better outcomes.[55]

UNDERSTANDING EFFECTS OF ROOM DESIGN

The single-family room (SFR) NICU was designed to improve medical and neurodevelopmental outcomes. SFRs enhance medical and neurodevelopmental outcomes for premature infants, foster parental interactions, and improve regulation of the environment, especially sound and light. Improvements in parent and staff satisfaction have been reported with the SFR concept.[71,72] Basic amenities a SFR should include are parent sleep space, individually controlled lighting, and private/secure storage for personal belongings.[73] The availability of SFRs encourages parental presence and infant interactions. Increased developmental support and maternal involvement, as evidenced by the provision of more SSC and direct infant care, was linked to increased weight at discharge, improved weight gain, fewer medical procedures, enhanced attention, and decreased stress and pain in SFR NICUs.[74] Privacy is improved in SFRs[72] as well as increased availability of mother's milk.[76] Exposure to human speech during the neonatal period, especially the mother's voice, adds linguistic value that can be crucial for the initial wiring of the brain for language acquisition. [77]

There are numerous benefits of SFRs; however, there is emerging confounding evidence that suggests that SFRs may not consistently lead to optimal neurodevelopmental outcomes across all infant populations. For example, it has been found that former premature infants at 2 years of age had compromised language development when compared with infants in open-bay units.[73,77] Abnormal language development may result from prolonged hospitalization in a SFR where lack of regular human speech is diminished if parents are not consistently present, thus increasing long periods of social isolation.[77]

***Clinical Application**: There are multiple factors that interact that may create either a positive healing environment or a neurotoxic environment. Light and sound are elements in the NICU that are easily modified in SFRs and have an important impact on neurodevelopmental outcomes. Clinicians should direct families to talk, read, and sing to their infants. Parents should be encouraged to stay with their infant as much as possible to fully participate in care in order to strengthen parental confidence and connectedness.*

FACILITATING NOISE REDUCTION AND PROMOTING AUDITORY DEVELOPMENT

The structural development of the human ear is complete by 24 weeks of gestation and becomes consistently functional after 28 weeks of gestation. Between 26 to 30 weeks of gestation, hair cells in the cochlea are adapted for exact frequencies and can transform acoustic vibrations into electrical stimuli that travel to the brainstem.[78] Hearing accuracy becomes nearly comparable with adult levels by 42 weeks of gestation.[79] Because the sensory receptors in the cochlea cover an area in the cortex much denser than in other sensory zones, it is highly vulnerable to afferent input. Modulating auditory input is essential in diminishing sensory overload and avoiding damage to the developing neural centers.[80,81,82]

The American Academy of Pediatrics (AAP) recommends sound levels less than 45 dB[79]; however, levels have been found to range between 7 dB to 120 dB.[79,81,83] Excessive environmental noise exposure in the developing premature infant leads to physiological instability, damaged hearing, poor neurodevelopmental outcomes, increased days on oxygen, and increased length of hospitalization.[79] Noise disturbs the autonomic nervous system, slows advancement to full enteral feeding and weight gain, and interrupts the sleep cycle.[81,84] High-frequency noise that reaches the immature cochlea may damage auditory pathways and impair language development.[85] Hearing loss is found in premature infants at a rate of 2% to 10% compared with 0.1% in the pediatric population.[81] Aside from excessive auditory input, hearing loss is associated with the synergistic use of aminoglycosides and incubator treatments, apneic spells, hypothermia, hyperbilirubinemia, and hypoxemia.[79]

Modifying the level of noise that reaches infants has been investigated. Sound levels are decreased when noise meters are used[86] or when implementing a "quiet hour."[84,87,88] In a small study examining a novel intervention, extremely low–birth-weight infants were randomized to wearing silicone earplugs or to a control group without plugs. Earplugs were placed at the time of randomization and used continuously until the infants attained 35 weeks PMA or were discharged (whichever happened first). Medical or social visits with family warranted removal of the earplugs. The control group received standard care. Mental Developmental Index (Bayley II) mean scores at 18 to 22 months corrected gestational age were significantly higher in infants with earplugs than in the control infants.[81,89]

Deprivation of biological maternal sounds that a developing fetus would normally hear in utero cause loss of significant acoustic input during a critical period of brain development. Parent communication and voice exposure is critical to infant auditory development. Researchers found that when premature infants born between 25 and 32 weeks of gestation were randomized in their first month of life to hear audio recordings of their mother's voice and heartbeat, they had a significantly larger auditory cortex bilaterally compared with infants who heard only typical NICU environmental sounds, demonstrating experience-dependent auditory plasticity.[90]

***Clinical Application**: Healthcare professionals should observe sound levels in the NICU, including the inside of incubators, and demonstrate mindful strategies to lessen noise such as lowering voices, decreasing volume of televisions, addressing alarm violations promptly and silencing them quickly, and closing incubator and cabinet doors with care. Use of overhead paging systems should be avoided, and alternative noiseless staff communication technologies should be employed. SSC provides an opportunity for an infant to hear parental biological sounds such as heartbeats or breathing sounds. Infants benefit from hearing conversations with human sounds and conversation. Parents should be encouraged to read aloud to their children and provide audio recordings of their voices for staff to play at appropriate decibel levels when they are not available.*

EDITORIAL COMMENT: There are, of course, multiple sources of noise in the neonatal intensive care unit (NICU), ranging from noises intrinsic to the NICU environment (incubator motors, respiratory equipment, alarms, etc.) to those from the broader hospital environment (building heating and cooling equipment, public address systems, etc.). A study at one large tertiary care NICU in which dBs were measured in seven areas for 1 week found that 99.99% of the levels were greater than the recommended level of 45 dB (CICSD 2010;37:69).

CONTROLLING LIGHTING AND VISUAL DEVELOPMENT

The visual system is the last sensory system to mature. Bright light and direct visual stimulation are often overwhelming. An understanding of neurodevelopmental vision progression will expose potential issues for vulnerable infants. At 25 weeks' postconceptual age (PCA), light stimulates the blink reflex,[91] and neurons of the visual cortex appear.[92] The pupillary light response may be elicited at 27 weeks' PCA, and vision is only a basic photometric reaction at this time.[91,93] Between 30 and 32 weeks' PCA, a bright light stimulates the eyelids to close promptly.[93] The premature infant can focus at 32 weeks and briefly track objects around 33 weeks, while showing visual preferences closer to 34 weeks.[94]

Lighting may enhance healing as well as potentially harm the growth and development of premature infants. Artificial and natural light transmits impressions, allows visual work of clinicians, impacts neonatal physiology and maturation, controls circadian rhythms, and provides neonatal therapy.[95] Cycled lighting should begin at 28 weeks PCA and be graded in terms of intensity and duration. In patient care areas, ambient lighting should have reasonable flexibility to address individualized needs of each infant and caregivers, and be easily adjusted by the healthcare team and families. Natural light offers significant psychological value for clinicians and families. In patient areas with access to natural light, be careful when infants are positioned close to windows because issues with radiant heat loss or gain and glare may occur.[96]

Clinical Application: *When performing a procedure or an examination, the infant's eyes should be shielded because premature infants may not have a mature pupillary reflex, so intense light may be unpleasant and damaging to the developing retina. Also, use ambient lighting instead of overhead bright light to create natural circadian cycling. Open-bay units present challenges for controlling light on the individual infant and require novel strategies and modifications.*

PROTECTING AND PROMOTING OLFACTION AND GUSTATION

Both olfactory and gustatory systems have important roles in feeding, metabolism, and digestion[97] as well as caregiver–infant attachment and pain management.[98] The olfactory system emerges between 8 to 11 weeks of gestation and is well developed by 24 weeks.[99,100,101] Taste receptors begin to emerge around 7 to 8 weeks of gestation and are fully functional by 18 to 20 weeks. Taste receptors are located throughout the entire oral–pharyngeal cavity, including the tongue, palate, pharynx, esophagus, and epiglottis.[101] When ingestion occurs, combined signals from olfactory and gustatory receptors communicate flavor to the brain. A fetus can detect flavors early in utero and have shown preferences to sweet solutions over bitter.[102] Fetal swallowing has been shown to increase in frequency with the introduction of sweet solutions into the amniotic fluid and decrease with bitter solutions.[102] This preference for flavor is also observed in 28-week preterm infants after birth, because they have been shown to recognize and prefer their mother's scent when presented with pads impregnated with maternal versus donor breast milk.[97] This sensory recognition benefits oral feeding, behavioral state regulation, and formation of affective neurological pathways.[103] Both olfaction and gustation are important in activation of anticipatory pathways that prepare the body for feeding and digestion known as the cephalic phase response.[50] This response increases gut motility and secretion of hormones and digestive enzymes that regulate blood glucose and enhance digestion.[50] Infants who require prolonged tube feedings demonstrate decreased time to full oral feedings and reduction in hospital stay when routinely exposed to maternal breast milk taste and odor three times a day between 28 to 34 weeks gestation.[104]

In terms of sensory modalities and pain management, the benefits of SSC and maternal breast milk decrease pain responses because of the olfactory properties in the familiar scent of the mother.[105] The use of sucrose or breast milk mitigates pain responses during routine skin-breaking procedures including intravenous line placement and blood draws.[106] Sensorial stimulation (SS) combines tactile, gustatory, auditory, and visual techniques that minimize pain responses.[106] A systematic review of 16 studies found that SS was more effective than sucrose alone in reducing pain.[106,107] Researchers are currently investigating the role of olfaction as a novel nonpharmacological agent that may contribute to this combined benefit of reducing pain.[108]

Regarding negative olfactory and gustatory experiences, exposure to detergents and disinfectants in the intensive care unit have resulted in decreased oxygenation and are noxious to the maturing infant.[109] Bitter medications, vitamins, hydrolyzed formulas, and gastroesophageal reflux negatively impact the afferent perceptions of smell and taste.[110,111,112]

Clinical Application: *Staff and parents should refrain from using scented lotions and other olfactory irritants. Allow hand sanitizer to dry before touching the infant or entering the incubator. Avoid scented bathing products and strong detergents. Provide a scented cloth from the mother (or father) in the isolette or crib. Encourage gentle application of colostrum or maternal breast milk to lips, and use during oral care. Incorporate sensory stimulation and provisions for the introduction of milk scent and taste surrounding early gavage feedings as part of prefeeding readiness routines. Combining sensory modalities of touch, taste, smell, and sound can promote positive associations supporting feeding progression, pain management, and bonding opportunities.*

Core Measure # 2: Partnering With Families

Improved health outcomes and enhanced family satisfaction result from family-centered collaboration (FCC) with the healthcare team. FCC is built on trust between families and the team of healthcare professionals.[113] It is important to view the infant's family unit as what the family perceives those bonds of family are[113] and to consistently integrate an appreciation of cultural, ethnic, and socioeconomic diversity.[114] Successful alliances between the healthcare team and families have demonstrated decreased lengths of stay, decreased parental stress, improved satisfaction for staff and parents, and better neurodevelopmental infant outcomes.[115,116] Researchers found that parents experienced less stress during the NICU hospitalization and less anxiety and depression after discharge when offered information and education.[117] Because of the stressful milieu of the NICU, healthcare organizations are cognizant to offer parents psychosocial assistance and support.[117]

The term *newborn intensive parenting unit (NIPU)* has been suggested to reflect abundant involvement of parents in their infant's care and consistent communication with the healthcare team.[118] An emerging infant care model known as family-integrated care suggests families are supported, educated, and empowered to offer as much direct infant care as possible. The NICU care team actively joins with families to educate, coach, and mentor them to assume primary responsibility for their infant's stay.[119] This method of care delivery incorporates mutual respect, information sharing, collaboration, confidence building, and joint decision-making.[119,120] An innovative approach targeted to meet educational and engagement needs of NICU families builds on digital resources including mobile devices, interactive learning platforms, and videoconferencing.[121] In addition to parent liaisons, support groups are an effective means to educate, engage, and empower families to interact with the healthcare team.[122] Throughout the NICU course and after discharge, infants and parents benefit from intervention programs that support the family unit and enhance infant outcomes.[123]

Clinical Application*: Parents are not visitors to the NICU, but rather vital to their infant's caregiving team and should be given 24-hour access to their infant. Families should be encouraged to participate in daily rounds. Ideally, these interdisciplinary rounds are at the bedside where parents have input along with the healthcare professionals about the plan of care for their child. Daily work rounds are a great opportunity to exchange information, educate families, and build a trusting collaborative relationship. If family members are not available for daily rounds, a phone call to parents may be used to update them on their infant's health status and the plan of care and to answer questions. Promoting direct care activities or assisting with tasks such as bathing, diapering, and feeding will help promote a healing environment.*

Core Measure #3: Positioning and Handling

General Positioning Goals

Developmentally supportive positioning and handling are cornerstones of developmental care. Ideal positioning for premature infants promotes symmetry, midline orientation, flexion, hands to mouth/face, containment, and comfort. Passive flexor tone develops naturally in utero during the third trimester. Flexion and containment enhance sensory input through mechanoreceptors located in tendons and joints, which promote proprioceptive mapping in the brain. This helps the infant develop muscle tone, motor coordination, and awareness of body position in space throughout life.[124] Premature infants miss the naturally occurring containment imposed by uterine walls in the third trimester. Even at term, maturing preterm infants do not achieve the same level of flexion as their term counterparts.[125] Flexor tone enhances head control, midline postures, and suck–swallow proficiency. Supportive positioning for the preterm infant attempts to achieve and promote flexor tone with alignment throughout the head/neck/trunk. Effective developmental positioning is evident when the infant demonstrates physiologic and behavioral stability, motor control, prolonged sleep, reduced stress cues, organized behavioral states, and enhanced self-regulation.[126] Swaddling and nesting with rolls or commercially available products often helps achieve these goals when used properly. Some infants may require positioning that varies from the general guidelines mentioned. Nurses and neonatal therapists work together to determine individualized positioning requirements for each patient when there are noted complications and/or specialized positioning is necessary, such as the need for prolonged immobilization or prevention of accidental extubation. The key to proper positioning is to recognize that infant's needs are dynamic and require frequent assessment and gentle weight shifts or position changes throughout the day based on their cues. The caregiver's role is to support and protect the infant while enabling natural opportunities for development.

Preventing Positioning Complications

Unlike the in utero fluid-filled environment, the extrauterine environment places prolonged periods of immobility and pressure on the soft, cartilaginous premature infant. The head is the body part that takes most of the unfortunate stress, absorbing the forces of pressure irrespective of position: supine, side lying, or prone.[127] Strong, preferential head turning to the right has been documented 45% to 79% of the time when infants are in supine.[129] Some researchers have associated these preferences with the influence of environmental factors and the dominance of right-handed caregivers.[128] Necessary medical interventions, especially the need for prolonged mechanical ventilation and endotracheal tube stability, have imposed sacrifices on positioning needs that can result in secondary musculoskeletal disturbances and asymmetry.[126] It should be mentioned that right-sided head preferences are cultural norms and may be associated with innate handedness. Typical in utero positioning during delivery is associated with right-side head orientation.[128] However, with significantly prolonged right-side preferences, especially in the premature population, infants may present with long-term adverse developmental outcomes including suboptimal reflexes and fine motor delays on the Bayley III.[129] It is unclear if the impact of positioning alone is responsible for the strong preferences; however, targeted early interventions can minimize pathological consequences that can occur if left untreated.

Plagiocephaly

In addition to head preference asymmetries, the incidence of misshapen heads has increased with younger survival rates and longer hospital stays in extremely premature and sick neonates. Estimated increases in identified plagiocephaly are fivefold since the 1990's "Back to Sleep Campaign,"[130,131] whereas reported incidences in some studies indicate the rate is as high as 30% to 46% at 2-month checkups.[130] Cranial deformities can have long-lasting sequelae and have been associated with atypical brain growth and specific changes in the cerebellar vermis, occipital lobe, and corpus callosum.[130,131,132]

Attempts to prevent such deformities require vigilant strategies or protocols to routinely adjust the infant's position throughout the day and across the weeks or months spent in the NICU. The goal of head repositioning and correct application of adaptive rolls and specialized products is to improve the amount of time spent in the midline position. Promoting time with the infant being held or engaged in supervised prone positions can assist with minimizing the negative effects of static positioning.[133] A few examples of interventions include rotating head of bed position, approaching the crib from both sides, slight weight shifts throughout the day, and modification of light sources or visual preferences. Intentional efforts to systematically adjust infant positioning throughout the day are of utmost importance in relieving excessive pressures on the developing skull and brain and decreasing the incidence of positional deformities. Inadequate positioning carries global consequences, and treatment for cranial molding may require head orthosis after discharge.[134,135] Likewise, long-term delays in motor, vision, facial, and sensory development have been associated with long-term positioning sequelae. Outpatient therapy is often necessary to address existing impairments or noted risk factors at discharge.[134]

Clinical Application: *Along with clinical observation, neurobehavioral and neuromotor assessments need to guide the nurse or developmental team in providing timely adjustments to infant positioning needs. Individualized awareness of the unique needs of each infant can prevent "cookie cutter" positioning that may impede proper development. Positioning can influence respiratory effort and should be considered in the overall assessment of oxygen needs. Screening assessments are helpful in revealing when therapy may be warranted because of significantly atypical, asymmetrical clinical presentations or with infants who are at high risk for impairments such as infants with prolonged intubation, extreme prematurity, lack of caregiver physical contact, or patients with known neurologic insult. Preventative programming and gentle frequent repositioning are primary goals of developmentally supportive interventions.*

Handling

Gentle handling of the infant involves contained, flexed, and slowly guided movements during direct interaction or care. Slow, deliberate movements in the very preterm infant help minimize surges in blood pressure that could potentially result in increased risks for intraventricular hemorrhage (IVH).[136] Diaper changes that minimize leg lifting and abdominal pressure are neuroprotective strategies that should be practiced especially in extremely premature infants less than 26 weeks of gestation. Studies have evaluated effects of midline position and handling routines in the first 72 hours of life and the subsequent impact on IVH. Although research showed modest evidence, most review articles do not support (or necessarily refute) practice changes.[136] A recent Cochrane Systematic Review did not support that the existing studies proved these interventions solely responsible for decreases in IVH.[137] However, it may be the synergistic effect of bundling strategies that have actually shown promise for diminishing IVH. Clinically, there are variations in adoption of midline positioning as a neuroprotective strategy. Individual units have implemented some or all of the previously mentioned strategies, as they are without overt risk and offer comfort to most infants.

Core Measure #4: Safeguarding Sleep

Preterm sleep–wake cycles have been identified as early as 30 weeks of gestation.[138] Sleep is necessary for optimal neuromotor development as well as enhanced autonomic functions associated with the release of growth hormones, weight gain, circadian rhythms, and immunological and gastrointestinal functions. Sleep patterns for developing premature infants vary greatly from their term counterparts. Term infants may spend about half of the time in rapid eye movement (REM) sleep or active sleep (which is characterized by a more active sleep with irregular heart rates, respiratory rates, and rapid ocular activity) and the other half of sleep spent in non-REM or quiet sleep.[139] This REM state will transition to a more mature and restful sleep closer to age 1. In contrast, premature infants spend almost 75% to 80% of their time sleeping in the active REM state. REM sleep is important for early cortical development, specifically the visual cortex, where non-REM sleep is necessary for memory, learning, and neuronal refinements.[139,140] Electroencephalograms (EEGs) have provided validating evidence on the nature of preterm infant's sleep and factors that interfere with quality sleep. Chronic lack of REM sleep can result in sensory, motor, and behavioral difficulties and depressed immune function, as well as impairment in cortical brain growth and plasticity.[35,141] Sleep disturbances have been associated with medications, pain, poorly timed care, noise, and other interruptions imposed by the NICU environment.[35,140]

Cue-based care is one method of attempting to coordinate nonemergent care among all interprofessional staff. Focusing on timing of care using infant cues without mandatory clock-based care or the clinician's timeline helps protect sleep. When possible, modifications to routine care should be based on observable, behavioral cues of the infant to determine if the pending interruptions are warranted or can be deferred to a later time.[7,35,141]

Therapeutic interventions such as gentle touch and massage, NIDCAP interventions, and soft music have documented results in improving sleep states.[142] Efficacy is often very specific to the individual infant and may not be generalizable to the entire premature cohort. Difficulty in assessing the impact of sleep interventions, via the preferred reporting items for systematic reviews and metaanalyses, has led researchers to accept moderate evidence, observational studies, expert opinion, and even parental input to establish individual sleep routines as well as unit practice guidelines.[143] NICUs need to provide periods of "protected sleep" and tools for clinicians to evaluate timing of interventions, such as routine blood draws. Uninterrupted sleep patterns are essential for brain development, neural plasticity, and generalized healing.[111] Because premature infants have diminished cues, behavioral sleep assessments are intended for use by nurses, developmental specialists, and other direct care clinicians to observe for trends in behaviors and dictate appropriateness of care, therapy, or nonurgent interventions.[144] Although it may appear as "common sense," having a simple yet systematic approach to recognizing, documenting, and protecting sleep serves to draw a conscious awareness and respect for this important activity of daily living.

Safe Sleep in the Neonatal Intensive Care Unit

In addition to protecting and promoting sleep, clinicians should be mindful of the AAP[145] position statement and recommendations for "safe sleep." Physicians and all staff should promote safe sleep guidelines in the NICU when medically appropriate as modeling is strongly correlated with compliance after discharge.[146]

The AAP recommends supine, or "back to sleep" position for infants greater than 32 weeks' PMA and all infants that are progressing toward discharge.[145] As the infant transitions to a point of "medical stability" and discharge is nearing, all positioning aids and modifications should conform with the AAP recommendations, and parents should demonstrate independence in positioning their infant accordingly. Consideration of a transition plan to reach this goal needs to be based on clinical recommendations that are developmentally aligned with individual infant needs.[147] During this time, exemptions can be made, with the clear indication for "therapeutic positioning needs." Therapists and nurses need to oversee the progression of infant needs and gradually work toward the supine position without need for positioning aids. There is a paucity of literature on defining medical stability and/or the appropriate manner to gradually transition infants that have extenuating behavioral or developmental needs to the supine position.[147] Researchers are developing algorithms and behaviorally based assessments to augment recommendations to support a more developmentally based transition. Despite the transition process, infants should be safely sleeping in the supine position before discharge, and staff should commit to modeling evidenced-based practices and consistent adherence to AAP recommendations to improve parent knowledge and compliance upon discharge.[145] Safe sleep audits, staff surveys, and staff/parent multimedia education have proven to be effective strategies in implementing consistent, safe sleep practices.[148,149]

Clinical Application: *Supportive positioning aids should be gradually removed from the crib except for infants who are not medically stable or who have significant developmental needs. In these cases, the healthcare team may use individual positioning informational cards, which can be posted at the bedside to inform caregivers and staff of the rationale for the temporary modification away from the supine position or to support specialized positioning aids. A plan for the eventual transition to the home going, supine sleeping position should involve parents, developmental team members, and nursing and the primary medical team.*

EDITORIAL COMMENT: Finland has one of the world's lowest infant mortality rates—1.7 deaths per 1000 live births in 2015, compared with 5.9 in the United States. A tradition in that country dating back to the 1930s is to give expectant mothers a box filled with sleep sacks, bathing products, diapers, and, most importantly, a small mattress that turns the box into a safe sleep environment. Several states, including Alabama, Ohio, and New Jersey, are now offering free baby boxes to all families of newborns. There are many factors involved in infant mortality, and randomized controlled trials are still enrolling patients, but with studies showing that many parents place their infants to sleep on nonrecommended sleep surfaces, one hopes that the baby box program can make a difference in reducing infant mortality (*Pediatrics.* 2016;138(3):e20161533).

Core Measure #5: Minimizing Stress and Pain

It has been estimated that infants in NICUs experience on average 10 painful procedures per day.[150] The most premature infants are those most at risk for alterations in neurodevelopment related to experiencing the highest number of painful procedures.[106] Like every other aspect of prematurity, pain pathways are not fully developed. Ascending pathways are developed first between 24 to 26 weeks of gestation; however, descending pathways remain immature until 6 to 8 months after birth.[151] The clinical implication is that at younger gestational ages, infants display hypersensitivity and difficulty in processing expected painful responses (i.e., heel sticks) and nonpainful touch (temperature assessment). Therefore it is important that NICUs have pain assessment tools (including behavioral assessments) in place not only for what is perceived painful but for routine care that may not be expected to be painful.[151] Poor sleep, the absence of nurturing touch, hunger, and gastrointestinal discomfort can often evoke what appears to be "painful" stress responses. Immaturity of the nervous system to process and modulate pain pathways impacts infant responses. When an infant is crying with motoric or physiological signs of pain/distress, it is important to consider and address both physical and social–emotional (lack of human or caregiver contact) etiologies[152] before offering pharmacological interventions. Pain-related stress has been linked to long-term consequences in children's somatosensory processing and altered perceptual processing and sensitization, as preterm infants have delayed functional maturation of the limbic, emotional areas of the brain, as well as pain pathways.[38,106] Long-term studies have demonstrated that prolonged and undermanaged pain in the neonatal population is associated with reduced cortical thickness and IQ at school age, abnormalities in white matter microstructure, and poor postnatal growth.[153] Infants experience different degrees of discomfort, stress, and pain related to direct patient care activities. Procedures that break the skin are especially pain provoking and increase in severity with repeated or chronic invasive procedures.[154] To assure that infants obtain sufficient pain relief, all NICUs should develop a pain and comfort management protocol.[155,156,157] A systematic approach integrates routine pain assessment and reduction of harmful stimuli and occurrence of painful procedures when possible.

Interventions recommended by the International Evidence-Based Group for Neonatal Pain have recognized several nonpharmacological interventions that should be used to mitigate pain. Nonpharmacological interventions include nonnutritive sucking, oral sucrose, music therapy, massage/comforting touch, swaddling, facilitated tucking, and SSC.[156,158] These strategies are more effective when they are combined[157,159,160] and present opportunities for parents to participate in the care of their child. Strong evidence supports parental presence and comfort during all procedures.[159] Because these interventions are noninvasive and build social connectedness with the caregiver, they should be integrated into pain prevention bundles and used in procedures that require direct patient contact.[159,161]

Several individual studies have suggested that strategies outlined by NIDCAP are effective in reducing behaviors associated with pain.[154] These developmental interventions include swaddling, direct touch, dim lights, pacing of the examination, and pacifier use. Eye examinations for assessment of retinopathy of prematurity (ROP) are perceived to be very distressing for infants.[162] Studies have looked at ways to reduce acute and long-term distress on eye examination days. In a recent randomized controlled trial (RCT), researchers studied infant behavior across two points of time to assess infant behavioral and cortisol stress responses at 30 and 60 min after the ROP examinations. Results indicated infants were able to recover faster behaviorally and demonstrated significantly lower salivary cortisol levels after NIDCAP interventions were used.[162]

In combination with nonpharmacological interventions, administration of oral sucrose has become a standard practice in most NICUs during routine ROP eye exams or other stress-inducing procedures. Delivery of a small bolus (0.1–1 mL per established protocol, or 0.2–0.5 mL/kg) of 24% sucrose administered gently into the oral cavity within 2 minutes of heel sticks and other invasive or "painful" procedures has been shown to diminish pain and stress responses. Oral sucrose administered on a pacifier is slightly less effective than the bolus method but more effective than a placebo.[163] In some cases, human milk appeared to provide the same benefits as sucrose.[164] Although sucrose has proven helpful for pain management, several studies revealed potential consequences of repeated sucrose administration. In a study of 107 preterm infants <31 weeks' gestation, greater than 10 doses in 24 hours was associated with poor motor and attentional abilities and diminished regulation of the HPA axis at 32, 34, and 36 weeks' gestation.[158] It is best to regulate use of sucrose and to combine this with other nonpharmacological treatments to maximize supportive interventions.[41]

Clinical Application: *Both pharmacological and nonpharmacological treatments should be combined for adequate and effective pain management. Clinicians should anticipate use of nonpharmacological methods for painful procedures, management of postoperative pain, and avoidance or improvement of continuous pain and stress surrounding frequently needed procedures (needle sticks, eye examinations, feeding tube insertion, dressing changes coordinating blood draws, etc.). Consider prudent and appropriate use of sucrose, pacifier, swaddling, and hands-on containment. Consider massage and utilization of parents or developmental team members to assist with providing nurturing touch during or after the procedure. Developmental specialists and therapists along with nurse champions should promote parents learning containment touch and daily massage routines through hands-on demonstration and practice.*

Core Measure #6: Protecting Skin and the Tactile System

"From a neurodevelopmental standpoint, the skin is the surface of the brain..."

Gibbins

In terms of sensory development, the tactile system is the first sensory system to fully mature and is functional at 24 weeks of gestation. It arises from the same ectodermal germ layer as the brain, and processes vital discriminatory, affective, and protective sensory input. The skin serves many important roles that affect neurodevelopment, such as thermoregulation, fat storage, insulation, fluid and electrolyte balance, defense against penetration and absorption of bacteria and toxins, sensation of touch, pressure, pain, and a communication channel for sensory information to travel the brain.[165] The goals of skin care in the premature population are to safeguard skin integrity, to decrease contact to possible toxic topical agents, and to optimize functionality of the skin as a barrier. Evidence-based practices should guide care for premature infants in the NICU for bathing, positioning, handling, emollient use, umbilical cord care, incubator humidification, and usage of adhesives and disinfectants.[165,55]

Although touch is critical for creating social bonds and improving overall maturation and healing, early touch experiences can be perceived as calming or irritating to premature infants. Oxygen desaturation, bradycardia, and behavioral distress have been associated with light touch and hands-on care in very preterm infants.[166] Touch that is light or random and applied to very preterm infants may be processed as painful and evoke stress behaviors that may be mapped as painful responses.[167] For example, a wet or soiled diaper could evoke behavioral responses similar to a painful procedure such a heel stick. This is as a result of immature pain and discriminative touch pathways.[168] Moderate pressure and static holding touch offer deeper proprioceptive input and are more organized, tolerable forms of touch.[142,169]

Clinical Application: *Research has demonstrated that moderate pressure touch or static touch is organizing and calming, versus light touch, especially in the very preterm infant. Before any care or procedure is provided, place hands on the infant for 5 seconds in a holding pattern to alert the infant to the caregiver's presence. This simple yet important gesture helps minimize stress, cortisol surges, and blood pressure spikes when infants are handled quickly and without intention.*

Core Measure #7: Optimizing Nutrition

Oral Feeding

Oral feeding, whether at the breast or with a bottle, is one of the most anticipated milestones for parents. It is one of the most complex tasks facing the maturing or high-risk infant and is a cornerstone for defining healthy outcomes and discharge readiness.[170] Successful oral feeding depends on maturation and integrity of the neurological system, coupled with positive oral experiences. Fetal swallowing begins around 11 weeks in utero, and sucking/swallow reflex and maturation of taste buds occur around 18 to 20 weeks of gestation. By 24 weeks in utero, a fetus will swallow up to 1 liter of amniotic fluid per day.[125] This sensory–gustatory process is interrupted in the premature infant at birth. The infant born at 24 weeks PMA is intubated and bombarded with atypical oral sensory experiences including gloved fingers, hygiene swabs, and oral suctioning.[141] The infant's new oral trajectory is now set on a different course and begins to entrain those atypical experiences and neural pathways in the brain. The act of synchronized suck–swallow–breathe coordination ex utero generally presents around 32 to 34 weeks PMA. The infant must now learn to regulate sucking and swallowing with breathing in an environment much different than the fluid-filled womb where smells and tastes are completely different.[125] Even though infants are set on this new course, many can adapt and prove successful in developing efficient oral feeding pathways with carefully timed introduction, guidance, and interventions that minimize stress, incoordination, and aspiration. In compromised infants with complicated medical courses, successful oral feeding will depend on a variety of factors that may require the help of specialized feeding teams.

Breastfeeding

Premature infants frequently are gavage fed until they can organize sucking with swallowing and breathing.[171] Around 28 weeks' corrected gestational age, mothers may offer their breasts that have been expressed to provide nonnutritive sucking opportunities.[172] Nonnutritive sucking on the breast that has recently been pumped may promote facial muscle development that facilitates direct breastfeeding when the infant is ready.[173,174] Around 32 weeks of gestation, many premature infants may initiate nutritive sucking at the breast.[175] However, many infant and maternal issues as well as clinical practices impact breastfeeding competence, not just gestational age.[176] Breastfeeding is often very difficult for premature infant–mother dyads because of infant morbidities.[177] Mothers encounter numerous challenges to maintaining an adequate supply for an extensive period of time before the infant is able to feed orally.[178] Mother–infant SSC should be promoted as soon as feasible after admission to the NICU and often may be viewed as the optimal strategy to set the stage for the beginnings of direct breastfeeding.[179] This interaction may accustom the infant to the maternal scent and familiarize the infant with sensations associated with direct breastfeeding. Daily SSC contact provides an opportunity for mothers and infants to "practice" breastfeeding when the premature is physiologically ready.[55]

Lactation management and breastfeeding support should be available upon admission to the NICU to minimize challenges that affect the delicate mother–infant connection and maternal milk supply. Opportunities to learn to breastfeed should be offered as soon as the premature infant is physiologically and developmentally ready.[55] Lactation consultants, nurses, feeding therapists, and developmental care specialists skilled in providing breastfeeding assistance enhance positive breastfeeding experiences and outcomes for premature infants.[175,180] Nurses are not only responsible for bedside care of infants but need to offer significant assistance, education, and support for the mother to establish and maintain her milk supply and to cultivate the maternal–infant relationship.[174,181] When providing breastfeeding support and education, the healthcare team should offer assistance and resources that are sensitive to diverse social, cultural, and linguistic lifestyles of individual families.[182] Support and guidance from knowledgeable and proficient nurses or lactation consultants are irreplaceable. Generally, the cross-cradle and football positions are optimal for learning to effectively breastfeed because they make it easier for mothers to provide head, neck, and shoulder support for premature infants.[55] An appropriately sized nipple shield may improve milk intake and duration of breastfeeding,[175] but this strategy is not without controversy.[176,177] Several researchers found infants who experienced their first oral feed as a breastfeeding opportunity went home receiving more mother's milk.[171,183,184,185] Mothers who are actively engaged in the breastfeeding process, which may promote maternal confidence and enhance parental caregiving skills, play a significant role in the NICU team.[178,183]

Benefits for lactating mothers who directly breastfeed or provide breast milk for their premature infants include decreased perceptions of anxiety and depression, less mood swings related to the positive effects of circulating hormones, enhanced emotional well-being, and lowered stress levels following breastfeeding when contrasted with bottle-feeding.[186] Evidence suggests that premature infants are more physiologically stable in relation to oxygen saturation, body temperature, and respiratory rate when breastfeeding than when bottle-feeding.[187] Mothers should be asked what their feeding goals are and if they plan to directly breastfeed. The healthcare team should verify that premature infants are effectively breastfeeding and that mothers are competent with the breastfeeding process and maintaining an adequate milk supply well before time of discharge.[55]

Clinical Application: *Professionals who are knowledgeable about lactation management issues and the breastfeeding process will help assure a positive breastfeeding experience for maternal–premature infant dyads. The healthcare team can offer timely, accurate education, consistent support, and individualized guidance throughout hospitalization to optimize short- and long-term infant health outcomes by improving the exclusivity and duration of human milk feeding. Physicians should understand the importance of their role in reinforcing benefits of breastfeeding and consider maternal goals in the overall nutritional plan of the infant. Clinicians such as lactation consultants or skilled nurses should be available to work with maternal–infant dyads to transition to effective breastfeeding-utilizing strategies to optimize milk transfer with sensitivity to infant physiologic and behavioral cues.*

Benefits of Breast Milk

Clinicians should strongly encourage mothers to provide their expressed milk or to directly breastfeed. Families need consistent support from all healthcare professionals to surmount the frequent challenges that mothers encounter to maintain the rigorous schedule of expressing their milk 8 to 10 times per day.[188] Mothers should ideally have continuous access to high-quality electric breast pumps in the NICU as well as at their home. Many insurance companies will cover the cost of an electric breast pump for home use.

Much evidence substantiates that human milk and breastfeeding provide optimal nutrition to promote infant brain development and long-term neurodevelopment.[189] Improved white matter mass, total brain volume, and test results were higher in children fed human milk when they were in the NICU. Human milk possesses several components to positively affect neurodevelopmental outcomes, particularly for premature infants whose underdeveloped brains are growing quickly during an important interval in the NICU in which white matter is vulnerable to inflammation, oxidative stress, and poor nutrition. Human milk offers optimal nutrition as well as bioactive mechanisms, such as antiinflammatory properties, antioxidants, growth factors, commensal bacteria, oligosaccharides, and stem cells that direct growth and development while halting or lessening the impact of biologic stresses.[184,190,191,192] Mental, motor, and behavior scores were significantly better at 18 months and 30 months of age for extremely premature infants fed mostly human milk. Confounding factors such as maternal age, education, marital status, race, and infant morbidities did not influence the findings.[190,193,194] Newer research findings indicate a significant dose-dependent relationship between increasing volumes of human milk ingested in the NICU and improved cognitive scores at 20 months of corrected age after adjusting for confounding variables.[6]

There are other numerous important short- and long-term positive outcomes for premature infants fed human milk, including decreased sepsis and necrotizing enterocolitis rates, enhanced immature host defense function,[196,197] a reduced number of hospital readmissions in the year following discharge from the NICU,[193,194] enhanced feeding tolerance,[193,194] decreased ROP rates,[198] decreased bronchopulmonary dysplasia,[199] and metabolic syndrome rates.[200]

In general, premature infants should receive human milk, fresh or frozen maternal milk when available, or pasteurized donor milk, and for those weighing less than 1500 g at birth, the human milk should be properly fortified.[201] Human milk enhances premature infant health as well as developmental outcomes; therefore healthcare team members should strongly support maternal efforts to provide their milk for their children.

Clinical Application: *Healthcare providers should educate mothers about the benefits of human milk, how to establish and maintain an adequate milk supply, and how to engage fathers or significant others to assist and support mothers with the milk expression process by applying identification labels, delivering expressed milk, or cleaning the breast pump. Consistent positive support from the healthcare team is important to sustain mothers' breast milk expression efforts.*

Cue-Based Feeding

Traditionally, feeding schedules are determined by volume targets and weight gain parameters based on the infant's birth weight or current weight. "Volume-driven feeds" depend on caloric intake, clock-based feeding schedules, and weight gain to dictate the course of feeding progression. Although this method has been shown to be successful in the very preterm infant less than 32 weeks of gestation, it can be less effective in the maturing infant over 34 weeks, resulting in longer transition times to full oral feeds and increased stress on the infant.[202] When maturing infants are expected to feed on rigid schedules with preset volumes that might not align with their cues, this creates stress on both the caregiver and infant.[203] However, because premature infants' cues may be unreliable and inconsistent, a semidemand schedule is often helpful as a transition from gavage and rigid volume-driven feeds to full cue-based feeding as the infant matures.[202] With advancing skill, increasing age, and maturation of all subsystems, infants that begin to show cues on a consistent basis should be considered ready for an oral feeding assessment. Infants presenting with readiness cues will be offered nutritive experiences on a continuum from prudent sensory tastes, via pacifier dipped in breast milk or formula, to suckling at the breast or a controlled bottle trial. Progression will depend on physiologic stability and suck–swallow–breathe coordination.

Identifying Cue-Based Clinical Behaviors

Cue-based feeding, or infant-driven feeding, is the method of assessing behavioral and physiological readiness of each individual infant to determine when to initiate and advance oral feeds. Infant cues guide the clinician across different points in the day of when to offer the feeding as well as through each individual feeding as to when to disengage. Medical stability and readiness variables include but are not limited to sustained quiet alert state, active muscle tone and vigor, nonnutritive suck search, less than 40% FiO_2 or <2 Liters per minute HFNC (high-flow nasal cannula), and respiratory rates less than 60 breaths per minute, or resting comfortably in baseline settings.[170] A Cochrane Systematic Review revealed a significant benefit of nonnutritive sucking (pacifier use) with emerging suck search. Nonnutritive sucking proved to be a strong predictor of oral feeding readiness and assists with quicker transition from gavage to full oral feeding.[204]

Instruments to Assess Readiness

Several studies have contributed to the evidence base in attempts to standardize readiness assessment tools, guidelines, and protocols for advancing cue-based oral feeding.[202,205,206] Although several algorithms exist, there are no care paths or assessment tools that have been universally agreed upon for the initiation of cue-based feeds. There are several published approaches in assessing readiness and quality of feed that should be evaluated when initiating a cue-based carepath.[207] Using a systematic protocol helps remove the random "trial-and-error" approach that relies too heavily on PCA and caregiver subjectivity in discerning when to start and how to progress oral feeds.[207,208]

Effectiveness of Cue-Based Feeding

Individual studies have demonstrated cue-based feeding regimens resulted in earlier discharges, improved weight gain, and less physiologic distress on the infant than volume-driven feeds.[209,210] To date, systematic reviews have been unable to validate the generalizable impact of cue-based feeding routines secondary to inconclusive evidence and poor methodological study designs.[211] However, in recent years, higher-quality randomized controlled trials have begun to capture the benefits of progressing feedings on infant behaviors and engagement cues as vital determinants in successful feeding outcomes.

When initiating cue-based feedings, clinicians should allow for variations in infant cues; however, objective measures should be in place to promote safety, nutritional intake, and weight gain[212]:

1. Feeding intervals should not exceed 4 hours.
2. Daily fluid minimums should be calculated versus per-feed volumes.
3. Routine assessment of growth of greater than 15 g/kg/day and total caloric intake of ~120 kcal/kg/day.
4. Semi-demand schedules for infants less than 2.5 kg (3-hour feed intervals or 4-hour intervals at night).
5. Glucose checks only with clinical suspicion or significant concern for hypoglycemia.

Readiness in Infants With Advancing Age and Moderate Respiratory Support

With ongoing advances in research and respiratory technology, decisions to initiate oral stimulation and controlled taste trials remain unclear in more complex infants.[213] Although this is not part of the standard care, some researchers have investigated the benefits of very prudent trials on high-flow nasal cannula (HFNC) or bubble continuous positive airway pressure (CPAP). The rationale for this considers infants with advancing age and at risk for deprivation-induced dysphagia. Some evidence exists regarding the importance of sensory experiences that aid in the development of reflexive neural pathways through stimulation of central pattern generators during critical windows of development.[213,214] In such cases, olfactory and gustatory stimulation has been shown to promote reflexive skill development, especially when combined with tactile (touch/massage) or kinesthetic movements.[214] Initiating oral feeding while on HFNC or CPAP continues to remain controversial and has been associated with increased risk of aspiration.

Generally, feeding specialists (occupational and/or speech therapists) should be consulted to assess and establish safe feeding trials. In many cases, specialized bottles, techniques, and protocols will be used to address complicated feeding situations. Controlling flow rate is a primary variable that can impact feeding performance and safe feeding opportunities.[215] Manipulation of contextual variables (volume, time of feed, method of presentation, flow rate of nipple) is often needed to support infant success and alignment with individual cues and needs.

Clinical Application: *Successful cue-based feeding requires synchronized interactions and bidirectional reciprocity between infant and feeder. Parental satisfaction, empowerment, and competence are reinforced when primary caregivers are taught to understand their infants' cues and respond to signs of stability, as well as signs of disengagement or distress. Parents benefit from learning to read their infant's cues instead of monitors and to respond to cues without the pressure of knowing a prescribed volume that must be taken. This reciprocity reinforces early social bonds and communication, and promotes a more co-regulated feeding experience that needs to continue well past discharge. Once the infant meets certain criteria in which oral feeding pathways are established, the medical team should consider manipulation of time, volume, and other contextual variables that are afforded to most term infants provided nutritional goals are being met. Infants that are advancing in chronologi-*

cal age, without the ability to engage in oral feeding opportunities (i.e., ventilated, CPAP, or HFNC), should be considered for a prudent oral stimulation program under the discretion of the medical team and guidance by the feeding therapist to maximize neural engramming and positive experiences during the critical windows of opportunity (32 to 44 weeks' PMA).

EVIDENCED-BASED THERAPEUTIC INTERVENTIONS

Aside from SSC, specific developmental interventions have shown promising results in independent studies and are often used by therapists trained more extensively in understanding their application to the premature population. Each intervention focuses not only on the convalescing infant but also on strengthening the infant–parent relationship. Three noninvasive interventions that improve parental confidence and short- and long-term infant benefits are massage, music therapy, and early literacy/communication-building activities.

Massage

The routine use of infant massage dates back over 2000 years in India, infants are engaged in massage from the moment of birth and throughout their first year of life.[142] In most studies, randomized controlled trials have demonstrated the effects of massage on weight gain as a primary or secondary outcome. Infants massaged with oils (e.g., safflower, coconut, medium-chain triglyceride oils, etc.) have improved weight gains over control groups.[142] Massage increases vagal tone, which is a proposed mechanism of action behind weight gain. Improved absorption of nutrients via transcutaneous absorption of natural, edible oils and production of the growth hormone (insulin-like growth factor 1) are also responsible for enhanced growth.[216] Additional massage studies have yielded improvements in circulation, gastric motility, pain responses, enhanced bone density, improved sleep states or alert states, improved immune responses, and enhanced caregiver attachment.[142] In terms of mitigating pain, massage provided 2 minutes before heel sticks on the ipsilateral leg showed lower scores on the neonatal pain scale than their nonmassaged peers.[61] Other studies found massage benefited both mothers and preterm infants, with mothers reporting less stress and anxiety after providing 8-minute massages on the days surrounding discharge.[217]

Methodological limitations in some studies have swayed researches from fully adopting massage as a standard of care; however, anecdotal, clinical findings often provide a strong testament to the benefits for a subset of maturing infants usually greater than 32 weeks' PMA. Despite research limitations, individual infants and parents share in the interactive, bonding benefits of massage irrespective of the statistical significance across the larger population.[218,219]

Music Therapy

Music therapy interventions consisting of live and recorded music and parent voices have shown physiological benefits as well as decreases in parental anxiety. Trained music therapists provide live music entrained to infant vital signs and with respect to the infant's auditory development and ambient noise level, ensuring that the infant's sensory system is not overstimulated. They also proactively teach parents the importance of the human voice, appropriate sound levels, and the beginnings of verbal communication with their infants. Studies have shown stabilizing effects on infant vital signs when a parent sings lullabies to their infant, particularly when their breath and lullaby is attuned to the infants' vital signs. In one study, infants were noted to sleep better over a 2-week period when instruments specially designed to mimic sounds of the womb and the mother's heartbeat were incorporated into live music therapy sessions. Live lullaby had positive, though less significant, impact on sleep, with the control group showing significantly diminished sleep quality compared to all intervention groups. Overall, quiet alert states, suck responses, and oxygen saturation, as well as perceived parent anxiety, all improved as a result of live music therapy sessions. A recent meta-analysis found evidence in favor of music therapy on infant vital signs, maternal stress, and maternal–infant bonding. With the culminating evidence on benefits of music therapy in the NICU, many highly ranked children's hospitals offer some form of live music therapy.

Early Language Skills

Developmental interventions have attempted to lessen the gap of the absent parent and/or isolation of the infant in the single-patient room by promoting reading interventions at the bedside. Therapists, nurses, volunteers, and parent representatives have been identified as available to assist in establishing "reading programs" or early-literacy initiatives in attempts to bridge this gap and promote enhanced cognitive skill development. A relatively newer area of study includes analyzing the effect of reading and spoken language in the presence of the premature infant. Studies have looked at the number of words spoken by an adult during a parent visit compared with no parent visiting with only staff interactions. Word analyzers were placed in private patient rooms for a set time period. Intelligible words were counted at two time points, 32 and 36 weeks' gestational age. The range of spoken words was significantly higher in the parent group and at the 36-week mark. In follow-up with these patients at 18 and 36 months, both groups of infants in the "no parent visiting group" experienced cognitive delays compared with their counterparts in standardized testing.[220] Likewise, infants that spent time in "high-quality developmental care units" scored higher in language acquisition at 18 months than infants in "low-quality units."[221]

THE HIGH-RISK NEONATE AND THE ROLE OF NEONATAL THERAPISTS

Aside from prolonged hospitalization associated with prematurity and a complicated medical course, many infants will have comorbid conditions that place them at high risk for neurodevelopmental delays. The AAP has defined guidelines that require a neonatal therapist (occupational or physical therapist) to be on staff in NICUs with level III or IV designation.[222] Infants with significant birth depression, neurological insults, such as IVH, hypoxic-ischemic encephalopathy and hydrocephalus, genetic or structural anomalies, narcotics abstinence syndrome, or severe bronchopulmonary dysplasia, are often referred to therapies as a result of observed clinical difficulties and risks associated with an altered developmental course.[223] Clinically, these infants often present with feeding difficulties, sensory abnormalities, atypical muscle tone and movement patterns, sleep and attentional disturbances, poorly modulated state or self-regulation, as well as diminished attachment to their primary caregiver.[224,225] These infants are usually referred to occupational, physical, and speech therapy for assessment and intervention during their NICU course. In addition to providing care along the rehabilitative continuum, neonatal therapists are included in preventive care and programming in many units.[223] This shift in care from rehabilitative to preventative helps identify early opportunities to improve positioning, caregiver engagement, feeding readiness, and other supportive care that minimizes stress on both the infant and family. Developmental neonatal therapists conduct neurobehavioral and developmental assessments that provide information that guides individualized interventions. Early identification and programming are essential in high-risk infants, as clinical symptoms often serve as warning signs for later delays.[225]

INTERPROFESSIONAL COLLABORATION

It is necessary that all clinicians and staff, regardless of their direct or indirect interaction with infants and families, understand the importance of creating a nurturing, healing environment and supportive culture of care. Administrators, physicians, clinicians, nurses, and support staff need to consider the impact that policies, procedures, and medical interventions have on the immature brain and family unit. Physicians, pharmacists, nutritionists, neonatal nurse practitioners, and nurses play critical roles in managing and providing direct medical care of these vulnerable infants. Lactation consultants promote, support, and protect breastfeeding and enhance human milk feeding. Neonatal occupational, physical, and speech therapists specialize in providing neurobehavioral, neuromotor assessments and interventions, feeding therapy, supportive touch/massage, cognitive, language, and sensory-based therapy as well as parent education. Social workers support families throughout their journey in the NICU as well as connect them with resources after hospital discharge. Child life specialists and music and art therapists are additional members of the team who contribute to the comprehensive culture of supporting family-centered developmental care. Parent liaisons are a relatively new addition to the team, providing direct support and mentoring to families.

DEMONSTRATED IMPACT OF "HIGH-QUALITY DEVELOPMENTAL CARE PROGRAMS"

Successful outcomes associated with developmental care approaches have yielded varying results over the years. The impact of such care is often difficult to assess, standardize, and measure. In 2012, Montirosso et al. proposed that the level of integrated developmental care practices might account for long-term variations in neurodevelopment. The researchers designed a prospective multicenter, longitudinal study measuring the relationship of varying levels of care from 25 NICUs with 178 very preterm infants (gestational age <29 weeks and/or birth weight <1500 g). Because there was no universally accepted measure of developmental care, the Neonatal Adequate Care for Quality of Life checklist was developed and used in conjunction with the standardized NICU Network Neurobehavioral Scale to evaluate the level of developmental care in each NICU and to assess infant neurobehavioral outcomes. The checklist measured level of parental involvement, nursing practices, and both pharmacological and nonpharmacological pain management.[227] Although the checklist serves as a global index and the synergy of the items constitutes the effect compared with any specific intervention, it was evident that greater use of developmental care practices and better pain control correlated with higher scores on the neurobehavioral assessment. Montessori's initial research led to additional studies demonstrating the impact of pain and behavioral problems at 18 months.[228] Additionally, infants from NICUs scoring high in developmental care showed better language skill development at 36 months and at 60 months than infants from lower-scoring units. Most interestingly is that even after controlling for socioeconomic status and parental distress, infants from highly engaged developmental care units had better health-related quality-of-life assessments at 5 years of age.[229]

To improve the quality of specialized caregiving, the National Association of Neonatal Nurses (NANN) outlined requirements for a developmental care specialist designation, which recognizes advanced training and testing for qualifying nurses and therapists. Likewise, in 2016, the National Neonatal Therapy Board Certification was established to recognize experienced occupational, physical, and speech therapists seeking advanced competency in neonatal therapy. Board certification assures credentialed therapists demonstrate evidence-based knowledge and have documented clinical expertise in providing safe and effective age-appropriate interventions.[125]

INSTITUTIONAL IMPLEMENTATION OF DEVELOPMENTAL NEUROPROTECTIVE CARE

Recognizing Joint Commission requirements to provide age-specific care across the life span, leading practitioners, researchers, and professional organizations have united to address core measures as the primary components for providing specialized, deliberate developmental care, and have published joint position statements for successful implementation across all NICUs.[230] The Canadian Association of Neonatal Therapists combined efforts with NANN[125] and the Council of International Neonatal Nurses to provide a detailed framework for the international institutional implementation of neuroprotective developmental care.[231] The roles of administrators, physicians, developmental specialists, and all intersecting interprofessionals are outlined in this guiding framework. Suggestions for adopting processes designed to sustain, promote, and standardize the culture of neuroprotective developmental care are clearly outlined.[230,231,232] Facilities interested in implementing high-level developmental care can use these guidelines with confidence.

SYSTEMATIC REVIEWS AND DEVELOPMENTAL CARE

Neurodevelopmental assessments along with advanced imaging techniques have attempted to assess the impact of developmental care in terms of capturing objective, neurological outcomes. Interventions such as SSC, nonnutritive sucking, facilitated tucking/containment, massage/nurturing touch, and parental involvement have shown good evidence in short- and long-term outcomes.[4,61,65,233,] Although review evidence has not been statistically significant in every area of developmental care to warrant universal acceptance, many individual studies have consistently demonstrated outcomes in favor of NIDCAP. In a review by Burke, six studies used EEG recordings as outcome measures and all found positive data favoring the NIDCAP intervention groups.[233] Developmental care research is continuing to evolve, with emphasis on improving many of the methodological limitations that currently limit inclusion in reviews.[4,233] It is difficult to assess interventions in a double-blind fashion and to keep the "spillover" effect from affecting control groups, as parents and staff are actively sharing information and modifying variables that ultimately provide comfort and perceived benefits.

RECOMMENDATIONS FOR FUTURE RESEARCH AND IMPLICATIONS FOR CLINICIANS

The advancement of evidence-based research supporting interventions in developmental care has increased in the past decade. Underpinnings in neuroscience, psychology, medicine, and embryology, among many other fields, are exploring the impact the NICU environment has on the developing brain and premature infant as well as the effectiveness of developmentally supportive interventions. It remains difficult to conduct high-validity, quantitative research with standard experimental design when trying to capture individualized and "humane" care that developmental paradigms suggest. Strategies to improve reliable and valid research include randomization with a large number of sites, assessing long-term outcomes with improved blind evaluation, and state-of-the-art neurologic imaging.[4] The continual advancements in clinical and diagnostic neuro-assessments, including noninvasive and highly sensitive imaging techniques, will allow researchers to analyze differences in preterm infants' brains on cellular levels. Recently, researchers have identified biochemical changes in nerve cell integrity using proton magnetic resonance spectroscopy. This specialized MRI technique analyzed molecules present in the cerebellum of preterm and full-term infants, identifying a correlation between diminished chemicals responsible for nerve integrity relating to neonatal infection. These promising imaging tools shed light into the finer workings of the brain and prove highly sensitive in analyzing dimensions of touch/comfort/attachment as well as infant stress and microchanges in brain architecture and functioning.[26]

DISCUSSION

Understanding and applying theoretical constructs and evidence-based knowledge surrounding developmental care is the responsibility of mindful practitioners. It is imperative that the culture of the NICU appreciates that nurturing human touch is impactful and necessary to healing, as well as critical in achieving optimal neurodevelopmental outcomes. The impact of the family and primary caregiver cannot be replaced or neglected and should be intentionally integrated into the culture of care. Clinicians should consider the potential epigenetic influences of routine, procedural, and stress-inducing interventions. Providing supportive developmental strategies as well as adapting medical care and the environment can minimize repeated stress on the maturing brain and compromised infant. Education of all practitioners should be embedded in standard orientation and competency training. Establishing qualitative assessments and outcomes is beneficial and impactful in buffering unnecessary stressors and enhancing the healing environment for patients, families, and primary caregivers.[36]

Emerging research is examining the impact the environment of care has on cortical growth, maturation, and neural plasticity as well as the relationship of human interaction/touch, attachment, and the developing brain. All clinicians interacting with premature and ill neonates need to receive education and training on techniques that can facilitate developing neural pathways. Strategies to create a healing, nurturing environment are the responsibility of the entire interprofessional team. Fostering an age-appropriate sensory environment, engaging the family in all dimensions of care, diminishing stress, and promoting developmentally supportive protocols will provide pathways for improved long-term qualitative outcomes. Expanding qualitative research and identifying improved outcome benchmarks could be used in conjunction with randomized controlled trials. Adopting guidelines for institutional implementation of neuroprotective developmental care, within the broader context of the highly sophisticated medical environment, can only serve to cultivate success and respect for all infants and families as they journey to healing and wellness.

The full reference list for this chapter can be found online at www.expertconsult.com.

CASE 8.1

Baby Sam was born at 25 and 1/7 weeks of gestation, with a birth weight of 760 g, to a 24-year-old primiparous single mother via spontaneous vaginal delivery. The infant has been emergently intubated and stabilized in the delivery room and is to be immediately transferred to an adjoining Level IV neonatal intensive care unit (NICU) for additional care in a transport isolette, supported and monitored by a team of physicians, respiratory therapist and nurses.

1. What is the recommended strategy to promote the development of a maternal–infant bond at this time?
Ideally, the resuscitation team may be able to take the infant to be viewed briefly by the parent in the transport isolette. Inquiries about the name of the child should be made to call the child by name when giving updates on infant status to the family. Families should be encouraged to visit the infant in the NICU soon, and mother should begin to express colostrum for her child.

2. As the premature infant arrives in the NICU, umbilical venous and arterial catheters need to be inserted. What interventions may limit the stress the premature infant may experience?
As the infant is examined and prepared for procedures, the infants' eyes should be shielded from bright lights. Clinicians should keep their voices low, briefly apply firm gentle touch as the infant is approached, address and silence monitor alarms quickly, and place positioning aids to maintain the infant's head in a midline position and extremities flexed. The lower extremities may be swaddled to stabilize infant position for the procedures as well as to comfort Baby Sam.

3. Baby Sam's mom started pumping her breasts about 2 hours after she delivered. She was able to collect several drops of colostrum with each breast milk expression session. The ventilator-associated pneumonia prevention bundle dictates that oral care should be provided every 4 hours. What substance should be used to provide oral care?
Colostrum should be used to provide oral care because oropharyngeal-associated lymphoid tissue can actually absorb some of the colostrum components to enhance the immune status of Baby Sam. Parents should be urged to assist with oral care after being educated on the procedure. Mom's efforts to provide breast milk should be supported. Tastes of colostrum may help the infant later on transition successfully to oral feeding.

4. On Day of Life 4, it is determined that a peripherally inserted central catheter (PICC) will be inserted. What are some pain management strategies that can be implemented for Baby Sam?
Baby Sam should be positioned using positioning aids, and the lower extremities may be swaddled, as arms may be the preferred site for the clinician to insert the PICC. An appropriate dose of an analgesic, such as morphine, should be administered before the procedure begins. An appropriately sized pacifier may be offered along with maternal colostrum or a 24% sucrose solution. The eyes should be shielded from bright lights needed for the procedure.

5. Mother will provide Baby Sam with skin-to-skin care (SSC). What are some supportive interventions that clinicians may provide to promote a safe and comfortable experience?
Educate Baby Sam's parents about the benefits of SSC and what to expect during the experience. Encourage them to provide SSC for at least 1 hour and to attend to their personal needs prior. Mother should pump her breasts before the SSC experience with Baby Sam; this way, she is comfortable. Use sufficient personnel to transfer the infant from the incubator to the parent's chest; generally a respiratory therapist can manage the respiratory equipment, the bedside nurse can transfer the infant on to the mother's chest, and another clinician may assist with IV and monitor lines. Baby Sam should have a hat on and be covered with a folded blanket after all tubes and lines are secure and correctly positioned. Parents can gently massage Baby Sam throughout the SSC episode, talk quietly, or sing to Baby Sam.

6. Mom of Baby Sam is very anxious about a particular procedure and the impact this is having on the entire family. What immediate resources and interventions could be used to engage the mother in care, and what are the expected benefits to mother and baby?
A clinician should sit down with the mother and ask open-ended questions in a compassionate, nonjudgmental, unhurried manner. Explain the benefits of medical interventions as well as the potential complications. Allow families to ask questions, and respect their input as an attempt to be part of the solution. Recognize that families cope in different ways based on their prior adverse life experiences and presence or absence of current life stressors, resources, and support system. Encourage mom to verbalize her concerns. Provide honest updates on the infant health status in terms Sam's mother can understand. Contact the NICU social worker to meet with mom to offer interventions and supports as indicated. Encourage mom to participate in Sam's ongoing care such as diaper changes or if she would like to provide SSC. Involve developmental team members to guide mom in activities that promote benefits to mom and Sam, such as infant massage. Encouraging meaningful interactions will empower mom to know that she is contributing to Sam's healing. If available, mom should be encouraged to "room-in" with Baby Sam in the NICU.

7. Baby Sam is now 31 weeks, weighs 1650 grams, has occasional self-resolved bradycardias and desaturations, has a nasogastric tube for gavage feedings, and is on a low-flow nasal cannula. Baby Sam enjoys sucking on his pacifier, his fingers, and nonnutritive sucking at the breast. When can oral feeds begin?
Establish nutritive neural connections and pathways by promoting prudent sensory tastes of maternal breast milk or formula to lips around 32 weeks. With consistent readiness cues, many infants can participate in oral feeding around 32 to 34 weeks. Initially, gavage feeding is established using traditional care paths that are centered on a predictable and consistent schedule and volume. When beginning oral feedings, an infant-led process, in which cues are systematically assessed and feedings are offered accordingly, is the ultimate goal and best method for achieving safe feedings and earlier attainment of full oral feeds. Volume and weight gain should be monitored but should not drive feeding progression in the maturing infant.

9

Respiratory Problems

Moira A. Crowley, Richard J. Martin

When one considers the complexity of the pulmonary and hemodynamic changes occurring after delivery, it is surprising that the majority of infants make the transition from intrauterine to extrauterine life so smoothly and uneventfully. Nonetheless, the staff working in the intensive care nursery spends a lion's share of their time caring for neonates with respiratory problems that are responsible for much of the morbidity and mortality in this period.

PHYSIOLOGIC CONSIDERATIONS

Normal Developmental Changes

Before birth, the lung is a fluid-filled organ receiving 10% to 15% of the total cardiac output. Within the first minutes of life, a large portion of the fluid is absorbed or expelled, the lung fills with air, and the blood flow through the lung increases eight- to tenfold. This considerable increase results from a decrease in pulmonary arterial tone and other physiologic changes that convert the circulation from a parallel arrangement to a series circuit.

The high vascular resistance in the fetal lung is caused by pulmonary arterial vasoconstriction. The pulmonary arterial vasodilation observed following delivery results in part from the large increase in oxygen tension, from the small decrease in CO_2 tension and the corresponding increase in pH, and from mechanical stretch associated with lung inflation at the onset of breathing.

At the same time, an adequate functional residual capacity (FRC = volume of air in the lungs at end expiration) is quickly attained. In healthy term infants, the first breaths are characterized by short deep inspirations and prolonged expirations through a partially closed glottis to ensure lung inflation. In preterm infants, continuous positive airway pressure (CPAP) enhances lung inflation.[1] By 1 hour, the distribution of air with each breath in the newborn is already similar to that observed in later life. Specifically, lung compliance (change in lung volume expressed in mL of air/change in pleural pressure expressed in cm of H_2O) and vital capacity increase briskly in the first hours of life, reaching values proportional to those in the adult.

Chemical control of respiration is, in general, similar in the newborn infant and the adult. As inspired (and arterial) pCO_2 is increased, both infants and adults increase their ventilation, although the neonatal ventilatory response is smaller. The ventilation of the newborn is also transiently increased when inspired gas mixtures contain less than 21% oxygen; this response suggests that the carotid body chemoreceptors are active at birth. The infant, however, differs from the adult in that if hypoxic exposure continues beyond about 1 minute, respiration is depressed during the first weeks of life. Hypoxia thus appears to depress the respiratory center, negating the hypoxic stimulation via peripheral chemoreceptors. This hypoxic respiratory depression in the newborn appears to depend on the presence of suprapontine structures in the brain. Even though hypoxic respiratory depression may be useful to the fetus (who maintains a normal PaO_2 of 20–25 mm Hg), persistence of this phenomenon into postnatal life may enhance vulnerability of neonatal respiratory control.

The effects of pulmonary stretch receptor activity on the timing of respiration (Hering-Breuer reflex) are more readily elicited in the newborn than in the adult. In infants, a sustained increase in FRC causes a marked slowing of respiratory rate by prolonging expiratory time.[2] In the first days of life, a brisk lung inflation causes a deep gasp (Head paradoxical gasp reflex) followed by apnea, which is, again, a manifestation of the Hering-Breuer inflation reflex. The deep gasp observed in the first day of life with low inflation pressures may explain the clinical observation that very low pressures (10–15 cm H_2O) are often effective in resuscitating the apneic newborn at birth by stimulating a gasp reflex.

The partial pressure of carbon dioxide (pCO_2) reflects the ability of the lung to remove CO_2. The HCO_3 concentration is controlled by the kidney. When the pH and CO_2 are determined, the HCO_3 can be calculated by using the Henderson-Hasselbalch equation:

$$pH = 6.1 + \log \frac{HCO_3}{pCO_2 \times 0.03}$$

If only the pH is measured, the cause of the acidosis or alkalosis cannot be determined. With metabolic acidosis, HCO_3 is decreased. To compensate for this, the infant hyperventilates, lowering arterial pCO_2. With respiratory acidosis caused by pulmonary disease, apnea, or hypoventilation, the arterial pCO_2 increases. The kidney attempts compensation by retaining HCO_3 and excreting hydrogen ions. Only by measuring the pCO_2 and pH and calculating HCO_3 can the cause of an abnormality in acid–base balance be determined. The normal newborn quickly regulates his or her pH to near adult values, although HCO_3 may be lower than normal adult values.

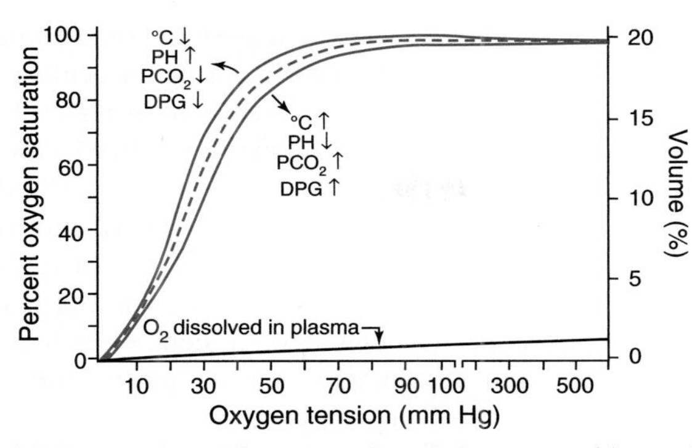

Fig. 9.1 Factors that shift oxygen dissociation curve of hemoglobin. Fetal hemoglobin is shifted to left as compared with that of adult. *DPG,* Diphosphoglycerate. (From Fanaroff AA, Martin RJ, Walsh MC, eds. *Neonatal-Perinatal Medicine.* 10th ed. Philadelphia, PA: Elsevier; 2015)

OXYGEN DELIVERY

Oxygen is carried in the blood in chemical combination with hemoglobin (Hb) and also in physical solution. The oxygen taken up by both processes depends on the partial pressure of oxygen (pO_2).

At ambient pressures, the amount of dissolved oxygen is only a small fraction of the total quantity carried in whole blood (0.3 mL O_2/dL plasma/100 mm Hg at 37°C). Most of the oxygen in whole blood is bound to Hb (1 g of Hb can maximally bind to 1.34 mL of oxygen at 37°C). The quantity of oxygen bound to Hb depends on the partial pressure and is described by the oxygen dissociation curve (Fig. 9.1). The blood is almost completely saturated (%sat. = mL O_2 bound to Hb/Hb (g) × 1.34X100) at an arterial oxygen tension (PaO_2) exceeding 90 mm Hg.

As an example, if the arterial pO_2 is 50 mm Hg, saturation is 90%, and Hb is 10 g/dL, then 9 g Hb is bound to oxygen. Thus the oxygen content of this 100-mL sample is 12.06 mL O_2 bound to Hb (1.34 × Hb 9) + 0.15 mL O_2 (0.3 × Hb 50/100) dissolved in plasma for a total of 12.21 mL O_2. Naturally, if the Hb is doubled, then for the same saturation, the O_2 transported by Hb is also doubled (1.34 × Hb 18 = 24.12 mL O_2) without changing the amount dissolved. The dissociation curve of fetal blood is shifted to the left and, at any PaO_2 less than 100 mm Hg, fetal Hb binds to more oxygen compared with adult Hb. The shift is the result of the lower affinity of fetal Hb for diphosphoglycerate. In contrast, the dissociation curve is shifted to the right by increasing acidosis and temperature. The clinical significance of the shift to the left for fetal Hb is that fetal blood will take up more oxygen at a given O_2 tension (pO_2). However, tissue pO_2 will need to decrease to a lower level to unload adequate oxygen. Thus oxygen delivery to the tissues is determined by a combination of cardiac output, total Hb concentration, and Hb oxygen affinity in addition to arterial pO_2 (Fig. 9.1).

The shift in the dissociation curve induced by fetal Hb makes clinical recognition of hypoxia (insufficient amount of oxygen molecules in the tissues to cover the normal aerobic metabolism) more difficult because cyanosis is observed at a lower oxygen tension. Cyanosis is first observed at saturations from 75% to 85%, which correspond to oxygen tensions of

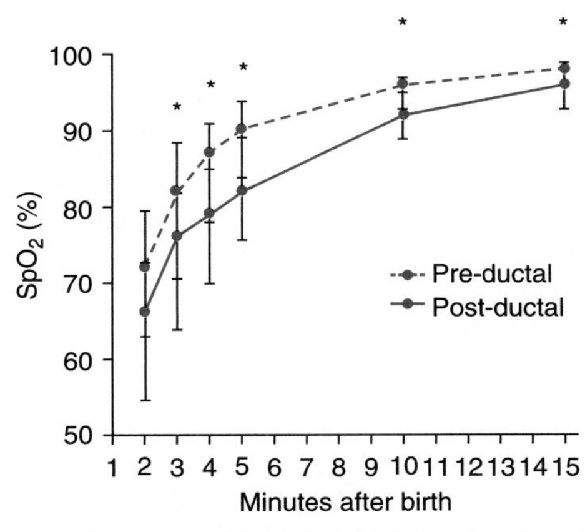

Fig. 9.2 Pre- and postductal SpO_2 levels during the first 15 minutes after birth (median, interquartile range [IQR]); IQR postductal SpO_2 levels were significantly lower than preductal SpO_2 levels at 3, 4, 5, 10, and 15 minutes (* <.05). (From Mariani G, Dik PB, Ezquer AJ, et al. Pre-ductal and post-ductal O_2 saturation in healthy term neonates after birth. *J Pediatr.* 2007;150(4):418.)

32 to 42 mm Hg on the fetal dissociation curve. Cyanosis in the adult is observed at higher tensions. The flattening of the upper portion of the S-shaped dissociation curve makes it almost impossible to monitor oxygen tensions above 60 to 80 mm Hg by following arterial oxygen saturation. Although the shape of the oxygen dissociation curve limits the usefulness of pulse oximetry to detect high PaO_2 values, keeping saturation measured via pulse oximeter between 92% and 95% is one of the most effective and practical ways of reducing the risk of hyperoxemia.

The pO_2 in arterial blood not only depends on the ability of the lung to transfer oxygen, but also is modified by the shunting of venous blood into the systemic circulation through the heart or lungs. Breathing 100% oxygen for a prolonged time partially corrects desaturation resulting from alveolar hypoventilation, diffusion abnormalities, or ventilation/perfusion inequality. Measurements of PaO_2 while breathing 100% oxygen are therefore useful diagnostically in determining whether arterial desaturation is caused by an anatomic right-to-left shunt, in which case oxygenation will fail to improve the condition (hyperoxia testing).

After birth, PaO_2 increases to between 60 and 90 mm Hg. During the first days of life, 20% of the cardiac output is normally shunted from right to left in either the heart or lungs. When the normal adult breathes 100% oxygen, PaO_2 increases to 600 mm Hg, compared with approximately 300 to 500 mm Hg in healthy neonates, which results from the substantial shunting in infants.

At the end of the first hour of life, perfusion of the lung is distributed in proportion to the distribution of ventilation. In the healthy newborn baby, oxygen saturations rise slowly over the initial few minutes of life; however, they approach 90% in the first 5 minutes. The postductal oxygen saturation levels are usually lower than the preductal measurements for as long as 15 minutes, indicating a persistence in elevated pulmonary vascular resistance for a significant period of time after birth (Fig. 9.2).[3] The speed with which pulmonary ventilation and perfusion is uniformly distributed is an indication of the remarkable adaptive capacities of the newborn infant for the maintenance of homeostasis.

EDITORIAL COMMENT: Dawson et al defined the reference ranges for pulse oxygen saturation (SpO_2) values in the first 10 minutes after birth for 468 infants who received no medical intervention in the delivery room. For all 468 infants, the 3rd, 10th, 50th, 90th, and 97th percentile values at 1 minute were 29%, 39%, 66%, 87%, and 92%, respectively; those at 2 minutes were 34%, 46%, 73%, 91%, and 95%; and those at 5 minutes were 59%, 73%, 89%, 97%, and 98%. It took a median of 7.9 minutes (interquartile range: 5–10 minutes) to reach an SpO_2 value of greater than 90%. SpO_2 values for preterm infants increased more slowly than those for term infants (see also Chapter 3).

(Dawson JA, Kamlin CO, Vento M, et al. Defining the reference range for oxygen saturation for infants after birth. *Pediatrics.* 2010;125:e1340.)

PRACTICAL CONSIDERATIONS

Oxygen Therapy

Oxygen supplementation is critical for the survival of many infants with respiratory problems. Previous restricted use resulted in an increase not only in mortality rate but also in neurologic handicaps. Additionally, recognition of the toxic effects of excessive or prolonged oxygen therapy is imperative when treating newborn infants. This has resulted in curtailed use of supplemental oxygen during neonatal resuscitation of both term and preterm infants (see Chapter 3). Therefore oxygen administration must be performed with great precision while carefully monitoring arterial oxygen tension or assessing oxygenation via noninvasive techniques.

Oxygen Administration

For spontaneously breathing infants who require supplemental oxygen, a small hood to provide supplemental oxygen prevents fluctuations in inspired oxygen when opening the incubator. This has been largely replaced by low-flow nasal cannulae to deliver gas mixtures. Because improper oxygen administration can be detrimental, the following practical considerations should be highlighted:

1. Peripheral cyanosis may be present in a neonate with a normal or high arterial oxygen tension.
2. Inspired oxygen concentration should be monitored in all infants receiving supplementary oxygen or assisted ventilation.
3. Oxygen therapy without concurrent assessments of arterial oxygen tension is dangerous. A noninvasive monitoring device to measure oxygen saturation by pulse oximetry or transcutaneous pO_2 should be used continuously in infants receiving any supplemental oxygen. In the presence of an arterial line during the acute phase of illness, consider measuring PaO_2 at least every 4 to 6 hours if the infant is receiving oxygen.
4. In preterm infants, arterial oxygen tension should be maintained between 50 and 80 mm Hg during the acute phase of respiratory failure. In the absence of available PaO_2 monitoring, SaO_2 should be kept in the 90% to 95% range.[4]
5. The development of retinopathy of prematurity (ROP) is related to high arterial oxygen tension levels, and these may rise above the normal range even with relatively low inspired oxygen concentrations. Whereas initial hyperoxia stunts retinal vascular development, later hypoxia appears to stimulate damaging vascular proliferation.
6. When infants receiving supplemental oxygen require bag-and-mask ventilation, both oxygen concentration and inflating pressures must be monitored closely.
7. Use of a nasal cannula for prolonged oxygen therapy allows greater mobility for the infant and enables oral feeding without manipulating oxygen concentration. Both inspired oxygen concentration and flow rate are precisely adjusted, and the infant's oxygenation is closely monitored, typically via pulse oximetry. Administration of oxygen by nasal cannula requires close monitoring because in active infants, the cannula is easily displaced from the nose. Also, changes in respiratory pattern and oral breathing may entrain different amounts of room air around the prongs, changing the true inspired oxygen concentration. Finally, high gas flows via nasal prongs are favored by some centers in select patients.
8. When the infant with respiratory distress syndrome (RDS) is improving, environmental oxygen should be lowered in small decrements while continuously monitoring oxygenation.
9. Any inspired oxygen concentration above room air can be damaging to pulmonary tissue if maintained over several days. Oxygen therapy is continued only if necessary.
10. All premature infants 30 weeks' gestation or less, or older if they had an unstable course or need for significant supplemental ventilation should be examined by an experienced ophthalmologist by the later of 31 weeks' postmenstrual age (PMA) or 4 weeks after birth for treatable ROP.[5]

Although oxygen targeting in extremely low–birth-weight infants has been under much investigation, the ideal saturation range for these most vulnerable infants remains unknown. Three recent international randomized controlled trials (RCTs) have addressed this clinical question, SUPPORT[4], BOOST-II[6], and COT[7], randomizing infants to low versus high saturation ranges and their effects on death and morbidities (ROP, necrotizing enterocolitis [NEC], bronchopulmonary dysplasia [BPD]). The results from these studies are conflicting, whereas SUPPORT and BOOST-II demonstrated higher mortality in the low saturation group with higher rates of ROP in the higher saturation group, the COT trial did not demonstrate any difference in their primary outcome of death or survival with one or more disabilities. A systematic review of the five available trials found an increase in relative risk of mortality in the lower saturation arm of 1.18 (95% confidence interval [CI]: 1.04–1.34).[8] A more recent review states that even though the infants randomized to higher saturation goals demonstrated higher survival rates, the quality of the evidence was low, thus making the conclusion that lower saturation goals are dangerous is premature.[9] Suffice it to say, at this time, a targeted saturation range of 90% to 95% may be safer than 85% to 89%, and has been widely adopted.

EDITORIAL COMMENT: The debate on the optimal oxygen concentration for extremely preterm infants rages on with the June 2018 publication of the results of the Neonatal Oxygenation Prospective Meta-analysis (NeOProM) collaboration. Analyzing data of approximately 5000 babies from five different trials, there was no significant difference in the composite outcome of death or major disability between higher or lower oxygen saturation groups. There was, however, a higher rate of death and necrotizing enterocolitis in the lower-saturation group and a higher rate of retinopathy of prematurity in the higher-saturation group. The competing outcomes suggest that it is prudent to maintain the oxygen saturation in the 90% to 95% range as indicated above. Recognize that this is easier said than done and saturation levels will fluctuate so that the babies are out of range, both high and low, for a significant period of time. Newer automatic controlling devices responding to oxygen levels may reduce these fluctuations and hopefully lessen complications (Askie LM, Darlow BA, Finer N, et al. Association between oxygen saturation targeting and death or disability in extremely preterm infants in the neonatal oxygenation prospective meta-analysis collaboration. *JAMA.* 2018;319(21):2190-2201).

NEONATAL PROBLEMS

Diagnosis

The initial objective is to establish an etiologic diagnosis for any observed respiratory symptoms. A major error in care can easily be made if other organ systems are not considered initially. Not every rapidly breathing infant has RDS or even respiratory disease. Hypovolemia, hyperviscosity (polycythemia), anemia, hypoglycemia, congenital heart disease, hypothermia, metabolic acidosis of any etiology, or even the effects of drugs or drug withdrawal may all mimic primary respiratory disorders. Appropriate care depends on the diagnosis. For example, rewarming should rapidly relieve respiratory symptoms in a mildly hypothermic infant; otherwise, sepsis must be strongly considered.

A working classification of some of these disorders is presented in Box 9.1. Whenever faced with these respiratory symptoms, the next steps (following a history and physical examination) should be to obtain the following:

- chest x-ray;
- white blood cell count with differential and hematocrit (peripheral hematocrits can be higher than intravascular hematocrits);
- blood sugar;
- assessment of blood gas status via an arterial stick or capillary blood gas. (A capillary blood gas reliably estimates $PaCO_2$ and pH, but not PaO_2.); and
- pulse oximetry to assess oxygenation.

The decision to catheterize the umbilical artery (see Appendix D) depends on the infant's condition. The umbilical artery and/or vein may need to be catheterized if significant metabolic acidosis or blood loss is suspected or if the infant remains severely distressed (as defined by continued hypoxemia and severe respiratory distress). On the other hand, if the infant has tachypnea and grunting with retractions but is active and pink, it is possible to withhold catheterization unless there is deterioration as manifested by marked respiratory distress and an oxygen requirement exceeding 40% to 50%.

BOX 9.1 Differential Diagnosis of Neonatal Respiratory Distress

Pulmonary Disorders

- Respiratory distress syndrome
- Transient tachypnea
- Meconium aspiration syndrome
- Pneumonia
- Air leak syndromes
- Pulmonary hypoplasia

Systemic Disorders

- Hypothermia
- Metabolic acidosis
- Anemia/polycythemia
- Hypoglycemia
- Pulmonary hypertension
- Congenital heart disease

Anatomic Problems of the Respiratory System

- Upper airway obstruction
- Airway malformations
- Space-occupying lesions
- Rib cage anomalies
- Phrenic nerve injury
- Neuromuscular disease

Although the newborn has a relatively larger cardiac output and a lower peripheral resistance and blood pressure than the older child and adult, measurements of blood pressure must be routine. It has been shown that hypotension in sick preterm infants may not be associated with hypovolemia. Hypothermia or acidemia results in severe peripheral vasoconstriction and will confound blood volume estimates from measurement of blood pressure. In a hypovolemic infant, blood pressure often declines only after acidemia and hypoxemia are corrected. Blood pressure can be measured with a blood pressure cuff of correct size placed on one or all extremities (if coarctation of the aorta is suspected), employing either oscillometric or Doppler ultrasound techniques. Alternatively, direct arterial measurements may be made via indwelling catheters. Normal blood pressures and ranges may be found in Appendix C.

If the initial hematocrit is less than 30% without blood incompatibility, or if the blood pressure is reduced, it is reasonable to assume blood loss (e.g., an acute fetomaternal hemorrhage) and consider immediate correction of blood volume. With acute blood loss, hypotension prevails over anemia, whereas after chronic blood loss, anemia dominates the clinical picture and perfusion is less compromised. Saline is initially used, and blood is requested, starting with a push infusion of 10 mL/kg, observing blood pressure, heart rate, and the infant's general condition. One must be extremely careful with rapid infusions of any solution in the critically ill premature infant because of the risk of increasing the incidence of intraventricular hemorrhage (IVH) by rapid volume expansion. Once a diagnosis has been made, it is necessary to determine whether the neonatal unit has all of the facilities that might be needed during the course of the illness. The following section discusses RDS in great depth, as this has been the primary model for understanding pathophysiology and management of neonatal respiratory disease.

Respiratory Distress Syndrome

RDS is still probably the most common initial problem in the intensive care nursery among premature infants weighing less than 1500 g. However, in preterm infants whose mothers have received antenatal steroids, and after postnatal intratracheal surfactant therapy, the characteristic clinical course for RDS may not be apparent. The following lists give the common symptoms, the physiologic abnormalities, and the pathologic findings.

Signs and Symptoms

- Difficulty in initiating normal respiration. The disease should be anticipated if the infant is premature, the mother has diabetes, or if the infant has suffered perinatal asphyxia.
- Expiratory grunting or whining (caused by closure of the glottis) is an important sign that sometimes may be the only early indication of disease; this maintains air in the immature lungs during expiration, and a decrease in grunting may be the first sign of improvement.
- Sternal and intercostal retractions (secondary to decreased lung and increased rib cage compliance)
- Nasal flaring
- Cyanosis (if supplemental O_2 is inadequate)
- Respirations—rapid (or slow when seriously ill)
- Extremities edematous—after several hours (altered vascular permeability)
- X-ray film showing reticulogranular ground glass appearance with air bronchograms

Physiologic Abnormalities

- Lung compliance reduced to as much as one-fifth to one-tenth of normal (Fig. 9.3)
- Large areas of lung not ventilated (right-to-left shunting of blood)[10]
- Large areas of lung not perfused
- Decreased alveolar ventilation and increased work of breathing
- Reduced lung volume

These changes result in hypoxemia, often hypercarbia, and, if hypoxemia is severe, metabolic acidosis.

Pathologic Findings (Anatomic, Biophysical, Biochemical)

- Gross—the lung is collapsed, firm, dark red, and liver-like
- Microscopic—alveolar collapse, with overdistention of the dilated alveolar ducts, pink-staining membrane on alveolar ducts (composed of products of the infant's blood and destroyed alveolar cells); hence the earlier term *hyaline membrane disease*
- Electron microscopic—damage and loss of alveolar epithelial cells (especially type II cells); disappearance of lamellar inclusion bodies
- Biophysical and biochemical—deficient or absent pulmonary surfactant,[11] especially phospholipid (surface tension lowering) component; abnormal pressure–volume curve, as shown in Fig. 9.3.

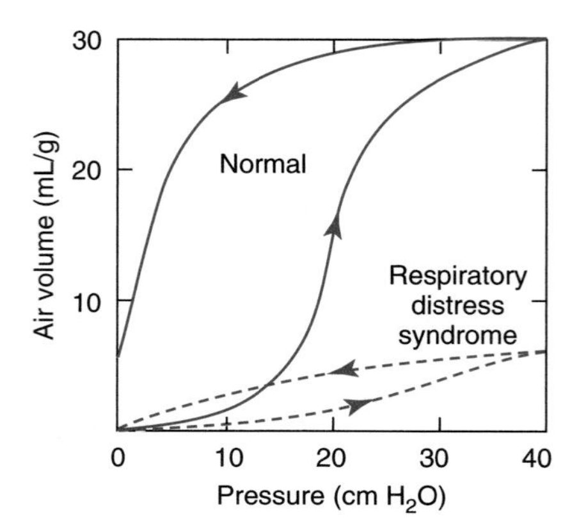

Fig. 9.3 Air pressure volume curves of normal and abnormal lung. Volume is expressed as milliliters of air per gram of lung. Lung of infant with respiratory distress syndrome *(RDS)* accepts smaller volume of air at all pressures. Note that deflation pressure volume curve closely follows inflation curve for the RDS lung.

Etiology

The distal respiratory epithelium responsible for gas exchange features two distinct cell types in the mature infant lung. Type I pneumocytes cover most of the alveolus, in close proximity to capillary endothelial cells. Type II pneumocytes have been identified in the human fetus as early as 22 weeks' gestation, but become prominent at 34 to 36 weeks of gestation. These highly metabolically active cells contain the cytoplasmic lamellar bodies that are the source of pulmonary surfactant. Surfactant synthesis is a complex process that requires an abundance of precursor substrates, such as glucose, fatty acid, and choline, and a series of key enzymatic steps that are regulated by various hormones, including corticosteroids.

Phosphatidylcholine is the dominant surface tension–lowering component of surfactant. In addition, surfactant-specific proteins have been characterized and their functions partially elucidated. Of particular interest is surfactant protein B, which is critical for minimizing surface tension and whose absence results in the phenotypic expression of lethal RDS at term.[12] Following secretion from lamellar bodies within the type II alveolar cells, the key phospholipid and protein components of surfactant are conserved by recycling and subsequent regeneration of surfactant. Exogenously administered surfactant appears to contribute to this recycling program by increasing surfactant pool size without inhibiting endogenous surfactant production.[11]

It is widely accepted that RDS is the result of a primary absence or deficiency of this highly surface-active alveolar

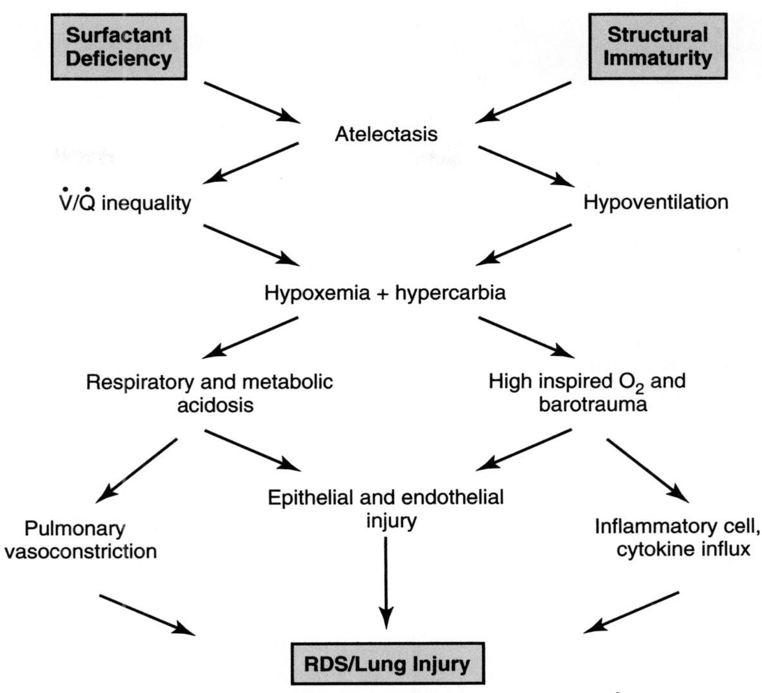

Fig. 9.4 Pathophysiology of neonatal respiratory distress syndrome *(RDS)*. V̇/Q̇, Ventilation-perfusion ratio.

lining layer (pulmonary surfactant). Surfactant, a complex lipoprotein rich in saturated phosphatidylcholine molecules, binds to the internal surface of the lung and markedly lessens the forces of surface tension at the air–water interphase, thereby reducing the pressure tending to collapse the alveolus. By equalizing the forces of surface tension in alveolar units of varying sizes, it is a potent antiatelectasis factor and is essential for normal respiration. Alteration or absence of the pulmonary surfactant would lead to the sequence of events shown in Fig. 9.4. This results in decreased lung compliance (stiff lung) and thus an increase in the work of breathing. The additional work would soon tire the infant, leading to a sequence of reduced alveolar ventilation, atelectasis, and alveolar hypoperfusion.

Asphyxia would induce pulmonary vasoconstriction; blood would bypass the lung through the fetal pathway (patent ductus arteriosus [PDA], foramen ovale), lowering pulmonary blood flow; and a vicious circle would be promoted. The resulting ischemia would be an added insult and may further reduce lung metabolism and surfactant production.

General Preventive Measures

A major effort in treating this disease should continue to focus on its prevention, including avoiding elective deliveries performed before 39 weeks' gestation unless medically indicated for either maternal or fetal reasons. The prolongation of pregnancy with bed rest or drugs that inhibit premature labor, as well as the induction of pulmonary surfactant with maternally administered steroids, plays an important role in reducing the incidence of this disease (see Chapter 2).

Antenatal steroids not only enhance surfactant production but also may improve pulmonary function (e.g., tissue elasticity) by nonsurfactant mechanisms.[13] Therefore the combined use of prenatal corticosteroids and postnatal surfactant therapy is complementary.[14] Antenatal steroids also reduce the incidence of IVH in preterm infants, possibly secondary to enhanced vascular integrity in the germinal matrix. Concern about the possibility of increased infection with antenatal steroids in the mother or infant appears unfounded. Therefore antenatal steroids are now standard of practice for pregnancies at risk of preterm delivery, although precise limits are still being defined.

Surfactant Therapy

Since the discovery that surfactant deficiency was a prominent feature of the pathophysiology of RDS, investigators have attempted to administer artificial aerosolized phospholipids to these infants.[15] Limited therapeutic success was encountered in these early studies. In contrast, animal models in which natural surfactant compounds were used yielded promising results. This stimulated Fujiwara et al to develop a mixture of both natural and synthetic surface-active lipids for use in humans.[16] The goal was to achieve alveolar stability with less potential risk for a reaction to foreign protein than would be the case with exclusively natural surfactant. When administered to an initial group of 10 preterm infants with severe RDS who were not improving despite artificial ventilation, a single 10-mL dose of surfactant instilled into the endotracheal tube resulted in a dramatic decrease in inspired oxygen and ventilator pressures. Other studies confirmed this initial success, employing calf and pig lung extract, pooled human surfactant obtained from amniotic fluid, and purely synthetic phospholipid preparation.[17]

Subsequent collaborative multicenter trials employed multiple doses of purely synthetic and mixed natural/synthetic

BOX 9.2 Surfactant Therapy for Respiratory Distress Syndrome

Resolved
- Greatest benefit when combined with antenatal corticosteroids
- Major surface tension–lowering ingredient: phosphatidylcholine
- Administration of fluid suspension requires endotracheal tube
- Improvement in arterial oxygenation
- Surfactant proteins enhance speed of action
- Exogenous surfactant enhances rather than inhibits endogenous surfactant synthesis
- Decrease in incidence of air leaks
- Improved mortality rate
- Prevention more effective than rescue up to <29 weeks

Unresolved
- Ideal preparation: role of surfactant proteins in improving respiratory function
- Role of ventilatory strategy in optimizing surfactant response—rapid wean to nasal continuous positive airway pressure (CPAP)
- Effect on incidence and severity of chronic lung disease
- Role of surfactant therapy in other neonatal respiratory disorders: meconium aspiration, pneumonia, pulmonary hypoplasia, congenital diaphragmatic hernia, pulmonary hemorrhage

preparations and confirmed clinical efficacy, leading in the 1990s to the widespread introduction of exogenous surfactant therapy into neonatal care. The most efficacious mixed surfactant products are all protein-containing preparations derived from bovine or porcine tissue. Of particular interest, as summarized in Box 9.2, is the ability of surfactant to decrease the number of deaths in low-birth-weight infants without significantly reducing the incidence of BPD in the smallest infants. The latter may be a consequence of the enhanced survival caused by surfactant administration to very preterm infants or to the multifactorial etiology of BPD.

Surfactant therapy currently requires the presence of an endotracheal tube, although less invasive techniques of administration, including instillation via catheter or aerosolization, are under study and gaining momentum. Multiple doses are occasionally needed for optimal benefit. The dramatic improvement in oxygenation is not accompanied by an immediate improvement in $PaCO_2$ or lung compliance unless ventilator settings are rapidly weaned.[18] Data suggest that the increase in lung volume, induced by surfactant, needs to be accompanied by ventilator and supplemental oxygen weaning. Hypotension and bradycardia may occur acutely during surfactant therapy; therefore caution must be exercised when using this treatment to avoid potential iatrogenic complications. Supplementation of surfactant with a single endotracheal instillation of steroid to diminish inflammation is an area of current interest and under study in both animal models and clinical trials.[19]

EDITORIAL COMMENT: The short-term outcome of the early inhaled budesonide trial favored the steroid group with a reduced rate of bronchopulmonary dysplasia. However, at 2 years of age, the rate of neurodevelopmental disability among surviving infants did not differ significantly between infants who received early inhaled budesonide for the prevention of bronchopulmonary dysplasia and those who received placebo. However, the mortality rate (19.9%) was higher among those who received budesonide than the placebo group (14.5%), negating any short-term benefits.[67]

(Bassler D, Plavka R, Shinwell ES, et al; NEUROSIS Trial Group. Early inhaled budesonide for the prevention of bronchopulmonary dysplasia. *N Engl J Med.* 2015;373:1497-1506.)

Because the genes that code for the surfactant proteins have been characterized, recombinant DNA technology will make production of modified human surfactant proteins possible. In combination with synthetic phospholipids, this will allow the widespread availability of a protein-containing artificial surfactant. Although no adverse immunologic consequences of foreign tissue protein administration have yet been reported in the recipients of natural surfactant therapy, close follow-up of these high-risk survivors of neonatal intensive care is always imperative.

Early treatment with CPAP is generally favored over initial prophylactic surfactant treatment as the initial support for extremely low–birth-weight infants. Finer et al randomly assigned 1316 immature infants to intubation and surfactant treatment (within 1 hour of birth) or to CPAP treatment initiated in the delivery room, with subsequent use of a protocol-driven limited ventilation strategy. Infants were also randomly assigned to one of two target ranges of oxygen saturation.[4] The primary outcome was death or BPD as defined by the requirement for supplemental oxygen at 36 weeks (with an attempt at withdrawal of supplemental oxygen in neonates who were receiving <30% oxygen). The rates of the primary outcome did not differ significantly between the CPAP group and the surfactant group (47.8% and 51.0%, respectively). Infants who received CPAP treatment, as compared with infants who received surfactant treatment, less frequently required intubation or postnatal corticosteroids for BPD ($P < .001$), required fewer days of mechanical ventilation ($P = .03$), and were more likely to be alive and free from the need for mechanical ventilation by day 7 ($P = .01$). The rates of other adverse neonatal outcomes did not differ significantly between the two groups. These data support consideration of CPAP as an alternative to intubation and surfactant in preterm infants.

GENERAL CLINICAL MANAGEMENT

The same principles of basic care for RDS can be applied to infants with many other neonatal pulmonary problems (see Table 9.1). During the acute phase, every maneuver is directed toward ensuring the infant's survival with minimal risk of chronic morbidity. The infant is placed in a neutral thermal environment (see Chapter 4) to reduce oxygen requirements and CO_2 production. To meet fluid and partial caloric requirements (dependent on environmental conditions, maturity, renal function, risk

TABLE 9.1 Supportive Care for Infants With Respiratory Distress Syndrome

Treatment	Logic
Trained staff nurses, respiratory therapists, and monitoring equipment. Available trained physicians, nurse practitioners.	Early management of complications and notification of change in course (e.g., apnea, bleeding from catheter)
Precise temperature control to maintain infant in neutral temperature	Maintains minimal oxygen consumption and carbon dioxide production
pH, PaO_2, $PaCO_2$, and HCO_3 measurements at least every 4–6 hours. Maintain PaO_2 at 50–80 mm Hg. Continuous PaO_2 or SaO_2 is optimal.	Permits continual assessment of infant's condition and limits toxic effects of oxygen or hypoxic injury
Monitor blood pressure.	Recognizes hypoperfusion, hypovolemia, patent ductus arteriosus
Attempt to keep pH >7.25. If $PaCO_2$ >60–65 or PaO_2 <50 mm Hg or >80 mmHg, change treatment.	Permits continual assessment of infant's condition and limits toxic effects of oxygen or hypoxic injury
Lower environmental oxygen slowly when RDS infant is still ill.	Prevents greater than expected decrease in PaO_2 when environmental oxygen is reduced (right-to-left shunt etiology?)
Surfactant therapy	Therapeutic approach to underlying etiology of respiratory distress syndrome (RDS)
Glucose-containing IV fluid 60–100 mL/kg first day, increasing daily with body weight determination for small infants to calculate if larger amounts of H_2O required. May require 150 mL/kg or more.	Need to balance fluid and partial caloric requirements while minimizing the risk of fluid overload problems (e.g., patent ductus arteriosus)
Controlled oxygen administration: via ventilatory support, cannula, or hood	Prevents large swings in environmental oxygen concentration
Continually monitor respiration, heart rate, and temperature as well as blood pressure.	Prevents hypoxemia and acidemia with apneic episodes
Frequent determinations of blood sugar, hematocrit, and electrolytes (Na, K, and Cl)	Necessary for calculating general metabolic requirements
Transfuse if central hematocrit <30–35 during acute phase of illness.	For adequate oxygen-carrying capacity
Urinary output, blood urea nitrogen, creatinine, and, when indicated, urinary pH, electrolytes, and osmolality	Evaluation of renal function and blood flow to the kidney. An increase in output occurs as the infant starts to improve.
Obtain blood culture; treat with ampicillin and gentamicin until cultures are available.	Cannot radiographically separate RDS from group B streptococcal (or other) pneumonia
Minimize routine procedures such as suctioning, handling, and auscultation.	Prevents iatrogenic decreases in PaO_2

for patency of the ductus arteriosus, and hydration), the infant is typically begun at 60 to 100 mL/kg/day of a 10% dextrose solution. This is increased to 120 to 160 mL/kg/day by the fifth day, recognizing that there is a high risk for either fluid overload or dehydration if clinical status, fluid balance, and electrolytes are not closely monitored in the smallest infants with RDS who may require more than 160 mL/kg/day. Administration of an amino acid solution should begin the first day, supplemented with small-volume feeds as is clinically appropriate. Respiration, heart rate, blood pressure, and oxygenation (via noninvasive techniques) are monitored continuously and complemented by blood gas sampling at least every 4 to 6 hours during the acute phase of illness, and perhaps more frequently in the immediate neonatal period after surfactant administration.

Most important in the prescription is skilled nursing and physician management. Vital signs must be noted and observations made in such a fashion as not to disturb the infant continually, yet the patient must always be observed. Modern electronic monitoring of heart rate, respiration, temperature, and oxygenation makes gentler care easier to administer. While basic care is being arranged (metabolic rate minimized, fluid and electrolyte needs met), the essentials of care involve maintaining an adequate PaO_2 and pH and closely observing for changes in the infant's state.

A general plan is to maintain the PaO_2 in the abdominal aorta between 50 and 80 mm Hg, $PaCO_2$ in the 40- to 60-mm Hg range, and pH above 7.20 to 7.25. Because clinical differentiation from group B streptococcal (or other bacterial) pneumonia is not possible, a blood culture and antibiotics should be considered and usually done for the first 36 to 48 hours. It is equally important to discontinue broad-spectrum antibiotics as soon as the possibility of infection is ruled out to prevent nosocomial fungal and bacterial infections.

Correction of severe metabolic acidosis with alkali has many theoretical physiologic benefits. With normalization of pH, myocardial contractility is increased, pulmonary vascular resistance is reduced, and the length of survival with asphyxia is prolonged. However, the rapid injection of hypertonic solutions such as $NaHCO_3$ is associated with a marked change in osmolality. Studies have revealed that excessive and rapid $NaHCO_3$ administration may be associated with an increased incidence of intracranial hemorrhage.[20–21] Current consensus is that $NaHCO_3$ administration is of very limited benefit[22] and has even been called useless therapy. Because administered $NaHCO_3$ is converted to CO_2 and is dependent on the lung for its removal, $NaHCO_3$ is contraindicated in the presence of respiratory acidosis without some form of controlled or assisted ventilation if it is to be administered.

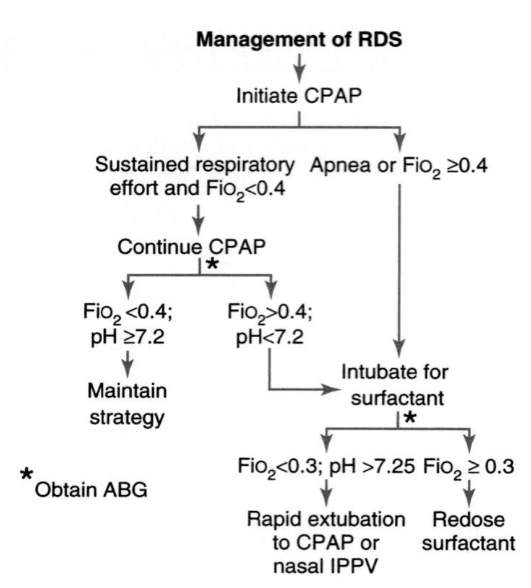

Fig. 9.5 Algorithm suggesting management strategy of respiratory distress syndrome *(RDS)*. Note that there is no uniform standard, and many accept higher oxygen concentrations than 40% prior to intubation for surfactant. *ABG,* Arterial blood gas; *CPAP,* continuous positive airway pressure; *FiO_2,* fraction of inspired oxygen; *IPPV,* intermittent positive pressure ventilation.

Almost all infants with RDS require ventilatory support in the form of CPAP. Some of these infants do not stabilize on CPAP and require ventilator support and surfactant therapy (Fig. 9.5). Possible indications for placing an infant on a ventilator include: respiratory acidosis with a pH of less than 7.20, apnea, and/or a need for a high concentration of inspired oxygen (i.e., ≥40%). Other criteria for a ventilator include increased work of breathing with grunting and/or severe retractions, and apnea complicating the course of RDS.

EDITORIAL COMMENT: The question of when to intubate a premature infant with RDS on CPAP is controversial. As noted by Manley, Yoder, and Davis, "[t]here is no universally accepted definition of CPAP 'failure.' Decisions to intubate take into account a number of factors including history, respiratory status, blood gases and x-rays. Studies such as the SUPPORT trial (>50% oxygen) and COIN trial (>60% oxygen) used differing intubation criteria. Prior to intubation, 'remediable' causes of CPAP failure such as secretions, improperly sized nasal prongs, and inadequate pressure should be corrected."

Manley BJ, Yoder BA, Davis P. Noninvasive ventilation of preterm Infants: an alternative to mechanical ventilation. In Bancalari, E, ed. *The Newborn Lung: Neonatology Questions and Controversies*, 3rd Ed. Philadelphia: Elsevier, 2019.

After 72 hours of age (or earlier after surfactant therapy), most infants with classic RDS start the recovery phase. Respiratory rate and retractions decrease, and PaO_2 increases without evidence of further CO_2 retention. This recovery phase is preceded by a period of spontaneous diuresis during which there is improved gas exchange, lung compliance, and FRC. Because the improved pulmonary function occurs after diuresis, it is important that the clinician anticipate the recovery phase and reduce ventilatory support to prevent barotrauma.

During this phase, expertise in oxygen management is required. Oxygen saturation via pulse oximetry is the mainstay of assessing oxygenation during recovery of respiratory distress. Levels are typically maintained between 90% and 95%.

In infants of very low birth weight, even in the absence of severe RDS, recovery may be prolonged. This may be attributed to impaired respiratory drive or respiratory muscle failure, persistent atelectasis not related to surfactant deficiency, nutritional compromise, intercurrent infection, congestive heart failure, or some combination of these interrelated factors.

Many very low–birth-weight infants require prolonged assisted ventilation and prolonged supplemental oxygen. Small volume gavage feeds, preferably of breast milk, can begin despite continuing ventilatory support and advanced as tolerated. This is a valuable adjunct to amino acid–glucose intravenous (IV) alimentation. As the infant recovers, apneic periods may be observed, but they do not have the ominous significance as when observed in the acute phase.

The complications of RDS may occur spontaneously or result from well-intended therapeutic interventions. Major problems may be a consequence of arterial catheter placement, oxygen administration, mechanical ventilation, and the use of endotracheal tubes, as discussed in Chapter 10. As the number of very low–birth-weight survivors grows, the time and effort devoted to preventing and treating respiratory morbidity in this population steadily increases.

During or following the recovery phase of RDS, cardiac failure secondary to a large left-to-right shunt through the PDA may occur as pulmonary vascular resistance declines. This may initially manifest as inability to wean oxygen or ventilator support. Bounding pulses, a wide pulse pressure, and a systolic murmur are most useful in making a clinical diagnosis. In most cases, conservative medical management with cautious fluid administration and diuretics will control the congestive heart failure, and the PDA will close as the infant grows. Although the PDA will close spontaneously in most cases, intervention to close it may reduce the risk of chronic pulmonary overflow, edema, and prolonged ventilator dependence. (Management of the PDA is considered in detail in Chapter 14).

Although cardiomegaly is often noted on x-ray examination, an enlarged liver and edema are not usually found with cardiac failure. Evaluation of the magnitude of shunting by echocardiography is usually indicated before initiating either pharmacologic or surgical closure of the ductus arteriosus (see Chapter 14). Prophylactic indomethacin administration appears to reduce the frequency of large left-to-right ductal shunts; however, there is no clear evidence that routine early indomethacin therapy reduces longer-term morbidity in susceptible infants. An additional benefit of prophylactic indomethacin may be to decrease the incidence of IVH. Ibuprofen therapy also promotes ductal closure and is less likely to impair renal blood flow and renal function when compared with indomethacin. Surgical closure should be a last resort, as infants subject to ductal ligation may be at greater risk for later neurodevelopmental impairment.

PERSISTENT PULMONARY HYPERTENSION OF THE NEWBORN

Persistent pulmonary hypertension of the newborn (PPHN), rather than the previous nomenclature, persistent fetal circulation, more aptly describes the syndrome characterized by pulmonary hypertension resulting in severe hypoxemia secondary to right-to-left shunting through the foramen ovale and ductus arteriosus in the absence of structural heart disease. Pulmonary hypertension in these infants is thought to result from pulmonary vasospasm, presumably because of altered pulmonary vasoreactivity, and at times it may be accompanied by an increase in muscle mass in the pulmonary vascular bed. The increase in pulmonary arterial smooth muscle tone may develop in response to intrauterine stress and can be associated with a decrease of a circulating (or local) pulmonary vasodilators such as nitric oxide (NO) or an increase in the amount of circulating (or local) pulmonary vasoconstrictors such as endothelin. This syndrome was initially described in term infants with respiratory distress and cyanosis without demonstrable cardiac, pulmonary, hematologic, or central nervous system disease. However, this same hemodynamic pattern can occur in preterm and term infants with primary pulmonary disease (e.g., surfactant deficiency, pneumonia, or meconium aspiration syndrome [MAS]), polycythemia, pulmonary hypoplasia (e.g., congenital diaphragmatic hernia [CDH]), or following neonatal asphyxia. Among preterm infants, pulmonary hypoplasia and sepsis appear to be associated with a higher incidence of pulmonary hypertension.[23] Sometimes no clear etiology for the PPHN or underlying lung disease can be assigned. The result is cyanosis, tachypnea, and acidemia, which can superficially resemble cyanotic congenital heart disease, primary pulmonary disease, or cardiomyopathy. The initial radiographic descriptions of PPHN stressed the absence of pulmonary parenchymal disease and decreased vascular markings; however, the chest x-ray study may instead reflect the concurrence of underlying pulmonary disease such as meconium aspiration or pneumonia. Echocardiography is invaluable as a guide to assessing elevated pulmonary artery pressure and pulmonary vascular resistance and, more importantly, as a means of excluding most anatomic cardiac malformations (see Chapter 14) and demonstrating right-to-left shunting at the level of the foramen ovale and ductus arteriosus.

The management of PPHN can be complex and very difficult because the severe hypoxemia may be poorly responsive to high-oxygen therapy or pulmonary vasodilators. Every attempt should be made to anticipate, and possibly prevent, the development of PPHN in patients with severe MAS or neonatal pneumonia, and early and aggressive treatment of hypoxemia should be provided. These babies are exquisitely sensitive to changes in environmental oxygen. Most require an environmental oxygen approaching 100% and may show little improvement without mechanical ventilation. Historically, some infants have benefited from modest alkalinization brought about by hyperventilation or the administration of $NaHCO_3$, which may relieve the intense pulmonary vasospasm and allow oxygenation to improve. This approach has mainly been abandoned, with the focus on improving oxygenation and decreasing pulmonary vascular resistance with inhaled NO (iNO). Similarly, PaO_2 is maintained at the upper recommended levels (60 to 100 mm Hg) to minimize hypoxic pulmonary vasoconstriction while minimizing barotrauma. Polycythemia, hypoglycemia, hypocalcemia, and hypotension should be treated if present. In fact, maintenance of systemic blood pressure at the high range of normal is often required to exceed excessively high pulmonary artery pressures and thereby counteract right-to-left shunting. Inotropic support (e.g., dopamine, dobutamine, milrinone, etc.) may be preferable to volume expansion because excessive fluids are poorly tolerated. Adequate sedation and, at times, muscle paralysis, may be necessary to combat the hypoxemia associated with agitation.

A major breakthrough in the treatment of PPHN has been the use of iNO at doses of 20 parts per million (ppm) or less to produce pharmacologic selective pulmonary vasodilation without producing significant systemic hypotension. Among preterm infants, the likelihood of a successful response to iNO increases with advancing gestational age.[23] Inhaled NO, together with other therapeutic approaches such as surfactant therapy and high-frequency ventilation, has been reported to significantly reduce the need for extracorporeal membrane oxygenation (ECMO).[24] More data suggest that sildenafil, an inhibitor of cyclic guanosine monophosphate (cGMP)–specific phosphodiesterase, may effectively induce pulmonary vasodilation by increasing endogenously released cGMP.[25] Nonetheless, ECMO remains a lifesaving treatment modality in infants who fail to respond to ventilatory and pharmacologic management of severe PPHN.[26] PPHN is a frequent association with hypoxic-ischemic encephalopathy. These infants often undergo hypothermia therapy; however, hypothermia therapy does not appear to significantly increase the prevalence of PPHN in this high-risk population.[27]

EDITORIAL COMMENT: Inhaled nitric oxide is effective at an initial concentration of 20 ppm for term and near-term infants with hypoxic respiratory failure who do not have a diaphragmatic hernia. It has significantly reduced the need for extracorporeal membrane oxygenation.

Sildenafil used for treatment of pulmonary hypertension has potential for reducing mortality and improving oxygenation in neonates, especially in resource-limited settings where iNO is not available. There is a need for randomized trials to compare sildenafil to other pulmonary vasodilators.

Overall, with these additions to our armamentarium, the outlook for babies with PPHN has improved remarkably.

MECONIUM ASPIRATION SYNDROME

Meconium is present in the amniotic fluid in 10% of all births, and its presence suggests that the infant may have suffered some asphyxial episode in utero. Evidence of this is derived from studies such as postmortem data demonstrating severe structural abnormalities in the muscular walls of the pulmonary arterial vascular bed, suggesting chronic in utero hypoxia in infants with fatal meconium aspiration.[28] It is doubtful that amniotic fluid alone can produce any airway obstruction. However, pulmonary disease is definitely observed in infants who have aspirated meconium (Fig. 9.6), and mortality and morbidity are significant without immediate aggressive management. Interestingly, the passage and subsequent aspiration of meconium are almost never seen before 34 weeks' gestation.

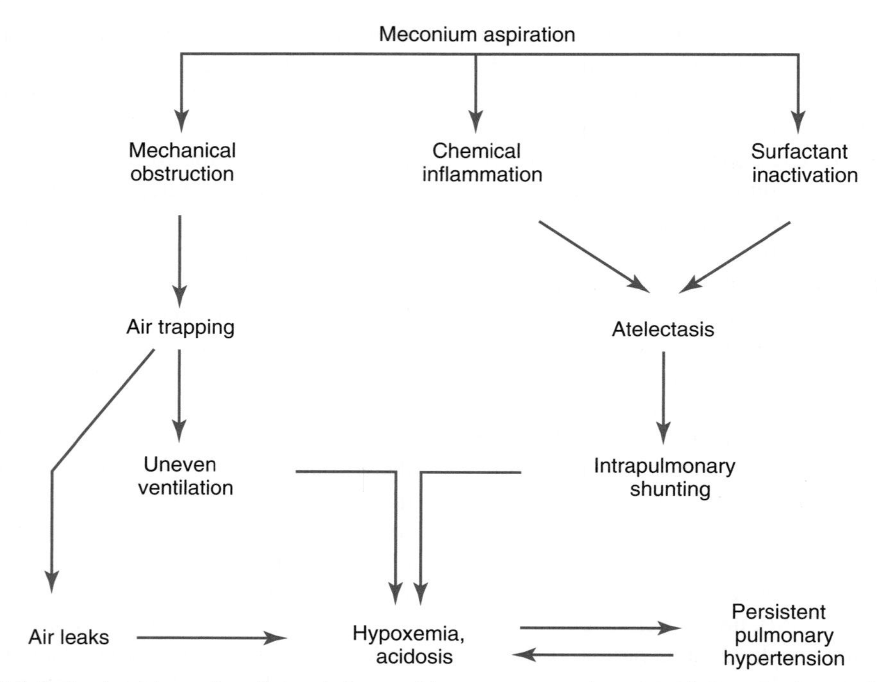

Fig. 9.6 Pathophysiology of cardiorespiratory problems accompanying meconium aspiration syndrome.

Because asphyxia is often the basis for the presence of meconium in the amniotic fluid, the infant who aspirates meconium at birth is often depressed and requires some resuscitation. Until recently, every nonvigorous infant born through meconium-stained fluid was intubated for suctioning of meconium from below the cords. However, there is no evidence to support this practice and its ability to prevent MAS. Thus the most recent Neonatal Resuscitation Program (NRP) guidelines do not advocate the practice of routine endotracheal suctioning of an infant born through meconium-stained fluid; rather, if the infant is depressed, immediate resuscitative steps should be started, including positive pressure ventilation in accordance to NRP guidelines.[29] Obstetricians have applied transcervical amnioinfusion in labor when meconium-stained amniotic fluid is present; however, a conclusive positive effect on neonatal outcome remains to be demonstrated.[30]

MAS is characterized by respiratory distress ranging from tachypnea to gasping respirations. Rales and wheezing may be heard. The infant may appear barrel-chested with an increase in the anteroposterior diameter of the chest. A chest radiograph shows areas of increased density and areas of overexpansion irregularly distributed throughout the lung; differentiation from pneumonia and retained lung fluid may be difficult.

The lung can remove meconium rapidly. Infants with mild cases usually recover after 48 hours of life. However, in sicker infants, respiratory compromise may be severe, with mechanical obstruction, hyperinflation, and atelectasis producing severe gas maldistribution with ventilation–perfusion mismatching. One complication of partially blocked, overexpanded areas of lung, occurring in 20% to 50% of infants with MAS, is the development of air leaks such as pneumothorax. Pneumothorax should be suspected if the clinical status of the infant deteriorates suddenly. Additional pulmonary pathology caused by meconium aspiration includes chemical pneumonitis, interstitial edema, and surfactant inactivation. Frequently, PPHN with severe superimposed hypoxemia develops in infants with significant MAS (see Fig. 9.6). Respiratory failure is associated with a significant mortality rate in these infants. Several studies have demonstrated that surfactant replacement therapy improves oxygenation, reduces pulmonary air leaks, reduces the need for ECMO, and improves outcome in infants with MAS.[31] Nevertheless, severe respiratory failure and hypoxemia may require additional treatment modalities such as high-frequency ventilation and NO administration, with ECMO therapy for those who fail to respond.

PNEUMOTHORAX

Pulmonary air leaks comprise a spectrum of disorders that includes pneumomediastinum, pneumopericardium, pulmonary interstitial emphysema (PIE), and pneumothorax. An asymptomatic pneumothorax is found in approximately 1% of all routine newborn chest radiographic examinations. Considering the high negative intrathoracic pressures recorded during the first minutes of life, it is surprising that pneumothorax does not occur more frequently. When air leak occurs, air from the ruptured alveolus dissects up the vascular sheath into the mediastinum and from there into the pleural space. In some series, as many as half of the symptomatic patients had aspirated meconium or blood. This suggests that obstruction with a ball-valve action may be the basis for the rupture. A pneumothorax frequently develops in infants with PIE in whom there is a tracking of air from ruptured alveoli into the perivascular pulmonary tissues, usually during prolonged assisted ventilation. Multiple studies of various exogenous surfactant preparations have demonstrated a significant reduction in pneumothorax among surfactant-treated infants.[32–33] Pneumothorax, manifesting with concurrent hypotension, is associated with increased risk of IVH, probably via impairment of venous return.

Pneumothorax should be suspected in any newborn with respiratory distress or in a baby on a respirator whose condition suddenly worsens. In infants with RDS, a pneumothorax may develop when the severity of disease is decreasing and lung compliance is increasing. Bilateral pneumothoraces are often observed in infants with hypoplastic lungs accompanying renal agenesis (Potter syndrome), other forms of renal dysplasia, midtrimester premature rupture of membranes, or CDH. In fact, the presence of otherwise unexplained extrapulmonary air in the early neonatal period should raise the question of an underlying renal or pulmonary malformation.

A high-intensity transilluminating light, using a fiberoptic probe, is especially helpful in quickly diagnosing a pneumothorax. If the infant's clinical condition is relatively stable, it is wise to check the diagnosis radiographically before treatment. An anteroposterior film may underestimate the size of a large anterior pneumothorax, in which case a horizontal-beam lateral film of the supine infant is helpful. A cross-table lateral film with the suspected pneumothorax side up will differentiate a pneumothorax from a pneumomediastinum.

Clinical findings include cyanosis, tachypnea, grunting, nasal flaring, or intercostal retractions. If the pneumothorax is unilateral and under tension, the cardiac impulse may be shifted away from the affected side, and ipsilateral breath sounds may be decreased. A distended abdomen with an easily palpable liver or spleen pushed down by the diaphragm is often a useful clinical feature signifying a tension pneumothorax. This may be useful in differentiating a left-sided tension pneumothorax manifesting in the delivery room from a (typically left-sided) CDH. Both are characterized by mediastinal shift to the right hemithorax; however, in the hernia patient, a scaphoid (rather than distended) abdomen is a presenting feature.

If the pneumothorax causes only minor symptoms, no specific therapy is necessary, but the infant's color, heart rate, respiratory rate, blood pressure, and oxygenation should be monitored. If severe respiratory distress is noted or the infant has underlying pulmonary disease, a thoracostomy tube should be placed. Lung perforation has been described following chest tube placement, and care should be exercised when guiding the catheter into the pleural space. Traumatic events may be reduced with a pigtail catheter. The catheter should be placed in the pleural space anterior to the lung. This is best achieved by insertion near the fourth intercostal space just lateral to the anterior axillary line. Occasionally, with a large area of rupture or bronchopleural fistula, chest tube placement may be required for several days. Pneumomediastinum does not require intervention, and asymptomatic pneumopericardium should be managed conservatively. Pneumopericardium may manifest with profound hypotension if there is accompanying gas tamponade, and pericardiocentesis will be lifesaving. Both pneumopericardium and PIE are almost invariably complications of assisted ventilation. In an attempt to avoid air leak and to manage air leak when present, mechanical ventilator pressures should be kept at a safe minimum. The use of high-frequency ventilation appears to be effective in treating air leak and may actually reduce the risk of development of air leak in preterm infants with severe respiratory failure[34] (see also Chapter 10).

TRANSIENT TACHYPNEA OF THE NEWBORN

Transient tachypnea of the newborn (TTN) often follows an uneventful delivery at (or close to) term. The major presenting symptom is a persistently high respiratory rate. Cyanosis may be present but is usually not of great significance, with few infants requiring more than 30% to 40% oxygen to remain pink. Air exchange is good, and therefore rales and rhonchi, expiratory grunting, and intercostal retractions are minimal; arterial pH and $PaCO_2$ measurements are usually within normal limits. The chest x-ray reveals central perihilar streaking because fluid remains in the periarterial tissue, often with fluid in the interlobar fissure, and occasionally there is a small pleural effusion; the cardiac silhouette may be slightly enlarged. If the radiologic picture includes patchy infiltrates, which probably reflect liquid-filled lobes, then TTN probably cannot be initially distinguished from infiltrates associated with meconium aspiration or pneumonia. The clinical picture of increased respiratory rate improves gradually during the first 5 days of life.

The pathogenesis appears to involve delayed resorption of fetal lung fluid, a process that requires activation of airway epithelial sodium channels.[35] In experimental situations, catecholamines have been found to stimulate fetal lung fluid resorption. Infants delivered by cesarean section without antecedent labor are found to have decreased catecholamine levels and an increased likelihood of development of transient tachypnea.[36] In fact, the respiratory morbidity associated with elective repeat cesarean delivery before 39 weeks is typically TTN.[37] Infants of diabetic mothers are also at increased risk of transient tachypnea, thought to be because of the interference by insulin on the β-adrenergic response of the lung.[38]

The presence of unabsorbed lung fluid produces decreased lung compliance, whereas the infant's increased respiratory rate attempts to minimize respiratory work. Ultrasound has been reported to demonstrate a unique difference in lung echogenicity between upper and lower lung areas in TTN.[39] The syndrome appears to be self-limited, and there have been no reported complications. The use of diuretics such as furosemide has not been found to be effective in decreasing the symptoms or duration of illness.[40]

EDITORIAL COMMENT: Neonatal respiratory distress is associated with changes in β-epithelial sodium channel (β-ENaC) and aquaporin (AQP_5) expression. The various roles of β ENaC and AQP_5 in respiratory distress and transient tachypnea of the newborn (TTN) serve as a reminder that it is not only surfactant, oxygen, and continuous positive airway pressure or mechanical ventilation that must be considered in the delivery room but also the shift in the function of the lung from secretion to absorption of fluid. AQP_5 expression enhances reabsorption of postnatal lung liquid and aids in the rapid recovery of infants with TTN. Transition for the fetus from a liquid environment with gas exchange through the placenta to air breathing must occur efficiently and effectively. Given all the physical and biochemical switching, it is a miracle that most babies accomplish this seemingly without effort. A key element in this transition is the clearance of lung fluid. This is accomplished by a combination of decreased secretion, increased absorption, and, to a lesser extent, excretion accompanying the big squeeze of the thorax during the birth process. The bulk of this fluid clearance is mediated by transepithelial sodium reabsorption through amiloride-sensitive sodium channels in the alveolar epithelial cells with only a limited contribution from mechanical factors and Starling forces. Disruption of this process can lead to retention of fluid in air spaces, setting the stage for alveolar hypoventilation. When infants are delivered late preterm, especially by cesarean section (repeat or primary) before the onset of spontaneous labor, the fetus is often deprived of these hormonal changes, making the neonatal transition more difficult.

Barker noted that the mechanisms for lung liquid clearance during the neonatal period develop gradually during the latter part of the third trimester of pregnancy, but the phenotypic switch of the lung epithelium from net secretion to net absorption triggered by events at birth is sudden. Although lung liquid absorption at birth is "a performance without rehearsal," the lung may be called on for an encore in later life when these same mechanisms are activated to clear accumulated edema liquid.

Bioelectrical studies of human infants' nasal epithelia demonstrate that TTN and respiratory distress syndrome (RDS) have defective amiloride-sensitive Na^+ transport. Neonatal RDS has, in addition to a relative deficiency in surfactant, defective Na^+ transport, which plays a mechanistic role in the development of the disease.

(Li Y, Marcoux MO, Gineste, et al. Expression of water and iron transporters in tracheal aspirates from neonates with respiratory distress. *Acta Paediatr.* 2009;98:17; Barker PM, Oliver RE. Lung edema clearance: 20 years of progress. Invited review. *J Appl Physiol.* 2002;93:1542.)

PULMONARY HEMORRHAGE

The signs of pulmonary hemorrhage range from blood-tinged tracheal or pharyngeal secretions to massive intractable bleeding. Most studies define significant pulmonary hemorrhage as bright red blood from the endotracheal tube in amounts that increase the need for ventilatory support or produce chest x-ray changes. Historically, pulmonary hemorrhage was associated with intrapartum asphyxia, infection, hypothermia, and defective hemostasis. Although occasionally manifesting in low-birth-weight infants who have previously appeared well, it more often affects infants who are already suffering from other life-threatening abnormalities or illnesses. The composition of the lung effluent in infants with massive pulmonary hemorrhage in most cases is a filtrate of plasma with a small admixture of whole blood, producing a hemorrhagic edema fluid, presumably formed because of increased pulmonary capillary pressure. Factors that might predispose infants to development of hemorrhagic pulmonary edema includes those favoring filtration of fluid (hypoproteinemia, overtransfusion), those causing damage to lung tissue (infection, RDS, and mechanical ventilation in high inspired oxygen), and abnormalities of coagulation.

In a retrospective cohort study, pulmonary hemorrhage was associated with the presence of a clinically significant PDA before or at the time of the hemorrhage.[41] In fact, left-to-right shunting through a PDA should be considered the primary etiology for pulmonary hemorrhage in a preterm infant who is often recovering from RDS. Surfactant therapy, by improving lung mechanics and decreasing pulmonary vascular resistance, may enhance the process. Pulmonary hemorrhage is probably not an indication to withhold surfactant therapy, because the blood products in the lung parenchyma may inactivate surfactant.[42] On rare occasions, aspiration of blood around the time of delivery may simulate pulmonary hemorrhage as a cause of neonatal respiratory distress when other risk factors for pulmonary hemorrhage are absent.[43] Pulmonary hemorrhage has also been seen in several neonates following treatment with extracorporeal life support.[44]

Pulmonary hemorrhage occurs most commonly on the second to fourth days of life. The usual mode of presentation is the development of bradycardia; apnea or slow, gasping respirations; and peripheral vasoconstriction. Blood-stained hemorrhagic edema is then seen welling from the trachea. Pulmonary hemorrhage can often be successfully treated by mechanical ventilation employing extra positive end-expiratory pressure and transfusion of blood products; occasionally, intratracheal epinephrine and high-frequency ventilation may be required.

BRONCHOPULMONARY DYSPLASIA/ NEONATAL CHRONIC LUNG DISEASE

In 1967, Northway et al first described BPD as a clinical syndrome associated with the use of assisted ventilation and high concentrations of oxygen.[45] Their patients had been on respirators using greater than 70% oxygen for longer than 5 to 6 days. During the prolonged recovery, the infants exhibited persistent respiratory difficulty and a characteristic radiographic progression that resulted in cystic lung changes. Increased concentrations of oxygen were required for several weeks before slow improvement was noted. Autopsy revealed that their lungs were diffusely involved with areas of emphysema and collapse, interstitial fibrosis, and changes in the epithelium of the airway.

The radiographic sequence of "classic" BPD initially described by Northway et al is no longer commonly seen, and

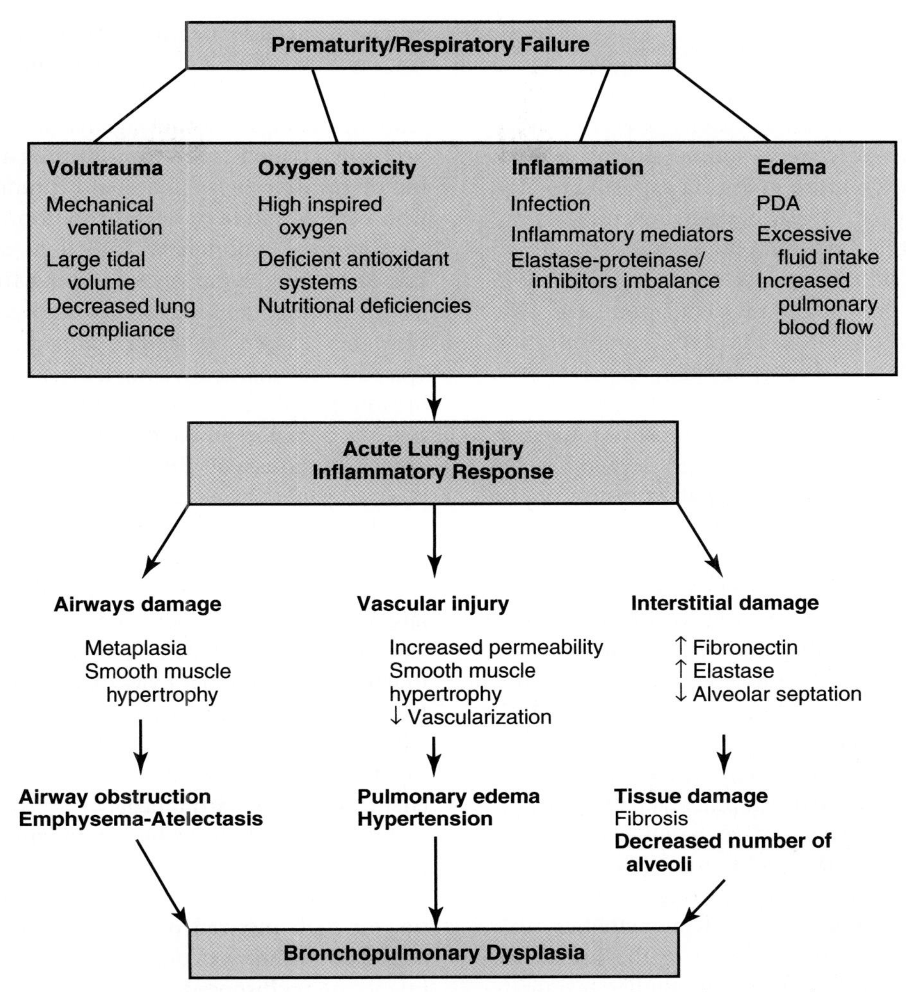

Fig. 9.7 Pathogenesis of bronchopulmonary dysplasia. *PDA,* Patent ductus arteriosus.

stage I is essentially indistinguishable from uncomplicated RDS. Dense parenchymal opacification, as seen in stage II BPD, may commonly simulate another process, such as congestive heart failure from a PDA or an infection. The bubbly pattern of stage III BPD is not necessarily seen, and when it does appear, it may not follow a period of parenchymal opacity. Finally, roentgenographic development of BPD (stage IV) may be more insidious than originally described. The characteristic picture of BPD ultimately appears at around 20 or 30 days of age. The major features of stage IV disease include hyperinflation and nonhomogeneity of pulmonary tissues, together with multiple fine, lacy densities extending to the periphery.

Since the original description of BPD by Northway et al, the problem of chronic respiratory disease in infants has steadily increased because of increased survival of very low–birth-weight infants. "New" BPD is characterized by alveolar hypoplasia and abnormal vascular organization seen on pathologic specimens.[46] Its pathogenesis is multifactorial in nature, and inflammation plays a major role. In the absence of clear diagnostic criteria for BPD, the following definitions for BPD are in current use: (1) oxygen dependence beyond 28 days of age with persistent chest x-ray changes after mechanical ventilation, and (2) oxygen dependence beyond 36 weeks' corrected postnatal gestational age.[47–48] Currently, there is an impetus to come up with a more useful predictive definition of BPD related in part to the multitude of infants receiving noninvasive ventilatory support (i.e., CPAP) in minimal or no supplemental oxygen.[49] BPD has been correlated with subsequent abnormal pulmonary findings at follow-up. It has been proposed that the more nonspecific term, *neonatal chronic lung disease*, be employed; however, BPD is still most widely used. Most very low–birth-weight infants who develop BPD may never have had severe RDS with high inspired oxygen or ventilator requirements. Laughon found that 68% of infants who develop BPD never required more than an FiO_2 of 30% in the first 7 days of life.[50]

Pathophysiologic and Clinical Features

Controversy surrounds the individual contributions of immaturity, inhaled oxygen, ventilator pressures, endotracheal tube injury, infection, and nutritional deficiencies to the overall pathologic picture of BPD (Fig. 9.7). Recent attention has focused on the role of a dysmorphic vascular structure that is prominent in animal models of BPD and the resultant marked decrease in alveolarization, as well as a role for genetics in contributing to BPD.[51]

Oxygen Toxicity

The lung is the organ exposed directly to the highest partial pressure of inspired oxygen. Although oxygen itself is essentially nonreactive, its potential for toxicity is derived from the formation of reactive oxygen species during normal cell metabolism, and even more so during exposure to high concentrations of oxygen. These oxygen-free radicals are cytotoxic because of their potential for interaction with all of the principal cellular components, resulting in inactivation of enzymes, lipid peroxidation in cellular and organelle membranes, and damage to DNA. The precise concentration of oxygen that is toxic to the lung probably depends on a large number of variables, including maturation, nutritional and endocrine status, and duration of exposure to oxygen and other oxidants. A safe level of inspired oxygen has not been established; it is even possible that exposure of the extremely immature lung to 21% oxygen may represent a cytotoxic challenge.

To combat the detrimental effects of oxygen toxicity, cells have evolved a complex system of antioxidant defenses to scavenge and detoxify reactive oxygen-free radicals. These antioxidant defenses include both chemical antioxidants, such as vitamin E, ascorbate, and glutathione, and the antioxidant enzyme system, consisting mainly of superoxide dismutase, catalase, and glutathione peroxidase. Studies have demonstrated a late gestational developmental pattern of pulmonary antioxidant enzyme maturation in numerous species. Therefore experimental animals, and presumably the human infant as well, if delivered prematurely, would be denied late gestational increases in antioxidant enzyme activities. This could partially explain the vulnerability of the premature infant to oxidant lung damage. Similarly, studies in rabbits have shown that the preterm rabbit is not capable of inducing a protective increase in antioxidant enzymes in response to hyperoxia exposure,[52] which may offer an additional explanation for the vulnerability of the premature infant to hyperoxic exposure.

Additional factors may contribute to the negative influence of hyperoxia on the neonatal lung. When the lung is continuously exposed to high oxygen, an influx of polymorphonuclear leukocytes containing proteolytic enzymes, such as elastase, occurs, resulting in proteolytic damage of structural elements in alveolar walls. Loss of mucociliary function may be an additional pathogenetic component in that exposure to 80% oxygen has resulted in a cessation of ciliary movement after 48 to 96 hours in cultured human neonatal respiratory epithelium. Finally, lung growth and development appear to be highly sensitive to oxygen exposure with reduced total alveolar number and lung internal surface area, as well as abnormal alveolar architecture in BPD infants.

Studies designed to enhance antioxidant capabilities in the human infant have yet to show any sustained benefit in terms of lung protection, although some show considerable promise. Clinical trials of vitamin E failed to demonstrate a lung protective effect. However, vitamin A (which may enhance lung development and repair via multiple mechanisms) has been shown to modestly reduce the primary outcome variable, death or BPD.[53] In addition, administration of antioxidant enzymes, particularly superoxide dismutase, might provide protection of the lung from oxidant damage.[54] Other agents that could potentially be protective include such iron-binding agents as deferoxamine or transferrin, which could function via reduction of iron-catalyzed free radical formation.

Abnormal pulmonary function is characterized by decreased lung compliance resulting from areas of fibrosis, overdistention, and atelectasis and increased pulmonary resistance caused by airway damage.[55] Wheezing may be episodic and markedly contribute to the increased work of breathing and oxygen requirement. Increased airway reactivity is a major problem at follow-up of preterm infants, especially those with BPD.[56–57] Chronic respiratory acidosis is accompanied by elevated bicarbonate and close to normal pH. This increase in serum bicarbonate is frequently exaggerated by chronic diuretic therapy.

Pulmonary edema is a prominent complication of BPD, largely caused by the increased pulmonary vascular pressure and permeability. Hypoxic pulmonary vasoconstriction and injury to the pulmonary vascular bed appear to be involved. Exacerbations of congestive heart failure may manifest with wheezing, fluid retention, and hepatomegaly. The underlying disease may mask the chest x-ray changes of pulmonary edema, including cardiomegaly.

Infection and the resultant inflammatory response frequently complicate the clinical course of chronic neonatal lung injury. Inflammatory mediators released by either infection or high inspired oxygen may aggravate the bronchoconstriction and vasoconstriction to which the lungs of these infants are predisposed.

Nutritional deficiencies and inadequate caloric intake can interfere with normal alveolar development and with the repair process of injured lung tissue. It can also negatively affect the antioxidant mechanisms. This problem is compounded by the increased work of breathing of these infants, which increases their oxygen consumption.[58]

Management

With skillful and patient management, most of these infants will recover, although abnormalities in pulmonary function may persist into childhood. Prolonged need for supplemental oxygen over several months is associated with a greater incidence of neurodevelopmental disorders when compared with infants with less severe lung disease.[59] The key to survival for infants with severe lung disease depends on close attention to details such as vigorous treatment of right-sided heart failure, precise fluid balance, use of diuretics, and gradual weaning from mechanical ventilation and raised environmental oxygen. The latter may need to occur in decrements of 1% to 2% of inspired oxygen. Oxygenation is typically monitored via pulse oximetry, and oxygen saturation is maintained in the low to mid-90s. Furosemide (Lasix), thiazide, and spironolactone are commonly used diuretics in preterm infants in the treatment of BPD to reduce pulmonary edema, which will improve oxygenation and lung compliance. However, long-term use has been associated with electrolyte anomalies and nephrocalcinosis.

These infants need to be closely watched for early signs of infection because pneumonia generally results in a setback. Bronchodilators are of benefit, especially when there are clinical signs of acute bronchospasm. They may be administered as systemic theophylline or as β-agonist inhalation therapy.[60] Controlled trials of both diuretic therapy and bronchodilator inhalation have revealed encouraging short-term improvements in airway resistance, even in the absence of wheezing.[61]

Steroids administered systemically or by inhalation have also been used to ameliorate BPD or to assist in weaning these infants from the ventilator[62]; however, reports of an increased incidence of cerebral palsy after postnatal systemic steroid use for BPD are of concern. This has led to considerable controversy as to the role, duration, and timing of postnatal systemic steroid therapy for BPD. Of particular concern is evidence that postnatal dexamethasone therapy may be associated with reduced cerebral tissue volumes as determined by follow-up magnetic resonance imaging.[63] Therefore hydrocortisone therapy has been proposed as an alternative to dexamethasone because hydrocortisone treatment for BPD may not be associated with the adverse neurobehavioral effects seen on follow-up of dexamethasone treatment.[64] An additional concern is a reported relationship between gastrointestinal perforation and indomethacin treatment for PDA in hydrocortisone-treated infants.[65] Current recommendations for postnatal steroid use in BPD include taking a cautious approach, avoidance of treatment in the first week of life or for a prolonged period, and tapering therapy over approximately 1 week.[66] The use of inhaled corticosteroids has also been proposed for the treatment of BPD. A recent RCT of early inhaled budesonide versus placebo demonstrated no difference in neurodevelopmental impairment among surviving extremely preterm infants at 18 to 22 months; however, they unexpectedly found a higher mortality rate in those infants receiving budesonide.[67]

Infants who develop severe BPD may also be afflicted with pulmonary hypertension; this needs to be carefully evaluated. In cases with an acute exacerbation of pulmonary hypertension, such as from an intercurrent pneumonia, there may be a role of a brief course of iNO. Sildenafil may also be a useful treatment for pulmonary hypertension associated with BPD.

Many of these infants require prolonged hospitalization, and a well-organized program of infant stimulation may help the child achieve maximum potential. Parents must be encouraged to assume some of the responsibility for medical procedures, such as chest physiotherapy, and, where possible, a consistent medical team should oversee the infant's care and be available for continuing parental support. Finally, adequate nutritional management is very important because malnutrition delays somatic growth and the development of new alveoli in these high-risk, labile infants.

EDITORIAL COMMENT: Despite a number of consensus conferences, there remains significant variation in the definitions of bronchopulmonary dysplasia (BPD). Also, there is inconsistency in the measurement of long-term pulmonary and neurodevelopmental outcomes of infants with BPD.

BPD continues to be the most frequently occurring significant morbidity for extremely preterm infants, yet highly effective therapies remain elusive. Promising new treatments such as mesenchymal stromal cell therapy are on the horizon, but well-designed clinical trials are needed to determine the true impact of these emerging therapies. Until then, the mainstays of therapy will be as outlined above, including more liberal use of human milk.

APNEA IN THE IMMATURE INFANT

Periodic breathing (short, recurring pauses in respiration) of 5 to 10 seconds' duration is common in the immature infant and should be considered a normal respiratory pattern at this age. Apnea, however, has been defined as either (1) a given time period with complete cessation of respiration (typically >15 to 20 seconds), or (2) the time without respiration after which functional changes are noted in the infant, such as a decrease in heart rate to about 80 beats per minute or oxygen saturation to about 80%. Although the use of a standard apneic duration appears to simplify routine nursery management, some small infants (usually <1000 g) appear to have oxygen desaturation if the apneic period extends beyond as little as 10 seconds. The problem increases substantially in incidence and severity with decreasing gestational age.

The relationship between apnea, desaturation, and bradycardia is not simple, as summarized in Fig. 9.8. Decreased central respiratory drive is the usual initiating event, with reflex bradycardia presumably triggered by the resultant desaturation. Excitation of inhibitory reflexes occasionally precipitates apnea and bradycardia.[68] A particularly perplexing problem is the frequent occurrence of oxygen desaturation and bradycardia in intubated, ventilated very low–birth-weight infants. In such infants, hypoventilation or ineffective ventilation with loss of lung volume is probably the initiating event.[69,70]

Hypoglycemia, fluid and electrolyte imbalance, temperature fluctuations, sepsis, anemia with or without a PDA, and severe brain lesions can be heralded by apneic spells and should be ruled out when apneic episodes first begin. In a small number of infants, usually close to term, apneic spells may be the manifestation of a seizure disorder. However, the majority of apneic periods occur in infants who are immature and have no organic disease. An exception is an apneic episode in an infant with severe RDS, which usually indicates the presence of hypoxia and acidemia or sepsis, and is a clear indication for immediate intervention, such as assisted ventilation.

The premature infant in whom specific causes for apnea have been reasonably excluded may be considered to have

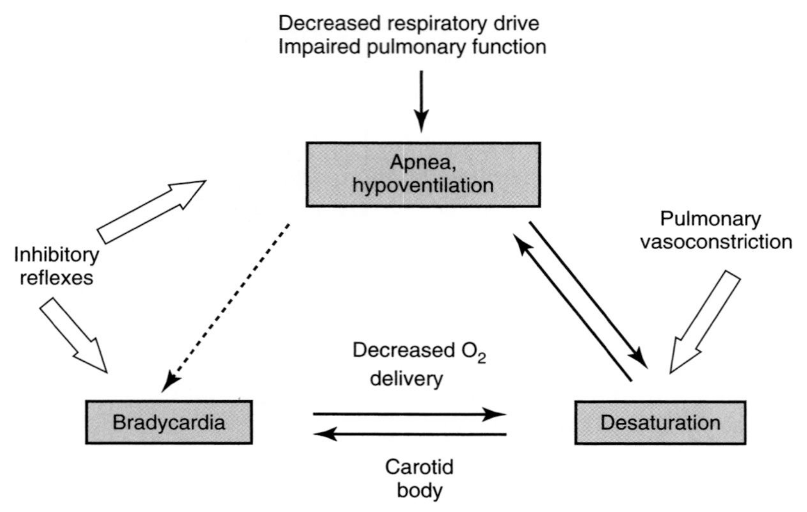

Fig. 9.8 Neonatal apnea, bradycardia, and desaturation.

TABLE 9.2 Factors Related to Apnea in the Immature Infant

Observation	Explanation
Hypoxemia causes respiratory depression and results in hypoventilation in neonates instead of sustained hyperventilation as in adults.	Hypoxemic depression of respiration in young infant is centrally mediated and appears to override stimulation from peripheral chemoreceptors.[a]
Hypercapnia causes hyperventilation as in adults, with diminished response in apneic versus nonapneic infants.	Decreased hypercapnic ventilatory response in apneic infants is probably secondary to immature central neural mechanisms.[a]
Obstructed inspiratory efforts may occur during apnea and may be misdiagnosed as primary bradycardia when breathing movements persist.[82]	Pharyngeal hypotonia and failure of upper airway respiratory muscles (genioglossus, alae nasi) to contract during inspiration may compromise upper airway patency.[a]
Apnea is more common during active sleep.	During active sleep, respiration is irregular; lung volume and oxygenation may decrease.

[a]Data from Davis PG, Schmidt B, Roberts RS, et al for the Caffeine for Apnea of Prematurity Trial Group. Caffeine for apnea of prematurity trial: benefits may vary in subgroup. *J Pediatr.* 2010;156:382; Schmidt B, Roberts RS, Anderson PJ, et al for the Caffeine for Apnea of Prematurity (CAP]) Trial Group. Academic performance, motor function, and behavior 11 years after neonatal caffeine citrate therapy for apnea of prematurity: an 11-year follow-up of the CAP Randomized Clinical trial. *JAMA Pediatr.* 2017;171:564–572; Ramanathan R, Corwin MJ, Hunt CE, et al. Cardiorespiratory events recorded on home monitors: comparison of healthy infants with those at increased risk for SIDS. *JAMA.* 2001;17:2199.

true idiopathic apnea of prematurity. Although no single physiologic or neurochemical explanation completely describes these apneic spells, Table 9.2 lists factors that singly or together make the immature infant more susceptible to apnea.[71–74]

EDITORIAL COMMENT: Although apnea of prematurity is more common in extremely premature infants, it certainly can occur in late preterm infants as well. When apnea occurs in term infants, a search for underlying causes such as seizure or infection may be indicated.

Treatment

Because prolonged apnea may cause clinically significant hypoxemia, and because these spells occur so commonly, hospitalized premature infants are typically continuously monitored until no clinically significant apneic episode has occurred for 3 to 7 days. Because apnea with an obstructive component (so-called *mixed apnea*) may not trigger a respiration alarm, simultaneous heart rate must always be monitored. In these infants, oxygen saturation is a useful adjunct to cardiorespiratory monitoring. Most episodes of 15 to 20 seconds' duration of apnea resolve spontaneously. Most of the remainder cease with gentle diffuse cutaneous stimulation. However, a bag and mask should be available near every monitored infant to be used if breathing does not begin promptly after stimulation. Inspired oxygen concentration depends on the infant's prior oxygen requirement.

A marked reduction in apnea has been noted with the use of CPAP and respiratory stimulants such as theophylline or caffeine.[75–77] Box 9.3 illustrates principles in the management of idiopathic apnea. The order in which these therapeutic steps are undertaken is based on the assessment of each individual patient.

Nasal CPAP at 3 to 5 cm H_2O is particularly effective in treatment of apneic episodes with an obstructive component.[77] The most probable mechanisms for the beneficial effect of CPAP include maintenance of upper airway patency, increase in FRC and PaO_2, and stabilization of the chest wall. The use of xanthine therapy (theophylline, caffeine) is widespread in the management of neonatal apnea. Theophylline is metabolized to caffeine in substantial amounts in neonates; their precise mechanism whereby either of these xanthine

BOX 9.3 Management of Idiopathic Apnea

- Diagnosis and treatment of specific causes (e.g., hypoglycemia, anemia, sepsis)
- Nasal continuous positive airway pressure
- Xanthine (caffeine or theophylline) therapy, commencing with a loading dose followed by maintenance therapy, and serum level monitoring, especially for theophylline
- Increased environmental oxygen as necessary to maintain adequate baseline oxygen saturation
- Assisted ventilation if all else fails

agents decreases apnea remains unclear.[78] Proposed mechanisms include generalized enhancement of central respiratory drive and a possible antiinflammatory effect via adenosine receptor antagonism. Although long-term sequelae from xanthine use have not appeared, care must be taken to avoid short-term side effects such as tachycardia and diuresis, probably more so with theophylline than with caffeine because the latter appears to have a greater margin of safety. Caffeine therapy does significantly shorten duration of supplemental oxygen administration and assisted ventilation.[79] Its use is associated with a transient increase in metabolic rate and impaired weight gain. It is unclear if very early initiation of caffeine, prolonged duration of therapy, and/or increased dose will favorably alter longer-term outcomes while ensuring optimal safety. Data suggest longer-term neurodevelopmental benefit from caffeine therapy.[80] At middle-school age, caffeine was not found to significantly reduce the combined rate of academic, motor, and behavioral impairments, but was associated with a reduced risk of motor impairment.[81]

Apnea may persist longer in preterm infants than was generally acknowledged. Such episodes may be accompanied by desaturation and/or bradycardia and often persist beyond 40 weeks of age in infants delivered before 28 weeks' postconceptional age.[82,83] Persistent apnea may also be asymptomatic in a large proportion of very low–birth-weight infants.[84] Prolonged apnea, often manifesting as bradycardia in these very low–birth-weight infants, is often associated with chronic neonatal lung disease. Persistence of symptomatic apnea and bradycardia prolongs the hospitalization of very premature infants and raises questions about the margin of safety for their discharge as well as about the indications for, and utility of, home apnea monitoring.[85]

What is the overall significance of these events in former preterm infants? Evidence does not link the persistence of these events to sudden infant death syndrome. Persistence of these cardiorespiratory events may be part of the spectrum of normal postnatal maturation. However, the possibility exists that they represent a subtle marker for neurodevelopmental or sleep disturbances, or other disorders of childhood. Data from several sources suggest that persistence of apnea of prematurity and accompanying bradycardia may be risk factors for later impairment in neurodevelopmental outcome.[86–88] Persistent hypoxic (but not bradycardic) events in extremely low–birth-weight infants have been associated with late death or disability.[89] However, establishment of a causal, rather than associative, relationship between these events and later outcome remains problematic.

QUESTIONS

True or False

As long as the arterial PaO_2 remains less than 100 mm Hg, there will be no retinal damage when using high concentrations of oxygen (>40%) for the treatment of RDS.

The answer is False. When PaO_2 is closely monitored and remains less than 100 mm Hg, retinal damage still develops in some very low–birth-weight infants. There are several possible explanations: (1) blood from a large right-to-left ductal shunt is directed to the sampling site in the lower aorta, whereas the retinal vessels receive unmixed blood with a higher PaO_2; (2) PaO_2 constantly fluctuates between arterial measurements; and (3) factors other than PaO_2 are involved in retinal injury. Continuous monitoring should help detect the PaO_2 fluctuations. Placing a skin pO_2 electrode or pulse oximeter on the right upper extremity to measure the saturation in the preductal blood should help detect any large right-to-left shunts and is useful to guide management in these situations. Nevertheless, even with continuous monitoring of the oxygen level, ROP still occurs. Any infant born at less than 30 weeks of gestation or having a birth weight less than 1500 g, or infants who do not fit those categories but have had a significant exposure to supplemental oxygen during their early life, should be examined by an experienced pediatric ophthalmologist at 4 weeks of age or a corrected age of 31 weeks' PMA, whichever is later, for ROP.

True or False

You are taking care of a 2-day-old, 1200-g male infant with moderate RDS. During the first 2 days of life, he has not been apneic and has maintained a reasonable pH, $PaCO_2$, and PaO_2 on 40% oxygen. However, the most recent PaO_2 measurement has decreased to 45 mm Hg (still on 40% oxygen). This environmental oxygen concentration should be left the same because raising it beyond 40% predisposes the infant to oxygen toxicity.

The answer is False. A decrease in PaO_2 to 45 mm Hg suggests worsening of the infant's condition. His condition may deteriorate rapidly if he remains on 40% oxygen. If the arterial oxygen is monitored closely (continually or at least every 4 hours), elevating the inspired oxygen concentration to maintain the PaO_2 between 50 and 80 mm Hg should not predispose the infant to lung or retinal injury, as appropriate readjustments to the inspired oxygen content can be made in response to an improved condition. Alternatively, the infant could be placed on CPAP, or if the infant is already on CPAP, the flow can be increased to increase the mean airway pressure, which, in turn, would lead to improved oxygenation. Also, evaluation of the underlying reason for the deterioration in PaO_2 would be important so the derangement can be rectified.

True or False

Maintaining the PaO_2 between 50 and 80 mm Hg will prevent pulmonary oxygen toxicity and lung injury.

The answer is False. Pulmonary oxygen toxicity is related to the inspired concentration of oxygen, not the arterial oxygen concentration, and any oxygen concentration more than room air can be damaging to pulmonary tissue. It should be noted, however, that oxygen toxicity is not the only contributor to neonatal lung injury. Other factors such as volutrauma, barotrauma, atelectrauma, and lung inflammation also play important roles in injury to the developing lung.

True or False

Your sister is 36 weeks pregnant and is scheduled for an elective cesarean section next week. You should be concerned because you believe that the infant may be at risk for developing respiratory distress?

The answer is True. RDS is the result of a primary absence of surfactant production, and affects most premature infants; however, in certain circumstances, it can affect term and near-term infants as well. Surfactant is produced by type II pneumocytes, which become a prominent cell in the alveolus at around 34 to 36 weeks of gestation. In general, surfactant secretion is increased during labor, and therefore if an infant is born via cesarean section before the onset of labor, they are at risk for decreased production and therefore respiratory distress after delivery. If elective delivery is to be pursued before 39 weeks' gestation, an explanation of the indication for the delivery must be documented in the chart, and recent data suggests that administering a course of betamethasone between 34 and 36 6/7 weeks' gestation my decrease the rates of RDS in this population.[90]

CASES

For each of the following cases, the blood gas information will be given in the following format: $pH/PaCO_2/PaO_2/HCO_3$. All information necessary will be given to you within the question.

CASE 9.1

Baby A is a 3900-g female with meconium aspiration syndrome. She is transferred to the neonatal intensive care unit (NICU) soon after birth, and umbilical venous and arterial catheters are placed. She is initially placed in an oxyhood for oxygen desaturation, and by 8 hours of age, she requires 70% oxygen.

At 8 hours of age, the baby's left leg turns dusky.

What should be done?

Initially, try warming the opposite extremity, which should cause a reflexive vasorelaxation in the extremity of interest. If the blanching does not improve quickly, then the umbilical arterial catheter must be removed immediately.

If the catheter is removed, how should the infant's oxygenation be managed?

There is no substitute for the combination of continuous oxygen monitoring (via pulse oximetry) and intermittent arterial blood sampling via an indwelling arterial catheter in an acutely ill neonate. Placement of a peripheral arterial line (e.g., radial artery line) should be attempted to continue arterial sampling in this patient to monitor pH, $PaCO_2$, and PaO_2.

When arterial catheterization is impossible, heel-stick or venous blood sampling can be used to monitor pH and $PaCO_2$, but not PaO_2. In that case, noninvasive oxygen monitoring is needed to control supplemental oxygen delivery.

The arterial gas obtained at 8 hours of age is: pH 7.16, $PaCO_2$ 60, PaO_2 50, and HCO_3 17.

How should this infant's ventilation and oxygenation be managed at this time?

Given this infant's respiratory acidosis and borderline oxygenation at a relatively high inspired oxygen concentration, the infant requires endotracheal intubation with mechanical ventilation. Arterial blood gases should continue to be monitored every 2 to 4 hours to adjust both ventilator and oxygen support required by the infant to resolve the respiratory acidosis and hypoxia. If the hypoxia is not resolving and it is thought that the infant has developed pulmonary hypertension, inhaled nitric oxide (iNO) should be added to the therapy. If this was a preterm infant with respiratory distress syndrome (RDS), placing the infant on continuous positive airway pressure (CPAP) would be an alternative to intubation. However, in a full-term infant, CPAP is not always well tolerated and could lead to a worsening of respiratory status and possibly cause a pneumothorax; placing a full-term infant in CPAP is done with extreme caution, and some would argue that intubation is the better choice of the two when treating a term infant with significant lung disease.

CASE 9.2

Baby B is a 2100-g, small-for-gestational-age, term male who has been grunting since birth. A chest x-ray shows no significant lung disease. The results of a blood gas at 30 minutes of life are: pH 7.14, $PaCO_2$ 35, PaO_2 30, and HCO_3 11.4. At that time, the infant is also noted to have a core body temperature of 34°C, heart rate of 140, respiratory rate of 60, and a mean arterial blood pressure of 39 mm Hg.

What are this infant's obvious problems?

This infant is hypothermic and hypoxemic and has a metabolic acidosis. The hypoxemia and acidosis may be the result of hypothermia because of inadequate thermoregulation after delivery. Infants, especially those who are small for gestational age, are at particular risk of hypothermia during the first hours of life because of their relatively large head-to-body surface area. However, sepsis must be a first consideration in the differential diagnosis of a hypothermic, acidotic infant.

How should these problems be handled?

The infant should be warmed by being placed under a radiant warmer or in an incubator. While the infant's body temperature is improving, the acidosis and hypoxemia should also be addressed. The infant should be placed on supplemental oxygen to treat the hypoxemia. Appropriate cultures should be obtained and antibiotics begun to treat the potential diagnosis of neonatal sepsis. Treating the infant's acidosis initially with bicarbonate is somewhat controversial. First, one could consider giving this infant a normal saline bolus (10 mL/kg) in anticipation of possible hypovolemia, and if the acidosis does not improve, repeat the bolus and then consider giving bicarbonate (2 mEq/kg). In addition, many would feel more comfortable intubating this hypoxic infant before giving bicarbonate to provide a controlled manner in which to ensure CO_2 elimination. The placement of an umbilical arterial catheter should be considered so that frequent blood gas samples can be drawn to monitor the infant's response to the interventions that have been made.

At 1 hour of age, after the infant has been in an incubator, placed on a nasal cannula at 1 liter per minute (LPM) with an FiO_2 of 0.4, and given a normal saline bolus of 10 mL/kg, the repeat arterial blood gas is: pH 7.28, $PaCO_2$ 36, PaO_2 90, and HCO_3 16.4. At this time, the core body temperature is 36°C, heart rate is 120, respiratory rate is 70, and the mean arterial blood pressure is 22.

What problem(s) does the infant have now?

This infant is now hypotensive. Hypoxemia or acidemia alone or in conjunction with one another can result in an elevation of blood pressure because of their effect on peripheral vasoconstriction. In this patient, partial correction of the metabolic acidosis and increasing the PaO_2 probably caused a decrease in peripheral vascular resistance, reflected as a decrease in the mean arterial blood pressure. The low blood pressure suggests a severely reduced blood volume, which should be expanded with isotonic fluid and/or blood products, if necessary. Of note, acidosis can worsen initially after fluid resuscitation, as the buildup of lactate in the tissue is now mobilized into the circulation, and large fluid replacement volumes may be necessary.

EDITORIAL COMMENT: Treatment of neonatal hypotension varies widely between institutions and individual practitioners, and pharmacotherapy for neonatal hypotension has changed over the past decade. However, hypotension is a broader concept than blood pressure alone, and the focus should not be just on correcting blood pressure, but also on improving end-organ perfusion, specifically cerebral perfusion. Unfortunately, few studies have incorporated the organ-relevant hemodynamic changes and long-term outcomes when assessing inotropic effects in neonates. In addition to fluid boluses, dopamine and dobutamine were the most frequently used inotropes. Their use has declined, and the use of hydrocortisone and vasopressin has increased.

CASE 9.3

Baby C is a 900-g female delivered at 27 weeks' gestation. Her Apgar scores are 1 and 7 at 1 and 5 minutes, respectively. She is initially placed on continuous positive airway pressure (CPAP) in the delivery room and transferred to the neonatal intensive care unit (NICU) for further management. A chest x-ray is consistent with the diagnosis of respiratory distress syndrome (RDS). Umbilical lines are placed, and an initial arterial blood gas result is: pH 7.19, $PaCO_2$ 55, PaO_2 60, HCO_3 19.5 on CPAP 5, and FiO_2 is 0.5. There have been no apneic episodes noted.

Should surfactant therapy be administered?

Over recent years, there has been a shift in neonatology practice from automatically intubating very low–and extremely low–birth-weight infants for surfactant administration to an approach of initially starting some of these infants on noninvasive modes of ventilation (i.e., CPAP, noninvasive positive pressure ventilation, etc.) in the delivery room. The question then becomes when, if ever, should these infants be treated with surfactant. Surfactant has improved survival, reduced the incidence of air leaks, and probably reduced the severity and incidence of chronic lung disease in infants with respiratory distress. In infants who have RDS and are not initially intubated, there are some guidelines available to help decide when and if a preterm infant should be intubated for surfactant, which takes into account gestational age, respiratory drive, and inspired oxygen concentration (see Fig. 9.5). In the case of this patient, although the infant has a strong respiratory drive, given the need for supplemental oxygen of 50%, surfactant should be considered.

At 5 hours of age, the infant is weaned from an FiO_2 of 0.6 to 0.27, and the blood gas is: pH 7.28, $PaCO_2$ 55, PaO_2, 62, and HCO_3 22.

Should surfactant be repeated?

There has been a great deal of flexibility with regard to the redosing of surfactant. However, given the fact that her pH is greater than 7.25 and her FiO_2 is less than 0.3, it would be reasonable to extubate this infant to either CPAP or another form of noninvasive ventilation and not to administer another dose of surfactant.

What are the complications of surfactant therapy?

Significant oxygen desaturation occurs in a small percentage of infants shortly after receiving surfactant therapy, which is usually quick to resolve as the surfactant is absorbed and ventilation and perfusion improve. There have also been concerns about pulmonary hemorrhage associated with surfactant administration. This appears to be a more significant problem in the most immature infants (those weighing <750 g and <25 weeks' gestation) and is likely because of changes in lung compliance in the face of an open ductus arteriosus. Also, there is a risk of developing a pneumothorax after surfactant administration as lung compliance improves if the inspiratory pressure used to inflate the less compliant lungs before surfactant administration is not decreased appropriately.

CASE 9.4

Baby D is a 2000-g male who has been grunting since birth. His chest x-ray reveals questionable respiratory distress syndrome (RDS). He is placed in 70% oxygen.

At 3 hours, a blood gas is obtained: pH 7.36, $PaCO_2$ 40, PaO_2 280, and HCO_3 22.2.

What should be done, if anything?

This infant is hyperoxic on 70% oxygen; thus the oxygen concentration should be decreased to 60% immediately, and pulse oximetry should be placed (if it has not been already) for rapid weaning of oxygen. Plan to decrease the oxygen by 2% to 5% every 5 to 10 minutes while maintaining a pulse oximeter reading of 90% to 95%. A repeat blood gas should be obtained in 2 to 4 hours or earlier if desaturation occurs.

At 5 hours of age, the repeat blood gas is: pH 7.36, $PaCO_2$ 43, PaO_2 45, and HCO_3 24 on an FiO_2 of 0.4.

What happened, and how should it be addressed?

The patient demonstrated a greater than expected decrease in PaO_2 when the oxygen concentration was weaned and is now hypoxic. This can generally be avoided with continuous monitoring. To resolve the problem, first return the oxygen to 60% to 70%. Second, transilluminate the chest to rule out the possibility of a pneumothorax, which can manifest as a sudden drop in the PaO_2; if transillumination is inconclusive, an x-ray should be obtained. Fifteen to 20 minutes after the FiO_2 has been increased, repeat the blood gas to determine what effect increasing the oxygen concentration has made.

The repeat blood gas after increasing the oxygen to 60% is: pH 7.37, $PaCO_2$ 45, PaO_2 70, and HCO_3 22.

What is the explanation for what happened between our first and last blood gases?

There is not a complete physiologic explanation underlying this phenomenon. It is assumed that, in some infants, the pulmonary vessels are particularly sensitive to changes in oxygen tension, and lowering the environmental oxygen results in pulmonary vasoconstriction and an increased right-to-left shunt. Under these circumstances, the PaO_2 decreases out of proportion to what might ordinarily be expected when the inspired oxygen concentration is reduced, thus explaining the decrease in the PaO_2 seen at 5 hours of age, which improved after increasing the oxygen.

CASE 9.5

Baby D is a 3000-g infant born at 41 weeks' gestation and is covered with thick meconium. Labor was complicated by late deceleration. Apgar scores are 2, 5, and 7 at 1, 5, and 10 minutes, respectively. The infant is bradycardic with poor respiratory effort after initial steps of resuscitation and requires positive pressure ventilation and intubation to improve the heart rate, and is transported to the neonatal intensive care unit (NICU) for further care. Chest x-ray shows bilateral patchy infiltrates. Umbilical lines are placed, and the infant is maintained on a ventilator and 100% oxygen.

At 6 hours of life, a blood gas is obtained: pH 7.35, $PaCO_2$ 34, PaO_2 32, and HCO_3 19.

What is the infant's main problem at this time?

The infant is markedly hypoxemic on 100% oxygen; however, the infant is not hypercarbic. It is unusual for such a degree of hypoxemia without CO_2 retention to be attributable solely to meconium pneumonitis. It appears that this infant's condition is compounded by persistent pulmonary hypertension secondary to neonatal asphyxia.

How should this be treated?

The response of the hypoxemia to ventilator support in such an infant is variable. Nonetheless, assisted ventilation should be continued with the goal to normalize the pH without maintaining the $PaCO_2$ below 40. The goal is to improve any acidemia because this can cause pulmonary vasoconstriction that will worsen hypoxia. If oxygenation fails to improve, other therapies such as increasing peripheral arterial blood pressure, sedation, surfactant, and inhaled nitric oxide (iNO) should be employed. Extracorporeal membrane oxygenation (ECMO) should be reserved for those infants who do not respond to maximal medical therapy.

The reference list for this chapter can be found online at www.expertconsult.com

10

Assisted Ventilation

Waldemar A. Carlo, Namasivayam Ambalavanan

But that life may, in a manner of speaking, be restored to the animal, an opening must be attempted in the trunk of the trachea, into which a tube or reed or cane should be put; you will then blow into this so that the lung may rise again and the animal take in air. Indeed, with a single breath in the case of this living animal, the lung will swell to the full extent of the thoracic cavity and the heart become strong and exhibit a wondrous variety of motions...when the lung long flaccid has collapsed, the beat of the heart and arteries appears wavy, creepy, twisting, but when the lung is inflated, it becomes strong again and swift and displays wondrous variations...as I do this, and take care that the lung is inflated at intervals, the motion of the heart and arteries does not stop.

Andreas Vesalius
De Humani Corporis Fabrica (1543)

The primary objective of assisted ventilation is to support gas exchange until the patient's ventilatory efforts are sufficient. Ventilation may be required during immediate care of the depressed or apneic infant, before evaluation and during treatment of an acute respiratory disorder, or for prolonged periods of treatment for respiratory failure. Trained personnel and equipment for emergency ventilation should be available in every delivery room and newborn nursery. Positive-pressure ventilation effectively stabilizes most infants who require resuscitation.

This chapter is an introduction to assisted ventilation. Before undertaking assisted ventilation of any form, it must be recognized that the techniques demand time, resources, and experienced personnel. Prolonged ventilation should only be used in units where trained nurses, respiratory therapists, and medical personnel are continuously available.

RESPIRATORY FAILURE

Hypercapnic respiratory failure is the inability to remove CO_2 by spontaneous respiratory efforts, which results in an increasing arterial P_{CO2} ($PaCO_2$) and a decreasing pH. Assisted ventilation is most commonly needed to treat hypercapnic respiratory failure. Hypoxemia is usually (but not invariably) present; in many instances, arterial oxygenation can be normalized if the inspired oxygen is increased. Infants with hypoxemic respiratory failure have a predominant problem of oxygenation, usually the result of right-to-left shunt or severe ventilation–perfusion ($\dot{V}/\dot{Q}$) mismatch. Respiratory failure can occur because of disease in the lungs or in other organs and systems (Fig. 10.1). Assisted ventilation is usually required when severe respiratory failure ensues (Box 10.1).

Clinical Manifestations of Respiratory Failure in the Newborn

The following are findings that should make the clinician suspect respiratory failure:

- worsening hypercapnia and/or hypoxemia;
- increase or decrease in respiratory rate;
- increase or decrease in respiratory efforts (grunting, flaring, retractions);
- periodic breathing with increasing prolongation of respiratory pauses;
- apnea; and
- decreasing blood pressure with tachycardia associated with pallor, circulatory failure, and ultimately bradycardia.

Cardiac Versus Pulmonary Disease

The clinician frequently needs to distinguish between cardiac and pulmonary disease in the sick newborn infant. Cyanotic heart disease may mimic respiratory disease. One possible way to differentiate between the two is to perform a hyperoxia test: place the infant in 100% oxygen for 10 minutes and then obtain an arterial Po_2 (PaO_2), or a pulse oximeter can be used, which is a less invasive means of performing a hyperoxia screening test.

In infants with pulmonary disease, PaO_2 usually increases to more than 100 mm Hg, whereas infants with cyanotic heart disease show little change in PaO_2. The hyperoxia test, although useful diagnostically, may also be misleading. In infants with severe pulmonary hypertension and right-to-left shunt, PaO_2 may not elevate with 100% oxygen. Alternatively, PaO_2 may increase more than 100 mm Hg early in life in infants with forms of cyanotic heart disease with high pulmonary blood flow (e.g., total anomalous pulmonary venous

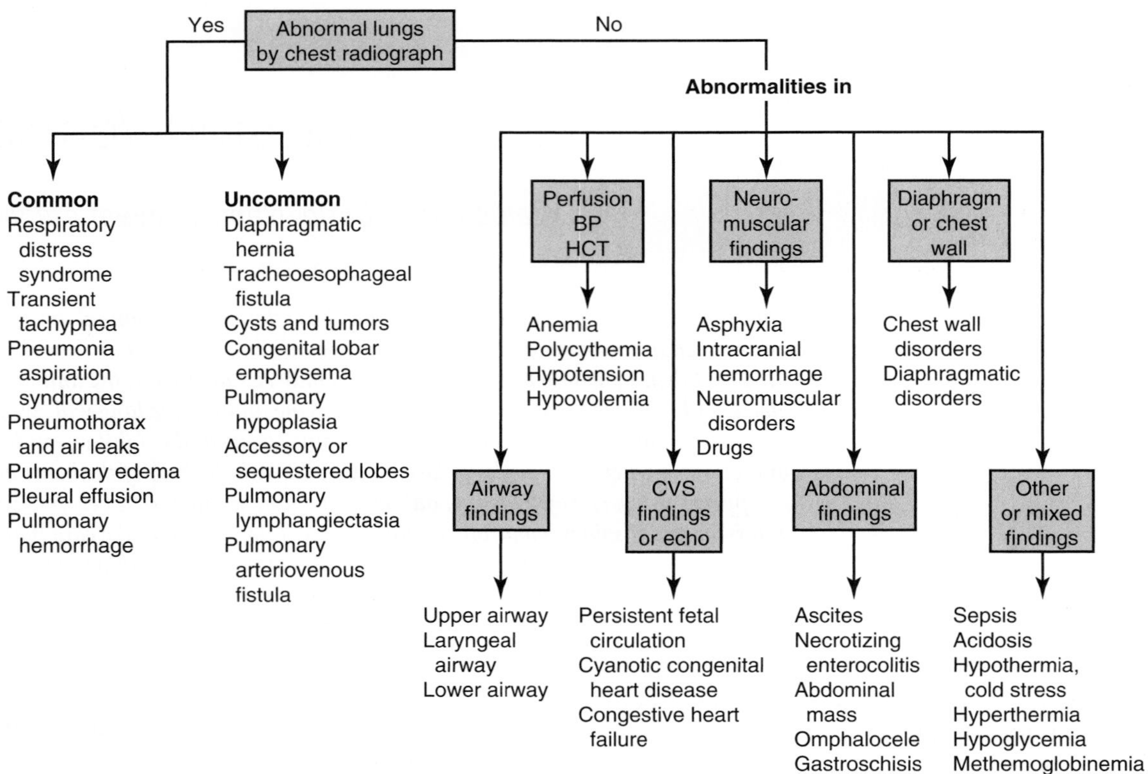

Fig. 10.1 Diagram of causes of respiratory distress in neonates. *BP,* Blood pressure; *CVS,* cardiovascular system; *echo,* echocardiogram; *HCT,* hematocrit.

BOX 10.1 General Indications for Assisted Ventilation

- Respiratory acidosis with pH <7.20–7.25
- Hypoxemia while on 100% oxygen or continuous positive airway pressure with 60%–100% oxygen
- Severe apnea

return). Echocardiography should be used to distinguish between cardiac and pulmonary disease when hypoxemia is unresponsive to ventilatory support.

ENDOTRACHEAL INTUBATION

Most infants should receive positive-pressure ventilation using bag and mask before attempting endotracheal intubation. This improves oxygenation and decreases $PaCO_2$, thereby decreasing the likelihood of bradycardia during endotracheal intubation. Positive-pressure ventilation using bag and mask is impractical for prolonged periods but can be used for the following:

- immediate resuscitation;
- stabilization before and after endotracheal intubation;
- ventilation in infants whose condition is deteriorating without obvious cause; and
- ventilation during transport to intensive care facilities when mechanical ventilation is unavailable.

Mechanical ventilation is an invasive therapy and is indicated only when the benefits outweigh the burdens.

Endotracheal Tube Size

It is preferable to use relatively small endotracheal tubes to prevent tracheal damage. The endotracheal tube should fit loosely enough to allow a leak of gas between tube and trachea when more than 10 cm H_2O inspired pressure is generated. Tube size can be related to infant size or gestational age. Recommended sizes are as follows in Table 10.1.

EDITORIAL COMMENT: The guideline of assuring a leak between the tube and the trachea is a good principal in larger infants and children, but because the resistance to airflow is inversely proportional to the fourth power of the inside radius of the tube, resistance becomes very great with very small tubes and the risk of obstruction is large. Therefore even though very small tubes may be somewhat easier to insert, we try to avoid tube diameters less than 2.5 mm.

–John Kattwinkel

Intubation

Insertion of an endotracheal tube should be performed with universal precautions under a radiant heat source to keep the infant warm. Free-flow oxygen should be administered as necessary.

Intubation can be a painful procedure, and so, premedication with an analgesic agent (morphine, fentanyl, or remifentanil) should be used for nonemergent intubations in neonates.[1]

TABLE 10.1 Endotracheal Tube Size by Gestational Age and Birth Weight

Gestational Age (week)	Birth Weight (g)	Endotracheal Tube Size (mm internal diameter)
<24	<500	2.0
24–28	500–1000	2.5
28–34	1000–2000	3.0
35–38	2000–3000	3.5
>38	>3000	3.5–4.0

TABLE 10.2 Endotracheal Tube Insertion Length by Infant Weight

Infant Weight (g)	Endotracheal Tube Insertion Length (tip to lip, cm)
500	6.5
1000	7
2000	8
3000	9
4000	10

A muscle relaxant (paralytic agent) should only be used with analgesia. Other agents that may be considered include sedatives (midazolam) and vagolytic agents (atropine). The ideal combination and sequence of premedications in neonates has not yet been established. Each unit should have protocols and lists of preferred medications to maximize safety.

The infant should receive positive-pressure ventilation and oxygen as needed between intubation attempts. The tip of the tube should be placed midway between the carina and the glottis. The following measurements in Table 10.2 can be used for endotracheal tube placement.

At these lengths, the distal end of the endotracheal tube should be at the midtrachea. It is easy to inadvertently pass the tube into the right mainstem bronchus, in which case the tube should be pulled back slowly until breath sounds are equal. Breath sounds should be equal bilaterally. A CO_2 detector should be used to confirm endotracheal placement. The tube should be secured well so that movement of the head and neck will not dislodge it. Lightweight plastic connectors can be used to prevent kinking the tube. The endotracheal tube position should be checked radiographically.

EDITORIAL COMMENT: I find that visual positioning of the distal stripe on the tube to be very valuable in initially assessing the appropriate depth of endotracheal tube placement. The stripe should be visible through the laryngoscope and should be place just proximal to the vocal cords. Also, if emergency access to the airway is required and endotracheal intubation expertise is not readily available, placement of a laryngeal mask airway (LMA) may be useful (see J. Wyllie, Perlman J, Kattwinkel J, et al. *Resuscitation.* 2015;95:e169–e201). The limitations are that even the smallest LMA version available may not be appropriate for babies weighing less than approximately 1800 g.

–John Kattwinkel

Oral Intubation

The advantages of oral intubation are the relative ease of insertion and that if necessary, a stylet can be used to aid insertion. Oral tubes should always be used in emergencies. The disadvantages of oral intubation are the increased tube mobility if the tube is inadequately secured and more difficulty in keeping the tube in position.

A laryngoscope with a Miller number 00 (small preterm), 0 (preterm), or 1 (term) blade inserted in the vallecula is used to pull upward to visualize the glottis while leaving the head in a neutral position. It is important not to traumatize the gums and tooth buds. The heart rate should be monitored continuously with auditory and visual signals during attempts at intubation. Continuous O_2 saturation or transcutaneous Po_2 monitoring is helpful because oxygenation can worsen abruptly. It is also helpful if the tube has been previously curved. To stiffen the tube for orotracheal intubation, it may be cooled or a stylet may be used.

Nasal Intubation

The advantage of nasal intubation is the improved stability with the reduced likelihood of slippage into the right mainstem bronchus or accidental extubation. The disadvantages are trauma to the nares and nasal septum, greater difficulty in insertion of the tube, and potential trauma to the developing eustachian tubes and sinuses. Nasotracheal intubation should always be performed as an elective procedure and should not be done in emergencies.

Using a laryngoscope blade, the lubricated endotracheal tube is inserted through the nares until it is visualized in the oropharynx. McGill forceps are used to guide the tube into the glottis. It is helpful if the endotracheal tube has been previously lubricated with a nontoxic, water-soluble lubricant. A stylet is never used for nasotracheal intubation.

Suctioning

Suctioning can be done if there are copious amounts of secretions or suspicion of endotracheal tube occlusion by secretions, but routine suctioning is not necessary. A strict sterile technique with disposable gloves and suction tubes is necessary. Closed systems for suction are available. The suction catheter should not be advanced past the distal end of the endotracheal tube. The infant should be allowed to recover between episodes of suctioning by maintaining stable O_2 saturations with increases in inspired oxygen concentrations and by reexpanding the lung with 10% to 20% more pressure than used for routine ventilation as needed. Saline can be instilled to facilitate removal of secretions when secretions are thick.

Although sometimes necessary, suctioning is potentially dangerous; it may cause a hypoxic episode owing to discontinuation of ventilation, extraction of gas from small airways, or atelectasis. Suctioning beyond the endotracheal tube may produce lesions in the trachea at the site of the suction catheter tip. Use of a special endotracheal tube connector allows mechanical ventilation during suctioning and prevents the catheter tip from going beyond the endotracheal tube.

> **EDITORIAL COMMENT:** Suctioning of the endotracheal tube will decrease oxygenation and pulmonary function. I would advocate being guided by pulse oximetry during the procedure, which may require transiently increasing inspired oxygen concentration by 10% to 15% immediately before and following the period of suctioning. I would also advocate avoiding the practice of "routine" suctioning except as secretions warrant.
>
> –John Kattwinkel

Changing an Endotracheal Tube

An endotracheal tube change is required only if the tube becomes dislodged or occluded or if the infant outgrows it. Routine change is not indicated.

APPLIED PULMONARY MECHANICS

The following principles are helpful in understanding mechanical ventilation. A pressure gradient between the airway opening and alveoli must exist to drive the flow of gases during both inspiration and expiration. The pressure gradient required to inflate the lungs is determined largely by the compliance and the resistance of the lungs.

Compliance

Compliance is a property of distensibility (i.e., of the lungs and chest wall) and is calculated from the change in volume per unit change in pressure:

$$\text{Compliance} = \frac{\Delta\text{Volume}}{\Delta\text{Pressure}}$$

The higher the compliance is, the larger the delivered volume per unit of pressure will be. Compliance in babies with normal lungs ranges from 3 to 6 mL/cm H_2O. Compliance in infants with respiratory distress syndrome (RDS) ranges from 0.1 to 1 mL/cm H_2O.

Resistance

Resistance is a property of the inherent capacity of the gas-conducting system (i.e., airways, endotracheal tube, and lung tissue) to oppose airflow and is expressed as the change in pressure per unit change in flow:

$$\text{Resistance} = \frac{\Delta\text{Pressure}}{\Delta\text{Flow}}$$

Resistance in babies with normal lungs ranges from 25 to 50 cm H_2O/L/second. Resistance is not dramatically altered in infants with RDS but is increased in intubated infants and ranges from 50 to 150 cm H_2O/L/second.

Time Constant

Time constant is a measure of the time (expressed in seconds) necessary for 63% of a step change (e.g., airway pressure gradient) toward equilibration. A step change in airway pressure occurs between the beginning and the end of a machine-delivered inspiration (during pressure-limited, time-cycled ventilation). The product of compliance and resistance determines the time constant of the respiratory system:

$$\text{Time constant} = \text{complex} \times \text{resistance}$$

For example, in an infant with normal lungs:

$$\begin{aligned}\text{One time constant} &= 0.005\ \text{L/cm}\ H_2O \\ &\times 25\ \text{cm}\ H_2O\text{/L/second} \\ &= 0.125\ \text{second}\end{aligned}$$

In an intubated infant with RDS:

$$\begin{aligned}\text{One time constant} &= 0.001\ \text{L/cm}\ H_2O \\ &\times 50\ \text{cm}\ H_2O\text{/L/second} \\ &= 0.050\ \text{second}\end{aligned}$$

It takes three time constants to achieve 95% of the pressure change to be equilibrated throughout the lungs; it takes five time constants for 99% equilibration. Thus, to allow for a fairly complete inspiration and expiration, inspiratory and expiratory times set on the ventilator should last about three to five time constants. In this example of an intubated infant with RDS, the duration of three to five time constants is 0.150 to 0.250 seconds. A very short inspiratory time can lead to inadequate tidal volume because ventilatory pressures may not equilibrate throughout the lungs (Fig. 10.2). A very short expiratory time can lead to gas trapping because exhalation may not be completed. Very long inspiratory or expiratory times are also not beneficial.

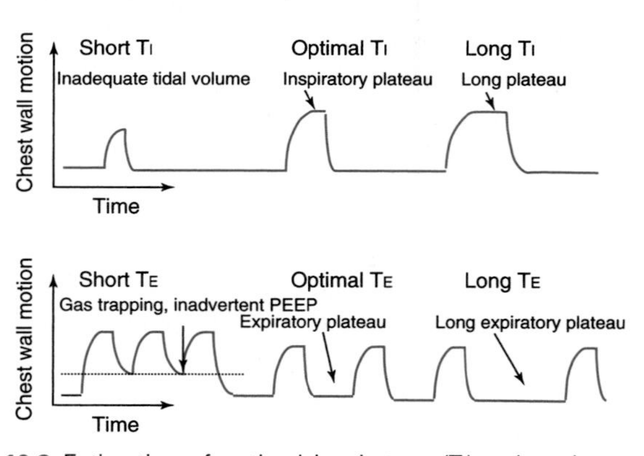

Fig. 10.2 Estimation of optimal inspiratory (T_I) and expiratory (T_E) times. Inspiratory and expiratory times are optimal when inspiration and expiration are complete, but the times are not too prolonged. (See text for further details.) *PEEP,* Positive end-expiratory pressure.

CONTINUOUS POSITIVE AIRWAY PRESSURE

Spontaneous breathing can also be assisted by expansion of the lungs with continuous distending pressure. This technique is valuable when respiratory drive is normal and pulmonary disease is not overwhelming. Continuous distending pressure can be applied with continuous positive airway pressure (CPAP) or continuous negative pressure around the chest wall. Because of the ease of delivery, CPAP is the usual mode of delivery of continuous distending pressure.

Surfactant deficiency in infants with RDS predisposes to alveolar collapse. The resulting atelectatic areas of the lungs are the sites of right-to-left shunting. Functional residual capacity increases when alveoli are prevented from closing by maintaining a continuous positive transpulmonary pressure throughout the respiratory cycle. In addition, ventilation of perfused areas of the lung increases, which reduces intrapulmonary shunt.

A simple system for CPAP was described by Gregory et al in 1971 (Fig. 10.3).[2] A suitable air–oxygen mixture passes through a humidifier. Gas passes through the tubing, which is attached to an endotracheal tube. The screw clamp on the reservoir controls the flow of gas and maintains a constant positive pressure within the system, as indicated on the pressure manometer. The side arm acts as an underwater safety valve by ending under a column of water. Nasal CPAP is simple and effective; it is usually applied with nasal or nasopharyngeal prongs, although other techniques for delivery can be used (Table 10.3). Problems with CPAP generally revolve around feeding difficulties, maintaining a good seal, and nasal trauma. Nursing and medical care are similar to those undertaken during mechanical ventilation.

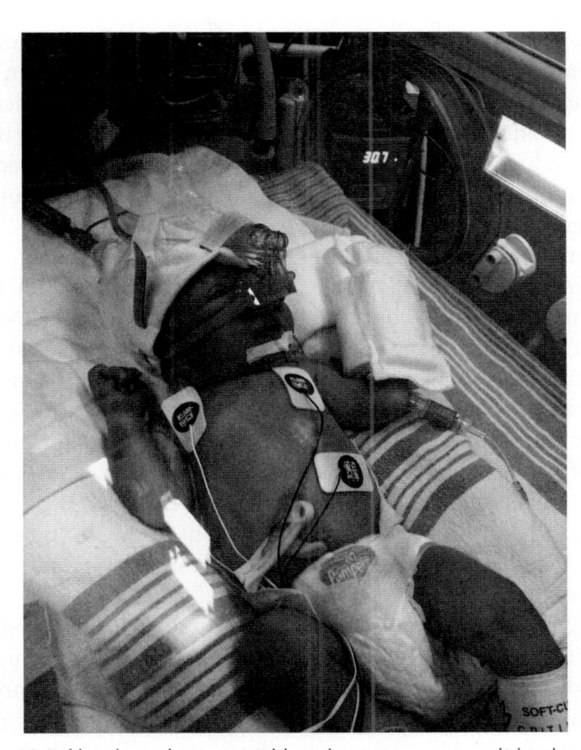

Fig. 10.3 Nasal continuous positive airway pressure unit in place on infant.

Trials performed before the era of surfactant showed that CPAP decreased death and the need for mechanical ventilation, but increased the risk for pneumothorax.[3] Subsequent surfactant trials showed that early surfactant treatment in the first 2 hours after birth compared with delayed treatment decreased air leaks and death or bronchopulmonary dysplasia (BPD).[4] However, the control infants in these trials received mechanical ventilation, and it is possible that mechanical ventilation without surfactant causes lung injury. More recent trials have compared the effects of CPAP to mechanical ventilation with surfactant administration.[5] Early CPAP, as compared with early intubation with surfactant, decreased BPD and/or death.[3,6] In bigger preterm infants, CPAP results in benefits comparable to that of surfactant.[7] Together, these studies indicate that CPAP is an effective alternative to intubation and surfactant in the treatment of RDS in most preterm infants.

General Guidelines for Continuous Positive Airway Pressure

1. CPAP should be initiated soon after birth in the most immature infants (<~29 weeks' gestation) with presumed RDS. In more mature infants, CPAP can be initiated when the infant requires more than 30% to 40% oxygen or when the infant has recurrent apnea.
2. Initially, nasal CPAP of 5 to 6 cm H_2O can be used. If there is no improvement, the pressure can be increased, usually in increments, up to 8 to 10 cm H_2O. Very high CPAP levels may overdistend the lungs, decrease their compliance, and increase the risk for pneumothorax. Nasal intermittent mechanical ventilation can be added to CPAP, which may reduce the need for intubation.[8] Nasal intermittent positive pressure added to CPAP also reduces the incidence of extubation failure and the need for reintubation.[9]
3. Continuous measurement of transcutaneous Po_2 and PCO_2 and oxygen saturation with a pulse oximeter can decrease the need for frequent blood gas measurements.
4. Because these positive pressures are not completely transmitted to the pleural space due to reduced lung compliance, venous return and cardiac output are usually not compromised. However, if $PaCO_2$ increases and PaO_2 decreases, a reduction in CPAP pressure should be considered.

TABLE 10.3 Techniques of Applying Continuous Positive Airway Pressure

Method	Advantages	Disadvantages
Nasal prongs	Simple	Trauma to turbinates and septum; excessive crying; variation in FiO_2; increased work of breathing
Nasopharyngeal prongs	Relatively simple, fixation easy	May become blocked or kinked
Endotracheal	Effective	Requires intubation; nursing and medical skills as for ventilator
Head box	Noninvasive	Neck seal a problem; suction difficult; nerve palsies
Face mask	Simple, inexpensive	Abdominal distention, pressure on face and eyes; CO_2 retention; cerebellar hemorrhage
Face chamber	Good seal, minimal trauma to face	Expensive; baby inaccessible
High-flow cannula	Easy to maintain in place; less trauma	Inconsistent delivery of pressure; leads to more failure compared to Nasal Prong CPAP

EDITORIAL COMMENT: Thoracic wall elastic recoil is almost nonexistent in extremely preterm babies (e.g., 29 weeks' gestation or less) so that the resting volume of the lung is very close to the collapsed volume. Also, the compliant chest wall tends to collapse as the diaphragm descends, resulting in an ineffective tidal volume. Early use of continuous positive airway pressure may improve the efficiency of ventilation in these very immature babies.

–John Kattwinkel

Weaning From Continuous Positive Airway Pressure

1. Inspired oxygen can be reduced in steps of 2% to 5% when the O_2 saturation is consistently within the targeted range.
2. CPAP can be reduced when the O_2 saturation is consistently within the targeted range and the inspired oxygen is consistently less than 30% to 40%.

EDITORIAL COMMENT: With small babies (<1500 g), if recurrent apneic spells are a problem, we may continue low-pressure continuous positive airway pressure (<5 cm H_2O) until inspired oxygen concentrations have been reduced to 21% to 30%.

–John Kattwinkel

See Chapter 9 for a discussion of the use of CPAP for apnea of prematurity.

MECHANICAL VENTILATION

Mechanical ventilation is one of the most important breakthroughs in the history of neonatal care. Mechanical ventilation allows the survival of previously nonviable infants, stimulating the development of a new era in neonatology.

Conventional mechanical ventilators achieve a pressure gradient between the airway opening and lungs, producing a flow of gas into the lung. This is usually created by intermittently building up a positive pressure in the proximal airway. Ventilators for infants are usually one of the following types:

1. Pressure-controlled ventilators. These ventilators deliver a preset peak inspiratory pressure (PIP), thus delivering a variable tidal volume depending largely on lung compliance. A constant flow of gas passes through the ventilator. Intermittently, the expiratory relief valve closes, and the gas flows to the infant. Pressure is limited to the desired magnitude. When the expiratory relief valve has been closed for the preset time, the valve opens, and inspiration ceases. Pressure-controlled ventilation is usually used with the technique of synchronized intermittent mandatory ventilation, which allows spontaneous breathing between ventilator breaths.
2. Volume-controlled ventilators. These ventilators deliver a preset tidal volume with a variable PIP depending largely on lung compliance. When this gas has been delivered by the piston, inspiration is terminated.

The tidal volume delivered by the ventilator must be adequate to normalize arterial oxygen and carbon dioxide. Important considerations are as follows:

- infant's tidal volume (4 to 6 mL/kg);
- compression loss in the ventilator tubing (if ventilator tubing volume is large, this may be appreciable); and
- volume losses by leaks from the tubing around the endotracheal tube.

Pressure-controlled ventilators have been the most frequently used types in neonates, but volume-controlled neonatal ventilators are being used as moderate-quality evidence from a meta-analysis of 20 randomized controlled trials, which shows that volume ventilation resulted in a reduction in death or BPD, pneumothorax, and intracranial hemorrhage.[10]

The clinician should learn preferably about and understand one or two types of ventilators rather than trying to be an expert in many types.

- Independent of the type of ventilator used, FiO_2 should initially correspond to the FiO_2 necessary to maintain an adequate oxygen saturation (90% to 95%). The clinician should watch for elevated oxygen saturations after starting mechanical ventilation because effective mechanical ventilation may result in a sudden reduction in oxygen requirement.

Ventilators have the following features:

1. Gas mixer (blender)—to allow easy adjustment of the inspired oxygen concentration between 21% and 100%.
2. Time adjustment—to allow altering of the inspiratory and expiratory times. This permits prolongation of inspiratory time in patients with a long inspiratory time constant or widespread atelectasis as well as its shortening if the time constant is short (see Fig. 10.2). Expiratory time should be prolonged when gas trapping is present or when the expiratory time constant is long. Expiratory time can be shortened when the respiratory time constant is short.
3. Expiratory relief valve—to limit the PIP. When used in combination with the inspiratory time adjustment, it allows the peak pressure to be held, generating a pressure plateau (see Fig. 10.2). A very long plateau is not beneficial. This valve also allows one to limit the peak pressure to reduce the likelihood of volutrauma or barotrauma.
4. Pressure gauge—to measure the applied airway pressures accurately. An adequate pressure monitor must be placed close to the endotracheal tube to measure correct peak inspiratory and positive end-expiratory pressures (PEEPs).
5. Alarms—to warn of inadvertent disconnections, pressure loss, high pressures, and failure of the ventilator to cycle at the proper time.
6. Humidification system—to saturate the inspired gases with water. The temperature of the inspired gas close to the endotracheal tube should be measured continuously and used to servo-control the humidification system.
7. PEEP—to maintain functional residual capacity.

8. Exhalation assist—to reduce the PEEP to desired levels when rapid rates are used. Inadvertent PEEP can be a problem with some pediatric ventilators because of a high expiratory resistance.

ALTERNATIVE MODES OF MECHANICAL VENTILATION

Technologic advances, including improvement in flow delivery systems, breath termination criteria, guaranteed tidal volume delivery, stability of PEEP, air leak compensation, prevention of pressure overshoot, pulmonary function monitoring, and triggering systems, have resulted in better ventilators. Patient-initiated mechanical ventilation, patient-triggered ventilation, synchronized intermittent mandatory ventilation, and noninvasive ventilation are increasingly being used in neonates.

1. Patient-triggered ventilation/synchronized intermittent mandatory ventilation. Patient-triggered ventilation uses spontaneous respiratory efforts to trigger the ventilator. Airflow, chest wall movements, airway pressures, esophageal pressures, or diaphragmatic electrical activity are used as indicators of the onset of the inspiratory effort. When the ventilator detects an inspiratory effort, it delivers a ventilator breath of predetermined settings (PIP, inspiratory duration, flow). Synchronized intermittent mandatory ventilation achieves synchrony between the patient and the ventilator breaths. Synchrony occurs easily in most neonates because strong respiratory reflexes during early life elicit relaxation of respiratory muscles at the end of lung inflation. Furthermore, inspiratory efforts usually start when lung volume is decreased at the end of exhalation. Synchrony may be achieved by nearly matching the ventilator frequency to the spontaneous respiratory rate or by simply ventilating at relatively high rates (60–120 breaths/minute). Triggering systems can be used to achieve synchronization when synchrony does not occur with these maneuvers.
2. Proportional assist ventilation. These ventilators reduce work of breathing. Both modes of patient-initiated mechanical ventilation discussed earlier (patient-triggered ventilation, synchronized intermittent mandatory ventilation) are designed to synchronize the onset of the inspiratory support. In contrast, proportional assist ventilation matches the onset and duration of both inspiratory and expiratory support and provides ventilation in proportion to the volume or flow of the spontaneous breath. Thus the ventilator can selectively decrease the elastic or resistive work of breathing. The magnitude of the support can be adjusted depending on the patient's needs. When compared with conventional and patient-triggered ventilation, proportional assist ventilation may reduce ventilatory pressures while maintaining or improving gas exchange.[11] Randomized clinical trials are needed to determine whether proportional assist ventilation leads to major benefits when compared with conventional mechanical ventilation.
3. Combination modes. Many of the newer-generation ventilators offer combinations of volume and pressure ventilation. Often these modes use pressure ventilation with a guarantee of a certain volume. No agreement among different ventilator manufacturers on terminology has been established, so similar modes have different names. To date, these combination modes have not been proven superior to the traditional modes.
4. Noninvasive ventilation. Noninvasive ventilation delivered nasally is being increasingly used to supplement nasal CPAP. Evidence from a meta-analysis of trials of early noninvasive ventilation with CPAP (nasal intermittent positive-pressure ventilation) demonstrated a reduction in the need for intubation without other benefits.[8] Evidence from a meta-analysis of trials on noninvasive nasal ventilation postextubation demonstrated a reduction in extubation failure and air leaks without an effect on death or BPD.[9] Noninvasive ventilation has been shown to reduce apnea and the need for ventilation. Further research is needed to determine efficiency and safety of this mode of ventilation.

EDITORIAL COMMENT: Neurally adjusted ventilator assist (NAVA) is a relatively new form of synchronization using a special nasogastric tube capable of detecting diaphragmatic electrical activity, which is then used to synchronize the ventilator breaths. Currently, NAVA is only available on one brand of ventilator, and studies are ongoing as to whether this form of ventilation will lead to better outcomes.

–John Kattwinkel

CARBON DIOXIDE ELIMINATION

CO_2 elimination largely depends on the amount of gas that passes in and out of the alveoli or alveolar ventilation (Fig. 10.4). The total amount of gas that passes in and out of the lungs (including alveoli and airways) is called *minute ventilation*. Minute ventilation may be calculated from the product of the tidal volume and respiratory frequency. Some of the tidal volume distributes to parts of the lungs (dead space) that are not involved in gas exchange (e.g., airways), so subtracting the dead space ventilation from the minute ventilation gives the alveolar ventilation. Thus increases in tidal volume (minus dead space) or frequency increase alveolar ventilation, increase CO_2 elimination, and decrease $PaCO_2$.

Tidal volume may be increased by increasing the pressure gradient between inspiration and expiration. This may be accomplished by increasing PIP or by decreasing PEEP. Tidal volume is usually independent of inspiratory and expiratory times. However, depending on the time constant of the respiratory system, very short inspiratory times may limit tidal volume delivery, and insufficient expiratory times leading to gas trapping may also limit minute ventilation.

Frequency is the other major determinant of minute ventilation. In addition to the frequency set on the ventilator, the infant may take spontaneous breaths because neonatal ventilators provide a continuous flow of gas during the expiratory phase.

Hypercapnia can be caused by hypoventilation or $\dot{V}/\dot{Q}$ mismatch. Hypoventilation is a very important cause of hypercapnia. Hypercapnia occurs when alveolar ventilation decreases. Hypercapnia caused by hypoventilation is easily managed with mechanical ventilation. Hypercapnia secondary to severe $\dot{V}/\dot{Q}$ mismatch may be more difficult to manage with mechanical ventilation. Optimal $\dot{V}/\dot{Q}$ matching occurs when the ratio of alveolar ventilation and alveolar perfusion is approximately 1.

OXYGENATION

Hypoxemia can be because of $\dot{V}/\dot{Q}$ mismatch, shunting, diffusion abnormalities, and hypoventilation.[12] $\dot{V}/\dot{Q}$ mismatch is a major cause of hypoxemia in infants with RDS and in neonates with other causes of respiratory failure. In these patients, the alveoli are poorly ventilated relative to their perfusion. In neonates with persistent pulmonary hypertension or cyanotic congenital heart disease, shunting is the predominant mechanism that leads to hypoxemia. Diffusion abnormality, typical of interstitial lung disease and other diseases that affect the alveolar–capillary interface, is not prominent in neonates with RDS and does not cause severe hypoxemia. Hypoventilation usually causes mild hypoxemia.

Unlike other causes of hypoxemia, shunting usually is unresponsive to oxygen supplementation and mechanical ventilation unless the shunt is reversed. Hypoxemia resulting from $\dot{V}/\dot{Q}$ mismatch can be difficult to manage but may be resolved if an increase in airway pressure reexpands atelectatic alveoli. Hypoxemia caused by impaired diffusion or hypoventilation usually responds to oxygen supplementation and mechanical ventilation.

In infants with RDS, oxygenation depends largely on the inspired oxygen concentration and the mean airway pressure (Fig. 10.5). Oxygenation increases linearly with increases in mean airway pressure, largely because functional residual capacity can be optimized with mean airway pressure adjustments resulting in improved $\dot{V}/\dot{Q}$ match but a very high mean airway pressure will lead to worsening of oxygenation and cardia output. Mean airway pressure is a measure of the average pressure to which the lungs are exposed during the respiratory cycle. Mean airway pressure may be calculated from the area under the curve divided by the duration of the cycle (Fig. 10.6). The equation is as follows.

$$\text{Mean airway pressure} = K\,(\text{PIP} - \text{PEEP})\,\frac{(T_I)}{(T_I + T_E)} + \text{PEEP}$$

where K is a constant that depends on the rate of increase of the airway pressure curve, PIP is peak inspiratory pressure, PEEP is positive end-expiratory pressure, T_I is inspiratory time, and T_E is expiratory time. Therefore mean airway pressure is increased by increasing any of the following (see Fig. 10.6):

1. PEEP
2. PIP
3. inspiratory-to-expiratory (I/E) ratio or inspiratory time
4. rate
5. inspiratory flow (increases K)

Although a direct relationship usually exists between mean airway pressure and oxygenation, several limitations follow:

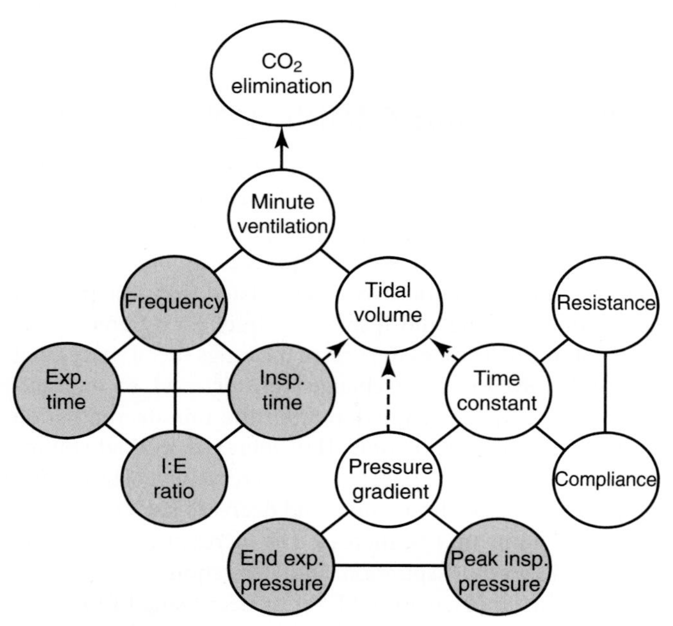

Fig. 10.4 Determinants of CO_2 elimination during pressure-limited, time-cycled ventilation. Ventilator-controlled variables are shaded. The relations between the circles that are joined by solid lines are described by simple mathematical equations. *Exp,* Expiration; *I/E,* inspiratory to expiratory; *insp,* inspiration. (Modified from Chatburn RL, Lough MD. Mechanical ventilation. In: Lough MD, Doerschuck C, Stern R, eds. *Pediatric Respiratory Therapy*. 3rd ed. Chicago, IL, Mosby Year Book; 1985:161.)

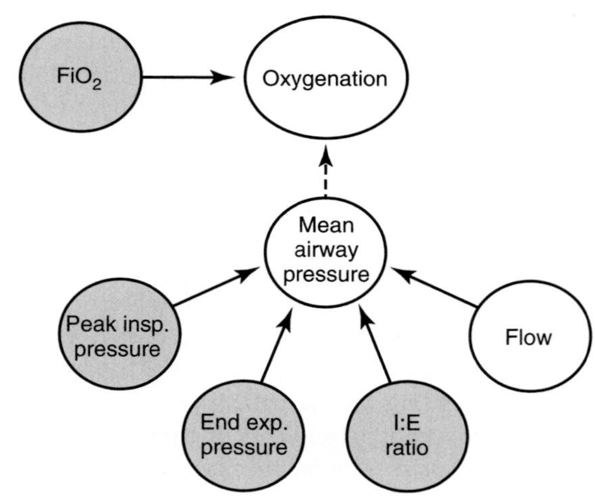

Fig. 10.5 Determinants of oxygenation during pressure-limited, timed-cycle ventilation. Circles depicting ventilation-controlled variables are shaded. Solid arrows represent mathematical relationships. *Exp,* Expiration; *I/E,* inspiratory to expiratory; *insp,* inspiration.

1. For the same change in mean airway pressure, increases in PIP and PEEP enhance oxygenation more than increases in I/E ratio.
2. Increases in PEEP are not as effective when an elevated level (>5–6 cm H_2O) is reached.
3. Very high mean airway pressure may cause lung overdistention, right-to-left shunting in the lungs (by redistribution of blood flow to poorly ventilated areas) or decreased cardiac output.
4. Long inspiratory times increase the risk for pneumothorax.

VENTILATOR SETTING CHANGES AND GAS EXCHANGE

From the earlier discussion, the effects of the changes in individual ventilator settings on blood gases can be extrapolated. The major effects are summarized in Table 10.4. Although effects may vary, these basic principles should serve as guidelines. However, when faced with an abnormal blood gas result, several alternative ventilator setting changes may be acceptable. Controversy still exists as to the optimal way to ventilate infants. It is generally preferred to provide an adequate tidal volume and then adjust the frequency to achieve sufficient CO_2 elimination. Mean airway pressure can then be changed to optimize oxygenation. The use of very high frequencies, in which short inspiratory time decreases tidal volume delivery or short expiratory time causes gas trapping and inadvertent PEEP, is not advocated.

In summary, major concepts of gas exchange in infants with RDS are that CO_2 elimination is proportional to alveolar ventilation and that oxygenation is related directly to mean airway pressure. Based on these concepts, ventilatory strategies have been developed that should provide an organized, logical, and consistent means of achieving desired blood gas results, thereby supporting the clinician in ventilator management decisions.[13] Studies in neonates with RDS, who were managed with such an algorithm, revealed more frequent correction of blood gas derangements and more appropriate efforts to wean the infant from ventilatory assistance.[12]

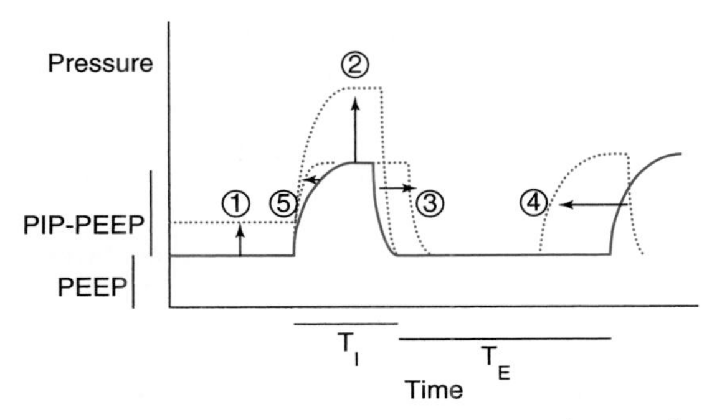

Fig. 10.6 Methods to increase airway pressure. Interventions: 1. Increase PEEP; 2. Increase PIP; 3. Increase I/E or T_I; 4. Increase rate; 5. Increase flow. *I/E,* Inspiratory-to-expiratory ratio; *PEEP,* positive end-expiratory pressure; *PIP,* peak inspiratory pressure; T_E expiratory time; T_I, inspiratory time.

MONITORING THE INFANT DURING MECHANICAL VENTILATION

During mechanical ventilation, the clinician undertakes the responsibility for the infant's gas exchange. Hence monitoring the patient's condition is vital and requires continuous observation.

The goal should be to maintain oxygen saturations between 90% and 95%, $PaCO_2$ at more than 40 mm Hg, and pH between 7.25 and 7.40. Continuous monitoring with a pulse oximeter and transcutaneous Pco_2 and Po_2 electrodes is invaluable during intubation, stabilization procedures, or weaning because blood gases can change abruptly. Because arterial CO_2 equilibrates with alveolar CO_2, quantitative end-tidal CO_2 monitoring can be used to estimate arterial CO_2. However, in patients with alveolar disease, there is incomplete equilibration of arterial and alveolar CO_2; therefore end-tidal

TABLE 10.4 Effect of Ventilator Setting Changes on Blood Gases

	Change	$PaCO_2$	PaO_2	Comments
PIP	↑↓	↓↑	↑↓	Use of high PIP increases risk of barotrauma (e.g., pneumothorax, interstitial emphysema)
PEEP	↑	↑	↑	An increase in PEEP prevents alveolar collapse and improves ventilation/perfusion relationship. A PEEP of 2 to 3 cm H_2O is physiologic. A higher PEEP is indicated in babies with RDS.
	↓	↓	↓	A decrease in PEEP may improve compliance and may improve CO_2 retention. Very high PEEP (e.g., >6 cm H_2O) is not very effective in increasing PaO_2.
Frequency	↑↓	↓↑	—	High ventilator frequencies may allow the use of low PIP and reduce the risk of pneumothorax. If I/E ratio is kept constant, frequency changes do not alter mean airway pressure and do not substantially affect PaO_2.
I/E Ratio	↑↓	—	↑↓	I/E ratio changes do not usually alter tidal volume or CO_2 elimination unless inspiratory time or expiratory time, or both, are too short.
Flow	↑↓	± ↓± ↑	± ↑± ↓	The effects of flow changes on blood gases have not been well studied in infants.

I/E, Inspiratory-to-expiratory ratio; *PEEP,* positive end-expiratory pressure; *PIP,* peak inspiratory pressure; *RDS,* respiratory distress syndrome.

CO_2 can underestimate arterial CO_2. Neonatal qualitative exhaled CO_2 monitoring is extremely useful in determining endotracheal versus esophageal tube placement because the diagnostic accuracy approximates 100%.[14]

Changes in Blood Gas Status: A Practical Approach

1. *A sudden decrease in PaO_2 accompanied by an increase in $PaCO_2$ associated with rapid clinical deterioration of the infant.* To differentiate whether the problem is with the ventilator or the infant, assess breath sounds by auscultation, listen over the stomach, and determine the position of the heart and trachea. Increase the PIP or tidal volume to see if chest rise and delivered tidal volumes improve.

   If the infant's condition improves, the problem is with lung compliance or tube patency. Then, decrease the PIP or tidal volume to see if the delivered tidal volume stays improved.

   If gas entry is diminished bilaterally, look for the following causes:

   - Decreased lung compliance. Lung compliance is very dynamic and can suddenly decrease. Action: increase PIP or tidal volume.
   - Tube displaced into nasopharynx. There may be gas entry heard over the stomach, and gas may be visibly escaping at the mouth or via a nasogastric tube with the end placed under water. Action: replace the tube.
   - Tube blocked. Tube blockage occurs especially after a few days of ventilation and afterward because of the increased accumulation of secretions. Action: suction tube briefly. If this has no effect, replace the tube.
   - Tension pneumothorax. Diminished breath sounds are heard on the affected side, and there may also be abdominal distention and an easily palpable liver and spleen; the condition is usually critical. Confirm that there is a pneumothorax using transillumination. Action: emergency relief of tension pneumothorax by inserting a chest tube or a 22-gauge catheter attached to a three-way stopcock and a 20-mL syringe into the third intercostal space at the midclavicular line or the fourth or fifth intercostal space at the anterior axillary line. Remove gas until the condition improves. If the infant has deteriorated, do not wait for a chest radiograph to perform the procedure. After stabilizing the infant, obtain a chest radiograph and consider inserting a chest tube.

   If gas entry is diminished unilaterally, check for the following causes:

   - Tube in mainstem bronchus. It is usually in the right mainstem bronchus, producing decreased gas entry on the left. Action: verify endotracheal tube measurement at the lip level. Withdraw tube 0.5 to 1 cm. Immediate improvement in gas entry will result. Recheck position by chest x-ray.
   - Unilateral pneumothorax. Radiologic confirmation of clinical diagnosis is obtained if the condition of the infant warrants a delay in initiating therapy. If not, treat as for tension pneumothorax.

   If the problem persists, try to manually inflate the lungs with a bag. If the condition improves, the problem is with the ventilator. Check the following:

   - concentration of inspired oxygen going to the ventilator
   - presence of leaks or disconnected tubing
   - mechanical or electrical failure

   If the tidal volumes have not decreased and gas entry is not diminished, lack of improvement suggests a nonrespiratory cause such as intraventricular hemorrhage, pneumopericardium, seizures, hypoglycemia, hypotension, or overwhelming sepsis. The incidence of intraventricular hemorrhage is greatly increased in infants who have a pneumothorax. The occasional occurrence of pneumoperitoneum, owing to forcing gas through the diaphragm in the periaortic spaces, can seriously mislead the clinician into the assumption that a ruptured viscus has occurred and abdominal surgery is indicated.

> **EDITORIAL COMMENT:** Airway sounds are easily transmitted across a small chest, and therefore evaluation of breath sounds can be terribly misleading in small infants. Even with "adequate" breath sounds, I would transilluminate the chest, check the placement of the endotracheal tube with a laryngoscope to be sure that the distal stripe can still be seen just proximal to the vocal cords, and perhaps replace the endotracheal tube before attributing the problem to a nonrespiratory etiology.
>
> **–John Kattwinkel**

2. *Gradual decrease in PaO_2 accompanied by an increase in $PaCO_2$ associated with gradual deterioration of the infant.* This suggests inappropriate ventilator settings. A decrease in PaO_2 suggests increasing intrapulmonary shunting resulting from progressive atelectasis.

   To improve PaO_2, consider the following measures:

   - Increase PIP.
   - Increase PEEP.
   - Increase tidal volume by 1 to 2 mL/kg (increases PIP; volume ventilator).
   - Increase the I/E ratio or the inspiratory time.
   - The responses to these maneuvers may vary, and blood gas analyses should be obtained.

3. *Gradual increase in $PaCO_2$ without gross changes in PaO_2.* A gradual increase in $PaCO_2$ is usually because of insufficient alveolar ventilation (insufficient tidal volume or frequency, or both). A gradual increase in $PaCO_2$ can also be caused by increased "anatomic" (i.e., airways, tubing) or "physiologic" (i.e., nonventilated but perfused alveoli) dead space. An increase in $PaCO_2$ is an indication for an increase in alveolar ventilation by increasing PIP or decreasing PEEP during pressure ventilation, by increasing tidal volume during volume ventilation, or by increasing cycling frequency. A reduction of anatomic dead space (e.g., shortening the endotracheal tube) may relieve hypercapnia.

To improve $PaCO_2$, increase minute ventilation by the following measures:

- Increase PIP by 2 to 5 cm H_2O (pressure ventilator).
- Increase tidal volume by 1 to 2 mL/kg (increases in PIP or tidal volume during volume ventilation).
- Increase ventilator rate by 5 to 10 breaths/minute.

4. *A decrease in $PaCO_2$ caused by overventilation.* A decrease in $PaCO_2$ is potentially dangerous because the lungs may be subjected to volutrauma if the low $PaCO_2$ is the result of ventilation with large tidal volumes. Also, alkalosis is associated with decreases in cerebral blood flow and tissue oxygen delivery. Hypocarbia is associated with periventricular leukomalacia as well as deafness. Hence a low $PaCO_2$ is an indication for a reduction in overall alveolar ventilation.
5. *Increase in PaO_2 unaccompanied by changes in $PaCO_2$.* This suggests a decrease in intrapulmonary shunting and reduction in degree of atelectasis. Because of the toxic effect of high inspired oxygen on lung tissue but the benefits of maintaining lung inflation, it is generally better to reduce the concentration of inspired oxygen to less than 40% to 70% before attempting to markedly reduce ventilator parameters.

Routine Care of the Infant

Monitoring of blood gases and respiratory status is an important aspect of supportive treatment, but attention must also be paid to temperature control, caloric and fluid intake, and metabolic balance. Clinicians should avoid excessive and unnecessary handling of the infant. Measures such as elevating the head of the bed 15 to 30 degrees, mouth care, daily assessments of readiness for extubation, and strict attention to hand hygiene may decrease the incidence of ventilator-associated pneumonia.

SPECIAL CIRCUMSTANCES

Pulmonary Interstitial Emphysema

Infants with severe RDS and those who have pulmonary interstitial emphysema (PIE) on chest x-ray may respond better to a rapid ventilating rate (60–150 breaths/minute), low peak pressure, low PEEP, and high-frequency ventilation.

Pulmonary Hypertension/Meconium Aspiration Syndrome

Infants with severe pulmonary hypertension with or without meconium aspiration syndrome may benefit from inhaled nitric oxide, a selective pulmonary vasodilator. Nitric oxide reduces the need for extracorporeal membrane oxygenation (ECMO) in neonates with pulmonary hypertension.[15] Other therapies include oxygen, surfactant, sedation, analgesia, and inotropic support, but there are limited data to support their clinical efficacy.

Neonatal Surgery

Intubation of the very low–birth-weight infant in the intensive care nursery and use of a ventilator during surgery are preferable. In this way, inspired oxygen and inspired gas temperature can be carefully controlled, as can pain management. Continuous oxygen saturation and intermittent arterial blood gas analyses are monitored throughout surgery to maintain the infant with adequate blood gases.

Drug Therapy

The use of muscle paralysis or sedatives may be useful in infants who "fight" the ventilator when $PaCO_2$ is increasing and PaO_2 is decreasing on "maximum" ventilation. A marked improvement in oxygenation may be observed, particularly in infants with pulmonary hypertension.

EDITORIAL COMMENT: Muscle paralysis for babies on ventilators must be viewed with caution. The histamine-releasing effect of competitive neuromuscular blocking agents (particularly curare) can cause hypotension and, rarely, bronchospasm. Some patients may require higher ventilator settings after paralysis as their own respiratory efforts are eliminated. Also, a system failure (e.g., extubation, tubing disconnection) in a paralyzed patient will be rapidly fatal.

–John Kattwinkel

Sedatives and analgesics are increasingly being used in the care of neonates requiring assisted ventilation. These agents may be used in combination with muscle paralysis. However, when it is desirable to preserve the patient's own respiratory effort, sedatives or analgesics may be used without muscle paralysis. Fentanyl and morphine sulfate are commonly used sedatives/analgesics. Sedatives and analgesics may decrease respiratory drive and should be used carefully. Routine opiate administration during conventional ventilation in neonates does not improve outcomes.[16]

Antibiotics should be used whenever a bacterial infection is suspected.

Preextubation systemic corticosteroids and postextubation racemic epinephrine reduces airway resistance when there is laryngeal edema. However, if the endotracheal tube is not too large, is well positioned, and is not mobile during ventilation, problems with the glottis following extubation are rarely observed.

Weaning From Ventilator

Ventilator weaning can be attempted when the concentration of inspired oxygen is approximately 50% or less. The PIP is gradually reduced as is the ventilator rate to allow the patient to contribute more to his or her ventilation. When the ventilator breaths elicit minimal chest rise, ventilator frequency is minimal (~10–20/minute), and the infant has adequate blood gases, the infant should be accomplishing almost all of the minute ventilation spontaneously. At this point, most infants can be successfully extubated to CPAP.

HIGH-FREQUENCY VENTILATION

Although conventional mechanical ventilation has contributed to a substantial reduction in neonatal mortality,

TABLE 10.5 Techniques for High-Frequency Ventilation

	High-Frequency Positive-Pressure Ventilation	Jet Ventilation	Flow Interruption	Oscillatory Ventilation
Tidal volume	> Dead space	> or < Dead space	> or < Dead space	< Dead space
Expiration	Passive	Passive	Passive	Active
Airway pressure waveform	Variable	Triangular	Triangular	Sine wave
Frequency	60–150/min	60–600/min	300–900/min	300–900/min

air leaks or BPD occurs in about 20% to 40% of ventilated very preterm infants. Although the precise pathophysiologic mechanisms underlying these forms of lung injury have not been determined, high ventilatory pressures and the resultant volutrauma are thought to be contributing factors.

High-frequency ventilation encompasses modes of assisted ventilation that employ smaller tidal volumes and higher frequencies than conventional techniques. The characteristics of the various high-frequency ventilators overlap (Table 10.5). High-frequency oscillatory ventilation can exchange gas adequately with small volumes (even smaller than dead space at times) at extremely high frequencies. Oscillatory ventilation is unique because exhalation is actively generated, as opposed to other forms of high-frequency ventilation in which exhalation is passive. High-frequency jet ventilation is characterized by the delivery of gases from a high-pressure source through a small-bore injector cannula. It is possible that the fast flows out of the cannula produce areas of relative negative pressure that entrain gases from their surroundings. High-frequency flow interruption also delivers small tidal volumes by interrupting a flow of pressure source, but in contrast to jet ventilation, it does not use an injector cannula. Furthermore, clinicians may employ widely varying ventilatory strategies. High-frequency ventilation may improve blood gases because, in addition to the gas transport by convection, other mechanisms may become active at high frequencies (for example, variable velocity profiles of gas during inspiration and exhalation, gas exchange between parallel lung units, increased turbulence, and diffusion may improve blood gases).

There has been extensive clinical use of the various high-frequency ventilators in neonates with RDS. High-frequency oscillator ventilation does not offer important advantages over conventional ventilation. High-frequency oscillator ventilation may decrease BPD, but it may increase air leaks.[17]

High-frequency positive-pressure ventilation employs standard ventilators modified with low-compliance tubing and connectors so that an adequate tidal volume may be delivered despite high ventilatory rates (60–150 breaths per minute) and short inspiratory times. When compared with conventional ventilation at rates of 30–40 breaths/minute for conventional mechanical ventilation with inspiratory times longer than 0.5 seconds, high-frequency positive-pressure ventilation reduced pneumothoraces, and there was a trend for reduction in mortality, but BPD was not affected.[18]

Air Leaks

High-frequency ventilation has been used to treat established air leaks. High-frequency positive-pressure ventilation in preterm infants with RDS prevents the development of pneumothoraces.[18] Jet ventilation in neonates with PIE may accelerate resolution of the air leak.[19] However, air leaks may be increased with oscillatory ventilation.[17]

EDITORIAL COMMENT: The technique of high-frequency ventilation requires major changes in the concept of gas flow in the lung. Currently it is believed that by vibrating the gas column, gas exchange is promoted by setting up asymmetric flow within the airways rather than by convection, which is the predominant mechanism of conventional ventilation. Studies suggest that high-frequency ventilation may improve ventilation/perfusion matching throughout the respiratory cycle, thus permitting lower peak inflation pressures and lower inspired oxygen concentrations. High pressure, high volume, and high oxygen have all been implicated in the development of bronchopulmonary dysplasia.

–John Kattwinkel

COMPLICATIONS OF ASSISTED VENTILATION

Despite major improvements in equipment and increased expertise in the applications of assisted ventilation, the care of smaller and sicker infants may result in many complications (Table 10.6). Pulmonary air leaks are one of the most common complications and occur in approximately 5% to 10% of ventilated patients. Pneumothorax may occur because of the lung disease or may result from the use of high PIP and inspiratory time, particularly in infants who "fight" the ventilator. However, spontaneous pneumothoraces are commonly observed, even in healthy neonates without lung disease. Transillumination of the chest is useful for immediate diagnosis, but radiographic confirmation should be obtained if the patient's status is not life-threatening. PIE is associated with gas trapping and impaired gas exchange and occurs in infants with severe pulmonary disease.

BPD, a form of chronic lung disease that occurs in neonates, is one of the most important complications associated with assisted ventilation. BPD was initially defined as an oxygen requirement and characteristic chest x-ray at 28 days of life. With the increasing survival of extremely low-birth-weight infants, the definition was changed to an oxygen

TABLE 10.6 Complications of Assisted Ventilation

Pulmonary air leaks	Pneumothorax, pneumomediastinum, pneumoperitoneum, pulmonary interstitial emphysema, pneumopericardium, pulmonary venous air embolism
Airway injury	Erosion, granuloma, palatal groove, subglottic stenosis, necrotizing tracheobronchitis
Endotracheal tube related	Dislodgement, extubation, atelectasis, occlusion, tracheal stenosis, vocal cord paralysis
Infection	Pneumonia, septicemia, meningitis
Miscellaneous	Volutrauma, bronchopulmonary dysplasia, hyperinflation, impaired cardiac output, intracranial hemorrhage, patent ductus arteriosus, retinopathy of prematurity

requirement at 36 weeks' postmenstrual age. The chest x-ray of infants with BPD often shows opacification of the lung fields, atelectasis, fibrosis, and overdistention. Although its precise pathophysiology remains obscure, immature and ill lungs as well as volutrauma appear to be contributing factors. The increasing incidence of BPD is largely as a result of improved survival rates of infants with immature or ill lungs. The incidence of BPD varies widely and may be as high as 50% in infants weighing less than 1000 g who require assisted ventilation from birth. Management of these patients must be multidimensional, with particular emphasis on prevention of further lung injury, maintenance of adequate oxygenation and nutrition, and prevention of infection and fluid overload. The effect of differences in care practices on the incidence of BPD suggests that optimal respiratory management of very low–birth-weight infants may decrease the incidence of BPD.[20] As discussed previously, clinical trials of early CPAP and minimal ventilation strategies have shown moderate reductions in the incidence of death and/or BPD.

EXTRACORPOREAL MEMBRANE OXYGENATION

ECMO is a technique whereby blood drains from the patient; then the blood passes through a membrane for extracorporeal exchange of oxygen and carbon dioxide and is then routed back to the patient. ECMO is particularly useful in neonates with transient pulmonary artery hypertension and severe hypoxemia resulting from a right-to-left shunt. Common conditions associated with pulmonary hypertension include meconium aspiration syndrome, RDS, idiopathic pulmonary hypertension of the neonate, pneumonia/sepsis, asphyxia, and congenital diaphragmatic hernia. Neonates with these and other conditions are considered candidates for ECMO if they have severe impairment of oxygenation. The alveolar-to-arterial oxygen gradient (A/aDO_2) is frequently used to evaluate impairment of oxygenation. An alveolar–arterial oxygenation gradient of 600 to 620 for 8 to 12 hours despite maximal therapy is usually considered an indication for ECMO. In the past, predicted survival rate for infants with such severe respiratory failure was as low as 20%. In marked contrast, following the introduction of ECMO, survival currently approximates 90% in these infants.

Complications during ECMO may be related to the primary disease or to technical aspects of the circuit. Intracranial hemorrhage and infarction, hemodynamic alterations, and hematologic disturbances occur occasionally. The improved survival rate has not been accompanied by an increase in permanent morbidity.

Inhaled Nitric Oxide

High pulmonary artery resistance is common in infants with pulmonary disease. Pulmonary artery vasodilators have been used in treatment of these infants, but the systemic vasodilatory effects have precluded efficacy and widespread use. Nitric oxide, a molecule produced endogenously by endothelial cells and other cell types, regulates pulmonary artery tone in utero and after birth. Exogenous nitric oxide reduces pulmonary vascular resistance during the perinatal period. Inhaled nitric oxide has been shown to improve oxygenation and reduce the need for ECMO in well-designed, large, randomized, controlled trials in term and late preterm neonates with severe hypoxemic respiratory failure.[21] However, inhaled nitric oxide has not been shown to have consistent benefits in preterm infants with RDS.[22]

SUMMARY

Survival of infants with severe pulmonary disease has dramatically improved with the improved used of techniques of assisted ventilation. Meticulous care is necessary with the following: strategies to optimize conventional ventilation and alternative modes of ventilation; placement of endotracheal tubes; frequent blood gas determinations; continuous monitoring of oxygen saturation, transcutaneous Po_2 and transcutaneous $PaCO_2$; and fluid, caloric, and thermal balance. However, most of the difficulty with adequately ventilating small infants resides not in the ventilator, but in the infant's extremely immature lungs and airways. The clinician should identify and correct atelectasis, increased dead space, and gas trapping, and treat the patient's pulmonary problems with appropriate ventilatory strategies rather than look for a better ventilator to solve the problems. Long-term morbidity associated with mechanical ventilation is still a major problem. Because assisted ventilation is a critical part of neonatal intensive care, a thorough understanding of pulmonary mechanics and gas exchange, as well as knowledge of the techniques and alternative modes of ventilation, is essential to optimize its use.

CASE 10.1

You are called to attend the delivery of a 26 weeks' gestational-age infant whose mother received a full course of antenatal steroids.

After resuscitation with bag-and-mask ventilation, the infant requires 30% FiO_2. A trial of continuous positive airway pressure (CPAP) is indicated in this infant. True or false?
CPAP used early in preference of mechanical ventilation reduces lung injury. The statement is true.

Surfactant should be given as soon as possible to this infant because it has been shown to improve outcomes. True or false?
Surfactant prophylaxis and early surfactant were shown to reduce mortality and air leaks when compared with intubation without surfactant. However, the trials of CPAP versus early surfactant have shown no benefits of prophylactic or early surfactant. The statement is false.

CASE 10.2

Before mechanical ventilation using a pressure-limited ventilator, the PaO_2 is 30 mm Hg, and the $PaCO_2$ is 60 mm Hg in 100% oxygen in a preterm baby. Thirty minutes after initiating therapy, a blood gas analysis is performed.

PaO_2 has risen to only 35 mm Hg, and $PaCO_2$ is still 60 mm Hg. It is advisable to switch to a volume-controlled ventilator because the lungs are too stiff to be adequately ventilated by a pressure-controlled machine. True or false?
The statement is false. The initial ventilator settings were probably somewhat subjective and should be adjusted to the infant's requirements. The high $PaCO_2$ indicates hypoventilation, and an attempt should be made to increase minute ventilation by increasing peak inspiratory pressure (PIP). The increase in PIP should also improve oxygenation. Adjustments should be made, checking blood gases until oxygen saturation is higher than 85% and $PaCO_2$ is less than approximately 50 mm Hg.

PaO_2 is only 35 mm Hg and $PaCO_2$ is 35 mm Hg. It might be helpful to increase positive end-expiratory pressure (PEEP) before increasing PIP further. True or false?
A PEEP of 5 to 6 cm H_2O will help prevent small airway closure. This may prevent atelectasis and reduce the degree of right-to-left shunt. The statement is true.

The PaO_2 has risen to 140 mm Hg. This is a dangerous level, and the concentrations of inspired oxygen should be reduced at once. True or false?
In immature infants, arterial oxygen tensions in that range have been associated with retinopathy of prematurity. The statement is true. Priority should be given to reducing the concentration of inspired oxygen in this situation versus altering other ventilator settings. Decrease inspired oxygen concentrations frequently and continuously monitor oxygen saturation.

CASE 10.3

A preterm infant born at 26 weeks' gestation with birth weight of 850 grams is admitted to the neonatal intensive care unit (NICU) on nasal continuous positive airway pressure (CPAP). His initial chest x-ray shows air bronchograms and a fine granular lung pattern consistent with respiratory distress syndrome (RDS). Over the past hour, his work of breathing has increased, and his oxygen requirement has risen from 25% to 35% to maintain oxygen saturations between 90% and 95%. The arterial blood gas pH is 7.25, and the P_{CO_2} is 59 mm Hg, Po_2 of 35 mm Hg, and HCO_3 of 14 mEq/L.

Which of the following should be the next step in the respiratory care of this infant?

1. Continue on CPAP.
2. Switch to high-flow nasal cannula.
3. Intubate and administer surfactant.
4. Briefly administer positive-pressure ventilation via bag-and-mask device, then place back on CPAP.

CPAP is effective to support extremely preterm infants with RDS when the FiO_2 is less than 40% to 50%. CPAP has been shown to be more effective in babies at this stage compared with high-flow nasal cannula and surfactant. In more mature infants, CPAP is also effective even when the FiO_2 is even higher.

CASE 10.4

A blood gas analysis is performed during mechanical ventilation on a preterm baby on 80% oxygen. There has been no change in the clinical condition of the infant since the previous estimation.

It is found that $PaCO_2$ has changed from 36 to 24 mm Hg, and pH has risen from 7.38 to 7.56. This is a sign that the infant is recovering and ventilator settings should remain unchanged. True or false?
A $PaCO_2$ of 24 mm Hg suggests overventilation. The resulting alkalosis is dangerous because it causes a reduction in oxygen delivery and cerebral blood flow and may be associated with lung injury. The $PaCO_2$ should be brought back to a more physiologic range by reducing minute ventilation (i.e., by reducing peak inspiratory pressure [PIP], tidal volume, or frequency). The statement is false.

The arterial oxygen tension is 30 mm Hg; pH is 7.30; and $PaCO_2$ is 45 mm Hg. The ventilator should not be changed. True or false?
$PaCO_2$ and pH are satisfactory, but oxygenation is too low. Positive end-expiratory pressure (PEEP) can be increased to increase mean airway pressure. The statement is false.

CASE 10.4—cont'd

The arterial oxygen tension is 56 mm Hg; pH is 7.23, and $PaCO_2$ is 26 mm Hg on low ventilator settings. Although the pH is within normal range, there is severe metabolic acidosis, which should be corrected with intravenous sodium bicarbonate. True or false?

Spontaneous hyperventilation on the ventilator may be as a result of compensation for a metabolic acidosis. Correction of severe metabolic acidosis may be indicated with intravenous bicarbonate. However, search should be made for the etiology of the acidosis, such as reduced cardiac output, anemia, sepsis, or pneumothorax, and the underlying cause corrected.

CASE 10.5

During mechanical ventilation, an infant becomes cyanotic. He is noted to be making very vigorous respiratory efforts, with considerable intercostal and sternal retractions out of phase with the ventilator.

This is a good indication for sedation and adjusting the ventilator to accommodate the infant's respiratory pattern. True or false?
Although "out of phase" respiration could account for this clinical picture, an obstructed endotracheal tube, a pneumothorax, or other major problem must first be excluded. The statement is false.

Gas entry is diminished over the left lung field. The diagnosis is pneumothorax, which should be relieved immediately. True or false?
Diminution of gas entry over the left lung field may be as a result of (1) the endotracheal tube slipping into the right mainstem bronchus, or (2) pneumothorax. The steps should be to check the endotracheal tube length of insertion (at the lip) and, if necessary, to withdraw the endotracheal tube slightly. If this fails to improve the infant's condition, a chest x-ray is indicated unless the infant is deteriorating rapidly and the left side of the chest is tympanic, transillumination is positive, and the heart is displaced. Emergency relief of a pneumothorax is then indicated. The statement is false.

A sample for blood gas estimation is obtained immediately, and resuscitative measures are started. When the blood sample is analyzed 1 hour later, the results show PaO_2 to be 127 mm Hg and $PaCO_2$ to be 8 mm Hg. This suggests that the infant had been crying before this cyanotic spell. True or false?
The most likely explanation for these bizarre blood gas findings is that an air bubble was left in the syringe, and equilibration has occurred between gas in the blood and gas in the air. The values tend to approximate the PaO_2 and $PaCO_2$ of room air. Samples drawn for blood gases must be bubble free, capped, iced, and analyzed in a timely manner. The statement is false.

Following prolonged mechanical ventilation and extubation, an infant may have some stridor and copious secretions. The stridor usually decreases spontaneously. True or false?
Despite the use of nontoxic endotracheal tubes, there can be some laryngeal edema. This, together with large quantities of secretions and impairment of tracheal ciliary function, may lead to some degree of upper airway obstruction, which decreases in 2 to 3 days. The statement is true.

CASE 10.6

A 1500-g male infant delivered precipitously after 31 weeks' gestation, whose mother had not received antenatal steroids, had signs of respiratory distress at birth. Apgar scores were 4 and 7 at 1 and 5 minutes, respectively. At initial assessment, the infant was tachypneic (60 breaths/minute) and had nasal flaring and retractions. Breath sounds were equal but diminished bilaterally. Dubowitz examination was consistent with maternal dates. Immediate chest x-ray showed diffuse granularity and air bronchograms. Blood sugar was 45 mg/dL, hematocrit 43%, blood pressure 50/32 (mean, 40 mm Hg), and temperature 36.3° C. In 55% oxygen by continuous positive airway pressure (CPAP), arterial blood gas values from an umbilical catheter were as follows: pH 7.15, P_{CO2} 55, and Po_2 40. The infant was intubated, given surfactant, and placed on a pressure-limited ventilator at peak inspiratory pressure (PIP) of 15 cm H_2O, positive end-expiratory pressure (PEEP) of 4 cm H_2O, frequency (rate) of 50 breaths/minute, inspiratory-to-expiratory (I/E) ratio of 1:5, and FiO_2 of 50%. The patient initially responded well, but 2 hours later, arterial blood gas values were as follows: pH 7.30, P_{CO2} 46, and Po_2 35.

Note: There may be several arterial blood gases and ventilator changes between each situation presented. Assume good breath sounds, chest rise, and blood pressure throughout, unless otherwise stated. Attempting to answer questions by looking at data subsequently presented is only confusing.

Select the best answer, although more than one answer may be acceptable.

What is the most appropriate ventilator setting change at this time?

1. Increase PIP.
2. Increase PEEP.
3. Increase frequency.
4. Decrease I/E ratio (e.g., 1:3 to 1:3.5).
5. Increase FiO_2.

The patient has hypoxemia with adequate ventilation and relatively low FiO_2. The best answer is to increase FiO_2.

At 12 hours of age, the ventilator settings and arterial blood gas values are pressure 20/4 cm H_2O, frequency 50 breaths/minute, I/E ratio 1:1.5, FiO_2 80%, pH 7.16, $PaCO_2$

Continued

CASE 10.6—cont'd

55 mm Hg, and PaO_2 135 mm Hg. What is the most appropriate change at this time?
1. Decrease PIP and decrease FiO_2.
2. Increase PEEP and decrease FiO_2.
3. Increase frequency and decrease FiO_2.
4. Increase I/E ratio and decrease FiO_2.
5. Decrease I/E ratio and decrease FiO_2.

The patient has hyperoxemia and mild respiratory acidosis. Of the alternatives given, increasing frequency is the most effective way to increase minute ventilation and resolve the respiratory acidosis. FiO_2 should be decreased.

At 18 hours of age, the ventilator settings and arterial blood gas values are pressure 20/5 cm H_2O, frequency 70 breaths/minute, I/E ratio 1:1, FiO_2 90%, pH 7.19, $PaCO_2$ 52 mm Hg, and PaO_2 35 mm Hg. What is the most appropriate change at this time?
1. Increase PIP.
2. Increase PEEP.
3. Increase frequency.
4. Increase I/E ratio.
5. Increase FiO_2.

Respiratory acidosis is still present but is now accompanied by hypoxemia. Increasing peak PIP is the best choice because the resultant increase in minute ventilation and mean airway pressure should improve $PaCO_2$ and PaO_2. Increasing frequency is also an acceptable alternative.

QUESTIONS

True or False

The most immature infants benefit from prophylactic and early intubation and surfactant treatment. True or false?
Randomized controlled trials have shown that even the most immature infants such as 24 to 25 weeks have a lower mortality with early CPAP when compared with early surfactant. The statement is false.

True or False

If you set a pressure-limited safety valve on a volume-controlled ventilator at 30 cm H_2O, a pneumothorax will not occur. True or false?
Although pneumothorax is particularly associated with high inflation pressures, it can occur at any time during either mechanical or spontaneous ventilation—even at low PIP. The statement is false.

True or False

The larger the volume of ventilator tubing, the less the compression volume at any given pressure.
During ventilation, a proportion of the gas delivered by the pump ("compression volume") does not reach the alveoli. The larger the volume of ventilator tubing, the greater the compression volume. Hence ventilator tubing should be low volume and nondistensible. The statement is false.

True or False

Condensation of water in ventilator inspiratory tubing can be reduced by placing as much tubing as possible inside the incubator.
A temperature gradient exists between air outside and inside the incubator. Water vapor condenses at lower temperatures, and droplets appear in tubing exposed to low temperatures. If water condensation occurs in the tubing, the gas delivered to the infant will have a water saturation lower than gas coming out of the humidifier. Heated ventilator tubing can also reduce condensation. The statement is true.

True or False

If a small leak develops between the trachea and the endotracheal tube during pressure-controlled ventilation, there will be adequate compensation by the ventilator.
A pressure-controlled ventilator delivers gas until a preset pressure is attained. Although it is possible to compensate for a small leak (e.g., around the endotracheal tube), a large leak may cause failure to reach the desired PIP. The statement is true.

True or False

During mechanical ventilation with 80% oxygen (for RDS), an increase in PIP may increase the PaO_2 to 200 mm Hg without altering $PaCO_2$ significantly.
When breathing a high concentration of oxygen, a low PaO_2 indicates venous admixture or shunting. This shunting is thought to occur primarily through areas of atelectatic lung. Effective ventilation may open some of these atelectatic areas, reducing the degree of shunting, with an ensuing increase in PaO_2. However, a large right-to-left shunt may not increase $PaCO_2$ markedly because the arteriovenous difference for CO_2 is only 4 mm Hg. Resolution of the shunt may not decrease $PaCO_2$, so the statement is true.

True or False

During mechanical ventilation, pH remains constant as long as the $PaCO_2$ does not change.
The pH depends on the $PaCO_2$ and the bicarbonate level. Metabolic and respiratory factors are often closely associated (e.g., a period of apnea is associated with an increase in $PaCO_2$ and a decrease in PaO_2, the latter leading to tissue anoxia and anaerobic metabolism). However, metabolic and respiratory factors may operate quite independently. The statement is false.

The reference list for this chapter can be found online at www.expertconsult.com.

11

Glucose, Calcium, and Magnesium

Richard A. Polin, David H. Adamkin

These infants are remarkable not only because like foetal versions of Shadrach, Meshach and Abednego, they emerge at least alive from within the fiery metabolic furnace of diabetes mellitus, but because they resemble one another so closely that they might well be related. They are plump, sleek, liberally coated with vernix caseosa, full-faced and plethoric… They convey a distinct impression of having had such a surfeit of both food and fluid pressed upon them by an insistent hostess that they desire only peace so that they may recover from their excesses. And on the second day their resentment of the slightest noise improves the analogy while their trembling anxiety seems to speak of intrauterine indiscretions of which we know nothing.

James W. Farquhar

The fetus receives a constant supply of glucose, calcium, and magnesium. Fetal plasma levels are closely regulated by maternal metabolic homeostasis, placental exchange, and fetal regulatory mechanisms. Abruptly at birth, termination of nutrient supply requires profound changes in energy and mineral metabolism. The provision of exogenous nutrients and the mobilization of endogenous fuel and mineral stores determine homeostasis. The result is the potential for rapid changes in plasma glucose and calcium levels during the first days of life. The infant who is premature, growth restricted, stressed, or born to a diabetic mother is at increased risk for problems with homeostasis, hypoglycemia, and hypocalcemia. As we will see, these issues are common and made even more challenging by the fact that most of these infants are asymptomatic. Therefore appropriate screening with protocols that look at identifying these infants along with a management plan is critical and will be reviewed particularly as it relates to diagnosis of hypoglycemia.

GLUCOSE

Fetal and Neonatal Energy Metabolism

An understanding of fetal and neonatal fuel metabolism has emerged from studies in animals and humans.[1] Fetal energy consumption is high, deriving from growth needs and energy storage as well as metabolic maintenance. Maternal glucose crosses the placenta via facilitated diffusion (primarily by the glucose transporters GLUT1 and GLUT3) and serves as the principal energy source for the fetus. There is a linear relationship between maternal and fetal glucose concentrations, with fetal concentrations 60% to 80% of maternal concentrations.[2] This linear relationship is present even during episodes of maternal hyperglycemia secondary to maternal diabetes or glucose infusions. Therefore in high-risk situations associated with maternal hyperglycemia, the neonate is born with approximately 70% of the maternal concentration at delivery.

Under normal circumstances, fetal gluconeogenesis is negligible; however, fetal gluconeogenesis may occur during episodes of prolonged maternal hypoglycemia or starvation. Glucose alone cannot account for the total oxygen consumption of the fetus. Other substrates such as lactate, free fatty acids (FFA), ketones, and amino acids cross the placenta and are potential energy sources for the fetus.

Energy is stored rapidly near term. Fat storage exceeds 100 kcal/day in the ninth month and accounts for 14% of total body weight at term.[3] Glycogen stores, a vital source of energy in the first hours of life, increase toward term to reach about 5% by weight in liver and muscle and up to 4% in heart muscle. These energy stores are compromised by prematurity and by intrauterine growth restriction. Acute perinatal distress or chronic fetal hypoxia can particularly diminish glycogen stores and predispose the infant to hypoglycemia after birth.

Insulin and glucagon do not cross the placenta and are present in the fetus by 12 and 15 weeks, respectively. The fetal insulin response to glucose infusion is poor very early in gestation. At the end of gestation, the insulin response is improved but remains blunted. Fetal blood insulin levels gradually rise toward term, whereas fetal glucagon levels remain low. The resulting high insulin-to-glucagon ratio promotes the accumulation of hepatic glycogen stores and suppresses gluconeogenesis, thus preparing the fetus for birth and maintenance of postnatal glucose homeostasis.

Insulin is an important hormone for fetal growth. The presence of maternal hyperglycemia and fetal hyperinsulinemia, as seen in the infant of a diabetic mother, is associated with macrosomia with elevated liver glycogen and total body fat stores.[4,5] Macrosomia in the presence of fetal hyperinsulinemia without maternal hyperglycemia is seen in infants with Beckwith-Wiedemann syndrome and in the rare infant with hyperinsulinemic hypoglycemia, which suggests that fetal insulin and not maternal hyperglycemia may be the important growth-promoting factor. Conversely, infants born with pancreatic aplasia and those with transient neonatal diabetes mellitus have little or no insulin present and demonstrate severe intrauterine growth restriction.

At birth, cold stress, work of respiration, and muscle activity cause increased energy demands. Because of the interrupted supply of maternal glucose, the newborn must call on stored fuels to maintain blood glucose levels. This transition at birth is facilitated by increased catecholamine and reversal of the insulin:glucagon ratio with increased glucagon, which promotes lipolysis and glycogenolysis. Decreased insulin levels and increased cortisol levels also facilitate glucose homeostasis at birth. Rapid glycogenolysis causes hepatic glycogen to fall to low levels within 24 hours in a fasted neonate. Gluconeogenesis is important in postnatal glucose homeostasis to supplement glycogenolysis. Lipolysis begins at birth, with the respiratory quotient decreasing from 1.0 in the fetus to less than 0.8 during the first day as most tissues switch to burning fat. Metabolism of FFA and ketones stabilizes blood glucose levels by sparing glucose utilization in heart, liver, muscle, and brain (ketones); and supporting hepatic gluconeogenesis by producing the reduced form of nicotinamide adenine dinucleotide.

Transitional Neonatal Hypoglycemia and Postnatal Glucose Homeostasis in Search of Hypoglycemia

The Pediatric Endocrine Society (PES) analyzed available data on this unique period that the first 48 hours is in all mammals, not just human babies.[6] This brief period of hypoglycemia is commonly observed in normal newborns during the transition from fetal to extrauterine life.

Using neuroendocrine and metabolic data, they determined that this 48-hour period was characterized by a relative hyperinsulinism, low ketone levels, inappropriate preservation of glycogen, and mean glucose level at the nadir of 55 to 65 mg/dL.[6] This resembles a known form of congenital hyperinsulinism, causing a lowering of the plasma glucose threshold for suppression of insulin secretion.[7] This 55 to 65 mg/dL range, which is the mean range at the nadir, turns out to be the same level below which adults and older children demonstrate neurogenic symptoms; therefore this observation, along with the rest of the metabolic profile, led the PES to suggest this was the critical range of glucose to maintain.[7] They further argued that this range is where the adult and older children activate mechanisms as seen in the neuroendocrine and metabolic profiles for brain protection.[7] The PES also reported on the fact that by 72 hours or so of life, the glucose levels rise to those similar to levels in older children and adults.[6] To summarize then, the PES using these endocrine-based mechanisms for determining critical levels of glucose found hyperinsulinemia accompanied by suppressed levels of ketones[8] and inappropriately large glycemic responses to glucagon and epinephrine,[9] suggesting the absence of alternative fuels, and the inappropriate preservation of glycogen in a newborn with low glucose levels, all consistent with a hypoketotic hyperinsulinemia.[2]

The American Academy of Pediatrics (AAP)[10] looked at the postnatal glucose homeostasis data and noted at birth that although the infant's blood glucose concentration is about 70% of the maternal level, it falls rapidly to a low nadir by 1 hour, as low at 20 to 25 mg/dL.[11] This nadir is prevalent in healthy neonates and is seen in all mammalian newborns. These levels are transient and begin to rise over the first hours and days of life. This observation is considered to be part of the normal adaptation for postnatal life that helps establish postnatal glucose homeostasis.[8,9,11] Are there advantages to having a lower blood glucose concentration compared with adults the first 48 hours? A decrease in glucose concentration soon after birth might stimulate physiologic processes that are required for survival, including promoting glucose production through gluconeogenesis and glycogenolysis.[12] Also, the decrease in glucose concentration enhances oxidative fat metabolism, stimulates appetite, and may help adapt to fast feed cycles.[9]

The AAP guideline, during the first hours of transition, uses the lower ranges of glucose values, not the mean from fetal and neonatal data.[9,13] It also emphasizes the clinical examination and condition of the infant. The AAP also looked at neurodevelopmental data to determine if there was any validated level of neuroglycopenia (the critical threshold of plasma glucose at which brain injury occurs).

The fundamental question of how best to manage asymptomatic newborns with low glucose concentrations remains unanswered. Balancing risks of overtreating newborns with low glucose concentrations who are undergoing normal transition following birth against the risks of undertreating those in whom low glucose concentrations are pathologic, dangerous, and/or a harbinger of serious metabolic disease remains a challenge.[14]

In the newborn, basal glucose production and utilization is 4 to 6 mg/kg/min. This high glucose utilization compared with the adult is primarily because of the higher ratio of brain weight to body weight in the newborn infant. During euglycemic conditions, most of the brain's metabolic needs are met by oxidation of glucose. When the availability of glucose is limited, alternative cerebral fuels such as lactate and ketone bodies may be used. Although these alternative fuels provide some protection to reduce the risk of hypoglycemia-induced brain injury in the newborn, the brain requires a continuous glucose supply; thus these alternative substrates are unable to completely replace glucose as a fuel for brain metabolism.

Blood glucose level at birth is 60% to 80% of the simultaneous maternal plasma concentration. Glucose concentrations normally decrease over 1 to 2 hours and stabilize at a nadir. Over the next 48 hours, the glucose levels increase, and by 72 hours or so, they more resemble adult levels than those levels associated with the first 48 hours of life.

Neurodevelopmental Outcome

The neurodevelopmental outcome approach is to find the critical threshold of plasma glucose associated with brain injury or where "neuroglycopenia" occurs in the newborn. In the adult, this is 50 mg/dL. Neuroglycopenia is the level at which there is an inadequate supply of glucose for the brain. This level is known for the newborn. This research was profoundly influenced by a multicenter nutrition study from the United Kingdom published in 1988.[15] The authors of the study evaluated blood glucose levels, drawn daily initially and then weekly, until discharge on 661 infants less than 1850 g at birth who were enrolled in a nutrition study looking at early diets and cognitive outcomes. They found that a critical glucose level less than 47 mg/dL would reliably predict adverse outcome.[15] The number of days below this value was strongly related to reduced scores for mental and motor development at 18 months' corrected age. Similar but less dramatic differences were found when the children were seen again as part of a larger study[16] when the children were 7 to 8 years old. These findings profoundly influenced neonatal care across the developed world ever since. This value, "47" mg/dL, became the worldwide standard and was applied to term healthy appropriate for gestational age (AGA) neonates as the gold standard "critical threshold," even though this study had no term infants in it. The authors themselves suggested in a letter that there is "difficulty providing causation when an observational approach is used" and remarked that "when such observations generate hypotheses or legitimate clinical concerns, this should stimulate future studies and randomized controlled trials."[17]

Almost 25 years later from the United Kingdom came a prospective trial including infants less than 32 weeks' gestation who had blood glucose levels measured daily for the first 10 days of life. A total of 47 had a blood glucose level less than 47mg/dL on at least 3 days of the first 10 days of life.[18] All were matched for appropriate variables with those who never had a value less than 47mg/dL. No differences were found in developmental progress or physical disability at 2 years of age.[18] Some 81% of the cohort were matched again at 15 years of age, and they were almost identical for full-scale IQ. The inclusion of children who had a level less than 47 mg/dL for greater than 4 days and another group less than 37 mg/dL on three occasions did not alter these results.[18] They concluded the study "found no evidence that recurrent low blood glucose levels (<47 mg/dL) in the first 10 days of life pose a hazard to preterm infants." This study does not imply that low blood glucose levels cannot be damaging in preterm infants.[18]

Studies from the Children with Hypoglycemia and Their Later Development (CHYLD) have added studies with serial follow-up and included use of glucose gel and subcutaneous glucose sensors. A large prospective of at risk-term and late preterm neonates defined hypoglycemia as less than 47 mg/dL. They identified 53% of 404 at-risk infants with hyperglycemia based on the four risk groups (late preterm, small-for-gestational-age [SGA] infants, large-for-gestational-age [LGA] infants, and infants of mothers with diabetes [IDM]). The fact that 53% of patients had glucose less than 47 mg/dL and 19% a level less than 36 mg/dL confirms the decision by the AAP to focus on these patients. They found no increase in risk for neurosensory impairment at 2 years of age with hypoglycemia. They also performed blinded interstitial glucose monitoring, and noted that intermittent blood sampling missed 25% of additional episodes of less than 47mg/dL. Even with aggressive treatment, including dextrose gel, nearly 25% of infants experienced 5 hours of glucose concentration less than 47 mg/dL. Risk of impairment was not increased, even in those infants with hypoglycemia that was unrecognized and therefore not treated (interstitial monitoring). Unexpected was the observation that higher glucose levels after treatment for hypoglycemia tended to be associated with neurodevelopmental impairment. Those infants who spent a larger proportion outside the central range of 54 to 2 mg/dL in the first 48 hours of life had worse outcomes.[19]

Next, 614 term and late preterm infants at risk for hypoglycemia were studied[20] using the same risk factors again as AAP.[10] The study included patients without hypoglycemia and both treated and untreated hypoglycemia. Hypoglycemia again defined as plasma glucose less than 47 mg/dL. Infants were screened and treated with the aim of keeping plasma glucose concentrations greater than 47mg/dL. Surprisingly, there were long and undetected periods of hypoglycemia detected only on interstitial monitoring. Almost one out of four had hypoglycemic episodes not detected on intermittent sampling.[20] Twenty-five percent of those undetected episodes lasted greater than 5 hours during the first week of life.[20] Further studies are underway to determine the utility of continuous glucose monitoring.[21]

Neurosensory impairment or processing difficulty at age 2 was reported among five subgroups, including a reference group who never had hypoglycemia, any episode of hypoglycemia greater than 3 days, or severe hypoglycemia (<36 mg/dL). There was no association between hypoglycemia and neurodevelopmental outcome at age 2 years.[20] However, data on the 4.5-year follow-up demonstrated executive function difficulties in those infants suffering more than one episode of hypoglycemia.[20] This was found only with continuous glucose monitoring,[20] not with intermittent sampling.

Revisiting transitional hypoglycemia is a unique perinatal cohort reported from Arkansas, which included 1400 infants at 10 years of age who had a single glucose level in the first hours of life correlated with fourth grade examinations from across the state.[22] Glucose levels of interest ranged from less than 30 to 45mg/dL. They found that a single episode of hypoglycemia, defined as less than 40 mg/dL that resolved by 3 hours of age, was associated with a 50% reduction in the odds of achieving proficiency in literacy and numeracy at age 10.[22] This group of patients represented all the births during a calendar year, so they were mostly made up of late preterm and term infants. As mentioned earlier, this was a single episode, so their levels were followed by a second value above the cutoff of less than 30, less than 40, and less than 45 mg/dL, respectively. An editorial reviewing this study suggest weaknesses include little information about the management strategies for hypoglycemia and no rates for breastfeeding.[23] Furthermore, they expressed concern whether the exposure group had a single episode of hypoglycemia because only the first two blood glucose levels were measured, and recurrent low glucose levels are common in at-risk infants, even throughout the first week.

As yet, there is no reason to assume that link between transitional neonatal hypoglycemia and subsequent poor academic performance is causal. It is possible that a brief period of hypoglycemia is a marker for other perinatal issues, perhaps including events during intrauterine development.

Should we now consider universal screening of all newborns because the Arkansas study suggests transient hypoglycemia may be associated with poorer academic achievement at 10 years of age? Screening is only justified when you can impact outcome with the result of the screening test. The brief period of hypoglycemia was diagnosed at 90 minutes of age, but the actual result was available 30 minutes after that. The second measurement showing resolution came 70 minutes after the first screen or at 3 hours of age. It is unlikely that any intervention could shorten the exposure to the brief period of "hypoglycemia."

Dextrose Gel and Continuous Glucose Monitoring

As mentioned in some of the CHYLD studies, dextrose gel can be a simple and inexpensive therapy administered directly to the buccal mucosa. A Cochrane review[24] that included two trials with 312 infants concluded that treatment of infants with neonatal hypoglycemia with 40% dextrose gel reduces the incidence of mother–infant separation for treatment and increases the likelihood of full breastfeeding after discharge compared with placebo gel. No evidence suggests occurrence of adverse effects during the neonatal period or at 2 years' corrected age.[24] Oral dextrose gel should be considered first-line treatment for infants with neonatal hypoglycemia.[24]

Also, the application of continuous interstitial glucose monitoring was used in many of the studies reviewed in the section on neurodevelopmental outcomes. A relatively large study included babies greater than 32 weeks who were at risk of hypoglycemia.[25] These infants were all admitted to the neonatal intensive care unit (NICU) and received routine treatment, including intermittent blood glucose measurements and blinded continuous interstitial monitoring. Continuous monitoring was well tolerated in 102 infants. There was good agreement between blood and interstitial glucose concentrations. Low glucose concentrations (<47 mg/dL) were detected in 32 babies (32%) with intermittent blood sampling and in 45 babies (44%) with continuous monitoring.[25] There were 265 episodes of low interstitial glucose concentrations, 215 (81%) of which were not detected with blood glucose measurement. One hundred seven episodes in 34 babies lasted greater than 30 minutes, and 78 (73%) were not detected with blood measurement.

They concluded that continuous interstitial glucose monitoring detects many more episodes of low glucose concentration than blood glucose measurement. The physiologic significance of these previously undetected episodes is unknown.[25]

Methodology

Sampling Problems

Several factors need to be considered when interpreting glucose concentrations. First, blood glucose concentrations are 10% to 15% lower than simultaneous plasma concentrations. This is particularly pronounced when the hematocrit is very high. Second, use of capillary samples from unwarmed heels may lead to an underestimation of venous glucose concentration because of stasis. Finally, glucose concentrations decline as much as 18 mg/dL/hour at room temperature while analysis is awaited. Thus all samples should be analyzed immediately or placed on ice.

Point-of-Care Testing

Although plasma glucose determination in the laboratory using the glucose oxidase reaction is the optimum method, point-of-care (POC) testing using reflectance glucometers offers the advantage of speed and small sample volumes, and permits quick clinical responses. The common thresholds for diagnosis of hypoglycemia with the low ranges of 35 mg/dL to 45 mg/dL and hyperglycemia at 170 mg/dL are at the limits of accuracy for many POC glucose analyzers. These should be looked at as screening devices and not the ultimate test for the diagnoses of hypoglycemia. The sensitivity for detecting hypoglycemia ranges from 80% to 100%, and the negative predictive values range from 80% to 96%, depending on the device and parameters used. Therefore confirmatory plasma glucose concentrations should be measured if hypoglycemia is detected using a POC device or if the infant has symptoms consistent with hypoglycemia, even if the POC test value shows a normal blood glucose concentration.

Hypoglycemia

Definition

Hypoglycemia in newborns is often asymptomatic. The most frequent symptoms are jitteriness and cyanosis. Other symptoms include convulsions, hypotonia, coma, poor feeding, apnea, congestive heart failure, high-pitched cry, abnormal eye movements, and temperature instability with hypothermia. In small, sick infants, symptoms may easily be missed. When symptoms are present, the age of onset is most commonly between 24 and 72 hours.

Because these symptoms are nonspecific, they often occur in newborns who are normoglycemic and have other problems. For example, jitteriness, the most common symptom, is found in up to 44% of normal newborns as well as in infants with a variety of other conditions (Box 11.1). Hypoglycemia must, therefore always be confirmed by chemical analysis and by response to treatment.

Recommendations for Screening and Management of Neonatal Hypoglycemia

The AAP Committee on Fetus and Newborn Medicine ratified, for another 5 years, their statement on postnatal glucose homeostasis, including an algorithm for screening and management of low glucose levels (Fig. 11.1).[10] Also, a reevaluation of transitional hypoglycemia has been published by the PES.[6]

A recent editorial called "Imperfect Advise" contrasts the two organizations' approaches as reviewed earlier in the chapter, and we will offer suggestions on how to combine the advice from both for management.[27] Also, critical to the PES recommendations is to make the diagnoses of persistent hypoglycemic syndromes before discharge.[7]

BOX 11.1 Differential Diagnosis of Jitteriness and Tremors in the Newborn

Metabolic disorders
- Hypoglycemia
- Hypocalcemia
- Hypomagnesemia
- Hyponatremia
- Hypernatremia

Neonatal drug withdrawal
- Opiates
- Selective serotonin reuptake inhibitors (SSRIs)
- Cocaine

Central nervous system disorders
- Malformations
- Hypoxic-ischemic encephalopathy
- Intracranial hemorrhage

Polycythemia

Sepsis, meningitis

The AAP clinical report is not inclusive of all preterm infants but focused on late preterm as well as specifically term SGA, LGA, and IDM at-risk patients. Of course, symptomatic infants are all screened.[10] All preterm infants were not included, based on the assumption that the vast majority of more premature infants would be cared for in intermediate care or in the NICU, where routine screening is already in place. The PES expands the list for screening to symptomatic, perinatal stress (birth asphyxia, cesarean section for fetal distress), maternal preeclampsia, meconium aspiration syndrome, premature or postmature, IDM, family history of genetic hypoglycemia, and congenital syndromes or abnormal physical features (Box 11.2).[7]

The PES does not offer screening times, nor does it discuss treatment or prevention. Its targets for therapy include less than 50 mg/dL in the first 48 hours, and then if intravenous fluids are required, a value greater than 60 mg/dL should be achieved.[7] It addresses the first 48 hours of life for these recommendations, then emphasizes the need for careful attention to not missing cases of persistent hypoglycemia (Box 11.2).

The AAP guidance applies to only the first 24 hours of life.[10] Actionable ranges of 25 to 40 mg/dL for the first 4 hours of life and then 35 to 45 mg/dL from 4 hours to 24 hours of age are the operational thresholds for the AAP.[10]

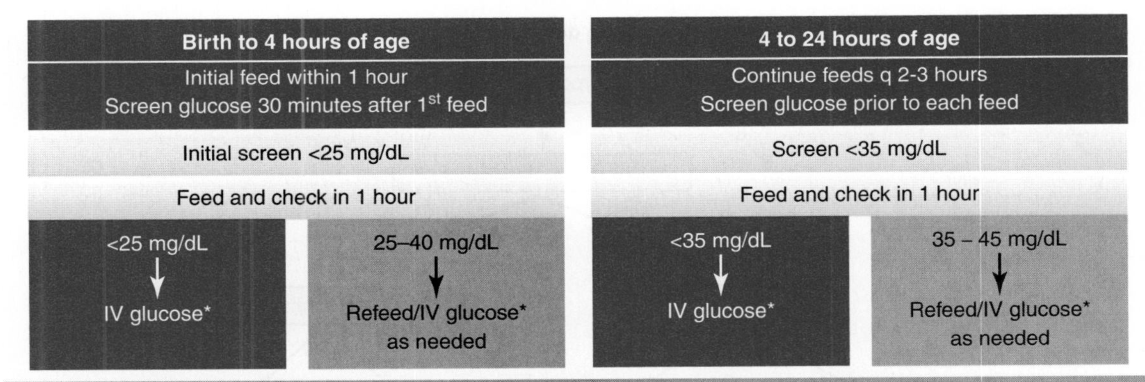

Screening and Management of Postnatal Glucose Homeostasis in Late Preterm and Term SGA, IDM/LGA Infants
[(LPT) Infants34 – 36 6/7 weeks and SGA (screen 0-24 hrs); IDM and LGA ≥34 weeks (screen 0-12 hrs)]
Symptomatic and <40 mg/dL → IV glucose
ASYMPTOMATIC
Birth to 4 hours of age
Initial feed within 1 hour
Screen glucose 30 minutes after 1st feed
Initial screen <25 mg/dL
Feed and check in 1 hour
<25 mg/dL
IV glucose*
25–40 mg/dL
Refeed/IV glucose* as needed
4 to 24 hours of age
Continue feeds q 2-3 hours
Screen glucose prior to each feed
Screen <35 mg/dL
Feed and check in 1 hour
<35 mg/dL
IV glucose*
35 – 45 mg/dL
Refeed/IV glucose* as needed
Target glucose screen ≥45 mg/dL prior to routine feeds
* Glucose dose = 200 mg/kg (dextrose 10% at 2 mL/kg) and/or IV infusion at 5–8 mg/kg per min (80–100 mL/kg per d). Achieve plasma glucose level of 40–50 mg/dL.
Symptoms of hypoglycemia include: Irritability, tremors, jitteriness, exaggerated Moro reflex, high-pitched cry, seizures, lethargy, floppiness, cyanosis, apnea, poor feeding.

Fig. 11.1 Screening for and management of postnatal glucose homeostasis in late-preterm (LPT]; 34–36 6/7 weeks) and term small-for-gestational age *(SGA)* infants and infants who were born to mothers with diabetes *(IDM)*/large-for-gestational age *(LGA)* infants. LPT and SGA (screen 0–24 hours), IDM and LGA greater than or equal to 34 weeks (screen 0–12 hours). *IV* indicates intravenous. (From Adamkin DH, Committee on Fetus and Newborn Clinical Report—postnatal glucose homeostasis in late-term and preterm infants. *Pediatrics.* 2011;127:175.)

BOX 11.2 Recognizing and Managing Neonates at Increased Risk for a Persistent Hypoglycemia Disorder

Neonates at increased risk of hypoglycemia and require glucose screening:

- Symptoms of hypoglycemia
- Large for gestational age (even without maternal diabetes)
- Perinatal stress
  - birth asphyxia/ischemia; cesarean delivery for fetal distress
  - maternal preeclampsia/eclampsia or hypertension
  - intrauterine growth restriction (small for gestational age)
  - meconium aspiration syndrome, erythroblastosis fetalis, polycythemia, hypothermia
- Premature or postmature delivery
- Infant of diabetic mother
- Family history of a genetic form of hypoglycemia
- Congenital syndrome (e.g., Beckwith-Wiedemann), abnormal physical features (e.g., midline facial malformations, microphallus)

Neonates in whom to exclude persistent hypoglycemia before discharge:

- Severe hypoglycemia (e.g., episodes of symptomatic hypoglycemia or need for intravenous dextrose to treat hypoglycemia)
- Inability to consistently maintain preprandial PG concentration greater than 50 mg/dL up to 48 h of age and greater than 60 mg/dL after 48 h of age
- Family history of genetic form of hypoglycemia
- Congenital syndromes (e.g., Beckwith-Wiedemann), abnormal physical features (e.g., midline facial malformations, microphallus)

From: Thornton PS, Stanley CA, DeLeon DD, et al. Recommendations from the Pediatric Endocrine Society for evaluation and management of persistent hypoglycemia in neonates, infants, and children. *J Pediatr.* 2015;167:238-245.

Glucose levels rise after the first 48 hours of life and should be similar to those of older children by 72 to 96 hours of age.[6] The AAP recommendation for treatment below the actionable range after feeding is based on individual risk assessment and examination of the infant.[10] Target glucose concentrations when intravenous fluids are required should exceed 45 mg/dL.[10]

What is clear with all recommendations is that the greater the glucose threshold set for screening and the more often these tests are done, the more often asymptomatic patients with low glucose levels will be identified. This could result in a neonatal intensive care admission, separation from mother for an asymptomatic infant, and provide a hindrance to successful breastfeeding.

Persistent Hypoglycemic Disorders

Some neonates can be identified by various clinical features as being high risk for severe hypoglycemia during the first 48 hours after delivery.[28,29] Also, some of these neonates are at risk for persistent hypoglycemia beyond 48 hours of life (Box 11.2). These include not only the rare infants with genetic hypoglycemic disorders, such as congenital hyperinsulinism or hypopituitarism, but also those with relatively more common prolonged neonatal hyperinsulinism (also referred to as perinatal stress hyperinsulinism) associated with birth asphyxia, intrauterine growth restriction, or toxemia.[30–32] Fig. 11.2 provides an algorithm showing how the major categories of hypoglycemia may be determined from the critical sample of beta-hydroxybutyrate, FFA, and growth hormone.[7]

The recommendations from the editorial to use the AAP and PES recommendations together include using the AAP

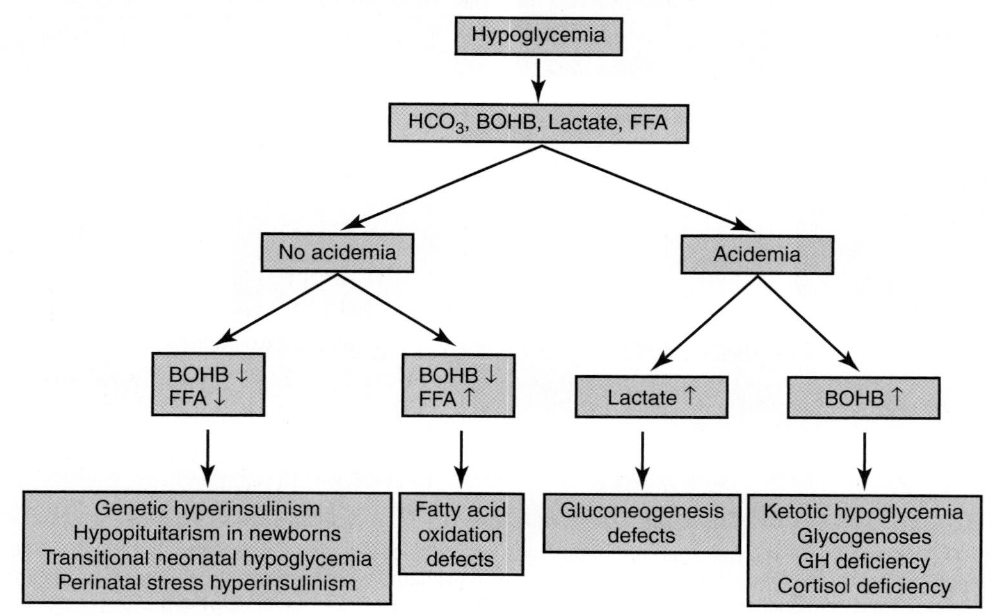

Fig. 11.2 Algorithm showing how the major categories of hypoglycemia can be determined with information from the critical sample. *BOHB,* Beta-hydroxybutyrate; *FFA,* free fatty acids; *GH,* growth hormone. (From Thornton PS, Stanley CA, DeLeon DD, et al. Recommendations from the Pediatric Endocrine Society for evaluation and management of persistent hypoglycemia in neonates, infants, and children. *J Pediatr.* 2015;167:238-245.)

BOX 11.3 Risk Factors for Neonatal Hyperglycemia

- Preterm birth
- Intrauterine growth restriction (IUGR)
- Increased stress hormone levels
- Increased catecholamine infusions
- Increased glucocorticoid concentrations (from use of antenatal steroids, postnatal glucocorticoid administration, and stress)
- Increased glucagon concentrations
- Early intravenous (IV) lipid infusion and high rates of infusion
- Higher-than-needed rates of IV glucose infusion
- Insufficient pancreatic insulin secretion (preterm and IUGR)
- Absence of enteral feedings, leading to diminished "incretin" secretion and action, which limits potential to promote insulin secretion

guidelines for the first 24 hours and then for 24 to 48 hours to use greater than 45 mg/dL.[27] To increase vigilance to diagnose possible persistent cases of hypoglycemia, consider delaying discharge from the nursery until infants who required intravenous fluids for symptomatic or asymptomatic low glucose levels or those with borderline low glucose levels demonstrate glucose levels after 48 hours greater than 70 mg/dL through several normal feed-fast cycles.[27] More data on the frequency and success of diagnosing persistent hypoglycemia will be necessary to support this strategy.

Hyperglycemia

Hyperglycemia (glucose concentration of >150 mg/dL) is a common, serious problem of very immature infants. Risk factors include low birth weight (especially when <1000 g), earlier gestational age, administration of intravenous glucose infusions (especially glucose infusion rates of >6 mg/kg/min), high illness severity, and glucocorticoid therapy (Box 11.3). Factors contributing to hyperglycemia in premature infants are reduced glucose-induced insulin secretion, immature insulin processing, and increased ratio of GLUT1 to GLUT2 in tissues.[33,34] Hepatic glucose release may fail to decrease when exogenous glucose is given. Stress from illness increases catecholamine release, which may further elevate glucose levels by inhibiting glucose use and insulin release.

Hyperglycemia has been associated with increased length of hospitalization, risk of death, and incidence of intraventricular hemorrhage.[35,36] The mechanism of injury may involve increases in plasma osmolarity (a glucose level of 450 mg/dL is equivalent to an additional 24 mOsm/L) and glucosuria leading to renal water and electrolyte losses and vascular fluid shifts.

Treatment and prevention are accomplished by adjusting the glucose infusion rate to that tolerated by each individual infant. Rates of 4 to 8 mg/kg/min are usually tolerated; however, lower glucose infusion rates may be needed. Glucose infusion rates should be expressed as milligrams per kilogram per minute because variations in either the volume or glucose content of the fluid result in alterations in actual delivery of glucose to the infant. Along with improving nitrogen balance, early amino acid administration at the time of birth in low-birth-weight infants decreases the incidence of hyperglycemia, possibly because of improved insulin release.[37,38] Occasionally, an insulin infusion starting at 0.01 U/kg/min but increasing to 0.1 U/kg/min if needed is indicated in those infants in whom decreasing the glucose infusion rate is inadequate or improved caloric intake is desired. Frequent monitoring of blood glucose concentration is crucial both to determine the adequacy of therapy and to avoid episodes of hypoglycemia.

EDITORIAL COMMENT Among very low–birth-weight infants, early neonatal hyperglycemia is common and is associated with increased risk of death and major morbidities. Sinclair et al. wished to assess effects on clinical outcomes of interventions for preventing hyperglycemia in very low–birth-weight neonates receiving full or partial parenteral nutrition.[39] They searched for randomized or quasi-randomized controlled trials of interventions for prevention of hyperglycemia in neonates with a birth weight of less than 1500 g or a gestational age of less than 32 weeks. They found only four eligible trials. Two trials compared lower and higher rates of glucose infusion in the early postnatal period. These trials were too small to assess effects on mortality or major morbidities. Two trials, one a moderately large multicenter trial,[40,41] compared insulin infusion with standard care. Insulin infusion therapy reduced hyperglycemia but increased death before 28 days and was complicated by hypoglycemia. Reduction in hyperglycemia was not accompanied by significant effects on major morbidities; effects on neurodevelopment are awaited. The authors concluded, "There is insufficient evidence from trials comparing lower with higher glucose infusion rates to inform clinical practice. Large randomized trials are needed, powered on clinical outcomes including death, major morbidities, and adverse neurodevelopment." With regard to insulin infusion, they noted that "the evidence reviewed does not support the routine use of insulin infusions to prevent hyperglycemia in very low-birth-weight neonates. Further randomized trials of insulin infusion may be justified. They should enroll extremely low-birth-weight neonates at very high risk for hyperglycemia and neonatal death."

Among 580 infants less than 27 weeks' gestation in Sweden,[42] a daily prevalence of hyperglycemia greater than 180 mg/dL (10 mmol/L) of up to 30% was observed during the first 2 postnatal weeks, followed by a slow decrease in its occurrence thereafter. Increasing parenteral carbohydrate supply with 1 g/kg/day was associated with a 1.6% increase in glucose concentration ($P < .001$).

Hyperglycemia was associated with more than double the 28-day mortality risk ($P < .01$). Insulin treatment was associated with lower 28- and 70-day mortality when given to infants with hyperglycemia, irrespective of the duration of the hyperglycemic episode ($P < .05$).

Neonatal Diabetes

Neonatal diabetes is a rare disorder. Most infants with neonatal diabetes are born at or near term, with marked intrauterine growth restriction reflecting low levels of insulin and insulin-like growth factor I. Weight loss, dehydration, hyperglycemia, and occasional ketosis usually appear in the first month of life. Seventy to eighty percent of cases involve an abnormality on chromosome band 6q24 caused by uniparental disomy of chromosome 6, duplication of paternal 6q24, or loss of methylation at the differentially methylated region at the 6q24 locus.[43,44] Treatment is with insulin, with a usual daily dose of 2 to 6 U.

The transient form of the disease usually resolves within a few months. However, many infants subsequently develop diabetes later in childhood or early adulthood. Approximately 50% of patients have permanent neonatal diabetes, and remission never occurs.[45] Permanent neonatal diabetes is associated with activating mutations to the K_{ATP} channel in the pancreatic beta cell, causing the channel to remain open and preventing insulin secretion. Some of these patients are responsive to sulfonylurea, which binds to the sulfonylurea receptor and helps close the K_{ATP} channel.[45,46,47]

MINERAL DISORDERS IN THE NEONATE

Fetal Calcium and Phosphorous Metabolism[48]

The placenta actively transports calcium to the fetus and maintains fetal total and ionized calcium levels at about 1 mg/dL above the respective maternal levels.[48] Between 28 weeks' gestation and term, fetal weight triples, but calcium content quadruples as bone mineral density progressively increases (Fig. 11.3). Fetal acquisition of calcium averages 150 mg/kg/day throughout this period. Although a full-grown adult contains about 1200 grams of calcium, calcium content is closely related to birth weight. A term infant has about 30 grams of calcium, most of which is acquired in the third trimester.

The placenta allows fetal bone calcification to proceed normally by actively transporting calcium and phosphorous. The principle regulator of fetal calcium transport is parathormone-releasing protein, which is produced by the placenta and fetal parathyroid glands.[50] The syncytiotrophoblasts of the placenta have mechanisms for calcium transport that are very similar to that found in the intestine. The transplacental calcium pump is regulated by parathyroid hormone (PTH)–related peptide, which is secreted by the placenta. Although not as well defined, transport of phosphorous may depend on a Na+ and pH–dependent active transport mechanism. The calcium drain causes a modest decrease in maternal calcium levels near term. Maternal parathyroid activity, 1,25-dihydroxyvitamin D levels, calcium absorption, and calcium mobilization from bone are all increased during pregnancy.[51] PTH and calcitonin do not cross the placenta; however, 25-hydroxyvitamin D (25OHD) does. Serum levels of 25OHD in the pregnant woman are not increased but vary with the mother's vitamin D intake, liver synthesis geography, and season. The human fetal parathyroid secretes PTH from about the 10th week of gestation, and intestinal receptors for 1,25 $(OH)_2D$ can be demonstrated by 13 weeks' gestation.[52,53] Fetal PTH levels are suppressed during gestation and play a minor role in transplacental calcium transfer. A comparison of fetal and maternal minerals and regulatory hormone levels are shown in Table 11.1.

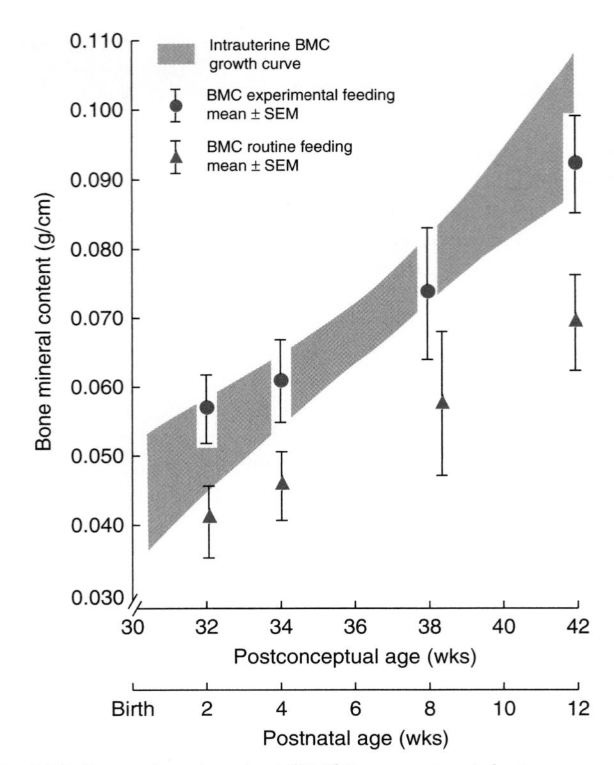

Fig. 11.3 Bone mineral content *(BMC)* in premature infants compared with intrauterine bone mineralization. The shaded area is the in utero rate of BMC increase and shows progressive bone mineralization during gestation until term. Premature infants fed Similac 20 (triangles) have diminished bone mineral accumulation; in contrast, infants fed formula with calcium (1260 mg/L), phosphorus (630 mg/L), and vitamin D (1000 U/L) (circles) have intrauterine rates of bone mineralization. These latter infants received calcium, 220 to 250 mg/kg/day, and phosphorus, 110 to 125 mg/kg/day. This calcium intake exceeds the in utero rate of calcium accumulation (150 mg/kg/day); the failure of BMC to exceed intrauterine rates in this group is possibly a result of fecal losses. *SEM,* Standard error of the mean. (From Steichen J, Gratton T, Tsang R, et al. Osteopenia of prematurity: the cause and possible treatment. *J Pediatr.* 1980;96:528.)

TABLE 11.1 Comparison of Serum Mineral Values Between the Fetus and Mother

Calcium	Fetus	>>	Mother	Late gestation
Phosphate	Fetus	>>	Mother	Late gestation
Magnesium	Fetus	>	Mother	Late gestation
iPTH	Fetus	<<	Mother	End of gestation
$1,25(OH)_2D$	Fetus	<	Mother	Late gestation
Calcitonin	Fetus	>	Mother	At term

iPTH, Intact parathyroid hormone; >, more than; >>, much more than;<, less than.

During pregnancy, maternal 25OHD crosses the placenta, and at term, fetal levels are 75% to 100% of maternal levels. The fetal kidneys can produce $1,25(OH)_2D$, but the synthesis is suppressed by the high serum levels of calcium and phosphorous and the low levels of PTH. There is likely some transfer of $1,25(OH)_2D$ from the maternal circulation.

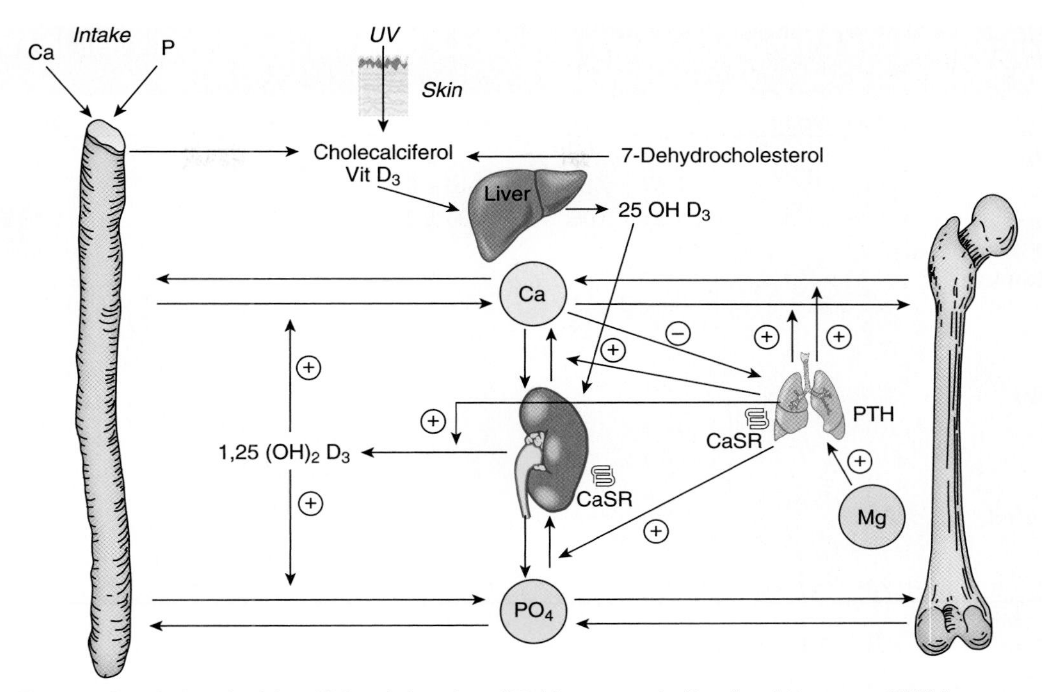

Fig. 11.4 Regulation of calcium (Ca) and phosphate (PO_4) homeostasis. Parathyroid hormone (PTH) increases Ca release from bone, Ca resorption in the kidney, and $1,25(OH)_2D_3$ excretion from the kidney. PTH production is stimulated by low Ca and inhibited by low Mg and high $1,25(OH)_2D_3$. Vitamin D increases Ca release from bone and Ca and PO_4 absorption from the intestine. Vitamin D production is stimulated by high PTH and low PO_4. *CaSR,* Calcium-stimulating response; *OH,* hydroxylase; *P,* phosphorus; *UV,* ultraviolet light; *Vit,* vitamin. (From Martin RJ, Fanaroff AA, Walsh MC, eds. Disorders of calcium, phosphorus, and magnesium metabolism in the neonate. In: *Fanaroff and Martin's Neonatal-Perinatal Medicine: Diseases of the Fetus and Infant.* 10th ed. Philadelphia, PA: Elsevier Saunders; 2014.)

Transitional Changes in Mineral Metabolism[54]

At birth, the constant placental calcium supply is interrupted. Although the premature baby has skeletal reserves of calcium, the maintenance of serum calcium concentration requires both rapid changes in endocrine function and the equilibrium between serum and bone. The factors affecting calcium in the neonate can be summarized as follows (Fig. 11.4):

PTH mobilizes calcium from bone, promotes calcium absorption from the gut, and increases renal phosphate excretion. Levels are low in cord blood, suppressed by the mild hypercalcemia caused by placental transport.[55] Postnatally, PTH concentrations rise for the first 48 hours in term infants and decrease by the end of the first week. Preterm infants have a more sustained rise in PTH. The rise in PTH levels is a physiologic response to decreasing calcium levels. However, the rise in PTH levels is somewhat deficient, resulting in the lower physiologic nadir for calcium levels (especially in preterm infants). Term babies usually achieve normal calcium levels by the second week of life; however, preterm infants may have lower calcium levels for an extended period of time. PTH secretion and function require magnesium.

1. Vitamin D is required for effective PTH action on both bone and gut. Fetal concentrations of 25OHD vary directly with gestational age and maternal plasma concentrations.[51] Newborn stores are usually adequate unless there is significant maternal dietary inadequacy or poor exposure to sunlight.[56] Levels of 1,25-dihydroxyvitamin D depend on both maternal plasma concentrations and synthesis in the fetal kidney.[56] Vitamin D supplementation during pregnancy can lessen the postnatal fall in serum calcium levels compared with unsupplemented women.
2. Calcitonin inhibits calcium mobilization from bone. Levels are elevated in neonates.[56] The placenta also produces calcitonin and supplies it to the fetus.[53]
3. Serum phosphate level increases after birth, and even more so after birth asphyxia.
4. Calcium is sensed in plasma via a specific calcium-sensing receptor (CaSR) complex.[58] The CaSR is present in the parathyroid chief cells and renal tubular cells, but also in bone cartilage and other tissues (including the brain).[54] The *CaSR* gene is located on chromosome band 3q13.3-21. When calcium binds to the extracellular domain of the CaSR, it alters PTH secretion via two second messengers. The CaSR monitors extracellular Ca^{2+} concentrations, allowing appropriate PTH secretion and renal tubular handling of calcium. Magnesium also binds the CaSR but is less potent. Several clinical disorders that result from molecular abnormalities of the CaSR leading to either loss or gain of function have been described. Heterozygous inactivating mutations result in familial benign hypercalcemia or familial hypocalciuric hypercalcemia (FHH). These mutations switch off PTH secretion at a higher concentration of calcium than normal and result in hypercalcemia. Homozygous mutations result in severe neonatal

TABLE 11.2 Early Life Changes in Serum Calcium, PTH, and Vitamin D Levels in Full-Term and Preterm Infants

	Cord Blood	24 hr	48 hr	96–120 hr	30 days
Calcium, nmol/L					
Full term	2.42 ± 0.08	2.17 ± 0.10	2.16 ± 0.08	2.22 ± 0.12	2.52 ± 0.08
Preterm	2.28 ± 0.09	1.91 ± 0.06	1.86 ± 0.07	2.08 ± 0.11	2.43 ± 0.06
Intact PTH, pg/mL					
Full term	5.1 ± 3	33 ± 8	30 ± 5	28 ± 16	
Preterm	4.5 ± 3	72 ± 17	56 ± 20	36 ± 14	
25(OH)D, ng/mL					
Full term	13 ± 3	12 ± 2		12 ± 2	17 ± 1
Preterm	10 ± 3	8 ± 2		12 ± 2	17 ± 2
1,25(OH)$_2$*D*, pg/mL					
Full term	38 ± 4	74 ± 9		100 ± 5	61 ± 4
Preterm	37 ± 6	62 ± 9		128 ± 29	108 ± 13

PTH, Parathyroid hormone.
From Hochberg Z, ed. *Vitamin D and Rickets. Endocrine Development,* Vol 6. Basel, Switzerland: Karger; 2003:34-49.

hyperparathyroidism. Activating mutations of the receptor result in hypocalcemia and hypercalciuria, a condition known as ADHR1.

At the end of gestation, the calcium levels (10–11 mg/dL) in fetal plasma (total and ionized) are higher than they are in the mother and are independent of the maternal concentrations (Table 11.2).[61] Phosphorous levels are also significantly higher in the fetus. There is normally a decrease in the serum calcium level in the first hours after birth that continues for 24 to 48 hours; serum calcium concentrations then rise and reach stable levels by 5 to 10 days of age. In healthy full-term infants, mean total calcium levels fall from 2.3 to 2.9 mmol/L (9.0–11.4 mg/dL) at birth to 1.9 to 2.6 mmol/L (7.8–10.2 mg/dL) at 24 hours. Mean ionized calcium levels fall from 1.3 to 1.6 mmol/L (5.2–6.4 mg/dL) at birth to 1.1 to 1.36 mmol/L (4.4–5.4 mg/dL) at 24 hours. Levels rise gradually, so that by 1 week of age mean ionized calcium levels reach 1.4 mmol/L (5.6 mg/dL). Healthy premature infants 33 to 36 weeks of age have lower calcium levels at 24 to 48 hours but otherwise are not different from term infants. Reference values for smaller preterm infants have not been well characterized.

After birth, the kidneys play a key role in regulating calcium and phosphorous homeostasis. Under normal circumstances, 98% of filtered calcium is reabsorbed in the tubules. Calcium excretion normally increases in the first 2 weeks of life. The kidney in preterm and term neonates responds normally to PTH.

Calcium is absorbed passively and through a vitamin D–dependent mechanism in the intestine. Serum levels of 25OHD and 1,25(OH)$_2$D are lower than maternal levels. Furthermore, infants born to mothers with vitamin D deficiency will have a diminished vitamin D status. Circulating 1,25(OH)$_2$D levels rise to adult levels in the first 2 days of life. In premature infants, most calcium absorption in the intestine is absorbed via nonvitamin D–dependent mechanisms. As the infant matures, vitamin D–dependent mechanisms become more important.

Calcium Measurements

Serum total calcium level, as routinely reported by clinical laboratories, represents the sum of protein-bound calcium (40%), diffusible but complexed calcium (e.g., citrate bound, 10%), and free ionized calcium (50%). Only the ionized calcium fraction, normally 1.10 to 1.36 mmol/L (4.4–5.4 mg/dL), is physiologically active, transported across membranes, and tightly regulated.

Variations in the two inert calcium fractions occur commonly because of alterations in serum protein level, albumin level, and pH.[59,60] In general, the plasma calcium concentration falls 0.8 mg/dL for every 1 g/dL decrease in the plasma albumin concentration. Correlation of total and ionized calcium is difficult. Various formulas have been used to estimate ionized calcium from total calcium by correcting for these alterations in serum albumin level, total protein level, and pH.[60,61] In general, these formulas have a low sensitivity and a high false-negative rate for predicting hypocalcemia in critically ill patients. Because most laboratories are currently able to measure ionized calcium in small blood volumes, direct determination of ionized calcium is the method of choice for evaluating calcium homeostasis in critically ill patients.

Hypocalcemia[62]

Classification of Hypocalcemia and Symptoms

Early neonatal hypocalcemia occurs in the first 2 to 3 days of life. Late-onset hypocalcemia occurs after day 2 or 3. Although overlap occurs, the age of onset is often helpful in determining the cause of neonatal hypocalcemia (Box 11.4).

Early hypocalcemia is most often asymptomatic, but late-onset hypocalcemia but may cause twitching, "hyperalertness," increased tone, hyperreflexia, jitteriness, and

BOX 11.4 Causes of Neonatal Hypocalcemia

Early Onset
- Prematurity
- Neonatal asphyxia and fetal distress
- Respiratory distress syndrome
- Hypoparathyroidism
- Maternal hyperparathyroidism
- Maternal diabetes
- Intrauterine growth restriction
- Maternal anticonvulsants
- Iatrogenic alkalosis
- Hypomagnesemia
- Citrated blood product administration
- Phototherapy

Late Onset
- Maternal hyperparathyroidism
- Transient congenital hypoparathyroidism
- Hypomagnesemia

Primary Hypoparathyroidism
- Transient congenital hypoparathyroidism
- DiGeorge syndrome and CATCH 22
- Familial X-linked, autosomal dominant and autosomal recessive (most common mutation of the calcium-sensing receptor gene)
- Pseudohypoparathyroidism

Vitamin D Deficiency
- Maternal anticonvulsant therapy
- Diet
- Malabsorption
- Renal insufficiency (↓ 1,25-dihydroxyvitamin D)
- Hepatic disease (↓ 25-hydroxyvitamin D)

Hyperphosphatemia
- Cow's milk–based formulas
- Excessive phosphate administration

Genetic Syndromes
- Kenny-Caffey syndrome
- Kearns-Sayre syndrome
- Long-chain fatty acyl CoA dehydrogenase deficiency

convulsions. Cyanosis, vomiting or intolerance of feedings, and a high-pitched cry have also been noted. Late-onset hypocalcemia may present with seizures. Like hypoglycemia, seizures secondary to hypocalcemia may be either focal, unilateral, or general. The Chvostek sign does not have value in premature infants and occurs in only 20% of hypocalcemic term or older infants. Because the symptoms of hypocalcemia are nonspecific and are commonly found in other high-risk infants as well as in those with hypoglycemia and other electrolyte abnormalities, hypocalcemia must be confirmed both by the laboratory and by response to specific treatment.

Serum calcium concentration should be determined daily for all infants at risk of hypocalcemia, and supportive treatment should be considered when low levels are encountered. The differential diagnosis of hypocalcemia is noted in Box 11.4.

Early Neonatal Hypocalcemia

Early neonatal hypocalcemia represents an exaggeration of the physiologic decrease in serum calcium level during the first 2 days of life. In 30% to 40% of low-birth-weight infants, chemical hypocalcemia develops. A smaller number of infants become symptomatic. The following factors identify infants at high risk:

- prematurity
- neonatal asphyxia and fetal distress
- respiratory distress syndrome
- maternal hyperparathyroidism
- maternal diabetes
- intrauterine growth restriction
- maternal anticonvulsants
- iatrogenic alkalosis
- hypomagnesemia
- citrated blood product administration

Early neonatal hypocalcemia generally represents a failure of calcium homeostatic mechanisms. Prematurity represents the most common association with early hypocalcemia, and is commonly asymptomatic.[63,64] The pathophysiology of hypocalcemia in that population includes interruption of placental calcium supply, transient parathyroid hypofunction, elevated calcitonin levels, and increased urinary losses accompanying high renal sodium excretion.[63] Infants with poor intrauterine growth most likely become hypocalcemic because of decreased transfer across the placenta.

Infants of diabetic mothers have depressed serum PTH concentrations, which may be secondary to higher calcium levels in utero. Infants of diabetic mothers may also have concurrent hypomagnesemia, which increases resistance to PTH and impairs hormone secretion.

Hypomagnesemia. Magnesium deficiency causes impaired PTH secretion and increases resistance to PTH action.[65] Hypocalcemia cannot be corrected with calcium therapy until hypomagnesemia has first been corrected. These infants can present with early or late hypocalcemia.

Birth asphyxia is commonly accompanied by hypocalcemia. It is believed to be secondary to hyperphosphatemia (resulting from tissue injury), elevated calcitonin levels, and decreased calcium intake. Bicarbonate therapy may aggravate hypocalcemia by decreasing calcium release from bone.

Maternal hyperparathyroidism. Maternal hypercalcemia leads to fetal hypercalcemia and suppression of neonatal PTH secretion.[66] The mother's disease is frequently clinically silent. Vague maternal symptoms, a history of pancreatitis or renal stones, or a history of having a previous infant with neonatal tetany may be present. Calcium and phosphorus determinations should be obtained from the mother whenever neonatal hypocalcemia is prolonged or resistant to treatment.

Late Neonatal Hypocalcemia

Classic neonatal tetany/hyperphosphatemia. Classic neonatal tetany occurs typically at 5 to 7 days of age. It is most commonly seen in infants fed cow milk or evaporated milk with a high phosphate content. Cow milk contains approximately 956 mg/L of phosphorus (molar Ca/P ratio of 1.0) compared with 150 mg/L in breast milk (molar

Ca/P ratio of 1.5 to 1.6). The high phosphate levels may antagonize PTH secretion or action, or promote calcium deposition in bones. Because current commercial formulas contain 280 to 360 mg/L of phosphorus (molar Ca/P ratio of 1.4–1.6), classic neonatal tetany has become rare. With breastmilk feeding, it should not occur.

Secondary Hypoparathyroidism

Transient or permanent hypoparathyroidism. Transient congenital idiopathic hypoparathyroidism is a benign, self-limited hypoparathyroid state persisting from 1 to 14 months and responding to calcium or moderate-level vitamin D supplements. PTH function is normal in the mothers of these infants.

Permanent hypoparathyroidism may be secondary parathyroid aplasia/hypoplasia or a genetic syndrome such as CATCH 22[67] and DiGeorge syndrome.[67] DiGeorge syndrome is classically characterized by conotruncal cardiac anomalies (truncus arteriosus, interrupted aortic arch, tetralogy of Fallot), thymic dysplasia, and hypocalcemia. Approximately 60% of patients develop hypocalcemia. Hypoparathyroidism may be transient in the neonatal period, permanent, or latent. Other associated features include dysmorphic facies and velopharyngeal incompetence. Many affected infants do not have congenital heart disease, which often results in a delay in the diagnosis until later infancy or childhood. Severe immunodeficiency occasionally occurs because of thymic aplasia. The majority of patients have a microdeletion in the chromosome 22q11 region.

CATCH 22 is a medical acronym for *c*ardiac defects, *a*bnormal facies, *t*hymic hypoplasia, *c*left palate, *h*ypocalcemia, and a variable deletion on chromosome band 22q11. CATCH 22 includes three syndromes with overlapping phenotypes: DiGeorge syndrome, velocardiofacial syndrome, and conotruncal anomaly face syndrome.

Several other familial forms of hypoparathyroidism have been described, including X-linked, autosomal dominant, and autosomal recessive forms. Autosomal dominant hypocalcemia with calciuria results from a gain in function in the CaSR causing inappropriate PTH response to hypocalcemia.

Other hypocalcemic syndromes. Severe maternal calcium and vitamin D deficiency can cause rickets in infants and neonatal hypocalcemia.[67] Maternal anticonvulsant therapy alters vitamin D metabolism, potentially leading to neonatal hypocalcemia.

Pseudohypoparathyroidism is a rare condition in which peripheral response to PTH is inadequate.[68] This condition can be autosomal dominant, autosomal recessive, or X-linked. Affected infants exhibit hypocalcemia, hypercalciuria, hyperphosphatemia, and elevated PTH levels with an inappropriately normal or low 1,25(OH_2) D level. Two forms of pseudohypoparathyroidism exist. Type I is associated with bony abnormalities. Other genetic causes of late hypocalcemia include Kenny-Caffey syndrome,[69] Kearns-Sayre syndrome,[70] and long-chain fatty acyl COA dehydrogenase deficiency.[71]

Maternal vitamin D deficiency: These neonates typically have low 25-hydroxy vitamin D levels, elevated parathyroid levels, and variable 1,25(OH_2) D levels.

Diagnosis of Hypocalcemia

Hypocalcemia is traditionally defined as total calcium levels below 2 mmol/L (8.0 mg/dL) in term infants and 1.75 mmol/L (7.0 mg/dL) in preterm infants. In term infants, ionized calcium concentrations below 1.1 mmol/L (4.4 mg/dL) should be considered abnormal. Although ionized calcium concentrations are not as well defined, levels below 1.0 mmol/L (4.0 mg/dL) are abnormal in preterm infants.

Most hypocalcemia is transient, and no workup beyond measuring total and serum ionized calcium levels is needed. The workup for infants with persistent severe hypocalcemia commonly includes.

- serum phosphorous levels
- serum magnesium levels
- serum PTH levels
- 25-hydroxy vitamin D levels
- spot urine for a calcium/creatinine ratio
- assessment of renal function

Treatment of Hypocalcemia

Who needs treatment?

Most infants with asymptomatic hypocalcemia recover with only nutritional support (early enteral feedings or addition of calcium to parenteral alimentation solutions).

Symptomatic treatment should treat both the acute hypocalcemia with correction of the underlying disorder.

Acute symptomatic hypocalcemia manifests as severe neuromuscular irritability or seizures. These infants are generally those who present with late neonatal hypocalcemia. Acute symptomatic hypocalcemia is treated by intravenous bolus infusions of 10% calcium gluconate (100–200 mL/kg). The dose can be repeated in 10 minutes if no response occurs. Calcium cannot be mixed with bicarbonate in intravenous solutions. Cardiac monitoring is required during calcium infusions. The hazards of intravenous calcium include bradycardia, cardiac arrest, cutaneous necrosis, cerebral calcifications, and intestinal gangrene. Calcium infusions should preferably be given through a central line. Administration of calcium using a peripheral venous line may result in skin sloughs from infiltration of the intravenous solution. Lines containing increased amounts of calcium should be labeled to avoid inadvertent flushing. Intraarterial calcium administration should always be avoided. Failure of hypocalcemia to respond to parenteral therapy suggests hypomagnesemia.

Following the bolus infusion, a continuous calcium infusion at a rate of 75 mg calcium/kg/day is indicated. If the infant is clinically stable and can tolerate enteral feedings, oral calcium therapy can be initiated and intravenous therapy tapered. Oral calcium salts, calcium gluconate (9 mg/mL elemental calcium), or calcium glubionate (23 mg/mL elemental calcium) can be initiated at 30 to 50 mg/kg/day of elemental calcium divided equally into four to six doses. In infants at risk of necrotizing enterocolitis or malabsorption, calcium gluconate is preferred to calcium glubionate because of its lower osmolarity (700 mOsm/L versus 2500 mOsm/L). After normocalcemia is achieved, treatment should be tapered. Often, therapy can be discontinued by 2 to 4 weeks.

In patients with hyperphosphatemia, the phosphate load needs to be reduced. Low-phosphorus formula (Similac PM 60/40 [Abbott Nutrition, Columbus, Ohio], phosphorus 190 mg/L, molar Ca/P ratio of 1.5) or breastmilk should be used. Additional oral calcium supplementation (10–20 mg elemental calcium/kg/day) helps further increase the relative absorption of calcium compared with phosphorus. Oral calcium supplementation can usually be discontinued beginning in 1 week and routine formula started in 2 to 4 weeks.

In patients with hypoparathyroidism, both oral calcium supplementation and vitamin D supplementation, usually in the form of calcitriol (1,25-dihydroxy vitamin D), is required.

Prognosis

Hypocalcemia with seizures may present an immediate threat to life in an infant with other problems with which to contend. Unlike with hypoglycemia, however, there seems to be no structural damage to the central nervous system. Thus hypocalcemia alone generally has a good prognosis. If hypocalcemia is complicating other serious conditions such as asphyxia, the prognosis is determined by the other disorders.

Hypercalcemia

Hypercalcemia is most often iatrogenic secondary to excessive calcium administration, excessive vitamin D administration, use of thiazide diuretics that reduce renal calcium excretion, or phosphate depletion usually caused by poorly constituted hyperalimentation solutions or human milk feedings. Primary neonatal hyperparathyroidism occurs both sporadically and by autosomal recessive inheritance.[59] It is because of abnormalities in CaSR function resulting in increased PTH levels. FHH[72] is a related disorder also caused by abnormalities in the CaSR, but is benign and inherited in an autosomal dominant pattern. PTH levels are normal with low to normal urinary calcium excretion in FHH. Individuals who are homozygous for the FHH gene mutation develop severe neonatal hyperparathyroidism. Secondary hyperparathyroidism occurs because of chronic maternal hypocalcemia (usually caused by maternal hypoparathyroidism), which leads to transient neonatal parathyroid overstimulation The hypercalcemia associated with subcutaneous fat necrosis[73] and Williams syndrome[74] may be related to increased 1,25-dihydroxyvitamin D synthesis. Other causes are listed in Box 11.5.

Hypercalcemia may be asymptomatic (especially with mild hypercalcemia (serum calcium 11.13 mg/dL) or present with nonspecific symptoms including poor feeding, ileus, failure to thrive, polyuria, dehydration, lethargy, and irritability. Severe hypercalcemia can cause lethargy or seizures. Infants with chronic hypercalcemia may present with failure to thrive. Chronic hyperparathyroidism may be associated with bone demineralization and fractures.

BOX 11.5 Causes of Hypercalcemia

- Neonatal hyperparathyroidism (transient vs. permanent)
- Maternal hypoparathyroidism
- Excessive calcium supplementation
- Excessive vitamin D supplementation
- Williams syndrome (↑ 1,25-dihydroxyvitamin D)
- Familial hypocalciuric hypercalcemia (inactivating mutation of the calcium sensing receptor gene)
- Phosphate depletion
- Aluminum toxicity
- Idiopathic infantile hypercalcemia
- Use of thiazide diuretics
- Adrenal insufficiency
- Subcutaneous fat necrosis
- Familial autosomal recessive hypophosphatasia
- Hypophosphatemia
- Primary chondrodystrophy (metaphyseal dysplasia)
- Blue Diaper syndrome

Initial treatment includes discontinuation of all calcium and vitamin D supplementation, and hydration with furosemide to increase calcium excretion. Other therapies include calcitonin, glucocorticoids, and dialysis. Specific treatment is directed to the underlying disorder.

Magnesium

Fetal and Neonatal Magnesium Metabolism

Magnesium is the second most abundant intracellular cation in the body. Adult humans contain 27 g of magnesium, whereas term newborn infants have only 0.8 grams. Magnesium is actively transported from mother to fetus, using a transport mechanism different from calcium. Furthermore, unlike calcium, this transfer is adversely affected both by placental insufficiency and by maternal magnesium deficiency caused by poor diet or disease. Approximately 65% of total body magnesium (vs. 99% of calcium) is contained in bone, 34% in the intracellular space, and 1% in the extracellular space. Only a minor fraction of magnesium in bone is freely exchangeable with extracellular magnesium. Because the fraction of magnesium in the extracellular fluid is low, plasma magnesium concentrations do not adequately reflect total body magnesium content. Parathyroid function has a small direct effect on serum magnesium levels. Magnesium, on the other hand, is critically necessary for normal parathyroid function.

The normal newborn serum magnesium concentration is 1.5 to 2.8 mg/dL (0.62–1.16 mmol/L) and is very similar to levels in older children or adults. In normal-term infants, the concentration of magnesium in umbilical cord blood is 1.6 (1.45–1.83) mg/dL. Those values do not vary with sex, race, season of birth, appropriateness of weight for gestation, or mode of delivery. Preterm infants exhibit slightly elevated concentrations (2.0 ± 0.4 mg/dL).[75] At 48 hours of life, serum magnesium concentrations decline in term and preterm infants and then increase over the first week of life. By the end of the first month, childhood levels are achieved. Maintenance of magnesium levels is generally regulated by the kidney. Eighty percent of total plasma magnesium is filtered at the glomerular membrane, most of which is reabsorbed by the thick ascending limb of the loop of Henle and less by the distal tubule, where there is an active transport mechanism.[76]

Short-term variations in magnesium concentrations affect parathyroid function. A short-term decrease in magnesium concentration results in an increase in PTH secretion, whereas short-term increase in magnesium concentrations leads to a reduction in PTH levels. PTH increase serum magnesium concentrations by mobilizing magnesium from bone and decreasing losses in the urine. Glucagon, insulin, PTH, vasopressin, and calcitonin increase the reabsorption of magnesium. Metabolic acidosis increases the excretion of magnesium.

Chronic magnesium deficiency results in decreased PTH secretion and a diminished action of PTH. Therefore magnesium deficiency can worsen hypocalcemia (see later). The release of magnesium from bone is decreased by calcitonin. Calcitonin also reduces the renal tubular reabsorption of calcium. Vitamin D does not play a major role in magnesium balance.

Serum magnesium levels are increased with severe hyperbilirubinemia and infants with generalized cellular injury or respiratory distress syndrome. Umbilical cord ionized magnesium levels are higher in preterm infants with acidosis, suggesting extracellular movement of magnesium.

Hypomagnesemia[77]

Magnesium levels of less than 1.5 mg/dL are encountered in the following conditions:

- maternal magnesium deficiency;
- intravascular volume expansion;
- in intrauterine growth restriction of any cause, including multiple gestation, or in association with maternal malnourishment;
- in association with maternal gestational diabetes and diabetes mellitus, in which it correlates with severity of the mother's disease;
- with hyperphosphatemia and after exchange transfusion (magnesium, like calcium, is subject to citrate complexing);
- in neonatal hypoparathyroidism (and maternal hyperparathyroidism);
- secondary to diarrhea or malabsorption states in older infants;
- in a specific intestinal magnesium malabsorption syndrome that is secondary to mutations in the transient receptor potential channel 6 (TRPM6) protein mapping to chromosome band 9q22[78];
- in association with hypercalciuria and nephrocalcinosis; and
- secondary to renal losses (primary[71] or induced by drugs, for example, amphotericin[72,79] B, loop diuretics and aminoglycoside antibiotics[80]).

Hypomagnesemia can cause symptoms similar to those caused by hypocalcemia but is unresponsive to calcium therapy.

Coexistence of Hypomagnesemia and Hypocalcemia

Hypomagnesemia and hypocalcemia, two metabolic problems, frequently coexist. They have common antecedents, such as maternal diabetes, hypoparathyroidism, malabsorption, exchange transfusion, and excess dietary phosphorus.

Magnesium deficiency causes failure of PTH release and of PTH's effect on serum calcium level. Treatment with calcium will not correct hypocalcemia until hypomagnesemia is corrected. Magnesium appears crucial for normal bone serum calcium homeostasis.

Treatment of Hypomagnesemia

Hypomagnesemia with tetany is treated with 25 to 50 mg/kg of magnesium sulfate administered intravenously or intramuscularly every 6 to 8 hours. A 50% magnesium sulfate solution is commonly used in which the recommended dose is 0.05 to 0.1 mL/kg. Magnesium given intravenously should be given over 30 to 60 minutes. Serum magnesium concentration should be rechecked every 24 hours. Hypermagnesemia with hypotonia may occur with overtreatment. Alternatively, magnesium may be given with feedings. The sulfate, gluconate, chloride, or citrate salt may be used in an initial dosage of 100 to 200 mg magnesium per kg per day given in divided doses every 6 hours. However, excessive dosages have a laxative effect.

Hypermagnesemia

Magnesium that crosses the placenta after treatment for toxemia or preterm labor may produce hypotonia, flaccidity, respiratory depression, poor suck, and decreased gastrointestinal motility. Prolonged maternal magnesium administration has been associated with abnormal bone mineralization. Hypermagnesemia may also occur during excessive magnesium administration with total parenteral nutrition. Treatment is expectant because magnesium levels decline by 48 hours. If severe symptoms are present, administration of calcium may reverse these effects, and forced saline diuresis may speed magnesium excretion.

CASE 11.1

You are called to see a 5-day-old infant because of irritability and jerking movements of the left arm and leg. He was the product of a full-term pregnancy and had a birth weight of 2800 g. Pregnancy was complicated by third-trimester bleeding. Delivery was by cesarean section because of placenta previa. One-minute Apgar score was 6; 5-minute Apgar score was 9. Feeding with evaporated milk formula was begun at 16 hours of age, and he did very well until a few hours ago when he became tremulous and fed poorly. Intermittent convulsions were noted. Examination reveals irritability but no other abnormalities. However, as the examination ends, the child has another seizure.

What diagnostic tests and procedures would you perform initially?

The symptoms shown by this baby are nonspecific. Central nervous system injury or infection is possible, and a lumbar puncture must be done. There is nothing in the case history to suggest hypoglycemia as a probable cause of the seizures, but some less common hypoglycemic syndromes (inborn error of metabolism, islet adenoma) may present this way, and glucose testing should be performed. Serum should be drawn for determination of electrolyte, calcium, blood urea nitrogen, and glucose levels.

Several features of this case suggest the possibility of hypocalcemia, notably stormy obstetric course, milk feedings, the age of onset of symptoms after the initially benign course, and irritability and tremulousness as cardinal symptoms. These features justify a trial with parenteral calcium after initial studies are done.

The therapeutic infusion is 2 mL/kg of 10% calcium gluconate over 10 minutes into an established intravenous line with electrocardiogram monitoring. Subsequent to immediate evaluation and treatment, the laboratory reports an ionized calcium level of 0.5 mmol/L and a phosphorus level of 11.5 mg/dL.

What factors may be important in the pathogenesis of the hypocalcemia?

The high serum phosphorus concentration indicates that dietary phosphorus load, relative hypoparathyroidism, and renal immaturity with retention of phosphate are important factors in the hypocalcemia.

What management should be instituted?

A low-phosphorus formula or formula with a favorable Ca/P ratio (Similac PM 60/40 or human milk) should be fed. Additional calcium supplementation (elemental calcium 20–80 mg/kg/day) can be used to increase the Ca/P ratio in the feedings to further decrease phosphate absorption.

What is the prognosis?

The prognosis is excellent. Supplemental calcium may be tapered and withdrawn at 3 to 4 weeks of age. Serum calcium level should be monitored at this time to be sure hypocalcemia does not recur. There should be no long-term sequelae.

CASE 11.2

You attend the delivery of an infant at 37 weeks' gestation. The mother has preeclampsia and has received magnesium sulfate for the last 24 hours. At the time of delivery, the infant is hypotonic and apneic, and requires intubation and positive pressure ventilation.

What is the most likely diagnosis and management?

Magnesium crosses the placenta, with fetal plasma concentrations directly correlating with maternal plasma concentrations. Maternal magnesium sulfate therapy leads to hypermagnesemia in the newborn infant. The diagnosis is most consistent with hypermagnesemia secondary to maternal therapy. Treatment is supportive. As long as urine output is adequate, magnesium levels will fall without further intervention.

CASE 11.3

A 1-day-old 1900-g infant born at 33 weeks' gestation to a diabetic mother has a focal seizure. Initial laboratory testing reveals an ionized calcium level of 0.5 mmol/L.

What is your initial treatment?

The initial treatment is 1.9 to 3.8 mL of 10% calcium gluconate infused intravenously over 10 minutes. Calcium should be added to the intravenous fluids to provide 75 mg/kg/day of elemental calcium.

A repeat ionized calcium concentration is 0.5 mmol/L. What is the most likely reason for the lack of response to therapy?

Premature infants and infants of diabetic mothers are at risk for hypomagnesemia. Magnesium is necessary for proper parathyroid hormone (PTH) secretion; therefore calcium concentrations will not increase if hypomagnesemia is present. Magnesium concentration should be checked, and if it is low, the infant should be treated with 25 to 50 mg/kg of magnesium sulfate.

CASE 11.4

Why is the infant in picture (A) below jittery?

1. Central nervous system (CNS) anomaly
2. Hypoglycemia
3. Hypothyroxinemia
4. Hypopituitarism

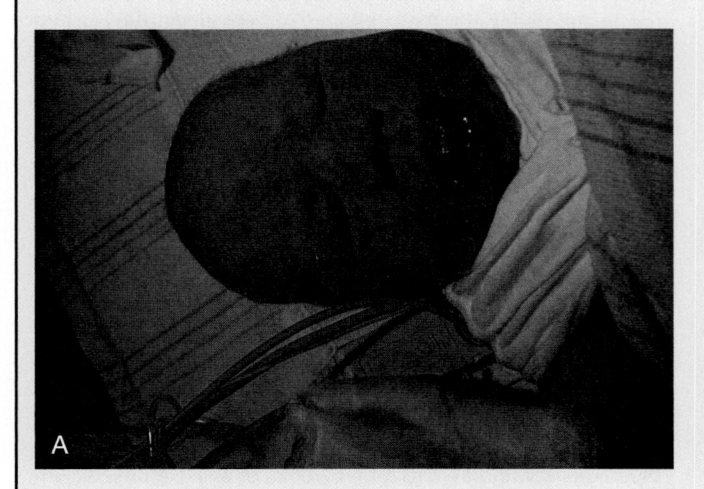

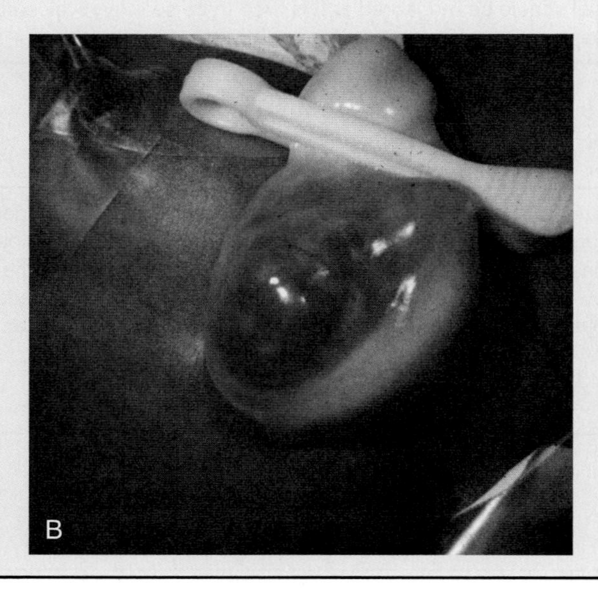

The jitteriness in this infant is probably because of hypoglycemia, which is common in Beckwith-Wiedemann syndrome. The hypoglycemia may be asymptomatic and usually resolves within the first 3 days of life. The big tongue (A) and omphalocele (B) on a large-for-gestational-age (LGA) infant points to the diagnosis of Beckwith-Wiedemann syndrome.

1. What are the ear anomalies in Beckwith Wiedemann syndrome?
2. What is the pathogenesis of the hypoglycemia in these infants?
3. What chromosomal anomaly is found in 20% of affected infants?

Answer

1. Pits and clefts
2. Hyperinsulinism
3. Uniparental disomy (UPD) 11P15.5

UPD occurs when an infant receives two copies of a chromosome, or part of a chromosome, from one parent and no copies from the other parent:

- Prader Willi syndrome and Angelman syndrome—both chromosome 15
- Beckwith-Wiedemann syndrome—chromosome 11
- Neonatal diabetes—chromosome 9 and also chromosome 14 and 7

Beckwith-Wiedemann Syndrome (Hyperplastic Fetal Visceromegaly)

Beckwith-Wiedemann syndrome (BWS) is an overgrowth syndrome associated with macrosomia (88% of cases), macroglossia (97% of cases), abdominal wall defects (80% of cases), usually an omphalocele (see picture B above), hypoglycemia in the neonatal period, and embryonal cancers of infancy and early childhood (4% of cases). The frequency of hypoglycemia in BWS is between 30% and 63%, and the hypoglycemia is caused by hyperinsulinism. Fewer than 5% of infants will have hypoglycemia beyond the neonatal period requiring either continuous feeding or, in rare cases, partial pancreatectomy. The genetics of BWS is complex and involves defects in imprinted gene expression in the 11p15 region. The majority of cases are sporadic but 10% to 15% occur in an autosomal dominant pattern, with maternal transmission associated with increased penetrance. The risk of BWS is higher after the use of assisted reproductive therapies.

QUESTIONS

Match the clinical scenarios with the following conditions and state the reasons for selection (more than one condition may be correct):

1. Hypoglycemia
2. Hyperglycemia
3. Hypocalcemia
4. Hypercalcemia

A 3400-g, 7-day-old infant with a large ventricular septal defect becomes jittery. Earlier in the day, the child's intravenous fluids were decreased from 20 mL/h to 11 mL/h because of congestive heart failure. The concentration of dextrose in the total parenteral nutrition was increased from 12.5% to 15%.

Although the concentration of dextrose in the intravenous fluids was increased, this did not offset the decrease in the rate of fluid administration. Therefore the glucose infusion rate decreased from 12.3 mg/kg/min to 8.1 mg/kg/min. An acute decrease in the glucose infusion rate may lead to hypoglycemia.

Although patients with DiGeorge syndrome often have cardiac disease, usually the lesions are conotruncal defects (e.g., interrupted aortic arch, truncus arteriosus, tetralogy of Fallot). Patients with isolated ventricular septal defects are unlikely to have DiGeorge syndrome. Patients with DiGeorge syndrome may have hypocalcemia. In addition to heart disease, patients with DiGeorge syndrome have recurrent infections because of T-cell deficiencies associated with an absent thymus. DiGeorge syndrome is because of a microdeletion 22q11.2.

Therefore the answer is 1 (hypoglycemia). This highlights the need to calculate glucose infusion rates in mg per kg per hour, and not to be seduced by the concentration, when assessing patients with hypoglycemia or hyperglycemia.

An 1800-g male infant is born at 40 weeks' gestation.

Infants with intrauterine growth restriction can have hypoglycemia, hyperglycemia, or hypocalcemia (answers 1, 2, and 3). Hypoglycemia may occur because of inadequate glycogen stores or hyperinsulinism. Infants with neonatal diabetes are hyperglycemic and growth restricted because of low intrauterine insulin concentrations. Intrauterine growth-restricted infants can be hypocalcemic secondary to low magnesium concentrations or fetal distress. Hypercalcemia is not usually associated with intrauterine growth restriction.

A 5-day-old infant shows jerking movements of the left arm and leg. On close evaluation, the child is also found to have some abnormal-appearing facies with mild hypertelorism, short philtrum, mildly low-set ears, micrognathia, and down-slanting palpebral fissures.

This infant has features consistent with DiGeorge syndrome. Hypoplasia of the parathyroid gland leads to hypoparathyroidism and hypocalcemia. Therefore the answer is 3 (hypocalcemia). Many patients with DiGeorge syndrome do not have cardiac disease and are therefore not diagnosed immediately after birth.

A 2600-g newborn has a hemoglobin level of 26 g/dL.

Hypoglycemia is frequent in plethoric infants. A high hemoglobin level may be a factor in hypoglycemia in infants of diabetic mothers and in those with Beckwith-Wiedemann syndrome. The answer is 1 (hypoglycemia).

A newborn exhibits jitteriness and seizures.

These symptoms are present with hypoglycemia and hypocalcemia. The answer is 1 and 3 (hypoglycemia and hypocalcemia). Box 11.1 lists many other conditions that have similar symptoms.

May be a clue to undiagnosed disease in the mother.

In a large-for-date infant, early hypoglycemia should be sought and may indicate unsuspected maternal diabetes. Neonatal hypocalcemia may be a clue to maternal hyperparathyroidism or familial hypocalciuric hypercalcemia (FHH). Neonatal hyperparathyroidism with hypercalcemia may be present when both parents have FHH and the infant is homozygous for the FHH gene mutation. The answer is 1, 3, and 4.

Associated with iatrogenic excessive administration of Vitamin D or A.

Excess vitamin D or vitamin A administration leads to hypercalcemia. The answer is 4 (hypercalcemia).

Cannot be corrected if hypomagnesemia is present.

Normal magnesium concentrations are necessary for normal parathyroid function. Hypocalcemia cannot be corrected in the presence of hypomagnesemia. Therefore the answer is 3 (hypocalcemia).

12

Neonatal Hyperbilirubinemia

Jon F. Watchko, M. Jeffrey Maisels

Care of the high-risk neonate usually refers to care of the low-birth-weight infant or the sick term newborn. Although hyperbilirubinemia is certainly a matter of concern in these infants, the decisions that must be made regarding jaundice in the high-risk neonate are, in general, less complex than those that must be made in the healthy full-term infant. For the term and late preterm infant, shorter hospital stays, the need for outpatient surveillance and management, and the occasional disturbing case of extreme hyperbilirubinemia and even kernicterus highlight the challenges clinicians face in the management of neonatal jaundice.

Bilirubin has both salutary and toxic effects. At physiologic levels, it exerts important antioxidant effects.[1] Although its toxic effects are well documented, there are also some concerns that aggressive use of phototherapy in extremely low-birth-weight (ELBW) infants may not be entirely innocuous.[2] Most neonatal jaundice is the result of a combination of events—an increase in the rate of bilirubin production, reabsorption of bilirubin into the plasma from the gut (the enterohepatic circulation), and inability of the liver to clear sufficient bilirubin from the plasma.

FORMATION, STRUCTURE, AND PROPERTIES OF BILIRUBIN

Bilirubin is the product of the catabolism of iron protoporphyrin, or heme, which comes predominantly from circulating hemoglobin (Fig. 12.1). Bilirubin is a tetrapyrrole compound with specific substitutions in the side chains of the four pyrrole rings (Fig. 12.2). The outer pyrrole rings are linked to the inner ones by methene bridges (containing one double bond each), but the two central rings are joined by a methane bridge (no double bond). Normally, the methene bridge oxidized in heme is in the alpha-position, and the resultant isomer is bilirubin IX-alpha (Fig. 12.3), the predominant isomer of bilirubin in the body. Although its structure is conventionally represented in linear fashion as shown in Fig. 12.2, the actual structure of bilirubin revealed by x-ray crystallography is like that shown in Fig. 12.3, in which the bilirubin molecule is stabilized by the presence of intramolecular hydrogen bonds (indicated by the dashed lines). In this conformation, the hydrophilic, polar COOH, and NH groups are not available for the attachment of water, whereas the hydrophobic hydrocarbon groups are on the perimeter, which makes the molecule insoluble in water but soluble in nonpolar solvents such as chloroform.

BILIRUBIN MEASUREMENT

Most laboratories today measure the unconjugated or indirect reacting bilirubin using the diazo technique. The unconjugated bilirubin is measured as that portion of the bilirubin that reacts poorly with the diazo reagent and requires the addition of an accelerant such as methanol or ethanol (which interferes with hydrogen bonding) to produce an immediate diazo reaction. This is the basis for measurement of indirect bilirubin by the van den Bergh reaction. On the other hand, a small portion of the bilirubin reacts "directly" with the diazo reagent without the need for an accelerant and is therefore known as the direct-reacting bilirubin. It is important to recognize, however, that conjugated bilirubin differs from direct-reacting bilirubin. Conjugated bilirubin is the result of the conjugation of unconjugated bilirubin with glucuronic acid and can be measured directly with the use of the BuBc slide method originally developed by Kodak[3] and now marketed as the Vitros technique (Ortho Clinical Diagnostics, Raritan, NJ, USA). When measured by this technique, conjugated bilirubin levels in the newborn are substantially lower than direct bilirubin levels.[4]

In the jaundiced newborn in whom the primary problem is excessive bilirubin formation or limited hepatic uptake and conjugation, unconjugated (i.e., indirect) bilirubin appears in the blood. When bilirubin glucuronide excretion is impaired (i.e., in cholestasis), conjugated bilirubin monoglucuronide and diglucuronide (direct-reacting bilirubin) accumulate in the plasma and, because of their solubility, also appear in the urine A fourth bilirubin fraction, known as *delta bilirubin,* which is formed nonenzymatically from conjugated bilirubin, is covalently bound to albumin, and reacts directly with the diazo agent.[5] Thus measurements of direct bilirubin include both conjugated as well as delta bilirubin. Delta bilirubin is only formed when there is an elevation in the conjugated bilirubin fraction, and generally plays no role in neonatal hyperbilirubinemia. Because of the strong covalent bond, the half-life of delta bilirubin is approximately 3 weeks and, as a result, an infant who is recovering from a hepatic insult may

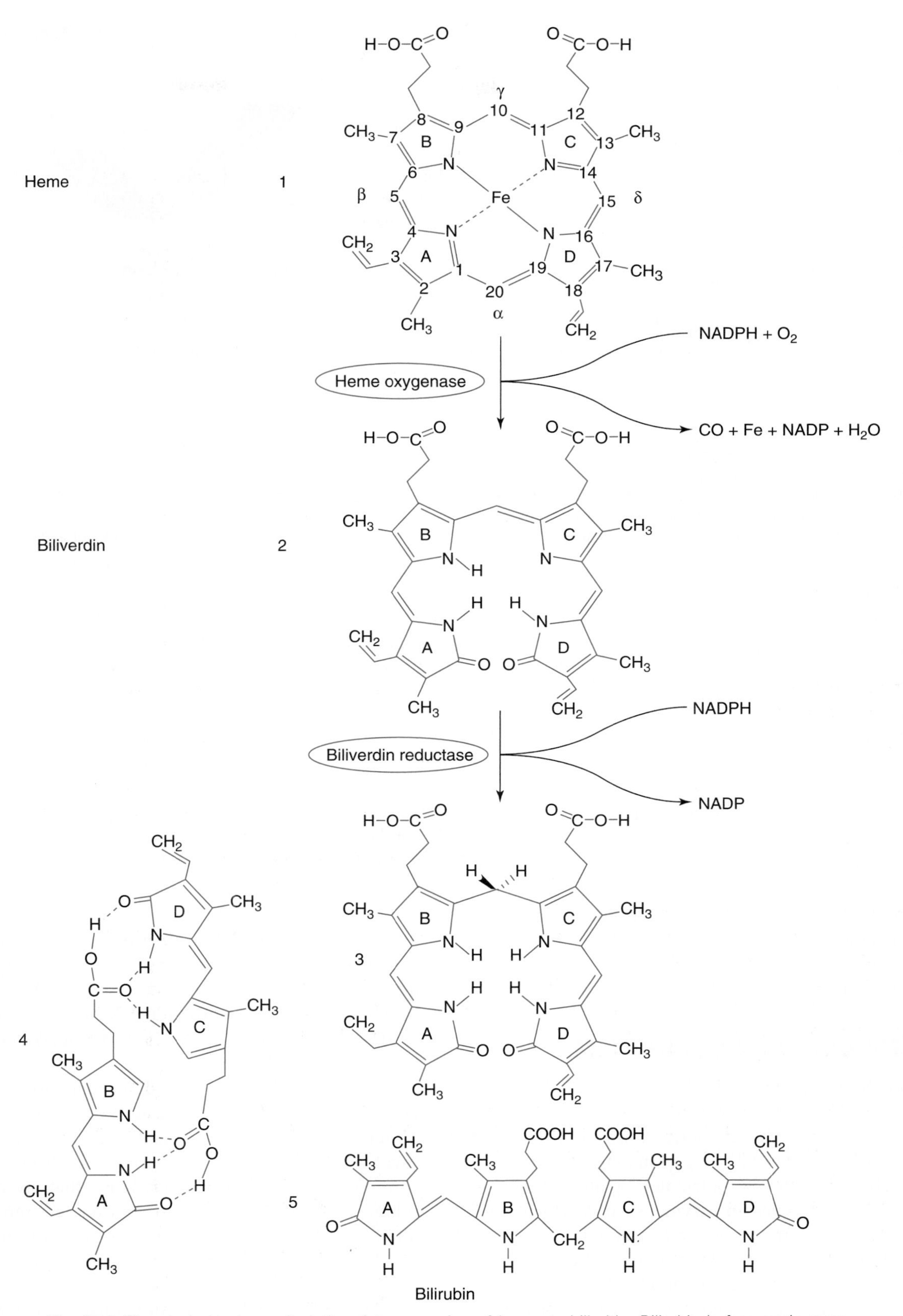

Fig. 12.1 Chemical structures depicting the conversion of heme to bilirubin. Bilirubin is frequently represented by any of the three structures (*3* to *5*) shown at the bottom. *NADP,* Nicotinamide adenine dinucleotide phosphate; *NADPH,* reduced form of nicotinamide adenine dinucleotide phosphate. (Modified from Gourley GR. Neonatal jaundice and disorders of bilirubin metabolism. In Suchy FJ, Sokol RJ, Balistreri WF, eds. *Liver Disease in Children.* 3rd ed. New York, NY: Cambridge University Press; 2007.)

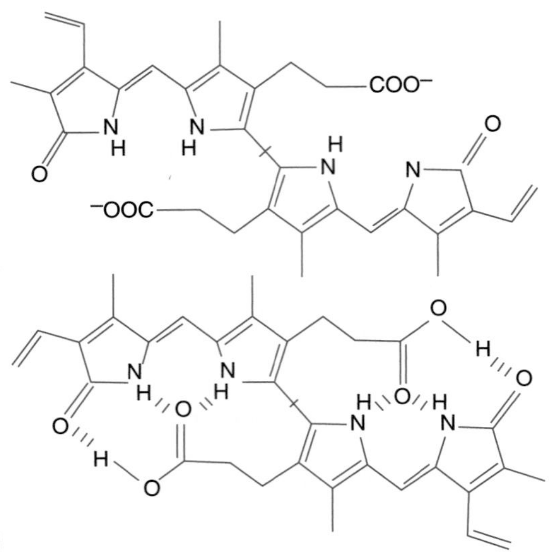

Fig. 12.2 Chemical Structure of Bilirubin. (A) Bilirubin dianion, with two free carboxyl groups; bilirubin monoanion has one free carboxyl group. (B) Bilirubin diacid, the predominant form of free bilirubin in plasma at physiologic pH. (From Brodersen R. Bilirubin transport in the newborn infant, reviewed in relation to kernicterus. *J Pediatr* 1980;96:349-356.)

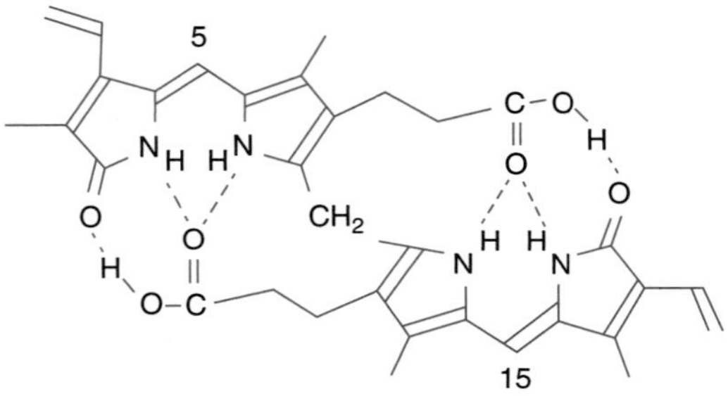

Fig. 12.3 X-ray crystallographic structure of bilirubin IX-alpha. *Dashed lines* indicate hydrogen bonding.

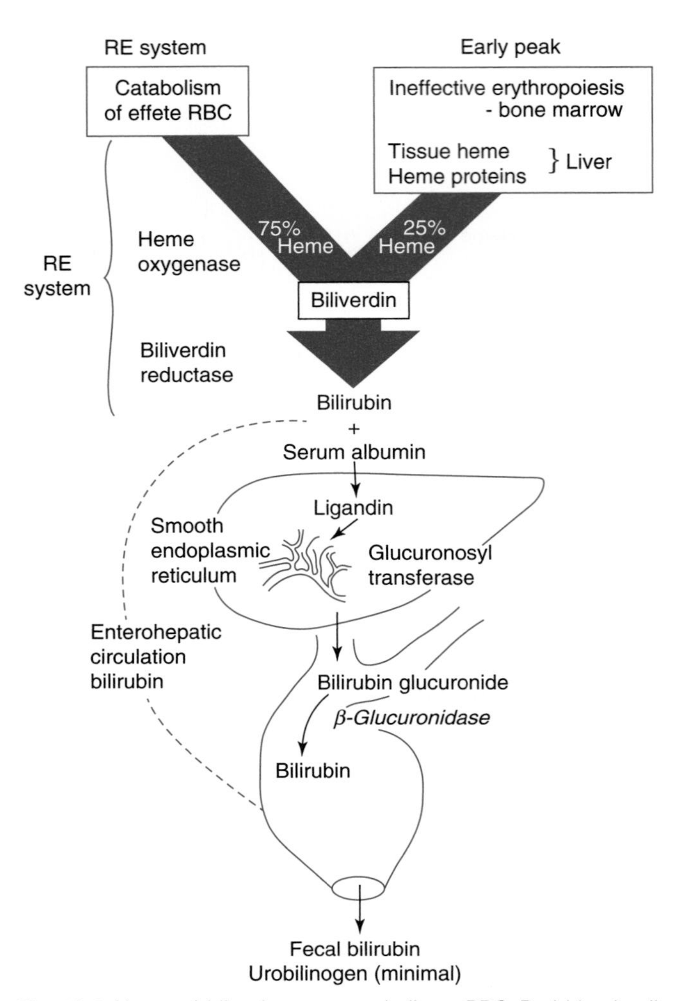

Fig. 12.4 Neonatal bile pigment metabolism. *RBC,* Red blood cell; *RE,* reticuloendothelial. (From Maisels MJ. Jaundice. In: Avery GB, Fletcher MA, MacDonald MG, eds. *Neonatology: Pathophysiology and Management of the Newborn*. Philadelphia, PA: JB Lippincott; 1999:765-819.)

continue to display an elevated direct bilirubin measurement when the conjugated bilirubin level has already returned to normal.[5] In the neonate, conjugated bilirubin (versus direct bilirubin) measurements are more precise and preferred.

NEONATAL BILIRUBIN METABOLISM

Heme degradation leads to bilirubin production from two major sources (Fig. 12.4). Approximately 75% of the daily bilirubin production in the newborn comes from senescent erythrocytes (the catabolism of 1 g of hemoglobin yields 35 mg of bilirubin), but 25% is contributed by nonhemoglobin heme contained in the liver (in enzymes such as cytochromes and catalases, and in free heme) and in muscle myoglobin, or comes from ineffective erythropoiesis in the bone marrow. Once it leaves the reticuloendothelial system, bilirubin is transported in the plasma and bound tightly to albumin, so that at physiologic pH, the solubility of bilirubin is very low (about 4 nm/L [0.24 mg/dL]). When the bilirubin-albumin complex encounters the hepatocyte, a proportion of the bilirubin, but not albumin, is transported into the cell, where it is bound to ligandin and then transported to the smooth endoplasmic reticulum for conjugation. Data suggest a role for solute carrier organic anion transporter 1B1 (SLCO1B1)[6] in facilitating hepatic bilirubin uptake. Gene polymorphisms of *SLCO1B1* that limit hepatic bilirubin uptake may contribute to hyperbilirubinemia.

Conversion of unconjugated bilirubin to its water-soluble conjugate must occur before it can be excreted; this is achieved when bilirubin is combined enzymatically with a sugar, glucuronic acid, which produces bilirubin monoglucuronide and diglucuronide pigments that are more water soluble and sufficiently polar to be excreted into the bile or filtered through the kidney. The enzyme catalyzing this reaction is uridine diphosphate glucuronosyltransferase, a single isoform of which (UGT1A1) accounts for almost all the bilirubin glucuronide in the human liver. The enzyme arises from the *UGT1A1* gene complex situated on chromosome 2 at 2q37. Mutations and amino acid substitutions at different loci on this gene are responsible for the inherited unconjugated hyperbilirubinemias: Crigler-Najjar syndrome types

I and II and Gilbert syndrome. Once conjugated, bilirubin is excreted via the bile canaliculi into the small intestine. A detailed review of the chemistry and metabolism of bilirubin can be found elsewhere.[7,8]

NORMAL SERUM BILIRUBIN LEVELS AND THE NATURAL HISTORY OF NEONATAL JAUNDICE

Unconjugated bilirubin is transported efficiently via the placenta from fetal blood into the maternal circulation by passive diffusion.[9] The mean total serum bilirubin (TSB) levels in cord blood range from 1.4 to 1.9 mg/dL (24–32 µmol/L), whereas maternal TSB levels are less than 1 mg/dL (17.1 µmol). For years, it has been taught that the TSB concentration in normal term infants increases from birth, reaches its apex on about the third or fourth day of life, and then declines, reaching normal levels by 7 to 10 days. When bilirubin levels are studied in large populations using transcutaneous bilirubin (TcB) measurements, however, it is clear that in those at or above the 50th percentile, the peak does not occur until about 96 hours and remains at that level through 120 hours (Fig. 12.5).[10] On the other hand, there are significant differences in the natural history in term and late preterm infants for each week of gestation.[11] In those with a gestational age of 40 weeks or longer, the peak TcB occurs at about 60 hours, whereas in those with a gestational age of 35 to 39 6/7 weeks, it does not occur until 96 hours or later (Fig. 12.6).[10,11] Because of intervention with phototherapy, no recent data are available on the natural history of bilirubinemia in infants of 34 weeks' gestation or less.

DEVELOPMENTAL JAUNDICE

The normal increase of TSB levels in the newborn has been termed *physiologic jaundice,* but there is good reason to consider abandoning this term.[12] Depending on ethnic characteristics, breast feeding, and other factors, there are significant differences in TSB levels in different populations so that what is physiologic for one infant may well be nonphysiologic for another. Particularly for low-birth-weight infants being cared for in the neonatal intensive care unit (NICU), the term *physiologic jaundice* has little meaning and is potentially dangerous. If no treatment is given, low-birth-weight infants have prolonged and exaggerated hyperbilirubinemia; the lower the birth weight, the higher the peak bilirubin level. A TSB of 10 mg/dL (171 µmol/L) on day 4 in a 750-g neonate is a normal bilirubin level for that infant and requires no investigation to identify a cause for the jaundice. Nevertheless, most neonatologists would treat this bilirubin level with phototherapy. Thus TSB levels well within the physiologic range are considered potentially hazardous and are commonly treated with phototherapy. The natural history of hyperbilirubinemia in this population is never observed, and defining these bilirubin levels as physiologic in such infants seems illogical and potentially dangerous.

A better term for this phenomenon is *developmental jaundice.*[12] The jaundice seen in almost every newborn results from a combination of mechanisms:

- The normal neonate produces about 6 to 8 mg/kg/day of bilirubin, which is about 2.5 times the rate of bilirubin production in the adult.[13]
- The newborn reabsorbs significant amounts of unconjugated bilirubin from the intestine (enterohepatic circulation). Unlike the adult, in early postnatal life, neonates have few bacteria in the small and large bowel, and they have greater activity of the deconjugating enzyme beta-glucuronidase. Thus conjugated bilirubin (which cannot be reabsorbed) is not converted to urobilinogen but is hydrolyzed to unconjugated bilirubin, some of which is reabsorbed, thus increasing the bilirubin load on the liver.
- There is a decrease in clearance of bilirubin from the plasma. This is the result of a deficiency in ligandin, the predominant bilirubin-binding protein in the hepatocyte, and a deficiency of UGT1A1, which, at term, approximates 1% of the activity found in the adult.

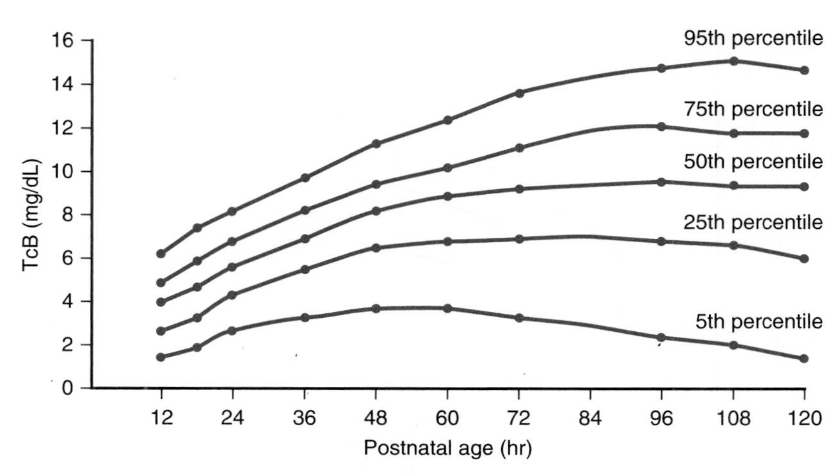

Fig. 12.5 Smoothed curves from 14,035 transcutaneous bilirubin *(TcB)* measurements in 2646 newborns (gestational age ≥35 weeks and birth weight ≥2000 g). (From Fouzas S, Mantagou L, Skylogianni E, et al. Transcutaneous bilirubin levels for the first 120 postnatal hours in healthy neonates. *Pediatrics.* 2009;125:e52.)

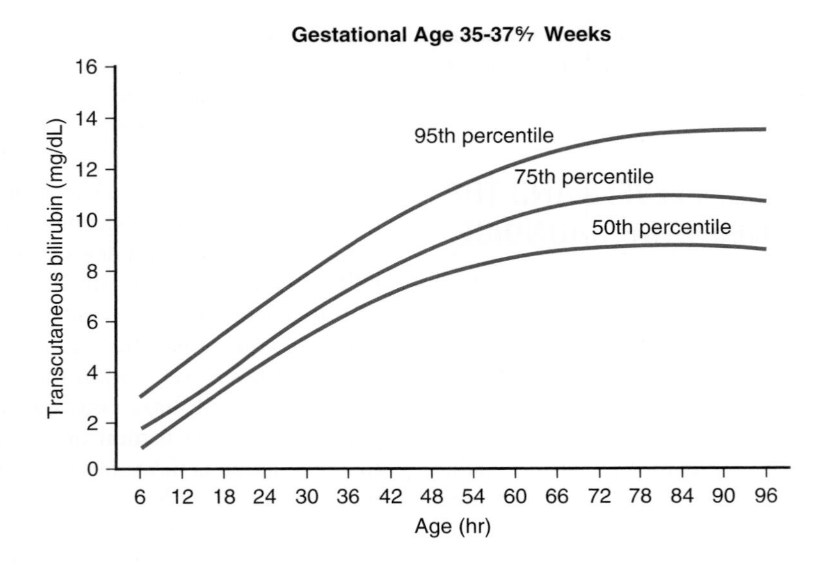

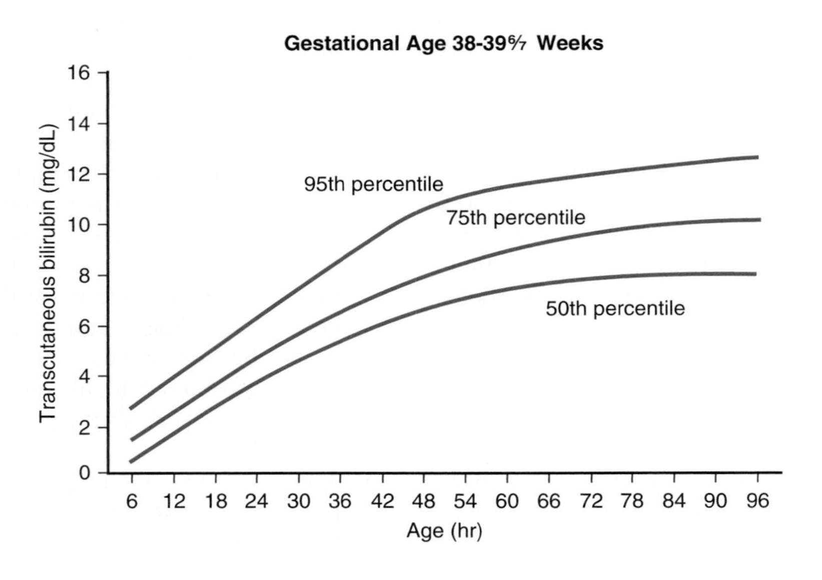

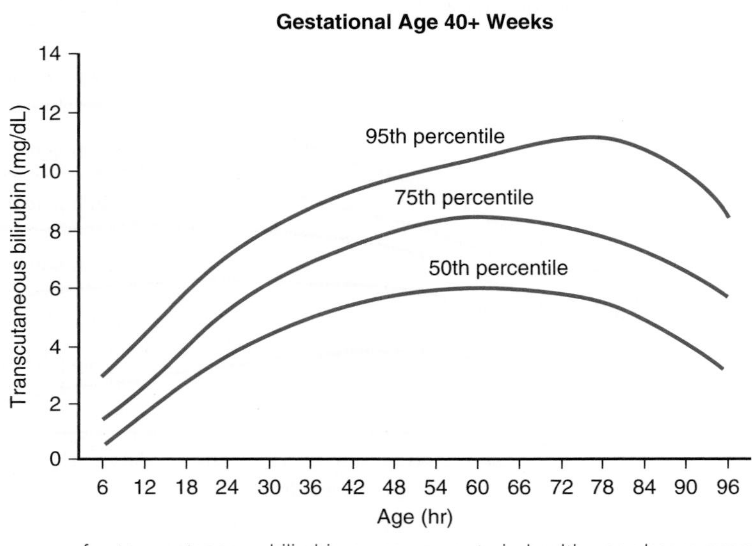

Fig. 12.6 Nomogram for transcutaneous bilirubin measurements in healthy newborns according to gestational age. (From Maisels MJ, Kring E. Transcutaneous bilirubin levels in the first 96 hours in a normal newborn population of 35 or more weeks' of gestation. *Pediatrics.* 2006;117:1169.)

BOX 12.1 Causes of Indirect Hyperbilirubinemia in Newborn Infants

Increased Bilirubin Production or Load on the Liver

Hemolytic Disease

Immune mediated

- Rh alloimmunization
- ABO and other blood group incompatibilities

Heritable

Red cell membrane defects

- Spherocytosis, elliptocytosis, stomatocytosis, pyknocytosis

Red cell enzyme deficiencies

- Glucose-6-phosphate dehydrogenase deficiency, pyruvate kinase deficiency, and other erythrocyte enzyme deficiencies

Hemoglobinopathies

- Alpha thalassemia, gamma-beta thalassemia

Unstable hemoglobins

- Heinz body hemolytic anemia

Other Causes of Increased Production

- Sepsis[a,b]
- Disseminated intravascular coagulation
- Extravasation of blood; hematoma; pulmonary, cerebral, or other occult hemorrhage
- Polycythemia
- Macrosomic infants of diabetic mothers

Increased Enterohepatic Circulation of Bilirubin

- Breast milk jaundice
- Pyloric stenosis
- Small or large bowel obstruction or ileus

Decreased Clearance

- Prematurity
- Glucose-6-phosphate dehydrogenase deficiency

Metabolic

- Crigler-Najjar syndrome types I and II, Gilbert syndrome
- Tyrosinemia[b]
- Hypermethioninemia[b]
- Hypothyroidism
- Hypopituitarism†

[a]Decreased clearance is also part of the pathogenesis of indirect hyperbilirubinemia.

[b]Elevation of direct-reacting bilirubin also occurs.

Modified from Watchko JF. Indirect hyperbilirubinemia in the neonate. In: Maisels MJ, Watchko JF, eds. *Neonatal Jaundice.* London, UK: Harwood Academic Publishers; 2000:52.

AN APPROACH TO THE JAUNDICED INFANT

The overwhelming majority of both preterm and term infants who are jaundiced are not jaundiced because of any pathologic process. Their jaundice is the result of developmental red blood cell, hepatic, and gastrointestinal immaturities unique to the neonatal period described above. The relevant clinical and laboratory risk factors for the development of severe hyperbilirubinemia in the term and late preterm infant are well documented.[14] The pathologic causes of indirect hyperbilirubinemia are listed in Box 12.1.

Who Is Jaundiced?

Jaundice is a clinical sign, and for years, clinicians have assessed the presence and intensity of jaundice and used this assessment to decide whether to obtain a serum bilirubin measurement. But the ability of clinicians to diagnose "clinically significant" jaundice varies widely, and this can lead to important errors in management.[15–17] In addition, whether the TSB level is "clinically significant" depends both on the actual TSB level and the infant's age in hours (Figs. 12.5–12.7). Currently, experts recommend that before birth hospitalization discharge, TSB or TcB should be measured in all newborns.[18,19]

EDITORIAL COMMENT:

- Conjunctival icterus is a largely neglected physical sign that may be helpful in identifying neonates with clinically relevant hyperbilirubinemia.
- Maisels presented preliminary blinded outpatient observations of neonates for conjunctival icterus as a function of transcutaneous bilirubin (TcB) measurements and confirmed a strong correlation between the presence of conjunctival icterus and elevated bilirubin levels.
- 98.2% of neonates without conjunctival icterus had TcB levels less than 15 mg/dL. So the absence of conjunctival icterus helps rule out significant hyperbilirubinemia.
- However, they noted conjunctival icterus in neonates at lower bilirubin levels than Azzuqa: 17% at TcB less than 10 mg/dL (171 umol/L) and 39.8% at TcB less than 15 mg/dL (257 umol/L), whereas Azzuqa reported babies with conjunctival icterus had bilirubins in the 50th to 75th percentile on the Bhutani nomogram with many above 17 mg/dL.

Maisels MJ, Coffey MP, Gendelman B, et al. Diagnosing jaundice by eye-outpatient assessment of conjunctival icterus in the newborn. *J Pediatr.* 2016;172:212-214.e1; Azzuqa A, Watchko JF. Conjunctival icterus—an important but neglected sign of clinically relevant hyperbilirubinemia in jaundiced neonates. *Curr Pediatr Rev.* 2017;13(3):169-175.

Noninvasive Bilirubin Measurements

TcB measurements are being used with increasing frequency as a screening tool in hospital nurseries, in outpatient settings, and in the NICU population.[10,20–31] They reduce significantly the number of TSB measurements needed in both the term nursery and the NICU, and they are invaluable in the outpatient setting.[22,25,32] TcB measurements provide instantaneous information while reducing the likelihood that a clinically significant TSB will be missed. The TcB value is a measurement of the yellow color of the blanched skin and subcutaneous tissues, not the serum bilirubin level, and should be used to help determine whether the TSB level should be measured. Because TcB measurements are noninvasive, they can be repeated several times during the birth hospitalization and provide useful information about the rate of rise of the bilirubin level. When plotted on a nomogram (see Figs. 12.5–12.7), TcB levels that are crossing percentiles indicate the need for additional observation and evaluation. Although TcB measurements provide a good estimate of the TSB level, they are not a substitute for TSB

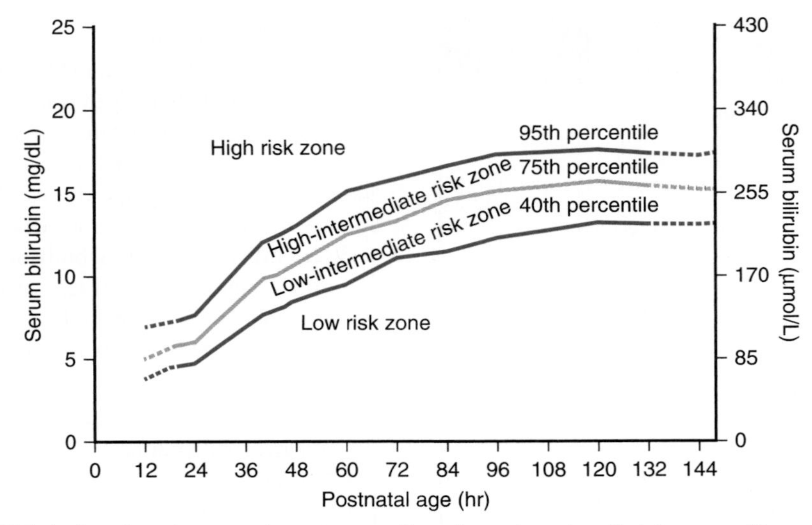

Fig. 12.7 Risk designation of term and near-term well newborns based on their hour-specific serum bilirubin values. (Dotted extensions are based on <300 total serum bilirubin values per epoch.) (From American Academy of Pediatrics, Subcommittee on Hyperbilirubinemia. Management of hyperbilirubinemia in the newborn infant 35 or more weeks of gestation. *Pediatrics*. 2004;114:4.)

TABLE 12.1 Discharge Diagnosis in 306 Infants Admitted With Severe Hyperbilirubinemia[a]

Diagnosis	Number	Percentage
Hyperbilirubinemia of unknown cause or breast milk jaundice	290	94.8
Cephalhematoma or bruising	3	1.0
ABO hemolytic disease[b]	11	3.6
Anti-E hemolytic disease	1	0.3
Galactosemia	1	0.3
Sepsis	0	

[a]Infants were readmitted after discharge as newborns. Mean age at admission was 5 days (range: 2–17 days), and mean bilirubin level was 18.5 ± 2.8 mg/dL (range: 12.7–29.1 mg/dL).

[b]Mother was type O, infant was type A or B, and direct Coombs test result was positive.

From Maisels MJ, Kring E. Risk of sepsis in newborns with severe hyperbilirubinemia. *Pediatrics* 1992;90:741.

values[32,33], and a TSB should always be obtained when therapeutic intervention is being considered.[19,20,32,33]

Laboratory Evaluation—Seeking a Cause for Jaundice

In the NICU, many neonates are jaundiced simply because they were born prematurely and have extremely limited UGT1A1 activity (0.1% of adult levels at 30 weeks' gestation). Even among term and late preterm infants who are readmitted to the hospital in the first 2 weeks of life with TSB levels of 18 to 20 mg/dL (308–340 μmol/L), only about 5% have an identifiable pathologic cause for jaundice (Table 12.1).[34]

The guideline of the American Academy of Pediatrics (AAP) recommends laboratory evaluation for the cause of hyperbilirubinemia in infants of 35 weeks' gestation or more whose TSB levels exceed the 95th percentile or in whom the rate of increase appears to be crossing percentiles.[14] In preterm infants, laboratory evaluation is indicated in any infant who meets the criteria for phototherapy. Table 12.2 provides an approach to the clinical and laboratory evaluation of the jaundiced newborn, and Box 12.1 lists the causes of indirect hyperbilirubinemia in the newborn.

The timing of the onset of jaundice is important; jaundice that appears within the first 24 hours or increases rapidly and crosses percentiles is because of excessive bilirubin production (hemolysis) until proven otherwise. Most newborns whose TSB levels exceed the 75th percentile on the Bhutani nomogram (see Fig. 12.7) have evidence of hemolysis.[11,14,29,35]

PATHOLOGIC JAUNDICE

Hemolytic Disease

Immune-Mediated Hemolytic Disease

The combination of antepartum and postpartum prophylaxis with Rh(D) immunoglobulin has dramatically reduced the incidence of erythroblastosis fetalis resulting from the Rh(D) antigen, and the incidence of Rh(D) hemolytic disease is currently estimated to be about 1 in 1000 live births. Nevertheless, infants born to sensitized mothers, whether the alloantibody is directed toward Rh(D), non-D Rhesus, or non-Rhesus red cell antigens, must be monitored closely for hyperbilirubinemia. Their potential to develop severe hyperbilirubinemia underscores the importance of reviewing maternal antierythrocyte antibody testing results in every obstetric patient and in characterizing the nature of each positive maternal antibody screen.[36]

ABO hemolytic disease occurs in infants of blood group A or B born to group O mothers. Because approximately 45% of Americans of Western European descent have type O blood and a similar percentage are type A, A-O incompatibility is

TABLE 12.2 Laboratory Evaluation of the Jaundiced Infant

Indications	Assessments
Jaundice in first 24 hr	Measure TcB and/or TSB
Infant meets criteria for phototherapy[a] or TSB rising rapidly (i.e., crossing percentiles [see Fig. 12.5])	Perform blood typing and Coombs test, if not done on cord blood. Perform complete blood count, reticulocyte count, and smear examination. Measure direct or conjugated bilirubin. Consider G6PD testing. Repeat TSB in 4–24 hr, depending on infant's age and TSB level.
TSB concentration approaching exchange levels or not responding to phototherapy	Perform investigations as above and G6PD testing and albumin level.
Elevated direct (or conjugated) bilirubin level	Do urinalysis and urine culture; evaluate for sepsis if indicated by history and physical examination.
Jaundice present at or beyond age 2–3 wk, or sick infant	Measure total and direct (or conjugated) bilirubin level. If direct bilirubin elevated, evaluate for causes of cholestasis. Check results of newborn thyroid and galactosemia screen, and evaluate infant for signs or symptoms of hypothyroidism.

[a]Because phototherapy is used at low TSB levels in low-birth-weight infants, these investigations are often unnecessary in low-birth-weight infants who meet the criteria for phototherapy.
G6PD, Glucose-6-phosphate dehydrogenase; *TcB*, transcutaneous bilirubin; *TSB*, total serum bilirubin.

the most common form of ABO incompatibility encountered in the United States.[37] Although about one of every three group A or B infants born to a group O mother has anti-A or anti-B antibodies attached to their red cells (as indexed by a positive direct antiglobin test), only one in five of those develops a modest to significant degree of hyperbilirubinemia. In an Israeli population of 162 direct antiglobulin test (DAT)-positive group A or B newborns born to group O mothers, 52% developed a TSB higher than the 95th percentile on the Bhutani nomogram.[38] Some 48% of O-B babies developed hyperbilirubinemia in the first 24 hours compared with 26% of O-A babies.[33] Of 258 Canadian infants who developed TSB levels of more than 425 μmol/L (24.9 mg/dL), 48 (16.7%) had ABO hemolytic disease.[39] There appears to be considerable variation in the frequency with which ABO hemolytic disease is responsible for severe hyperbilirubinemia (see Table 12.1). O-B heterospecificity is associated with greater hyperbilirubinemia risk than O-A, particularly in neonates whose mothers are of African genetic heritage.

The diagnosis of ABO hemolytic disease as opposed to ABO incompatibility should generally be reserved for infants who have a positive DAT finding *and* clinical jaundice within the first 12 to 24 hours of life (icterus praecox).

BOX 12.2 Criteria for Diagnosing ABO Hemolytic Disease as the Cause of Neonatal Hyperbilirubinemia

- Mother group O, infant group A or B

and

- Positive result on DAT
- Jaundice appearing within 12–24 hr
- Microspherocytes on blood smear
- Negative DAT result but homozygous for Gilbert syndrome mutation

DAT, Direct antibody test.

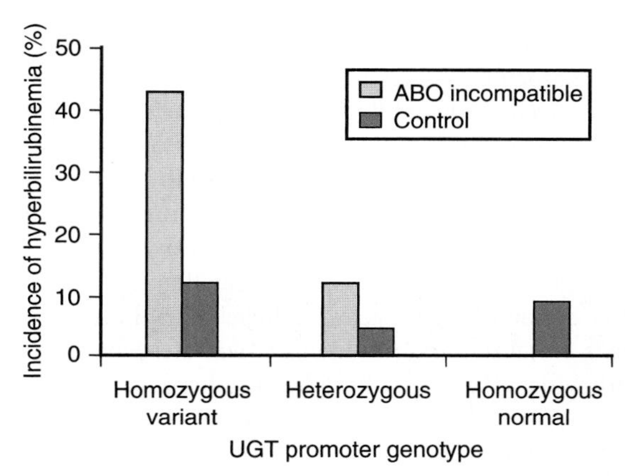

Fig. 12.8 Incidence of hyperbilirubinemia defined as total serum bilirubin level of 15 mg/dL (256 μmol/L) in ABO-incompatible direct antibody test (DAT)-negative and ABO-compatible (control) infants according to the uridine diphosphate glucuronosyltransferase *(UGT)* promoter genotype. ABO-incompatible DAT-negative infants who were also homozygous for the variant UGT promoter (Gilbert syndrome) had a significantly higher incidence of hyperbilirubinemia than did ABO-incompatible DAT-negative infants who were homozygous normal for the UGT promoter. The former subgroup also had a significantly greater incidence of hyperbilirubinemia than any of the three UGT promoter genotype subgroups in the control (ABO-compatible) infants. (From Kaplan M, Hammerman C, Renbaum P, et al. Gilbert's syndrome and hyperbilirubinaemia in ABO incompatible neonates. *Lancet* 2000;356:652.)

Reticulocytosis and the presence of microspherocytes on the smear support the diagnosis (Box 12.2). Underscoring the importance of a positive DAT result in support of the diagnosis of ABO hemolytic disease, Herschel et al concluded that in DAT-negative newborns of ABO-incompatible mother-infant pairs who have significant hyperbilirubinemia, a cause other than isoimmunization should be sought,[40] a conclusion supported by the observations of Kaplan and associates.[41] They found that 43% of DAT-negative, ABO-incompatible infants who were homozygous for the variant *UGT1A1* promoter associated with Gilbert syndrome had a TSB level of 15 mg/dL (256 μmol/L) or higher compared with none of the ABO-incompatible DAT-negative infants who were homozygous normal (for the promoter element) (Fig. 12.8). There was no difference between ABO-incompatible and ABO-compatible DAT-negative newborns, as long as the ABO-incompatible neonates did not have Gilbert syndrome. This observation suggests that ABO incompatibility holds some modest icterogenic potential, even when the DAT is negative that becomes manifest when coupled with the impaired bilirubin-conjugating capacity and increase in red cell turnover seen in Gilbert syndrome.[41,42] There are other possible explanations for the finding of ABO hemolytic disease in the absence of a positive DAT result. Some cases may reflect the insensitivity of the DAT or may occur in infants who have a paucity of A and B antigens on their red cells or unusually efficient absorption of serum antibody by A and B antigen epitopes present in body tissues and fluids.

Heritable Causes of Hemolysis

Red cell membrane defects associated with neonatal hyperbilirubinemia include hereditary spherocytosis, elliptocytosis, stomatocytosis, and infantile pyknocytosis. Newborns, however, frequently exhibit substantial variations in red cell size and shape, and it is not always easy to establish one of these diagnoses. Spherocytes are not usually seen on red cell smears and, when present, suggest the diagnosis of hereditary spherocytosis or ABO hemolytic disease. A recent observation suggests that a mean corpuscular hemoglobin concentration divided by the mean corpuscular volume of 0.36 or more is a useful marker to identify neonates who might have spherocytosis.[43] Because hereditary spherocytosis frequently has an autosomal dominant inheritance pattern, a family history can often be elicited. In addition, the presence of severe jaundice in neonates with hereditary spherocytosis is closely related to an interaction with the Gilbert syndrome allele, a phenomenon also observed as noted earlier in ABO hemolytic disease and in infants with glucose-6-phosphate dehydrogenase (G6PD) deficiency.[44]

Red cell enzyme deficiencies. G6PD deficiency is a problem that affects hundreds of millions of people around the world. Nevertheless, many neonatologists in the United States do not (but should) think about this enzyme deficiency as a likely cause of significant neonatal hyperbilirubinemia. Although G6PD deficiency occurs in approximately 12% of African American males and 4% of African American females,[45] severe hyperbilirubinemia does not develop in most G6PD-deficient newborns. Nevertheless, G6PD deficiency is a frequent cause of bilirubin encephalopathy and uniformly overrepresented among kernicterus cases relative to its background frequency across several populations worldwide. In the United States, G6PD deficiency–related extreme hyperbilirubinemia and kernicterus risk is highest among infants of African American descent.[46] In the kernicterus registry, G6PD deficiency was the cause of the hyperbilirubinemia in 21% of cases, two-thirds of whom were African American.[46] G6PD deficiency is an X-linked disorder, and hemolysis can occur following exposure to an oxidative challenge. Agents potentially involved include naphthalene (a component of mothballs), dyes, and infection, but more often than not, no offending agent is identified. Interestingly, in some, but not all, G6PD-deficient infants in whom severe hyperbilirubinemia develops, there are no signs of overt hemolysis (anemia and reticulocytosis)[47,48] suggesting that abnormal bilirubin clearance together with some degree of hemolysis is the cause of the hyperbilirubinemia. Others disagree with this view and assert that overt signs of hemolysis are not found because the hemolysis is self-limited and extravascular, and involves an older fraction of the red cell population.[49]

The identification of a molecular marker for Gilbert syndrome in the promoter region of the *UGT1A1* gene has demonstrated a remarkable association between hyperbilirubinemia, G6PD deficiency, and Gilbert syndrome. The most common genetic polymorphism encountered in whites with Gilbert syndrome is an additional TA insertion in the TATA box of the *UGT1A1* gene promoter. Affected individuals are homozygous for the variant promoter and have seven repeats—$(TA)_7$ TAA (7/7) instead of the more usual six repeats—$(TA)_6$ TAA (6/6). Heterozygotes have one allele each of the wild-type and variant promoter (6/7). In Israel, of G6PD-deficient infants with TSB levels of 15 mg/dL (257 μmol/L) or more, only 10% were homozygous for the normal *UGT1A1* promoter (6/6), whereas 50% were homozygous for the variant Gilbert *UGT1A1* promoter (7/7). TSB levels of 15 mg/mL or more did not develop in either the neonates with G6PD deficiency alone or in those with only the variant *UGT1A1* promoter (7/7).[44]

Pyruvate kinase deficiency is an autosomal recessive disorder that is less common than G6PD deficiency but may present with significant jaundice, anemia, and reticulocytosis. In particular, pyruvate kinase deficiency should be considered in hyperbilirubinemic neonates of Amish descent.

Unstable hemoglobins. The term *unstable hemoglobins* is applied to hemoglobins exhibiting reduced solubility or higher susceptibility to oxidation of amino acid residues within the individual globin chains.[50] More than 100 structurally different unstable hemoglobin mutants have been documented, and the clinical syndrome associated with unstable hemoglobin disorders is often called *congenital Heinz body hemolytic anemia.* Some of these infants can manifest severe hemolytic anemia and hyperbilirubinemia.

OTHER CAUSES OF INCREASED BILIRUBIN PRODUCTION OR LOAD ON THE LIVER

The hemoglobinopathies rarely manifest themselves as jaundice in the neonatal period, although such cases have been described occasionally. Cephalohematomas, intracranial or pulmonary hemorrhage, or any occult bleeding may lead to an elevated TSB level from breakdown of the extravascular erythrocytes. In some studies, the presence of intraventricular hemorrhage has been associated with an increase in TSB levels in very low-birth-weight infants, but others have not found this association. Polycythemia is usually listed as a potential cause of hyperbilirubinemia because the catabolism of 1 g of hemoglobin produces 35 mg of bilirubin. Nevertheless, mean bilirubin levels and the incidence of hyperbilirubinemia were similar in polycythemic infants receiving partial exchange transfusions and in those receiving symptomatic treatment.[51]

Any small or large bowel obstruction, ileus, or delayed passage of meconium exaggerates the enterohepatic circulation of bilirubin (this is also thought to be the mechanism for hyperbilirubinemia associated with pyloric stenosis). In any of these conditions, correction of the obstruction produces a prompt decline in bilirubin levels. Macrosomic infants of mothers with insulin-dependent diabetes are at an increased risk of hyperbilirubinemia, probably as a result of increased bilirubin production.

Decreased Bilirubin Clearance

Inherited Unconjugated Hyperbilirubinemia—Inborn Errors of Bilirubin UGT1A1 Activity

UGT1A1 accounts for almost all of the bilirubin glucuronidation activity in the human liver, and three degrees of inherited UGT1A1 deficiency are recognized. Crigler-Najjar syndrome type I is inherited in an autosomal recessive pattern with marked genetic heterogeneity, and more than 30 different genetic mutations have been identified. Infants with this condition have virtually complete absence of bilirubin UGT1A1 activity, severe jaundice develops in the first 2 to 3 days of life, and intensive phototherapy and, often, exchange transfusions are required.[52] Unless these children receive a liver transplant, which is curative, they are committed to lifelong phototherapy, which becomes less and less effective as they get older.

Type II Crigler-Najjar disease, also known as *Arias syndrome,* has a pattern of inheritance that is usually autosomal recessive, but it may also be autosomal dominant. The disorder is characterized by low but detectable activity of bilirubin UGT1A1, and the hyperbilirubinemia usually shows some response to phenobarbital therapy likely related to the presence of a phenobarbital response element in the *UGT1A1* gene promoter sequence. Although jaundice is generally less severe than in patients with Crigler-Najjar syndrome type I, marked hyperbilirubinemia develops in some children with Crigler-Najjar syndrome type II, and kernicterus can also occur.[52]

At one time, the diagnosis of Gilbert syndrome was never made until adolescence, when it manifests as a mild, benign, chronic unconjugated hyperbilirubinemia with no evidence of liver disease or overt hemolysis. Gilbert syndrome affects approximately 9% of the population, and both autosomal dominant as well as recessive inheritance patterns have been found. The identification of the genetic basis for this disorder (a variant promoter for the gene encoding *UGT1A1*) has permitted its identification in the newborn. Newborns who are homozygous for the A(TA)7TAA polymorphism have somewhat higher TSB levels in the first days of life than do heterozygous or normal infants, although the effect is modest.[53] The Gilbert syndrome genotype is also an important contributor to the prolonged indirect hyperbilirubinemia found in some breast-feeding infants. Twenty-seven percent of breast-fed infants who had TSB levels of more than 5.8 mg/dL (100 μmol/L) at age 28 days had the Gilbert syndrome genotype, and 16 of 17 breast-fed Japanese infants with prolonged jaundice had at least 1 mutation of the *UGT1A1* gene,[54] primarily of the G71R type.[55] The association of the Gilbert genotype with significant jaundice in G6PD-deficient infants, ABO-incompatible, DAT-negative infants (see Fig. 12.8), and infants with hereditary spherocytosis has been discussed earlier.

BOX 12.3 Causes of Prolonged Indirect Hyperbilirubinemia

- Breast milk jaundice
- Hemolytic disease
- Hypothyroidism
- Extravascular blood
- Pyloric stenosis
- Crigler-Najjar syndrome
- Gilbert syndrome genotype in breast-fed infants

Other Inborn Errors of Metabolism

Jaundiced infants who have vomiting, excessive weight loss, hepatomegaly, and splenomegaly should be suspected of having galactosemia. In galactosemia, the hyperbilirubinemia during the first week of life is almost exclusively unconjugated, but the conjugated fraction tends to increase during the second week, which probably reflects liver damage. A test of the urine for reducing substances using alkaline copper sulfate reagent tablets (Clinitest, Bayer Corp., Elkhart, Ind.) helps make the diagnosis. Infants with tyrosinemia and hypermethioninemia are jaundiced primarily because of neonatal liver disease so that indirect hyperbilirubinemia is generally accompanied by some evidence of cholestasis. Prolonged indirect hyperbilirubinemia is one of the clinical features of congenital hypothyroidism, a condition that should be identified by routine metabolic screening programs currently used for newborns. Other causes of prolonged indirect hyperbilirubinemia are listed in Box 12.3.

Breast Feeding and Jaundice

A strong association between breast feeding and an increased incidence of neonatal hyperbilirubinemia has been found in most[46,56–58] but not all studies.[59] The primary contributors to jaundice associated with breast feeding are a decreased caloric intake in the first few days of life and an increased enterohepatic circulation.[60] Breast-fed infants ingest much lower volumes of milk and therefore receive fewer calories in the first days after birth than do those fed formula,[61] and caloric deprivation itself appears to enhance the enterohepatic circulation of bilirubin. Increasing the frequency of breast feeding significantly reduces the risk of hyperbilirubinemia, which provides further support for the important role of caloric deprivation and the enterohepatic circulation in the pathogenesis of breast-feeding jaundice. The stools of breast-fed infants weigh less, and the cumulative wet and dry stool output of breast-fed infants is lower than that of formula-fed infants.[62]

Mixed Forms of Jaundice

Sepsis

Jaundice is one sign of bacterial sepsis, but septic infants almost always have other signs of infection. Unexplained indirect hyperbilirubinemia as the only sign of sepsis is rare (see Table 12.1), and lumbar punctures or blood and urine cultures in jaundiced infants who otherwise appear well are

BOX 12.4 Most Likely Causes of Cholestasis in Infants 2 Months of Age or Younger

Obstructive Cholestasis

- Biliary atresia
- Choledochal cyst
- Gallstones or biliary sludge
- Algille syndrome
- Inspissated bile
- Cystic fibrosis
- Congenital hepatic fibrosis/Caroli disease

Hepatocellular Cholestasis

Idiopathic neonatal hepatitis

Viral infection

- Cytomegalovirus
- HIV

Bacterial infection

- Urinary tract infection
- Sepsis
- Syphilis

Genetic/metabolic disorders

- Alpha-1 antitrypsin deficiency
- Tyrosinemia
- Galactosemia
- Hypothyroidism
- Progressive familial intrahepatic cholestasis (PFIC)
- Cystic fibrosis
- Panhypopituitarism

Toxic/secondary disorders

- Parenteral nutrition-associated cholestasis

From Moyer V, Freese DK, Whitington PF, et al. Guideline for the evaluation of cholestatic jaundice in infants: recommendations of the North American Society for Pediatric Gastroenterology, Hepatology and Nutrition. *J Pediatr Gastroenterol Nutr.* 2004;39:115.

not recommended.[34] On the other hand, those who appear sick or have direct hyperbilirubinemia or other findings in the physical examination or laboratory evaluation that are out of the ordinary should be evaluated for possible sepsis. Other infectious causes of mixed forms of jaundice include congenital syphilis, the TORCH (*t*oxoplasmosis, *o*ther infections *r*ubella, *c*ytomegalovirus infection, *h*erpes simplex) group of intrauterine infections, and Coxsackie B virus infection.

Cholestatic Jaundice

Cholestasis refers to a reduction in bile flow and is the term used to describe a group of disorders associated with conjugated (or direct reacting) hyperbilirubinemia. Such jaundice indicates inadequate bile secretion or biliary flow. Although it is frequently transient in sick low-birth-weight infants, particularly those receiving parenteral nutrition, a pathologic cause must always be ruled out. For a detailed discussion of the causes and management of cholestatic jaundice, refer to a review of this subject.[63] Conditions most likely associated with conjugated hyperbilirubinemia in the neonatal period are listed in Box 12.4 and documented in a recent Northern California cohort.[4] Cholestasis occurs in about 1 in 2500 infants and can be categorized as obstructive or hepatocellular. Most cases of conjugated hyperbilirubinemia in early infancy are the result of neonatal hepatitis or biliary atresia. Neonatal hepatitis is characterized by prolonged conjugated hyperbilirubinemia without any obvious evidence of bacterial or viral infection or the other causes listed in Box 12.4. Extrahepatic biliary atresia occurs when there is obliteration of the lumen of part of the biliary tract or absence of some or all of the extrahepatic biliary system. Extrahepatic biliary atresia occurs in 1 in 10,000 to 19,000 newborn infants, and it is important to make the diagnosis expeditiously before irreversible sclerosis of the intrahepatic ducts occurs,[63] particularly if the biliary atresia is a component of the biliary atresia splenic malformation syndrome or is the cystic form of biliary atresia (see later discussion). The identification of cholestatic jaundice and initiation of the necessary diagnostic investigations will occur in a timely fashion if every infant who is clinically jaundiced beyond the age of 2 to 3 weeks undergoes measurement of direct-reacting bilirubin (Tables 12.2 and 12.3, and Fig. 12.9).[63] Earlier laboratory investigations are mandatory in any jaundiced infant who has pale stools or dark urine (the urine of most newborns is nearly colorless). This simple approach ensures timely evaluation and treatment of infants with extrahepatic biliary atresia. Some institutions perform a total and direct (or conjugated) bilirubin measurement on all jaundiced newborns, and some studies have shown that infants with biliary atresia already have elevated direct bilirubin measurements in the first few days.[64,65]

The initial treatment of extrahepatic biliary atresia is a portoenterostomy or Kasai procedure in which a loop of small intestine is anastomosed to the porta hepatis following excision of the atretic ducts. About one-third of patients who undergo the Kasai procedure survive for longer than 10 years without liver transplantation.[66] About one-third have adequate bile drainage, but complications of cirrhosis develop, and liver transplantation is necessary before the age of 10 years. The remaining one-third require earlier liver transplantation because bile flow is inadequate following portoenterostomy, and progressive fibrosis and cirrhosis develop. Overall survival of these children, including those undergoing liver transplantation, is now about 90% at age 4 years.[67] Portoenterostomy must be done before there is irreversible sclerosis of the intrahepatic bile ducts, but the effect of the timing of the Kasai procedure on outcome remains controversial.[66,68] Although recent data from France suggest that the outcome following this procedure is best when the procedure is performed before age 31 days,[66] data from the United Kingdom show no difference in outcome of isolated biliary atresia regardless of whether the Kasai procedure is performed before 40 days or between 41 and 60 days.[68] On the other hand, there is a major deleterious effect of delaying surgery in those infants whose biliary atresia is a component of the biliary atresia splenic malformation syndrome (splenic malformation, situs inversus, preduodenal portal vein, absence of the vena cava) and in those with cystic biliary atresia.[68]

TABLE 12.3 Recommended Approach to the Identification and Evaluation of Cholestasis in Infants

Recommendation	Level of Evidence
It is recommended that any infant noted to be jaundiced at 2 weeks of age be clinically evaluated for cholestasis with measurement of total and direct serum bilirubin. However, breast-fed infants who can be reliably monitored and who have an otherwise normal history (no dark urine or light stools) and physical examination may be asked to return at 3 weeks of age, and if jaundice persists, total and direct serum bilirubin are measured at that time.	C
Retest any infant with an acute condition or other explanation for jaundice whose jaundice does not resolve with appropriate management of the diagnosed condition.	D
Ultrasonography is recommended for infants with cholestasis of unknown cause.	A
Liver biopsy is recommended for most infants with cholestasis of unknown cause.	A
Measurements of gamma-glutamyl transpeptidase and lipoprotein X are not routinely recommended in the evaluation of cholestasis in young infants.	C
Scintigraphy and analysis of duodenal aspirate are not routinely recommended but may be useful in situations in which other tests are not readily available.	A
Magnetic resonance cholangiopancreatography and endoscopic retrograde cholangiopancreatography (ERCP) are not routinely recommended, although ERCP may be useful in experienced hands.	C

Level A: Recommendation based on two or more studies that compared the test with a criterion standard in an independent, blind manner in an unselected population of infants similar to those addressed in the guideline. Level B: Recommendation based on a single study that compared the test with a criterion standard in an independent, blind manner in an unselected population of infants similar to those addressed in the guideline. Level C: Recommendation based on lower-quality studies or studies for which inadequate information is provided to assess quality, together with expert opinion and consensus of the committee. Level D: No studies available; recommendation based on expert opinion and consensus of the committee.
From Moyer V, Freese DK, Whitington PF, et al. Guideline for the evaluation of cholestatic jaundice in infants: recommendations of the North American Society for Pediatric Gastroenterology, Hepatology and Nutrition. *J Pediatr Gastroenterol Nutr* 2004:39:115.

By far the most common association with cholestasis in the NICU is prolonged use of intravenous alimentation. When total parenteral nutrition (TPN) is used for 2 weeks or longer, and particularly when such use is exclusive of enteral feedings, cholestatic jaundice may appear. Cholestasis develops in as many as 80% of infants who receive TPN for longer than 60 days, and 50% of those with birth weights of less than 1000 g are affected. The pathogenesis of TPN-associated cholestasis is not clear, but it is thought to be related to a combination of factors, including immaturity of bile secretion in preterm infants, a decrease in bile flow that occurs with no enteral feeding, the use of omega-6 poly unsaturated fatty acids, and potential toxicity of both trace elements and amino acids.

The term *neonatal hepatitis,* which implies an inflammatory or infectious process, is a misnomer. The term *transient neonatal cholestasis* is preferred because the clinical and biopsy findings are the result of a combination of factors, including: (1) immaturity of bile secretion associated with prematurity; (2) chronic or acute ischemia-hypoxia of the liver following intrauterine growth restriction, acute perinatal distress, or lung disease; (3) liver damage caused by perinatal or postnatal sepsis; and (4) decrease in bile flow resulting from delays in enteral feeding.

An approach to the evaluation of infants with cholestatic jaundice is provided in Fig. 12.9. Imaging findings may permit some shortcuts and even avoid the necessity for liver biopsy in some cases. Magnetic resonance cholangiography provides visualization of the extrahepatic bile ducts. Failure to see the bile ducts is highly suggestive of biliary atresia. Other studies suggest that identification of the "triangular cord" (a triangular or tube-shaped echogenic density just cranial to the portal vein bifurcation on a transverse or longitudinal ultrasound scan) can distinguish infants with extrahepatic biliary atresia (in whom the triangular cord is present) from those who have other causes of cholestasis.[69,70] The cord represents the fibrous remnant in the porta hepatis, and when it is seen, the authors recommend prompt laparotomy without further investigation. When it is absent, hepatic scintigraphy is done.[69,70]

Treatment of cholestasis. The treatment of neonatal cholestasis involves treating the cause, although some pharmacologic agents have been used to stimulate bile flow. Phenobarbital increases the uptake of bilirubin by the liver, induces conjugation, enhances bile acid synthesis, and increases bile flow. The administration of phenobarbital before performance of hepatic scintigraphy has helped improve the reliability of this diagnostic test, but the therapeutic use of phenobarbital to improve bile flow and lower serum bilirubin concentrations in conditions such as TPN-associated cholestasis has been disappointing.

The use of ursodeoxycholic acid (UDCA) appears to offer more promise. UDCA is a hydrophilic bile acid with a significant choleretic effect. It appears to be a relatively safe agent when used in children who do not have a fixed obstruction to bile flow. It has been used in the treatment of cholestatic jaundice in infants with cystic fibrosis, as well as in erythroblastosis fetalis. UDCA may also be of value in the treatment of extreme hyperbilirubinemia in older children with Crigler-Najjar syndrome.[71] The mechanism of action of UDCA is not well understood, but it may affect the enterohepatic circulation of endogenous bile salts and increase hepatic bile flow.

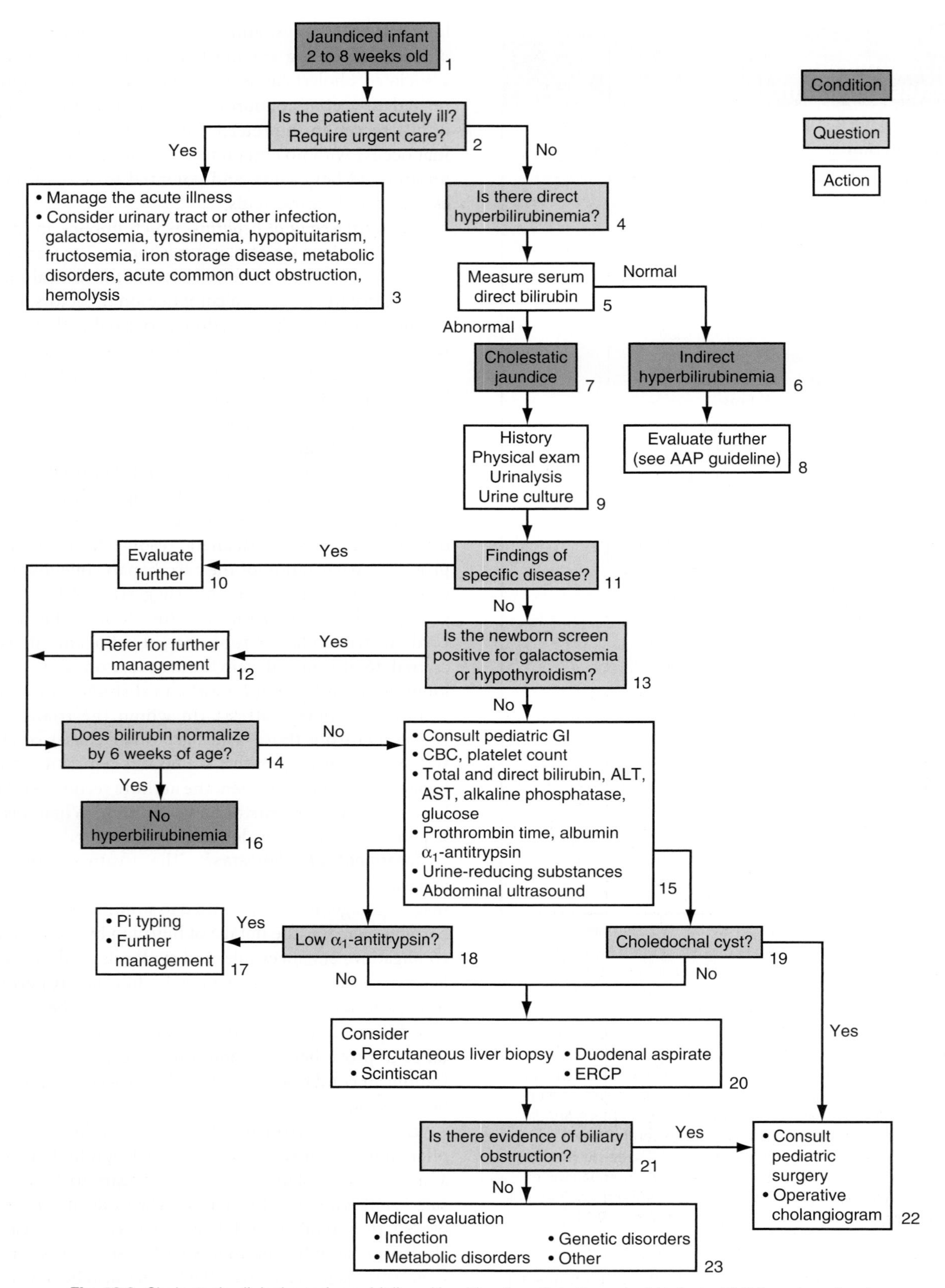

Fig. 12.9 Cholestasis clinical practice guideline. Algorithm for a 2- to 8-week-old-infant. *AAP,* American Academy of Pediatrics; *ALT,* alanine aminotransferase; *AST,* aspartate aminotransferase; *CBC,* complete blood count; *ERCP,* endoscopic retrograde cholangiopancreatography; *GI,* gastroenterology; *Pi,* protease inhibitor. (From Moyer V, Freese DK, Whitington PF, et al. Guideline for the evaluation of cholestatic jaundice in infants: recommendations of the North American Society for Pediatric Gastroenterology, Hepatology and Nutrition. *J Pediatr Gastroenterol Nutr.* 2004;39:115.)

BILIRUBIN TOXICITY

The presence of bilirubin pigment at autopsy in the brains of infants who were severely jaundiced was observed more than 100 years ago, and the term *kernicterus* was applied to infants who died and demonstrated bilirubin staining of the "kern," or nuclear region of the brain. The areas of the brain most commonly affected are the basal ganglia, particularly the subthalamic nucleus and the globus pallidus (Fig. 12.10); the hippocampus; the geniculate body; various brain stem nuclei, including the inferior colliculus, oculomotor, vestibular, cochlear, and inferior olivary nuclei; and the cerebellum, especially the dentate nucleus and vermis.[72] Neuronal necrosis is the dominant histopathologic feature after 7 to 10 days of postnatal life.

The areas of neuronal injury explain the clinical sequelae of bilirubin encephalopathy. In classic kernicterus, markedly jaundiced infants pass through three clinical phases. Initially, the infant becomes lethargic and hypotonic and sucks poorly. Subsequently, hypertonia, fever, and a high-pitched cry develop. The hypertonia is characterized by backward arching of the neck (retrocollis) and trunk (opisthotonos). After about a week, the hypertonia subsides and is replaced by hypotonia. In those who survive, extrapyramidal disturbances (choreoathetosis), auditory abnormalities (auditory neuropathy spectrum disorders including sensorineural hearing loss most severe in the high frequencies), gaze palsies, and dental enamel hypoplasia develop. The presence of retrocollis and opisthotonos (the acute intermediate phase of bilirubin encephalopathy) was thought to represent irreversible damage, but with urgent intervention using phototherapy and exchange transfusion, a normal outcome is possible in some cases.[73,74]

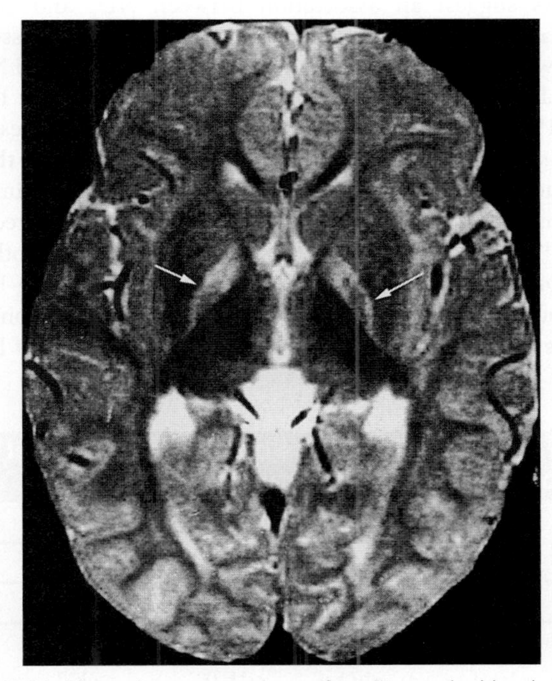

Fig. 12.10 Magnetic resonance image for a 21-month-old male infant who had erythroblastosis fetalis and manifested extreme hyperbilirubinemia and clinical signs of kernicterus at age 54 hours. Note the symmetric, abnormally high-intensity signal from the area of the globus pallidus on both sides (arrows). (From Grobler JM, Mercer MJ. Kernicterus associated with elevated predominantly direct-reacting bilirubin, *S Afr Med J.* 1997;87:146.)

The diagnosis of kernicterus can be confirmed by magnetic resonance imaging (MRI)[75,76] (see Fig. 12.10). Bilateral symmetrically increased T2 signal (or T2 FLAIR signal) in the globus pallidus and subthalamic nucleus of an infant with a history of hyperbilirubinemia is the neuroimaging hallmark of kernicterus and consistent with the neuropathology of this condition.[75,76] Although early in postnatal life, MRI of at-risk infants frequently show increased T1 signal in these regions, this may represent a false-positive finding because of the presence of myelin in these structures.[75,76] Cranial ultrasonography cannot be relied on to identify bilirubin-induced brain damage. Nevertheless, hyperechogenicity has been seen in the basal ganglia and globus pallidus in term and preterm infants who subsequently manifested signs of kernicterus.[75]

Although there is no doubt about the relationship between hazardous bilirubin levels and acute bilirubin encephalopathy leading to kernicterus as characterized by severe motor and auditory dysfunction, it is possible that this outcome is only the most obvious and extreme manifestation of a spectrum of bilirubin toxicity. Acknowledging that kernicterus can be symptomatically diverse, Le Pechon and colleagues propose the use of the term kernicterus spectrum disorders (KSDs) to encompass all of the neurological sequelae of bilirubin neurotoxicity, subclassifying KSDs on the basis of the principal disabling motor and auditory features.[77] At one end of the spectrum might lie more subtle forms of bilirubin-induced neurodevelopmental impairment that occur at lower bilirubin levels and in the absence of any obvious clinical findings in the neonatal period,[77,78] a premise that has been challenged by others.[79,80]

Kernicterus in the Term and Late Preterm Newborn

Kernicterus remains a significant problem in the developing world and still occurs in the United States, Canada, and Western Europe.[46,81–88] Contrary to the experience in the 1940s and 1950s, however, these are generally not infants with Rh hemolytic disease; rather, most are term and late preterm newborns who are apparently healthy at the time of discharge but who subsequently develop extreme to hazardous hyperbilirubinemia (usually a TSB level of >30–35 mg/dL).[46,79,80,89,90] Such bilirubin levels occur in only about 1 in 10,000 infants, and the risk of kernicterus at these TSB levels varies between approximately 8.5% to 27%.[79,89,91] Some of the factors that appear to have contributed to this situation are short hospital stays and inadequate follow-up for newborns, increased incidence of hyperbilirubinemia related to an increase in breast feeding, less concern by pediatricians about jaundice, and failure to interpret bilirubin levels according to the baby's age in hours, not days.

Short Hospital Stays for Newborns

There is evidence that early discharge is associated with an increased risk of significant hyperbilirubinemia. The AAP recommends that infants discharged at less than 72 hours be seen within 2 days of discharge unless the risk of hyperbilirubinemia is very low.[19,92] A recent commentary provides detailed guidelines for risk assessment and follow-up (see later discussion).[19] Figs. 12.5–12.7 make one thing clear: If newborns leave the hospital before they are 36 hours old, their peak bilirubin level will usually occur after they are discharged. Thus jaundice is now primarily an outpatient problem, and monitoring and surveillance following discharge are essential if extreme hyperbilirubinemia is to be prevented.[14,19,92]

Hemolytic Disease and Outcome

Initial observations in the late 1940s and early 1950s showed a strong relationship between increasing TSB levels (particularly levels of >20 mg/dL [>342 μmol/L]) and the risk of kernicterus in infants with Rh hemolytic disease. Hsia et al reported that the incidence of kernicterus in their erythroblastotic population was 8% for those with TSB levels of 19 to 24 mg/dL (325–410 μmol/L), 33% for those with TSB levels of 25 to 29 mg/dL (428 to 496 μmol/L), and 73% for those with levels higher than 30 mg/dL (513 μmol/L).[93] Subsequent studies, however, found strikingly different outcomes. In a study of 129 infants born between 1957 and 1958, all of whom had indirect bilirubin levels of more than 20 mg/dL (342 μmol/L), neurodevelopmental damage was seen in only 2 of 92 (2%) who underwent detailed psychometric, neurologic, and audiologic evaluations at 5 to 6 years of age.[94] The presence of hemolysis is considered to be a risk factor for bilirubin encephalopathy, although the reason for this is not clear. Recent studies have shown that infants with TSB levels of 25 mg/dL (428 μmol/L) or more and a positive DAT result are at greater risk for low IQ scores at ages 5 to 8 years.[66,79,94,95]

Outcome in Infants Without Hemolytic Disease

The relationship between hyperbilirubinemia and poor developmental outcome in full-term and late preterm infants who do not have hemolytic disease has been studied extensively.[96–99] When analyzed as a whole, the data tend to demonstrate that in otherwise healthy neonates without hemolytic disease, TSB levels that do not exceed approximately 25 mg/dL (428 μmol/L) do not place these infants at risk of neurodevelopmental impairment (NDI). In such infants, there has been no convincing demonstration of any adverse effect of these bilirubin levels on IQ, definite neurologic abnormalities, or sensorineural hearing loss.[79,80,89,90,95,100,101]

A relationship has been described between neurologic and psychometric abnormalities and the duration of exposure to elevated TSB levels. In a Turkish study, exposure to TSB levels of more than 20 mg/dL (342 μmol/L) for fewer than 6 hours was associated with a 2.3% incidence of neurologic abnormality. The incidence increased to 18.7% if exposure lasted 6 to 11 hours and to 26% with 12 or more hours of exposure.[102] In contrast, the large National Institute of Child Health and Human Development (NICHD) collaborative phototherapy trial, a 6-year follow-up of 224 control group infants who did not receive phototherapy and who had birth weights of less than 2000 g show no association between IQ and duration of exposure to elevated bilirubin levels.[103]

Hyperbilirubinemia and the Preterm Infant

Compared with term infants, sick, very low-birth-weight infants are at greater risk of developing kernicterus as well as autopsy-proven "low bilirubin kernicterus," the latter representing bilirubin-induced brain damage at TSB levels not thought to pose a neurotoxicity risk, i.e., those below recommended exchange transfusion thresholds. Although pathologic kernicterus in premature newborns is now rare, it has not disappeared completely, and whether modest elevations of TSB cause brain damage in preterm infants is controversial.[104] Two studies of large populations of ELBW infants suggest an association between NDI and small increases in TSB.[2,105] Higher peak TSB levels were associated with an increased risk of death, hearing loss, and NDI in ELBW infants (<1000 g birth weight) born between 1994 and 1997.[105] In a randomized controlled trial of aggressive versus conservative phototherapy for ELBW infants, there was no difference between treatment groups in the primary outcome of death or NDI at 18 to 22 months of corrected age.[2,106] Among survivors, however, aggressive phototherapy produced a significant decrease in NDI, hearing loss, profound impairment, and athetosis compared with conservative phototherapy (see Table 12.4 for the details of how

TABLE 12.4 Criteria for Initiating Phototherapy and Exchange Transfusions in the National Institute of Child Health and Human Development Neonatal Research Network Trial

	AGGRESSIVE MANAGEMENT			CONSERVATIVE MANAGEMENT			
	Phototherapy Begins	Exchange Transfusion		Phototherapy Begins		Exchange Transfusion	
Birth Weight		mg/dL	μmol/L	mg/dL	μmol/L	mg/dL	μmol/L
501–750 g	ASAP after enrollment	≥13.0	≥222	≥8.0	≥137	≥13.0	≥257
751–1000 g	ASAP after enrollment	≥15.0	≥257	≥10.0	≥171	≥15.0	≥257

Enrollment is expected within the period 12–36 hr after birth, preferably between 12 and 24 hr.
From Morris BH, Oh W, Tyson JE, et al. Aggressive vs conservative phototherapy for infants with extremely low birth weight. *N Engl J Med.* 2008;359:1885.

phototherapy was used in this study). Mean TSB levels in infants with hearing loss were 6.5 ± 1.7 mg/dL versus 5.5 ± 1.5 mg/dL in those with no hearing loss ($P < .001$). Peak TSB levels in infants with NDI were 8.6 ± 2.3 versus 8.3 ± 2.3 in unimpaired survivors ($P = .02$). Whether these small differences in TSB levels or the use of aggressive phototherapy was responsible for the outcomes is difficult to say.

Sugama et al documented hypotonia and choreoathetosis, together with the classical MRI findings of kernicterus at follow-up, in two preterm infants of 31 and 34 weeks' gestation.[107] Neither of these infants was acutely ill in the newborn period, and their peak TSB levels were 13.1 mg/dL (224 μmol/L) and 14.7 mg/dL (251 μmol/L). In a study from the Netherlands, classical MRI findings of kernicterus were found in five sick preterm infants (25–29 weeks' gestation), with peak TSB levels ranging from 8.7 to 11.9 mg/dL (148–204 μmol/L).[75] Serum albumin levels in these infants were strikingly low (1.4–2.1 g/dL).

Unbound or Free Bilirubin

Recognition that a peak TSB level, by itself, is a rather poor predictor of the likelihood of NDI or kernicterus raises the question of whether measurements of unbound or "free" bilirubin (B_f) or the ratio of bilirubin to albumin may better predict bilirubin neurotoxicity risk.[99,108–111] Bilirubin (B) is transported in the plasma as a dianion bound tightly but reversibly to serum albumin (A):

$$B^{2-} + A \leftrightarrow AB^{2-}$$

Most bilirubin in the circulation is bound to albumin, and a relatively small fraction remains unbound. The concentration of B_f is believed to dictate the biological effects of bilirubin in jaundiced newborns, including its neurotoxicity. Elevations of B_f have been associated with kernicterus in sick preterm infants. In addition, elevated B_f concentrations are more closely associated than TSB with transient abnormalities in the brain stem auditory-evoked potential in both term and preterm infants.[109,111] Although a B_f level of more than 1.0 ug/dL may predict the presence or absence of NDI in preterm neonates with high sensitivity and specificity, there is no agreement about what constitutes the neurotoxic B_f threshold[91]; that is, the threshold at which B_f produces changes in cellular function culminating in permanent cell injury and cell death. In addition, clinical laboratory measurement of B_f is not generally available, although efforts to bring B_f and related indices to the clinical arena are ongoing.[109–113]

The ratio of bilirubin (in milligrams per deciliter) to albumin (in grams per deciliter) does correlate with measured B_f in newborns, has been used as an approximate surrogate for the measurement of B_f, and is endorsed by the AAP as a metric to consider in making decisions to perform an exchange transfusion in hyperbilirubinemic neonates.[92] Indeed, in an Egyptian population, an elevated B/A ratio exceeding the AAP exchange transfusion (ExT) threshold was a strong predictor of bilirubin neurotoxicity risk including the progression of ABE severity, neurologic impairment, and kernicterus.[114] In the presence of significant hypoalbuminemia, the B/A ratio becomes an increasingly relevant index of bilirubin neurotoxicity risk as exemplified by the phenomenon of low-bilirubin kernicterus, where the CNS bilirubin exposure is neurotoxic and oftentimes related to an abnormally low serum albumin. In the low-bilirubin kernicterus case series of Govaert et al,[115] serum albumin levels ranged from 1.3 to 1.9 g/dL, and every neonate demonstrated an elevated B/A ratio that met or exceeded recommended B/A ratio ExT thresholds. Thus a modestly elevated TSB coupled with marked hypoalbuminemia represents a risk of bilirubin neurotoxicity dictated by the very low serum albumin alone, independent of any abnormality in albumin-bilirubin binding affinity,[113] although, in some circumstances, poor albumin-binding affinity can play a role as well.[116] Although a randomized controlled trial in the Netherlands (the BARTrial)[117] reported no benefit on neurodevelopmental outcomes of using the B/A ratio in conjunction with the TSB to determine hyperbilirubinemia treatment (phototherapy and/or exchange transfusion), few were treated based on the B/A ratio.[118] The latter reflected in part the limited number of subjects with low albumin concentrations.

It must also be recognized that albumin-binding capacity varies significantly among newborns, is impaired in sick infants, and increases with increasing gestational age and postnatal age. A recent study of very low-birth-weight infants confirmed that bilirubin-binding capacity was lower and unbound bilirubin higher in unstable neonates than in stable neonates.[119] An increase in unbound bilirubin was associated with higher rates of death or NDI. TSB levels were also associated with an increased risk of death or NDI but only in unstable and not in stable infants.[119] In fact, in stable infants, an increase in TSB levels was associated with a decrease in death or cerebral palsy, a puzzling and currently unexplained finding.[119] In the NICHD phototherapy trial involving 224 infants who were born between 1974 and 1976 with birth weights of less than 2000 g and who were evaluated at age 6 years, no relation was seen between measures of bilirubin-albumin binding and IQ scores at follow-up.[120]

Crucially important in the measurement of B_f is the bilirubin-albumin binding constant k, a term whose numeric value actually may vary considerably depending on conditions, including, among other factors, sample dilution, albumin concentration, and the presence of competing compounds.[99,108,121] Moreover, the risk of bilirubin encephalopathy is likely not simply a function of the B_f concentration alone or the TSB level but of a combination of several factors—namely, the total amount of bilirubin available (the miscible pool of bilirubin), the tendency of bilirubin to enter the tissue (the B_f concentration), and the susceptibility of the cells of the central nervous system to be damaged by bilirubin.[122] Clarifying and defining clinically germane B_f concentrations, B/A ratios, exposure conditions, and exposure durations, as well as improving, standardizing and validating B_f measurements, are important lines of clinical and translational research.[112]

In calculating the risks of bilirubin toxicity, factors that affect the binding of bilirubin to albumin should be taken into account. One of these factors is the concentration of free fatty acids that compete with bilirubin for its binding to albumin, although this does not occur until the molar ratio of free fatty acids to albumin exceeds 4:1. Such ratios are generally not achieved with doses of up to 3 g/kg of intralipid given over 24 hours. Some studies have shown that the binding of bilirubin to albumin is not affected by changes in serum pH,[123,124] although the correction of neonatal acidosis in 11 sick newborns decreased the serum free bilirubin concentration.[125] A decrease in pH, however, does increase the binding of bilirubin to cells and partitioning to extravascular tissue and therefore its deposition in the central nervous system.[126,127]

Drugs can affect bilirubin-albumin binding both singly and in combination. Because of their bilirubin-displacing capabilities, drugs that should be avoided in the period immediately after birth, or at least until serum bilirubin levels are less than 5 mg/dL (85 μmol/L), include ethacrynic acid, azlocillin, carbenicillin, cefotetan, ceftriaxone, moxalactam, sulfisoxazole, and ticarcillin.[128,129]

Entry of Bilirubin Into the Brain

Under normal circumstances, there is a constant flux of bilirubin in and out of the brain, and changes in the brain stem auditory-evoked response can be demonstrated at modest elevations of serum bilirubin. These changes reverse as the bilirubin level decreases. Bilirubin also enters the brain when there is a marked increase in the serum level of unbound bilirubin. Even bilirubin bound to albumin can enter the brain when the blood–brain barrier is disrupted, and in all of these situations, acidosis increases deposition of bilirubin in brain cells.

Neurotoxicity of Bilirubin

It is not known exactly how bilirubin exerts its toxic effects, and no single mechanism of bilirubin intoxication has been demonstrated in all cells.[130,131] Bilirubin lowers membrane potential, decreases the rate of tyrosine uptake and dopamine synthesis in dopaminergic striatal synaptosomes, and impairs substrate transport, neurotransmitter synthesis, and mitochondrial functions in neurons.[130] Unconjugated bilirubin also activates glial cells with the release of proinflammatory cytokines such as tumor necrosis factor, interleukin-1 beta, and interleukin-6, which suggests that inflammatory processes can contribute to the toxic effects of bilirubin on nerve cells.[131]

CLINICAL MANAGEMENT

Prevention of Severe Hyperbilirubinemia in the Term and Late Preterm Newborn

Risk Assessment

Because severe hyperbilirubinemia in the term and late preterm newborn now occurs predominately, but not exclusively, in infants who have been discharged following birth, a systematic evaluation of the potential risk of subsequent severe hyperbilirubinemia should be carried out before discharge for all term and late preterm newborns. Box 12.5 lists factors that are most consistently associated with an increase in the risk of severe hyperbilirubinemia and should be used in conjunction with Fig. 12.11 in performing a risk assessment before discharge.

BOX 12.5 Risk Factors for Severe Hyperbilirubinemia to be Considered With the Gestational Age and the Predischarge Total Serum Bilirubin or Transcutaneous Bilirubin Level[a]

- Exclusive breast feeding, particularly if nursing, is not going well and/or weight loss is excessive (>8%–10%)
- Isoimmune or other hemolytic disease (e.g., glucose-6-phospate dehydrogenase deficiency, hereditary spherocytosis)
- Previous sibling with jaundice
- Cephalohematoma or significant bruising
- East Asian race

From Maisels MJ, Bhutani VK, Bogen D, et al. Hyperbilirubinemia in the newborn infant >35 weeks' gestation: an update with clarifications. *Pediatrics*. 2009;124(4):1193.

Universal Newborn Bilirubin Screening

First described by Bhutani et al in 1999,[38] measurement of a predischarge TSB or TcB level has been shown in different populations to be a good predictor of the risk of an infant subsequently developing or not developing hyperbilirubinemia.[132–135] Evidence suggests that combining predischarge measurement of the TSB or TcB with evaluation of clinical risk factors will improve the accuracy of this prediction.[136,137] In addition, measurement of the TSB or TcB, when interpreted using the hour-specific nomogram (see Fig. 12.7), provides a quantitative assessment of the degree of hyperbilirubinemia and indicates the need (or lack of) for additional testing to identify the cause of hyperbilirubinemia and for additional TSB measurements (see Table 12.2).[14,19]

Because the measurement of predischarge TSB or TcB combined with assessment of clinical risk factors currently provides the best prediction of the risk of subsequent severe hyperbilirubinemia, a predischarge TSB or TcB value should be obtained for every infant.[19] The TSB can be measured on the same sample that is drawn for the metabolic screen, which saves an additional heel-stick. The TSB or TcB is plotted on the nomogram to determine the risk zone and combined with the previously determined and relevant clinical risk factors (see Box 12.5) to assess the risk of subsequent hyperbilirubinemia and to formulate a plan of management and follow-up (see Fig. 12.11).[19] When combined with the risk zone, the factors that are most predictive of hyperbilirubinemia risk are lower gestational age and exclusive breast feeding. The lower the gestational age, the greater the risk of hyperbilirubinemia.[136,137] When two or more successive TSB or TcB measurements are obtained, it is helpful to plot these data on the nomogram to assess the rate of rise. Hemolysis is likely if the

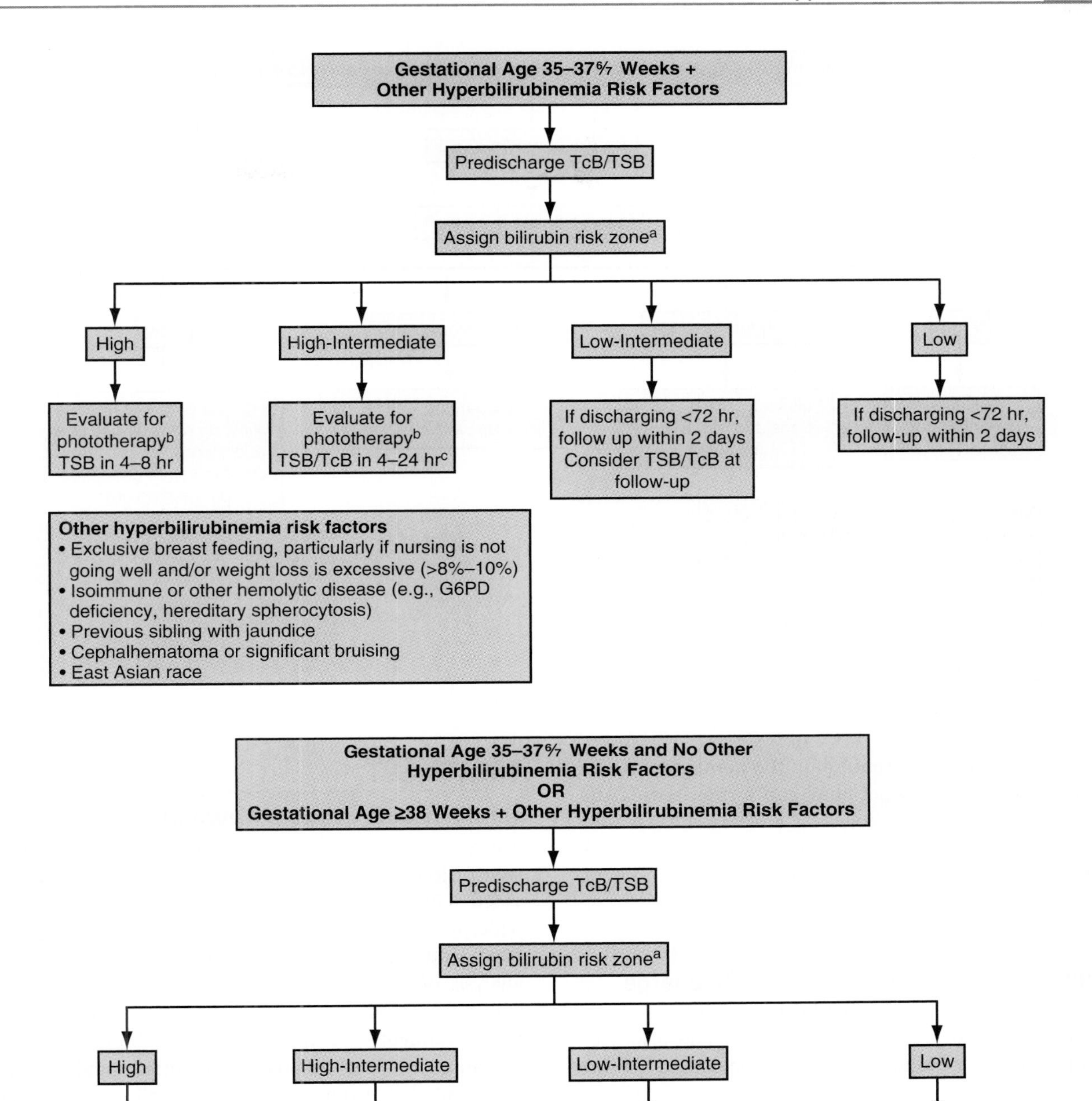

Fig. 12.11 For legend, see following page algorithm providing recommendations for management and follow-up according to predischarge bilirubin measurements, gestational age, and other risk factors for subsequent hyperbilirubinemia. [a]See Fig. 12.7. [b]See Fig. 12.12. [c]In hospital or as outpatient. [d]Follow-up recommendations can be modified according to level of risk for hyperbilirubinemia; depending on the circumstances, in infants at low risk, later follow-up can be considered. *G6PD,* Glucose-6-phosphate dehydrogenase; *TcB,* transcutaneous bilirubin; *TSB,* total serum bilirubin. (From Maisels MJ, Bhutani VK, Bogen D, et al. Hyperbilirubinemia in the newborn infant ≥35 weeks' gestation: an update with clarifications. *Pediatrics.* 2009;124[4]:1193.)

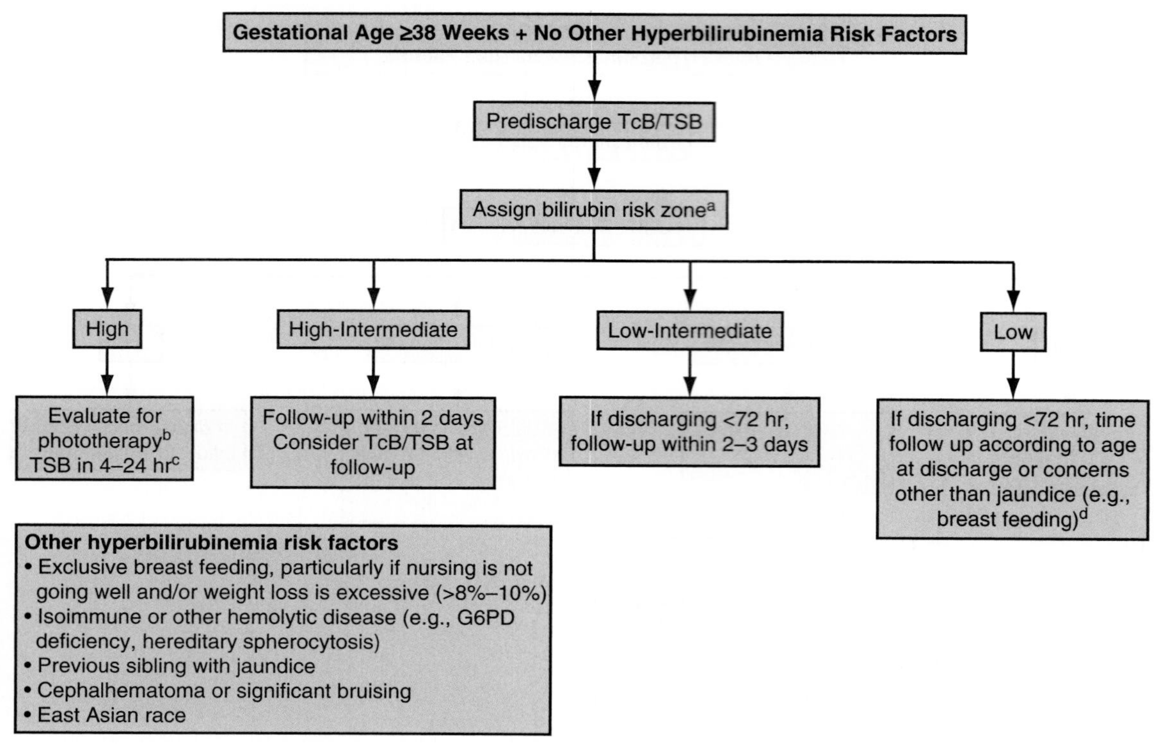

Fig. 12.11 cont'd

TSB or TcB is crossing percentiles on the nomogram or the rate of rise exceeds 0.2 mg per hour, and further testing and follow-up are needed (see Table 12.2 and Fig. 12.11). Note that even with a low predischarge TSB or TcB value, the risk of subsequent hyperbilirubinemia is not zero, so appropriate follow-up should always be provided (see Fig. 12.11).[136]

Response to Predischarge Total Serum Bilirubin Measurements and Follow-Up after Discharge

Fig. 12.11 provides a guideline for management and follow-up according to predischarge screening and also provides suggestions for evaluation and management at the first follow-up visit.[19]

Measuring Bilirubin Production

When heme is catabolized, carbon monoxide (CO) is produced in equimolar quantities with bilirubin, and measurements of blood carboxyhemoglobin levels or end-tidal CO, corrected for ambient CO ($ETCO_c$), provide the only available methods for quantifying hemolysis.[138] Although routine measurement of $ETCO_c$ at 30 ± 6 hours of life does not improve the prediction of subsequent hyperbilirubinemia, measurement of $ETCO_c$ in infants with TSB levels above the Bhutani 75th percentile suggests that most have increased red cell turnover (or hemolysis).[35,139] A recent study suggests that combining measurement of $ETCO_c$ with a TSB rate of rise greater than 2 mg/dL per hour may prove useful in identifying infants who have increased bilirubin production as well as those with a limited capacity to clear the bilirubin load, placing them at risk for subsequent severe hyperbilirubinemia.[35,139]

TREATMENT

Term and Late Preterm Newborns

The AAP guidelines for the use of phototherapy and exchange transfusion in infants of 35 weeks' gestation or more are provided in Figs. 12.12 and 12.13. These guidelines have achieved widespread acceptance and are used throughout the United States and in many other countries. Nevertheless, a recent analysis of the phototherapy guidelines suggests that they could be modified to decrease the number of infants who need treatment.[140] There is little doubt, however, that if significantly jaundiced infants were identified, and these guidelines and the recommendations for follow-up consistently implemented, kernicterus would be extremely rare. Effective use of phototherapy in these infants is described later (see "Phototherapy: Effective Use of Phototherapy").

Breast-Fed Infants

Of infants who have TSB levels high enough to require phototherapy and who do not have evidence of isoimmunization or other obvious hemolytic disease, 80% to 90% are fully or partially breast fed,[34] and the entity of jaundice in the breast-fed infant has recently been reviewed.[141,142] Much of this hyperbilirubinemia is associated with inadequate breast feeding, and attention to increasing the frequency of breast feeding during the first few days after birth will decrease TSB levels. Supplemental feedings of water or dextrose water should not be provided to breast-fed infants because this does not lower their TSB levels. If supplementation is deemed necessary in an infant with hyperbilirubinemia, human milk or formula

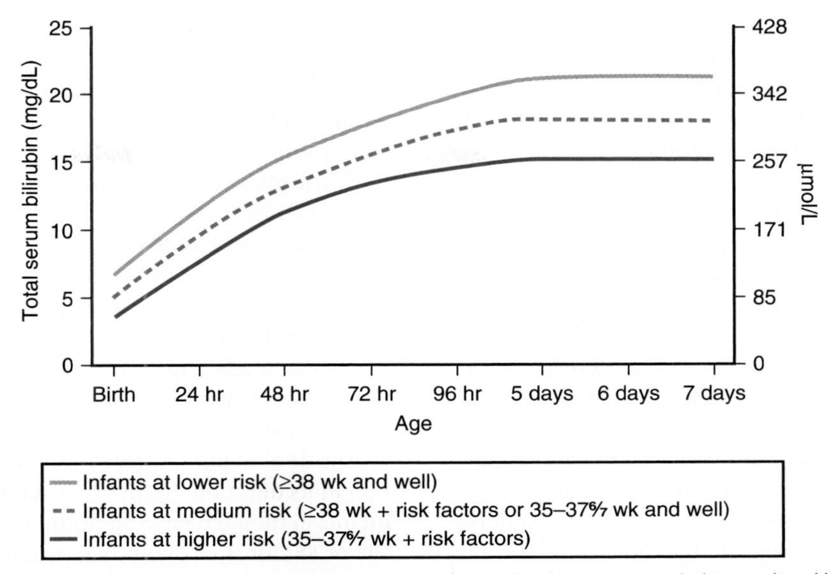

Fig. 12.12 Guidelines for phototherapy in hospitalized infants of 35 or more weeks' gestation. Note: These guidelines are based on limited evidence, and the levels shown are approximations. The guidelines refer to the use of intensive phototherapy, which should be used when the total serum bilirubin (TSB) level exceeds the line indicated for each category. Infants are designated as "higher risk" because of the potential negative effects of conditions affecting albumin binding of bilirubin, the blood–brain barrier, and the susceptibility of the brain cells to damage by bilirubin. "Intensive phototherapy" implies irradiance in the blue-green spectrum (wavelengths of approximately 430–490 nm) of at least 30 µW/cm^2/nm (measured at the infant's skin directly below the center of the phototherapy unit) and delivered to as much of the infant's surface area as possible. Note that irradiance measured below the center of the light source is much greater than that measured at the periphery. Measurements should be made with the spectroradiometer specified by the manufacturer of the phototherapy system. A TSB level that does not decrease or continues to rise in an infant who is receiving intensive phototherapy strongly suggests the presence of hemolysis. (From American Academy of Pediatrics, Subcommittee on Hyperbilirubinemia. Management of hyperbilirubinemia in the newborn infant 35 or more weeks of gestation., *Pediatrics.* 2004;114:297.)

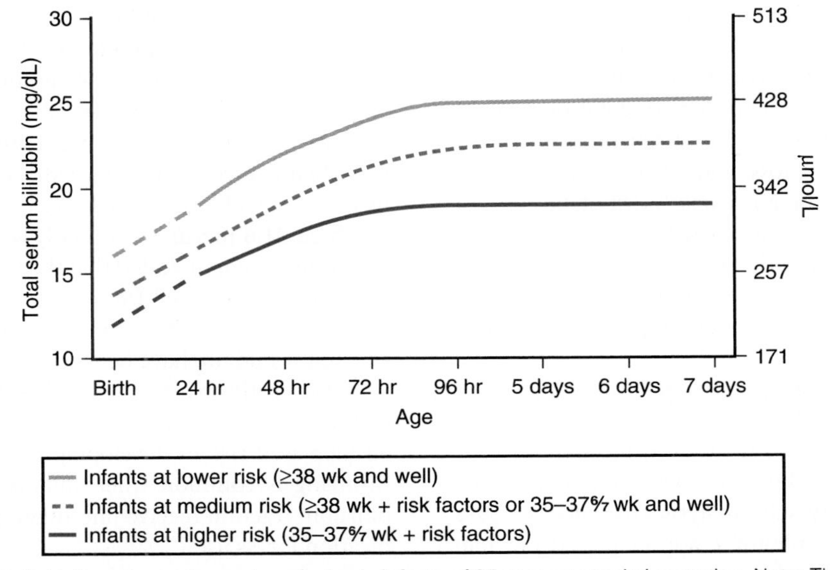

Fig. 12.13 Guidelines for exchange transfusion in infants of 35 or more weeks' gestation. Note: These guidelines are based on limited evidence, and the levels shown are approximations. During birth hospitalization, exchange transfusion is recommended if the total serum bilirubin (TSB) rises to these levels despite intensive phototherapy. For readmitted infants, if the TSB level is above the exchange level, repeat TSB measurement every 2 to 3 hours and consider exchange if the TSB remains above the levels indicated after intensive phototherapy for 6 hours. The following bilirubin-to-albumin ratios can be used together with, but in not in lieu of, the TSB level as an additional factor in determining the need for exchange transfusion.

should be provided. It is always undesirable to interrupt nursing, and when the TSB level in a breast-fed infant reaches a level at which phototherapy is being considered, breast feeding should be continued while the infant undergoes treatment with intensive phototherapy (see "Phototherapy").

Low-Birth-Weight Infants

In the last three decades, there appears to have has been a remarkable decrease in the incidence of kernicterus found at autopsy in infants who died in the NICU, although, as noted above, kernicterus in surviving NICU infants is still being seen in high-resource countries. Some of the decrease in kernicterus at autopsy could be the result of liberal use of phototherapy, but it is also true that there has been a substantial decrease in the number of autopsies performed. Phototherapy has dramatically decreased the necessity for exchange transfusion in low-birth-weight infants so that these procedures are becoming increasingly rare in the NICU.[2,143] In the NICHD Neonatal Research Network study,[2] only 5 of 1974 ELBW infants (0.25%) required an exchange transfusion. Table 12.5 provides an approach to the use of phototherapy and exchange transfusion based on gestational age.[19] There is no solid evidence base for the recommendations provided. The recommended treatment levels are based on operational thresholds or therapeutic normal levels (a level beyond which specific therapy will likely do more good than harm).[144] In the NICHD Neonatal Research Network study,[2] 974 ELBW infants were randomly assigned at age 12 to 36 hours to receive either aggressive or conservative phototherapy.[2] The protocol used in that study is shown in Table 12.4. In infants assigned to the aggressive phototherapy group, the mean TSB levels were lower than those in the conservative phototherapy group (4.7 ± 1.1 versus 6.2 ± 1.5 mg/dL). There was no difference between the groups in the primary outcome (death or NDI), but in survivors at 18 to 20 months of corrected age, aggressive phototherapy was associated with a significant decrease in NDI, profound impairment (mental or psychomotor developmental index of ≤50 or severe gross motor impairment), severe hearing loss, and athetosis. The authors noted that the reduction in NDI was "attributable almost entirely to there being fewer infants with profound impairment in the aggressive phototherapy group." These results suggest that aggressive phototherapy, as used in this trial, significantly reduced the risk of neurodevelopmental handicap in surviving infants.[2]

On the other hand, in the aggressive phototherapy group, there was a 5% increase in mortality in the infants with birth weights of 501 to 750 g who had received mechanical ventilation.[145] Although this difference was not statistically significant, a post hoc Bayesian analysis estimated an 89% probability that aggressive phototherapy increased the rate of deaths in the subgroup.[145] The reasons for these findings are not clear, but these tiny infants have gelatinous, thin skin through which light will penetrate readily, reaching more deeply into the subcutaneous tissue. There is evidence that phototherapy produces DNA damage,[146] oxidative injury to cell membranes,[147,148] and heat deposition, and such injury could have a negative effect on these tiny infants.[147,149] The investigators planned to use a "target irradiance level" of 15 to 40 μW/cm²/nm, and the mean irradiance levels achieved were 22 to 25 μW/cm²/nm.[2] Because phototherapy in this study, and in almost all infants of this birth weight, is used in a prophylactic mode (with the goal of preventing further elevation of the TSB level), it is quite likely that lower irradiance levels (i.e., a lower dose of phototherapy) could be equally effective and perhaps less harmful. In view of the observed increase in mortality, it seems prudent, at least in infants with birth weights of less than 750 g, to initiate phototherapy at lower irradiance levels and to increase these levels, or to increase the surface area of the infant exposed to phototherapy, only if the TSB level continues to rise.

The dose of phototherapy can also be reduced by a reduction in its duration. In the Neonatal Research Network Study, infants in the aggressive phototherapy group received an average of 88 hours of phototherapy compared with 35 hours in the conservative group. DNA damage increases linearly with the duration of phototherapy,[146] and Hansen has suggested that the increased duration of phototherapy could be related to the increase in mortality.[150] Preliminary data suggest that the duration of phototherapy can be reduced by as much as 75% by using intermittent or cycled phototherapy with no negative effect on peak TSB levels.[151]

Infants with Elevated Direct-Reacting or Conjugated Bilirubin Levels

There are no good data to guide the clinician in dealing with the occasional infant who has a high TSB level as well as a significant elevation in direct-reacting bilirubin. Kernicterus has been described in infants with TSB levels of more than 20 mg/dL (340 μmol/L) but in whom, because of significant elevations in direct bilirubin levels, the indirect bilirubin levels were well below 20 mg/dL (340 μmol/L).[152,153] Elevated direct bilirubin levels may decrease the infant's albumin-binding capacity. The magnetic resonance image shown in Fig. 12.10 was obtained from an infant with Rh erythroblastosis fetalis in whom a TSB level of 45.2 mg/dL (773 μmol/L) developed, of which 31.6 mg/dL (514 μmol) was direct reacting.[153] It is commonly recommended that the direct bilirubin concentration not be subtracted from the total bilirubin level unless it exceeds 50% of the TSB concentration.[14] This seems reasonable but would not have benefitted the aforementioned infant with Rh erythroblastosis.[153] It has been suggested, but not confirmed, that infants with the bronze baby syndrome are at an increased risk of developing bilirubin encephalopathy.[154] Bronzing is common when infants with an elevated direct bilirubin fraction receive phototherapy but is not a contraindication for its use.

Infants With Hemolytic Disease

Infants with hemolytic disease are generally considered to be at a greater risk for the development of bilirubin encephalopathy than are nonhemolyzing infants with similar bilirubin levels, although the reasons for this are not clear. In

TABLE 12.5 Suggested Use of Phototherapy and Exchange Transfusion in Preterm Infants Less Than 35 Weeks' Gestational Age

	Phototherapy	Exchange Transfusion
Gestational Age (wk)	Initiate Phototherapy Total Serum Bilirubin (mg/dL)	Total Serum Bilirubin (mg/dL)
<28	5–6	11–14
28 0/7–29 6/7	6–8	12–14
30 0/7–31 6/7	8–10	13–16
32 0/7–33 6/7	10–12	15–18
34 0/7–34 6/7	12–14	17–19

- This table reflects recommendations for operational or therapeutic total serum bilirubin (TSB) thresholds—bilirubin levels at, or above which, treatment is likely to do more good than harm.[58] These TSB levels are not based on good evidence and are lower than those suggested in recent UK[11] and Norwegian[5] guidelines.
- The wider ranges and overlapping of values in the exchange transfusion column reflect the degree of uncertainty in making these recommendations.
- Use the lower range of the listed total serum bilirubin levels for infants at greater risk for bilirubin toxicity, e.g., lower gestational age; serum albumin levels <2.5 g/dL; rapidly rising TSB levels, suggesting hemolytic disease; and those who are clinically unstable.[31] When a decision is being made about the initiation of phototherapy or exchange transfusion, infants are considered to be clinically unstable if they have one or more of the following conditions: blood pH <7.15, blood culture–positive sepsis in the previous 24 hours, apnea and bradycardia requiring cardiorespiratory resuscitation (bagging and or intubation) during the previous 24 hours, hypotension requiring pressor treatment during the previous 24 hours, and mechanical ventilation at the time of blood sampling.[31]
- Recommendations for exchange transfusion apply to infants who are receiving intensive phototherapy to the maximal surface area but whose TSB levels continue to increase to the levels listed.
- For all infants, an exchange transfusion is recommended if the infant shows signs of acute bilirubin encephalopathy (e.g., hypertonia, arching, retrocollis, opisthotonos, high-pitched cry), although it is recognized that these signs rarely occur in very low-birth-weight infants.
- Use total bilirubin. Do not subtract direct reacting or conjugated bilirubin from the total.
- For infants less than or equal to 26 weeks' gestation, it is an option to use phototherapy prophylactically starting soon after birth.
- Use postmenstrual age for phototherapy (e.g., when a 29 0/7-week infant is 7 days old, use the TSB level for 30 0/7 weeks.
- Discontinue phototherapy when TSB is 1–2 mg/dL below the initiation level for the infant's postmenstrual age.
- Discontinue TSB measurements when TSB is declining and phototherapy is no longer required.
- Measure the serum albumin level in all infants.
- Measure irradiance at regular intervals with an appropriate spectroradiometer.
- The increased mortality observed in infants ≤1000 g who are receiving phototherapy[17,25,37] suggests that it is prudent to use less-intensive levels of irradiance in these infants. In such infants, phototherapy is almost always prophylactic—it is used to prevent a further increase in the TSB, and intensive phototherapy with high irradiance levels usually is not needed. In infants ≤1000 g, it is reasonable to start phototherapy at lower irradiance levels. If the TSB continues to rise, additional phototherapy should be provided by increasing the surface area exposed (phototherapy above and below the infant, reflecting material around the incubator). If the TSB nevertheless continues to rise, the irradiance should be increased by switching to a higher-intensity setting on the device or by bringing the overhead light closer to the infant. Fluorescent and light-emitting diode (LED) light sources can be brought closer to the infant, but this cannot be done with halogen or tungsten lamps because of the danger of a burn.

From Maisels MJ, Watchko JF, Bhutani VK, Stevenson DK. An approach to the management of hyperbilirubinemia in the preterm infant less than 35 weeks of gestation. *J Perinatol.* 2012;32:660-664.

Rh hemolytic disease, phototherapy should be used early, as soon as there is evidence of a rapidly increasing bilirubin level. The AAP guidelines (Figs. 12.12 and 12.13) provide for earlier institution of phototherapy and exchange transfusion in the presence of isoimmunization.[11] Recent studies have confirmed the wisdom of this approach.[95,114,155] In infants with TSB concentrations of more than 25 mg/dL, the presence of isoimmunization (a positive DAT result) significantly increases the risk of a low IQ score.[95] The use of intravenous gamma-globulin (IVIG) has been shown to reduce the need for exchange transfusions in both Rh and ABO hemolytic disease,[112] although two recent randomized controlled trials involving several affected infants with Rh disease did not show any benefit from IVIG administration,[156,157]and a Cochrane review concluded that the routine use of IVIG cannot currently be recommended.[156,158] In these trials, IVIG was only used when phototherapy had failed to control the rise in TSB, but it is possible that IVIG could have been effective if it had been used earlier.[159] Tin-mesoporphyrin will decrease TSB levels in preterm infants, breast-fed infants, those with Coombs-positive ABO incompatibility, and in G6PD deficiency, but this drug is not yet

TABLE 12.6 Radiometric Quantities Used

Quantity	Dimensions	Usual Units of Measure
Irradiance (radiant power incident on a surface per unit area of the surface)	W/m^2	W/cm^2
Spectral irradiance (irradiance in a certain wavelength band)	$W/m^2/nm$ (or W/m^2)	$\mu W/cm^2/nm$
Spectral power (average spectral irradiance across a surface area)	W/m	mW/nm

From Maisels MJ. Why use homeopathic doses of phototherapy? *Pediatrics.* 1996;98:283–287.

approved for use by the U.S. Food and Drug Administration (FDA) (see "Pharmacologic Treatment").[160]

Infants With Hydrops Fetalis

The pathogenesis of hydrops fetalis is not fully understood. In the fetal sheep model, acute severe anemia leads to hydrops associated with increased venous pressure and placental edema, whereas the same degree of anemia produced over a longer period does not. Thus high-output failure resulting from anemia is probably not the primary mechanism for hydrops. Profound extramedullary hematopoiesis occurs in the fetus with erythroblastosis fetalis, and this leads to both portal hypertension and disruption of normal liver function. It is likely that these are the primary mechanisms responsible for the development of hydrops in iso-immune hemolytic disease. Infants with hydrops are commonly hypoxic and severely anemic, and they demand immediate treatment. Exchange transfusion of 50 mL/kg of packed cells soon after birth increases the hematocrit to about 40%. Phlebotomy should not be performed routinely on these infants because they are usually normovolemic, and their blood volume should not be manipulated without appropriate measurements of hemodynamic status. In addition, before therapeutic decisions are made, acidosis, hypercarbia, hypoxemia, and anemia must be corrected. Serum glucose levels must be monitored carefully because hypoglycemia is common.

PHOTOTHERAPY

Phototherapy works in much the same way as do drugs: the absorption of photons of light by bilirubin molecules in the skin produces a therapeutic effect similar to the binding of drug molecules to a receptor. Whereas drug doses are conveniently measured in units of weight, photon doses are more difficult to measure and are expressed in less familiar terms. Table 12.6 defines the radiometric quantities used in assessing the dose of phototherapy, and Table 12.7 lists the major factors that influence the dose, and therefore the efficacy, of phototherapy. Several recent comprehensive reviews are recommended.[147,161,162]

Light Spectrum

Bilirubin absorbs light most strongly at wavelengths of 475 to 478 nm, so light in the blue-green region of the spectrum from 460 to 490 nm is effective in reducing bilirubin levels.[147] The penetration of tissue by light increases markedly with increasing wavelength.[116] The optical properties of bilirubin and skin determine the light wavelengths that most effectively lower bilirubin level; these are wavelengths that are predominately in the blue-green spectrum.[161] Light of wavelengths outside of this range is predominantly absorbed by hemoglobin, does not effectively reduce bilirubin, and generates unnecessary heat.[147] Note that none of the light systems used in phototherapy emit any significant amount of ultraviolet (UV) radiation, and UV light is never used for phototherapy.[147] A small amount of UV light is emitted by fluorescent tubes, but this UV light is of longer wavelengths (>320 nm) than those that cause erythema, and in any case, almost all UV light produced is absorbed by the glass wall of the fluorescent tube and by the Plexiglas cover of the phototherapy unit. Light-emitting diodes (LEDs) do not emit UV light.

Irradiance

There is a direct relationship between the efficacy of phototherapy and the irradiance used, and irradiance is inversely related to the distance between the light source and the infant (Fig. 12.14). The irradiance in a certain wavelength band is called the spectral irradiance and is expressed as $\mu W/cm^2/nm$ (see Table 12.6). As shown in Fig. 12.14, there is a strong inverse relationship between the light intensity (measured as spectral irradiance) and the distance from the light source. Thus the closer the phototherapy lamp is to the infant, the more effective it is. Note that halogen or tungsten lamps cannot be put close to the infant because of the risk of burn.

Spectral Power

The spectral power is the product of the skin surface irradiance and the spectral irradiance across this surface area. Calculations of spectral power permit comparisons of the dose of phototherapy received by infants using different phototherapy systems.

Mechanism of Action and Where Phototherapy Acts

Although the conversion of some bilirubin to photoisomers during phototherapy takes place in the skin (producing a "bleaching" of the jaundiced infant), this has no effect on the TSB level. The bilirubin-lowering effect of phototherapy is produced by the action of light on bilirubin bound to albumin in the superficial skin capillaries.[163] Donneborg et al demonstrated that although phototherapy reduced both

TABLE 12.7 Factors That Affect the Dose and Efficacy of Phototherapy

Factor	Technical Terminology	Rationale	Clinical Application
Type of light source	Spectrum of light (nanometers)	Blue-green spectrum is most effective at lowering total serum bilirubin (TSB); light at this wavelength penetrates skin well and is absorbed strongly by bilirubin.	Use special blue fluorescent tubes or light-emitting diodes or another light source with output in blue-green spectrum for intensive PT.
Distance of light source from patient	Spectral irradiance (a function of both distance and light source) delivered to surface of infant	↑ Irradiance leads to ↑ rate of decline in TSB. Standard PT units deliver 8–10 μW/cm²/nm; intensive PT delivers ≥30 μW/cm²/nm.	If special blue fluorescent tubes are used, bring tubes as close as possible to infant to increase irradiance. (Do *not* do this with halogen lamps because of danger of burn.) Positioning special blue tubes 10–15 cm above infant will produce an irradiance of at least 35 μW/cm²/nm.
Surface area exposed	Spectral power (a function of spectral irradiance and surface area)	↑ Surface area exposed leads to ↑ rate of decline in TSB.	For intensive PT, expose maximum surface area of infant to PT. Place lights above and below[a] or around[b] the infant. For maximum exposure, line sides of bassinet, warmer bed, or incubator with aluminum foil.
Cause of jaundice		PT is likely to be less effective if jaundice is caused by hemolysis, if cholestasis is present (direct bilirubin is increased), or if haemoglobin and haematocrit are elevated.[208,209]	When hemolysis is present, start PT at a lower TSB level and use intensive PT. Failure of PT to lower TSB suggests that hemolysis is the cause of the jaundice. When direct bilirubin is elevated, watch for bronze baby syndrome or blistering.
TSB level at start of PT		The higher the TSB, the more rapid the decline in TSB with PT.	Use intensive PT for higher TSB levels. Anticipate a more rapid decrease in TSB when TSB >20 mg/dL.

[a]Commercially available sources for light below include special blue fluorescent tubes available in the Olympic Bili-Bassinet (Natus Medical, San Carlos, Calif.), BiliSoft fiberoptic LED mattress (GE Healthcare, Wauwatosa, Wisc.), NeoBLUE Cozy mattress (Natus Medical).
[b]The Mediprema Cradle 360 (Mediprema, Tours Cedex, France) provides 360-degree exposure to special blue fluorescent light.
PT, Phototherapy.
From Maisels MJ, Watchko JF. Treatment of hyperbilirubinemia. In: Buonocore G, Bracci R, Weindling M, eds. *Neonatology: A Practical Approach to Neonatal Diseases*. Milan, Italy: Springer-Verlag; 2009.

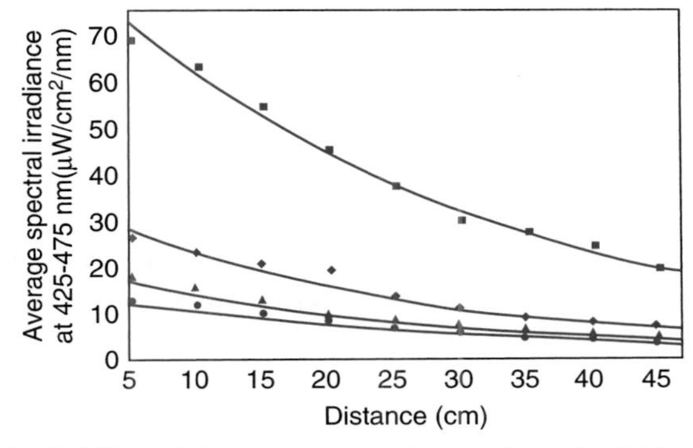

Fig. 12.14 Effect of light source and distance from the light source to the infant on average spectral irradiance. Measurements were made across the 425- to 475-nm band using a commercial radiometer (Olympic Bilimeter Mark II). The phototherapy unit was fitted with eight 24-inch fluorescent tubes. □ Special blue, General Electric 20-W F2012/B blue tube, Δ, daylight blue, four General Electric 20-W F20T12/D blue tubes and four Sylvania 20-W F20T12/D daylight tubes; ●, daylight, Sylvania 20-W F20T12/D daylight tube. Curves were plotted using linear curve fitting (True Epistat, Epistat Services, Richardson, TX). The best fit is described by the equation y = AeBX. (From Maisels MJ. Why use homeopathic doses of phototherapy? *Pediatrics*. 1996;98:283. Copyright 1996 by the American Academy of Pediatrics.) *TSB*, Total serum bilirubin

the transcutaneous and the serum bilirubin levels, rotation of the infant from prone to supine or supine to prone (thus exposing the unblanched skin to the light) had no effect on the rate at which phototherapy lowered the serum bilirubin levels. This study confirmed what had previously been observed repeatedly: rotation of the infant does not improve the efficacy of phototherapy.[164–167] In addition, photoisomers can be detected in the blood within 15 minutes of initiating phototherapy,[168,169] far too soon to be accounted for by isomerization in the skin. Phototherapy detoxifies bilirubin by converting it to photoproducts that are more lipophilic than bilirubin and can bypass the conjugating system of the liver and be excreted without further metabolism.[161] Absorption of light by albumin-bound bilirubin induces a fraction of the pigment to undergo several photochemical reactions that occur at very different rates. These reactions generate yellow stereoisomers of bilirubin and colorless derivatives of lower molecular weight.

Bilirubin Photochemistry

During phototherapy, bilirubin absorbs light, and photochemical reactions occur.[147,161] The relative contributions of the various reactions to the overall elimination of bilirubin are unknown, although in vitro and in vivo studies suggest that photoisomerization is more important than photodegradation. Bilirubin elimination depends on the rates of formation as well as the rates of clearance of the photoproducts.

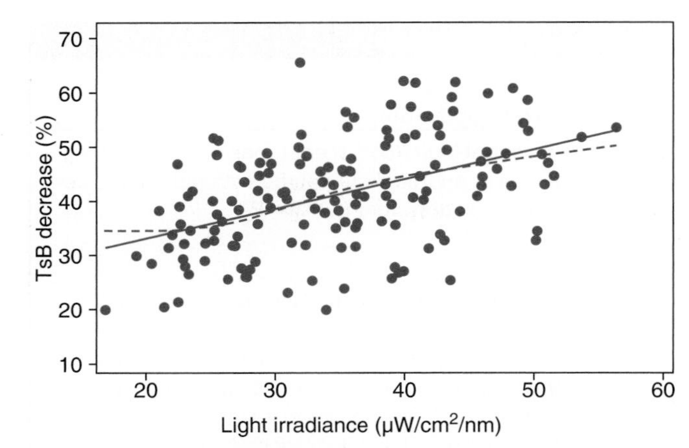

Fig. 12.15 Linear relationship between light emitting diode phototherapy irradiance in the range of 20 to 55 μW/cm²/nm and decrease in total serum bilirubin after 24 hours of therapy with no evidence of a saturation point. Solid line indicates linear regression, and dashed line indicates smooth regression. (From Vanborg PK, Hansen BM, Greisen G, Ebbesen F. Dose-response relationship of phototherapy for hyperbilirubinemia. Pediatrics 2012; 130:e352-e357, Copyright © 2012 by the AAP. With permission).

Photoisomerization occurs rapidly during phototherapy, and isomers appear in the blood long before the level of plasma bilirubin begins to decline.[168,169] The radiometric quantities used and the important factors that influence the dose and efficacy of phototherapy are listed in Table 12.7.

Clinical Use and Efficacy

Phototherapy is an effective mechanism for the prevention and treatment of hyperbilirubinemia and dramatically reduces the need for exchange transfusion. Multiple controlled trials confirm the efficacy of phototherapy.[56] Some idea of the magnitude of the effect of phototherapy can be gauged from the following: when phototherapy was not used, 36% of infants with birth weights of less than 1500 g required an exchange transfusion.[170] In the NICHD Neonatal Research Network study, 5 of 1974 infants (0.25%) with birth weights of 1000 g or less required an exchange transfusion.[22]

Dose–Response Relationship and the Maximum Dose of Phototherapy

Fig. 12.15 shows that there is a clear relationship between the dose of phototherapy and the decline in the TSB level.[171,172] Because the conversion of bilirubin to executable photoproducts is partly irreversible and follows first-order kinetics, there is a direct relationship between the irradiance used and the rate at which the TSB declines.[171,172] Previous studies suggested that there was a saturation point beyond which an increase in irradiance produced no added efficacy,[172] but a recent study could not define such a saturation point,[171] so the maximum effective dose of phototherapy is currently unknown. Table 12.7 lists the factors that determine the dose of phototherapy. The initial TSB level is also an important factor that influences the rate of decline of serum bilirubin level, with the rate being proportional to the initial bilirubin concentration. Because configurational isomers formed during light treatment revert to natural unconjugated bilirubin in the intestine after hepatic excretion, reabsorption of natural bilirubin occurs via the enterohepatic circulation and contributes to the bilirubin load to be cleared by the liver. Both of these phenomena account for the fact that light treatment is most effective during the first 24 hours of therapy, after which the efficacy decreases.

Types of Light

Fluorescent Tubes

Daylight, white, and blue fluorescent tubes are now less widely used fluorescent light sources, as they are less effective than special blue fluorescent tubes, which provide significantly more irradiance in the blue spectrum (see Fig. 12.14). Special blue tubes are labeled F20T12/BB (General Electric, Westinghouse) or TL52/20W (Phillips). These are different from regular blue tubes (F20T12/B), which provide only slightly more irradiance than daylight or white tubes (see Fig. 12.14). Compact special blue fluorescent bulbs (Osram 18W) are also effective and are cheaper than standard fluorescent bulbs.[173] Systems have been developed that provide special blue fluorescent light above and below the infant as well as a 360-degree configuration (see footnote to Table 12.7).

Halogen Lamps

High-pressure mercury vapor halide lamps provide reasonably good output in the blue range and have the advantage of being much more compact than lamps containing standard fluorescent tubes. An important disadvantage, however, is that, unlike fluorescent lamps, they cannot be brought close to the infant (to increase the irradiance) without incurring the risk of a burn. Furthermore, the surface area covered by most halogen lamps is small, and the spectral power is therefore less than that produced by a bank of fluorescent lamps.

Fiberoptic Systems

Fiberoptic phototherapy systems contain a tungsten-halogen bulb that delivers light via a fiberoptic cable to be emitted by the sides and ends of the fibers inside a plastic pad. These systems provide a convenient way of delivering phototherapy above and below the infant simultaneously. But the original fiberoptic pads covered only a small surface area, which significantly reduced the spectral power achieved. New designs that combine an LED light source with fiberoptic pads have overcome this problem (see footnote to Table 12.7).

Light-Emitting Diodes

The use of high-intensity gallium nitride LEDs permits higher irradiance to be delivered in the spectrum of choice (e.g., blue, blue-green) with minimal heat generation.

An LED unit is a low-weight, low-voltage, low-power, portable device that provides an effective means of delivering intensive phototherapy.[174] An LED light source and fiberoptic pads have now been combined to create pads that are much larger than the original fiberoptic pads and deliver a high irradiance (see footnote to Table 12.7).

Effective Use of Phototherapy

Term and Late Preterm Infants

In the NICU, phototherapy is used primarily as a prophylactic measure to prevent slowly increasing serum bilirubin concentrations from reaching levels that might require an exchange transfusion. In the days when full-term infants remained in the hospital for 3 to 5 days, phototherapy was also commonly used to treat modestly jaundiced infants. Currently, of full-term and late preterm infants who need phototherapy, about 66% receive phototherapy during their birth hospitalization, and 33% are those who have left the hospital and are readmitted on days 4 to 7 for treatment of severe hyperbilirubinemia.[175] Such infants need a therapeutic dose of phototherapy (sometimes termed *intensive phototherapy*) to diminish the bilirubin level as soon as possible.[14] The AAP defines intensive phototherapy as an irradiance of at least 30μW/cm^2/nm delivered to as much of the surface area of the infant is possible.[14] If special blue fluorescent tubes are used, they should be no farther than 10 to 15 cm from the infant and should be brought as close as possible to the infant (see Fig. 12.14). To do this, a term or late preterm infant must be in a bassinet, not an incubator (the top of the incubator prevents the light from being brought sufficiently close to the infant). When necessary in low-birth-weight infants or infants in the NICU, the special blue fluorescent lights can be placed between the radiant warmer and the warmer bed. In either case, the light should be no further than 10 to 15 cm from the infant. At this distance, special blue fluorescent tubes provide an average spectral irradiance of 40 to 50 μW/cm^2/nm (see Fig. 12.14). This configuration does not produce significant warming of naked full-term infants, and if slight warming does occur, the lamps can be elevated slightly. Halogen phototherapy lamps cannot be positioned closer to the infant than recommended by the manufacturers without incurring the risk of burn.

LED lights are also effective for intensive phototherapy.[174] Their only potential disadvantage is that they produce almost no heat, so most naked infants will need to be placed in an incubator or under a radiant warmer.

The use of fiberoptic or LED-fiberoptic pads has made it easy to increase the surface area of the infant exposed to phototherapy, and this type of "double phototherapy" is significantly more effective than single phototherapy in preterm and term infants.[176,177]

Using these techniques, particularly in infants with extreme hyperbilirubinemia, a decline of 30% to 40% in TSB concentrations can be achieved within 24 hours.[73,178]

Low-Birth-Weight Infants

Use of phototherapy in low-birth-weight infants is described earlier (see "Treatment: Low-Birth-Weight Infants").

Measurement of Phototherapy Dose

Because phototherapy is a drug, like all drugs, the dose should be measured to ensure that a therapeutic level is being achieved and that excessive levels of irradiance are not being used when they are not required. The radiometric quantity most commonly reported in the literature is the spectral irradiance (see Table 12.6). In the nursery, spectral irradiance can be measured by using commercially available spectroradiometers. These instruments take a single measurement across a band of wavelengths, typically 425 to 475 or 400 to 480 nm, and provide a readout in microwatts per square centimeter per nanometer. Unfortunately, there is no standardized method for reporting phototherapy doses in the clinical literature, so it is difficult to compare published studies on the efficacy of phototherapy. In addition, different radiometers and spectroradiometers produce markedly different results when measuring irradiance from the same phototherapy system.[149] Thus it is important to use the spectroradiometer recommended by the manufacturer for use with a given phototherapy system.

The measured irradiance varies widely depending on where the measurement is taken. Irradiance measured below the center of the light source is much greater than that measured at the periphery, but the recommendations issued by the AAP and given in this chapter refer to irradiance levels measured directly below the center of the light source.[14]

In the past, it was not thought necessary to measure spectral irradiance daily, but there is no longer any reason why this should not be done. It is recommended that irradiance from all phototherapy units be measured at least daily and documented in the medical record, as should the type of phototherapy system being used and the surface area of the infant being exposed.

Intermittent Versus Continuous Therapy

Because light exposure increases bilirubin excretion (compared with darkness), continuous phototherapy should be more efficient than intermittent phototherapy. However, clinical studies comparing these two methods in term and late preterm infants have produced conflicting results.[179] Nevertheless, recent preliminary data suggests that intermittent or cycled phototherapy in ELBW infants is as effective as continuous phototherapy in maintaining low TSB levels and can potentially reduce the duration of exposure to phototherapy by as much as 75%.[151] If bilirubin levels are very high, intensive phototherapy should be administered continuously until a satisfactory decline in the TSB level has occurred. On the other hand, in most circumstances, phototherapy does not need to be continuous. It should certainly be interrupted during feeding or parental visits, and eye patches must be removed to allow appropriate parent-infant contact.

Hydration

Because some of the lumirubin produced during phototherapy is excreted in urine, maintaining adequate hydration and a good urine output helps improve the efficacy of phototherapy. However, supplementation (with dextrose water) is not necessary for an infant receiving phototherapy unless there is evidence that the infant is dehydrated. In such infants, it makes more sense to provide both supplemental calories and fluids using a milk-based formula because formula inhibits the enterohepatic circulation of bilirubin and helps lower the bilirubin level.

Biological Effects and Complications

Even though phototherapy has been used on millions of infants for more than 30 years, reports of acute clinically recognized toxicities are exceptionally rare. Nevertheless, there is good evidence in the human infant of DNA damage that is strongly correlated with the length of exposure to phototherapy[146] and oxidative stress[148] that also leads to an increase in CO production in the skin and possibly internal organs.[180] Bilirubin is a photosensitizer and, in some circumstances, can act as a photodynamic agent in the presence of light and produce damage.[181] In infants with congenital erythropoietic porphyria, phototherapy produces severe blistering and photosensitivity,[182,183] and congenital porphyria is an absolute contraindication to the use of phototherapy. All of the affected infants had significant direct hyperbilirubinemia and elevated plasma porphyrin levels.[184] Significant accumulation of coproporphyrin has also been described in infants with bronze baby syndrome, which occurs exclusively in phototherapy-exposed infants who also have cholestasis. In the bronze baby syndrome, dark grayish-brown discoloration develops in the skin, serum, and urine in infants with cholestatic jaundice who are exposed to phototherapy.[185] The pathogenesis of this syndrome is not fully understood. If phototherapy is necessary, however, an elevated direct-reacting bilirubin level is not a contraindication to its use, even if bronzing results.

Complications associated with the use of fiberoptic phototherapy blankets have been reported in extremely premature infants (≤25 weeks' gestation) who had conditions that might reduce skin integrity, such as birth trauma, hypotension, poor perfusion of the skin, or bacterial contamination of the incubator or bed, and have included extensive erythematous denuded areas of skin resembling a partial-thickness burn as well as purplish red necrotizing lesions.[186,187] It is important to note that the skin of extremely premature infants is remarkably fragile.

Because light can be toxic to the retina, the eyes of infants receiving phototherapy should be protected with appropriate eye patches.[188]

Conventional phototherapy can produce an acute change in the infant's thermal environment, leading to an increase in peripheral blood flow and insensible water loss.[189] This issue has not been studied for LED lights, but because of their relatively low heat output, they should be much less likely to cause insensible water loss. In term infants who are nursing or feeding adequately, additional intravenous fluids are usually not required.

Phototherapy decreases the expected postprandial increase in blood flow velocity in the superior mesenteric artery and might also increase cerebral blood flow velocity in preterm infants of 32 weeks' gestation or less. Phototherapy also increases the likelihood of a patent ductus arteriosus in very low-birth-weight infants.

In the NICHD Neonatal Research Network randomized, controlled study, there was a 5% increase in mortality in infants with birth weights of 501 to 750 g in the "aggressive phototherapy" group[2] (see "Treatment: Low-Birth-Weight Infants" discussed earlier).

A 6-year follow-up of children in the NICHD collaborative phototherapy study showed no differences between the phototherapy and control groups in any aspect of growth or developmental outcome.[103] Nevertheless, until very recently, there has been a complete absence of adequate long-term studies on large populations of infants treated with phototherapy. Two such studies now suggest a rare but important association between infant phototherapy (n = 178,000) and myeloid leukemia and kidney cancer in the first year of life [190] (number needed to harm ≈ 10,000) as well as subsequent early childhood epilepsy in 52/1,830 boys who received phototherapy (hazard ratio 1.98 [CI: 1.40–2.78]) but not in girls.[191]

EXCHANGE TRANSFUSION

Exchange transfusion (ExT) removes bilirubin-laden blood from the circulation and replaces it with donor blood. The efficacy in clearing bilirubin from the plasma and extravascular space is a direct function of the mass of albumin exchanged. It follows that the ideal replacement fluid should have both a high plasma volume and a high albumin concentration to optimize the amount of bilirubin-free albumin introduced into the infant's circulation during the exchange. Accordingly, washed packed red blood cells mixed with thawed adult fresh frozen plasma to a hematocrit approximating 40% is the preferred exchange transfusion replacement product. The fresh frozen plasma provides a high albumin concentration and the hematocrit of 40%, a high plasma volume; in combination, they assure a high albumin content for ExT. In addition to removing bilirubin, when used in the treatment of immune-mediated hemolytic disease, ExT also accomplishes the following goals:

- removal of antibody-coated red blood cells;
- correction of anemia;
- removal of maternal antibody; and
- removal of other potential toxic by-products of the hemolytic process.

A double-volume ExT (approximately 170 mL/kg) removes about 85% of the infant's red blood cells and 110% of the circulating bilirubin (extravascular bilirubin enters the blood during the exchange), but because at least 50% of the infant's bilirubin is in the extravascular compartment, only one-third to one-half of the total body bilirubin is removed.[192] Postexchange bilirubin levels are about 60% of preexchange levels, and the reequilibration that occurs between the vascular and extravascular bilirubin compartments produces a rapid rebound of TSB levels (within 30 minutes) to 70% to 80% of preexchange levels. A detailed description of the basic indications for, and contraindications to, performing exchange transfusions as well as the technique for and complications of the procedure has been provided elsewhere.[192,193]

As discussed previously, very few ExTs are currently being done. The prevention of Rh hemolytic disease with Rh immunoglobulin and the effective use of intensive phototherapy has led to a dramatic decline in the number of

BOX 12.6 Potential Complications of Exchange Transfusion

Cardiovascular
- Arrhythmias
- Cardiac arrest
- Volume overload
- Embolization with air or clots
- Thrombosis
- Vasospasm

Hematologic
- Sickling (donor blood)
- Thrombocytopenia
- Bleeding (overheparinization of donor blood)
- Graft-versus-host disease
- Mechanical or thermal injury to donor cells

Gastrointestinal
- Necrotizing enterocolitis

Biochemical
- Hyperkalemia
- Hypernatremia
- Hypocalcemia
- Hypomagnesemia
- Acidosis
- Hypoglycemia

Infectious
- Bacteremia
- Virus infection (hepatitis, cytomegalovirus infection)
- Malaria

Miscellaneous
- Hypothermia
- Perforation of umbilical vein
- Drug loss
- Apnea

From Watchko JF. Exchange transfusion in the management of neonatal hyperbilirubinemia. In: Maisels MJ, Watchko JF, eds. *Neonatal Jaundice*. London, UK: Harwood Academic Publishers; 2000:169-176.

ExTs performed.[2] As fewer of these procedures are done, it is likely that the risks and complications will increase. A list of potential complications is provided in Box 12.6. An overall mortality rate of 0.3 in 100 procedures has been reported, but in term and near-term infants who are relatively well, the risk of death is low.[194] Jackson reported a 15-year experience of exchange transfusion (1980–1995) in 106 infants.[195] A total of 81 infants were healthy, and there were no deaths in these infants, although severe necrotizing enterocolitis requiring surgery did develop in one child. There were 25 sick infants, of whom three (12%) experienced serious complications from the exchange transfusion, and two (8%) died. There were three additional deaths that were considered "possibly" a result of the ExT. Thus the total number of deaths in sick infants, possibly as the result of the exchange, was 5 of 25 (20%). Adverse events associated with ExTs were reviewed at two perinatal centers in Cleveland, Ohio, between 1992 and 2002.[194] Over a 10.5-year period, only 67 infants were identified and had ExTs for hyperbilirubinemia—an average of about three ExTs per year in each institution. The gestational ages ranged from less than 32 weeks ($n = 15$) to term ($n = 22$). Adverse events occurred in 74% of the exchanges, with thrombocytopenia (44%), hypocalcemia (20%), and metabolic acidosis (24%) being the most common. There were only two serious adverse events, both in infants who had other preexisting, serious neonatal morbidities. The one infant who died was a critically ill 25-weeks' gestation infant with a birth weight of 731 g. The investigators also found that ExTs performed using umbilical venous and arterial catheters were significantly more likely to be associated with adverse events than those done through the umbilical vein alone or via other routes.[194] ExT also carries the usual risk of infection associated with any blood transfusion, although this risk is currently very low.[196]

PHARMACOLOGIC TREATMENT

For a recent detailed review of this topic, please see Cuperus et al.[197]

Acceleration of Normal Metabolic Pathways for Bilirubin Clearance

Phenobarbital induces conjugation and excretion and increases bile flow and, when given to mothers and infants, can lower TSB levels in the first week of life. However, because of concerns about long-term toxicity, it is rarely used.

Decreasing Bilirubin Production

The metalloporphyrins are inhibitors of heme oxygenase, the enzyme necessary for the conversion of heme to biliverdin, one of the first steps in the formation of bilirubin from hemoglobin. In a series of controlled clinical trials, the use of tin-mesoporphyrin was shown to be effective in reducing TSB levels and the requirement for phototherapy in full-term and preterm infants as well as in infants with G6PD deficiency.[160,198–201] The only side effect seen has been a transient, non–dose-dependent erythema that disappeared without sequelae in infants who received phototherapy after administration of tin-mesoporphyrin,[200] but the use of this drug is not yet approved by the FDA. As noted above, although, some controlled trials documented that the administration of IVIG to infants with Rh and ABO hemolytic disease significantly reduced the need for exchange transfusion,[102,202,203] more recent studies have not confirmed this.[156,157] In these trials, however, IVIG was only used when phototherapy had failed to control the rise in TSB, but it is possible that IVIG could have been effective if it had been used earlier.[204] The potential mechanism of action of IVIG is unknown, but it is possible that it might alter the course of hemolytic disease by blocking Fc receptors and thus inhibiting hemolysis. Several observational studies, however, suggest an association between the use of IVIG in term and late preterm infants with Rh and ABO hemolytic disease and the diagnosis of necrotizing enterocolitis,[205–207] although it is possible that this complication could be related to the product used.[207]

Binding of Bilirubin to Detergents

UDCA, a bile salt, has been used to treat cholestatic jaundice and, under some circumstances, could be beneficial in ameliorating indirect hyperbilirubinemia as well.[71] The mechanism for this is not fully understood, although bile salts might capture unconjugated bilirubin in the intestinal lumen and decrease the enterohepatic circulation.[197]

CASE 12.1

A 37 2/7-weeks' gestation male infant is born following an uncomplicated pregnancy and delivery. He is breast fed by his mother and appears to be nursing adequately. At age 40 hours, a physical examination reveals no jaundice, and the transcutaneous bilirubin (TcB) concentration is 6.7 mg/dL (low-risk zone). He is discharged home at the age of 42 hours, and the mother is instructed to bring him back to the pediatrician's office in 10 days. On the morning of the sixth day, he is brought to the office because the mother has noticed that he was increasingly jaundiced over the previous 2 days and had nursed poorly. He had refused the breast completely for the past 12 hours, was lethargic, and had a weight loss of 14% of his birth weight. On closer questioning, the mother acknowledges that he had never nursed very well. Upon examination, the infant appears extremely jaundiced but is otherwise alert and responsive and had no posturing or arching of back. A stat serum bilirubin level is 29.4 mg/dL (50 μmol/L), and he is admitted to the hospital. The attending pediatrician asks the resident to start phototherapy and requests that a repeat bilirubin level be obtained in 8 hours. The infant is placed under daylight phototherapy lamps that produce an irradiance of 9 μW/cm²/nm in the blue spectrum (420–480 nm). The resident asks about sending blood for typing and cross-matching for a possible exchange transfusion, and the attending pediatrician responds, "Unless we find evidence of hemolytic disease, this sounds like typical breast milk jaundice, and these babies never get into trouble. But let's get a type and Coombs anyway." The resident complies. The baby's blood type is A Rh-positive with a weakly positive result on direct Coombs test. The mother's blood type is group O Rh-positive, and her antibody screen is negative.

Do you agree with the attending pediatrician's orders?

There are several problems with the way this baby is being treated. The attending pediatrician's assertion that these infants "never get into trouble" is not true. Kernicterus is well described in apparently healthy term (≥37 weeks' gestation) and late preterm (34–36 6/7 weeks' gestation) breast-fed newborns. A bilirubin level of 29.4 mg/dL (503 μmol/L) is a medical emergency and demands immediate and intensive phototherapy. Under these circumstances, standard phototherapy lights are inadequate, and intensive phototherapy must be used. A phototherapy source that delivers light in the 460- to 490-nm blue region of the spectrum and that can deliver an irradiance of at least 30 μW/cm²/nm should be used, and lights should be placed above and below the infant. The sides of the bassinet can be lined with aluminum foil to further optimize the surface area of the infant exposed to phototherapy. Typing and cross-matching for blood for exchange transfusion must be performed as soon as possible because the cause of this extreme hyperbilirubinemia is unknown, and if a subsequent total serum bilirubin (TSB) level remains the same or even increases despite appropriate phototherapy, an emergent exchange transfusion should be performed. Because it is essential to know which way the bilirubin level is moving, a repeat TSB level should be obtained within 2 to 3 hours and certainly no later than 4 hours. In addition, the baby should be given formula in an attempt to reduce the enterohepatic circulation. Because the rate of decline of the TSB level with phototherapy is directly related to the initial TSB level (the higher the level, the more rapid the decline), a decrease of at least 2 to 3 mg/dL (and often more) can be expected in the first 4 hours. In addition to limiting the enterohepatic circulation, formula gives needed calories as well as additional fluid. Because the structural isomer lumirubin is excreted in the urine, maintaining a good urine output helps lower the TSB level more rapidly.

Does this infant have ABO hemolytic disease?

It is hard to be sure. His TcB was only 6.7 mg/dL at age 40 hours, and although there is A-O incompatibility with a positive DAT result, more typically, ABO hemolytic disease is characterized by clinical jaundice within the first 24 hours and certainly by 36 hours. It is quite likely that this infant has a combination of increased bilirubin production from ABO incompatibility together with breast feeding–associated hyperbilirubinemia related to a low caloric intake and exaggeration of the enterohepatic circulation.

A major error in the care of this infant was scheduling a follow-up visit at age 10 days in a newborn discharged at age 42 hours. As emphasized earlier, such infants should always be seen within 2 days of discharge, particularly if the baby is breast fed and younger than 38 weeks' gestation, as was the case here.

What other tests should be ordered for this infant?

In addition to the blood typing and Coombs test, a complete blood count with smear, reticulocyte count, and glucose-6-phosphate dehydrogenase (G6PD) determination should be performed. Measurement of serum albumin level would be helpful. In selected infants with very low serum albumin levels and therefore less ability to bind bilirubin, earlier exchange transfusion might be considered.

How could this extreme hyperbilirubinemia have been prevented?

Follow-up of this infant within 2 days of discharge would likely have identified an infant who was becoming progressively jaundiced. A TSB level would have been obtained, the mother would have been counseled to improve breast-feeding efforts, and, if necessary, phototherapy would have followed.

CASE 12.2

A healthy full-term female infant is brought to the pediatrician's office at age 3 weeks. The baby is being breast fed, has had an excellent weight gain, and has perfectly normal examination results except that she is slightly jaundiced.

What questions should be asked of the mother?

The most important information needed is the color of the baby's stool and urine. If the urine is pale yellow and nearly colorless and the stool is a normal brownish color, the likelihood of cholestatic jaundice is slim.

The mother reports that the baby's stools and urine are normal. What should be done?

For any infant who is jaundiced at 3 weeks of age or older a total *and* direct bilirubin level *must* be measured to rule out cholestatic jaundice and the possibility of extrahepatic biliary atresia.

The total serum bilirubin (TSB) level is 8.2 mg/dL, and the direct bilirubin level 0.5 mg/dL. Do you need to do anything else?

Although it is overwhelmingly likely that this baby has breast milk jaundice, any baby with prolonged indirect hyperbilirubinemia should undergo an evaluation of thyroid function because hypothyroidism is one cause of prolonged indirect hyperbilirubinemia. This can easily be accomplished without further testing by referring to the hospital chart (or the state laboratory results) and confirming that the metabolic screen was done and that the thyroid function was normal.

The mother comes back when the baby is 10 weeks old, and the baby is still jaundiced. The TSB level is 7.5 mg/dL (130 μmol/L), and the direct bilirubin level is 0.4 mg/dL (7 μmol/L). What should the mother be told?

Indirect hyperbilirubinemia up to age 12 weeks is well within the limits of the breast milk jaundice syndrome; reassure the mother that she need not be concerned.

Are there additional questions that should be asked of the mother?

Ask the mother whether there is any history of mild, unconjugated hyperbilirubinemia in her family (Gilbert syndrome). There is a strong association between prolonged indirect hyperbilirubinemia in breast-fed infants and the $(TA)_7$ [*UGT1A1*28*] dinucleotide variant allele within the $A(TA)_nTAA$ repeat element of the *UGT1A1* TATAA box promoter,[3] which differs from the wild-type $A(TA)_6$ TAA promoter. Individuals with Gilbert syndrome are homozygous for the *UGT1A1*28* allele.

CASE 12.3

A 40-weeks' gestation African American female breast-fed infant, birth weight 3400 g, was discharged home at 36 hours of age with no evidence of jaundice and a predischarge transcutaneous bilirubin (TcB) value of 7.6 mg/dL (low intermediate risk zone). The mother is a 26-year-old O Rh-positive, antibody screen–negative, multiparous woman who breast fed her two previous children. The infant was seen in the pediatrician's office 2 days after discharge and during that visit was noted to show marked signs of jaundice, including scleral icterus. The mother reported that her daughter had fed poorly that morning and has been less active. A total serum bilirubin (TSB) concentration is 24.7 mg/dL. The infant is directly admitted to a local neonatal intensive care unit (NICU) for further evaluation, and intensive phototherapy is started on arrival. The infant's admission weight is 3200 g, and she is noted to be lethargic but otherwise neurologically intact. On admission, the TSB level is 28.8 mg/dL, the infant's blood type is O Rh-positive, and the direct antiglobulin test (DAT) result is negative. The hemoglobin and hematocrit are 14 g/dL and 42%, respectively, the reticulocyte count is 2%, and red blood cell morphology on smear is unremarkable.

What is the most likely explanation for this infant's extreme hyperbilirubinemia?

Of the major risk factors for subsequent severe hyperbilirubinemia, only breast milk feeding is evident. However, by report, the infant had been feeding well until the morning of admission, and the infant's weight has declined only approximately 6% from birth. The blood type and DAT result rule out an immune-mediated hemolytic process. The TSB level is rising quickly, and an alternative cause must be sought.

The most likely cause of this infant's extreme hyperbilirubinemia is glucose-6-phosphate dehydrogenase (G6PD) deficiency. Although the disorder is X-linked and is more prevalent in male infants, homozygous and heterozygous females may be affected. The prevalence of G6PD deficiency in African American females is 4.1%. The absence of overt anemia, reticulocytosis, and abnormal red cell morphology on smear do not exclude this diagnosis.

What would you anticipate the TSB trajectory to be in response to phototherapy?

Although hyperbilirubinemia in the context of G6PD deficiency is often responsive to intensive phototherapy, one cannot be assured of this. The marked increase in TSB from 24.7 mg/dL to 28.8 mg/dL in the period between the drawing of the bilirubin sample at the office visit and the measurement of TSB on NICU admission suggests active hemolysis, which may not be responsive to phototherapy alone. Appropriately, a blood sample is sent to the blood bank on NICU admission for typing and cross-matching of blood for a possible double-volume exchange transfusion. Indeed, repeat TSB measurement 3 hours after admission is 31.2 mg/dL despite intensive phototherapy, and the infant undergoes a double-volume exchange transfusion. A G6PD assay and genotyping are performed on the first aliquot of the infant's blood removed during the double-volume exchange transfusion.

After the exchange transfusion, the TSB level is 21.2 mg/dL, but the infant is noted to have posturing, both retrocollis and opisthotonos. What should be done?

The infant should undergo a second double-volume exchange transfusion. The presence of advanced clinical signs of acute bilirubin encephalopathy is an indication for immediate exchange transfusion irrespective of the TSB level.

Prompt institution of the second double-volume exchange transfusion is associated with a further decrease in TSB to 16.7 mg/dL and resolution of bilirubin encephalopathy signs. Magnetic resonance imaging (MRI) results and auditory brain stem response before discharge are both normal.

The pediatric resident states that the infant is most likely a homozygous G6PD-deficient female, given the infant's hyperbilirubinemia course. The attending neonatologist is not so sure.

CASE 12.3

The results of the quantitative G6PD enzyme assay is 7.6 IU/g hemoglobin (normal: 7.0–20.5 IU/g hemoglobin), and on genotype, the infant is heterozygous for the *G6PD A-* mutation. Female neonates heterozygous for the *G6PD* mutations represent a unique at-risk group. X inactivation results in a subpopulation of G6PD-deficient red blood cells in *every* female heterozygote; that is, each heterozygous female is a mosaic with two red blood cell populations including one that is G6PD deficient. A heterozygous female may be reported as enzymatically normal yet harbor a sizable population of G6PD-deficient, potentially hemolyzable red blood cells that represent a substantial reservoir of bilirubin. When this pool undergoes acute hemolysis, hazardous hyperbilirubinemia can evolve rapidly, as seen in this infant. There is no reliable biochemical assay to detect G6PD heterozygotes; only DNA analysis can provide this information. No apparent trigger for hemolysis (e.g., naphthalene in mothballs, sepsis) was identified as is frequently the case.

It should be noted that in the presence of acute hemolysis, the G6PD level can be normal, even in homozygotes, because older red blood cells are destroyed, and the remaining younger cells have higher levels of G6PD. In such a case, if G6PD deficiency is suspected, the G6PD level should be measured again in 2 to 3 months. In a homozygous G6PD-deficient infant, the G6PD level will then be low.

The reference list for this chapter can be found online at www.expertconsult.com

13

Infections in the Neonate

Ankita P. Desai, Ethan G. Leonard

INTRODUCTION

The fetus and the newborn are susceptible to multiple infections: bacterial, viral, and fungal. This susceptibility is multifactorial and stems from maternal risk factors, obstetrical complications, the postnatal environment, prematurity, and the immature host defenses of the newborn. Throughout this chapter, we will review common pathogens to which the neonate may be exposed, as well as briefly discuss newer congenitally-acquired infections.

BACTERIA AND FUNGI

Epidemiology, Risk Factors, and Presentation

Neonatal sepsis is defined as a systemic inflammatory response syndrome secondary to infection. The age of onset of sepsis reflects the likely mode of acquisition, microbiology, and clinical presentation with consequent implications on morbidity and mortality. Worldwide, it is estimated that more than 1.4 million neonatal deaths per year are caused by invasive infections.[1] Epidemiologically, neonatal sepsis is divided into the following categories: early-onset sepsis (EOS), late-onset sepsis, and very late–onset sepsis.

EOS is a systemic, multiorgan disease that presents in the first week of life and usually within the first 72 hours of life. Infection is most often acquired before delivery. Perinatal factors contribute to the development of infection and include rupture of membranes prematurely (before onset of labor) or a prolonged period (>18 hours) before delivery, chorioamnionitis, maternal fever, maternal urinary tract infection, and infant prematurity or low birth weight. These infants have a fulminant onset of respiratory symptoms, usually due to pneumonia, poor perfusion, temperature instability, and acidosis. The microbiologic features of EOS reflect maternal genitourinary and gastrointestinal colonization.

In the Active Bacterial Core Surveillance in four states from 2005 to 2008, as assessed by the Centers for Disease Control and Prevention (CDC), the overall rate of EOS in the United States was estimated at 0.77 per 1000 live births with a case fatality rate of 10.9%.[1] Before the adoption of intrapartum antibiotic prophylaxis (IAP) against group B *Streptococcus* (GBS), this pathogen caused the overwhelming majority of EOS. Today, GBS still causes most cases of EOS; however, enteric bacilli such as *Escherichia coli* have become more prevalent in term infants and are as likely as GBS to cause EOS in very low-birth-weight premature infants.[2,3] GBS is estimated to be responsible for 0.29 infections per 1000 live births with case fatality rate of 7%, and *E. coli* is responsible for 0.19 infections per 1000 live births with a case fatality rate of 25%.[1] Although GBS a enteric bacilli cause the preponderance of EOS, a third pathogen, *Listeria monocytogenes,* can cause EOS, although decreasing in incidence. Unlike GBS and the gram-negative pathogens, which usually are acquired through asymptomatic maternal colonization, *L. monocytogenes* generally causes a flulike or gastrointestinal illness in the mother. This organism is mostly acquired from animal products: unpasteurized milk, cheese, delicatessen meats, and hot dogs. The importance of this organism will become clear in the discussion of empiric antibiotic therapy.

Late-onset sepsis is defined as the infections that occur beyond the first week of life but before 30 days of life. Very late–onset sepsis occurs beyond 30 days of life. Although intrapartum complications may be identified, these are not typical. Late-onset disease is more likely to reflect infection with gram-positive organisms acquired in the nursery: coagulase-positive staphylococci, *Staphylococcus aureus*, and enterococci. Invasive candidiasis is also an emerging cause of late-onset diseases. Very late–onset disease includes infections caused by GBS, gram-negative bacilli, and *Streptococcus pneumoniae.*

The high incidence of gram-positive infection in the hospitalized infant usually reflects the combination of lower gestational age and low birth weight and the consequent need for the insertion of central venous catheters for supportive care.[3] Although many of these infants will manifest poor feeding, temperature instability, and lethargy, they are more likely to have localized disease: urinary tract infection, osteoarthritis, or soft tissue infection. Meningitis is common. Presentation may be slowly progressive or fulminant. Mortality is lower than with EOS but may still be 20% to 40%.

The widespread use of IAP in the United States has been shown to have decreased the incidence of EOS by 70% to 0.44 cases per 1000 live births, an incidence equivalent to that of late-onset sepsis.[4] Of importance is that the improved survival of very low-birth-weight infants has put them at increased risk of systemic nosocomial infection.

The most important risk factors for the development of neonatal sepsis are low birth weight and prematurity. The incidence of sepsis is inversely proportional to the gestational age or birth weight of the infant. Sepsis is the most common cause of death in infants under 1500 g.[5] Other independent risk factors for sepsis include immature immune function, exposure to invasive procedures, hypoxia, metabolic acidosis, hypothermia, and low socioeconomic status; all aforementioned factors are associated with low birth weight and prematurity. In a multicenter survey of GBS disease carried out by the CDC, 13.5 cases per 1000 live births were diagnosed among black infants compared with 4.5 cases among 1000 white infants, and EOS was twice as common among black infants as among white infants.[6] Although males have a higher incidence of sepsis, once respiratory distress syndrome is accounted for, they are not at a significantly higher risk of sepsis, contrary to the results of older studies.[1,7] It is generally felt that sepsis is more common among the firstborn of twins. Infants with galactosemia are more likely to become infected with gram-negative organisms, in particular, *E. coli.* The administration of iron for anemia appears to increase risk because iron may be a growth factor for a number of bacteria. Finally, the widespread use of broad-spectrum antibiotics may cause a shift in the nursery to a higher prevalence of resistant bacteria that are also more invasive, as well as yeast. This phenomenon informs the need for better antimicrobial stewardship. Prevention of healthcare-associated infections through antimicrobial stewardship, limiting use of invasive devices and standardization of catheter procedures, and improved hand hygiene are important ways to decrease late-onset disease.

Evaluation and Management of Neonatal Sepsis

Definitive diagnosis of bacterial infection is predicated on the recovery of a pathogen from a normally sterile body site such as blood, urine, or cerebrospinal fluid (CSF). Although many indirect indices of infection have been identified and studied, including total white blood cell count, absolute neutrophil count, C-reactive protein level, procalcitonin level, and levels of a variety of inflammatory cytokines, taken individually, these tests are nonspecific and are not adequately sensitive to confirm or exclude systemic infection.

In infants with suspected EOS, cultures of blood should be drawn, and, if the infant is in a hemodynamically stable condition, spinal fluid should be obtained, and the infant should be started on intravenous antibiotics. The need for lumbar puncture in the first 24 to 72 hours of life has been a topic of some controversy.[8] Data suggesting that lumbar puncture is unnecessary in these infants comes primarily from retrospective studies of asymptomatic infants. The poor correlation between the results of neonatal blood cultures and CSF cultures underscores the need for lumbar puncture. Several studies report that bacterial meningitis would be missed in approximately one-third of very low-birth-weight neonates on the basis of blood culture results alone.[9,10] Antibiotic regimens should cover GBS, gram-negative bacilli, and *L. monocytogenes.* The most commonly used regimens are ampicillin and cefotaxime or ampicillin and gentamicin. Both regimens are quite effective against GBS. Unfortunately, *E. coli* has increasingly become resistant to ampicillin. In many institutions, more than half of the *E. coli* isolates are resistant to ampicillin. A search of the Cochrane database for evidence suggesting that one regimen is superior to another does not yield a conclusion.[11] Regardless of the regimen used, ampicillin should be included because the cephalosporins have no activity against *L. monocytogenes,* and gentamicin monotherapy would be ineffective.

The data for empirical therapy in late- and very late–onset disease are not definitively in favor of any one regimen.[12] Given the prevalence of staphylococcal species, many clinicians would include vancomycin in the empiric treatment of a hospitalized neonate with signs of sepsis beyond the seventh day of life. If the infant is being admitted from the community, the regimen should include coverage for GBS, *E. coli,* and *S. pneumoniae.* Commonly cited guidelines for the evaluation of febrile children without a focus of infection who are between 30 and 60 days of life include obtaining blood and urine samples for culture and performing a lumbar puncture before administration of antibiotics.

Group B Streptococcus Infection

Streptococcus agalactiae, or GBS, is the most common cause of vertically transmitted neonatal sepsis. It is a significant cause of maternal bacteriuria and endometritis, and a major cause of serious bacterial infection in infants up to 3 months of age. Ten serotypes of GBS have been identified on the basis of differing polysaccharide capsules: Ia, Ib, II, and III through IX. Epidemiologically, the serotypes responsible for neonatal disease shifted significantly in the 1990s. Type Ia, Ib, III, and V cause 95% of cases in infants in the United States.[13–15] Type III still causes the majority of late-onset disease and neonatal meningitis.[16] Antibodies against specific serotypes of GBS are protective but not cross-reactive.

Although GBS can cross the placenta, the primary mode of transmission is after rupture of membranes and during passage through the birth canal. Approximately 20% to 40% of women are colonized in their genital tract, but the primary reservoir of GBS is the lower gastrointestinal tract. High genital inoculum at delivery increases the likelihood of transmission and the consequent rate of early-onset GBS (EOGBS). Half of infants born to colonized women will themselves be colonized with GBS. Of these, 98% will be asymptomatic, whereas 2% will have evidence of invasive disease. Before the use of IAP targeted against GBS, the incidence of EOGBS ranged from 1 to 3 cases per 1000 live births. By definition, EOGBS presents in the first 6 days of life, and close to 90% of cases present within 24 hours of life. The vast majority of these infants demonstrate systemic illness by 12 hours.

In 1986, Boyer and Gotoff published the first randomized, controlled trial showing the effectiveness of IAP in reducing neonatal colonization and EOGBS.[17] In 1996, the CDC published the first set of guidelines for the prevention of perinatal GBS disease. The guidelines endorsed two approaches to IAP: (1) women with vaginal or rectal cultures positive for GBS should receive IAP; or (2) women with any of the following risk factors—delivery before 37 weeks' gestation, membrane rupture 18 hours or longer before delivery, or maternal fever of 38 C or higher—should receive IAP. In addition, any woman who had a history of GBS bacteriuria or who had previously delivered an infant with EOGBS was to receive IAP. In addition to the administration of IAP, the guidelines provided for the evaluation of the infant after delivery. These strategies reduced the incidence to

0.34–0.37 cases per 1000 live births in 2010.[18,19] Ongoing active surveillance of GBS demonstrated that the screening-based approach was superior to the risk-based approach in preventing EOGBS.[20] In 2010, the CDC published revised guidelines that promoted the universal screening of all pregnant women between 35 and 37 weeks' gestation using rectovaginal cultures, and recommended that all women with positive culture results receive IAP.[18] The guidelines also recommended IAP for mothers who had any history of GBS bacteriuria during the pregnancy, who had suspected chorioamnionitis, or who had previously delivered an infant with EOGBS. These guidelines also clarified the antibiotic dosages for IAP and provided alternatives for mothers with penicillin allergy, and the management of an exposed newborn (Fig. 13.1).

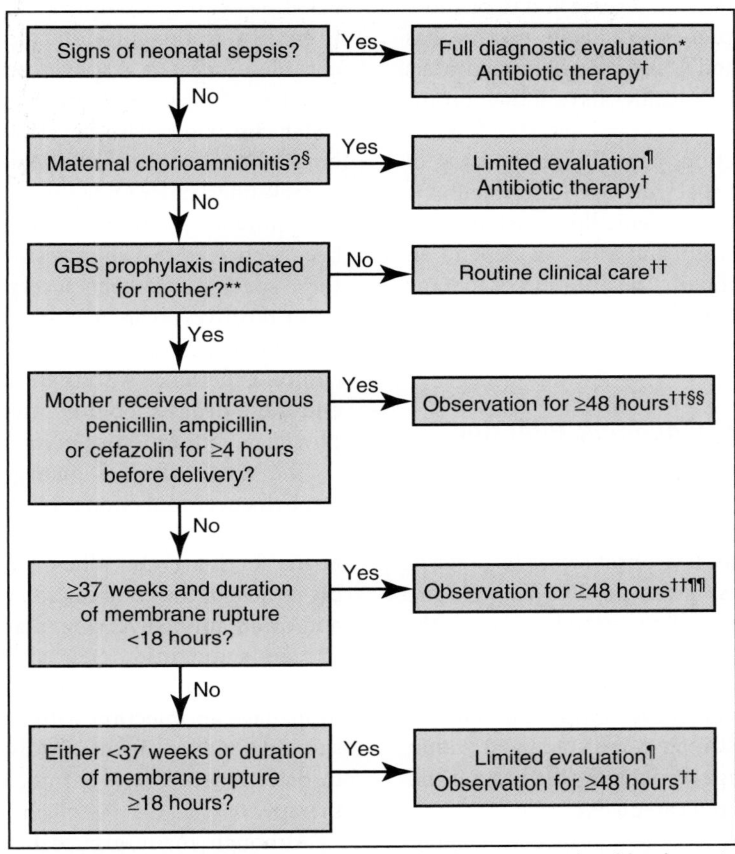

• Full diagnostic evaluation includes a blood culture, a complete blood count (CBC) including white blood cell differential and platelet counts, chest radiograph (if respiratory abnormalities are present), and lumbar puncture (if patient is stable enough to tolerate procedure and sepsis is suspected).

† Antibiotic therapy should be directed toward the most common causes of neonatal sepsis, including intravenous ampicillin for GBS and coverage for other organisms (including *Escherichia coli* and other gram-negative pathogens) and should take into account local antibiotic resistance patterns.

§ Consultation with obstetric providers is important to determine the level of clinical suspicion for chorioamnionitis. Chorioamnionitis is diagnosed clinically and some of the signs are nonspecific.

¶ Limited evaluation includes blood culture (at birth) and CBC with differential and platelets (at birth and/or at 6–12 hours of life).

** See table 3 for indications for intrapartum GBS prophylaxis.

†† If signs of sepsis develop, a full diagnostic evaluation should be conducted and antibiotic therapy initiated.

§§ If ≥37 weeks' gestation, observation may occur at home after 24 hours if other discharge criteria have been met, access to medical care is readily available, and a person who is able to comply fully with instructions for home observation will be present. If any of these conditions is not met, the infant should be observed in the hospital for at least 48 hours and until discharge criteria are achieved.

¶¶ Some experts recommend a CBC with differential and platelets at age 6–12 hours.

Fig. 13.1 Algorithm for secondary prevention of early-onset group B streptococcal (GBS) disease among newborns. (From Centers for Disease Control and Prevention. *Prevention of Perinatal Group B Streptococcal Disease: Revised Guidelines* from CDC, 2010. MMWR 2010; 59(No. RR-10):1–32.

As of 2003, the incidence of EOGBS was down to 0.3 cases per 1000 live births.[21] Although effective, the screening-based approach incurs the costs of testing, IAP, and management of the exposed infant. Although to date, no studies have shown an association between penicillin and ampicillin IAP and the emergence of antibiotic resistance in other bacteria, this risk remains a concern. An immunization-based strategy targeting pregnant women has the potential to prevent EOGBS, late-onset disease, and some maternal disease and to be more cost-effective. A multivalent protein conjugate vaccine has proved effective in a murine model, and several human trials of individual serotype conjugate vaccines have shown promise.[22–25]

For documented GBS infection, penicillin is the drug of choice and is the most narrow-spectrum agent. Ampicillin is an acceptable alternative agent. No penicillin resistance has been reported to date. The dosages and intervals depend on the postgestational age of the infant. The duration of therapy is 10 days for bacteremia without a focus, 14 days for uncomplicated meningitis, and up to 4 weeks for septic arthritis, endocarditis, or ventriculitis.[26]

Coagulase-Negative *Staphylococcus* Infection

For several decades, coagulase-negative staphylococci have been the most common cause of nosocomial bloodstream infections in the neonatal intensive care unit and are responsible for the majority of cases of late-onset sepsis in preterm neonates. Infections with these gram-positive bacteria are most often associated with indwelling central venous catheters. These bacteria are part of normal human skin flora. *Staphylococcus epidermidis* is the most common species of coagulase-negative staphylococci recovered from human skin and mucous membranes. Most infants are colonized within the first week of life from passage through the birth canal and repeated exposure from colonized caregivers.

The major virulence factor for coagulase-negative staphylococci is its ability to adhere to plastic and other foreign bodies by producing a biofilm. The biofilm consists of multiple layers of bacteria surrounded by an exopolysaccharide matrix or slime. This biofilm protects the bacteria from host phagocytic cells and interferes with the ability of many antimicrobial agents to effectively eliminate infection. This affinity for plastic foreign bodies explains the high recovery rate of these organisms from infected catheters, ventricular shunts, endotracheal tubes, and artificial vascular grafts and cardiac valves.

Neonatal infections with coagulase-negative staphylococci typically present without localizing signs with fever, new-onset respiratory distress, or a deterioration in respiratory status. Other common nonspecific signs of coagulase-negative staphylococcus sepsis include apnea, bradycardia, poikilothermia, poor perfusion, poor feeding, irritability, and lethargy. Indolent infection is more common than fulminant disease, with mortality generally under 15%. Coagulase-negative staphylococci infections, however, are a major source of morbidity, leading to increased antibiotic exposure, length of stay, and hospital costs.

Treatment of coagulase-negative staphylococci often requires the use of vancomycin. More than 80% of strains acquired in the hospital are resistant to beta-lactam antibiotics.[27] Resistance is typically attributable to altered penicillin-binding proteins and beta-lactamase production. Unfortunately, these types of resistance can be inducible and therefore may not be detected by routine microdilutional methods. If a strain is reported as penicillin sensitive, consultation with the hospital microbiologist is recommended to confirm testing for inducible resistance. More than 50% of coagulase-negative staphylococci are resistant to clindamycin, trimethoprim-sulfamethoxazole, gentamicin, and ciprofloxacin. Coagulase-negative staphylococci isolated from hospitalized patients show varying rates of resistance to the tetracyclines, chloramphenicol, rifampin, and newer-generation quinolone antibiotics. Some *S. epidermidis* isolates have been recovered that show resistance to vancomycin; however, these species have been susceptible to the newer agents for gram-positive organisms: linezolid, quinupristin–dalfopristin, and daptomycin.[28,29] Pharmacokinetic (PK) data and clinical experience with these agents in neonates are limited, and these drugs should be used only in consultation with a physician with expertise in infectious diseases.

The most effective management of coagulase-negative staphylococci infections is the combination of systemic antimicrobial therapy and, whenever possible, the removal of the foreign body. When a foreign body cannot be feasibly removed, the combination of vancomycin with rifampin, and/or an aminoglycoside, may be used. In the case of ventricular shunt infections, antibiotics may be administered both systemically and intraventricularly. If an attempt is made to manage an infection without foreign body removal, consultation with an infectious disease expert would be advised to determine the best antimicrobial agents and duration of therapy.

Although many groups have proposed different strategies to prevent neonatal catheter infections, few studies have yielded promising results. Several groups have studied the use of prophylactic antibiotics in neonates with indwelling catheters. The Cochrane Neonatal Group found no evidence to support this practice for neonates with umbilical arterial or venous catheters,[30,31] nor did they find evidence to support routine use of vancomycin in preterm infants to prevent nosocomial sepsis.[32] The use of a vancomycin–heparin lock solution to prevent nosocomial bloodstream infection showed promise in a small randomized, controlled, double-blinded study in critically ill neonates with peripherally inserted central venous catheters[33]; however, larger studies are needed. The use of antibiotic- or silver-impregnated catheters has not been studied in neonates. In 2002, the CDC recommended against the routine use of antimicrobial prophylaxis for patients with central venous catheters.[34] In 2006, the Cochrane Neonatal Group began a systematic review of the use of systemic antibiotics to reduce morbidity and mortality in neonates with central venous catheters. Although prophylactic systemic antibiotics reduced the rate of proven or suspected septicemia, there was no significant difference in overall mortality.

There was a lack of data pertaining to selection of resistant organisms or long-term neurodevelopmental outcomes; thus this is not routinely recommended.

Staphylococcus Aureus Infection

S. aureus is a gram-positive bacteria that is morphologically indistinguishable from the coagulase-negative staphylococci by light microscopy. *S. aureus* is part of normal skin flora. This organism causes a much wider and potentially more invasive spectrum of disease than that caused by coagulase-negative species. This pathogen is a common cause of superficial pustular disease and localized cellulitis, and is the most frequent cause of surgical site infection in infants and adult patients. The production of numerous toxins, enzymes, and binding proteins facilitates its ability to establish aggressive, life-threatening pyogenic infection. Small-inoculum colonization or infection can produce catastrophic, toxin-mediated disease such as scalded skin syndrome or toxic shock.

Over the last two decades, *S. aureus* has shown an increasing resistance to beta-lactam antibiotics, as documented by methicillin susceptibility testing[35]; these methicillin-resistant strains (MRSA) are resistant to all penicillins, penicillin–beta-lactamase inhibitor combination drugs, cephalosporins (except for newer fifth-generation cephalosporin [ceftaroline]), and carbapenems. Most hospital-acquired strains are resistant to clindamycin. Until recently, these resistant strains were not inherently more virulent. Unfortunately, however, over the last several years, community MRSA strains have acquired an additional virulence factor, Panton-Valentine leukocidin. This factor has contributed to a significant increase in invasive, pyogenic infection by MRSA. Several outbreaks in preterm and term neonates, as well as nosocomial transmission from caregivers, equipment, and toys in neonatal intensive care units, have been reported.[36–40] In an ill, hospitalized neonate who develops suspected or documented infection with gram-positive cocci, vancomycin should be included in the empirical antibiotic regimen. As discussed earlier, bloodstream infections caused by coagulase-negative species are much more prevalent than bacteremias from *S. aureus;* however, many clinicians would elect to start vancomycin for any gram-positive bloodstream infection in a hospitalized neonate because of the high rate of resistance to beta-lactam antibiotics in the coagulase-negative strains and the potential consequences of not treating MRSA. Other drugs are available with activity against MRSA, including older drugs like tetracyclines and trimethoprim–sulfamethoxazole, but these drugs are typically avoided in neonates. Several newer drugs—quinupristin–dalfopristin, linezolid, daptomycin, dalbavancin, and ceftaroline—have activity against MRSA. MRSA infections in neonates should be managed by an individual with expertise in the pharmacodynamics (PDs) and PKs of these drugs.

Candidiasis

The survival of fragile, very low-birth-weight neonates has led to increased infections because of candidiasis in the nursery. *Candida* species are responsible for 2.4% of early-onset infections in newborns, but, more importantly, they cause 10% to 12% of late-onset infections. Overall, infections with these fungi are among the three most common infections in the neonatal intensive care unit.[5,41,42]

Although *Candida albicans* once caused 75% of invasive candidal infections, infections involving nonalbicans species are now becoming more common, approaching 40% to 45% of infections. The incidence of *Candida parapsilosis* infection, relatively unique to the newborn, has risen more than tenfold, and this species now causes 25% of fungal infections in the newborn. Also of note, the incidence of *Candida tropicalis* and *Candida glabrata* infection has nearly doubled during the same time period.[43,44] The reported mortality attributable to *C. albicans* infection varies widely but may be as high as 20% to 40%.[45,46] The mortality from *C. parapsilosis* is certainly significant, but tends to be lower than that attributable to *C. albicans.*

Vertical transmission from mother to infant usually occurs during passage through the birth canal, especially in the presence of vaginitis. This is most often seen with *C. albicans* and *C. glabrata.* Congenital infections may rarely be seen and have been attributed both to ascending infection from the vagina and transplacental infection. *C. parapsilosis,* however, is frequently transmitted horizontally and is the most common fungal organism isolated from the hands of healthcare workers. This fungus is not commonly found in the genitourinary tracts of mothers. Colonization appears to occur more readily among very low and extremely low-birth-weight infants than among term infants, and occurs in up to 25% of these infants in the first week of life.[47] One-fourth of intubated infants demonstrate respiratory colonization.

A large number of predisposing factors have influenced the rate of dissemination. One of the primary factors is the prolonged and frequent use of broad-spectrum antibiotics that suppress the growth of bacteria in the gastrointestinal tract and consequently allow candidal overgrowth. In particular, the use of third-generation cephalosporins seems to increase the risk of gastrointestinal colonization and subsequent candidemia.[45,48] Eventually, penetration of the epithelial barrier leads to disseminated disease. The likelihood of mucosal penetration and dissemination are proportion to the density of the colonization. *C. albicans* has been shown to adhere to the mucosa of the preterm infant better than to that of the term infant. Dense colonization of the gastrointestinal tract increases the chances of translocation of the yeast across the mucosa. Intestinal ischemia, necrotizing enterocolitis, and spontaneous perforation of the intestine, common in the preterm infant, are all highly associated with candidemia. Delayed enteral feeding has also been associated with infection.[48] The use of histamine 2 blockers raises the pH of the stomach and increases colonization, particularly of *C. parapsilosis.*[49] Disrupted integument, such as that which occurs after abdominal and cardiac surgeries, increase risks in term infants. In a similar fashion, candidal organisms readily penetrate the relatively poor barrier provided by the immature skin of the preterm infant, and that skin also readily breaks down during ordinary care. Colonized infants are more likely to be delivered vaginally than by cesarean section.[47,50] The use of topical petrolatum for skin care of extremely low-birth-weight infants may increase the risk. Catheters, as well as all other indwelling tubes (endotracheal, chest, urinary, ventriculoperitoneal), may become infected. The longer the duration of an indwelling catheter, particularly if used for total parenteral nutrition or infusion of intravenous lipids, the greater the risk is to the infant.[49] Immature immune defenses provide yet another set of risk factors. Neutrophils ingest and kill *Candida* intracellularly, but neutropenia is also common in very low-birth-weight infants. Theophylline may inhibit the candidacidal activity of neutrophils. Steroids inhibit the immune response, induce hyperglycemia, and, in the mouse, increase the adherence of the yeast to the intestinal mucosa.

Congenital candidiasis is extremely rare. In the term infant, infection results in an erythematous, macular eruption that then becomes pustular and desquamates.[51] These same skin infections become burn-like in the preterm infant and then develop a sheetlike desquamation, becoming superficial erosions. Intrauterine infection is highly associated with the presence of genital tract foreign bodies, in particular, cerclage, but has not been associated with maternal diabetes or urinary tract infections. The diagnosis in the newborn can be made with skin scrapings and blood and CSF cultures. In the term infant with only cutaneous infection, survival is the rule. These infants do not require treatment, although many clinicians will administer topical therapy to relieve symptoms and to decrease the mass of organisms the infant has to clear. In contrast, in the preterm infant weighing less than 1500 g, or in any infant with respiratory symptoms signifying aspiration and pneumonia, mortality is the rule unless systemic treatment is begun.

Mucocutaneous infection (thrush or a monilial diaper rash) is the most likely infection after birth, seen in 4% to 6% of newborns and occurring as early as 4 to 5 days after birth but peaking at 3 to 4 months. Thrush manifests as white, curd-like, pseudomembranous plaques on the oropharynx or posterior pharynx, whereas the diaper dermatitis produces an erythematous, scaly lesion with satellite papules or pustules in the intertriginous areas. The latter may be repetitively reinfected by a gastrointestinal tract reservoir. Therapy in those areas is local. Oral nystatin may be given to treat the thrush. Gentian violet works as efficaciously, but its propensity to stain makes it less popular. For the skin lesions, topical nystatin alone works well, although occasionally it should be combined with oral nystatin to reduce the gastrointestinal tract reservoir and to prevent spillage onto the groin. Once the rash starts spreading beyond the usual area in the diaper, systemic therapy should be administered.

Invasive candidiasis is a leading cause of morbidity and mortality in infants of less than 1000 g. Incidence in neonatal centers ranges from 2% to 28%.[52] Systemic disease in these infants, unlike in adults, results in multiple foci of infection. Onset is delayed, usually occurring at several weeks of life, and the duration of candidemia, even with treatment, averages 7 days. Most infants have several positive blood culture results, and 10% experience candidemia for longer than 14 days.[48,53] Infants have a multitude of signs and symptoms, including, in order of frequency, respiratory deterioration, apnea and bradycardia, hyperglycemia, a necrotizing enterocolitis–like picture without pneumatosis, skin involvement, temperature instability, and hypotension.[54] Meningitis, once reported in half of infants with systemic candidiasis, now occurs in only 5% to 9%,[48,55] probably because of more aggressive diagnosis and treatment. Roughly half of infants with meningitis will have negative blood culture results, and half will have normal CSF parameters.[51,55] Endophthalmitis, once seen in half of infants, again is now relatively uncommon, occurring in fewer than 1%.[56,57] Prognosis is excellent if the infection is treated. However, fungal sepsis in extremely low-birth-weight infants may be associated with increased frequency of threshold retinopathy of prematurity.[58,59] Endocarditis, which may be the source of infected thromboemboli, is associated with the presence of central venous catheters. The prognosis for osteoarthritis or osteomyelitis is also good with treatment. Cutaneous manifestations may include a generalized erythema or subcutaneous abscesses. Infants may be neutropenic or have an extreme leukocytosis. Continued thrombocytopenia is often an indication of ongoing disease. Pneumonitis presents with respiratory deterioration and a bronchopulmonary dysplasia–like picture on chest radiograph. Other infants may develop abdominal distension, guaiac-positive stools, and feeding intolerance but no pneumatosis intestinalis. A few will have hepatic abscesses, diarrhea, or perforation. Mortality is extremely high in those with candidal peritonitis. Urinary tract involvement is found in over half of infants with systemic candidiasis and ranges from a bladder infection to renal abscesses or renal papillary necrosis to a mycetoma or fungal ball in the renal pelvis, possibly resulting in a flank mass. Disease of the urinary tract may be entirely silent or present with hypertension or acute renal failure with oliguria or anuria. Mortality is usually in the range of 20% to 50%, but death or disability ensues in as many as 73% of extremely low-birth-weight infants.[48] Compared with age-matched controls, there is a higher incidence of periventricular leukomalacia, chronic lung disease (CLD), severe retinopathy of prematurity, and adverse neurologic outcome at 2 years corrected age.[60]

Candidal species grow readily in cultures of blood or urine or specimens from other normally sterile sites, and yeast or hyphae can be seen on urinalysis. Given the propensity for dissemination, the patient should undergo ultrasonography of the kidneys, echocardiography, and a retinal examination. Fungal stains of skin scrapings can be helpful. A complete blood count and C-reactive protein level may give indirect evidence of infection. A lumbar puncture if the infant is stable enough to tolerate the procedure, together with culture, gram staining, and cytologic analysis, is imperative. Overall, it is important to have a high index of suspicion.

Consideration should also be given to the removal of possibly contaminated medical devices, particularly central intravascular catheters. Amphotericin B has been the standard for antifungal therapy for years, but many other agents have been introduced, and few data are available to indicate the advantages of one drug over another, let alone safety, efficacy, dosages, or duration of treatment. CSF penetration of amphotericin B, although better than in adults, is highly variable. This has led a few to suggest the use of 5-fluorocytosine or fluconazole, both of which have good penetration of the CSF, in combination with amphotericin B. Others have successfully treated meningitis with amphotericin B alone. There are three lipid formulations approved by the U.S. Food and Drug Administration for use in adults: amphotericin B lipid complex, amphotericin B colloidal dispersion, and liposomal amphotericin B (AmBisome). Because higher dosages may be used without toxicity, these preparations may be appropriate for the infant with renal disease or severe nephrotoxicity.[61–63] A few studies have shown fluconazole to be efficacious in the treatment of invasive disease in neonates, equivalent to treatment with amphotericin B.[64,65] Unfortunately, resistance to fluconazole in certain Candida species, such as *Candida glabrata* and *Candida krusei,* are climbing. Fluconazole monotherapy is only recommended in neonates after identification of the fungal organism and determination of its susceptibility. The echinocandins are a newer antifungal drug class that is fungicidal against most candidal species. Newer literature supports the safety of use of this class of antifungals in the neonatal population. Caspofungin and micafungin have been studied in the neonatal population, and case report series show clinical efficacy and tolerability among these critically ill patients.[66] Newer second-generation triazoles, such as voriconazole, posaconazole, and isavuconazole, have been developed with broad spectrum of activity against medically important yeast. Clinical trials to evaluate the safety and PK/PD in infants has not been done for these agents, and therefore use is not recommended until further study.[67]

Prevention is clearly the best treatment for neonatal systemic candidiasis, yet this is also the area of greatest controversy. Treatment of maternal candidal infections may limit vertical transmission to the neonate. Prevention of horizontal transmission is more difficult. Hand washing does not reduce the recovery of *C. albicans* from medical workers' hands.[68] Removal of artificial fingernails may help. Careful attention to central lines is of benefit, as is attention to limiting exposure to drugs that increase the risk of disease. No consensus has been reached on the use of fluconazole prophylaxis. Some studies have shown a decrease in the incidence of colonization, invasive disease, or mortality.[69–73] Finally, concern remains regarding the risk of isolates developing resistance. A recent meta-analysis of three trials involving over 1600 infants found a decrease in the risk of invasive fungal infection in very low-birth-weight infants with oral–topical antifungal prophylaxis but warned about the major methodologic weaknesses in trials to date.[74] Also, one recent trial comparing fluconazole and nystatin oral prophylaxis had to be halted early because of a significant increase in deaths not related to fungal infections among the nystatin-treated infants.[75] Reports do exist of increased resistance among infants with *C. parapsilosis* infection, a rising form of candidiasis.[76,77]

Multidrug-Resistant Gram-Negative Pathogens

Gram-negative bacilli responsible for neonatal LOS mainly include *E. coli*, *Klebsiella* sp., *Enterobacter* sp., and *Pseudomonas* sp. The use of broad-spectrum antimicrobial therapy in the past decades have contributed to overall increase in multidrug-resistant gram-negative (MDRGN) pathogens. These organisms account for approximately 20% of bacteremia cases and are associated with 2.8-fold increase in neonatal mortality rate compared with nonresistant strains.[78] These resistant strains may be acquired from the mother during labor, particularly in the setting of prolonged rupture of membranes, during direct care, or indirectly through contact after birth. Nosocomial transmission of these resistant pathogens occur readily because of prolonged survival on hands of healthcare workers, medical devices, and sinks and inanimate surfaces. Premature neonates may acquire these infections through the hospital environment, mechanical ventilation, vascular catheters, administration of breast milk or formula, skin care, or surgical intervention. Choice of empiric first-line therapy for early- and late-onset sepsis is critical and should be informed by known colonization with MDRGN pathogens. Infants known to have infection or colonization with multidrug-resistant pathogens should be maintained on contact isolation to reduce transmission to other infants.[79]

Gonococcal Infections

Neisseria gonorrhoeae is frequently asymptomatic in women and may therefore be unknowingly transmitted to neonates. Endocervical screening samples should be sent for mothers in the first trimester of pregnancy, and, for women at high risk, a second culture should be performed late in the third trimester. Gonococcal infection, whether or not overt clinical symptoms are present, may cause vaginitis, cervicitis, salpingitis, and pelvic inflammatory disease. These conditions may result in neonatal morbidity and mortality directly by infection of the neonate or indirectly by precipitation of preterm labor with its consequent complications.

The most common manifestation of neonatal infection is ophthalmia neonatorum, a severe bacterial ocular infection. Before the routine use of silver nitrate, tetracycline, or erythromycin topical eye preparations, an infant born to a mother with *N. gonorrhoeae* endocervical infection had approximately a 30% chance of developing ocular disease. A premature infant or an infant born after a prolonged period after membrane rupture has an even greater risk of developing infection. Signs of infection typically manifest by 48 to 96 hours of life but may occur within hours. Classically, the infant has bilateral lid edema, chemosis, and purulent drainage. Without treatment, the infection can result in permanent corneal damage and panophthalmitis with vision loss.

Rarely, disseminated infection with *N. gonorrhoeae* occurs in neonates secondary to bacteremia. The majority of systemically infected infants in the United States are born to mothers who were inadequately screened and who have asymptomatic infection. The most common presentation of disseminated neonatal *N. gonorrhoeae* infection is pyogenic polyarthritis. The infant may have a pseudoparalysis of the affected limb.

Even in disseminated disease, meningitis has rarely been reported. Interestingly, the hallmark skin manifestations of disseminated *N. gonorrhoeae* infection seen in adults are not common in bacteremic infants. Localized cellulitis at breaks in the skin do occur. In the United States, most systemically infected infants do not have ocular disease because of the universal use of topical prophylaxis. The diagnosis of infection at any site is best made by gram staining and culture of purulent material on appropriate media.

Prevention of neonatal infection is accomplished through appropriate maternal screening, treatment of infected pregnant mothers, and universal ophthalmic prophylaxis. Pregnant women found to have *N. gonorrhoeae* infection should be treated according to current CDC guidelines (available at cdc.gov). Universal ophthalmic prophylaxis effectively prevents ocular disease in over 95% of infants born to infected mothers; however, as noted, the topical therapy does not prevent systemic illness. Infants born to mothers with known *N. gonorrhoeae* infection should receive standard ocular prophylaxis and a single dose of 125 mg of intravenous or intramuscular ceftriaxone. In preterm or low-birth-weight infants, the dose should be 25 mg to 50 mg/kg with a maximum dose of 125 mg.

For any infant with suspected infection, cultures should be performed on blood and CSF as well as samples from any exudate—ocular, skin abscess, or articular. Most infants should be hospitalized to ensure evaluation and therapy. Gonococcal ophthalmia neonatorum should be treated with a single dose of intravenous or intramuscular ceftriaxone at 25 to 50 mg/kg up to a maximum dose of 125 mg. In addition, infants should receive frequent eye irrigation with saline until the discharge has resolved. Topical therapy alone is insufficient to treat established infection and is unnecessary with systemic therapy. In infants with bacteremia or septic arthritis, ceftriaxone or cefotaxime therapy should be administered for 7 days. If cultures of CSF give positive results, the duration of therapy should be 10 to 14 days.[80]

Any infant with documented gonococcal disease should also be evaluated for other common sexually transmitted diseases: syphilis, *Chlamydia trachomatis* infection, HIV infection, and hepatitis B.

Chlamydia Trachomatis Infection

C. trachomatis is an obligate intracellular bacterium. *C. trachomatis* infection is the most common reportable sexually transmitted disease in the United States. The high prevalence of maternal infection, coupled with the lack of efficacy of the topical agents recommended as universal ocular prophylaxis for neonates, makes *C. trachomatis* the most common cause of ophthalmia neonatorum. A few of the at least 18 identified serotypes are responsible for the majority of genital infections in women and, consequently, in neonates. Transmission is primarily from infected genital secretions but has been reported in infants born via cesarean section to mothers with intact membranes. Infants born to mothers with untreated infection have a 50% likelihood of acquiring infection, with the nasopharynx being the most frequently colonized site. Once colonized, infants have between a 25% and 50% chance of developing conjunctivitis and between a 5% and 20% chance of developing pneumonia.

Conjunctivitis typically appears within a few days to weeks after birth, but the timing of infection cannot reliably distinguish *C. trachomatis* infection from gonococcal disease. The symptoms tend to be similar to, although milder than, those seen in gonococcal disease: lid edema, erythema, and purulent exudate. Treatment results in resolution of symptoms within 1 to 2 weeks without permanent sequelae. No treatment or inadequate therapy can result in symptoms for up to a year with the potential for conjunctival scarring or micropannus formation. Diagnosis is confirmed by culture of cells from conjunctival specimens. The test depends on the collection of epithelial cells because *C. trachomatis* is an intracellular pathogen. Consultation should be undertaken with the hospital microbiologist or infectious disease expert to determine the most appropriate collection methods and culture media. Staining will reveal intracytoplasmic inclusion in more than 90% of neonatal ocular specimens, with confirmation of *C. trachomatis* infection by species-specific monoclonal antibody staining.

Pneumonia caused by *C. trachomatis* typically presents from the late neonatal period through the first 4 months of life with a mild to moderate respiratory illness characterized by persistent staccato cough, tachypnea, and nasal congestion without fever. Physical examination often demonstrates tachypnea and rales but no wheeze. Half of infants with *C. trachomatis* pneumonia have evidence of conjunctivitis. Classically, chest radiography demonstrates bilateral interstitial infiltrates with hyperinflation. Diagnosis of *C. trachomatis* pneumonia is largely clinical. Although in many affected infants, cultures of nasopharyngeal specimens will be positive for the organism, the absence of a positive culture finding in samples from this site does not eliminate the possibility of *C. trachomatis* as the responsible pathogen. Elevation of *C. trachomatis*–specific immunoglobin M (IgM) to a titer of 1:32 or higher is diagnostic, but this assay is not always readily or rapidly available. Interestingly, IgM levels do not typically increase in infected infants with isolated ocular disease.

Infants with chlamydial conjunctivitis should be treated with oral erythromycin base or ethylsuccinate, 50 mg/kg/day divided into four doses for 14 days or azithromycin 20 mg/kg as a single daily dose for 3 days. Pneumonia may be treated with erythromycin in the same manner as ocular disease or may be treated with azithromycin 20 mg/kg/day for 5 days. Outside of the period immediately after birth, sulfonamides may be used if the infant cannot tolerate erythromycin therapy. Up to 20% of treated infants will require a second course of antibiotics. In infants younger than 6 weeks of age, erythromycin therapy has been associated with hypertrophic pyloric stenosis. The American Academy of Pediatrics (AAP) continues to recommend that neonates with chlamydial disease be treated with erythromycin pending further studies of other potentially effective agents and further delineation of the association between erythromycin and pyloric stenosis.[81] If neonates are treated with erythromycin, the physician should inform the parents of this association and its warning signs.

Disease prevention efforts target screening of all pregnant women, treatment of those infected, and documentation of cure. Despite the high likelihood of neonatal infection for infants born to untreated or inadequately treated mothers, the routine use of systemic erythromycin therapy for exposed infants is not recommended given the association with the drug and hypertrophic pyloric stenosis. *C. trachomatis* disease, as discussed, is generally not associated with significant morbidity or mortality. Infants should be observed for clinical signs of infection and treated if such signs are present.

Syphilis

After World War II, the number of cases of acquired and, consequently, of congenital syphilis declined steadily until the late 1980s and early 1990s, when an epidemic occurred. This epidemic coincided with an increase in the incidence of HIV infection, crack cocaine use, and the poverty rate. During 2000–2016, the rise in primary and secondary syphilis was attributed to increased cases among men, and specifically, men who have sex with men. By 1998, aggressive public health measures led to a decline in congenital syphilis cases to low levels of fewer than 500 cases per year, until an increase in 2013, with continued upward rise (Fig. 13.2).[82] The 2013 rate of congenital syphilis marked the first increase since 2008. During 2013–2014, rate increased 27.2%, it increased by 6% in 2014–2015, and it again increased by 27.6% in 2015–2016.

The causative organism, *Treponema pallidum*, can cross the placenta at any time during pregnancy and during any stage of maternal disease. Among newly infected women, 40% of pregnancies result in stillbirth, spontaneous abortion, or perinatal death. Women with untreated primary or secondary syphilis have a 60% to 90% chance of transmitting infection to the fetus. Women with early latent and late latent infection have a 40% and 8% chance of transmission, respectively.

By definition, congenital syphilis is a hematogenously spread infection and therefore lacks a primary stage. More than half of infected newborns are asymptomatic at birth. Conventionally, infection that is detected before a child is 2 years old is referred to as early disease, and infection discovered after 2 years of age is classified as late disease. Early-onset disease typically manifests before an infant is 3 months old.

When symptomatic, infected infants manifest multiorgan involvement consistent with their hematogenously disseminated infection. Neurologic symptoms are usually absent even when the CSF is markedly abnormal. The CSF shows signs of elevated protein or pleocytosis in 50% of symptomatic infants and in up to 10% of asymptomatic infants. Some infants may have pseudoparalysis of an extremity secondary to bony involvement. Long bone radiographs show abnormalities in 95% of symptomatic infants and 20% of asymptomatic infants.[83] The chronic, erosive rhinorrhea of syphilis, "snuffles," is no longer commonly seen. If present, the nasal discharge is highly infectious. Highly symptomatic infants may present with respiratory distress and pulmonary infiltrates referred to as *pneumonia alba.* Nearly all symptomatic infants have hepatomegaly with elevations in serum alkaline phosphatase level. Generalized lymphadenopathy is also common. Many symptomatic infants develop an erythematous, maculopapular rash that becomes coppery and frequently involves their palms and soles. Infants, unlike children and adults with skin involvement, may develop vesicles or bullous lesions, known as *pemphigus syphiliticus,* that tend to rupture and contain numerous infectious organisms. Leukocytosis, anemia, or thrombocytopenia is present in the majority of symptomatic infants.

Late-onset disease presents in children older than 2 years of age. Bony malformations secondary to chronic osteomyelitis include frontal bossing, saber shins, and saddle nose deformity. Dental abnormalities include abnormal molars and notched, small central incisors classically described as *Hutchinson teeth.* Interstitial keratitis presents as unilateral or bilateral photophobia with lacrimation that occurs after the fifth year of life. The symptoms are followed within weeks to months by vascular opacification of the cornea and consequent blindness. Eighth nerve involvement can present at any age with vertigo, progressive hearing loss, and ultimately permanent deafness. The high proportion of asymptomatic infected neonates and the devastating consequences of late-onset disease underscore the importance of screening all women in early pregnancy. All 50 states require serologic testing of women at the beginning of prenatal care.

The definitive diagnosis of syphilis is made by darkfield microscopic identification of spirochetes in exudate or tissue

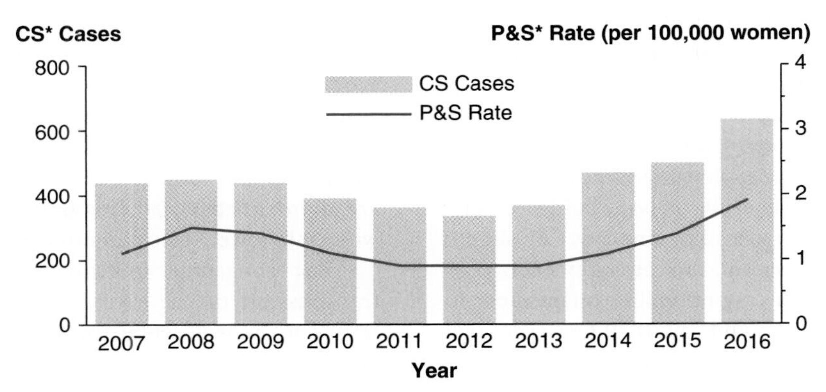

Fig. 13.2 Reported cases by year of birth and rates of primary *(P)* and secondary *(S)* syphilis among women, United States, 2007–2016. **CS,* Congenital syphilis. From Centers of Disease and Control and Prevention. *Sexually Transmitted Disease Surveillance 2016.* Atlanta: U.S. Department of Health and Human Services; 2017.

or direct fluorescent antibody testing of such material. These tests can be performed on the placenta or umbilical cord. Unfortunately, neither procedure is particularly sensitive or practical. Serologic screening is generally performed using nontreponemal tests: the rapid plasma reagin (RPR) test and the Venereal Disease Research Laboratory (VDRL) test. These tests detect immunoglobin G (IgG) and IgM to lipoidal antigen from *T. pallidum*. These tests, however, are not specific enough to make a definitive diagnosis. False-positive results can be seen in pregnancy, intravenous drug use, a variety of connective tissue diseases, and viral infection. Nontreponemal antibodies generally appear within 8 weeks of infection and are seen in 100% of patients with secondary or latent syphilis. False-negative results can occur if specimens are drawn too early after infection or if antibody concentrations are extremely high and cause a prozone effect. Titer testing can be performed using serial dilution to provide useful quantitative data about a patient's response to therapy. The same nontreponemal test should be used to follow a patient's titer. The titers typically show a fourfold decrease within 6 months of successful therapy for primary or secondary infection, and antibodies are undetectable after a year. Unfortunately, most untreated patients, including those with congenital infection, will become seronegative by nontreponemal testing within 2 years. Only the VDRL test has been approved for detecting spinal fluid infection.

Treponemal tests—the fluorescent treponemal antibody absorption test and the microhemagglutination assay–*T. pallidum*—are more specific for *T. pallidum* and should be performed to confirm a diagnosis of syphilis in patients with positive results on nontreponemal tests. These tests are qualitative, and results remain positive for life. They are therefore not used to ascertain the treatment status or clinical response of a patient.

An infant born to a mother with a history of syphilis or serologic evidence of syphilis should undergo the same test of nontreponemal antibodies as the mother so that titers can be compared. If the mother's titer has increased fourfold, if the infant's titer is four times higher than the mother's titer, or if the infant has signs or symptoms of infection, further evaluation is warranted. Cord blood is not reliable for serologic diagnosis. Further evaluation should also be initiated if documentation of maternal therapy is unavailable, if insufficient serologic follow-up is available to assess adequacy of therapy, if syphilis during pregnancy was treated with a nonpenicillin regimen,[84] or if syphilis during pregnancy was treated less than 1 month before delivery. In any infant with signs and symptoms of infection, nontreponemal titers four times higher than those of the mother, or positive results on body fluid testing by darkfield microscopy or fluorescent examination, CSF should be sent for VDRL testing, cell count, and measurement of protein concentration. In addition, asymptomatic infants born to inadequately treated mothers should have their CSF examined even if their nontreponemal titers are the same as or less than four times higher than the mother's titer.

Any infant with evidence of infection, positive results on placental or umbilical cord testing by darkfield microscopy or fluorescent technique, a fourfold higher nontreponemal titer than the mother, or positive VDRL results for CSF should be treated with parenteral penicillin G for 10 days. If infection cannot be excluded, the evaluation cannot be completely performed, or follow-up is not ensured, the infant should be treated for 10 days. A negative CSF VDRL result does not exclude congenital neurosyphilis; pleocytosis and elevated protein level should be considered signs of infection. In the case of an asymptomatic infant born to an inadequately treated mother, if physical examination findings, results of laboratory evaluation including CSF testing, and radiographic findings are normal and appropriate follow-up is expected, some experts would treat with a single intramuscular dose of benzathine penicillin.

The AAP recommends that exposed infants undergo nontreponemal serologic follow-up testing at 2 to 4 months, 6 months, and 12 months after treatment or until the titers decline fourfold or are nonreactive. The titers should be nonreactive by 6 months in infants who have been adequately treated or who were uninfected but had transplacentally acquired maternal antibody. Persistently positive titers or increasing titers warrant complete evaluation and 10 days of intravenous penicillin G therapy. Neonates with positive results on VDRL tests of CSF or uninterpretable CSF results should have repeat examinations of their CSF every 6 months until negative.[85] Fig. 13.3 shows the algorithm for evaluation and treatment of infants born to mothers with reactive serologic tests for syphilis.

VIRUSES

Congenital Cytomegalovirus Infection

Cytomegalovirus (CMV) is the most frequent congenital infection in humans.[86] The virus is endemic worldwide without any seasonal pattern. Typically, after a primary infection, virus is shed for weeks to years before becoming latent. Prevalence of infection is largely dependent on socioeconomic factors including crowding, maternal parity, and number of sexual partners. In the United States, seropositivity is much higher among African-American and Asian women. Among infants in the United States and Western Europe, seropositivity rates are between 0.5% and 2%; however, among young women, seropositivity rates are much higher, between 50% and 85%. In developing countries and among lower socioeconomic groups, seropositivity rates in young women may approach 90%. Another way to estimate the neonatal impact is to examine seroconversion rates. In upper- or middle-class women in the United States, annual seroconversion rates are approximately 2%. This number increases to 6% among women in lower socioeconomic groups.[87]

Most congenital infection results from transplacental transmission of the virus. A primary maternal infection results in transplacental transmission rates of 30% to 40%. Ten percent to 15% of these neonates will develop symptomatic infection. The later in pregnancy that maternal seroconversion occurs, the higher the likelihood of neonatal infection. Seventy-five percent of infants become infected in

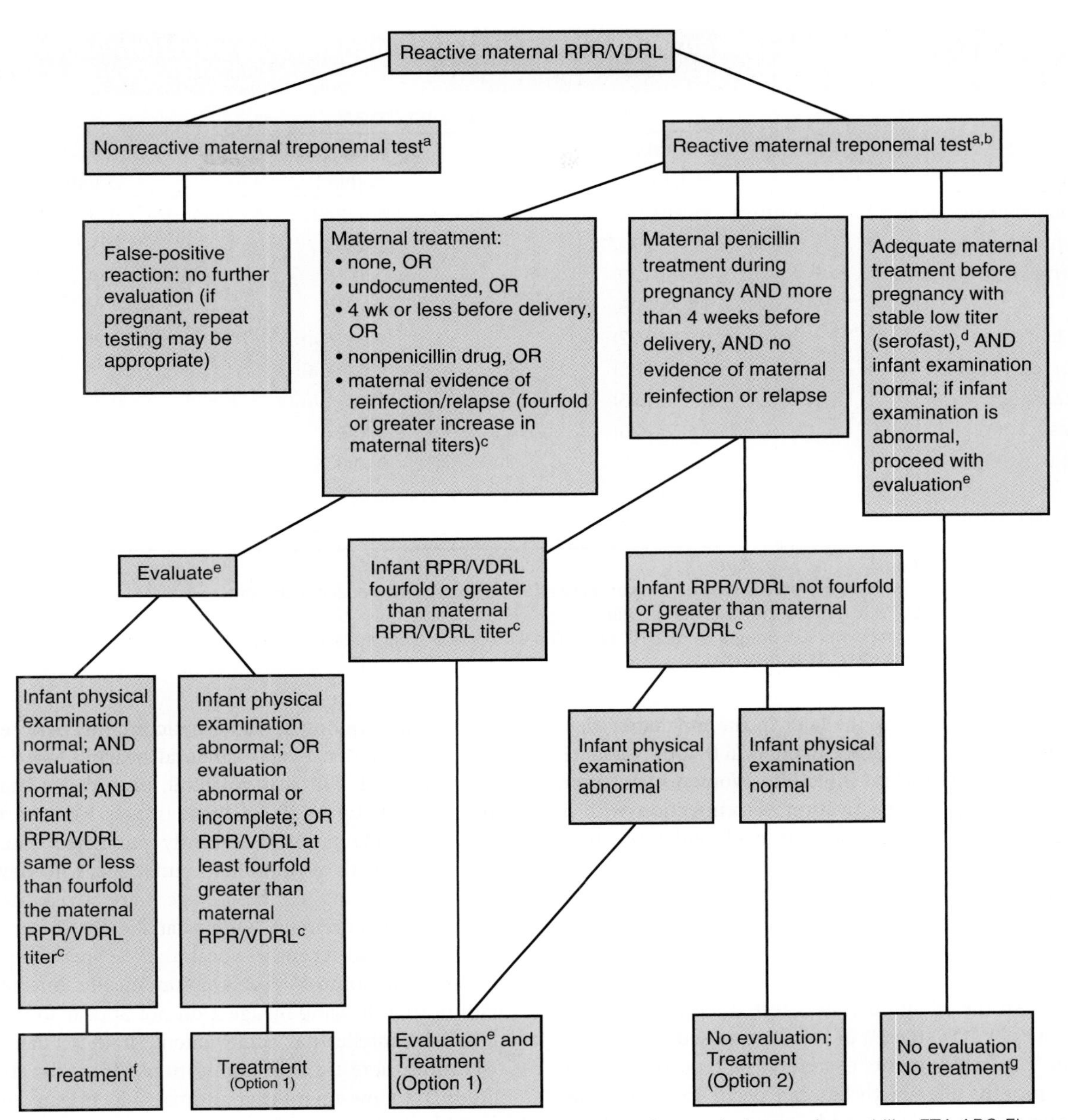

Fig. 13.3 Algorithm for evaluation and treatment of infants born to mothers with reactive serologic tests for syphilis. *FTA-ABS,* Fluorescent treponemal antibody absorption; *MHA-TP,* microhemagglutination test for antibodies to T. pallidum; *TP-EIA,* T. pallidum enzyme immunoassay; *RPR,* rapid plasma reagin; *TP-PA, Treponema pallidum* particle agglutination; *VDRL,* Venereal Disease Research Laboratory. From American Academy of Pediatrics. Syphilis. In: Kimberlin DW eds. *Red Book: 2015 Report of the Committee in Infectious Diseases.* 30th ed. Elk Gove Village, IL: American Academy of Pediatrics; 2015: 755–768.

[a]TP-PA, FTA-ABS, TP-EIA, or MHA-TP.

[b]Test for human immunodeficiency virus (HIV) antibody. Infants of HIV-infected mothers do not require different evaluation or treatment for syphilis.

[c]A fourfold change in titer is the same as a change of two dilutions. For example, a titer of 1:64 is fourfold greater than a titer of 1:16, and a titer of 1:4 is fourfold lower than a titer of 1:16. When comparing titers, the same type of nontreponemal test should be used (e.g., if the initial test was an RPR, the follow-up test should also be an RPR).

[d]Women who maintain a VDRL titer 1:2 or less or an RPR 1:4 or less beyond 1 year after successful treatment are considered serofast.

[e]Complete blood cell (CBC) and platelet count; cerebrospinal fluid (CSF) examination for cell count, protein, and quantitative VDRL; other tests as clinically indicated (e.g., chest radiographs, long-bone radiographs, eye examination, liver function tests, neuroimaging, and auditory brainstem response).

[f]Treatment (Option 1 or Option 2, below), with most experts recommending Treatment Option 1. If a single dose of benzathine penicillin G is used, then the infant must be fully evaluated, full evaluation must be normal, and follow-up must be certain. If any part of the infant's evaluation is abnormal or not performed, or if the CSF analysis is rendered uninterpretable, then a 10-day course of penicillin is required. [g]Some experts would consider a single intramuscular injection of benzathine penicillin (Treatment Option 2), particularly if follow-up is not certain.

Treatment Options:

1. Aqueous penicillin G, 50,000 U/kg, intravenously, every 12 hours (1 week of age or younger) or every 8 hours (older than 1 week), or procaine penicillin G, 50,000 U/kg, intramuscularly, as a single daily dose for 10 days. If 24 or more hours of therapy is missed, the entire course must be restarted.
2. Benzathine penicillin G, 50,000 U/kg, intramuscularly, single dose.

TABLE 13.1 Sequelae in Children With Congenital Cytomegalovirus Infection According to Type of Maternal Infection[93]

Sequela	TYPE OF MATERNAL INFECTION Primary % (No.)	Recurrent % (No.)	*p*-Value
Sensorineural hearing loss	15 (18/120)	5.4 (3/56)	0.05
Bilateral hearing loss	8.3 (10/120)	0 (0/56)	0.02
Speech threshold ≥60 dB[a]	7.5 (9/120)	0 (0/56)	0.03
IQ ≤70	13.2 (9/68)	0 (0/32)	0.03
Chorioretinitis[b]	6.3 (7/112)	1.9 (1/54)	0.20
Other neurologic sequelae[c]	6.4 (8/125)	1.6 (1/64)	0.13
Microcephaly	4.8 (6/125)	1.6 (1/64)	0.25
Seizures	4.8 (6/125)	0 (0/64)	0.08
Paresis or paralysis	0.8 (1/125)	0 (0/64)	0.66
Death[d]	2.4 (3/125)	0 (0/64)	0.29
Any sequela	24.8 (31/125)	7.8 (5/64)	0.003

[a]For the ear with better hearing.
[b]Three of the seven children with chorioretinitis (43%) in the primary infection group had visual impairment.
[c]Four of the eight children (50%) had more than one abnormality.
[d]After the newborn period. From Fowler KB, Stagno S, Pass RF, et al. The Outcome of Congenital Cytomegalovirus Infection in Relation to Maternal Antibody Status. *N Engl J Med.* 1992; 326(10):663–7.

the third trimester. However, the later in the pregnancy that the infection occurs, the lower the likelihood that the neonate will have clinically significant infection. Women may suffer recurrent infection from reactivation or reinfection with a different viral strain.[88] In these cases, transplacental infection occurs in approximately 1% of infants, and, among this 1%, it causes symptomatic disease in only 1%.

Postnatal infection also occurs. Among women with active infection, polymerase chain reaction (PCR) methodology can detect CMV excretion in breast milk in 70%–90% of women when the whey portion is tested. Perinatal transmission occurs in 40% to 60% of infants exposed to infected breast milk.[89] Infected infants excrete virus typically from 3 weeks to 3 months after birth but can occur for as long as a year. Transmission occurs readily among young children, particularly in daycare settings, where salivary exposure is presumed to be the culprit. Seroconversion may be as high as 15% to 45% among parents of children attending daycare, and teachers have an 11% rate. Subsequent pregnancies account for nearly a quarter of symptomatic congenital infections in the United States. In contrast, likely reflecting adherence to basic contact precautions, healthcare workers do not have a seroconversion rate above community baseline. Nosocomial transmission may incur in the nursery, related to contaminated hands of providers or other fomites. Finally, nosocomial infection can result from blood transfusions or exchange transfusions. These cases may be significantly decreased by using seronegative donors, leukocyte filtration, or deglycerolized packed red blood cells.

Nearly 90% of congenital infections are asymptomatic, and the infants are not growth restricted or premature. However, 10% to 15% of these infants are still at risk of later developmental abnormalities, which typically appear in the first 2 years of life. Among asymptomatic infants, between 7% and 25% will experience sensorineural hearing loss.[90,91] Half of these neonates will have bilateral, progressive hearing loss. In one study, up to 2% of these infants went on to require cochlear implantation.[91] Recently published data describe that infants with asymptomatic infection who develop sensorineural hearing loss before age 2 are at risk for impaired academic achievement with statistically lower full-scale intelligence and receptive vocabulary scores compared with noninfected controls.[92] Asymptomatically infected infants with normal hearing by age 2 do not appear to demonstrate decreased intellectual achievement. If these data stand up over time, there are clear implications for the duration of longitudinal follow-up for asymptomatically infected infants.

Table 13.1 summarizes the occurrence of symptoms in infants based on maternal antibody status.[93] Infants born to mothers with early primary infection have a mortality rate of 20% to 30% related to liver failure, hemorrhage, disseminated intravascular coagulation (DIC), and secondary bacterial infection. Some deaths may occur after the neonatal period as a result of neurologic sequelae. Half of symptomatic infants have intrauterine growth restriction, and 33% are born prematurely. Approximately 50% will have microcephaly, with some demonstrating the characteristic periventricular calcifications. Splenomegaly closely followed by hepatomegaly are the two most common findings in symptomatic newborns. Two-thirds will develop clinically apparent hyperbilirubinemia that can be persistent and typically demonstrates a rise both in indirect and direct bilirubin levels. The majority of symptomatic infants will have a transaminitis. Thrombocytopenia because of megakaryocyte suppression may be severe. Petechiae and purpura are seen in over half of symptomatic infants. Less common complications include seizures,

Coombs-negative hemolytic anemia, and diffuse interstitial pneumonitis. Disruption of enamel of primary teeth may be seen in infants, leading to significant caries. Male infants have a higher frequency of inguinal hernias.

Sensorineural hearing loss is found in over 30% of symptomatic infants. Chorioretinitis, optic atrophy, and strabismus occur in approximately 20% of symptomatic infants. Retinitis in these infants is more likely to be macular compared with infected adults.[94] Overall outcomes are poor, with 90% of infants developing at least one neurologic abnormality. Although microcephaly is a strong predictor of intellectual impairment, intracranial calcifications on computerized tomographic images suggest a risk as high as 90% along with accompanying progressive, severe bilateral hearing loss, optic atrophy, and neuromuscular abnormalities. Ultrasound can detect calcifications, but magnetic resonance imaging may detect additional prognostically significant findings such as polymicrogyria, hippocampal dysplasia, and cerebellar hypoplasia.[95]

As previous noted, perinatal infection may develop in an infant after passage through the birth canal or from breast milk. In the term infant, this infection is typically asymptomatic with little effect on developmental outcome. Few of these infants will develop diffuse interstitial pneumonitis, but morbidity and mortality are low. Preterm infants are at higher risk. Transfusion of infected packed red blood cells may result in a systemic inflammatory response syndrome with pneumonia, organomegaly, thrombocytopenia, and neutropenia with a morality as high as 50%. Breastfeeding of preterm infants by seropositive mothers does not usually result in this acute presentation or seem to carry long-term developmental sequelae.[96]

Viral isolation in tissue culture, from urine or saliva, remain the most sensitive and specific test for diagnosis in the infant. To differentiate congenital infection in the neonate from perinatal infection, virus must be isolated in the first 2 weeks after birth. With hyperimmune sera or monoclonal antibodies, detection may occur within 24 hours. Because IgG is transplacentally transferred, its detection is not helpful without paired sera. Measure of serum IgM is associated both with false positives and negatives. PCR amplification for detection of viral DNA has been found to be extremely sensitive for diagnosis in a large range of tissues and secretions, particularly blood and saliva.[97] A newer technique involves the use of a nested PCR to detect viral DNA in dried blood spots that are obtained for metabolic tests as part of newborn screening.[98] The dried blood spots are not infectious, and samples can be shipped and stored for years.

Maternal and prenatal diagnosis is more complicated. Mothers are usually asymptomatic; therefore infection does not arouse clinical suspicion. Screening thus becomes more important. The detection of IgG does not distinguish primary versus recurrent infection in the mother. IgM responses are variable, and the antibody may be detected for 16 weeks or longer after primary infection. An IgG avidity assay, based on the determination that antibody in the first months following an infection is of lower avidity, is effective as a negative predictor up to 21 weeks of pregnancy but less so later. The critical issue is whether or not the fetus is infected and whether an infection is symptomatic. Cordocentesis for fetal blood testing will miss many infected fetuses. IgM appears after 20 weeks' gestation and is only detectable in half of cases. Viral DNA can be detected, but the test has a low sensitivity. Quantitative PCR of amniotic fluid has become the gold-standard assay.[99] Ultrasonographic abnormalities may be associated with, but are not diagnostic of, infection. These findings include microcephaly, intracranial calcifications or cysts, intrauterine growth restriction, oligohydramnios or polyhydramnios, pericardial effusions, pleural effusions, hepatic lesions, and other hyperechoic abdominal masses.

Because disease is often present for a prolonged period in the fetus and has already had deleterious effects, treatment does not prevent many of the adverse outcomes. The best "treatment" is therefore prevention of fetal infection. Vaccines continue to be explored, but none are currently available. One study provided 31 pregnant women who had primary infection with hyperimmune globulin; only 3% of the treated mothers versus 50% of untreated mothers had symptomatic infants with consequent sequlae.[100] Of note, treatment also resulted in improvements in placental thickness that occurs with primary infection.[101] Passive protection after birth would be unlikely to be of benefit. Although prevention is key, infected infants can benefit from antiviral therapy. In a randomized, controlled trial of intravenous ganciclovir in 100 infants with central nervous system (CNS) disease, the therapy prevented worsening hearing loss at 6 months and 1 year of age.[102] Fewer developmental delays at 6 and 12 months of age, as measured by Denver developmental tests, were also seen among infants receiving intravenous ganciclovir therapy than among control infants.[103] In 2015, Kimberlin et al conducted a randomized placebo-controlled trial of valganciclovir therapy in neonates with symptomatic congenital CMV disease, comparing 6 months of therapy with 6 weeks of therapy. They concluded that valganciclovir for 6 months, compared with 6 weeks, did not improve hearing in the short term, but did improve hearing and developmental outcomes at 24 months.[104] This has changed the landscape of treatment for congenital CMV considerably, as the tolerability and ease of administration for oral valganciclovir is much improved over intravenous ganciclovir. Treatment of congenital CMV in infants with CNS disease should be considered but needs to be initiated in the first month of life. Infants need to be monitored closely for toxicity, particularly neutropenia. A role for antiviral therapy has not been established for congenitally infected, asymptomatic infants despite a known incidence of neurological consequences. Most neonatologists and infectious disease specialists believe that vaccine development will be critical in eliminating harm from this virus.

Herpes Simplex Virus

There are two types of herpes simplex virus (HSV) that cause disease: HSV-1 and HSV-2. Both types cause disease in neonates. HSV-1, the common cause of gingivostomatitis and orolabial disease, now accounts for a majority of genital infection. HSV-2 is most commonly associated with genital infection. Both types are ubiquitous. Approximately 26% of U.S. children demonstrate serological evidence of HSV-1 infection by age 7.[105] Approximately 20% to 25% of adults in the United States have genital HSV-2 infection.[106,107] Approximately 2% of women seroconvert during pregnancy.[108,109] Approximately two-thirds of women who acquire infection during pregnancy remain asymptomatic. As is true for CMV and other viruses in the herpes family, HSV is able to enter a latent state after primary infection. The facial ganglion and the sacral ganglion are the two most common locations for HSV-1 and HSV-2, respectively, to establish latency. This latency allows the viruses to cause recurrent disease despite the presence of both cellular and humoral immunity. In immunologically normal hosts, recurrent infections typically cause more mild disease. The aforementioned acquisition rate during pregnancy suggest that recurrent infections are the most common cause of genital HSV during pregnancy.

Neonatal infection is overwhelmingly acquired during the intrapartum period; infection during this time accounts for 85% of transmission from fetal exposure to infected maternal genital secretions. Only 5% of infections are acquired in utero. There are five factors known to influence transmission of HSV from mother to neonate.[110,111]

- type of maternal infection (primary versus recurrent);
- maternal HSV antibody status;
- duration of rupture of membranes;
- integrity of mucocutaneous barriers (e.g., use of fetal scalp electrodes); and
- mode of delivery (cesarean versus vaginal).

Infants born to mothers who have a first episode of genital HSV infection near term and are shedding virus are at much greater risk of developing neonatal herpes than are infants whose mothers have recurrent genital herpes.[112] Among women with a first episode of genital HSV, 57% of exposed neonates developed HSV disease when infection was primary and 25% when nonprimary. In contrast, in women with recurrent genital HSV, only 2% of exposed neonates developed disease. Some protection is afforded by preexisting neutralizing antibodies. Most infected neonates are born to women with clinically unapparent infection at the time of delivery and have neither a past history of genital herpes or a sexual partner reporting a history of genital HSV. The use of invasive monitoring provides a site for viral entry into the fetus, and this site is often the location of initial lesions. Rupture of membranes longer than 6 hours before delivery in a mother with active lesions is an additional risk factor. Mothers with active lesions should ideally undergo cesarean section before rupture of membranes and within 6 hours of rupture. Cesarean section reduces the risk of fetal infection from 7.7% to 1.2%, but does not eliminate the risk entirely.[113]

Intrauterine infection is relatively rare and may result from either ascending infection from the birth canal or transplacental infection. It may also occur in either primary or recurrent maternal infection. These infants are severely affected and have a combination of skin vesicles with scarring, hydranencephaly or microcephaly, and keratoconjunctivitis. The third route of neonatal transmission occurs postnatally. Virus may be transmitted if breastfeeding from an infected breast or being kissed by an individual who has orolabial herpes. In the United States, surveillance data indicate that 2200 cases of neonatal disease are diagnosed annually.

Unlike children and adults who acquire HSV and in contrast to infants congenitally infected with CMV, neonates rarely experience asymptomatic infection with HSV-1 or HSV-2. Neonatal disease is classified into localized skin, eye, and mouth (SEM); meningoencephalitis (CNS); and disseminated disease. These presentations occur with approximately equal frequencies. Although indistinguishable clinically, normal neurologic outcomes with therapy occur more frequently in infants infected with HSV-2 (41%) than those infected with HSV-1 (23%).[114]

Symptoms of SEM disease typically appear at 7 to 10 days of life. The most easily recognized skin lesion is the vesicle. The vesicle may progress into a cluster of vesicles that may coalesce to form bullae. Lesions are most commonly found on the head, especially if there had been scalp monitoring, but may also be found on the trunk or extremities. Lesions in the mouth presumably are caused by swallowed contaminated amniotic fluid and maternal secretions. Keratoconjunctivitis, chorioretinitis, and cataracts may develop. Although initially limited to the skin, if untreated, will frequently progress to systemic disease. Even with acyclovir therapy, 50% of neonates with SEM will have a recurrence of skin lesions.[115]

Isolated CNS disease in the newborn probably represents retrograde axonal transport of the virus in infants who have acquired transplacental neutralizing antibody, which possibly has not allowed hematogenous spread of the virus.[116] In these infants, the infection becomes apparent at a slightly older age, after the first week of life—often in the second or third week, but even as late as 6 weeks of life. Nonspecific signs may include temperature instability, lethargy, irritability, and poor feeding. HSV encephalitis should always be considered in the presence of focal or generalized seizures, particularly if refractory, associated with tremors, a bulging fontanelle, pyramidal tract signs, or focal neurologic deficits. Skin lesions often are absent. CSF may be normal initially or show subtle abnormalities. Many infants will have bloody CSF. CSF analysis may demonstrate low glucose with a mononuclear pleocytosis. CSF protein may be normal early in the course but rises significantly over time. Computed tomography may show localized or multifocal areas of hemorrhage, edema, or infarction. An electroencephalogram may also help determine the extent of the disease. Untreated, 50% of infants will die. Even with therapy, a significant percentage of survivors have neurologic sequelae by 1 year of age.[117]

Most infants with disseminated HSV disease are born to mothers with primary infection and lack transplacental antibody. The resulting viremia in the infant spreads the disease to all organs, usually in the first week of life but also in the first 24 hours. Adrenal hemorrhage and shock with fulminant hepatitis may be prominent. There may be a systemic inflammatory response syndrome–like picture with metabolic acidosis, respiratory distress, DIC, direct hyperbilirubinemia, thrombocytopenia, neutropenia, transaminitis, and seizures. A vesicular rash is not usually present at onset and may be entirely absent in 70% of neonates. The majority of these neonates develop meningoencephalitis. Others may develop interstitial pneumonia, hemorrhagic pneumonia, or necrotizing enterocolitis with pneumatosis intestinalis. This group of infants have the highest mortality, over 80% if untreated, but as high as 30% even with appropriate treatment.

In suspected infection, viral isolation by culture remains the standard. Swab specimens for viral isolation should be taken from all skin lesions, the nasopharynx, urine, stool, and conjunctivae. Isolation of the virus from the skin or nasopharynx in the first 24 hours of life may represent transient contamination from birth; therefore swab specimens should be taken at 24 hours of life in infants born vaginally to mothers with genital lesions or known shedding. Viral typing is important for prediction of survival and neurological outcome. CNS analysis and molecular diagnostics of CSF should be performed. PCR of CSF is highly sensitive and specific. Skin lesions should be examined either by immunofluorescence or PCR testing. Regardless of classification, infants with disease should undergo neuroimaging and audiological and ophthalmologic examinations.

Intravenous acyclovir is the appropriate therapy for all forms of disease. The dose should be 60 mg/kg/day in three divided doses. Infants with SEM should be treated for 14 days to prevent dissemination. CNS and disseminated disease are treated for 21 days; however, patients with CNS disease should have repeat CSF testing and additional therapy if PCR remains positive. Adequate hydration is important to prevent tubular nephrotoxicity. If ophthalmic disease present, ocular therapy should be used. Current recommendations include placing all infected infant on 6 months of oral acyclovir prophylaxis. Data suggest improved neurologic outcomes and a decrease in skin outbreaks. Prophylactic dosing is 300 mg/m^2/dose orally three times daily. Absolute neutrophil counts should be measured at 2 and 4 weeks following initiation of suppressive therapy and then monthly.

In 2013, the AAP published an updated algorithm for managing asymptomatic neonates born to women with active genital herpes lesions. The algorithm provides directions for obstetrical and neonatal testing and treatment (Fig.13.4).[118]

Human Immunodeficiency Virus Infection

In the early 1980s, acquired immunodeficiency syndrome (AIDS) was first described in infants and children. Children younger than 13 years infected with human immunodeficiency virus (HIV) account for fewer than 1% of the total number of infected people in the United States. More than 90% of these cases resulted from vertical transmission from infected mothers. Since 1992, the CDC has reported a 90% decrease in new infection in children younger than 13 years of age. Only 166 new cases in this age group were reported in 2005, down to 122 in 2016.[119,120] As will be discussed, this nadir was achieved by improved prenatal screening, management of pregnant mothers, and postpartum prophylaxis.

HIV is an RNA retrovirus of the genus *Lentivirus*. The virus primarily targets $CD4^+$ lymphocytes, where it incorporates itself as a provirus into the host cells' genome and is replicated as part of normal host cell DNA replication. Infection is therefore lifelong. Even in the presence of potent combination antiretroviral therapy and reduction in HIV RNA serum levels below detectability, latent virus has been demonstrated in peripheral blood monocytes. In active infection, virus can be isolated from a variety of cells, organs, and bodily fluids; however, epidemiologic studies have only demonstrated infectivity from blood, breast milk, cervical secretions, and semen.

Neonatal infection is generally clinically silent. Infants may have nonspecific physical examination findings of hepatosplenomegaly or lymphadenopathy. Oral candidiasis in a neonate, as previously discussed, does not arouse suspicion for pathologic T-cell dysfunction. Refractory, recurrent oral candidiasis, encephalopathy, developmental delay, poor growth, chronic diarrhea, and parotitis are relatively common findings in infected infants during the first year of life; again, none of these symptoms are particularly specific for HIV infection. Before the improvement in identification of infected mothers, use of highly active antiretroviral therapy (HAART), and initiation of appropriate postnatal prophylaxis for viral and opportunistic infections, pneumonia caused by *Pneumocystis jiroveci* (formerly *Pneumocystis carinii*) accounted for the majority of AIDS-defining illness in the first year of life; the peak incidence occurred between ages 3 and 6 months.[121] Many infants, however, do not have AIDS-defining opportunistic infection, but rather may experience both recurrent common or serious bacterial infections, including otitis media, sinusitis, pneumonia, septic arthritis, bacteremia, or meningitis. Although a single occurrence of these infections does not raise suspicion about immunodeficiency, their recurrence should alert the clinician to evaluate the infant's immune system. In general, the likelihood of serious bacterial infection or opportunistic infection correlates inversely with infants' $CD4^+$ count. If HAART is not initiated, these counts begin to decline around 3 months of age.[122]

Diagnosis of HIV infection in infants can be made in several ways. Serologic testing is not diagnostic in a neonate because a positive result on an enzyme immunoassay may simply reflect maternal serologic status because of passive transplacental transfer of IgG antibody. Antibody tests may yield false-negative results if the mother was infected late in pregnancy and had not yet seroconverted. In infants born to HIV-infected mothers, blood should be sent for either HIV DNA PCR testing or HIV RNA PCR assay during the first 48 hours of life. If results are positive, a second sample should be sent for PCR assay to confirm the diagnosis. Once infection has been established, HIV RNA PCR testing is used to monitor the efficacy of therapy because this test yields a quantitative result or viral load in copies per milliliter. There are several ways to rule out infection. A negative result on two PCR samples obtained after 1 month and 4 months of life rules out infection. Two negative antibody test results separated by 1 month obtained after 6 months of life or a single

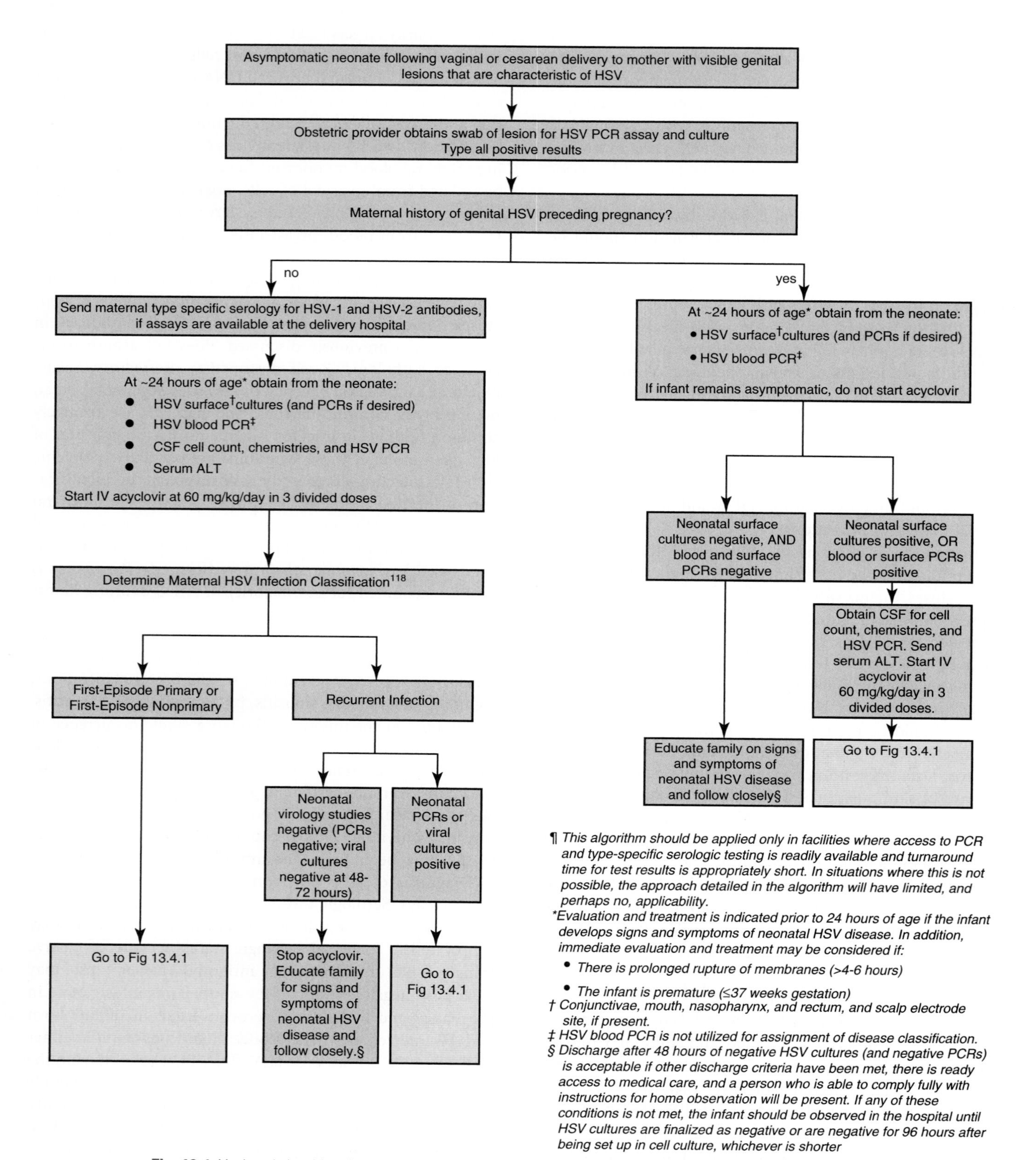

Fig. 13.4 Updated algorithm for managing asymptomatic neonates born to women with active genital herpes lesions. *ALT,* Alanine transaminase; *CNS,* central nervous system; *CSF,* cerebrospinal fluid; *HSV,* herpes simplex virus; *PCR,* polymerase chain reaction; *SEM,* skin, eye, and mouth. From Kimberlin DW, Baley J, Committee on Infectious Diseases and Committee on Fetus and Newborn. Guidance on Management of Asymptomatic Neonates Born to Women with Active Genital Herpes Lesions. *Pediatrics* 2013;131(2):e635–e646.

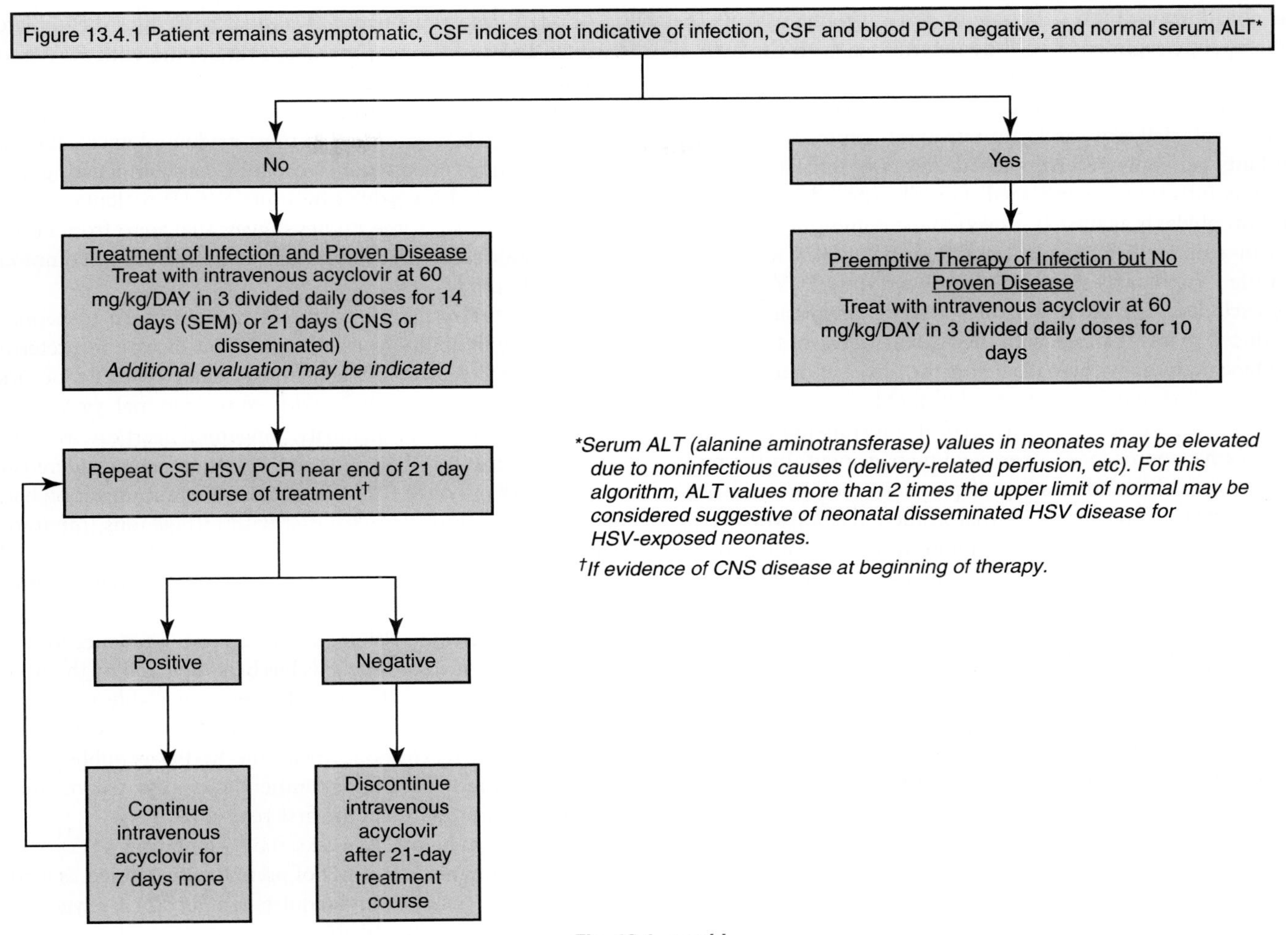
Figure 13.4.1 Patient remains asymptomatic, CSF indices not indicative of infection, CSF and blood PCR negative, and normal serum ALT*
No
Yes
Treatment of Infection and Proven Disease
Treat with intravenous acyclovir at 60 mg/kg/DAY in 3 divided daily doses for 14 days (SEM) or 21 days (CNS or disseminated)
Additional evaluation may be indicated
Preemptive Therapy of Infection but No Proven Disease
Treat with intravenous acyclovir at 60 mg/kg/DAY in 3 divided daily doses for 10 days
Repeat CSF HSV PCR near end of 21 day course of treatment†
Positive
Negative
Continue intravenous acyclovir for 7 days more
Discontinue intravenous acyclovir after 21-day treatment course
*Serum ALT (alanine aminotransferase) values in neonates may be elevated due to noninfectious causes (delivery-related perfusion, etc). For this algorithm, ALT values more than 2 times the upper limit of normal may be considered suggestive of neonatal disseminated HSV disease for HSV-exposed neonates.
†If evidence of CNS disease at beginning of therapy.

Fig. 13.4, cont'd

negative antibody test result after 12 to 18 months of life excludes infection.[123]

As noted earlier, interruption of vertical transmission has greatly reduced the number of infected children in the United States. In 1994, the Pediatric AIDS Clinical Trials Group Protocol 076 trial demonstrated a 67% reduction in perinatal HIV transmission with use of a zidovudine regimen for mother and infants.[124] Currently, the CDC recommends universal screening of all pregnant women in the first trimester with repeat testing in the third trimester for women felt to be at high risk of infection. Numerous subsequent studies have looked at a variety of simple and complex regimens testing different antiretroviral agents, timing, and duration, and have examined their efficacy and side effects in pregnant women and their offspring. The routine use of HAART starting in 1996 has made it possible to greatly suppress viral burden in infected patients. Several studies have demonstrated the benefit of viral suppression in mothers in preventing vertical transmission to their infants.[125] The CDC currently recommends that pregnant women receive HAART, containing zidovudine, if possible, if they require it for their own health or if they have HIV RNA levels of more than 1000 copies/mL.[126] As noted earlier, the virus can be detected in peripheral monocytes even when undetectable in plasma. Therefore there is no absolute viral threshold that reduces the risk of transmission to zero, and consequently, the CDC urges consideration of this regimen for pregnant women even if they have HIV RNA levels of less than 1000 copies/mL. Several studies have shown that elective cesarean delivery in HIV-infected women who have not received HAART, if performed before rupture of membranes and onset of labor, reduces the rate of vertical transmission by 50%.[127,128] Whether the benefits outweigh the risks for cesarean section in women receiving HAART who have RNA viral loads of less than 1000 copies/mL is controversial, and therefore cesarean section is not recommended for those women. Worldwide, breastfeeding has been a major mechanism for vertical transmission. Studies estimate that between 15% and 40% of vertical transmission worldwide occurs through breast milk. Since 1985, the CDC has recommended that women with HIV avoid breastfeeding if they have access to safe, affordable formula[129]; the World Health Organization made a similar recommendation in 2000.[126]

Any infant born to an infected mother should receive antiretroviral therapy as soon as possible after delivery. Antiretroviral therapy administered beyond 48 hours of life is not likely to impact the rate of vertical transmission. The therapeutic regimen should be determined with the help of a pediatric infectious disease specialist because of the need to take into account the mother's viral load, CD4+ count, mode of delivery, and antiretroviral exposure. Exposed infants generally receive antiviral therapy for 4 to 6 weeks unless infection is confirmed. For all exposed infants, chemoprophylaxis against *P. jiroveci,* most commonly trimethoprim–sulfamethoxazole, should be initiated at 4 to 6 weeks of life. Prophylaxis should be continued until HIV infection is excluded. The likelihood of vertical transmission can be reduced to less than 1% with the aggressive use of HAART to reduce maternal viral loads below the limits of detection and the use of neonatal antiretroviral prophylaxis.

The efficacy of disrupting vertical transmission has led to aggressive approaches to perinatal management. In the most recent guidelines for testing of pregnant mothers and neonates, the CDC recommends that women in labor whose HIV status is unknown be offered rapid antibody testing. If the results are positive, the woman should be offered antiretroviral therapy and cesarean section without waiting for confirmatory test results.[130] This aggressive approach reflects clinical consensus that the risk of exposing an uninfected mother or child to antiretroviral therapy and/or surgery is outweighed by the ability to prevent vertical transmission of this incurable infection. Infants with documented HIV infection should be evaluated and treated by an experienced pediatric infectious disease physician who can monitor response to therapy as well as medication toxicities. Current guidelines suggest that all children younger than 1 year of age receive HAART regardless of viral load or immune status. *Pneumocystis* prophylaxis should be continued until the infant is 12 months of age and has CD4+ counts appropriate for age. The need for chemoprophylaxis against infection with other opportunistic agents, including *Mycobacterium avium–intracellulare* complex, *Toxoplasma gondii*, and various herpes viruses, are determined by the patients' CD4+ counts and clinical conditions. A discussion of specific HAART regimens is beyond the scope of this chapter. HAART has dramatically increased the life expectancy of infants and children with HIV infection. In the absence of a cure, HIV-infected children may require lifelong therapy with drugs that have been associated with premature coronary artery disease, insulin resistance, and bone fragility. The personal and societal costs of prolonged HAART therapy underscore the current aggressive focus on HIV prevention.

Respiratory Viruses

Respiratory infections may be common in neonates, but many are asymptomatic. It is possible that these infections are asymptomatic as a result of maternal transplacental and breast-milk antibodies.[131] Respiratory viruses, however, can be causes of acute respiratory illnesses in preterm infants, leading to rehospitalization, increased healthcare burden, and long-term morbidity. Human metapneumovirus (HMPV), rhinovirus, and respiratory syncytial virus (RSV) have been associated with asthma and recurrent wheezing, which are common long-term pulmonary complications of prematurity.

HMPV infections occur in annual epidemics during late winter and early spring months, overlapping with RSV and influenza viruses. The peak of HMPV is typically 1–2 months after the peak of RSV. The prevalence of HMPV infection is second after RSV according to most epidemiological studies. Viral infections are often not recognized as complicating factors in neonatal intensive care unit (NICU) patients, except during outbreaks. Some studies suggest that apart from nosocomial outbreaks, viral respiratory infections are uncommon in the NICU.[132]

RSV is the respiratory virus of most concern to neonatologists, with ability to cause significant disease in preterm infants. RSV season in the United States typically occurs from November to March, with some regional variability. Infant with CLD of prematurity, congenital heart disease, and infants born at less than 29 weeks' gestation are considered at highest risk of severe RSV disease. Passive immunization had been employed for decades, first with intravenous immunoglobulin, then high-titer respigam, until finally monoclonal Palivizumab was licensed in June 1998 for the reduction of serious lower respiratory tract infection caused by RSV in children at increased risk for severe disease. Guidance for the use of palivizumab prophylaxis has been updated by the AAP multiple times as further data becomes available regarding the greatest risk of hospitalization attributable to RSV infection. The most recent policy from the AAP was published in 2014, with the following recommendations for palivizumab prophylaxis for infants in the first year of life[133]:

- Infants born before 29 weeks, 0 days gestation.
- Preterm infants with CLD of prematurity defined as birth <32 weeks, gestation and requirement for >21% oxygen for at least 28 days after birth.
- Hemodynamically significant heart disease.
- Clinicians may administer up to a maximum of five monthly doses of palivizumab (15 mg/kg per dose) during the RSV season for infants who qualify during the first year of life.
- Providers may choose to continue for second year of life in infants with CLD and continued need for medical support (supplemental oxygen, chronic corticosteroids, diuretic therapy).
- Prophylaxis should be discontinued in infants who have breakthrough RSV disease.
- Other conditions in which prophylaxis may be considered include certain pulmonary or neuromuscular diseases that impair ability to clear secretions and profound immunocompromising conditions.

Hepatitis B and C

Together, hepatitis B and C are responsible for most of the 1.4 million annual deaths attributed to viral hepatitis. There is growing concern for perinatal transmission of hepatitis C virus (HCV) in the United States, most pronounced in areas with HCV incidence increasing among young adults and women of childbearing age. Maternal IV drug use is the major risk factor for HCV infection. There is immediate need to increase HCV screening among those at risk and increase testing, particularly in infants born to HCV-infected mothers. Vertical transmission of HCV occurs in 5.8% of infants born to women infected with HCV; transmission is higher in women also coinfected with HIV or with high HCV viral loads. Risk of transmission is very low if mother does not have detectable HCV RNA at time of delivery. Risk may also increase with prolonged rupture of membranes or internal fetal monitoring. Breastfeeding does not appear to increase the risk of transmission.

One study reported that national rates of HCV detection among women of childbearing age increased by 22% during 2011–2014. HCV testing among children <2 years of age increased by 14%, and the proportion of infants born to HCV-infected mothers increased by 68%, from 0.19% to 0.32%.[134] There is a need for improved testing for HCV in at-risk pregnant women, testing guidelines for children born to HCV-positive mothers, and standard perinatal HCV case definition to improve early identification and linkage to care to prevent HCV-related sequelae.

Diagnosis of HCV infection in infants is made by positive HCV RNA on two or more occasions. The hepatitis C antibody is not useful in diagnosis until after 18 months of age because of possibility of passive maternal antibody transfer. Testing for HCV RNA is typically recommended around 2–3 months of age and again around 6 months of age. Chronic infection is defined as persistence of HCV RNA for at least 6 months. Disappearance of HCV RNA defines resolution of infection. Most children with infection are asymptomatic with minor abnormalities such as hepatomegaly or abnormal live enzymes. In children with vertical transmission, clearance rates are variable, ranging from 10%–55% overall.[135]

There are currently no licensed treatments for infants or children with HCV infection. Combination therapy with ribavirin and interferon has been reported, but side effects can be severe, such as influenza-like symptoms, hematologic abnormalities, neuropsychiatric symptoms, thyroid or ocular abnormalities, and growth disturbances. Because children often remain asymptomatic during childhood and histologic progression is slow, treatment may be delayed until after age 3, or even adulthood. Infected children should be counseled regarding natural history of disease, treatment options, and infectivity.

In contrast to low transmission rates of HCV, the perinatal transmission rate of hepatitis B virus (HBV) is quite high. If a mother is hepatitis B e antigen (HBeAg) positive, the transmission rate is 70%–90%.[136] This rate, less than 10%, is much lower if mother is hepatitis B surface antigen (HBsAg) positive but HBeAg negative. If perinatally infected, the infant has a 90% chance of becoming a chronic carrier and subsequent 15%–25% risk of dying from cirrhosis or liver cancer in adulthood. Perinatal or early childhood transmission accounts for more than one-third of chronic infections.[137] Early identification and prophylaxis given to infants born to mothers with HBV is 85%–95% effective in reducing the acquisition of infection. All pregnant women should be screened for HBV, and those with ongoing risk should have repeat testing during labor. In 2017, the AAP recommended that healthy newborns receive the first hepatitis B vaccine dose in the first 24 hours. Infants of mothers who are positive for HBsAg as well as infants less than 2 kg whose maternal HBsAg status is unknown should receive hepatitis B immunoglobulin (HBIG) and hepatitis B vaccine within 12 hours of life. If HBsAg status is unknown, infants greater than 2 kg should receive hepatitis B vaccine within 12 hours of birth, and HBsAg should be sent from mother. If the mom is found to be positive, HBIG should be given as soon as possible. Exposed infants should complete the recommended hepatitis B vaccine series by 6 months of age. Infants who are less than 2000 gm should receive the recommended birth dose as above, but this initial dose does not count as part of the three-part vaccine series. The next dose should be given at 1 month of age and proceed with the vaccine series. The infant will therefore receive a total of four doses of hepatitis B vaccine. After completion of the vaccine series, infants born to mothers with HbeAg positivity should be tested for hepatitis B surface antibody (anti-HBs) and HBsAg between 9–18 months of age. Infants with anti-HBs levels <10 should be revaccinated with the three-part vaccine series. Pregnant women who are identified to be positive for HBsAg should be referred to an appropriate subspecialist for evaluation and management of chronic HBV infection. Recent literature supports use of lamivudine to decrease the risk of in utero transmission in the last months of pregnancy. Tenofovir and telbivudine have also been shown to be safe for use in pregnancy, but lamivudine has been used the longest with the most safety data. There is currently not enough evidence to support the need for cesarean delivery to prevent perinatal transmission of HCV to infants, nor is breastfeeding contraindicated in infants that received the recommended regimen of HBIG and hepatitis B vaccine.[137]

Zika Virus

Zika virus is a flavivirus in the family Flaviviridae. It is transmitted in a human–mosquito–human transmission cycle. It was isolated on several occasions from the *Aedes africanus* mosquito after its discovery in 1947. Initially, there was no concern for human disease. However, seroprevalence studies indicate that it was present in a broad geographic distribution in much of Africa and Southeast Asia, suggesting that human infection was common. Reports of outbreaks in Micronesia and French Polynesia were noted. It was first identified in the Americas in March 2015, when an outbreak of an exanthematous illness occurred in Bahia, Brazil. By December 2015, an estimated 1.3 million cases had been identified. As of March 2016, the virus had spread to at least 33 countries and territories in the Americas.[138]

In the fall of 2015, Brazilian investigators noted an increase in infants born with microcephaly in the areas that Zika virus was first reported. Substantial evidence indicates that Zika virus can be transmitted from mother to fetus during pregnancy. Zika virus RNA has been identified in the amniotic fluid of mothers whose fetuses had cerebral abnormalities detected by ultrasound, and viral antigen and RNA have both been identified in brain tissue and placenta of infants born with microcephaly, and also tissues from miscarriages.

Transmission through breast milk has not been documented to date. It can be transmitted sexually, and also through blood or tissue donation.

The incubation period for Zika virus is unknown, but it is believed to be less than a week. Common symptoms in a cohort of pregnant women include maculopapular rash, fever, arthritis or arthralgia, nonpurulent conjunctivitis, myalgia, headache, retroorbital pain, edema, and vomiting. The full spectrum of fetal outcomes resulting from fetal Zika virus infections is yet to be determined. There is strong evidence linking microcephaly to maternal Zika virus infection. The greatest risk seems to be during the first trimester, but some cases occurred as late as 18 weeks of gestation. Early fetal loss and ocular abnormalities (microphthalmia, cataracts, optic nerve hypoplasia) have also been noted among infants. Other brain anomalies include absent corpus callosum, hydrocephaly, cerebral calcifications, ventricular dilation, brain atrophy, and abnormal gyration. Neurologic sequelae include hypertonia, hypotonia, irritability, tremors, hearing loss, and swallowing dysfunction.[139]Diagnosis is made by detection of viral nucleic acid by RT-PCR and the detection of IgM antibodies. Diagnosis by reverse transcription (RT)-PCR is possible within 1 week of symptoms. In contrast, viral RNA has been detected in serum of pregnant women whose fetus had evidence of congenital infection for approximately 10 weeks after infection. IgM typically appears within the first week of symptoms and will persist for several months. Recommended laboratory testing for possible congenital Zika virus includes testing for Zika virus RNA in serum and urine, as well as Zika IgM antibodies in serum. If CSF is obtained, RT-PCR and IgM testing should be performed. Presently, specimens go to a reference laboratory.

Treatment is typically considered supportive for symptoms, as there is no specific antiviral treatment currently available. Prevention and control measures center on avoiding mosquito bites, reducing sexual transmission, and controlling the mosquito vector. Pregnant women are encouraged to avoid areas with ongoing Zika virus transmission and unprotected sexual contact with partners at risk for Zika virus infection, and to use methods to avoid mosquito bites such as insect repellent, permethrin treatment of clothes, bed nets, window screens, and air conditioning.[138] Couples who have possible Zika exposure and are considering pregnancy should postpone pregnancy for 6 months following potential exposure or diagnosis of Zika. Pregnant women who report illness consistent with Zika virus within 2 weeks of returning from area with Zika transmission should be tested for Zika virus.

Clinical management of infants born with clinical findings consistent with congenital Zika infection includes Zika laboratory testing as listed above, ultrasound of the head, comprehensive ophthalmology evaluation, and hearing screen by age 1 month. Referral to a developmental specialist, early intervention services, neurology, genetics, and infectious diseases may also be warranted. Infants born without clinical findings consistent with congenital Zika infection, but born to mothers with laboratory evidence of possible infection during pregnancy, should still undergo the same evaluation recommended for infants with clinical findings, and should be monitored for symptoms that may develop over time, such as hearing problems, developmental delays, and impaired visual function.[139]

CASE 13.1

An infant is born vaginally at 39 weeks to a mother with known gonococcal and chlamydial cervicitis. The mother's human immunodeficiency virus (HIV) status, hepatitis B status, and Venereal Disease Research Laboratory (VDRL) status are unknown. The baby receives 0.5% erythromycin ocular ointment and intramuscular vitamin K.

Which of the following is (are) true?

1. The infant has a 30% chance of developing ophthalmia neonatorum from *N. gonorrhoeae* and a 25% chance of developing it from *C. trachomatis.*
2. The infant should receive a 25 to 50 mg/kg dose of intramuscular ceftriaxone.
3. The infant should receive oral erythromycin therapy for 2 weeks.
4. The infant should be given hepatitis B vaccine and hepatitis B immunoglobulin (HBIG) within 12 hours of birth.

The correct answer is 2.

Standard ocular prophylaxis with 0.5% erythromycin, 1% tetracycline, or 1% silver nitrate is more than 95% effective in preventing gonococcal ophthalmia neonatorum. In the absence of prophylaxis, the neonate would have approximately a 30% likelihood of developing gonococcal disease. This prophylaxis, however, is ineffective in preventing chlamydial disease. Approximately 50% of infants born to mothers with *Chlamydia* infection will have nasopharyngeal infection; half of these infected children will go on to develop ophthalmia neonatorum. Infants born to a mother known to be infected with *N. gonorrhoeae* should receive standard ocular prophylaxis as well as a single dose of intramuscular ceftriaxone at 25 to 50 mg/kg to a maximum dose of 125 mg. This therapy effectively prevents gonococcal ophthalmia neonatorum and disseminated gonococcal disease. *Chlamydia* does not cause disseminated infection. Although 10% of infants born to mothers with chlamydial infection will develop pneumonia, *Chlamydia* does not disseminate or cause acute, vision-threatening ophthalmic disease. The association between neonatal erythromycin exposure and hypertrophic pyloric stenosis combined with the relatively indolent consequences of chlamydial infection preclude the prescription of erythromycin as a prophylactic. In cases of documented neonatal chlamydial infection, the benefits of erythromycin outweigh the risks.

Although hepatitis B is readily transmitted vertically, the vaccine is fairly effective in preventing disease. Infants greater than 2 kg should receive the vaccine within 12 hours of birth while the mother is tested for hepatitis B surface antigen (HBsAg). If she is found to be positive for the antigen, the infant then should receive HBIG. In addition, the mother should be tested for syphilis and HIV infection. Only infants of mothers that are positive for HBsAg or infants less than two kilograms whose maternal HBsAg status is unknown should receive HBIG and Hepatitis B vaccine within 12 hours of life.

CASE 13.2

A 3-week-old male infant is brought to the emergency department with vesicular lesions on his thigh and abdomen. The vesicles appear to contain cloudy fluid and are surrounded by an erythematous base. The infant is afebrile and otherwise well appearing.

Which of the following is (are) true?

1. The vesicles should be unroofed to obtain specimens for viral and bacterial culture.
2. The absence of a maternal history of genital herpes simplex virus (HSV) infection makes this cause unlikely.
3. Mothers with active, recurrent genital herpes pose the highest risk of vertical transmission.
4. Exudate from the lesions is inadequate to test for HSV.

The correct answers are 1 and 4.

The differential diagnosis for vesicular lesions includes bacterial impetigo and HSV or varicella–zoster virus infection. If these lesions are prominent in the diaper area, *C. albicans* is also a possibility. Some 60% to 80% of infants with neonatal HSV infection are born to mothers without a clinical history of HSV disease. Although mothers with active, recurrent HSV infection give birth to the majority of infected infants, the risk of transmission to the infant is greatest in a mother with a first-episode primary infection. The latter situation implies a mother without any protective antibodies to HSV. Both culture and antigen testing for HSV rely on the recovery of cells. The base of the vesicle should be scraped for diagnosis.

Gram staining of a sample from a lesion gives a negative result. A direct fluorescent antibody test is positive for HSV-2.

Which of the following is (are) true?

1. The infant should undergo lumbar puncture.
2. The infant should be admitted to the hospital for at least 2 weeks of intravenous acyclovir therapy.
3. This patient will likely show an elevation of transaminase levels.
4. If a lumbar puncture is performed and the results are negative, the infant can be managed with oral therapy.

The correct answers are 1 and 2.

Neonatal HSV infection is classically divided into three clinical presentations. The most severe and earliest to present is disseminated disease. This usually manifests in the first week of life with systemic illness and multiorgan involvement, and carries a high mortality. The majority of these patients have significant hepatitis. The next most serious presentation is that of meningoencephalitis. This presentation typically occurs around 3 weeks of age and has clinical manifestations that can be as subtle as fever without a focus or as obvious as severe alterations in mental status and seizures. The gold standard for making this diagnosis has become polymerase chain reaction (PCR) testing of the cerebrospinal fluid (CSF). HSV infection is clearly in the differential diagnosis of any neonate with an "aseptic" meningitis. The patient in this case description has the most indolent type of neonatal HSV–skin, eye, and mouth (SEM) disease. The patient should undergo a lumbar puncture because a positive PCR result on the CSF would have prognostic implications and would extend the duration of therapy. Even if they have a well appearance, if they are not treated systemically, infants with this presentation develop disseminated disease 70% of the time. Acyclovir should be administered intravenously for 2 weeks because of its exceedingly poor oral bioavailability. The dosing and efficacy of newer, more bioavailable antiviral agents for treatment of these infants have not been adequately studied.

CASE 13.3

The mother of a 42-day-old, 32-weeks' gestation preterm infant asks you about the appropriate timing of immunizations and the need for prophylaxis for respiratory syncytial virus (RSV) infection. The infant currently weighs 2700 g and, after going home, will continue to receive supplemental oxygen via nasal cannula for chronic lung disease.

Which of the following is (are) true?

1. The infant should receive the same immunizations as any 6-week-old infant.
2. The infant should receive a single 0.25-mL dose of influenza vaccine in January and a second 0.25-mL dose a month later.
3. Whether treatment with monoclonal RSV antibody (palivizumab) is needed in infants such as this 32-week gestation premature infant is controversial.
4. The immunizations should be given when the infant reaches a corrected age of 6 weeks.

The correct answer is 1.

Inactivated polio, conjugate pneumococcal, *Haemophilus influenza* B, and DTaP (diphtheria, tetanus, and acellular pertussis) vaccines are all safe and immunogenic in this population. The infant should be immunized as any other infant. If the infant has not already received the first dose of hepatitis B vaccine, it would be appropriately given at this point. If an infant weighing less than 2000 g received the first dose of hepatitis B at birth because of maternal risk factors, that dose would not be counted toward the three doses necessary to complete the series. The first counted dose can be given anytime after 4 weeks of age.

Inactivated influenza vaccine should not be administered before 6 months of life. The first time it is to be administered to a child younger than 3 years, the doses would be split up, as described in the case description.

Although controversy exists about the need for palivizumab in a healthy infant born after 32 weeks' gestation, consensus exists that infants younger than 2 years of age with chronic lung disease of prematurity who require therapy within 6 months of the start of RSV season should receive antibody prophylaxis for at least the first season.

14

The Heart

Christina M. Phelps, Philip T. Thrush, Clifford L. Cua

Congenital heart disease remains the most common cause of infant death because of a congenital malformation in the United States.[1] Infant mortality rates arising from congenital malformations has declined in the decade from 2005 to 2014.[2] Critical congenital heart disease (CCHD) occurs in 25% of newborns with congenital heart disease and is defined as disease requiring surgery or procedural intervention in the first year of life. In 2011, CCHD was added to the recommended screening panel for newborns by the U.S. Department of Health and Human Services (HHS). Between 2007 and 2013, the death rate of infants with congenital heart disease in mandatory screening states fell from 8 to 6.4 per 100,000 births.[3] During this time period, death from CCHD decreased by 33% in states with mandatory screening compared with states without screening and historical rates in screening states.[3] Not all congenital or neonatal acquired heart disease will be found with the current screening methods. Thus care for newborns demands an awareness of the prevalence of cardiac defects and the ability to differentiate infants with cardiac disease from other critically ill newborns. In 2000, the prevalence of congenital heart disease found by a population study in Quebec was 11.89 per 1000 among children and 5.78 per 1000 in the general population. By contrast, the prevalence of severe congenital heart disease was 1.45 per 1000 children and accounted for 12% of all congenital cardiac lesions in children.[4] The most recent reported birth prevalence in North America was 6.9 per 1,000 live births compared with 8.2 in Europe and 9.3 in Asia.[5] Advances in fetal and neonatal ultrasonographic screening allow identification of an increasing number of children with congenital heart disease and, more importantly, appropriate counseling for their parents. Sixty to seventy percent of newborns admitted to large pediatric cardiac intensive care units have an established diagnosis at the time of birth.[6] Increased rates of prenatal diagnosis have not consistently translated to improved outcomes over the past decade.[7–9] Although some studies indicate an important benefit of fetal diagnosis in terms of morbidity and mortality, the unintended result is that in some centers, postnatal acute presentations of congenital heart disease are becoming more rare, and this may be detrimental by assuaging fears of congenital heart disease in symptomatic newborns and thus causing delay in care and potentially increased morbidity and mortality. Additionally, fetal diagnosis of heart disease increases maternal anxiety and unhappiness during pregnancy, creating psychologic dysfunction and distress that can persist in both parents for months after birth.[10–13] Historically, up to 25% of children with congenital heart disease were not diagnosed until after discharge from the newborn nursery, and misdiagnosis was found to occur in up to 7 per 100,000 live births in the United States.[14–16]

Careful evaluation of the history, physical examination findings, laboratory data (including the response of upper and lower body blood gas concentrations and arterial oxygen saturation in an enriched oxygen environment), radiographic findings, and results of electrocardiography, echocardiography, and occasionally additional imaging such as cardiac computerized axial tomography (CAT), magnetic resonance imaging (MRI), or invasive cardiac catheterization allow the physician to delineate the specific congenital cardiac defect. When a neonate suspected of having congenital heart disease is being examined, it is important to frame physical and laboratory findings within the context of the transition from fetal to neonatal circulation. This chapter considers the physiology and pathophysiology of the fetal and neonatal cardiovascular systems in newborns with and without heart disease.

PHYSIOLOGY AND PATHOPHYSIOLOGY

Fetal and Neonatal Circulations

Newborns undergo dramatic changes in the pulmonary and systemic circulations following birth. In the fetus, oxygen-rich blood from the placenta reaches the right atrium via the umbilical vein and shunts preferentially across the foramen ovale to the left ventricle, providing increased oxygen content to the myocardium and brain (Fig. 14.1). A smaller portion of the highly oxygenated blood passes from the right atrium to the right ventricle and bypasses the lungs via the ductus arteriosus to flow to the lower body. Because of this parallel circulation, individual organs may receive blood from both ventricles, and thus the output of the fetal heart is expressed as combined ventricular output (CVO). Advances in fetal ultrasonographic techniques have enabled a more accurate determination of human fetal blood flow than was previously available using fetal lamb studies. In the normal human fetus, CVO has been documented by echocardiographic studies to be 450 mL/kg/min.[17]

Approximately 45% (200 mL/kg/min) of this blood perfuses the placenta for oxygen uptake and returns via

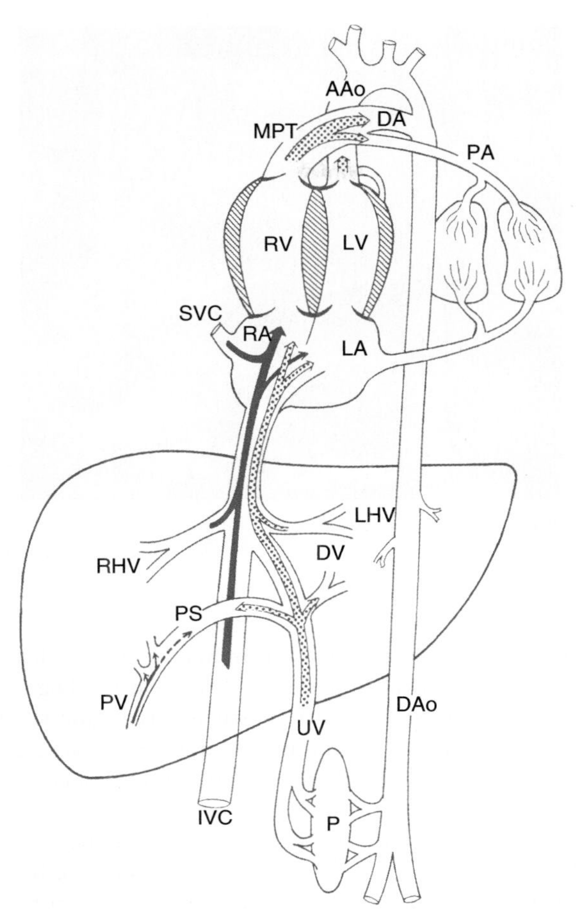

Fig. 14.1 Diagrammatic representation of normal fetal circulation. *AAo,* Ascending aorta; *DA,* ductus arteriosus; *DAo,* descending aorta; *DV,* ductus venosus; *IVC,* inferior vena cava; *LA,* left atrium; *LHV,* left hepatic vein; *LV,* left ventricle; *MPT,* main pulmonary trunk; *P,* placenta; *PA,* pulmonary artery; *PS,* portal system; *PV,* portal vein; *RA,* right atrium; *RHV,* right hepatic vein; *RV,* right ventricle; *SVC,* superior vena cava; *UV,* umbilical vein.

the umbilical veins. Approximately one-half of umbilical venous return enters the inferior vena cava directly through the ductus venosus, thereby bypassing the hepatic microcirculation; the remainder passes primarily through the left lobe of the liver and enters the inferior vena cava via the left hepatic vein. Venous return from the lower body, ductus venosus, and hepatic veins pass into the thoracic inferior vena cava, where there is incomplete mixing. Preferential streaming occurs into various cardiac chambers, with blood from the ductus venosus and left hepatic veins passing preferentially across the foramen ovale into the left atrium. In the normal fetal circulation, oxygenated blood crossing the foramen ovale comprises 76% of the left ventricular output and 33% of combined cardiac output, supplying the cerebral and myocardial circulations.[18] Thus the streaming of blood from the inferior vena cava to the left heart increases the efficiency of oxygen delivery to the most actively metabolizing area of the fetus, the brain. Venous drainage from the right hepatic veins and the abdominal inferior vena cava tends to stream preferentially to the right atrium and right ventricle. Similarly, desaturated superior vena caval return from the cerebral circulation is preferentially directed to the right ventricle through the tricuspid valve. The right ventricle ejects much of this relatively undersaturated blood via the ductus arteriosus back to the placenta. The remainder of the right ventricular output passes into the pulmonary vascular bed. The proportion of CVO to the lungs increases throughout gestation by 60% from 20 to 38 weeks, with pulmonary blood flow accounting for 11% of the CVO.[18,19] Thus although the circulations are not completely separated, each ventricle primarily performs its postnatal function—the left ventricle delivers blood for oxygen utilization, the right for oxygen uptake.

The left and right ventricles do not eject similar volumes in the fetus. The right ventricle has been shown to be dominant in fetal lamb studies, ejecting almost twice the blood volume ejected by the left ventricle. In human fetuses, the stroke volume of the right ventricle is approximately 28% greater than that of the left ventricle.[17] Left ventricular output is distributed mainly in the upper body, including the brain (~20% of CVO) and the myocardium (3%); the remainder (~10%) crosses the aortic isthmus to the lower body.

In the fetus, the ductus arteriosus is part of a specialized system of oxygen-sensitive organs and tissues in the body. Blood flow across the ductus arteriosus is 78% of the right ventricular cardiac output and 46% of the CVO.[18] In comparison with the aorta and the pulmonary arteries, it is thicker walled, with a medial layer composed of longitudinal and spiral layers of smooth muscle fibers within concentric layers of elastic tissue and an intimal layer of smooth muscle and endothelial cells.[20–22] Continued patency of the ductus arteriosus throughout gestation is controlled by the relatively low fetal oxygen tension and the inhibition of procontractile mechanisms by vasodilators.[23,24] The vasodilators primarily responsible for ductal patency include prostaglandin and prostacyclin, which interact directly with ductal prostanoid receptors, and to a lesser extent carbon monoxide and nitric oxide.[24–26]

Fetal Echocardiography

Fetal echocardiography has significant clinical implications postnatally.[27] As described later in the chapter (see section on echocardiography of the newborn), all echocardiographic techniques can be performed with a fetal echocardiogram. A fetal study is usually performed between 18 to 22 weeks' gestation for optimal imaging. Studies earlier in gestation can be performed, but a repeat study may be needed to clarify images. Indications for a fetal study can be as a result of either maternal or fetal indications (Table 14.1).[28]

Aside from cardiac anatomic diagnosis, analysis of fetal blood flow patterns in the ductus venosus, umbilical artery, and umbilical vein can provide information on the overall cardiovascular well-being of the fetus.[29] Fetal echocardiography may also have prognostic implications in patients with congenital diaphragmatic hernia (CDH) and twin-twin transfusion syndrome.[30–33] From a cardiac standpoint, fetal echocardiography can accurately diagnose most forms of

TABLE 14.1 Indications for Fetal Echocardiogram

Maternal Indications	Fetal Indications
• Family history of congenital heart disease • Metabolic disorders • Exposure to teratogens • Exposure to prostaglandin synthase inhibitors • Rubella infection • Autoimmune disease (systemic lupus erythematosus [SLE], Sjögren syndrome, etc.) • Familial inherited disorders (Marfan, Noonan syndrome, etc.) • In vitro fertilization	• Abnormal obstetrical ultrasound screen • Extracardiac abnormality • Chromosomal abnormality • Arrhythmia • Hydrops • Increased first-trimester nuchal translucency • Multiple gestation and suspicion of twin-twin transfusion syndrome

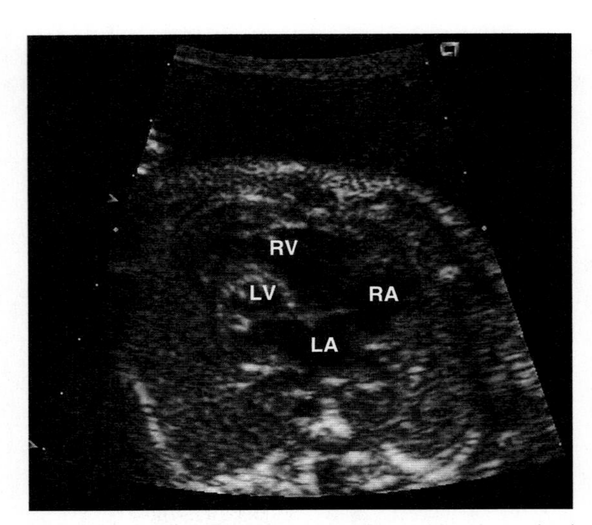

Fig. 14.2 Fetal echocardiogram of an infant with a hypoplastic left heart. *LA*, Left atrium; *LV*, left ventricle; *RA*, right atrium; *RV*, right ventricle.

congenital heart defects and their evolution in utero (Fig. 14.2).[34] This may improve the postnatal morbidity and mortality, especially in ductal dependent cardiac defects.[27,35,36] Level of parental psychological stress, however, appears to be related to the severity of the cardiac defect and not to a prenatal versus postnatal diagnosis.[12] Another recent use of fetal echocardiography is in conjunction with interventional techniques.[37,38] Interventions have been reported in fetuses with hypoplastic left heart syndrome and restrictive atrial septum,[39] severe aortic stenosis,[40,41] and pulmonary stenosis/atresia.[42] Fetal echocardiography is essential for assisting in these procedures.

Fetal Heart Failure

The parallel nature of the fetal circulation makes it uniquely equipped to tolerate most structural abnormalities of the heart that are life-threatening after birth. Even in cases of significant obstruction and falling unilateral ventricular output, the unaffected side of the heart is able to increase its output, and fetal blood flow is redistributed so that the unaffected ventricle can produce most, if not all, of the cardiac output.[43] As a result, cardiac shunts, pulmonary overcirculation, and anatomic causes of systemic hypoperfusion generally do not become noteworthy until the infant is born. There are a limited number of cardiovascular causes of fetal distress that may result in the development of hydrops, including arrhythmias, myocardial disease, severe atrioventricular (AV) or semilunar valve insufficiency, and premature constriction of the ductus arteriosus with a restrictive atrial septum. All of these conditions share a final common pathway of elevated ventricular end-diastolic pressure, increased atrial and central venous pressure, and movement of fluid from the capillary bed into fetal tissue.[43]

Sustained tachyarrhythmias (over 200 beats per minute) for more than 12 hours continuously or bradycardia associated with congenital heart disease are not well tolerated. Tachyarrhythmias may be controlled by administering antiarrhythmic medications to the mother, including digoxin, beta-blockers, sotalol, flecainide, and amiodarone. Digoxin is a first-line therapy for short ventriculoatrial supraventricular tachycardia (SVT) and atrial flutter in the absence of hydrops and is associated with an 80% to 85% success rate in the treatment of fetal SVT and a 60% to 65% success rate for atrial flutter.[44,45] Sotalol is another first-line therapy with a 72% conversion rate.[46,47] Arrhythmia control is likely to be successful if treatment is initiated before the development of hydrops. Successful treatment of supraventricular tachyarrhythmias in the presence of hydrops is more complex and typically requires the use of at least two medications and a longer therapeutic course. Incessant fetal SVT warrants an attempt at conversion with intraumbilical administration of antiarrhythmic medications. Even with successful treatment, there is an 8% to 30% reported risk of fetal or neonatal mortality.[48–50]

Fetal bradycardia may be associated with significant intrauterine mortality. The outcome for bradycardia in the fetus is determined by the cause. Sinus or low atrial bradycardia is seldom symptomatic and does not require treatment. Persistent and asymptomatic bradycardia is most commonly associated with long corrected QT interval (QTc).[51,52] No treatment is necessary for the fetus unless there is associated ventricular tachycardia or torsades.[51] Another etiology of fetal bradycardia, AV block, is estimated to occur in 1 in 22,000 live births.[53] AV block is caused by maternal autoantibodies in approximately 45% to 48% of cases and can present as early as 18 weeks' gestation.[54,55] There have been reports of successful treatment of early low-grade heart block, with improvement in outcomes by administration of fluorinated steroids to the mother, but there have been no randomized studies with adequate follow-up.[55–57] Beta-sympathomimetic agents, intravenous immunoglobulins, and direct fetal pacing are also being used as therapies for autoimmune-mediated fetal AV heart block. Another 45% to 55% of fetal AV block is associated with structural heart disease (most commonly left atrial isomerism and congenitally corrected transposition of the great arteries [TGA]).[58] Unfortunately, even with aggressive intervention, survival of infants with AV block associated with structural heart disease is particularly dismal, with a 75% to 90% incidence of fetal or neonatal demise.[54]

Structural heart disease is the most common cause of fetal heart failure and may lead to significant mortality without intervention. Some fetuses with severe semilunar valve stenosis are candidates for an attempt at intrauterine valvuloplasty to stabilize the patient's condition and ideally improve long-term surgical options.[40,41] Technical success is increasing, and there has been success in altering the natural history of the disease.[59] Early delivery with immediate intervention is often the best management strategy for fetuses who show symptoms associated with specific structural heart defects such as ductus arteriosus restriction, Ebstein anomaly of the tricuspid valve, or tricuspid valve dysplasia with significant tricuspid insufficiency.[54]

Circulatory Changes After Birth

By the end of the third trimester, the fetal pulmonary circulation begins to demonstrate vasoreactivity and responsiveness to maternal hyperoxygenation.[60] The onset of breathing produces a dramatic increase in pulmonary blood flow (from 11% of the CVO to a full cardiac output) and a decrease in pulmonary vascular resistance (PVR). With the onset of ventilation, air replaces intra-alveolar fluid, and local oxygen concentration increases markedly, both of which may directly dilate the pulmonary vascular smooth muscle or cause the release of vasodilating substances. Bradykinin, a potent pulmonary vasodilator, is released when the lungs are exposed to oxygen; bradykinin, in turn, stimulates endothelial cell production of nitric oxide, a potent vasodilator. Prostacyclin (prostaglandin I_2), a pulmonary vasodilator derived from the metabolism of arachidonic acid, is released when the lung is mechanically ventilated (not necessarily oxygenated) or exposed to other vasoactive substances such as bradykinin or angiotensin II. Inhibiting prostaglandin production by administering a cyclooxygenase inhibitor (such as indomethacin) attenuates the normal ventilation-induced decline in PVR, which further supports the role of these vasoactive substances in the establishment of a normal pulmonary circulation after birth. Clamping the umbilical cord removes the low-resistance placental circulation and immediately increases the infant's systemic vascular resistance (SVR).[61] The increase in pulmonary blood flow greatly alters the venous return to the left atrium and consequently the left ventricular preload. Left ventricular cardiac output increases from an estimated 179 mL/min/kg to approximately 240 mL/min/kg within the first 2 hours after birth because of increased stroke volume.[62] As the ductus arteriosus closes and the left-to-right shunt diminishes, left ventricular output falls to approximately 190 mL/min/kg.[62]

The initial dramatic decrease in PVR is secondary to relaxation of the resistance vessels. There is then a slow, progressive decline over the next 2 to 6 weeks of life as these pulmonary arterioles remodel from their fetal pattern, in which a large amount of smooth muscle is present in the medial layer, to the adult pattern, with very little muscle in the media. The development of the "physiologic anemia" that normally occurs during this time decreases the viscosity of the blood perfusing the lungs, which decreases shear stress and also contributes to the overall decrease in PVR.

Closure of the foramen ovale. Functional closure of the foramen ovale occurs after the placenta is removed from the circulation. With clamping of the umbilical cord, blood flow through the inferior vena cava to both atria decreases dramatically. Initiation of breathing increases blood flow through the pulmonary bed to the left atrium. These changes result in a left atrial pressure that now exceeds the right atrial pressure, which causes the valve-like flap of the foramen ovale to close. Although functional closure of the foramen ovale occurs in most infants, anatomic closure is not always complete. As a result, any action that raises right atrial pressure to the point that it equals or exceeds left atrial pressure can result in a right-to-left shunt across the foramen ovale. Likewise, in conditions that have large left-to-right shunts, such as a large patent ductus arteriosus (PDA) or ventricular septal defect (VSD), the left atrium may become dilated, which results in stretching of the atrial septum and incompetence of the foramen ovale and a left-to-right shunt. In many adults, despite the events leading to functional foramen closure, a probe-patent foramen may persist.

Closure of the ductus arteriosus. Closure of the ductus arteriosus is a more complex phenomenon. The media of the ductus arteriosus contains smooth muscle in a spiral configuration that is maintained in a relaxed state, primarily by the action of prostaglandins. Constriction and closure after birth reflect removal of the stimuli that maintain relaxation and the addition of factors that produce active constriction. Circulating prostaglandin E_2 (PGE_2) concentrations in the fetus are high because of the very low pulmonary blood flow. With clamping of the placenta, the source of PGE_2 is removed. With inspiration, there is a dramatic increase in pulmonary blood flow and an abrupt increase in oxygen tension that inhibits ductal smooth muscle voltage-dependent potassium channels and results in an influx of calcium and ductal constriction.[24] In addition, the remaining PGE_2 is almost completely metabolized as it passes through the pulmonary circulation, which results in a rapid decrease in serum levels of PGE_2 and allows active constriction of the ductus arteriosus to be unopposed. The ductus arteriosus constricts rapidly; in mature infants, functional closure generally occurs within 10 to 15 hours after birth. Permanent closure by intimal cushion formation, intimal proliferation, fibrosis, and thrombosis may take several weeks.

Myocardial Performance and Cardiac Output

Fetal myocardium differs from neonatal and adult myocardium in several important ways. The primary fuel for fetal myocardium is almost exclusively glucose in contrast to the adult heart, which can use fatty acids as a significant energy source. In addition, especially early in gestation, the fetal heart grows by hyperplasia of the myocardial cells in contrast with the newborn heart, in which the myocardium grows by hypertrophy. Fetal myocardium also functions distinctly by developing less active tension for a given stretch than does adult myocardium and therefore has less ability to contract. Thus ventricular output can be increased only modestly by volume loading and only at relatively low atrial pressures; unlike in the adult, output increases only slightly at levels more than 2 to 4 mm Hg above baseline. Inotropic stimulation of the fetal myocardium also increases cardiac output relatively little. This inability to respond to changes in preload and in the inotropic state is related in part to immaturity of muscle structure. Early in gestation, there are relatively fewer contractile elements, an immature sarcoplasmic reticulum with lower affinity for calcium binding, and a somewhat chaotic overall arrangement of fibers with considerable interstitial tissue. Infants born preterm have been shown to have persistent abnormalities of their myocardium.[63] Toward term, more contractile elements are present, and these are more mature and are arranged in a more orderly fashion. Another factor limiting fetal myocardial performance is incomplete sympathetic innervation, which limits response to inotropic stimulation. The fetus is best able to increase ventricular output by increasing its heart rate. There is a linear relationship between ventricular output and heart rate up to about 250 beats per minute; thereafter, ventricular output reaches a plateau and even starts to decline. As heart rate goes below the normal range, ventricular output decreases dramatically because of the limited ability to increase stroke volume. As a result, the fetal myocardium is operating under a high-volume load and responds poorly to any increase in ventricular afterload. Although adrenergic support can be supplied either by circulating catecholamines or through neural pathways, the overall quantitative response may be less than in the adult. The control of cardiac rate and the distribution of cardiac output are the major mechanisms for maintenance of circulatory function.

As discussed previously, the left ventricular cardiac output increases dramatically within the first 2 hours after birth and remains elevated for several weeks before decreasing to approximately 190 mL/min/kg.[62] Because of the high resting values in the period immediately after birth, ventricular output can be increased only modestly by volume loading or inotropic stimulation with dopamine and dobutamine. The neonatal myocardium remains sensitive to the administration of the calcium ion and responds positively to the lusitropic effects of milrinone. After the initial newborn period, resting values decrease progressively, and ventricular output can be increased much more effectively.

Normal Physiologic Data in the Newborn

The normal physiologic values in the heart and great vessels are shown in Fig. 14.3. Pulmonary arterial pressures (PAPs) in the newborn are variable but generally decrease to half of systemic pressure within 8 to 12 hours and to one-third of systemic pressure within a day or so. Over the next 4 weeks, there is a further slow, progressive decline to adult levels.

The oxygen saturation on the right side of the heart is approximately 60% to 70%; that on the left side of the heart is

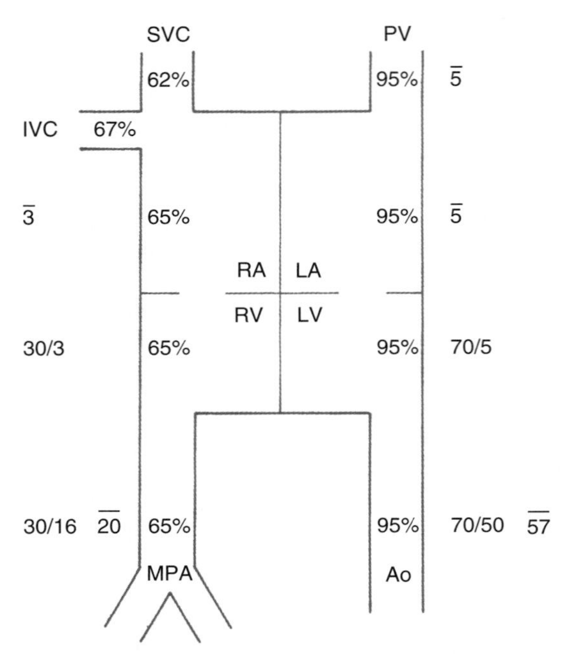

Fig. 14.3 Representative blood oxygen saturation (%) and pressure (mm Hg) in various cardiac chambers and vessels in the normal newborn infant. *Ao*, Aorta; *IVC*, inferior vena cava; *LA*, left atrium; *LV*, left ventricle; *MPA*, main pulmonary artery; *PV*, pulmonary vein; *RA*, right atrium; *RV*, right ventricle; *SVC*, superior vena cava.

92% to 95%. The oxygen saturations may be used to determine the direction of shunting within the heart or great vessels. For example, an increased saturation in the right atrium suggests a left-to-right shunt at the atrial level; a decreased saturation in the left atrium in a neonate with otherwise healthy lungs indicates a right-to-left shunt at the atrial level.

Physical Factors that Control Blood Flow

Flow (*Q*) through a vascular bed is governed by the resistance to flow (*R*) and the pressure decrease across the bed (ΔP) (Ohm's law).

$$Q = \frac{\Delta P}{R}$$

Furthermore, by application of Poiseuille's law, resistance to flow is directly related to the viscosity of the blood and inversely related to the cross-sectional area of the bed (radius).

An appreciation of the general relationship of pressure, resistance, and flow is important in understanding the pathophysiology and natural history of various congenital heart defects.

Blood flows where resistance is least.

Vascular resistance is calculated from the formula

$$Q = \frac{\Delta P}{R}$$

For the systemic circulation, the ΔP (pressure decrease) is systemic arterial pressure (SAP) minus systemic venous pressure (SVP); for the pulmonary circulation, the ΔP is PAP minus pulmonary venous pressure (PVP).

$$PVR = \frac{PAP - PVP}{\text{Pulmonary flow}}$$

$$SVR = \frac{SAP - SVP}{\text{Systemic flow}}$$

If the pressure decrease is measured in millimeters of mercury and the flow is measured in liters per minute per square meter, then the calculated vascular resistance is considered in *resistance units.* One resistance (or Wood) unit is equal to 80 dyne • sec/cm^5. The maximum normal PVR is 2.5 to 3 units, and the maximum normal SVR is 15 to 20 units.

Peripheral vascular resistance is not the only type of resistance that will affect flow. For example, a narrowed valve provides more resistance to blood flow than does a wide-open valve; a small VSD provides more resistance to blood flow than does a large VSD; and a thick, noncompliant ventricular chamber provides more resistance to blood flow than does a thinner, more compliant ventricular chamber.

If two similar cardiac chambers or arteries (one left-sided or systemic and the other right-sided or pulmonary) communicate with each other and the opening between them is so large that there is little or no resistance to blood flow, the defect is considered nonrestrictive. The pressures on each side of the opening are fully transmitted and approximately equal. If the opening is small (restrictive), there is resistance to blood flow, and the pressures are not fully transmitted. In the presence of a nonrestrictive defect, the resistances to outflow (downstream resistance) from each of the two communicating chambers determine the direction of blood flow. For example, with a large VSD in which ventricular pressures are equal, PVR is usually lower than SVR, and pulmonary blood flow is greater than systemic blood flow; that is, a left-to-right shunt is present (Fig. 14.4A). Because the flows and shunting pattern depend on the relationship of the downstream pulmonary and SVRs, these are called *dependent shunts.* When the two resistances are equal, no shunt occurs (Fig. 14.4B). When resistance to outflow of the right ventricle exceeds that of the left ventricle (Fig.14.4C)—as might occur with the development of pulmonary vascular disease or, more commonly, when there is an associated pulmonic stenosis (tetralogy of Fallot)—right-to-left shunting is present. When there is a communication between the two sides of the heart at different anatomic levels (e.g., arteriovenous malformation, left ventricular–right atrial communication), the pressure difference between the two chambers or vessels, rather than downstream resistance, dictates the magnitude of the shunt; these are called *obligatory shunts.* For example, in a left ventricular–right atrial shunt, blood shunts continuously through the defect because the left ventricular pressure is always higher than right atrial pressure, regardless of the distal pulmonary and SVRs.

It is customary to relate the cardiac outputs and pressures in each side of the heart. Thus if there is three times as much flow into the pulmonary artery as into the aorta, there is a 3 to 1 pulmonary-to-systemic flow ratio. If the pressure in the pulmonary artery is 60 mm Hg and that in the aorta is 90 mm Hg, pulmonary hypertension is at two-thirds of the systemic level.

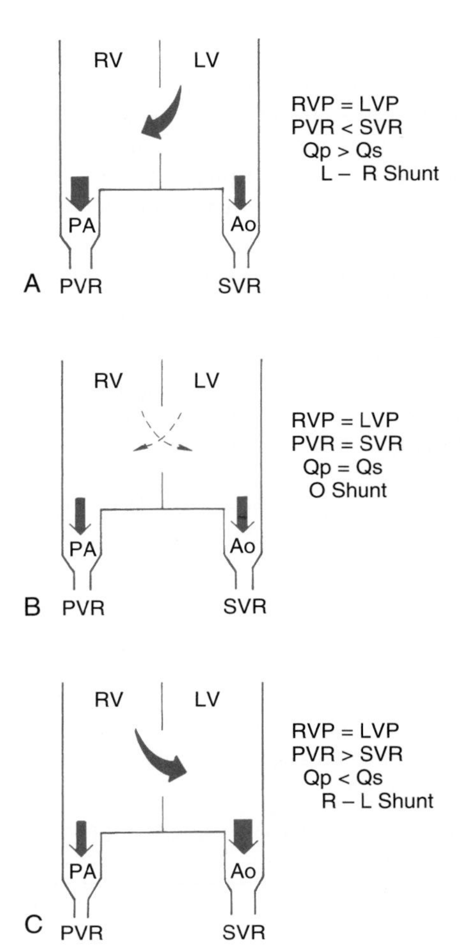

Fig. 14.4 Diagrammatic representation of intracardiac shunting patterns as related to outflow resistances of the two sides of the heart. See text for description of (A), (B), (C). *Ao,* Aorta; *L,* left; *LV,* left ventricle; *LVP,* left ventricular pressure; *PA,* pulmonary artery; *PVR,* pulmonary vascular resistance; *Qp,* pulmonary blood flow; *Qs,* systemic blood flow; *R,* right; *RV,* right ventricle; *RVP,* right ventricular pressure; *SVR,* systemic vascular resistance.

PHYSICAL EXAMINATION

It is imperative to perform a complete physical examination of all neonates and to monitor for ongoing changes suggestive of pathologic conditions. In 2010, HHS Secretary's Advisory Committee on Heritable Disorders in Newborns and Children recommended screening for congenital heart disease be added to newborn screening programs. The screening targeted ductal-dependent lesions with high mortality and morbidity without accurate diagnosis. A 2017 study demonstrated a 33% decrease in deaths from CCHD in states with mandatory screening.[3] As of December 2017, 47 states and the District of Columbia mandated pulse oximetry screening for congenital heart disease. Although pulse oximetry screening is a valuable tool in identifying infants with CCHD, the remainder of the physical examination should not be neglected, and the infant in extremis should be considered with a wide differential. An infant with known heart disease remains susceptible to other disease processes, including bacterial sepsis, anemia, and pulmonary disease. Acutely ill infants may have several simultaneous working diagnoses while caregivers are stabilizing their physiologic condition. In these instances, some additional factors may suggest cardiac abnormalities. Dysmorphic or syndromic features in any neonate should prompt the clinician to pay particular attention to the cardiovascular system as the infant transitions to postnatal life.

> **EDITORIAL COMMENT:** From an analysis of 21 studies including half a million screened babies, Plana concluded that of 10,000 apparently healthy late preterm or full-term newborn infants, 6 will have critical congenital heart defects. Screening by pulse oximetry will detect 5 of these infants as having CCHD and will miss one case. In addition, screening by pulse oximetry will falsely identify another 14 infants out of the 10,000 as having suspected CCHD when they do not have it. Fewer false positives were noted when pulse oximetry was performed longer than 24 hours after birth. They concluded that pulse oximetry screening is highly specific and a moderately sensitive test for detection of CCHD with very low false-positive rates. Current evidence supports the introduction of routine screening for CCHD in asymptomatic newborns before discharge from the well-baby nursery. Many of the so-called false positives have respiratory problems or sepsis, so the test is extremely valuable.
> (Plana MN, Zamora J, Suresh G, Fernandez-Pineda L, Thangaratinam S, Ewer AK. Pulse oximetry screening for critical congenital heart defects. *Cochrane Database Syst Rev.* 2018;3:CD011912.)

Cyanosis

Central cyanosis indicates a reduced arterial blood oxygen saturation and is generally visible when reduced hemoglobin in the blood exceeds 5 g/dL (saturation ≤85% in patients with a normal hemoglobin level). If the lungs are functioning normally, the level of systemic arterial blood oxygen saturation depends entirely on the effective pulmonary blood flow—that is, the amount of blood oxygenated by the lungs that subsequently passes into the systemic arterial circulation. Neonates frequently experience acrocyanosis that is unrelated to heart disease. The best method of assessing for central cyanosis in an infant is to look at the tongue. Other diagnostic procedures are needed to determine the cause of the cyanosis. Comparing arterial blood oxygen saturation or Po_2 above and below the ductus arteriosus may be beneficial. In addition, the "hyperoxia" test, or ventilation with a high inspired oxygen concentration, is frequently considered a valuable diagnostic tool. An increase of more than 50 mm Hg (and often much higher) in systemic arterial Po_2 is seen in infants with primary pulmonary problems (especially because high levels of oxygen tend to dilate the pulmonary arterioles and decrease the PAPs). A PaO2 of less than 100 mm Hg in an enriched oxygen environment indicates congenital heart disease until proven otherwise and should prompt an echocardiographic examination and the initiation of PGE_2 therapy. Frequently, the practicalities adhere less to the textbook: a significant increase in systemic arterial blood oxygen tension or saturation can occur in cyanotic heart disease as long as effective pulmonary blood flow is reasonable. Therefore a PaO2 of 100 to 250 mm Hg may be suggestive of congenital heart disease and warrants additional investigation. A PaO_2 above 250 mm Hg makes life-threatening cyanotic heart disease less likely. If a hyperoxia test is performed, direct oxygen measurements should be made simultaneously in the upper and lower body to exaggerate any potential difference and thus help delineate the presence of a right-to-left ductal shunt. The measurement of upper and lower body saturation during crying can also help exaggerate potential differences because of ductal shunting.

> The pulse oximeter is your friend. It is readily available, and measuring upper- and lower-limb pulse oximetry can give a lot of valuable information, particularly when combined with a hyperoxia test.

Respiratory Distress

Most infants with mild arterial oxygen desaturation are tachypneic because of chemoreceptor stimulation but show little or no respiratory distress. Congenital heart disease that presents with respiratory distress is very difficult to diagnose in infants: their symptoms are usually more insidious and less dramatic than cyanosis, the differential diagnosis is broader, and the yield of heart disease is much less, which lowers one's index of suspicion. When a physician sees a newborn lying in a crib, blue and comfortable, the diagnosis is almost always cardiac disease; when the infant is acyanotic, tachypneic, and showing retractions, it is usually not. Infants with respiratory distress usually have modest degrees of systemic blood oxygen desaturation, depending on the type of circulatory derangement and the severity of pulmonary edema. The respiratory distress is related to decreased lung compliance in these patients, and interstitial fluid is usually present. Thus even with a normal separation of circulations, some degree of hypoxemia is present.

Cardiac Examination

Palpation

The cardiac impulse should be palpated. Obvious cardiac malposition in the right chest should be documented and warrants additional evaluation. The right ventricular impulse is dominant in a newborn.

Auscultation

Heart sounds in most newborns with significant congenital heart disease are abnormal. The rapid heart rates of most neonates can make this determination difficult even for the experienced practitioner. Multiple studies have assessed the skill of pediatric cardiologists and general pediatricians in detecting heart disease in inpatient neonatal settings and have found sensitivity rates of 80% to 83% for congenital heart disease.[64–66] A single-second sound after the first 12 hours may indicate atresia of a semilunar valve or transposition of the great arteries. The presence of a pulmonary systolic ejection click may be normal in the first hours, but after that, any systolic ejection click is abnormal, indicating an abnormal pulmonary or aortic valve, an enlarged pulmonary artery or aorta, or truncus arteriosus. If the infant has pulmonary disease without congenital heart disease and has a narrowly split- or single-second sound, then a high PVR is expected. Although systolic murmurs are more easily distinguished than the first and second heart sounds, they are common during the neonatal period and have historically been reported in up to 60% of healthy newborns.[67] Studies have demonstrated a higher incidence of congenital heart disease in infants with murmurs in the neonatal period. In a study of 7204 consecutively examined newborn infants, fewer than 1% of the neonates were found to have cardiac murmurs. All neonates with cardiac murmurs were referred for echocardiography, and an underlying cardiac malformation was diagnosed in 54% of them.[68] A retrospective review of 20,323 live births over a 3-year period in a hospital in Israel found 170 newborns with an isolated finding of a heart murmur who were referred for echocardiography. Of those infants, 147 (86%) were found to have structural heart defects, including isolated VSD (37%), PDA (23%), and combined VSD and PDA (7%); abnormalities creating left-to-right shunts comprised 66% of the diagnoses.[69] Certain murmurs noted in the neonatal period are nearly diagnostic. An S_4 gallop is always abnormal.

EDITORIAL COMMENT: Whereas the echocardiogram and pulse oximeter are trending to make the stethoscope obsolete, there is still much to be learned from careful observation of color, palpation of all the pulses, and auscultation, as described above.

Abdominal Examination

Hepatomegaly is a nonspecific finding that may be indicative of increased central venous pressures. It can be associated with cardiac lesions that volume-load the right side of the heart (such as a systemic arteriovenous malformation, anomalous pulmonary venous return, or right-sided valve insufficiency, as seen with Ebstein anomaly and absent pulmonary valve syndrome). Hepatomegaly may also be associated with low-output states such as myocarditis, cardiomyopathy, cardiogenic shock following ductal constriction in a ductal dependent systemic lesion, and tachyarrhythmias.

Peripheral Examination

It is imperative to palpate femoral and radial pulses in all newborns. Bounding pulses are typically associated with a widened pulse pressure and may be found in congenital abnormalities with increased diastolic pulmonary blood flow. Diminished femoral pulses or brachial–femoral delay may be associated with coarctation of the aorta, hypoplastic left heart syndrome, or an interrupted aortic arch. Inability to palpate pulses in all extremities should prompt the examiner to palpate the right carotid or temporal artery. If these pulses remain intact, the diagnosis would include an aberrant subclavian artery in addition to aortic arch obstruction. If all pulses are severely diminished, the obstruction to blood flow is at the aortic valve or within the left ventricle. Diminished femoral pulses should prompt the clinician to initiate therapy with prostaglandin infusion while awaiting confirmatory imaging or transfer to another center.

IMAGING IN THE NEONATAL INTENSIVE CARE UNIT

Accurately diagnosing the anatomy and physiology of the cardiac defect is the cornerstone for pediatric cardiology. To accomplish these goals, multiple imaging modalities are available. Currently, the most frequent techniques for imaging in the NICU are echocardiography, CAT scans, MRI, and cardiac catheterization. The decision to obtain one or more of these studies will depend on the history, clinical exam, and clinical course of the patient. With the use of these imaging techniques, a complete assessment of the cardiac defect can be obtained to aid for an optimal clinical outcome. This section will focus specifically on the uses of these techniques in the NICU.

Echocardiography

Echocardiography remains the main imaging technique in pediatric cardiology.[70–72] An echocardiogram is likely the first cardiac imaging technique that will be obtained to rule in or out a cardiac abnormality (Table 14.2). Most clinical and surgical decisions can be made purely from the echocardiographic exam. Advantages of echocardiography include its portability, noninvasive nature, real-time information, safety,

TABLE 14.2 Indications for Initial Echocardiographic Examination

Syndromes	Trisomy 13 Trisomy 18 Trisomy 21 CHARGE association VACTERL association DiGeorge syndrome Noonan syndrome Turner syndrome William syndrome
Nonsyndromes	Congenital diaphragmatic hernia Omphalocele Midline abnormality workup Tracheoesophageal fistula
Other	Unexplained hypoxemia Abnormal cardiac exam Perinatal asphyxia Persistent positive blood cultures Genetic abnormalities not otherwise specified

CHARGE, Coloboma of the eye, heart disease, atresia choanal, mental retardation, genital anomalies, ear anomalies; *VACTERL,* vertebral anomalies, anal atresia, cardiac anomalies, tracheoesophageal fistula, renal anomalies, limb anomalies.

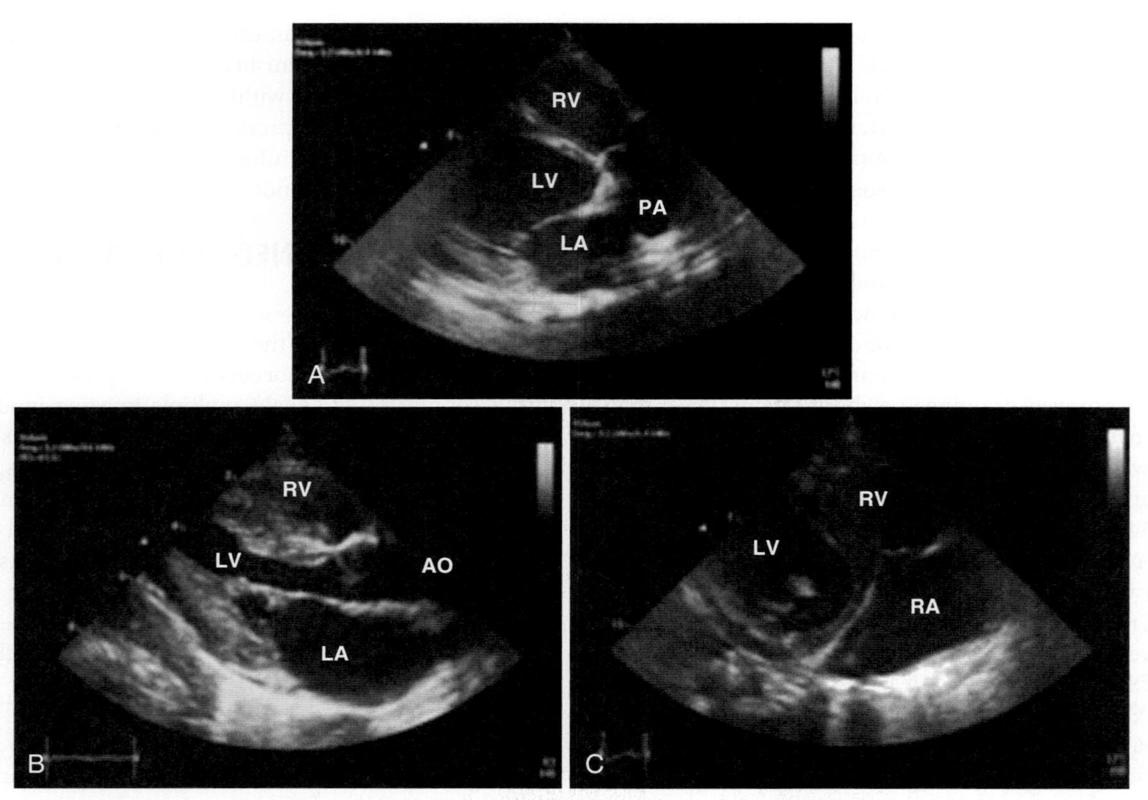

Fig. 14.5 Echocardiogram in the parasternal long-axis view sweeping anterior (A) to posterior (C) through the heart. *Ao,* Aorta; *LA,* left atrium; *LV,* left ventricle; *PA,* pulmonary artery; *RA,* right atrium; *RV,* right ventricle.

and overall ease of use. Disadvantages of echocardiography include limitations in imaging because of some clinical scenarios and only fair ability to accurately diagnose certain complicated extracardiac vascular anomalies.

Echocardiography is the application of ultrasound to obtain an image via reflected sound waves. Higher-frequency probes, usually 5 MHz or higher, are used in the NICU because minimal penetration of the sound wave into the patient is needed, and the shorter wavelengths allow for clearer resolution of the images. Scatter of the ultrasound wave, which inhibits image quality, usually occurs between interfaces of material that have disparate density. Bone and air, when adjacent to soft tissue or fluid, produces significant artifacts, whereas soft tissue next to fluid produces minimal artifact. As such, clinical scenarios, such as a pneumothorax or bronchopulmonary dysplasia (BPD), may minimize image quality.

A complete and standardized approach is needed for the initial echocardiographic evaluation of the neonate. The usual examination consists of the probe placed just to the left of the sternum to obtain parasternal long (Fig. 14.5A–C) and short axial images (Fig. 14.6A–C) at the apex of the heart to obtain an apical four-chamber view (Fig. 14.7A–C), subxiphoid to obtain subcostal coronal (Fig. 14.8A–C) and sagittal images (Fig. 14.9A–C), and in the suprasternal notch to obtain suprasternal long- (Fig. 14.10A,B) and short-axis views (Fig. 14.11A–B). More views may be obtained depending on the complexity of the anatomy. If the heart is displaced, as in the case of dextrocardia or CDH, adjustments of probe position are required. Numerous sweeps with application of M-mode, two-dimensional analysis, Doppler, and color Doppler allow for an inclusive examination that will give anatomical, physiologic, and functional data. For a complete review, the reader is referred to recent textbooks *Echocardiography in Pediatric and Adult Congenital Heart Disease*, eds. Eidem BW, Cetta F, and O'Leary PW; or *Echocardiography in Pediatric and Congenital Heart Disease: From Fetus to Adult*, eds. Lai WW, Mertens LL, MS Cohen, and Geva T.

M-Mode Echocardiography

M-mode echocardiography was one of the earliest techniques for evaluating cardiac structures. A single line of interrogation is obtained and plotted over time (Fig. 14.12). Two-dimensional echocardiography has largely replaced this modality, but M-mode is still used mainly to calculate shortening fraction and measure wall thickness and chamber size, though guidelines are always updated.[73] This is usually obtained in the parasternal short-axis view at the level of the papillary muscle (Fig. 14.13). Shortening fraction is defined as (left ventricular end-diastolic dimension–left ventricular end-systolic dimension)/left ventricular end-diastolic dimension. A normal value is anything above 28%. Limitations of M-mode include the fact that it involves only a single plane to estimate global function; thus regional wall abnormalities may be missed. It is also fairly preload dependent and does not measure intrinsic myocardial contractility per se. Shortening fraction also assumes normal electrical conduction and a

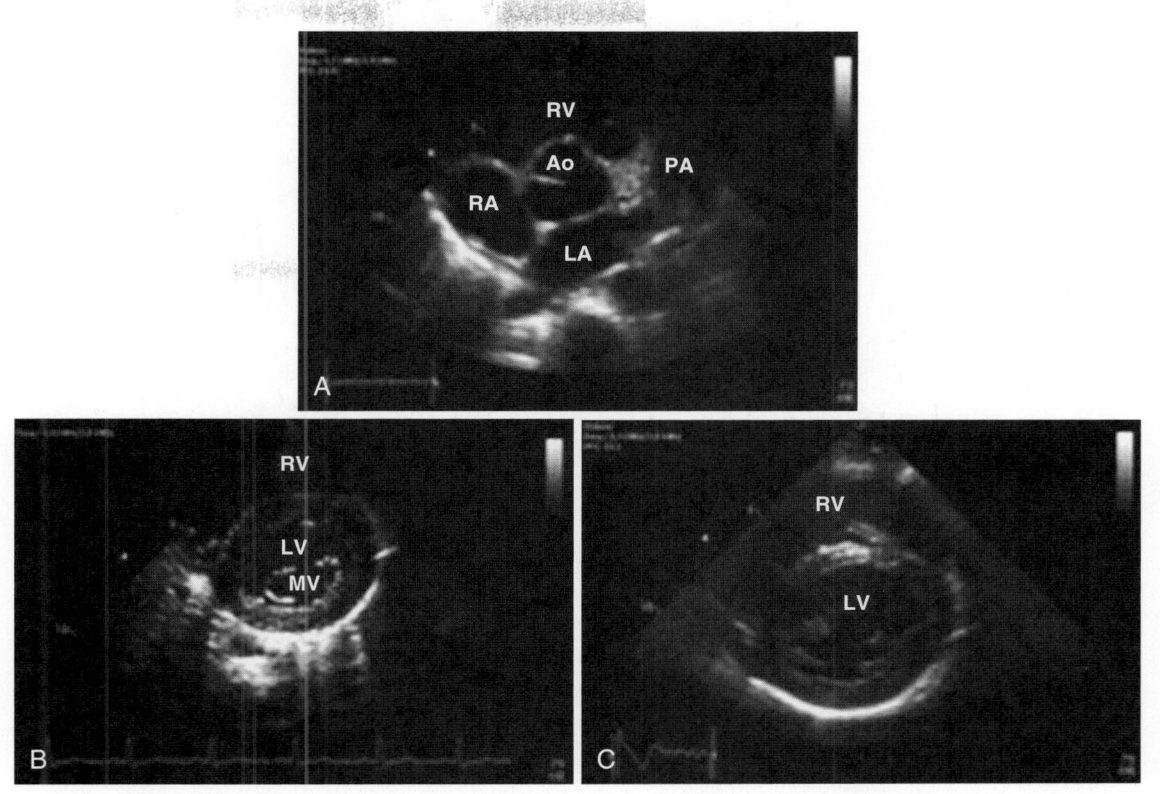

Fig. 14.6 Echocardiogram in the parasternal short-axis view sweeping from the base (A) to the apex (C) of the heart. *Ao,* Aorta; *LA,* left atrium; *LV,* left ventricle; *MV,* mitral valve; *PA,* pulmonary artery; *RA,* right atrium; *RV,* right ventricle.

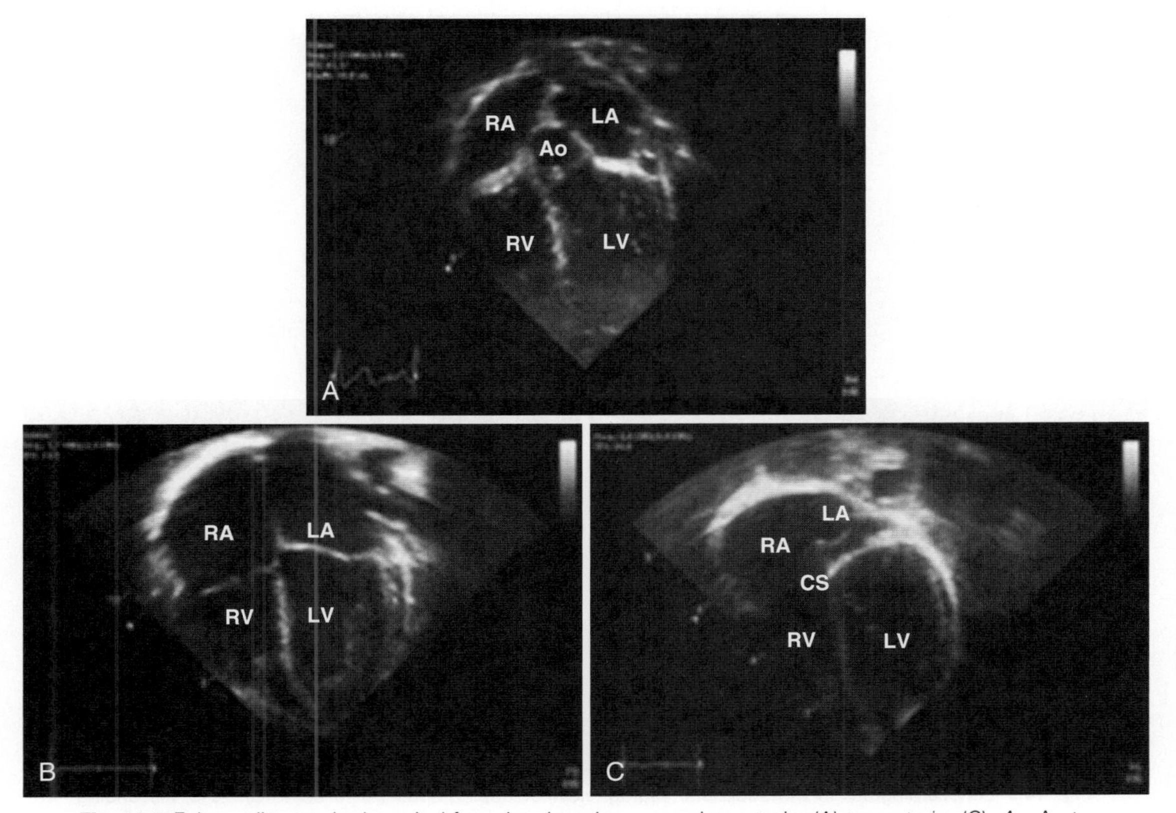

Fig. 14.7 Echocardiogram in the apical four-chamber view sweeping anterior (A) to posterior (C). *Ao,* Aorta; *CS,* coronary sinus; *LA,* left atrium; *LV,* left ventricle; *RA,* right atrium; *RV,* right ventricle.

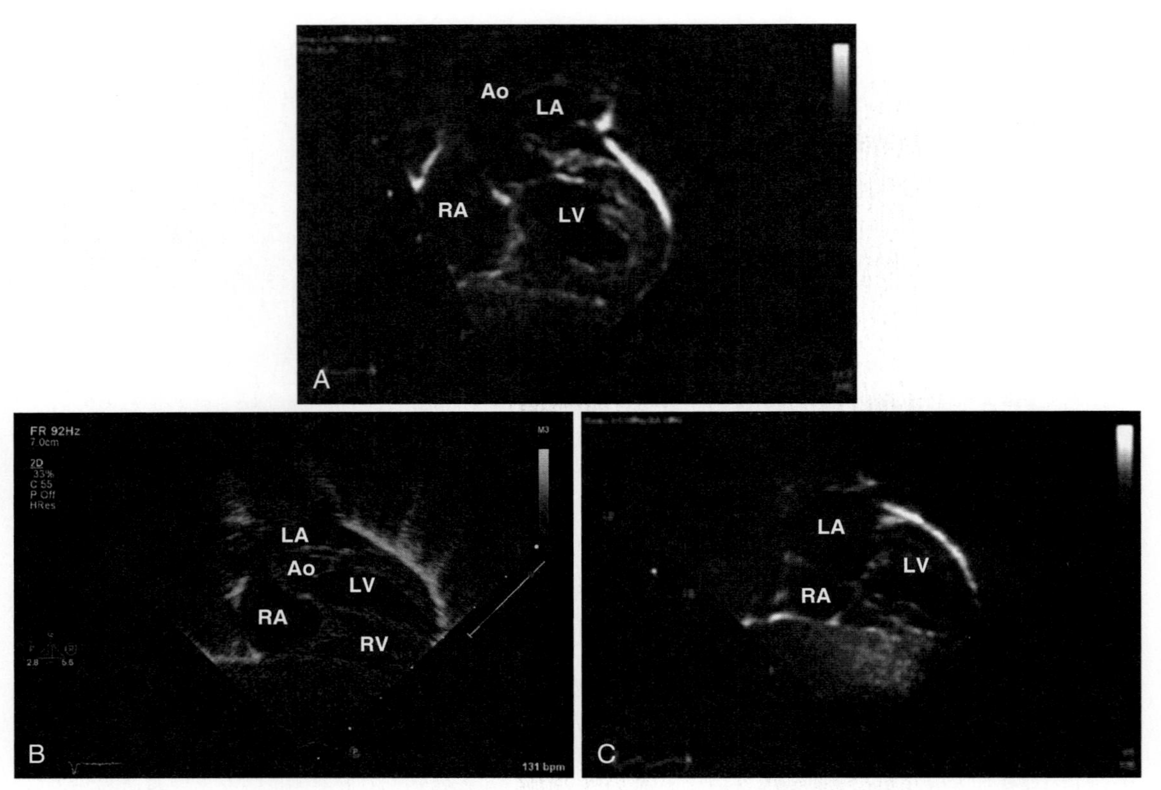

Fig. 14.8 Echocardiogram in the subcostal coronal view sweeping anterior (A) to posterior (C). *Ao*, Aorta; *LA*, left atrium; *LV*, left ventricle; *RA*, right atrium; *RV*, right ventricle.

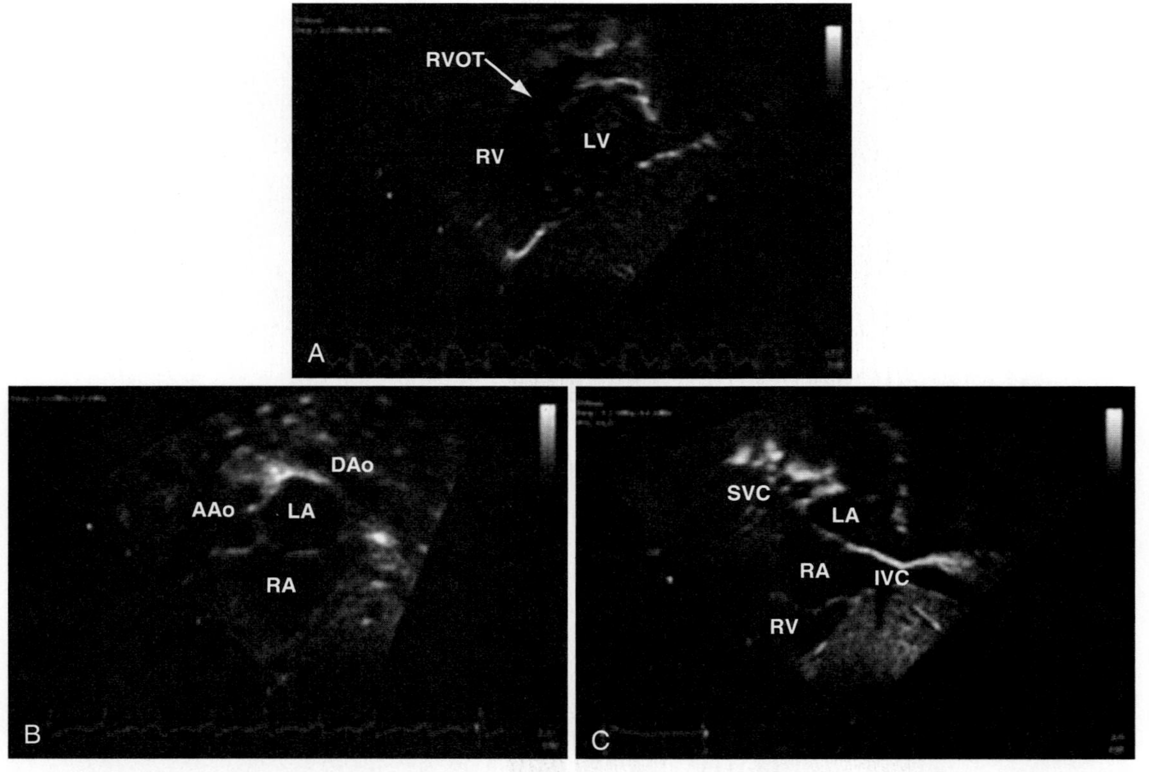

Fig. 14.9 Echocardiogram in the subcostal sagittal view sweeping apex (A) to base (C). *AAo*, Ascending aorta; *DAo*, descending aorta; *IVC*, inferior vena cava; *LA*, left atrium; *LV*, left ventricle; *RA*, right atrium; *RV*, right ventricle; *RVOT*, right ventricular outflow tract; *SVC*, superior vena cava.

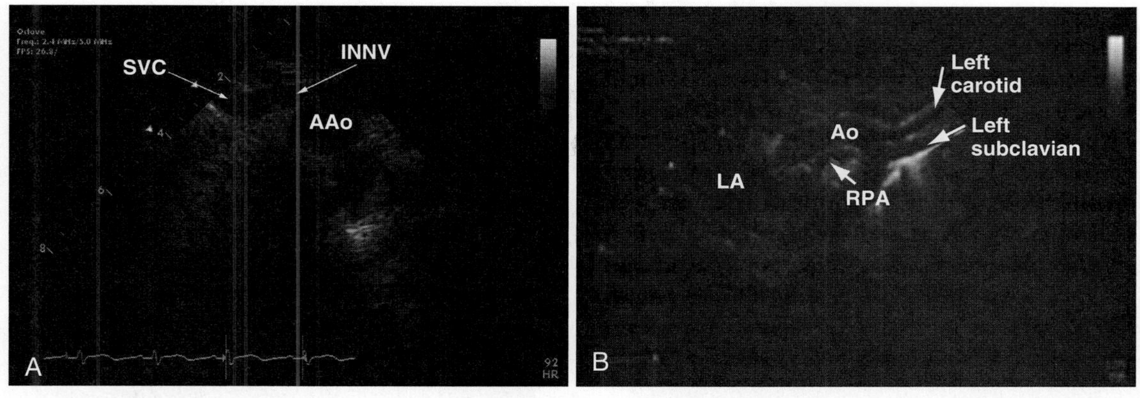

Fig. 14.10 Echocardiogram in the suprasternal long-axis view sweeping from the patient's right (A) to left (B) side, assuming a left aortic arch. *AAo,* Ascending aorta; *Ao,* aorta; *INNV,* innominate vein; *LA,* left atrium; *RPA,* right pulmonary artery; *SVC,* superior vena cava.

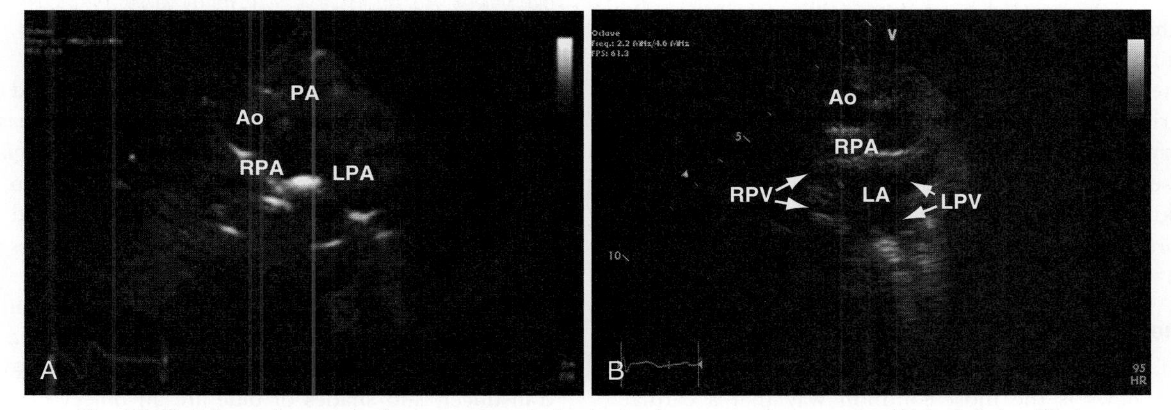

Fig. 14.11 Echocardiogram in the suprasternal short-axis view sweeping superior (A) to inferior (B) *Ao,* Aorta; *LA,* left atrium; *LPA,* left pulmonary artery; *LPV,* left pulmonary vein; *PA,* pulmonary artery; *RPA,* right pulmonary artery; *RPV,* right pulmonary vein.

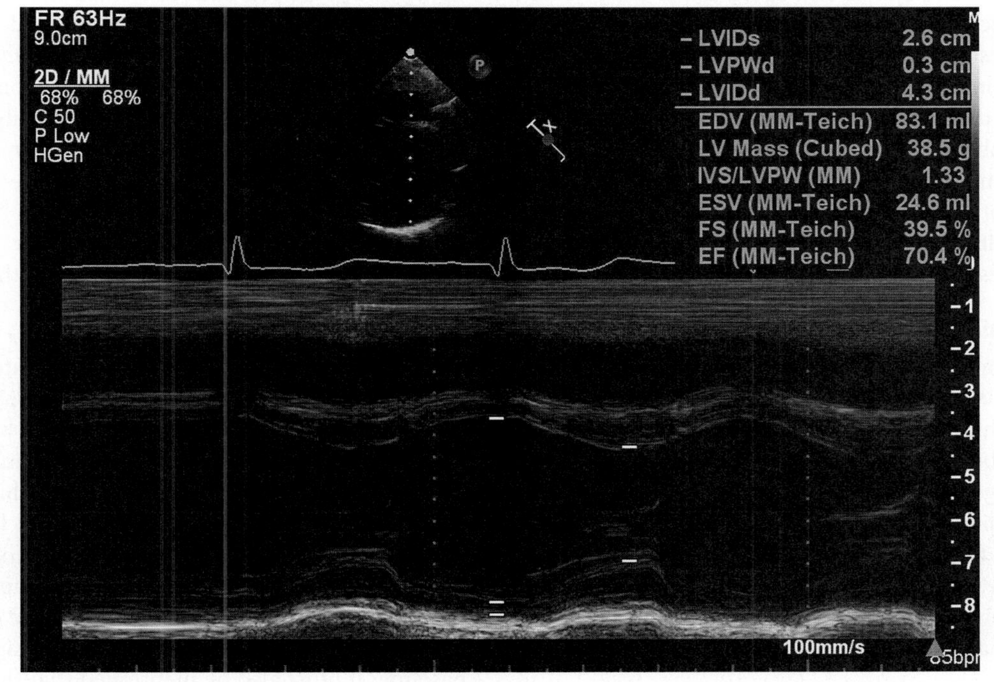

Fig. 14.12 M-mode analysis through the left ventricle with a normal shortening fraction of 39%. *EF,* ejection fraction; *EDV,* end diastolic volume; *ESV,* end systolic volume; *FS,* fractional shortening; *IVS/LVPW,* interventricular septum / left ventricular posterior wall; *LVIDd,* end-diastolic left ventricular internal dimension; *LVIDs,* end-systolic left ventricular internal dimension; *LVPWd,* end-diastolic left ventricular posterior wall thickness.

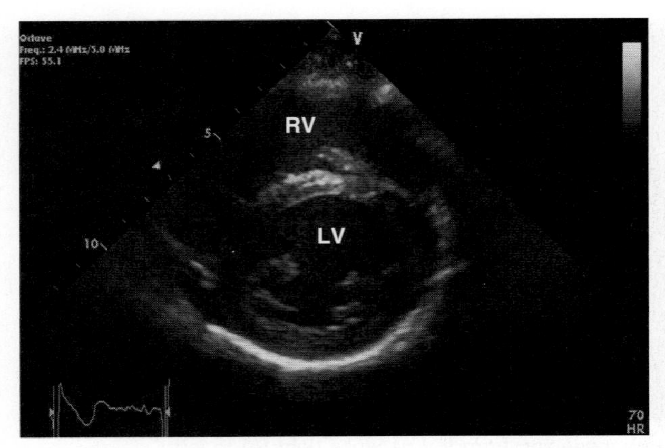

Fig. 14.13 Parasternal short axis at the level of the papillary muscle. *LV,* Left ventricle; *RV,* right ventricle.

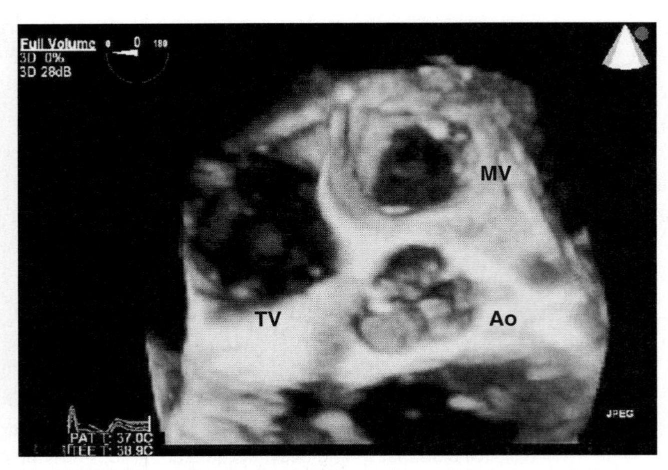

Fig. 14.14 Three-dimensional echocardiographic image of the cardiac valves. *Ao,* Aortic valve; *MV,* mitral valve; *TV,* tricuspid valve.

circular shape of the left ventricle. Conduction abnormalities or flattening of the interventricular septum that may occur with dilated right ventricular volumes because of shunts or elevated right ventricular pressures attributed to persistent pulmonary hypertension of the newborn (PPHN) may invalidate these measurements. Normative data are available for wall thickness and chamber sizes and are usually referenced to a *z*-score. A *z*-score is simply a standard deviation, and if a *z*-score is within ± 2, it is considered normal.

Two-Dimensional Echocardiography

As stated, use of two-dimensional echocardiography via numerous views is the most common way that a cardiac anatomical diagnosis is made. Systolic function can also be qualitatively and quantitatively obtained. Tracing the left ventricular chamber in end systole and end diastole can give an estimate of ventricular volume, and thus an ejection fraction can be calculated similarly to shortening fraction. In general, an ejection fraction above 50% is considered normal. In addition to anatomic diagnosis and function analysis, secondary changes to chamber sizes may give physiologic clues. For example, a PDA may be large by dimensions, but if left-sided structures are not enlarged, there may be minimal left-to-right shunt, possibly because of PPHN or not enough time has passed for these changes to be noted.

Three-Dimensional Echocardiography

The ability to render real-time three-dimensional imaging has been a relatively new advancement in technology. The benefit of this technology includes the ability to improve spatial relationships between structures versus trying to mentally construct an image via two-dimensional images (Fig. 14.14). Although three-dimensional imaging continues to improve, practical uses in the NICU are minimal at this time. This modality may be more useful for neonates with congenital heart disease. This modality's usefulness for neonates with structurally normal hearts has yet to be defined.

Doppler Echocardiography

Use of the Doppler principle enables the determination of direction and velocity of moving objects being interrogated. Currently, measurement of blood flow velocity and direction is the main use for Doppler analysis, although measurement of myocardial velocity, termed *tissue Doppler imaging (TDI)*, has recently been introduced as another way to quantify systolic and diastolic function. Color, pulse, and continuous-wave Doppler are the three main techniques used for analysis.

Color Doppler simply transforms the image being examined into color pixels within the interrogated area. By convention, shades of red signify an object moving toward the transducer, and shades of blue are an object moving away from the transducer. Color Doppler does not necessarily give quantitative information, but it is extremely helpful for identifying minor defects such as a small muscular VSD or PDA that might not be easily seen by standard two-dimensional echocardiography (Fig. 14.15). Color analysis also aides in the qualification of regurgitant jets based on the width of the regurgitant jet. Stenotic areas are also easily seen with color analysis because the solid red/blue color usually becomes multicolor because of the abrupt increase in velocities that occur in those areas (Fig. 14.16).

Pulse and continuous-wave Doppler are simply two technical ways to measure the velocity of the object of interest. Pulse Doppler enables interrogation of a specific area and definition the velocity at that point. The drawback is that high-velocity objects cannot accurately be measured because they will exceed the pulse Doppler capabilities. Continuous-wave Doppler can measure high-velocity signals because it is continuously measuring signals, but it cannot pinpoint the area where the change of velocity occurs. This is important because the area where the change in velocity occurs is usually where a stenosis is located. By convention, objects moving away from the transducer have velocities designated below a baseline, and objects with flow toward the transducer have velocities designated above the baseline. It must also be mentioned that the line of interrogation should be as close to parallel to the object of interest, or else velocities will be underestimated and thus also gradients.

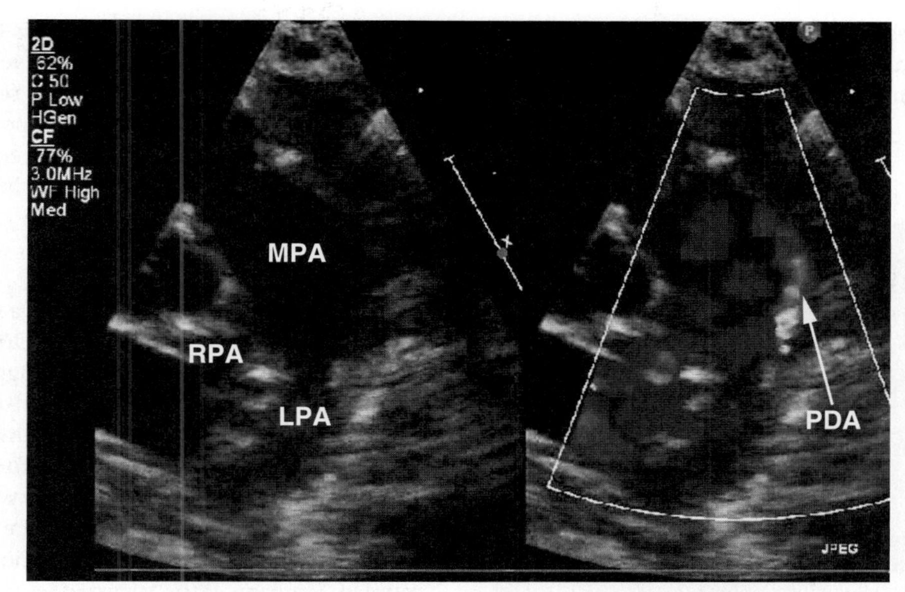

Fig. 14.15 Image of a small patent ductus arteriosus *(PDA)* obtained using color Doppler echocardiography. *LPA,* Left pulmonary artery; *MPA,* main pulmonary artery; *RPA,* right pulmonary artery.

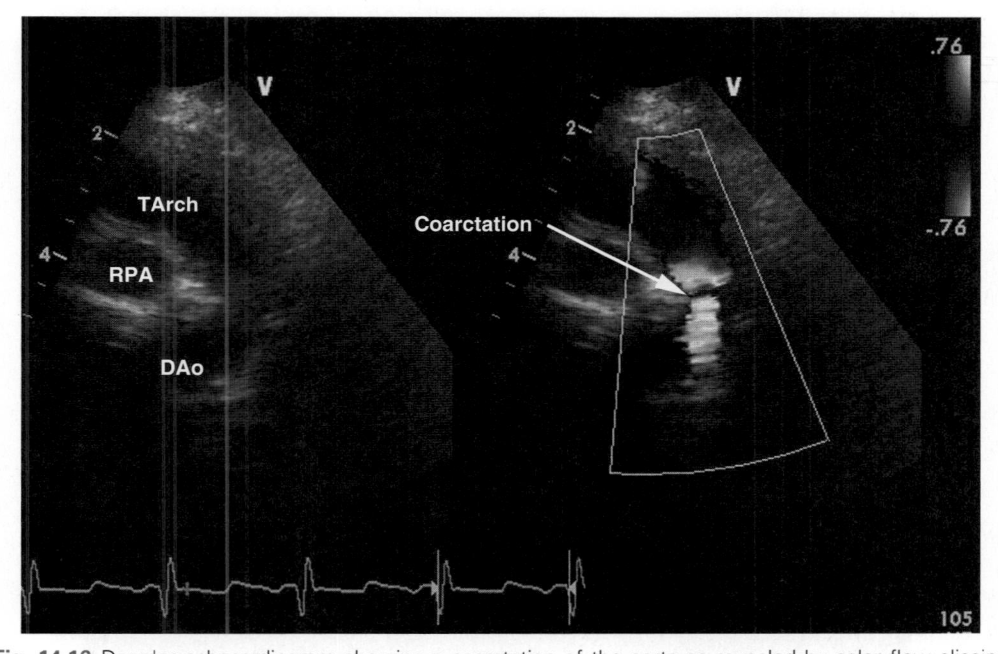

Fig. 14.16 Doppler echocardiogram showing a coarctation of the aorta as revealed by color flow aliasing at the coarctation site. *DAo,* Descending aorta; *RPA,* right pulmonary artery; *TArch,* transverse aortic arch.

TDI is a newer technique that measures the velocity of the myocardium via Doppler. The area interrogated is usually the free wall at the level of the AV valves. Three waves are usually obtained via TDI, e′ wave corresponding to early ventricular relaxation, a′ wave corresponding to atrial contraction, and an s′ wave corresponding to ventricular systolic function (Fig. 14.17). The e′ and a′ waves quantify diastolic function, and the s′ wave quantifies systolic function.[74] This technique is less preload dependent and therefore may be more useful than other previously described values. TDI has been used in infants with BPD,[75,76] infants of diabetic mothers,[77,78] and infants with CDH[79,80] to help assist in quantifying right ventricular function. Differences in cardiac function have been noted between various neonatal groups with and without a specific medical condition, as noted above. The prognostic ability of this modality has yet to be determined on a consistent basis, but preliminary studies are encouraging. This technique will likely continue to grow in use as more normative data become available and if its prognostic ability is established.[81–87]

Estimation of pressure gradients between two separate areas is obtained by measuring the blood velocity across the site and using the Bernoulli equation:

$$\Delta P = 1/2\, \rho \left(v_2^2 - v_1^2\right) + \rho \, f(dv/dt) \; *ds + R(\mu)$$

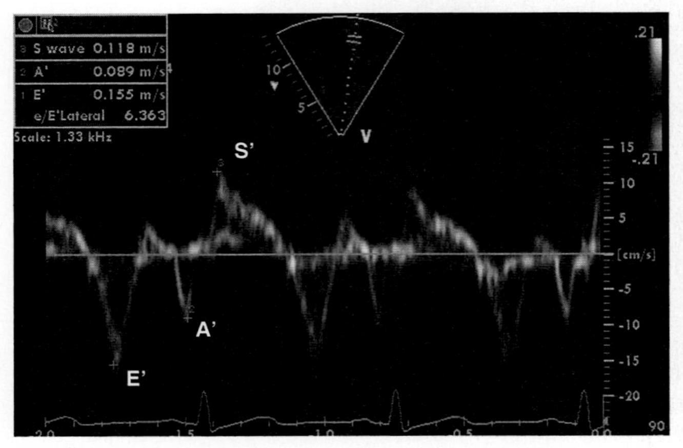

Fig. 14.17 Tissue Doppler analysis of the left ventricular free wall at the level of the mitral valve annulus. See text for details.

ΔP is the pressure difference across the stenotic area, ρ is the density of blood, v_1 and v_2 are the velocities proximal and distal to the stenosis, R is the viscous resistance, and μ is the viscosity of the fluid. The three components of the formula account for kinetic energy, loss of energy through acceleration and deceleration of blood, and viscous forces. This formula can be simplified to

$$\Delta P = 4\, v^2$$

assuming minimal proximal velocity, a discrete stenosis, and minimal viscosity. By using all three Doppler techniques and the Bernoulli equation, the physiology can be thus determined (Fig. 14.18). For example, a left-to-right shunt is seen via color Doppler through a PDA with a peak velocity of 3.5 m/s by continuous-wave Doppler. The pressure difference between the aorta and main pulmonary artery is 3.5 m/s X 3.5 m/s X 4 = 49 mm Hg. Furthermore, the right ventricular systolic pressure can be calculated as aortic systolic pressure—49 mm Hg. Similarly, if the tricuspid jet is 2.5 m/s, the pressure difference between the right atrium and right ventricle is 25 mm Hg. Assuming a normal right atrial pressure is 5 mm Hg, the right ventricular systolic pressure is approximately 30 mm

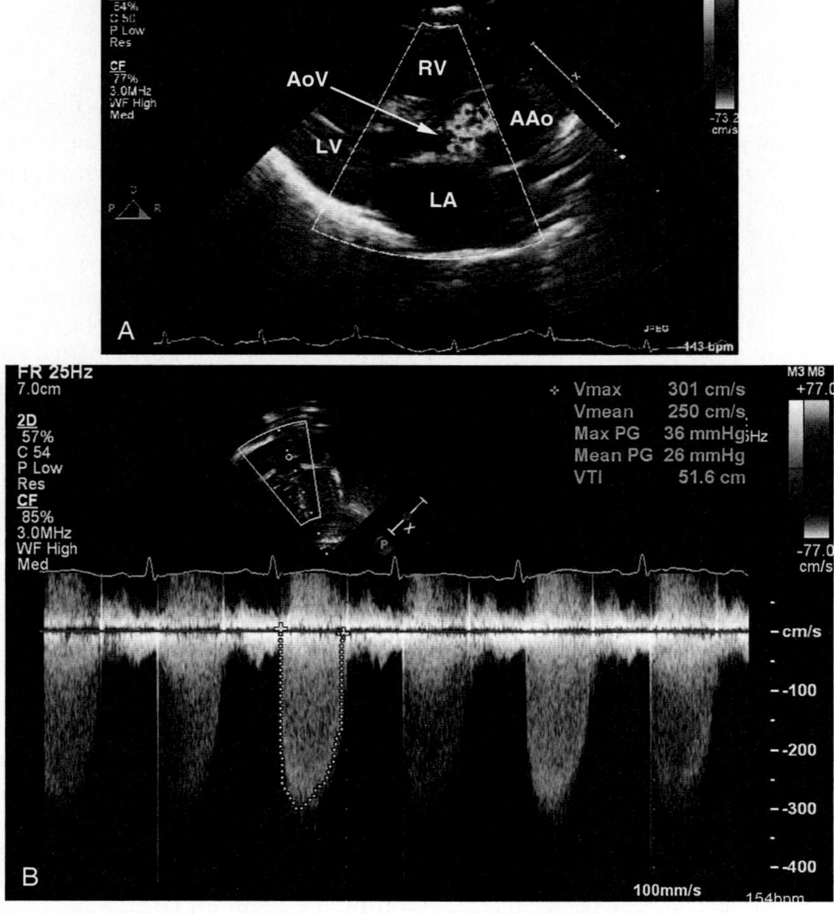

Fig. 14.18 Color flow aliasing at the level of a stenotic aortic valve (A) with a peak velocity of 3 m/sec by continuous wave Doppler echocardiography estimating a 36-mm Hg gradient (B). *AAo*, Ascending aorta; *AoV*, aortic valve; *LA*, left atrium; *LV*, left ventricle; *RV*, right ventricle.

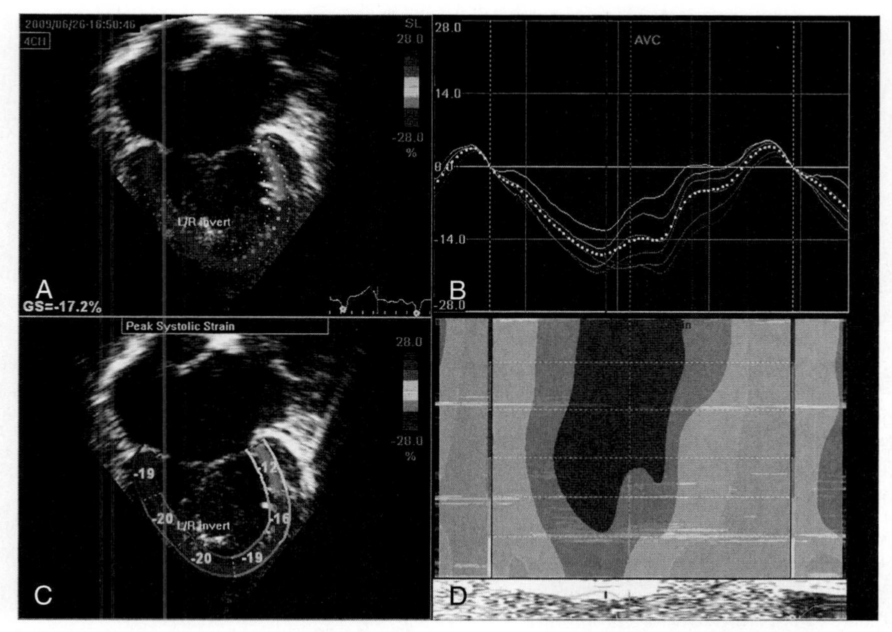

Fig. 14.19 Strain analysis based on echocardiographic imaging in a patient with hypoplastic left heart syndrome. Segments are color-coded as follows: yellow= basal interventricular septum, light blue = mid interventricular septum, green = apical interventricular septum, red = basal right ventricular free wall, dark blue = mid right ventricular free wall, purple = apical right ventricular free wall. (A) Strain curve with global right ventricular strain value. (B) Color-coded segmental strain curves with global right ventricular. Dashed white line = strain curve. (C) Segmental strain values. (D) Curved M-mode.

Hg. Numerous calculations are thus performed to quantify the physiology present. This equation will underestimate the gradient if there is a long segment stenosis or if polycythemia is present because of the simplification. Conversely, if there is a significant proximal stenosis in series such as a stenotic aortic valve and a coarctation of the aorta, the proximal velocity must be taken into account, or else the distal gradient will be overestimated. In general, a velocity of 1 m/s or less can be ignored.

Strain and strain rate (deformation analysis). Strain (ε) is defined as the deformation of an object relative to its original length and is expressed as a percentage. Strain rate is the local rate of deformation or strain (ε) per unit of time and is expressed in 1/sec. These values can be obtained via TDI or via speckle-tracking technology using echocardiography. These parameters are probably the least preload-dependent values obtained via echocardiography and thus, theoretically, the best values to quantify contractility and relaxation. This technique does not use geometrical assumptions and therefore is ideal for quantifying function in patients with complex congenital anatomy (Fig. 14.19). Even less data for deformation than TDI currently exist in pediatrics, especially in the NICU setting, but similar to TDI, this technique will likely continue to gain acceptance over time as more normative data are obtained and its prognostic ability is established.[82,88–94] Obtaining these values is a little more time-consuming than the other quantitative measures previously mentioned, and this may be one of the major issues in limiting this technique's use in the clinical setting.

Transesophageal Echocardiography

Transesophageal echocardiography (TEE) is simply the application of all the above noted echocardiographic techniques via a probe inserted down the esophagus. It is rarely indicated in the NICU setting because most, if not all, the images can be obtained with a transthoracic echocardiogram. Neonates would likely need to be intubated for this procedure to secure an airway. If needed, probes are currently available for neonates weighing as small as 2.5 kg. TEE is most often performed in neonates in conjunction with a cardiac catheterization or surgical intervention to give real-time information and aid in the intervention being performed (Fig. 14.20).[95,96]

Computerized Axial Tomography/Magnetic Resonance Imaging

CAT scans or MRIs may add additional information that the echocardiogram cannot provide. As stated before, complex extracardiac abnormalities dealing with pulmonary arteries, pulmonary veins, and the aortic arch may not be well delineated via echocardiogram. Cardiac defects such as mixed total anomalous pulmonary veins and tetralogy of Fallot with multiple aortopulmonary collaterals are just two examples where CAT scans and MRIs are superior to echocardiography for defining extracardiac abnormalities (Figs. 14.21 and 14.22). In addition to anatomic information, both modalities have the ability to provide hemodynamic data, with MRI being superior to a CAT scan in that respect.

In general, MRI is preferable to CAT scans because of the lack of radiation exposure. Because many of these children

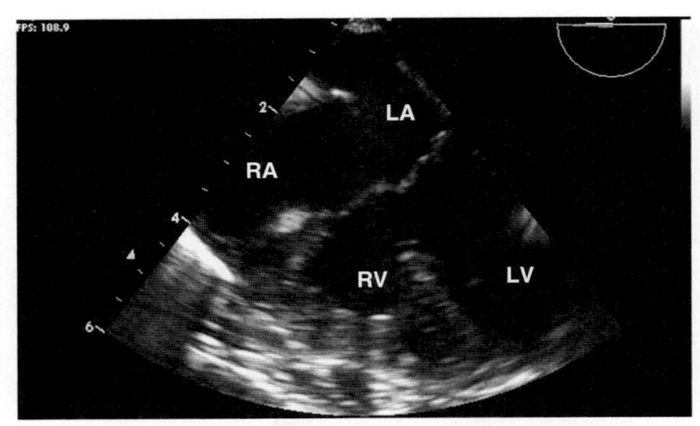

Fig. 14.20 Transesophageal echocardiogram of a patient with an atrioventricular septal defect. Note the common atrioventricular valve and the large central defect. *LA,* Left atrium; *LV,* left ventricle; *RA,* right atrium; *RV,* right ventricle.

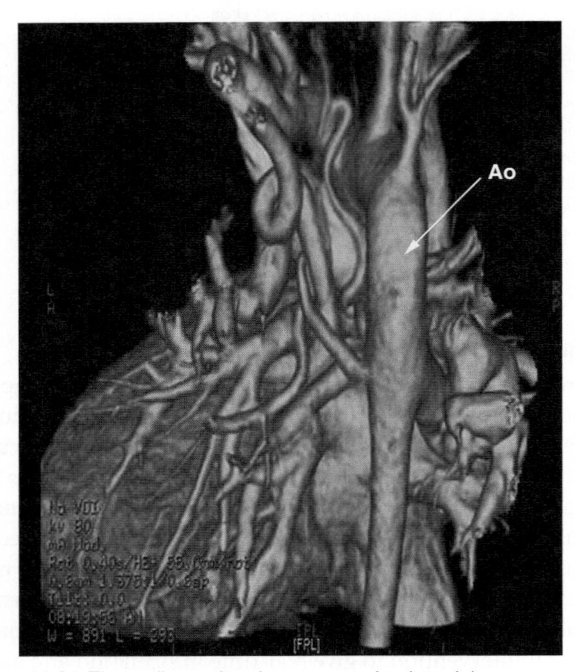

Fig. 14.21 Three-dimensional computerized axial tomographic scan reconstruction for a patient with tetralogy of Fallot, pulmonary atresia, and multiple aortopulmonary collaterals. This left posterior oblique view shows multiple collateral vessels arising from the aorta and supplying blood to the small pulmonary arteries. *Ao,* Aorta.

with complex cardiac anatomy may undergo multiple imaging and catheterization procedures over a lifetime, minimization of radiation exposure is warranted. CAT scans customarily require contrast, so it is a relative contraindication in patients with renal insufficiency (Table 14.3). There have also been some concerns raised with MRI and gadolinium contrast use in patients with renal insufficiency associated with nephrogenic systemic fibrosis.[97,98] Because of this concern, gadolinium use is probably best not used in those patients until more data are available. CAT scans are quicker in obtaining images than MRIs; thus in an unstable patient, a CAT scan may be preferable to an MRI. CAT scan imaging is also not as affected by artificial material such as stents, coils, and so on, compared

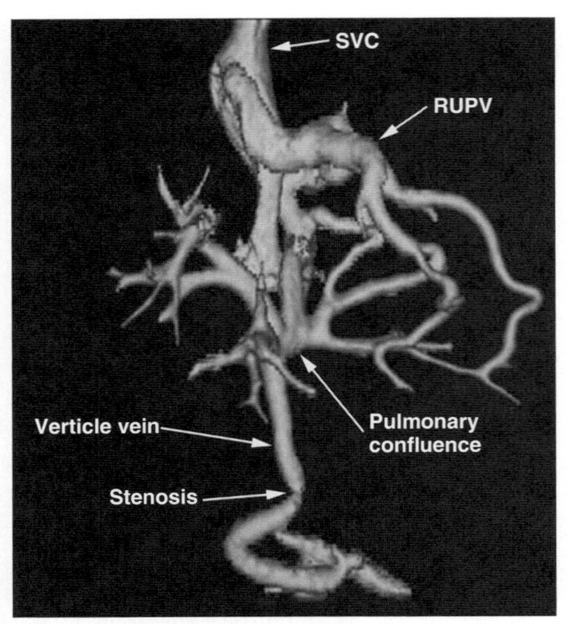

Fig. 14.22 Three-dimensional computerized axial tomographic scan reconstruction (posterior view) for a patient with mixed total anomalous pulmonary venous return. The right upper pulmonary vein *(RUPV)* drains into the superior vena cava *(SVC),* with the other veins draining into a confluence, then down via a vertical vein into the hepatic veins. Note the narrowing in the vertical vein where a stenosis is present.

with an MRI. As technology advances, more devices have become MRI compatible. It is essential that whenever a patient may undergo an MRI, screening for device compatibility is performed (www.mrisafety.com). Cardiac MRI may not be readily available at some institutions, so the decision of imaging may be a driven by practical considerations.

Cardiac Catheterization

Similar to CAT/MRI studies, catheterization images give excellent images of extracardiac structures. Nonetheless, most anatomical, physiological, and functional data can be obtained via the imaging modalities previously described. It would be extremely rare to perform a catheterization procedure purely for imaging purposes. A catheterization is usually performed in the neonate because an intervention is required such as a balloon atrial septostomy or a valvuloplasty.[99] Disadvantages of catheterization include its invasive nature and the radiation and contrast exposure involved (Table 14.3).

In summary, multiple imaging techniques are available in the NICU. Echocardiography will likely remain the main modality for the reasons stated above, but other techniques may give additive information depending on the clinical situation. Imaging technology will undoubtedly improve over time, but the goal will always remain the same: complete and accurate assessment of anatomy, physiology, and function of the cardiac defect.

DIAGNOSTIC GROUPS OF CONGENITAL HEART DISEASE

The spectrum of neonatal congenital and acquired heart disease is conventionally divided into broad categories based on

TABLE 14.3 Advantages and Disadvantages of Imaging Techniques

	Echocardiography	CAT scan	MRI	Cardiac Catheterization
Portable	Yes	No	No	No
Noninvasive	Yes	Yes	Yes	No
Intracardiac structures	+ + + +	+ + +	+ + + +	+ +
Hemodynamic assessment	+ + +	+ +	+ + +	+ + + +
Extracardiac structures	+ + +	+ + + +	+ + + +	+ + + +
Contrast exposure	No	Yes	No	Yes
Radiation exposure	No	Yes	No	Yes
Interventional capability	No	No	No	Yes

CAT, Computerized axial tomography; *MRI,* magnetic resonance imaging.

presentation, unifying pathologic features, and anticipated course. Practically, there can be significant variation in the duration of neonatal transition, which impacts the observed physiology of a given lesion. Ideally, lesions can be classified by their primary presenting features: (1) cyanosis caused by obstruction to pulmonary blood flow or poor mixing, (2) hypoperfusion and shock caused by obstruction to systemic blood flow, or (3) mild or no cyanosis with tachypnea and increased pulmonary blood flow. This section discusses these types of presentation, the most common lesions in each, the diagnostic tests necessary to distinguish among the lesions, subsequent therapy, and the differential diagnosis of noncardiac disease.

Mild or No Cyanosis With Respiratory Distress and Increased Pulmonary Blood Flow

Infants with a primary presentation of tachypnea secondary to cardiac disease can be categorized into two major subgroups: (1) those with pure left-to-right shunts, in whom the shunt solely consists of pulmonary venous return being directed back to the pulmonary arterial circulation, so that any arterial desaturation is secondary to alveolar fluid or an intrapulmonary shunt; and (2) those with bidirectional shunts (complete mixing lesions), in whom systemic venous blood is also directed back to the systemic arterial circulation, which directly causes some arterial desaturation. Both groups may have elevated PVPs or pulmonary blood flow that causes interstitial edema, at which point respiratory distress becomes apparent.

Some of the most common defects in congenital heart disease, including simple left-to-right shunt lesions (atrial and VSDs, PDA, endocardial cushion defect, arteriovenous malformations, and aortopulmonary window) as well as more complex complete mixing lesions such as anomalous pulmonary venous connection and truncus arteriosus, present with respiratory distress in infancy. Often these neonates are asymptomatic immediately after birth. As the PVR falls, infants may begin to manifest signs of increased pulmonary blood flow, including tachypnea, tachycardia, diaphoresis, hepatomegaly, and eventually failure to thrive. An exception to this situation is the preterm infant, in whom there may be hemodynamically significant left-to-right shunting within a few days following delivery that contributes to earlier onset of symptoms. When the lung, particularly the pulmonary vascular bed, is underdeveloped or damaged, such as with diaphragmatic hernia, omphalocele, or chronic lung disease, a small shunt seems much larger because of the reduced size of the pulmonary vascular bed in these infants.

The differential diagnosis of infants with respiratory distress includes parenchymal lung disease, an aspiration syndrome, diaphragmatic hernia, pneumonia, and PPHN. The premature infant with resolving respiratory distress syndrome who requires increasing respiratory support may have either an increasing ductal shunt or the onset of interstitial lung disease. Thus several days of careful evaluation may be required before the presence of heart disease is fully appreciated.

Ventricular Septal Defect

An isolated VSD accounts for between 30% and 40% of all congenital heart disease. The majority of isolated VSDs are very small and restrictive. In these infants, the resistance to flow between the left and right ventricles allows the pulmonary vessels to mature normally into adult-type vessels. With a rapid decrease in PVR, there is a corresponding decrease in right ventricular pressure, and a left ventricular–right ventricular pressure gradient will arise. Therefore a left-to-right shunt can develop quickly, resulting in a loud (grade 3–4/6) systolic murmur that is often present in the newborn period. Despite the low PVR, the resistance to flow at the VSD prevents large-volume left-to-right shunting, which averts symptoms of congestive heart failure. Infants with this defect rarely demonstrate pulmonary overcirculation. As a result, most of these defects follow their natural history and close spontaneously, and the remainder rarely require surgical intervention because the defect and resulting additional pulmonary blood flow do not contribute to the development of additional abnormalities.

In a large, nonrestrictive VSD (Fig. 14.4), the pressure in the right ventricle and pulmonary artery is at systemic levels. If the thick-walled pulmonary vessels matured normally, the vascular resistance would decrease rapidly, and there would be a large left-to-right shunt with left ventricular failure and pulmonary edema. Such a series of events is unusual. In fact, when a large VSD is present, a heart murmur is not usually heard, even in the newborn period. The left-to-right shunt does not develop rapidly because the pulmonary resistance vessels remain heavily muscular for a longer period than normal, and the decrease in PVR is delayed. The variation in PVR from one child to the next is considerable. In some infants, the resistance decreases considerably; in others, hardly at all. When there is a large defect, the shunt is usually maximal by 2 to 3 weeks of age, so that congestive heart failure, when it occurs, is usually present by 4 weeks of age.

Patent Ductus Arteriosus

Persistent patency of the ductus arteriosus beyond the first few days of life accounts for 10% to 15% of all congenital heart defects. Premature infants comprise the majority of patients with persistent patency of the ductus arteriosus. The proportion increases with lower gestational age and weight, with up to 70% of infants born less than 28 weeks of age demonstrating ductal patency. Patency of the ductus arteriosus may result from adverse events such as hypoxia or acidosis in the newborn. The exact mechanisms for persistent patency in premature infants are not clear. In premature animal models, the ductus arteriosus is less responsive to the constricting effects of oxygen, the relaxing effects of PGE_2 and prostacyclin are greater, and the metabolism of PGE_2 is not efficient. As a result, even the small circulating concentrations of PGE_2 that may be present in the immature infant can cause the ductus arteriosus to remain in a partially relaxed state. The principles discussed for VSD also apply to PDA. However, because there is length to the ductus arteriosus as well as caliber, resistance to flow is greater. A nonrestrictive PDA is less common, so that systemic-level pulmonary hypertension is also less common.

In a full-term infant with a PDA, the outcome depends on the size of the channel. With the gradual decrease in postnatal PVR, a left-to-right shunt develops from aorta to pulmonary artery, which produces excessive pulmonary blood flow, increased pulmonary venous return, and left atrial and ventricular dilatation. A small PDA produces only the typical continuous machinery murmur and full pulses. A moderate to large PDA may produce signs of congestive heart failure as well as a typical continuous murmur and wide pulse pressure (bounding pulse), often in the second month of life. In the healthy term infant, only rarely does heart failure occur in the newborn period.

Patent ductus arteriosus in preterm infants. As noted earlier, preterm infants, and particularly very low-birth-weight infants, have a significantly increased incidence of persistent PDA compared with their term peers. The PDA of the preterm infant warrants specific discussion because it may seriously complicate the management of RDS and is by itself associated with mortality.[100] Although the left ventricle is capable of maintaining near-normal systemic blood flow even with a large left-to-right shunt in the premature infant, the increased intravascular blood volume and the associated increase in interstitial fluid aggravate the respiratory distress already present. If left ventricular oxygen demand exceeds supply, the left ventricle may begin to fail, which raises PVP and further increases interstitial fluid production. In addition, PAPs may be elevated because of the nonrestrictive PDA itself or because of pulmonary venous hypertension, which may further decrease lung compliance and exacerbate the pulmonary dysfunction. Thus a PDA in the presence of RDS may seriously affect pulmonary function by a variety of mechanisms.

The diagnosis of a PDA may be difficult in that tachycardia, and an intermittent systolic murmur may be the only auscultatory findings. A wide pulse pressure is often present, as is increased precordial activity. Ventilator therapy and continuous positive airway pressure may mask not only the clinical findings but also the radiographic findings of a PDA. When the chest radiograph shows a large heart and pulmonary venous congestion in the presence of signs of a PDA and a large liver, there is no problem in diagnosis. However, for many reasons, the heart may not be very large, and severe RDS may obscure radiographic findings of cardiomegaly and pulmonary edema. In the premature infant with pulmonary disease, impaired oxygen exchange in the lung may maintain an elevated PVR, which masks the presence of PDA. Improvement in the pulmonary disease permits the pulmonary resistance to fall, and signs of a left-to-right ductal shunt to ensue. Thus a PDA must be suspected in all infants with severe RDS when the illness is protracted, blood gas concentrations suddenly deteriorate and require manipulation of ventilation, or apneic episodes are intensified. Fluid balance must be closely monitored because excess fluid administration may exacerbate the physiology of a PDA and induce congestive heart failure. Infants must undergo auscultation for murmurs several times each day during the illness and should be briefly removed from the ventilator to permit proper auscultation. Echocardiography and Doppler imaging are diagnostic. Color-flow Doppler mapping can detect even a small, hemodynamically insignificant PDA. In the past, a large left atrium-to-aortic ratio, bulging of the atrial septum from left to right indicating increased left atrial pressure, a dilated left ventricle, and the need for severe fluid restriction and diuresis together with failure of aggressive ventilatory management, were considered sufficient to suggest that the ductus was hemodynamically significant. Studies have determined that conventional echocardiographic markers do not predict outcome or neurodevelopment at 2 years.[101–103] As a result, several studies have used biomarkers, including troponin T, brain natriuretic peptide (BNP), and N-terminal pro-BNP, to distinguish a hemodynamically significant PDA.[104–107] The question remains whether infants undergoing treatment for a hemodynamically significant PDA, as identified by these markers, have improved outcomes compared with peers whose PDAs are identified as significant by conventional methods.[108,109]

Part of the challenge in identifying infants with a significant PDA is that the management approach to these infants remains controversial. The approach to PDA has evaded a one-size management plan and has generated scoring systems aimed at identifying infants whose ductus warrants closure.[108,110] Constriction of the ductus arteriosus in premature infants has been achieved by pharmacologic manipulation using inhibitors of prostaglandin synthesis or by surgical ligation. Permanent closure of the ductus arteriosus requires both effective muscular constriction to block luminal blood flow and anatomic remodeling to prevent later reopening. In the last few years, multiple investigators have looked for ways to determine the appropriate treatment strategy for premature infants with a PDA. To ascertain which patients require treatment, investigators must clearly show a morbidity or mortality risk associated with a PDA in this patient group. Several studies have linked a ductus arteriosus in premature infants with increased risk of chronic lung disease, necrotizing enterocolitis, intraventricular hemorrhage, diminished regional cerebral oxygen saturation,[111,112] and overall poor neurodevelopmental outcome and mortality.[100,111,113,114] Both indomethacin and ibuprofen have been studied extensively, and they have been determined to be equally effective in closing a PDA.[101,106,115] However, confounding the decision to close the duct are additional data from several studies linking treatment with indomethacin to necrotizing enterocolitis, platelet dysfunction, and renal failure, and ibuprofen to pulmonary hypertension and hemorrhage.[111] Although these risks may be acceptable to physicians facing the significant morbidities associated with intraventricular hemorrhage or necrotizing enterocolitis, a Cochrane review demonstrated that administration of indomethacin at less than 24 hours of life, regardless of PDA status, is associated with a reduction in the risk of severe intraventricular hemorrhage but has no impact on mortality or severe developmental disability at 18 to 36 months.[116] As a result, several recent studies have challenged the idea that premature neonates should receive prophylactic treatment. With conservative management, a cohort of infants born before 28 weeks determined that spontaneous ductal closure occurred 73% of the time and that conservative management is feasible.[117] Because of the risk factors and failures associated with medical management, some centers have pursued percutaneous ductal closure in the cardiac catheterization laboratory in instances where conservative management fails.[118] From 2011 until 2015, 747 infants less than 6 kg underwent transcatheter attempt at PDA closure with a 94% success rate. Weight less than 2 kg was associated with higher risk of device embolization and arterial injury.[119] Despite medical, catheter, and surgical options, there remains large center-specific practice variability in the screening and treatment of the preterm infant with a PDA.

EDITORIAL COMMENT: Bixler et al reviewed the changes in patent ductus arteriosus (PDA) diagnosis and treatment from 829,091 infants between 23 and 30 weeks' gestation entered in the Pediatrix Clinical Data Warehouse. The diagnosis of PDA declined from 51% to 38% ($P < .001$), use of indomethacin or ibuprofen decreased from 32% to 18%, and PDA ligation decreased from 8.4% to 2.9% (both $P < .001$).

Several short-term benefits (decreased intraventricular hemorrhage [IVH], pulmonary hemorrhage, and ligation) may result from prophylactic indomethacin or prophylactic treatment of the PDA, but there is little evidence to suggest that delaying treatment for the first few days after birth has any detrimental effects on later morbidities In contrast, there is growing evidence that delaying treatment of a moderate/large PDA beyond the first week may contribute to the development of bronchopulmonary dysplasia (BPD) and BPD/death. (Bixler GM, Powers G, Clark RH, et al. Changes in the diagnosis and management of patent ductus arteriosus from 2006 to 2015 in United States neonatal intensive care units. *J Pediatr.* 2017;108:105.)

Aortopulmonary Window

An aortopulmonary widow is a relatively uncommon communication between the ascending aorta and the pulmonary trunk differing from a truncus because of the presence of two semilunar valves. The defect, although variable in size, is very proximal and, unlike a PDA, does not have length; thus flow is determined simply by the difference in systemic and pulmonary resistances. As a result, a large left-to-right shunt may develop early in life. Classic cardiac examination findings include a systolic murmur with mid-diastolic rumble secondary to increased blood flow across the mitral valve. The electrocardiograph (ECG) typically demonstrates left or biventricular hypertrophy. The classic chest radiographic findings include cardiac enlargement with prominence of pulmonary artery and pulmonary vasculature. Because of the magnitude of the shunting that can occur, these patients are often referred for surgical repair at the time of diagnosis to avoid the development of pulmonary vascular disease.

Combined Shunt Defects

Although an isolated VSD, PDA, or atrial septal defect (ASD) rarely causes symptoms of heart failure in the full-term newborn, combinations of these are more likely to do so. For example, in a term infant with the clinical features of VSD, if cardiac failure and respiratory distress develop in the first week or two of life, an additional shunt or another cardiac or vascular abnormality might be present. In infants beyond the first day of life, it is important to remember that the closing ductus arteriosus may unmask another lesion such as a coarctation or arch interruption that causes an infant in stable condition to abruptly become symptomatic.

Complete Atrioventricular Septal Defect (Endocardial Cushion Defect)

Endocardial cushion defects are composed of atrial and VSDs as well as a common AV valve orifice. Endocardial cushion defects are commonly associated with trisomy 21 and an ECG with left axis deviation. In isolation, these lesions are rarely associated with cardiac failure in the newborn, as shunting is dependent on the fall of PVR. Patients with signs of early failure may have a more complex lesion with associated left-sided heart obstruction, valvular insufficiency, or less commonly, left ventricular-to-right atrial shunting that causes an obligatory shunt (not dependent on PVR).

Truncus Arteriosus

Truncus arteriosus is characterized by a single arterial trunk that arises from the heart and gives rise to the aorta, the pulmonary arteries, and the coronary arteries. It occurs in 1% of cases of congenital heart disease and may be fatal by a mean age of 2.5 months if untreated.[120,121] The pathophysiology is variable, but generally, as PVR falls in the first days of life, torrential pulmonary blood flow ensues, and the patient rapidly develops significant pulmonary overcirculation and symptoms of heart failure, including tachypnea, failure to thrive, feeding difficulties, and sweating. Because of the excessive pulmonary blood flow, infants with truncus arteriosus may present as only minimally cyanotic and frequently develop oxygen saturation levels above 90%. If there is proximal pulmonary artery stenosis, the described clinical presentation may be delayed. In the newborn period, classic physical examination findings include a hyperdynamic precordium, a left precordial bulge, a loud single S_2 with an early systolic ejection click, and a systolic ejection murmur along the left sternal border. If the truncal valve is insufficient, an early diastolic decrescendo murmur may be noted at left midsternal border accompanied by signs of heart failure immediately after birth. As pulmonary blood flow increases, the patient develops a wide pulse pressure and bounding pulses because of continuous diastolic flow into the pulmonary arteries and an apical rumble from increased flow across the mitral valve. The ECG frequently demonstrates right, left, or biventricular hypertrophy and should be used to rule out the unusual scenario of myocardial ischemia. Medical management can be extremely challenging if there is no obstruction to pulmonary blood flow and is focused on alleviating symptoms with diuresis, inotropic support to augment cardiac output, and ventilatory support until the patient can undergo definitive surgical repair. Mortality in the first year of life may be higher than 80% without repair.[121] Thus early identification of neonates with truncus arteriosus can be critical to their long-term survival.

Total Anomalous Pulmonary Venous Return

In total anomalous pulmonary venous return (TAPVR), also known as *total anomalous pulmonary venous connection,* both systemic and pulmonary venous flows return to the right atrium, where they mix. There is an obligate right-to-left shunt across the atrial septum that is the only preload to the left side of the heart and provides the systemic cardiac output. Oxygen saturations in all cardiac chambers are identical and are determined by the relative amount of pulmonary blood flow. TAPVR types are classified according to the manner in which blood from the confluence returns to the heart: supracardiac (~50% of cases), cardiac (~25%), infradiaphragmatic (~15%), and mixed (~10%). The location of the defect and the degree of obstruction dictates the presentation of an infant with TAPVR.

The majority of infants with unobstructed venous return have a dramatic increase in pulmonary blood flow as vascular resistances fall over the weeks after birth. As a result, it is not uncommon for pulmonary blood flow to be three or more times that of the preserved systemic circulation. As a result, oxygen saturation percentages are typically in the upper 80s and low 90s, and there is no clinically apparent cyanosis. Instead, these infants manifest tachypnea, poor feeding, repeated "respiratory infections," failure to thrive, and clinical signs of heart failure. On physical examination, there is a prominent right ventricular impulse, a widely split S_2 with an accentuated pulmonary component, and an S_3 gallop. There may be a systolic murmur along the left upper sternal border, reflective of increased pulmonary blood flow across the pulmonic valve and relative pulmonary stenosis. The ECG characteristically demonstrates a tall, peaked P wave in lead II, right axis deviation, and right ventricular hypertrophy. The chest radiograph shows signs of increased pulmonary blood flow with enlarged right atrium and ventricle, prominent pulmonary artery, and in the case of supracardiac veins draining into the left innominate vein, the "snowman sign" created by the large supracardiac shadow.

Obstructed TAVPR, which is more common in the infradiaphragmatic type, manifests after the first 6 hours of life with progressive increased work of breathing, feeding failure, and cardiorespiratory collapse. The differential diagnosis at the time of presentation often includes PPHN, RDS, pneumonia, pulmonary lymphangiectasia, meconium aspiration, and hypoplastic left heart syndrome. Cardiovascular findings are minimal. The right ventricular impulse is not increased, and S_2 is normally split. There may be a soft blowing murmur in the pulmonic area, but the remainder of the cardiac examination yields normal finding. Hepatomegaly is almost always present. The ECG demonstrates right ventricular hypertrophy with qR in V_3R but may be without tall, spiked P waves. The chest radiograph demonstrates pulmonary venous obstruction with diffuse densities in a reticular pattern fanning out from the hilum and obscuring the cardiac borders. The heart is not enlarged. Infants with this defect must be symptomatically supported until a cardiac surgeon is available. Most undergo surgical repair within a few hours of diagnosis. All children with very severe respiratory distress who are candidates for extracorporeal support should undergo echocardiography before initiation of support. The presentations of severe meconium aspiration lung disease and severe obstruction in TAPVR are similar and easily confused. This form of TAPVR remains one of the few cardiac surgical emergencies in the newborn.

The most severe form of anomalous venous return is complete atresia of the common pulmonary vein with no definitive egress of blood from the lungs. These infants become profoundly cyanotic immediately after birth and have markedly diminished pulmonary blood flow. There are no significant cardiac examination findings, and the chest radiograph demonstrates severe venous obstruction. Most infants with atretic pulmonary veins die within a few days of life.

Additional Defects

Interference with inflow to the left ventricle, as in congenital mitral stenosis or cor triatriatum, may lead to severe pulmonary venous congestion and respiratory distress but may not compromise systemic perfusion in the newborn period. Congenital mitral stenosis may be related to parachute mitral valve or double-orifice mitral valve with chordae that are shortened and deformed and valve leaflets that are thickened and dysplastic. Infants are typically small with growth failure and have wheezing and dyspnea. The cardiac examination demonstrates a rumbling diastolic murmur with an opening snap. Chest radiograph demonstrates left atrial enlargement and pulmonary venous congestion. Infants with cor triatriatum have a similar presentation and in many instances have been diagnosed as having chronic lung disease and have undergone treatment for many months before a congenital cardiac malformation is suspected.

Cyanotic Heart Disease

Central cyanosis indicates reduced arterial blood oxygen saturation and is generally visible when the level of reduced hemoglobin in the blood exceeds 5 g/dL. The typical picture of the infant with cyanotic heart disease is the development of cyanosis in the first few hours of life, which may be noted initially only with crying or feeding, and the absence of respiratory distress. As the ductus arteriosus begins to close, the cyanosis may become progressively more obvious.

There are two major subgroups of lesions that feature cyanosis as the primary finding: (1) lesions with obstruction to pulmonary blood flow, and (2) lesions with normal or increased pulmonary blood flow but with separation of the pulmonary venous return from the systemic arterial circulation. In both subgroups, effective pulmonary blood flow is low. The differential diagnosis of these infants includes mild pulmonary disease, PPHN, abnormalities of the central nervous system, and methemoglobinemia. The initial evaluation usually directs the physician to strongly suspect cardiac disease. The history of the cyanotic infant with heart disease is generally benign and the pregnancy and delivery uneventful. In contrast, the infant with PPHN often has a history of perinatal distress or meconium aspiration. An exception in the cardiac group is tricuspid insufficiency resulting from myocardial ischemia, in which a history of perinatal asphyxia is common. Additional testing may be beneficial in differentiating pulmonary and cardiac abnormalities. Simultaneous upper- and lower-extremity pulse oximetry measurements can be diagnostic. If the oxygen saturation in the upper body is lower than that in the lower body, the infant most likely has dextro-transposition with pulmonary hypertension or coarctation of the aorta. In contrast, infants with PPHN have elevated PVR, and the ductus arteriosus, if patent, shows right-to-left ductal shunting with subsequent lowering of the blood oxygen saturation or Po_2 in the descending aorta. Chest radiographs taken in the first few days of life usually show normal heart size. Most cyanotic lesions are associated with either a diminutive pulmonary artery (e.g., pulmonary atresia) or one that is transposed to the right; thus the normal pulmonary artery contour at the upper left region of the cardiac silhouette is absent. In addition, the aortic arch should be visualized because the aorta may descend to the right of the spine in right-sided obstructive lesions (especially if associated with DiGeorge syndrome). Finally, an attempt should be made to evaluate the pulmonary vascularity. Although assessment of pulmonary vascularity radiographically depends on the quality of the image and lung expansion, if there are diminished markings on a good-quality radiograph with normally inflated lungs in the absence of PPHN, there is almost always heart disease.

If the patient is not at a facility where echocardiography can be performed, immediate transfer is mandatory. Stabilization before the transport is of utmost importance: metabolic requirements must be reduced to a minimum to provide adequate substrate delivery, and if oxygen delivery is borderline (measured blood oxygen saturation is ≤80%, Po_2 is ≤30 to 35 mm Hg, or metabolic acidosis is present), prostaglandin E_1 infusion started at 0.02 μg/kg/min and increased to 0.04 μg/kg/min should be initiated. Prostaglandin E_1 effectively dilates the ductus arteriosus to provide adequate pulmonary or systemic blood flow, and the infant's condition can then be stabilized and carefully evaluated if a duct-dependent lesion is present. It is appropriate to administer prostaglandin E_1 to any infant in whom the diagnosis of cyanotic congenital heart disease is strongly suspected, even before a complete evaluation is performed. Prostaglandin E_1 has well-defined side effects, such as apnea, jitteriness or even frank seizures, hypotension with peripheral vasodilatation, and a possible increased risk of infection that should be expected by the treating physician. Fluid administration may be necessary after initiation of prostaglandin E_1 treatment to maintain the arterial blood pressure if there is significant systemic vasodilatation, and intubation may be necessary if significant apnea occurs.

Abnormalities of the Tricuspid Valve

Tricuspid atresia is a complete mixing lesion. Because of the atretic valve, there is no outlet from the right atrium except across the patent foramen ovale to the left atrium. Blood flow reaches the right ventricle via a VSD that is typically unrestrictive in the neonate. Tricuspid atresia may be associated with normally related or transposed great arteries, and saturations and blood flow depend on the relationship of the great arteries, the size of the VSD, and the presence or absence of semilunar valve stenosis. If pulmonary blood flow is unobstructed, patients may have tachypnea and early heart failure with minimal to no cyanosis. The physical examination is significant for an increased left ventricular impulse (in contrast to other cyanotic heart diseases with increased right ventricular impulses). Depending on the anatomy, the second heart sound may be single (with atresia of one of the great arteries), normal (in normally related great arteries), or diminished (in transposed great arteries). A murmur may or may not be present depending on restriction of blood flow through the VSD and the semilunar valves. The ECG may demonstrate left axis deviation and right atrial enlargement. Echocardiography should be performed and, in addition to confirming the diagnosis, will concentrate on assessing the stability of the circulation in the absence of a PDA.

Ebstein anomaly of the tricuspid valve is characterized by the downward displacement of the valve leaflets into the right ventricular cavity. The severity of disease is often dependent on the degree of displacement and the ability of the remaining portion of the right ventricle to generate sufficient force to eject blood into the pulmonary vessels. Newborns may have massive cardiomegaly, marked cyanosis, holosystolic murmurs, a gallop rhythm, hydrops, and pulmonary artery hypoplasia. The ECG will demonstrate right atrial hypertrophy, and there may be associated Wolff-Parkinson-White (WPW) syndrome (short PR interval and a delta wave). The chest radiograph frequently demonstrates significant cardiomegaly, or "wall-to-wall heart." Infants with severe disease will require prostaglandin to maintain pulmonary blood flow until PVR has fallen and the adequacy of the right ventricle and pulmonary valve can be assessed. Many cardiologists adopt a "watch and wait" strategy with these infants in an effort to avoid early surgical intervention and the associated mortality.

Abnormalities of the Right Ventricular Outflow Tract

Tetralogy of Fallot is the signature lesion associated with cyanosis because of decreased pulmonary blood flow. The symptoms and presentation depend on the degree of subpulmonary or pulmonary valve obstruction. Infants with mild obstruction may manifest primarily symptoms of heart failure from the large VSD. Other infants may have severe cyanosis on closure of the ductus arteriosus. "Tet spells" may be associated with vigorous crying—infants are initially hyperpneic and restless with increasing cyanosis. The murmur becomes softer and may disappear entirely during a spell because of the lack of pulmonary blood flow. If untreated, the infant may have a syncopal episode. Treatment for an acute spell involves knee-to-chest positioning, oxygen supplementation, sedation, and/or analgesia, administration of beta-blockers, and surgical repair to provide a consistent form of pulmonary blood flow.

In cases of absent pulmonary valve syndrome, the hemodynamic pattern is similar to that in tetralogy of Fallot, but there is often severe respiratory distress. The massively dilated pulmonary arteries that are present in this syndrome compress the airways and cause respiratory embarrassment.

Pulmonary atresia with a VSD is a more severe form of tetralogy of Fallot that presents with severe cyanosis shortly after birth. The infant with pulmonary atresia and VSD lacks the prominent pulmonary murmur present in tetralogy of Fallot. The S_1 may be associated with an ejection click secondary to a dilated aortic root. If the patient has additional pulmonary blood flow in the form of collateral vessels from the descending aorta (which may be identified by continuous murmurs auscultated over the patient's back), the infant may have a stable form of pulmonary blood flow. All other infants require treatment with PGE_2. The ultimate surgical treatment depends on the presence or absence of the native pulmonary arteries and their size.

Neonates with pulmonary atresia with an intact ventricular septum have severe cyanosis that progresses as the ductus arteriosus closes. The S_2 is single and loud. Often there are no other murmurs (or a continuous murmur from the ductus). This defect is dependent on the ductus for pulmonary blood flow. Because of the high-pressure right ventricle, there may be associated coronary artery abnormalities that affect whether surgical palliation via the single ventricle route or orthotopic heart transplantation is recommended.

Transposition of the Great Arteries

Infants with TGA show severe cyanosis immediately after birth. Left untreated, these infants rapidly progress from cyanosis to tissue hypoxemia, acidosis, and, if the disorder is unrecognized, death. Unlike infants with other cyanotic congenital heart lesions, these infants have a normal volume of blood passing through the pulmonary bed. However, because the heart is arranged in parallel, infants with TGA have very low effective pulmonary blood flow (deoxygenated blood from the systemic circulation that reaches the pulmonary bed) and effective systemic blood flow (oxygenated blood that perfuses the systemic bed). The degree of mixing between the separate circulations depends on the number and size of the anatomic connections. Blood may shunt at the atrial, ventricular (if a VSD is present), or ductal level. The typical infant with TGA and an intact ventricular septum becomes progressively more hypoxemic as the ductus arteriosus closes secondary to inadequate mixing at the foramen ovale. Frequently, these infants are given prostaglandin E_1 until the atrial communication can be enlarged. Although it is unusual to have sufficient mixing at the ductal level, the increased pulmonary blood flow provided by the PDA dilates the left atrium, which allows a larger anatomic left-to-right shunt across the stretched foramen ovale and increased systemic oxygen delivery. Often, this is sufficient to avoid acidosis and tissue oxygen debt. Frequently, however, patients with TGA will undergo balloon atrial septostomy either in the cardiac catheterization laboratory or at the bedside. Clinically, the infant with TGA is likely to be male and appear cyanotic but healthy, with a weight appropriate for gestational age. Auscultatory findings may be unremarkable except for a single loud S_2. A nonspecific systolic murmur may be present. Reverse differential cyanosis is rare but is indicative of TGA with a PDA and an associated aortic arch abnormality or pulmonary hypertension. ECG findings may vary considerably, with findings of the initial study often normal for age. In the neonate with TGA and an intact ventricular septum, the chest radiograph may demonstrate a narrowed superior mediastinum with an egg-shaped cardiac silhouette ("egg on a string"), mild cardiomegaly, and increased pulmonary vascular markings. Surgical repair (arterial switch operation) is often undertaken in the first week of life, and most patients are expected to survive to adulthood and lead a normal life.

In summary, an infant with cyanosis and little respiratory distress usually has cardiac disease and requires prompt evaluation and stabilization. When the initial evaluation cannot exclude cardiac disease, it is important to proceed with a complete cardiovascular evaluation. With the dramatic improvements in neonatal surgery and the advent of prostaglandin E_1 therapy, infants with cyanotic heart disease are now expected to survive to lead a more normal life.

Systemic Hypoperfusion

The third common type of presentation of critical heart disease in the newborn is shock because of hypoperfusion. Hypoperfusion is secondary to inadequate ejection of blood into the systemic arterial system, resulting in hypotension and progressive metabolic acidosis. This typically occurs as the ductus arteriosus constricts in a patient with a ductal-dependent systemic circulation but may also be found in infants with lesions in which the function of the left ventricle is seriously impaired without underlying obstruction. The course may be rapidly progressive over the first few hours of life or insidious in onset over the first few weeks. Cardiac lesions in this category include functional abnormalities of the left ventricle such as endocardial fibroelastosis, dilated cardiomyopathy, hypertrophic cardiomyopathy, left ventricular noncompaction, left ventricular outflow tract obstruction, aortic valve stenosis, interruption of the aortic arch, coarctation of the aorta, Shone complex, and hypoplastic left heart syndrome. Systemic hypoperfusion may also be caused by arrhythmias that severely decrease cardiac output in the neonate. Hypoperfusion syndromes often have associated findings, including lethargy, a mottled appearance with pallor and poor pulses, and a degree of systemic arterial desaturation caused by mixing of systemic and pulmonary venous return, and most are associated with respiratory distress secondary to elevated PVPs.

The differential diagnosis of primary noncardiac hypoperfusion is broad and includes sepsis, adrenal insufficiency, anemia, hypovolemia, inborn errors of metabolism, and neurologic instability. In practice, all of these typically have a component of poor cardiac function that improves as the underlying disease is correctly diagnosed and treated. While working toward a unifying diagnosis for a hypoperfused state, it is important to consider conditions that are most life-threatening if missed. The most frequent misdiagnosis in an infant with heart disease and hypoperfusion is sepsis. Because overwhelming infection is associated with high mortality, it is reasonable to perform a workup for sepsis and even begin specific therapy in any infant with signs of low output, but it is important to consider cardiac disease as well. The most important decision immediately following the diagnosis of left-sided heart disease is to determine whether the left ventricle can sustain systemic cardiac output. If there is any question, the infant should receive prostaglandin therapy to ensure continued patency of the ductus arteriosus until a more thorough assessment can be made.

The history can help distinguish between cardiac and noncardiac disease and differentiate among the specific cardiac lesions. In general, the timing of presentation depends on the role of the ductus and the timing of its closure. There is sometimes a history of perinatal problems. A history of recent viral infection in the mother may be elicited in infants with myocarditis. Fetal hydrops occurs in intrauterine SVT, cardiomyopathy, premature closure of the foramen ovale, and, on rare occasions, aortic stenosis or hypoplastic left heart syndrome. Maternal diabetes suggests diabetic cardiomyopathy, and a familial history might suggest other forms of cardiomyopathy.

The physical examination uniformly shows a pale, tachypneic, and lethargic infant. It is critical to differentiate sinus tachycardia in a severely stressed infant from an underlying conduction disturbance resulting in poor function. Some arrhythmias may be easily distinguished on telemetry, although a full 12-lead ECG should be obtained to confirm the diagnosis and guide treatment. Peripheral pulses are decreased in low-output states, but a differential pulse or blood pressure between the upper and lower extremities can be diagnostic. In patients with obstruction along the aortic arch or descending aorta (i.e., interrupted aortic arch or coarctation of the aorta), the lower limb pressures will be low in the absence of a nonrestrictive ductus arteriosus. It is important to realize that the left subclavian artery frequently arises at the origin of the coarctation and thus should not be used to represent ascending aortic pressures in coarctation (Fig. 14.23). Similarly, the right subclavian artery may arise aberrantly from the descending aorta in 0.5% to 2% of the population, which makes assessment of the ascending aorta difficult.[122] However, a difference in intensity between the carotid or temporal artery pulse and the extremity pulses can be a clue to this diagnosis. The precordial impulse is often nonspecific, usually showing a right ventricular heave. The S_2 is single in hypoplastic left heart syndrome, but because of the tachycardia in low-output states, it is often difficult to appreciate a split sound in any of the lesions. Murmurs rarely help the diagnosis in this group: in the presence of severe heart failure, most lesions are not associated with murmurs or have nonspecific ones. Coarctation of the aorta in which a VSD or subaortic stenosis is present is an exception, but critical aortic stenosis may be associated with little or no murmur when the left ventricular output is low. Rales are heard in most low-output states as a result of elevated PVPs.

Arterial blood gas values often indicate a metabolic acidosis at the time of diagnosis. Differential pulse oximetry measurements between the right hand and foot may be helpful. In coarctation or interruption of the aorta, the saturation in the foot will be lower if the ductus is patent because there will be right-to-left shunting from the pulmonary artery to the descending aorta. Conversely, if the saturation is higher in the descending aorta, transposition with PPHN or transposition with interrupted arch should be considered. The chest radiographic study often shows cardiomegaly and interstitial edema in both cardiac and noncardiac lesions once there is severe heart failure, and thus is not useful for diagnosis. The ECG is helpful in identifying several lesions. For example, left-sided forces are absent in hypoplastic left heart syndrome (Fig. 14.24A); the regular rapid heart rate of SVT is diagnostic; there are signs of an anterolateral ischemia or infarction in an anomalous left coronary artery (Fig. 14.24B); endocardial fibroelastosis is characterized by prominent Q and R waves in the precordial leads; there usually is marked right ventricular hypertrophy in coarctation of the aorta or critical aortic stenosis; ST-T wave abnormalities are present in myocarditis. The echocardiogram is diagnostic in the obstructive lesions; however, occasionally an isolated aortic coarctation can be masked after the administration of prostaglandin E_1 because the presence of a large PDA decreases the flow through the area. Also, in some patients, ductal tissue wraps around the aorta (so-called *ductal sling)*, causing the obstruction when it contracts and the ductus arteriosus closes. This area can be dilated by administration of prostaglandin E_1, which makes diagnosis problematic in its presence. The echocardiogram is also useful in assessing ventricular performance and the response to therapeutic interventions.

Therapy must be prompt. Once deterioration begins, it is usually rapidly progressive. Initial measures must be directed at the metabolic derangements: partial correction of the metabolic acidosis; maintenance of adequate substrate, hemoglobin, and blood volume; and prompt inotropic support with rapidly acting agents such as dopamine or epinephrine. Prostaglandin E_1 administration is of utmost importance when obstructive lesions are considered; maintaining ductal patency ensures that the lower body will be perfused with

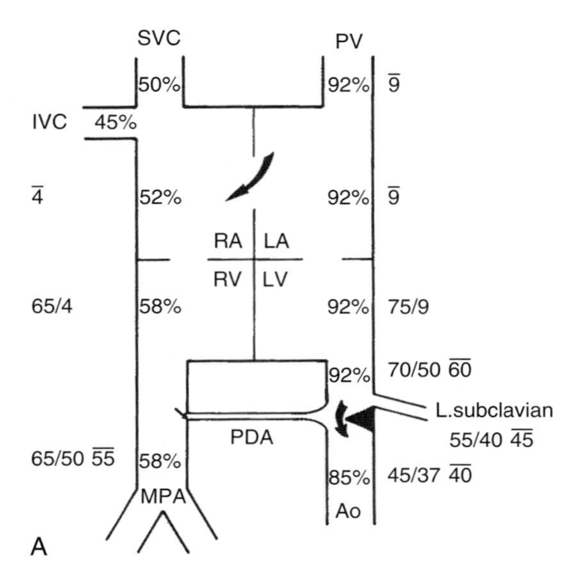

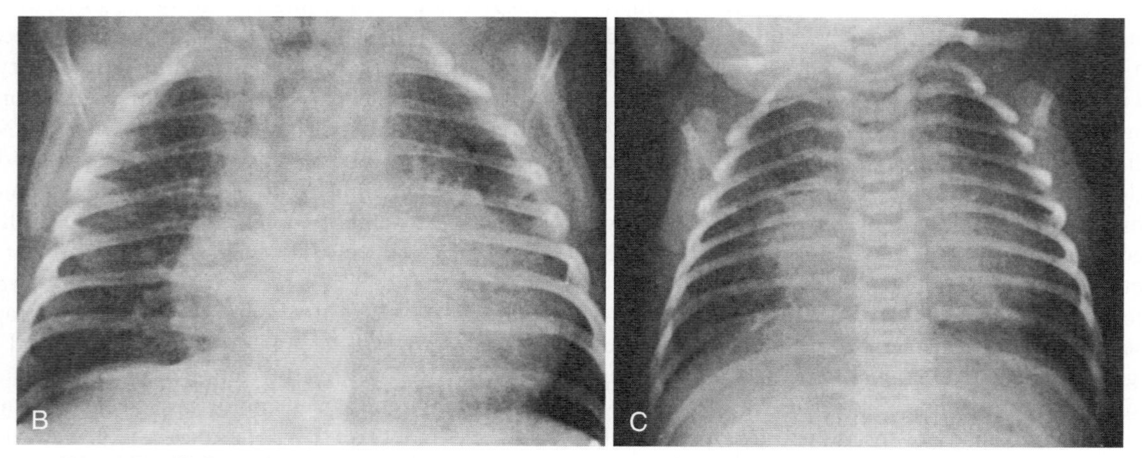

Fig. 14.23 (A) Representative blood oxygen saturation (%) and pressure (mm Hg) in an infant with coarctation of the aorta. (B) Chest radiograph of an infant with coarctation of the aorta. (C) Chest radiograph of an infant with hypoplastic left heart syndrome. Chest radiographs usually cannot differentiate between left-sided obstructive lesions. *Ao,* Aorta; *IVC,* inferior vena cava; *LA,* left atrium; *LV,* left ventricle; *MPA,* main pulmonary artery; *PDA,* patent ductus arteriosus; *PV,* pulmonary vein; *RA,* right atrium; *RV,* right ventricle; *SVC,* superior vena cava.

blood ejected from the right ventricle through the pulmonary artery. The entire body can be perfused by this route in critical aortic stenosis and hypoplastic left heart syndrome. In left ventricular obstructive lesions, the infant can be maintained on prostaglandin E_1 before surgery. If the diagnosis is in doubt, antibiotics should be instituted after a sepsis workup, and corticosteroids should be considered if adrenal insufficiency is a possibility.

EDITORIAL COMMENT: Sudden collapse with hypotension and acidosis in a term infant requires prompt evaluation and intervention. As noted above, it is imperative to rule out sepsis, often viral infections, critical cardiac lesions, and inherited metabolic disorders. Careful examination with four-extremity blood pressure measurements, blood and viral cultures, blood gases, serum ammonia, echocardiogram, chest x-ray, and ECG are all essential components of the initial evaluation.

ARRHYTHMIAS IN THE NEONATE

Neonatal Arrhythmias

Neonatal arrhythmias are not infrequent, but the clinical significance can vary greatly depending on the diagnosis, which can be difficult, especially distinguishing sinus tachycardia from tachyarrhythmias. Neonatal arrhythmias occur in 1% to 5% of newborns during the first 10 days of life.[123] Neonatal arrhythmias can be classified using various schemes, including origin of focus, bradycardia versus tachycardia, and benign versus nonbenign. No single scheme encompasses all aspects of arrhythmias, and often, an expanded classification system must be used. Below we address the various arrhythmias encountered in the neonate.

Extrasystoles

Premature atrial contractions (PACs) and ventricular contractions (PVCs) are also common findings in the fetal

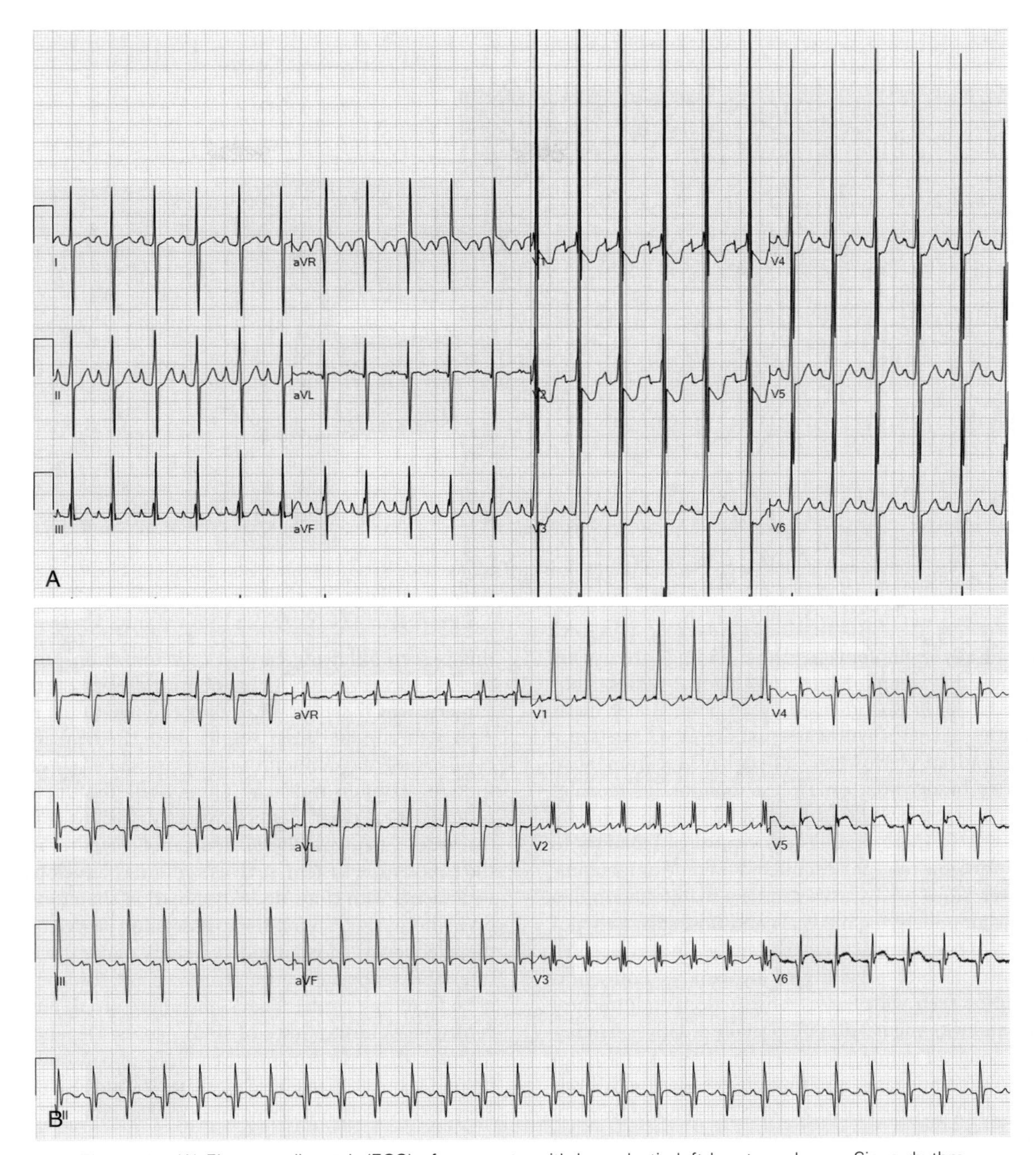

Fig. 14.24 (A) Electrocardiograph (ECG) of a neonate with hypoplastic left heart syndrome. Sinus rhythm with right atrial enlargement and right ventricular hypertrophy. (B) ECG in anomalous left coronary artery from the pulmonary artery (ALCAPA) with prominent Q waves in lead V6.

and newborn period, with PACs being the most common arrhythmia seen in the neonatal period. PACs can be normally conducted, aberrantly conducted, or blocked (Fig. 14.25). Distinguishing between PACs and PVCs can prove difficult for various reasons. The P wave can be superimposed on the preceding T wave, QRS prolongation can be subtle in the newborn, and aberrantly conducted PACs are common. Blocked PACs may mimic sinus bradycardia when atrial bigeminy is present and the P waves are superimposed on the antecedent T wave. These extrasystoles rarely produce symptoms and become less frequent with time. In patients with central venous lines, it is important to ensure that the catheter is not producing right atrial mechanical irritation resulting in PACs. In this case, withdrawal of the catheter from the right atrium should result in termination of the arrhythmia.

Sinus Bradycardia, Sinus Pauses, and Junctional Escape Beats

Sinus bradycardia, sinus pauses, and junctional escape beats are very common findings in neonates, reported in 19% to 90% of infants.[124] However, this is likely an underestimation, as only hospitalized infants are monitored; these patients are

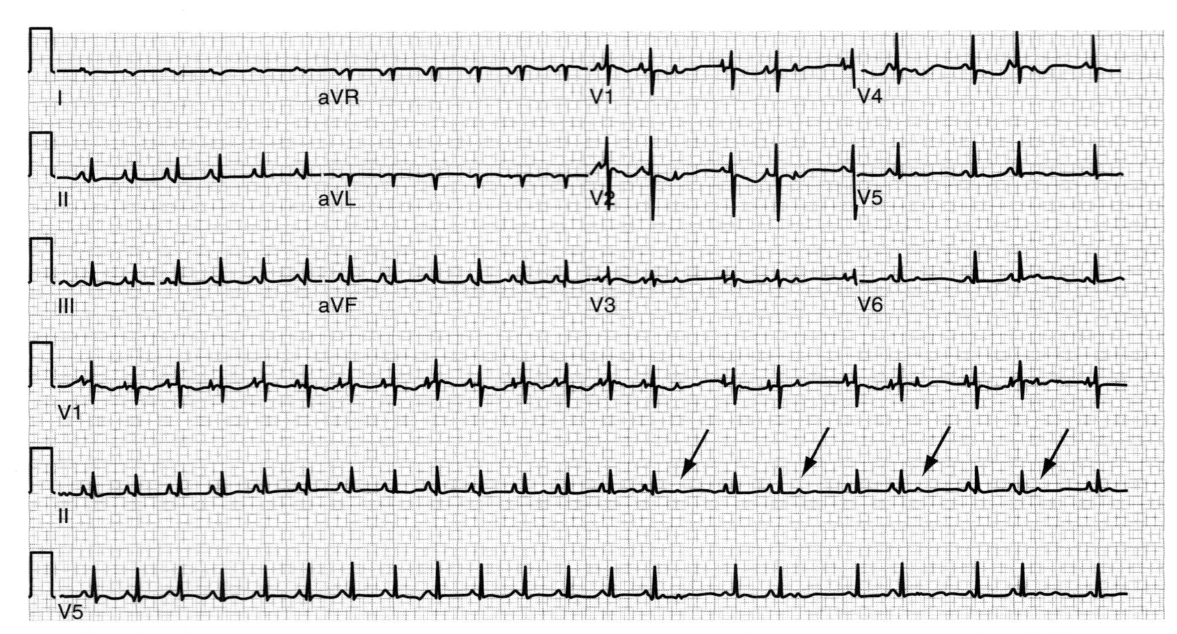

Fig. 14.25 Sinus rhythm with blocked premature atrial contractions in an asymptomatic 1 day old. Sinus rhythm preceding atrial trigeminy. Solid arrows indicate blocked premature atrial contractions.

almost universally asymptomatic. These findings are usually transient and rarely symptomatic. In previous studies, sinus bradycardia has been documented by 24-hour Holter monitor in healthy neonates with rates as low as 42 beats per minute while asleep.[124] However, others have recommended defining sinus bradycardia on Holter monitor in neonates as 60 beats per minute while asleep and 80 beats per minute while awake.[125,126] These findings are typically secondary to increased autonomic tone and require no therapy or intervention. However, sinus bradycardia can be a manifestation of a more significant underlying medical condition, such as hypothyroidism, hypoglycemia, hyperkalemia, hypercalcemia, increased intracerebral pressure, or hypoxia.[127] Sinus bradycardia can be seen with airway obstruction, endotracheal intubation, and with medications, especially sedatives. Finally, infants with long QT syndrome have been shown to have significantly slower sinus rates, and thus any neonate with sinus bradycardia should be evaluated for long QT syndrome.[128]

Treatment for sinus bradycardia is usually directed toward the underlying etiology. However, in symptomatic infants, temporary chronotropic and inotropic support may be warranted and can be achieved pharmacologically utilizing various drugs, including isoproterenol, epinephrine, and atropine. Temporary pacing is rarely necessary, and efforts should remain focused on addressing the underlying etiology.

Sinus Node Dysfunction

Sinus node dysfunction can be secondary to direct injury to the sinus node or intrinsic sinus node disease. Sinus node dysfunction often manifests as slow resting heart rates, decreased heart rate variability, decreased peak heart rate, and prolonged sinus pauses. True congenital sinus node dysfunction, either with or without structural heart disease, is rare and is most likely secondary to sodium channelopathies.[129] More often, this is seen following cardiac catheterization procedures or cardiac surgery, such as balloon atrial septostomy or ASD surgery, which can result in direct injury to the sinus node. Although surgery often results in permanent dysfunction, cardiac catheterization procedure–associated sinus node dysfunction is often transient. Sinus node dysfunction can be acquired as seen in cardiomyopathy, various inflammatory diseases (e.g., myocarditis), and genetic syndromes affecting the conduction system, such as sodium channelopathies.

Patients with sinus node dysfunction should be evaluated by 24-hour Holter monitor to assess for degree of bradycardia, frequency and duration of sinus pauses, average heart rate, and associated atrial tachycardias. Escape beats can arise from any cardiac focus, including atrial, junctional, or ventricular, during times of sinus pauses. Depending on the findings, these patients may benefit from pacemaker implantation. Associated atrial tachycardias should also be appropriately treated with antiarrhythmic medications.

Atrioventricular Block

First-Degree Atrioventricular Block

First-degree AV block, also called first-degree heart block, is defined as a PR interval greater than the upper limit of normal for a patient's age. The PR interval upper limit of normal in the first 24 hours of life is 160 msec and 140 msec at 1 month of age, although this is variable during the first month of life and continues to vary throughout childhood.[130] The PR interval can be prolonged because of delay in conduction from the sinus node through the atrium, from the atrium to depolarization of the bundle of His, or from depolarization from the bundle of His to initiation of ventricular depolarization. First-degree AV block is typically caused by delayed conduction at the level of the AV node. First-degree AV block may be associated with congenital heart disease or may be secondary to an inflammatory process, such as viral myocarditis. Various autoimmune inflammatory disorders, muscular dystrophies, trauma, and pharmacologic therapies (including tricyclic antidepressants, clonidine, and digoxin) can cause a prolonged PR, but these are rare in neonates. First-degree AV block is often considered a normal variant and does not produce symptoms. No therapy is typically indicated.

Second-Degree AV Block (Type I and Type II)

Second-degree AV block is present when there is intermittent failure to conduct atrial impulses to the ventricular conduction system. Second-degree AV block can be further subclassified into Mobitz type I (Wenckebach) and Mobitz type II block. Mobitz type I is defined by progressive lengthening of the PR interval with eventual loss of conduction to the ventricle of one beat. The PR interval of the subsequent conducted atrial impulse is always shorter than the PR interval of the last conducted ventricular beat. Mobitz type II is defined by abrupt failure to conduct one or more atrial impulses to ventricles without preceding PR prolongation. This block is typically occurs below the AV node and can progress acutely to complete heart block.[131] The pattern of type II second-degree AV block can be regular and is described as 2:1, 3:1, and so on. High-grade second-degree AV block is considered 3:1 or higher. This differs from complete heart block by the presence of R-R interval variation or R-R intervals that are multiples of the atrial cycle length.

Type I second-degree AV block is often considered a normal variant and can be seen during periods of sleep in older children. Etiologies of type I second-degree heart block are similar to those of first-degree heart block. High-grade second-degree heart block has a variety of causes, only a handful of which are seen in the neonatal period, including viral myocarditis, tuberous sclerosis, cardiac surgery, cerebral edema, and certain medications such as antiarrhythmics and digoxin. High-degree second-degree AV block may also be associated with congenital heart disease, typically AV septal defects, l-TGA, and left atrial isomerism in patients with heterotaxy syndrome. High-grade AV block may also be caused by mutations in the cardiac transcription factors *TBX5* and *NKX2.5*.[132–134]

Therapy is not necessary for Mobitz type I or asymptomatic Mobitz type II second-degree heart block. The mainstay of therapy for patients with symptomatic high-grade heart block is pacemaker implantation, which will be discussed below with complete AV block.

Third-Degree or Complete AV block

Third-degree or complete AV block is characterized by a complete lack of conduction of atrial impulses to the ventricles (Fig. 14.26). The P-P intervals are typically constant on electrocardiogram, although they can display some variability as a result of respirations and vagal tone. The R-R intervals are fixed as well, with no association to the P waves. As opposed to surgical complete heart block, congenital complete heart

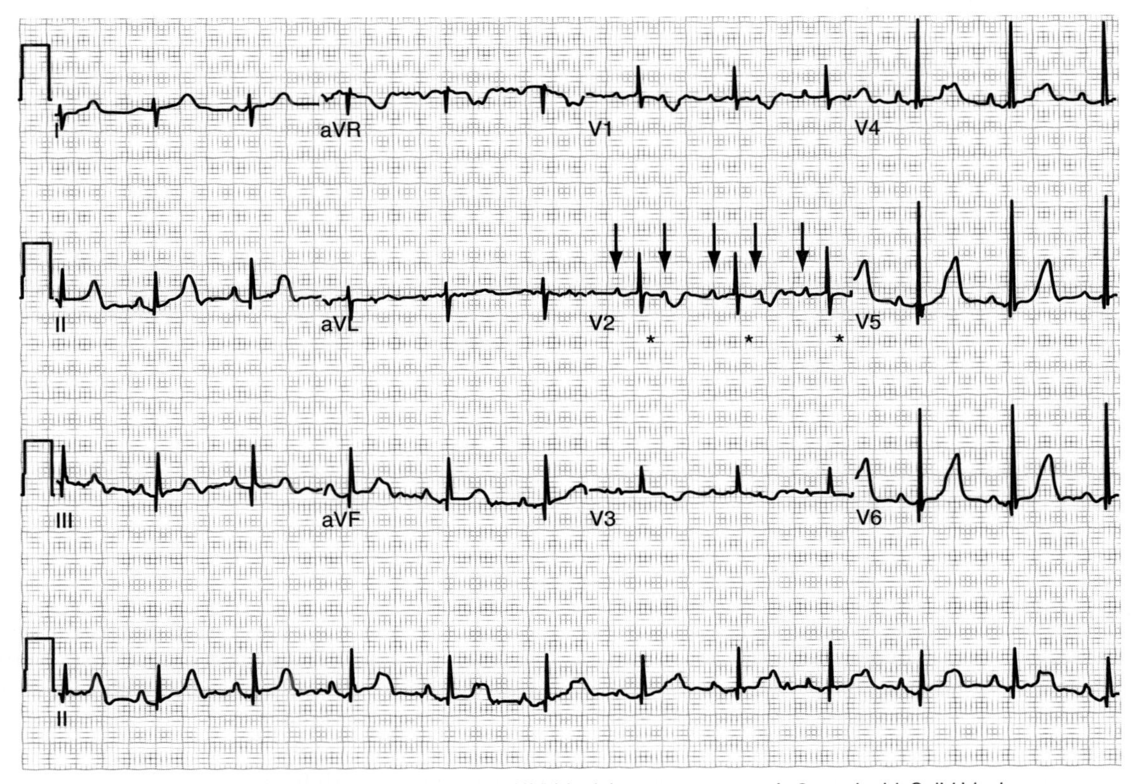

Fig. 14.26 Congenital complete atrioventricular (AV) block in an asymptomatic 3 week old. Solid black arrows indicate underlying atrial rate of 167 beats per minute. Asterisks (*) denote narrow complex junctional escape rhythm with rate of 83 beats per minute.

block can display some variability in the escape rhythm, depending on the physiologic conditions.

Complete AV block occurs in ~1 of every 20,000 pregnancies.[135] Major etiologies of complete AV block include autoimmune complete AV block secondary to maternal antibodies and congenital anatomical abnormalities. In 91% of affected neonates, complete AV block is secondary to neonatal lupus erythematosus.[136] This is secondary to transplacental passage of maternal anti-Ro/SSA and/or anti-La/SSB antibodies—autoantibodies often seen in mothers with systemic lupus erythematosus (SLE) and Sjögren syndrome. In this entity, complete AV block is thought to be a result of an immune-mediated inflammatory cascade resulting in fetal myocardial fibrosis and thus complete heart block. It is important to recognize that the mother may be completely asymptomatic and the birth of an affected neonate may be the initial sign of maternal SLE. After an initially affected child, the risk of subsequent children with complete AV block is up to 25%. Anatomical abnormalities have been reported in 14% to 42% of cases, including AV septal defects, left atrial isomerism, and TGA.[137]

Although complete heart block is the most concerning electrocardiographic finding in neonatal lupus erythematosus, these infants and neonates can display first- and second-degree AV block as well. Neonates can manifest heart block as early as 16 to 18 weeks' gestation, and first-degree heart block can rapidly progress to complete heart block. The fetus with complete AV block can present with *hydrops fetalis*, and the fetal mortality rate ranges from 15% to 30%.[55] The mortality during the first year of life because of dilated cardiomyopathy is 12% to 41%.[56] Thus efforts have focused on early identification via fetal echocardiography to identify those infants with early, low-grade heart block. The use of fluorinated steroids, that is, betamethasone or dexamethasone, are not metabolized by the placenta and have been shown to prevent progression of first-degree AV block to complete heart block in fetuses of mothers with anti-Ro/SSA and/or anti-La/SSB antibodies.[55,56]

Although congenital complete heart block is universally irreversible once present, postoperative AV block may be transient or persistent. Although older studies have recommended waiting 10 to 14 days for return of AV conduction, more recent reports suggest that AV conduction is unlikely to return after 7 to 8 days. Current guidelines recommend delaying pacemaker implantation for 7 days from surgery to evaluate for return on AV conduction.[138]

After delivery, all neonates with complete heart block or known exposure to maternal autoantibodies deserve electrocardiographic evaluation. All patients with high-grade second-degree AV block or complete AV block ultimately will require permanent pacemaker implantation. Based on current guidelines from the American College of Cardiology, the American Heart Association, and the Heart Rhythm Society, current class I indications for permanent pacing in neonates with congenital complete AV block include: (1) congenital third-degree AV block with a wide QRS escape rhythm, complex ventricular ectopy, or ventricular dysfunction; (2) congenital third-degree AV block in the infant with a ventricular rate less than 55 beats per minute; and (3) congenital third-degree AV block with congenital heart disease and a ventricular rate less than 70 beats per minute. Class IIb indications for these neonates include asymptomatic neonates with congenital third-degree AV block with an acceptable rate, narrow QRS complex, and normal function.[138]

Prolonged QT

A prolonged QT interval is general considered greater than 460 msec. However, it is important to correct the QT interval for heart rate. This is termed the *QTc*, and it can be determined by several formulas but is generally calculated using Bazett's formula:

$$\text{QTc} = \text{QT interval}/\sqrt{(\text{R} - \text{R interval})}$$

where the R-R interval is the R-R interval preceding the measured QT interval. Prolonged QTc (≥470 msec) can occur after stressful delivery but usually resolves within 48 to 72 hours.[139] Otherwise, QTc prolongation is typically either secondary to a genetic long QT syndrome or medications. The QTc can also be prolonged in the presence of hypocalcemia, hypokalemia, and hypomagnesemia. There are several forms of long QT syndrome, including Jervell-Lange-Nielsen syndrome, Romano-Ward syndrome, and long QT syndromes 1 to 8. These have been mapped to multiple loci and can affect multiple genes. All are inherited in an autosomal dominant pattern except for Jervell-Lange-Nielsen syndrome, which is autosomal recessive. A prolonged QTc places neonates at risk for bradycardia, torsades de pointes, ventricular tachycardia, and sudden death.

Treatment is aimed at preventing arrhythmias associated with long QT syndromes. All electrolytes should be corrected as necessary and any QTc-prolonging medications discontinued if possible. A current list of QTc-prolonging medications can be found at www.qtdrugs.org. Asynchronous cardioversion and magnesium are useful for treatment of torsades de pointes, although cardioversion may not prevent reinitiation of the arrhythmia. The mainstays of therapy for patients with long QT syndromes are beta-blockers. Implantable cardiac defibrillators are also warranted in high-risk patients and those with torsades de pointes despite beta-blocker therapy.

Narrow QRS Complex Tachycardia

Sinus Tachycardia

Sinus tachycardia is a normal variant in neonates and children. In neonates, this can be difficult to differentiate from arrhythmias because of the ability of the neonatal conduction system to conduct normal at rates upwards of 230 beats per minute. Therefore it is imperative to differentiate this from an arrhythmia before initiation of any therapy. Sinus tachycardia is a sign of any condition that requires increased cardiac output. In the newborn, this may include pain, fever, infection, anemia, opiate withdrawal, hyperthyroidism, dehydration, and potential certain drugs. Treatment should be directed toward the underlying cause.

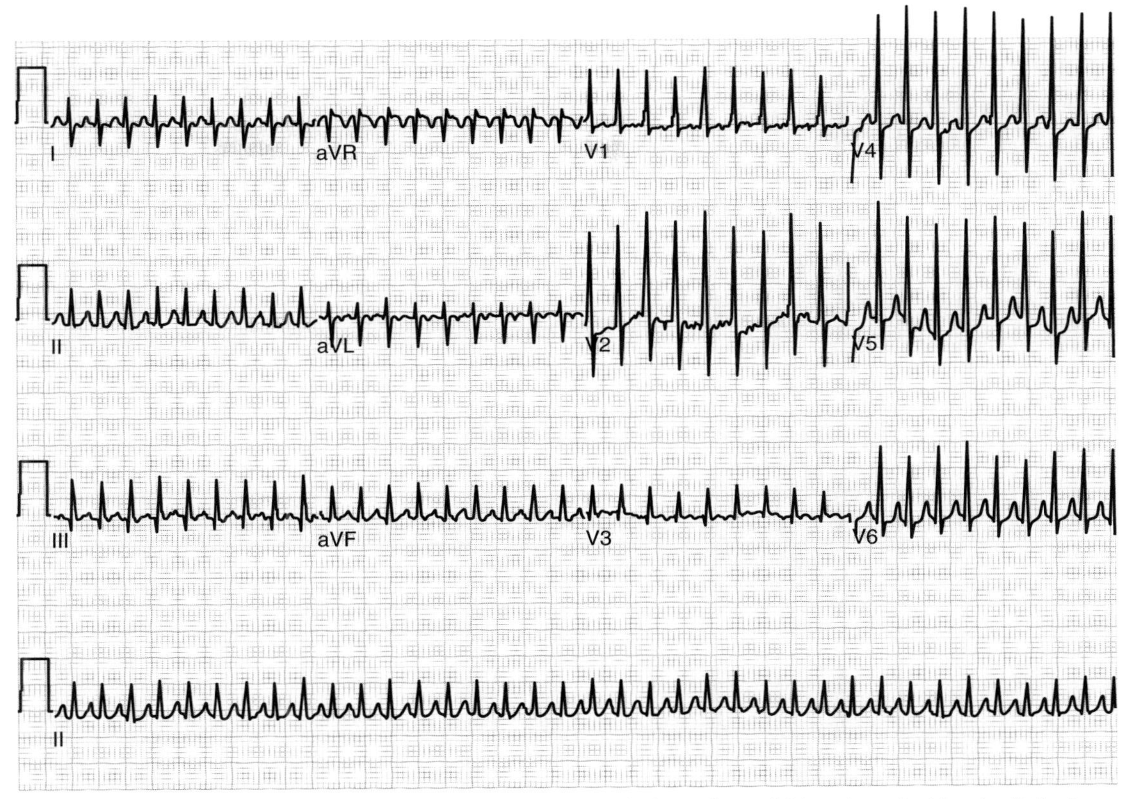

Fig. 14.27 Atrioventricular reentrant tachycardia (supraventricular tachycardia) in a 4-week-old male. Patient presented with manifestations of decreased cardiac output over preceding 24 hours and mild left ventricular dysfunction by echocardiogram. Note the retrograde P waves are difficult to discern and are buried in the T waves.

Supraventricular Tachycardias

Atrioventricular Reentrant Tachycardia. Supraventricular tachycardia is a generalized term that encompasses multiple distinct electrophysiologic tachyarrhythmias, two of which are AV reentrant tachycardia (AVRT) and AV nodal reentrant tachycardia, which is uncommon in the neonatal period.

AVRT is the most common cause of tachycardia in the newborn period. AVRT is the most likely abnormal SVT encountered in the NICU. AVRT is characterized by sudden onset and termination, typically normal QRS complexes, and fixed cycle length (R-R interval). The P wave is usually identified following the QRS complex but can be buried in the T wave. It usually has a retrograde morphology (negative in leads II and aVF) (Fig. 14.27). In the presence of a bundle branch block or when using the accessory pathway as the antegrade limb of the reentrant circuit, the QRS can be prolonged (aberrant conduction), and it can be extremely difficult to distinguish from ventricular tachycardia. There is typically a 1:1 A-V relationship. AVRT is usually seen in a structurally normal heart but can be associated with Ebstein anomaly of the tricuspid valve, congenitally corrected TGA, and hypertrophic cardiomyopathy.

AVRT is typically well tolerated for short periods of time in the neonate. Neonates may be relatively asymptomatic until prolonged tachycardia results in decreased ventricular function. Symptoms can include palpable tachycardia, irritability, tachypnea, poor oral intake, diaphoresis with feeds, and respiratory distress. When decreased ventricular function is present, it is usually resolved with adequate treatment of the arrhythmia.

AVRT can be terminated by a multitude of mechanisms. In the hemodynamically stable patient in AVRT, vagal maneuvers can be attempted. This can include applying ice to the face for 20 to 30 seconds to elicit the dive reflex, gagging the patient, or insertion of a rectal thermometer. Applying pressure over the eye or the carotid sinus should be avoided, as the prior can result in retinal detachment and the later can result in unilateral occlusion of cerebral blood flow. All of these maneuvers increase vagal tone, resulting in decrease in AV node conduction. In the event these maneuvers are unsuccessful, an intravenous bolus of adenosine can be used as this results in block of the AV node conduction. The initial dose of adenosine is 100 mcg/kg with subsequent doses of 200 mcg/kg and 400 mcg/kg. It is important to immediately follow the rapid IV bolus with an adequate saline flush to ensure the medication reaches the central circulation quickly, given the short half-life of adenosine. This can be accomplished with both syringes directly inserted in the same hub or by use of a three-way stopcock. A common cause for failure of adenosine to break SVT is inadequate administration. It is equally important to record the rhythm throughout the administration of adenosine. This allows for assessment of the underlying atrial rhythm, as well as the mechanism of reinitiation of arrhythmia if it were to occur. If the initial dose of adenosine successfully converts AVRT to sinus rhythm but

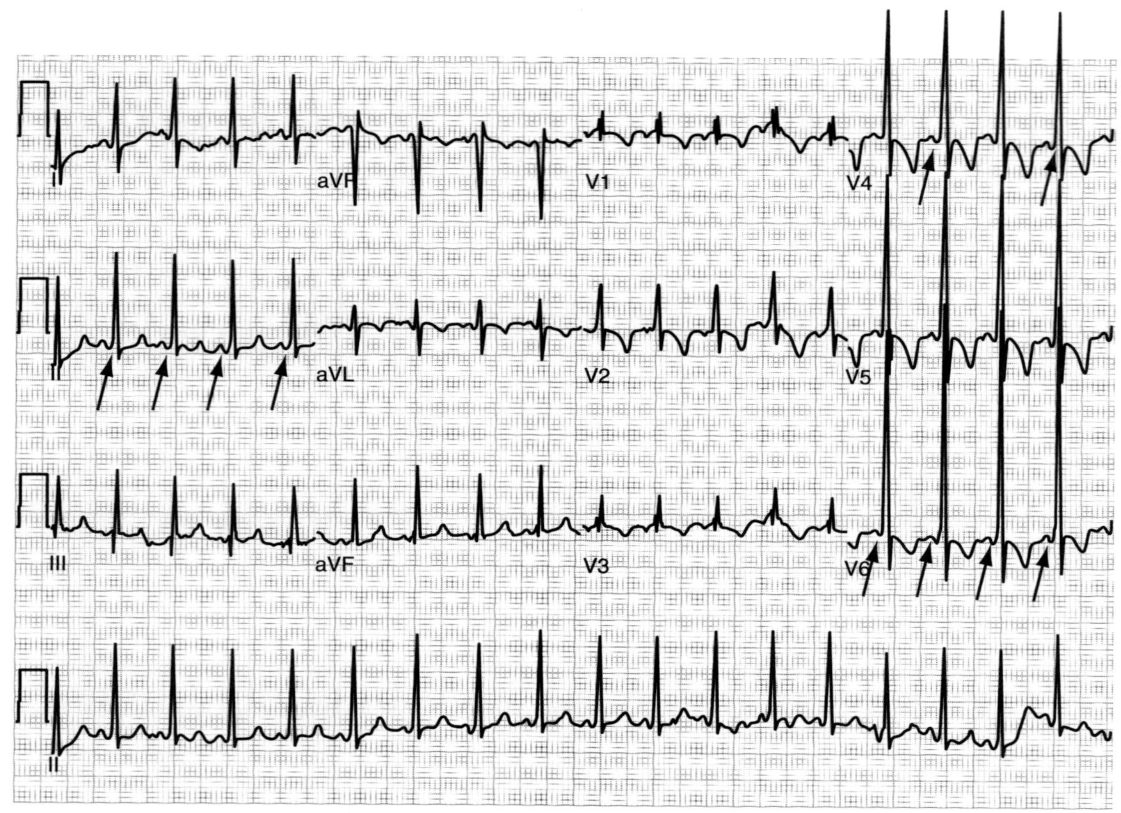

Fig. 14.28 Wolff-Parkinson-White syndrome. Patient from Fig. 14.25 demonstrated preexcitation (solid black arrows) at baseline after conversion to sinus rhythm following administration of adenosine.

the arrhythmia recurs, additional doses of adenosine at escalating doses are unlikely to result in sustained sinus rhythm, and additional antiarrhythmic medication is required. Tachycardia can also be terminated by overdrive atrial pacing. This can be accomplished by placing a transesophageal pacing probe and atrially pacing at a rate 10% higher than the SVT rate for around 20 seconds. In hemodynamically unstable patients, synchronized cardioversion should be immediately employed to terminate the arrhythmia.

There are multiple therapies available for AVRT. Current first-line therapies for AVRT include digoxin and beta-blockers, such as propranolol. Digoxin should be avoided in neonates with WPW syndrome, as this can potentiate conduction down the accessory pathway by decreasing its refractoriness, resulting in ventricular arrhythmias.[140–142] In the event digoxin and/or propranolol are unsuccessful, flecainide, amiodarone, and sotalol have been used with success.[143] As the antiarrhythmic properties increase, so do the side effects, and additional monitoring is required. Calcium channel blockers should be avoided in neonates because of reports of hemodynamic collapse following administration. Only in extreme cases is intracardiac electrophysiology study and accessory pathway ablation necessary. The prognosis for neonates with AVRT is excellent, and most do not require further treatment past 6 to 12 months of age.

Following conversion of SVT to normal sinus rhythm, a baseline electrocardiogram should be obtained to assess for evidence of ventricular preexcitation manifested on the electrocardiogram as a delta wave. This is referred to as WPW syndrome (Fig. 14.28). This is important for initial medical management decisions as outlined previously. The prevalence of WPW syndrome is 0.4 to 1 per 1000 in infants and children and 60% presenting before 2 months of age.[144] Although patients who present with WPW syndrome during the neonatal period and infancy have a 60% to 90% chance of resolution during the first year of life, one-third will experience recurrence of symptoms during the first decade of life, typically around 4 to 6 years of age.[123] Patients demonstrating WPW syndrome should have screening echocardiograms to assess for associated congenital heart disease.

Persistent junctional reciprocating tachycardia. Persistent junctional reciprocating tachycardia (PJRT) is a relatively rare form of reentrant tachycardia. This is an incessant orthodromic tachycardia with anterograde conduction over the AV node and retrograde conduction via an accessory pathway with slow and decremental conduction.[145] This arrhythmia can present in utero, in the neonatal period, during childhood, or during adulthood in slower forms of PJRT. Over a long period of time, the incessant tachycardia can lead to tachycardia-induced cardiomyopathy, although this is reversible with rate control. Infants with cardiomyopathy may present because of symptoms of heart failure. During episodes of PJRT, the P wave is characteristically inverted in the inferior leads but may be normal during the brief periods of sinus rhythm. These periods of sinus rhythm are typically no more than a few beats. Because of the risk

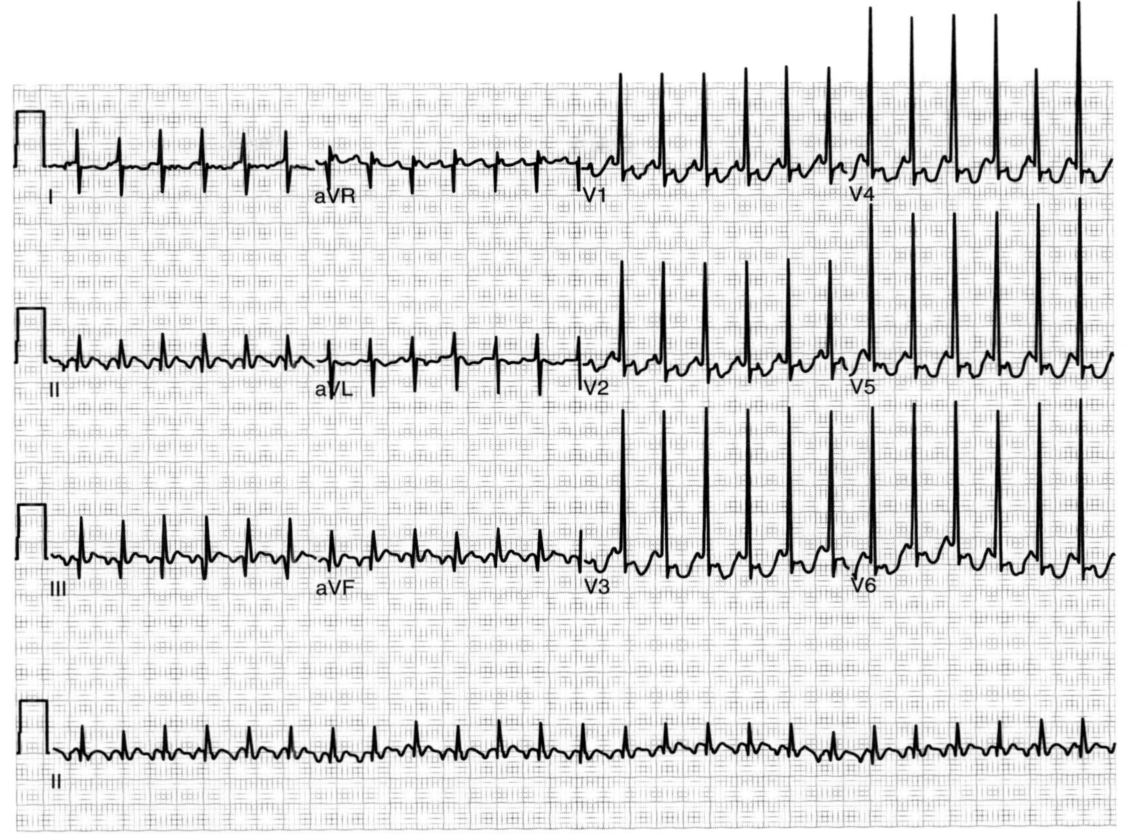

Fig. 14.29 Atrial flutter with 2:1 Atrioventricular conduction in a 1 day old. Note the sawtooth flutter wave pattern, most evident in the rhythm strip, at a rate of around 380 beats per minute and a ventricular rate of around 190 beats per minute.

of tachycardia-induced cardiomyopathy, aggressive therapy should be initiated for PJRT. Beta-blockers have been used with some success but may be inadequate. There have been reports of success rates of 80% using amiodarone and verapamil to achieve arrhythmia suppression.[146] PJRT may also spontaneously resolve, although not as frequently as AVRT. Vaksmann et al found resolution in 22% of their cohort and in 25% of those patients less than1 year of age. Unfortunately, the range for resolution of tachycardia was 2 months to 16 years with a median of 5.4 years.[146]

Ectopic/chaotic atrial tachycardia. Ectopic atrial tachycardia (EAT) is a primary atrial tachycardia resulting from localized automatic foci located in the atria. This accounts for 5% to 20% of SVT in pediatrics and can be present in paroxysmal and permanent forms.[143,147] In this arrangement, there is no reentrant circuit. EAT is usually chronic and incessant. The tachycardia tends to have a gradual onset and resolution as opposed to the abrupt onset and resolution of reentrant tachycardias. EAT typically manifests with heart rates at or just above the upper limit of normal for age. However, the resting heart rate is often more elevated than expected, and there is an exaggerated response to exercise.[139] EAT can be distinguished from sinus tachycardia by abnormal P-wave morphology on electrocardiogram. The permanent form can frequently lead to congestive heart failure; otherwise, the symptoms can be very subtle, and the clinician must have a high degree of suspicion. Class Ic (propafenone and flecainide) and class III (sotalol, amiodarone) have been shown to provide effective rhythm control in multiple studies.[148–151] In the case of medication failure, catheter ablation of the automatic focus is a therapeutic option. EAT has a 75% to 95% chance of spontaneous resolution during the first year of life according to previous reports.[148] One study looked specifically at those patient diagnosed with EAT before 3 years of age (range 1 day to 2 years, median 7 days) and found that 78% of patients in this group had spontaneous resolution.[152]

Chaotic atrial tachycardia is defined as an atrial tachycardia with at least three P-wave morphologies. The tachycardia rates vary significantly with irregular P-P intervals. Chaotic atrial tachycardia is not typically associated with congenital heart disease. However, it has been frequently associated with respiratory illness, especially respiratory syncytial virus bronchiolitis.[153,154] As with EAT, prolonged arrhythmia can result in decreased cardiac function. Treatment options are similar to those for EAT.

Atrial flutter. Atrial flutter is uncommon in the neonatal period and accounts for around 3% of neonatal arrhythmias.[155] It is caused by a macroreentry circuit within the atrial muscle. Atrial flutter is characterized by regular, rapid atrial tachycardia with sawtooth flutter waves (Fig. 14.29).

These are typically best appreciated in the inferior leads and tend to have atrial rates of 300 to 600 beats per minute. AV block is typically present with 2:1 block, and thus the R-R interval is an integer of the atrial rate. However, the conduction can vary. In the neonatal presentation, atrial flutter is typically not associated with congenital heart disease, but was seen in conjunction with an ASD in one study.[156] As with other tachyarrhythmias, neonates in atrial flutter for prolonged periods of time can present with depressed ventricular function. Spontaneous conversion to normal sinus rhythm in infants with atrial flutter is common, occurring in almost 25% of patients. For those who fail to convert to sinus rhythm, direct current (DC) cardioversion and transesophageal pacing are effective in converting to sinus rhythm. Previously, digoxin has been the antiarrhythmic medication of choice, but its efficacy has become debatable because of the widely variable time between initiation of digoxin therapy and conversion to sinus rhythm.[156,157] Given the likelihood of spontaneous conversion, it is reasonable to monitor the asymptomatic infant for a period of several hours, but cardioversion should be the treatment of choice in symptomatic neonates. As atrial flutter is a self-limited process with a low risk of recurrence; once sinus rhythm has been established, no further antiarrhythmic medication may be necessary following initial cardioversion.

Junctional ectopic tachycardia. Junctional ectopic tachycardia (JET) is an uncommon narrow–complex automatic tachycardia originating in or near the AV node that is typically seen in the early postoperative period in infants and children with congenital heart disease. However, JET can also be seen as congenital form in patients who have had no prior surgery. JET is characterized by a narrow–complex tachycardia with rates typically 180 to 240 beats per minute with AV dissociation and a slower atrial rate.[158] Appropriately timed atrial beats conduct normally through the AV node, and this can be an important clue to the diagnosis. Transesophageal atrial electrocardiogram may be necessary to confirm the diagnosis. In postoperative patients with JET, the atrial electrogram can often be obtained from temporary atrial pacing wires. Congenital nonoperative JET can present at any age, but when it presents in in the first 6 months of life, it is associated with a 4% mortality.[159] The etiology of congenital JET is poorly understood, but postoperative JET is thought to be secondary to surgical trauma. The hemodynamic significance of JET warrants aggressive therapy. JET is refractory to overdrive pacing, DC cardioversion, and adenosine. Class III antiarrhythmics, particularly amiodarone, have been relatively successful in controlling the rhythm. Additional management should focus on withdrawal of inotropic agents when possible and modest cooling. A study demonstrated that therapeutic hypothermia resulted in a significant decrease in JET rate and subsequent restoration of AV synchrony either via return to sinus rhythm or the ability to successfully atrially pace above the JET rate.[160] In patients with persistent JET or failure of amiodarone, it is reasonable to pursue either radiofrequency ablation or cryoablation of the automatic focus. Both modalities have similar success rates (82%–85%) and recurrence rates (13%–14%).[159] These procedures may lead to inadvertent high-grade second-degree or complete heart block necessitating pacemaker implantation.

Wide QRS Complex Tachycardia

Accelerated Idiopathic Ventricular Rhythm

This is a benign arrhythmia occasionally seen in the neonatal period. It is characterized by wide–complex tachycardia with rates no greater than 20% of the preceding sinus rate. Most of these rhythms will be less than 200 beats per minute. The QRS will be prolonged above the upper limit of normal for age and generally has a left bundle branch morphology. Fusion beats are commonly seen at the onset and termination of the accelerated ventricular rhythm because of the similar rate compared with the sinus rate. There is no association with congenital heart disease, and it results in no hemodynamic compromise. No further evaluation or therapy is necessary.

Ventricular Tachycardia

Ventricular tachycardia (VT) is defined as three or more consecutive ventricular beats that occur with a rate greater than 20% above the preceding sinus rhythm (Fig. 14.30). VT is a wide-QRS complex tachycardia, but it is important to distinguish VT from aberrantly conducted SVT, whether because of rate or antegrade conduction down an accessory pathway, such as in WPW syndrome. VT can be distinguished by the presence of fusion beats, AV dissociation, and morphology similar to PVCs. Unfortunately, neonates and infants tend to have 1:1 retrograde conduction. This means that AV dissociation may not be seen in VT in this population. VT can be monomorphic (a single morphology) or polymorphic (more than one morphology), such as torsades de pointes. It can also be nonsustained, lasting between 3 and 30 beats, or sustained, greater than 30 beats. VT can progress to ventricular fibrillation if left untreated.

The presence of VT requires a thorough evaluation for possible causes. These can include myocarditis, cardiomyopathy, tumors (including hamartoma and rhabdomyomas), myocardial infarction (secondary to anomalous origin of the left coronary artery from the pulmonary artery, maternal cocaine use, and thromboembolism), electrolyte abnormalities, metabolic abnormalities, drug intoxication, and long QT syndrome, to name a few. Initial evaluation should consist of an electrocardiogram, echocardiogram, and possibly cardiac MRI to aid in the diagnosis of cardiac tumors not seen by echocardiogram.

The morphology of VT can also be a clue to the underlying diagnosis. Polymorphic VT tends to occur in myocarditis and myocardial infarctions. Incessant VT, defined as VT greater than 10% per 24-hour period, is often associated with myocarditis and hamartomas.[161]

In patients with sustained VT and hemodynamic compromise, synchronized DC cardioversion is the treatment

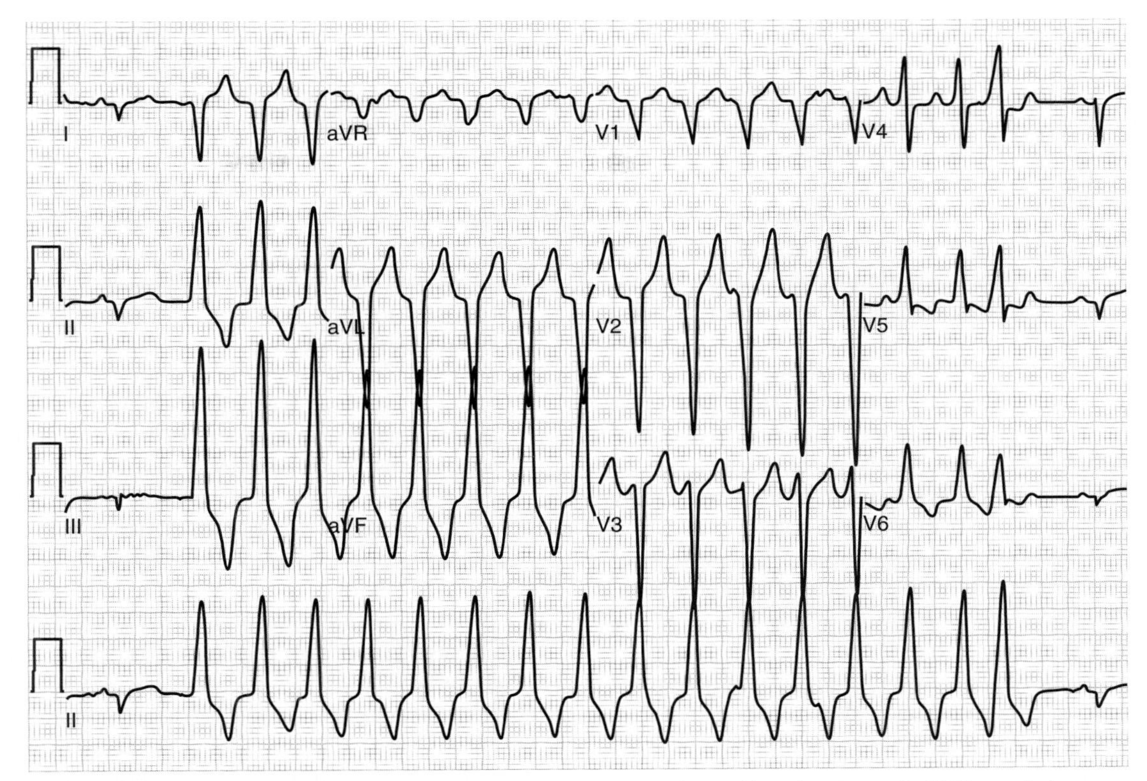

Fig. 14.30 Ventricular tachycardia with a rate of 140 beats per minute. Note the change in QRS morphology compared with the sinus beats.

of choice. In patients who remain hemodynamically stable, initial management may consist of either intravenous procainamide or lidocaine, but pharmacologic therapy is typically initiated after conversion to sinus rhythm. In patients with asymptomatic, nonsustained VT, no underlying etiology, and a structurally normal heart, spontaneous resolution is expected, and therefore therapy may not be indicated once converted to sinus rhythm.[162] For sustained, incessant, or rapidly conducting nonsustained VT, class I, class II, and class III antiarrhythmic drugs have been used with varying success. An implantable cardioverter defibrillator is typically not indicated in the neonatal period.

Arrhythmias are a common problem in the neonatal period. Although AVRT is the most common arrhythmia encountered, most other forms of SVT and VT are rare. The electrocardiogram remains crucial for accurate diagnosis and in proper therapeutic intervention. Echocardiographic evaluation is warranted in all neonatal arrhythmias, but most are not associated with congenital heart disease. Finally, although some neonatal arrhythmias, such as PJRT and incessant VT, can be recalcitrant to treat, most are responsive to antiarrhythmic medications and are "outgrown" during the first year of life.

Practical Hints

All of the following hints should be used in conjunction with additional data to make a diagnosis of cardiac disease. The adequacy of systemic perfusion, arterial oxygen tension, and results of the cardiac examination should be used in conjunction with heart size, respiratory pattern, and other findings to point toward a diagnosis.

1. Heart sounds are usually abnormal in newborns with a serious congenital heart disease. A single S_2 after the first 12 hours often indicates heart disease, although with rapid heart rates, this can be difficult to verify. A well-split S_2 is always abnormal and suggests TAPVR. The presence of a pulmonary systolic ejection click may be normal in the first hours, but after that, any systolic ejection click is abnormal, indicating an abnormal pulmonary or aortic valve, an enlarged pulmonary artery or aorta, or truncus arteriosus. If the infant has pulmonary disease without congenital heart disease and has a narrowly split or single S_2, then a high PVR is expected.
2. Visible central cyanosis in the early newborn period usually indicates a very low arterial oxygen tension. Even when the clinical judgment is that of only questionable cyanosis, the arterial Po_2 may be very low.
3. Peripheral cyanosis (acrocyanosis) is normal and must be differentiated from central cyanosis. A suspicion of hypoxemia must be verified by arterial blood gas determinations.
4. Measurement of systemic arterial blood gas concentrations while the infant breathes room air and while supplemental oxygen is administered may be helpful in

differentiating pulmonary from cardiac cyanosis. A PaO_2 of less than 100 mm Hg in an enriched oxygen environment indicates congenital heart disease until proven otherwise and is an indication for echocardiography and the initiation of PGE_2 therapy. A PaO_2 of 100 to 250 mm Hg is suggestive of congenital heart disease and warrants additional investigation. A PaO_2 above 250 mm Hg makes life-threatening cyanotic heart disease less likely. In questionable cases, hypoxemia without significant hypercapnia (CO_2 retention) tends to suggest primary cardiac disease. However, pulmonary venous congestion may result in considerable CO_2 retention.

5. Blood gas concentrations determined from heel-stick specimens do not provide accurate measures of the arterial Po_2. However, the error is always on the low side, so that in cyanotic congenital heart disease, a reasonably high Po_2 on a heel-stick sample is reassuring.
6. Transcutaneous Po_2 or oximetric measurements are inaccurate at low levels and in the presence of hypoperfusion. They are valuable for monitoring trends or comparing upper and lower body oxygenation.
7. Oximetric measurements may be beneficial in determining the type of congenital heart disease. Measurements should be taken simultaneously in the right upper and either lower extremity. Cyanosis–desaturation that is equal in the upper and lower extremities can indicate right-sided heart obstruction or TAPVR. Cyanosis–desaturation that is worse in the lower extremity indicates left-sided heart obstruction or suprasystemic pulmonary artery pressures in the face of a PDA. Cyanosis–desaturation that is worse in the upper extremity is diagnostic for dextro-TGA with elevated PVR or coarctation until proven otherwise.
8. Femoral or pedal pulses must be carefully and repeatedly palpated in all newborn infants. The pulse may be palpable, even with significant coarctation of the aorta while the ductus arteriosus is open, disappearing when the ductus arteriosus closes. Observation of diminished or absent femoral pulses by any examiner requires additional investigation.
9. A high index of suspicion is required to diagnose congenital heart disease early. Careful history taking, physical examination, and laboratory studies—including chest radiographs, ECG, and blood gas or oximetric studies in an enriched oxygen environment—often help establish the diagnosis. However, two-dimensional echocardiography permits accurate and definitive diagnosis, accomplished without delay.
10. Life-threatening congenital heart disease is sooner or later associated with respiratory distress or frank cyanosis, or both.
11. The presence of a large liver usually indicates systemic venous congestion but does not necessarily point to congestive heart failure. Many conditions in the neonatal period can produce an enlarged liver.
12. On occasion, in the presence of RDS and a PDA, congestive heart failure may be diagnosed without cardiomegaly.

CASE 14.1

On the day of discharge, the physical examination findings for a full-term baby are significant for a harsh murmur at the lower left sternal border. The examination before this was unremarkable. The child is acyanotic, and the murmur is typical of a ventricular septal defect (VSD) with left-to-right shunt.

Is a VSD possible? Why?

A VSD is possible. The left ventricular pressure is not transmitted to the right side through the small, restrictive VSD. Therefore nothing impedes the normal decrease in PVR. As the pulmonary vascular resistance decreases, the right ventricular pressure decreases as it would normally. Therefore there is a large pressure gradient between the ventricles, and an early left-to-right shunt is possible.

Is the defect likely to be small or large?

The shunt rarely becomes large because of the high resistance to flow through the small defect. The major key to suspecting that the defect is small is the early onset of the loud, typical murmur. Also, large defects should not produce a murmur because the pressure equalizes between the right and left ventricle when a large VSD is present.

Is eventual congestive heart failure likely?

Heart failure is not likely when the left-to-right shunt is small.

If the defect was larger, what symptoms would the infant manifest, and how would it best initially be managed?

In the setting of a moderate to large defect that permits significant left-to-right shunting, infants manifest several symptoms. Because of the increased pulmonary blood flow, these patients are tachypneic, although they rarely display respiratory distress at rest, and their oxygen saturation is usually 99% to 100% unless they have significant pulmonary flow to produce interstitial edema. They may have minimal to mild retractions. The liver may be felt below the right costal margin. During feedings, these infants may become more tachypneic or diaphoretic, or develop respiratory distress. Because of increased energy demands, they may also demonstrate poor weight gain.

CASE 14.2

A 40-year-old mother has just delivered a term infant boy. She had little prenatal care and no prenatal testing or ultrasonography. The infant does well and goes to the newborn nursery. On examination, the infant is found to have multiple features consistent with trisomy 21. The cardiac examination is unremarkable, but because occasional premature atrial contractions (PACs) are noted on a monitor, an electrocardiograph (ECG) is obtained. This ECG shows normal sinus rhythm with occasional PACs and a leftward/northwest axis.

Given the findings described, does this infant have congenital heart disease?

Yes. The finding of a leftward or northwest axis on ECG is very suspicious for an atrioventricular (AV) septal (endocardial cushion) defect. The PACs are insignificant and are a common finding in the neonatal period.

Assuming the infant has a complete AV septal defect (AVSD), does the lack of a murmur surprise you?

No. In this clinical situation, the pulmonary pressures have not fallen, and thus there may be minimal shunting at the level of the VSD component. In patients with trisomy 21, this fall in pulmonary pressures can be delayed or may not occur. Murmurs are not typically heard because of shunting through the atrial septal defect (ASD), but in the setting of a large left-to-right shunt at the atrial level, there may be a diastolic rumble associated with relative tricuspid stenosis at the lower left sternal border or a systolic ejection murmur associated with relative pulmonary stenosis at the left upper sternal border caused by increased flow across either valve. The degree of atrial-level shunting is determined by the ventricular compliance, so in a patient on the first day of life, there is likely minimal shunting because the right ventricle is still relatively stiff and noncompliant.

Echocardiography confirms a balanced complete AVSD with moderate-sized atrial and VSD components. As this infant grows, how will the infant's heart disease manifest?

Manifestations will depend on the right-sided pressures. If the pulmonary pressures remain elevated, the infant will be unlikely to develop overcirculation and will remain relatively balanced. The infant may be mildly cyanotic at baseline because of bidirectional shunting at the ventricular level, or may become more cyanotic with transient increases in the right-sided pressure, such as during crying. If pulmonary pressures and right-sided pressures fall, the patient is likely to develop VSD-type physiology with increased pulmonary circulation. In this situation, the patient would manifest symptoms similar to those discussed in Case 1 and may require anticongestive therapy.

CASE 14.3

A 36-weeks' gestation infant is born to a 20-year-old primigravid mother. The mother received minimal prenatal care. The mother's labor was prolonged with rupture of membranes 18 hours before delivery. There is meconium in the fluid, and the infant undergoes suctioning for meconium aspiration following vaginal delivery. He is intubated because of respiratory distress and taken to the neonatal intensive care unit for further management, where oxygen saturation measured on his right hand is 75%. An oxygen saturation probe on his left foot reads 90%.

What is the difference between differential cyanosis and reverse differential cyanosis?

Differential cyanosis is present when the preductal oxygen saturation is higher than the postductal oxygen saturation. Reverse differential cyanosis is present when the preductal oxygen saturation is lower than the postductal oxygen saturation. A patent ductus arteriosus (PDA) is necessary for either form.

What form of differential cyanosis does this patient have, and what clinical situations result in this finding?

The patient has reverse differential cyanosis. This type of cyanosis can be seen in transposition of the great arteries (TGA) with either a significant coarctation or interrupted aortic arch. Obtaining oxygen saturation measurements from the left upper extremity can be helpful in determining the site of either coarctation or interruption. Reverse differential cyanosis can also occur in TGA with supersystemic pulmonary pressures that result in right-to-left shunting across the PDA.

How can these three distinct entities best be identified?

In the neonatal period, echocardiography should be sufficient to determine the presence of coarctation or interruption. Pulmonary pressures can accurately be estimated, and flow across the PDA can be determined by color in color flow Doppler echocardiography.

What clinical scenarios can result in differential cyanosis (not reverse)?

Normally related great arteries with a hypoplastic aortic arch, severe coarctation, or interruption can result in differential cyanosis. Also, pulmonary hypertension of the newborn (PPHN) with normally related great arteries can result in differential cyanosis.

What should be the initial management of this patient with reverse differential cyanosis?

A common theme in all cases of reverse differential cyanosis is the presence of TGA. Initial management should include initiation of prostaglandin E_1 infusion to maintain ductal patency. Additional management may include balloon atrial septostomy to insure adequate mixing before surgical repair or supplemental oxygen or inhaled nitric oxide to help with management of PPHN if appropriate.

CASE 14.4

A 38-weeks' gestation girl was born to a 30-year-old mother via cesarean section. Pregnancy was uncomplicated. A grade 3/6 systolic ejection murmur heard best at the midleft sternal border and right sternal border was noted on examination while the infant was in the nursery. Because the infant was feeding well, she was discharged home at 2 days of age on Friday with instructions for follow-up with the pediatrician on Monday. She did well through the weekend, feeding every 3 hours, but on Monday morning, she became more irritable, pale, and tachypneic. She was taken immediately to her pediatrician, who noted poor pulses, tachycardia, respiratory distress, hepatomegaly, a hyperdynamic right ventricular impulse, and a systolic ejection murmur. The infant was subsequently transferred to the emergency department of a tertiary care pediatric hospital.

Can a diagnosis be suggested?

The location of the murmur in the nursery raises suspicion of aortic stenosis. The progression of symptoms is indicative of critical aortic stenosis with duct-dependent systemic blood supply.

What are the effects of aortic valve stenosis in utero on the left ventricle?

Aortic valve stenosis results in increased left ventricular pressure and left ventricular hypertrophy. Increased left ventricular hypertrophy results in decreased left ventricular compliance, which may lead to decreased flow through the left side of the heart if severe enough. If flow through the left side of the heart is too restricted, it can affect the development of "downstream" structures, including left ventricular chamber size, aortic valve annulus size, and the size of the ascending aorta.

Explain the cardiac collapse when this patient was taken to the pediatrician.

The findings this infant exhibited are characteristic of a patient whose left ventricle is unable to handle the entire cardiac output. In this situation, the infant is dependent on the patent ductus arteriosus (PDA) for systemic circulation. The symptoms of circulatory collapse can occur abruptly as the ductus closes. Inadequate systemic circulation results in poor peripheral pulses. The respiratory symptoms are secondary to pulmonary venous congestion. Tachycardia is a manifestation of the infant's attempt to increase cardiac output (cardiac output = stroke volume × heart rate).

In a patient such as this with severe aortic stenosis, what would one expect to see on the electrocardiograph (ECG)?

Patients with aortic valve stenosis typically demonstrate voltage changes that meet the criteria for left ventricular hypertrophy, although approximately one-third of patients with severe aortic stenosis may have a normal ECG. However, the findings of left ventricular hypertrophy, ST depression, and T-wave inversion are fairly specific for severe aortic stenosis.

What initial steps should be taken to stabilize this patient's condition?

This patient is clearly duct dependent, and prostaglandin E_1 infusion should be initiated immediately to restore systemic circulation. Metabolic acid–base derangements must be managed, and the hemoglobin level should be optimized. Echocardiography is essential to accurately establish the diagnosis and identify any associated lesions. This is also important to determine whether the patient may need a two-ventricle repair.

15

The Kidney

Scott T. McEwen, Beth A. Vogt

Advances in neonatology, perinatology, and molecular genetics have defined new disease processes and continue to raise exciting questions in the field of nephrology. Prenatal maternal-fetal care and ultrasound imaging continue to improve the diagnosis of many urinary tract anomalies, which allows for improved prenatal and perinatal care. The use of invasive vascular catheters introduced new complications, including renal artery and aortic thrombosis. The administration of loop diuretics and steroids to infants with bronchopulmonary dysplasia (BPD) has significantly increased rates of neonatal hypertension and nephrocalcinosis (NC). Simultaneously, genetic similarities among children whose conditions were formerly considered phenotypically distinct are redefining congenital anomalies of the kidneys and urinary tract (CAKUT).

This chapter reviews the anatomic and physiologic development of the kidney, outlines the recommended approach to evaluation of the neonate with suspected kidney disease, and comments on the more common nephrologic and urologic problems seen in preterm and term neonates.

ANATOMIC DEVELOPMENT

Mammalian kidney development begins at 5 weeks' gestation, and the fetal kidney begins to produce urine by 10 weeks. This developmental process continues until approximately 36 weeks' gestation and stops at birth, even in preterm babies born before 36 weeks.[1] Formation of the metanephric kidney is complex and requires coordinated development from three separate embryological processes: branching morphogenesis, epithelial-mesenchymal transformation, and angiogenesis.[1] Disruptions in normal kidney development can lead to CAKUT, which accounts for 40% to 50% of chronic kidney disease (CKD) worldwide and 36% of end-stage renal disease (ESRD) in children.[1]

Formation of the renal collecting system begins as an outgrowth of the mesonephric duct called the ureteric bud.[2] The ureteric bud elongates and interacts with the surrounding metanephric mesenchyme through a coordinated process that requires several well-characterized signaling interactions. The ureteric bud then undergoes several rounds of branching, giving rise to the renal pelvis, calyces, and collecting ducts. The length of the ureteric bud proximal to the first branch matures to become the ureter. Abnormal development of the renal collecting system can result in defects such as renal agenesis, dysplasia, and urinary obstruction (Table 15.1).[3]

The nephrons of the definitive kidney arise from a separate process of epithelial-mesenchymal transformation.[1] The developing ureteric bud invades and undergoes reciprocal signaling with the surrounding metanephric mesenchyme, inducing mesenchymal cells to condense into epithelial vesicles.[4] These vesicles then use genetic signals to pattern themselves into an elongated S-shaped vesicle with proximal, middle, and distal portions that will mature into the definitive nephron segments.[2] Finally, the renal vesicles fuse with the ureteric bud, becoming the junction of the distal tubule and collecting duct of the mature nephron (Fig. 15.1). Failure of this complex process of nephrogenesis can result a wide variety of congenital anomalies, including renal agenesis, hypoplasia, dysplasia, or cyst development (Table 15.1).[3,5]

The glomerulus also arises from the metanephric mesenchymal cells and forms by the same mechanisms as other capillary beds.[1] This process involves both vasculogenesis (creating new blood vessels) and angiogenesis (sprouting from existing vessels). The development of glomerular cells is intimately linked to the developing nephron segment that will become the podocytes of Bowman's capsule and requires regulation by several molecular signals.[6] Interestingly, glomeruli appear to retain some developmental potential after preterm birth, offering an exciting potential target for regenerative science and possible future therapies for preterm infants with prematurely arrested renal development.[7,8]

PHYSIOLOGICAL DEVELOPMENT

During fetal development, the kidneys play a minor role in regulating salt and water balance, as this function is performed by the placenta. The fetal kidneys primarily function to produce large amounts of urine to provide adequate amniotic fluid. With the loss of placental function at birth, the kidneys quickly adapt to the extrauterine environment and assume the role of regulating water and mineral balance. Rapid maturation of renal blood flow, glomerular filtration, and tubular handling of solutes occurs in the first 2 to 3 postnatal weeks. This physiological maturation then continues slowly for the first 2 years of life, after which these functions reach adult levels.

TABLE 15.1 Confirmed Causative Genes Associated With Congenital Anomalies of the Kidneys and Urinary Tract Phenotypes

Developmental Process	Associated CAKUT Phenotype	Associated Genes
Ureteric bud initiation and elongation	Renal agenesis Renal dysplasia Vesicoureteral reflux	*RET* *BMP4* *PAX2* *GATA3* *SIX1* *SIX2* *EYA1* *SALL1* *ROBO2*
Branching morphogenesis	Renal dysplasia	*AGT* *AGTR*
Epithelial-mesenchymal transformation	Renal agenesis Renal dysplasia Renal hypoplasia	*FGF20* *WNT4*
Genetic patterning of nephron	Cystic kidney disease	*UMOD*
Unassigned but known to cause CAKUT in humans	Renal agenesis Renal dysplasia Renal hypoplasia Cystic dysplasia Vesicoureteral reflux UPJ obstruction Horseshoe kidney VACTERL association	*REN* *HNF1B* *CHD1L* *DSTYK* *KAL1* *SIX5* *SOX17* *TNXB* *TRAP1* *UPK3A* *MUC1*

CAKUT, Congenital Anomalies of the Kidneys and Urinary Tract; *UPJ,* ureteropelvic junction; *VACTERL,* vertebral defects, anal atresia, cardiac defects, tracheoesophageal fistula, renal anomalies, and limb abnormalities.
Modified from Vivante A, Kohl S, Hwang DY, Dworschak GC, Hildebrandt F. Single-gene causes of congenital anomalies of the kidney and urinary tract (CAKUT) in humans. *Pediatr Nephrol.* 2014;29(4):695.

RENAL BLOOD FLOW

The mature kidney receives a large percentage of cardiac output relative to its small size, which is necessary to continually regulate the extracellular fluid (ECF) composition. At birth, renal blood flow represents 4% to 6% of the cardiac output, and this value increases quickly during the first postnatal week, reaching the adult value of 20% to 25% by the end of the first year (Table 15.2).[9] Renal blood flow is initially low because of high renal vascular resistance caused by elevated levels of circulating vasoconstrictor hormones such as renin, angiotensin, aldosterone, endothelin, and catecholamines that counteract fetal prostaglandins. Renal blood flow increases as concentrations of these hormones decrease and systemic mean arterial pressure and cardiac output increase, more than doubling renal blood flow during the first postnatal week. The increase in renal blood flow is attenuated and delayed in preterm infants.[10]

In addition to the increase in overall renal blood flow, there is a marked change in distribution of blood flow within the neonatal kidney in the postnatal period. Because of a preferential decrease in vascular resistance in the outer cortex, there is a pronounced increase in blood flow to the outer cortex, which is the site of most glomerular filtration.[11]

GLOMERULAR FILTRATION RATE

Glomerular filtration rate (GFR) in the fetal kidney is significantly lower than adult values and increases with gestational age. By 34 weeks' gestation, a GFR of approximately 14 mL/min/1.73 m^2 is achieved, and the rate further increases to 20 to 30 mL/min/1.73 m^2 at term (Table 15.2). In preterm infants, the GFR is even lower, especially in very low-birth-weight infants and infants with NC.[12] The GFR continues to increase postnatally, achieving adult values of 120 mL/min/1.73 m^2 by 2 years of age.

Several factors account for the marked increase in GFR in the first postnatal weeks. The primary determinant of GFR is renal blood flow, so the GFR increases in parallel. Second, higher mean arterial pressure increases glomerular hydrostatic pressure, which increases GFR. The subsequent rise in GFR during the first 2 years results from continued increases in renal blood flow and glomerular pressure as well as maturation of superficial cortical nephrons, which expands the glomerular filtration surface area.[9]

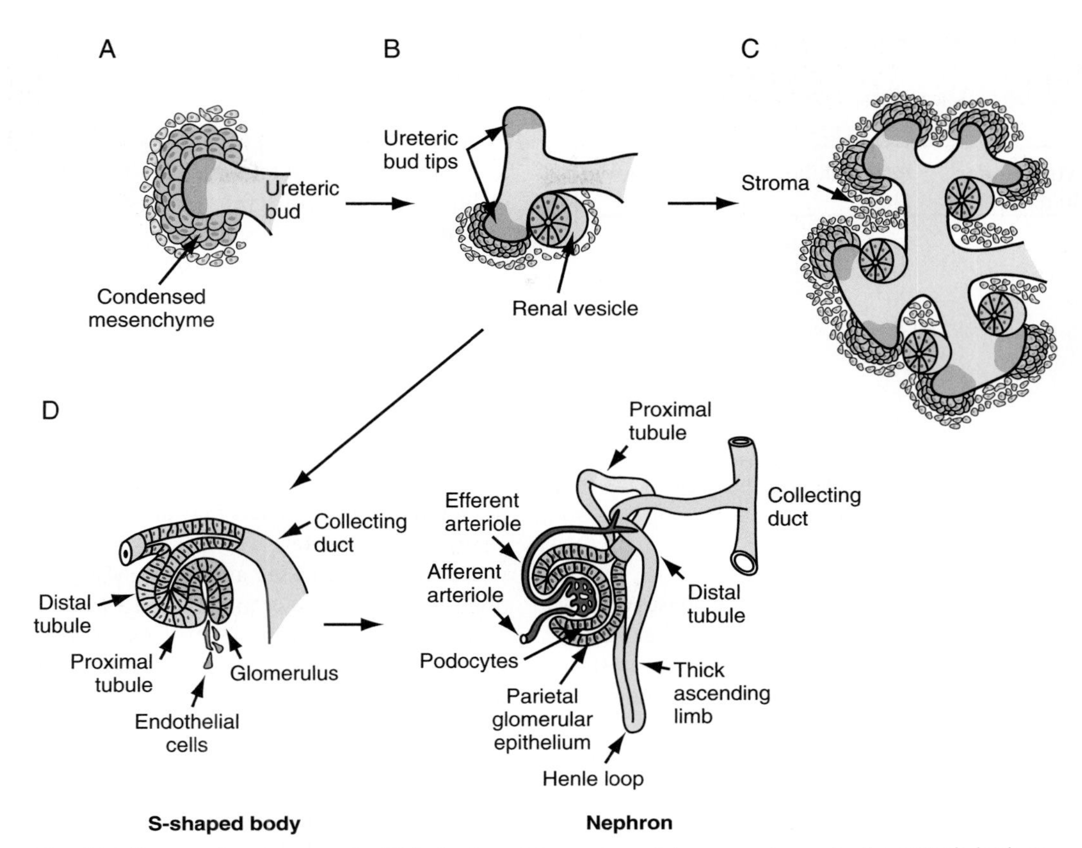

Fig. 15.1 Stages of nephrogenesis. (A) Induction of the metanephric mesenchyme by the ureteric bud promotes aggregation of condensed mesenchyme around the tip of the ureteric bud. (B) Renal vesicles form as the mesenchyme transitions to epithelium. (C) Fusion of renal vesicles occurs with the collecting ducts. (D) A cleft forms in the renal vesicle, giving rise to the comma-shaped body and with formation of a second proximal cleft the S-shaped body forms. Invasion of the proximal cleft by angioblasts leads to formation of the glomerulus. (Modified from Dressler GR. The cellular basis of kidney development. *Annu Rev Cell Dev Biol.* 2006;22:509-529.)

TABLE 15.2 Normal Values for Renal Function

Age	Glomerular Filtration Rate (mL/min/1.73 m^2)	Renal Blood Flow (mL/min/1.73 m^2)	Maximal Urine Osmolality (mOsm/kg)	Serum Creatinine (mg/dL)	Fractional Excretion of Sodium (%)
Newborn					
32–34 wk gestation	14 ± 3	40 ± 6	480	1.3	2–5
Full Term	21 ± 4	88 ± 4	800	1.1	<1
1–2 wk	50 ± 10	220 ± 40	900	0.4	<1
6 mo–1 yr	77 ± 14	352 ± 73	1200	0.2	<1
1–3 yr	96 ± 22	540 ± 118	1400	0.4	<1
Adult	118 ± 18	620 ± 92	1400	0.8-1.5	<1

Modified from Avner ED, Ellis D, Ichikawa I, et al. Normal neonates and maturational development of homeostatic mechanism. In: Ichikawa I, ed. *Pediatric Textbook of Fluids and Electrolytes*. Baltimore, MD: Williams & Wilkins; 1990.

During the first week of postnatal life, an infant's GFR passes through three distinct phases to maintain fluid and electrolyte homeostasis.[12] The prediuretic phase, which occurs in the first 24 hours of life, is characterized by a transient increase in GFR followed by a return to low baseline GFR and minimal urine output regardless of salt and water intake. This phase may extend up to 36 hours of life in the preterm infant. The diuretic phase follows, in which the GFR increases rapidly and the infant experiences diuresis and natriuresis regardless of salt and water intake. The postdiuretic phase typically begins around day 4 to 5 of life, at which time the GFR begins to increase slowly with maturation, with salt and water excretion varying according to intake.

TABLE 15.3 Change in Body Water With Maturation

	PERCENT BODY WEIGHT		
Age	**Extracellular Fluid**	**Intracellular Fluid**	**Total Body Fluid**
Gestational			
14 wk	65	27	92
28 wk	55	25	80
40 wk	45	30	75
Postnatal			
14 wk	25	40	65

Modified from Sulyok E. Postnatal adaptation. In: Holliday MA, Barratt TM, Avner ED, eds. *Pediatric Nephrology*. Baltimore, MD: Williams & Wilkins; 1994.

Importantly, the duration and timing of these phases differ among infants, so that individualization of fluid and electrolyte therapy is required. If insensible fluid losses are overestimated during the prediuretic phase, excess fluid intake may result in dilutional hyponatremia. On the other hand, a deficiency in fluid intake during the diuretic phase may lead to dehydration and hypernatremia.

FLUID DISTRIBUTION

The change in distribution of intracellular fluid (ICF) and extracellular fluid (ECF) in the fetus and newborn infant is summarized in Table 15.3. In the healthy term infant, ECF volume decreases and ICF volume increases in the first few days of life, with a net loss of total body water that manifests clinically as weight loss after birth.[13] This diuresis and ECF fluid loss is often delayed in neonates with respiratory distress syndrome (RDS). The change in ICF during the first week of life is variable and dependent on total energy intake. In preterm infants, the ICF volume increase can be attenuated so that more than a 10% loss in body weight during the first week of life may represent only ECF contraction without an increase in ICF.

Water movement between the vascular and interstitial fluid compartments is also higher in the neonatal period than it is later in life, which leads to a relatively large interstitial fluid compartment. This phenomenon may be attributed to a number of factors, including increased hydrostatic pressure, decreased intravascular osmotic pressure, and increased levels of atrial natriuretic peptide (ANP), vasopressin, and cortisol. The relatively large interstitial fluid compartment can partially replace lost vascular volume and enables the neonate to better tolerate hemorrhage or physiological diuresis, but it also reduces the ability to excrete a free water load.

SODIUM HANDLING

Serum sodium concentration is maintained in a tight physiological range that does not differ between neonates and adults, and renal excretion is the only active mechanism of regulation. Although neonates retain approximately 1 mEq/kg/day of sodium because of somatic growth of new tissues, in general the renal excretion of sodium adjusts to account for a range in daily intake. Healthy term neonates have basal sodium handling with a fractional excretion of sodium (FE_{Na}) around 1%; this can be slightly higher in formula-fed babies than in those fed on human milk because of the difference in the sodium content of these solutions.[14] Urinary sodium losses may be increased in certain conditions, including renal dysplasia, hypoxia, respiratory distress, hyperbilirubinemia, acute tubular necrosis (ATN), polycythemia, and the use of theophylline or diuretics. Pharmacologic agents, such as dopamine, labetalol, propranolol, captopril, and enalaprilat, that influence adrenergic neural pathways in the kidney and the renin-angiotensin axis may also increase urinary sodium losses in the neonate.

Renal sodium losses are inversely proportional to gestational age, and the FE_{Na} may exceed 3% in infants born before 28 weeks' gestation (Fig. 15.2).[13] As a result, preterm infants younger than 35 weeks' gestation may display early negative sodium balance and hyponatremia because of high renal sodium losses and inefficient intestinal absorption. Sodium deficiency in early postnatal life leads to early and sustained growth retardation, and intake of 4 to 5 mEq/kg/day may be necessary in preterm infants to offset these renal losses during the first weeks of life.[13]

The mechanisms responsible for increased urinary sodium losses in the preterm infant are multifactorial. Compared with adults, neonates have decreased sensitivity to angiotensin and aldosterone, and their kidneys have increased sensitivity to ANP, all of which promote sodium excretion.[13] Inappropriate sodium wasting occurs during glomerulotubular imbalance, the condition where the GFR exceeds the reabsorptive capacity of the renal tubules. This imbalance occurs in preterm neonates because of tubular immaturity, large extracellular volume, and reduced oxygen availability necessary for active transport.

PLASMA OSMOLARITY AND FREE WATER HANDLING

Control of plasma osmolarity is necessary to maintain cellular volume and is especially critical for brain function and homeostasis. The regulation of serum osmolarity relies on the kidney to respond to antidiuretic hormone (ADH) and regulate free water excretion through the concentration or dilution of urine. As noted in Table 15.2, the maximum renal concentrating ability is low at birth and progressively increases following delivery from about 600 milliosmoles (mOsm)/kg H_2O in the first 2 weeks of life to adult values of 1200 mOsm/kg H_2O by 2 years of age. This improvement in the ability to concentrate urine is primarily due to the maturation of the renal medulla, which contains the loop of Henle and collecting ducts. With age, these structures lengthen, which allows for increased medullary interstitial sodium and urea concentration.[15] Also, the sensitivity of the collecting

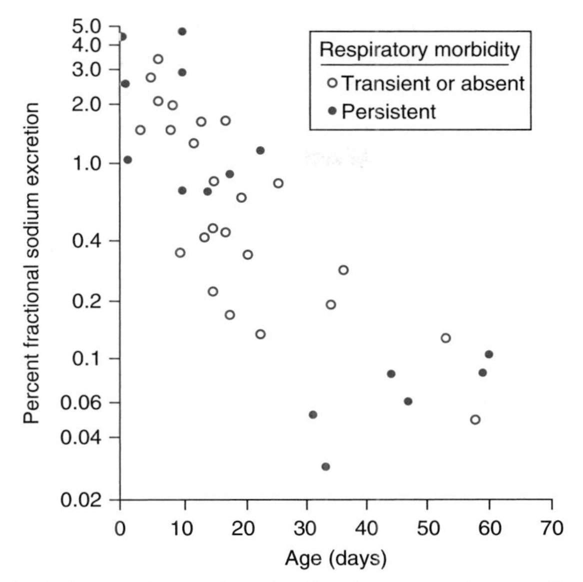

Fig. 15.2 Fractional excretion of sodium in neonates born at 28 to 33 weeks of gestation during the first 2 months of life. (From Ross B, Cowett RM, Oh W. Renal functions of low birth weight infants during the first two months of life. *Pediatr Res.* 1997;11:1162.)

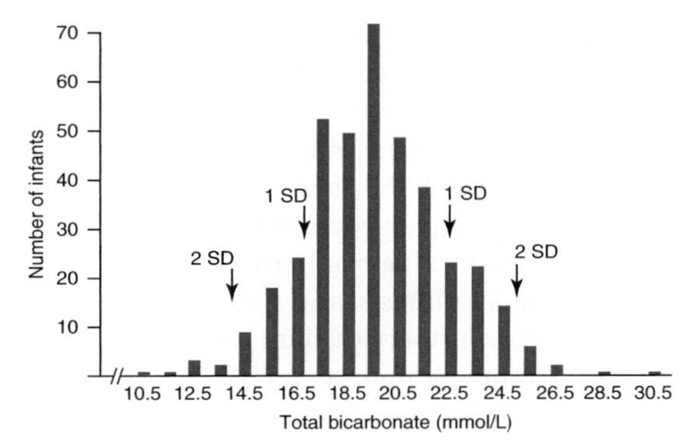

Fig. 15.3 Frequency distribution of serum total bicarbonate level in low-birth-weight neonates during the first month of life. (From Schwartz GJ, Haycock GB, Chir B, et al. Late metabolic acidosis: a reassessment of the definition. *J Pediatr.* 1979;95:102.)

duct to ADH improves, allowing water movement along the medullary osmolarity gradient.[16]

Similarly, the ability of the neonatal kidney to excrete excess free water by diluting the urine is limited compared with the adult kidney. Term and preterm newborns can dilute their urine to an osmolality of 70 mOsm/kg and 100 mOsm/kg, respectively, whereas adults can dilute their urine to 50 mOsm/kg. This inability to maximally dilute the urine is as a result of the reduced GFR and immaturity of transporters in the early distal tubule (diluting segment) and can predispose neonates to hyponatremia.

ACID–BASE BALANCE

Regulation of the extracellular pH is tightly controlled by both the lungs and kidneys as well as extracellular buffers. The role of the kidney is primarily to regulate the excretion of buffers, especially bicarbonate and titratable acids such as ammonia. The range of neonatal serum bicarbonate levels is lower than that of adults, and healthy infants maintain a mild metabolic acidosis (Fig. 15.3).

The limitation in acid–base homeostasis seen in neonates, particularly preterm infants, is related to immaturity of both proximal and distal tubular function. The proximal tubular bicarbonate transport threshold is much lower in neonates than in adults, leading to incomplete bicarbonate reabsorption. Proximal tubular bicarbonate wasting is more pronounced in preterm infants, resulting in an expected transient renal tubular acidosis.[17] Limited distal tubular excretion of titratable acid and incomplete development of tubular ammonia production also contribute to the relative metabolic acidosis of the newborn. Treating neonates acutely with intravenous bicarbonate for metabolic acidosis provides little benefit because of renal bicarbonate wasting, adds risks of intraventricular hemorrhage and cardiac deterioration, and can worsen intracellular acidosis.[18]

EDITORIAL COMMENT: Historically, neonates with metabolic acidosis were routinely given sodium bicarbonate despite the lack of evidence to support the practice. As noted in a seminal commentary by Drs. Aschner and Poland, cleverly titled "Sodium Bicarbonate: Basically Useless Therapy," the detrimental effects of the therapy often outweigh the benefits, and instead the focus should be on "understanding and treating the underlying cause of the acidosis" (*Pediatrics* 2008;122:831).

In the first 24 hours of life, an early combined respiratory and metabolic acidosis may develop as a result of stress during birth and disturbances in cardiopulmonary adaptation. Late metabolic acidosis, on the other hand, develops after the first week of life because of net excess of acid intake compared with the capacity for acid excretion. Late acidosis is more pronounced in preterm neonates and those receiving parenteral nutrition[17] but usually resolves by the end of the first month of life with renal maturity; if persistent, late acidosis can result in poor weight gain or skeletal growth.

An important consequence of chronic metabolic acidosis in the newborn is enhanced urinary calcium loss and negative calcium balance, which may contribute to the bone demineralization and osteopenia of prematurity.[17] The mechanism for this process is multifactorial. Acidosis causes release of calcium from bones, increases parathyroid hormone secretion, inhibits intestinal calcium absorption, impairs activation of vitamin D, and increases urinary calcium excretion. Therefore chronic metabolic acidosis should usually be corrected with enteral supplementation with a goal of achieving a serum bicarbonate level of greater than 18 mEq/L.

CALCIUM AND PHOSPHORUS BALANCE

Within 24 to 48 hours after birth, the serum calcium concentration decreases, a phenomenon that is most pronounced in preterm infants.[17] Although the mechanism of neonatal hypocalcemia is not completely known, it appears to be as a result of suppressed parathyroid hormone secretion and elevated serum phosphate concentration. In most neonates, the ionized calcium level remains above a physiologically acceptable concentration, and the infant experiences no clinical symptoms. Symptomatic hypocalcemia may occur, however, in neonates stressed by illness or in the presence of aggressive fluid administration, diuresis, and sodium supplementation, all of which increase urinary calcium losses.

The normal serum phosphorus level in the newborn ranges from 4.5 to 9.5 mg/dL, which is significantly higher than that of adults and is necessary for positive phosphorus balance needed for bone and cellular growth. Factors leading to the higher neonatal serum phosphorus level include the generous phosphorus content of cow's milk formulas, low GFR, and higher tubular reabsorption of phosphorus. Phosphorus reabsorption is lower, however, in preterm infants, which can lead to relative phosphate wasting and can contribute to inadequate bone mineralization and osteopenia.[17] Therefore supplementation of phosphorus and calcium is often needed in preterm infants to promote adequate bone development.

EVALUATION

The evaluation of a newborn with suspected kidney disease must be comprehensive and begins with a careful history and physical examination. Selected laboratory studies may be useful in determining the cause and severity of renal dysfunction. Focused radiologic evaluation may be useful in clarifying renal anatomy or function and detecting complications of vascular catheters.

HISTORY

When neonatal kidney disease is suspected, the medical history should focus on identifying prenatal risk factors that aid diagnosis as well as pre- and postnatal factors that influence therapy and prognosis. The cause of congenital kidney disease cannot always be determined, but genetically inherited conditions and nephrotoxic teratogens are becoming increasingly identified.

Review of the family medical history should include information on any prior fetal or neonatal deaths, or family history of kidney disease, congenital renal malformations, or recurrent urinary tract infection (UTI) that may signal urinary reflux or obstruction. When syndromes involving multiple organ systems are being considered, additional information about familial hearing loss, vision loss, cleft lip/palate, limb or vertebral skeletal malformations, congenital heart defects, or renal malignancy such as Wilms tumor should be elicited. It is increasingly recognized that most forms of CAKUT have a genetic etiology, even though affected family members may have significantly different pathology from the same genetic variant (e.g., mother with vesicoureteral reflux [VUR] has a child with unilateral renal agenesis).[3,5] Thus, information about any structural, cystic, or congenital kidney disease is significant.

The maternal antenatal history should be reviewed, with particular attention given to medications, toxins, or unusual exposures during the pregnancy. Many prescribed medications have known teratogenic effects and are commonly prescribed to women of childbearing age.[19] Treatment for conditions such as hypertension, acne, seizures, malignancy, autoimmune disease, and many psychiatric diseases commonly use such medications, and presence of these conditions should prompt a detailed history of current and past medication usage.

Results of prenatal ultrasonography should be reviewed with attention to kidney size, echogenicity, malformations, amniotic fluid volume, and bladder size and shape. The presence of small or enlarged kidneys, renal cysts, hydronephrosis, bladder enlargement, or oligohydramnios may suggest significant renal or urologic abnormalities. Also, developmental anomalies of other structures, such as skeletal or cardiac malformations, should raise suspicion for syndromes that may include renal malformations.

PHYSICAL EXAMINATION

Evaluation of blood pressure and volume status is critical in the newborn with suspected kidney disease. Hypertension is often present in neonates with autosomal recessive polycystic kidney disease (PKD), acute kidney injury (AKI), or renal thromboembolism. Hypotension, on the other hand, may suggest volume depletion, hemorrhage, or sepsis, which may lead to renal ischemia and AKI. Edema or anasarca may be seen in oliguric AKI, hydrops fetalis, or congenital nephrotic syndrome. Isolated ascites may be seen with urinary tract obstruction with rupture of the bladder or renal pelvis, so-called "urinary ascites."

The lower pole of both kidneys should be palpable on abdominal examination because of the reduced abdominal muscle tone of the neonate. The majority of neonatal abdominal masses are genitourinary in origin, so an abdominal mass in a newborn should be assumed to involve the urinary tract until proven otherwise.[19] The most common renal cause of an abdominal mass is hydronephrosis followed by multicystic dysplastic kidney (MCDK). Less common causes include PKD, renal vein thrombosis, ectopic or fused kidneys, renal hematoma or abscess, and renal tumors. The newborn bladder is often palpable just above the pubic symphysis, but a lower urinary tract obstruction should be suspected when the bladder is enlarged. Absence or laxity of the abdominal muscles may suggest Eagle-Barrett (prune belly) syndrome.

A number of associated anomalies should raise suspicion for underlying renal defects. Because the genital and urinary systems are derived from a common developmental precursor, any anomaly of genital structures should elicit evaluation of the kidneys and bladder. Other features associated with disrupted development of the urinary system include small or malpositioned ears, aniridia or coloboma, microcephaly, spinal cord dysraphism and neural tube defects, pectus excavatum, hemihypertrophy, limb deformities, imperforate anus, and congenital heart disease. There appears to be an association between presence of a single umbilical artery and underlying renal anomalies. Historically, these newborns received a thorough evaluation with labs and imaging studies, but that approach has fallen out of favor with improvements in prenatal ultrasonography, and newer data showing only 2% of neonates with an isolated single umbilical artery have clinically significant renal anomalies.[19]

A constellation of physical findings called Potter syndrome can be seen in neonates with fetal deformation by uterine wall compression. Characteristic facial features include wide-set eyes, depressed nasal bridge, beaked nose, receding chin, and posteriorly rotated, low-set ears. Although it was originally described in babies with bilateral renal agenesis, this syndrome can occur in any infant with a history of severe oligohydramnios, most commonly resulting from obstructive uropathy and cystic kidney diseases.[19] This condition has a high mortality from associated pulmonary hypoplasia, and surviving infants often have significant morbidity because of the underlying renal disease and associated anomalies such as a compressed chest wall and arthrogryposis.

URINALYSIS

Some 98% of full-term infants void in the first 30 hours of life, with as many as 25% doing so in the delivery room. A delay in urination can be normal and should not cause immediate concern in the absence of an enlarged bladder, abdominal mass, or other indications of renal disease. Failure to urinate in the first 48 hours should prompt further investigation for structural or obstructive urinary tract anomalies and may necessitate placement of a urinary catheter.

Evaluation of the urine is a vital part of the examination of any neonate suspected of having a urinary tract abnormality. Collection of an adequate, uncontaminated specimen is difficult in the neonate. A specimen collected by cleaning the perineum and applying a sterile adhesive plastic bag enables analysis of urinary blood, protein, or electrolytes. For cultures, bladder catheterization produces a reliable specimen but may be technically difficult in preterm infants. Suprapubic bladder aspiration has been considered the collection method of choice in infants without intraabdominal abnormalities or bleeding disorders, although few clinicians choose this approach. A noninvasive clean-catch technique relying on external bladder stimulation to generate a urine stream is gaining popularity and appears to have contamination rates similar to urethral catheterization.[20]

> **EDITORIAL COMMENT:** Point-of-care ultrasound (POC US) is increasingly available in the neonatal intensive care unit (NICU) for use by the neonatal team. Some studies, such as cardiac ultrasound, require significant training and experience to obtain proficiency. A relatively simple study is the use of POC US to evaluate the bladder before a catheter or suprapubic tap procedure to evaluate urine volume.

Analysis of the urine should include inspection of color and clarity, dipstick testing, and microscopic analysis. The urine of newborns is usually clear and nearly colorless. Cloudiness may be caused by either UTI or the presence of crystals. A dark yellow-orange color may be as a result of conjugated bilirubin but occasionally indicates simply concentrated urine in newborns. Urate crystals and certain drugs may stain the urine pink and be confused with bleeding. Brown urine suggests glomerular hematuria, hemoglobinuria from hemolysis, or myoglobinuria from muscle breakdown.

Urine dipstick evaluation can detect the presence of heme-containing compounds (red blood cells, myoglobin, and hemoglobin), protein, and glucose. The presence of leukocyte esterase and nitrites should raise suspicion of UTI, and a culture should be obtained for confirmation. Microscopic urinalysis should be performed if the urinary dipstick result is abnormal to assess for the presence of red blood cells, casts, white blood cells, bacteria, and crystals.

LABORATORY EVALUATION

Clinical evaluation of neonatal renal function begins with measurement of serum creatinine. Normal values for serum creatinine vary with gestational and postnatal age because of differences in GFR discussed previously (Table 15.2). The serum creatinine level is relatively high at birth and reflects maternal levels because of placental transfer. Creatinine decreases after birth as renal blood flow and GFR increase, reaching a nadir that reflects true neonatal GFR after 2 to 3 weeks, but this decline can be prolonged after preterm birth. In general, serum creatinine inversely correlates with GFR so that a doubling of the creatinine represents a 50% reduction in GFR. Although directly measuring the GFR is possible using radioisotopes or ionic contrast agents, these methods are generally difficult to accomplish and aid little in the clinical care of neonates. The "bedside" Schwartz formula uses serum creatinine and body length and often suffices for the care of preterm and term infants despite validation only in children older than 12 months.[21] This equation estimates GFR standardized to body surface area:

$$\text{Estimated GFR (mL/min/1.73 m}^2\text{)} = 0.413 \times \frac{\text{Height (cm)}}{\text{Creatinine (mg/dL)}}$$

RADIOLOGIC EVALUATION

Renal ultrasonography is the initial imaging modality of choice in infants with suspected renal disease. It offers a noninvasive anatomic evaluation of the urinary tract without the use of contrast agents or radiation exposure. Ultrasound provides useful information about the size and morphology of the kidneys and bladder and can detect the presence of hydronephrosis, cysts, stones, NC, masses, and abscesses. Doppler evaluation with ultrasound can illuminate renal parenchymal blood flow defects in cases of pyelonephritis and infarction. Doppler investigation of the renal vessels and aorta is useful in cases of neonatal hypertension where thromboembolism or vascular stenosis is suspected.

Voiding cystourethrography (VCUG) is the procedure of choice to evaluate the urethra and bladder and to detect VUR. The most common indications for this procedure are the evaluation of hydronephrosis or investigation following a UTI. VCUG is the gold-standard study for evaluation of suspected bladder outlet obstruction such as posterior urethral valves. This study involves urinary catheterization and fluoroscopy and thus confers a small infectious risk and radiation exposure. VCUG should be performed in all neonates with suspected urinary tract obstruction, those with severe hydronephrosis, and following UTI.

Other radiologic tests may occasionally be used for diagnostic purposes in the neonate. The radiolabeled isotope mercaptoacetylglycine (MAG-3) is cleared by the kidney, and imaging its rate of excretion after giving a diuretic is the preferred method to diagnose urinary tract obstruction. This test may be useful in an infant with clinically significant hydronephrosis with a normal VCUG. Dimercaptosuccinic acid is a radionuclide that is taken up by the kidney rather than excreted, making it useful to identify renal scarring or pyelonephritis. Computed tomography (CT) may be helpful in evaluating suspected renal abscess, mass, nephrolithiasis, or any condition where detailed anatomic information is needed.

SPECIFIC PROBLEMS

HEMATURIA

CASE 15.1

At 60 days of age, a former 900-g 27-week infant with a history of BPD passes reddish-brown urine. Urinalysis shows 3+ blood with more than 250 red blood cells/mm^3, no protein, positive leukocyte esterase, and nitrite. Urine culture grows greater than 50,000 *Escherichia coli*, and renal ultrasonography is normal with no NC or hydronephrosis. The infant is treated with IV antibiotics with resolution of macroscopic hematuria.

Hematuria can be classified into two categories: microscopic and macroscopic. Microscopic hematuria is defined as greater than or equal to five red blood cells on high-powered examination without visible urine discoloration. Macroscopic hematuria is defined as visibly discolored (red or brown) urine with greater than or equal to five red blood cells on high-powered examination. When a neonate is suspected of having macroscopic hematuria, it is important to rule out conditions mimicking hematuria. Urate crystals, bile pigments, and porphyrins may discolor the urine, but in these conditions the urinary dipstick test is negative for blood, and the microscopic examination reveals no red blood cells. Infants with myoglobinuria because of inherited metabolic myopathy, infectious myositis, or rhabdomyolysis may have red or brown urine and test dipstick positive for blood, but the microscopic examination of the urine reveals no red blood cells. Similarly, infants with hemoglobinuria because of hemolytic disease such as ABO incompatibility will have a positive urinary dipstick for blood but no red blood cells on microscopic examination. Vaginal bleeding or skin breakdown from diaper dermatitis can mimic gross hematuria.

Once it is determined that an infant has hematuria, there is a broad differential diagnosis.[22] UTI should be suspected in infants with fever or other signs of instability. ATN or cortical necrosis should be considered in infants with a history of perinatal asphyxia. Renal vein thrombosis should be considered in infants with risk factors such as birth to a diabetic mother, cyanotic congenital heart disease, volume depletion, or an indwelling umbilical venous catheter. Coagulopathy related to hemorrhagic disease of the newborn should be considered in at-risk infants who have not received vitamin K prophylaxis. Urolithiasis or NC should be suspected in infants with a history of chronic lung disease and loop diuretic use. Other causes of hematuria include trauma from bladder catheterization or suprapubic aspiration, obstructive uropathy, and tumors. Glomerulonephritis, a common cause of hematuria in older children and adolescents, is an unlikely cause of hematuria in the neonate.

Evaluation of the neonate with hematuria includes formal urinalysis with microscopic examination, catheterized urine culture, complete blood count (CBC), serum electrolytes, creatinine, and kidney/bladder ultrasound. Further evaluation may include coagulation profile, urine calcium-to-creatinine ratio, abdominal CT scan, or urologic evaluation.

PROTEINURIA

CASE 15.2

A 1900-g male infant is delivered at 34 weeks' gestation to consanguineous parents. An enlarged placenta is noted at the time of delivery. At 5 days of age, the infant develops periorbital and peripheral edema as well as abdominal distension. Urinalysis shows 4+ protein and no blood, and serum albumin falls to 1.5 gm/dL. Serum creatinine is 0.4 mg/dL, and blood pressure is normal.

Proteinuria is defined as a urinary dipstick value of at least 1+ (30 mg/dL), with a specific gravity of 1.015 or less, or a urinary dipstick value of at least 2+ (100 mg/ dL), with a specific gravity of more than 1.015. Normal urinary protein-to-creatinine ratio is less than 0.5 mg/mg in infants and toddlers younger than 2 years of age. Nearly any form of renal injury can result in a transient increase in urinary protein excretion, including ATN, fever, dehydration, cardiac failure, high doses of penicillin, and recent administration of a contrast agent. Persistent heavy (4+) proteinuria, edema, and hypoalbuminemia in a neonate should prompt the consideration of congenital nephrotic syndrome, an autosomal recessive disorder characterized by massive proteinuria, failure to thrive, a large placenta, and CKD. Proteinuria associated with glucosuria, hypokalemia, hypophosphatemia, and metabolic acidosis raises concern for Fanconi syndrome, a rare condition characterized by generalized proximal tubular dysfunction; possible causes include cystinosis, Lowe syndrome, galactosemia, and mitochondrial disorders. False-positive urinary dipstick values for protein may be the result of highly concentrated urine, alkaline urine, infection, and detergents.

ACUTE KIDNEY INJURY

CASE 15.3

A 2300-g female infant is delivered after a 36-week uncomplicated pregnancy. Fetal decelerations were noted before delivery, and a tight nuchal cord is present. Apgar scores are 1 at 1 minute and 4 at 5 minutes. The infant is resuscitated using intubation, compressions, and epinephrine. Arterial blood gas analysis shows a pH of 7.02, Pco_2 of 54 mm Hg, and Po_2 of 73 mm Hg. Initial laboratory work reveals normal electrolyte levels and a serum creatinine concentration of 0.9 mg/dL.

Over the next 3 days, the infant becomes oliguric, and laboratory results are as follows: Na 127 mmol/L; K 6.5 mmol/L; Cl 106 mmol/L; HCO_3 15 mmol/L; blood urea nitrogen 36 mg/dL; and creatinine 3.0 mg/dL. Urinalysis shows hematuria (2+) and proteinuria (1+). Renal ultrasonography shows hyperechoic parenchyma without evidence of renal dysplasia or obstruction. Peritoneal dialysis is initiated for supportive treatment of presumed acute tubular necrosis (ATN). After 10 days, dialysis is discontinued as the infant's renal function recovers. The infant is discharged home at 21 days of age with a serum creatinine concentration of 1.0 mg/dL. Follow-up laboratory work 3 months later shows the serum creatinine level to be 0.7 mg/dL.

AKI is a common condition in the neonatal intensive care unit (NICU), ranging from mild renal dysfunction to complete anuric kidney failure. AKI is characterized by a sudden decline in kidney function over hours to days, resulting in derangements in fluid, electrolyte, and acid–base balance. There has been difficulty in establishing a standardized definition of AKI in neonates because of a number of factors, including maturational differences in kidney function at different gestational ages, the overall low GFR of neonates, and the fact that serum creatinine reflects maternal creatinine for days to weeks after birth. A consensus definition for neonatal AKI was recently established and termed the neonatal modified KDIGO (Kidney Disease: Improving Global Outcomes) criteria.[23] These criteria define neonatal AKI in infants under 120 days of age as an increase in serum creatinine of 0.3 mg/dL (or higher) or 50% or more from the previous lowest value and/or urine output less than 0.5 mL/kg/h. Three stages of neonatal AKI are defined by relative changes in serum creatinine from baseline (Box 15.1). Biomarkers including neutrophil gelatinase-associated lipocalin, urinary interleukin-18, and cystatin C may show promise in the earlier detection of neonatal AKI, potentially identifying earlier stages of kidney injury that occur before the elevation of serum creatinine.[24]

Neonatal AKI is a common occurrence, occurring in 30% of critically ill neonates recently evaluated in a large multicenter retrospective cohort study.[25] The incidence of AKI varied by gestational age group, occurring in 48% of infants at 22 to 29 weeks' gestation, 18% of infants at 29 to 36 weeks' gestation, and 37% of infants 36 weeks' or higher gestation.[25]

BOX 15.1 Neonatal Modified Kidney Disease: Improving Global Outcomes Criteria for Acute Kidney Injury

Stage	SCr	Urine output
0	No change in SCr or rise <0.3 mg/dL	≥0.5 mL/kg/h
1	SCr rise ≥0.3 mg/dL within 48 h or SCr rise ≥1.5–1.9 x reference SCr within 7 days	<0.5 mL/kg/h for 6–12 h
2	SCr rise ≥2.0–2.9 x reference SCr	<0.5 mL/kg/h for ≥12 h
3	SCr rise ≥3.0–2.9 x reference SCr or SCr >2.5 mg/dL or receipt of dialysis	<0.3 mL/kg/h for ≥24 h or anuria for ≥12 h

SCr, Serum creatine.
From Selewski DT, Charlton JR, Jetton JG, et al. Neonatal acute kidney injury. *Pediatr.* 2015;136(2):e463-473.

Neonates are at high risk of developing AKI because of their intrinsically low GFR, immaturity of renal tubules, increased susceptibility to impaired renal perfusion, frequent exposure to nephrotoxic agents including indomethacin and aminoglycosides, and frequent use of umbilical catheters with potential for thrombosis.[23] Within the NICU population, certain groups at heightened risk of developing AKI include term and late-preterm neonates with perinatal asphyxia, very low-birth-weight and extremely low-birth-weight infants, and infants requiring cardiac surgery or extracorporeal membrane oxygenation (ECMO) support.

Clinical signs of AKI include oliguria, systemic hypertension, evidence of fluid overload or volume depletion, cardiac arrhythmia, decreased activity, seizure, vomiting, and poor feeding. Laboratory findings include elevated serum creatinine and blood urea nitrogen, hyperkalemia, metabolic acidosis, hypocalcemia, hyperphosphatemia, and a prolonged half-life for medications excreted by the kidney (e.g., aminoglycosides, vancomycin, theophylline). The causes of neonatal AKI are multiple and can be divided into prerenal, renal, and postrenal categories (Box 15.2).

Prerenal Acute Kidney Injury

Prerenal azotemia is the most common type of AKI in the neonate and may account for up to 85% of all cases. Prerenal azotemia is characterized by inadequate renal perfusion, which is followed by improvements in renal function and urine output if promptly treated. The most common causes of prerenal azotemia are hypotension, volume depletion, hemorrhage, septic shock, necrotizing enterocolitis, patent ductus arteriosus, and congestive heart failure. Administration of medications that

BOX 15.2 Causes of Acute Kidney Injury in the Neonate

Prerenal
- Volume depletion
- Hypotension
- Hemorrhage
- Sepsis
- Necrotizing enterocolitis
- Congestive heart failure
- Drugs: angiotensin-converting enzyme inhibitors, angiotensin receptor blockers, nonsteroidal antiinflammatory agents, amphotericin

Renal (Intrinsic)
- Acute tubular necrosis
- Renal dysplasia
- Polycystic kidney disease
- Renal vein thrombosis
- Uric acid nephropathy

Postrenal (Obstructive)
- Posterior urethral valves
- Bilateral ureteropelvic junction obstruction
- Bilateral ureterovesical junction obstruction
- Neurogenic bladder
- Obstructive nephrolithiasis

reduce renal blood flow, such as indomethacin or ibuprofen, angiotensin-converting enzyme (ACE) inhibitors, and phenylephrine eye drops, can result in prerenal azotemia.

Renal (Intrinsic) Acute Kidney Injury

The most common cause of intrinsic AKI in neonates is ATN. Risk factors for ATN include a prolonged prerenal state, perinatal asphyxia, sepsis, neonatal cardiac surgery, need for ECMO support, and nephrotoxic drug administration (acyclovir, aminoglycoside antibiotics, amphotericin B, ACE inhibitors, nonsteroidal antiinflammatory drugs [NSAIDs], radiocontrast agents, and vancomycin). The pathophysiology of ATN is complex and appears to involve interrelationships among renal tubular cellular injury, hypoxia, and altered glomerular filtration and hemodynamics. Other causes of intrinsic AKI in the newborn include renal dysplasia, autosomal recessive PKD, and renal arterial or venous thrombosis. Glomerulonephritis, although a common cause of AKI in older children and adolescents, is very uncommon in the neonatal population.

Postrenal (Obstructive) Acute Kidney Injury

Neonatal obstructive AKI may be caused by several congenital urinary tract conditions, including posterior urethral valves, bilateral ureteropelvic or ureterovesical junction (UVJ) obstruction, obstructive urolithiasis, and neurogenic bladder. Rarer causes of obstructive AKI include extrinsic compression of the ureters or bladder by a tumor such as a sacrococcygeal teratoma or intrinsic obstruction by renal calculi or fungus balls. Although relief of obstruction may yield improvement in urine output and GFR, many infants will develop CKD because of variable degrees of associated renal dysplasia.

BOX 15.3 Diagnostic Indexes in Acute Kidney Injury

Test	Prerenal AKI	Intrinsic AKI
BUN/Cr ratio (mg/mg)	>30	<20
FE_{Na} (%)	≤2.5	≥3.0
Urinary Na (mEq/L)	≤20	≥50
Urinary Osm (mOsm/kg)	≥350	≤300
Urinary specific gravity	>1.012	<1.014
Ultrasonography	Normal	May be abnormal
Response to volume challenge	U/O >2 mL/kg/h	No increase in urinary output

AKI, Acute kidney injury; *BUN*, blood urea nitrogen; *Cr*, creatinine; *FE_{Na}*, fractional excretion of sodium; *Osm*, osmolality.

Evaluation of Acute Kidney Injury

A careful history should focus on prenatal ultrasound abnormalities, history of perinatal asphyxia, pre- or postnatal administration of nephrotoxic medications, and a family history of kidney disease. The physical examination should focus on signs of volume depletion or volume overload, the abdomen, genitalia, and a search for other congenital anomalies or signs of the oligohydramnios (Potter) syndrome. Laboratory evaluation may include electrolytes, blood urea nitrogen, creatinine, calcium, phosphorus, albumin, and uric acid. Urine should be sent for urinalysis, culture (when the etiology is unclear), and sodium and creatinine levels. The FE_{Na}, as well as other diagnostic indexes, may be useful in differentiating prerenal from intrinsic AKI (Box 15.3).

Neonates with a FE_{Na} value of more than 3% generally have intrinsic AKI, whereas those with a FE_{Na} value of less than 2.5% have prerenal AKI. Baseline normal FE_{Na} values in preterm neonates may be as high as 5% at birth,[26] so the FE_{Na} measurement may be less helpful in distinguishing intrinsic versus prerenal AKI in that population. Renal ultrasound is helpful in the identification of congenital renal disease and urinary tract obstruction.

Prevention of Acute Kidney Injury

The prevention of AKI in newborn infants requires maintenance of an adequate circulatory volume, careful fluid management, and prompt diagnosis and treatment of hemodynamic or respiratory abnormalities. Nephrotoxic medications such as acyclovir, aminoglycoside antibiotics, amphotericin B, ACE inhibitors, NSAIDs, radiocontrast agents, and vancomycin should be used judiciously in neonates at high risk for AKI. Prophylactic theophylline (5 mg/kg IV) given within the first hour of life has been shown to reduce the incidence of AKI in asphyxiated neonates, although its use must be weighed against potentially harmful neurologic side effects.[27] Therapeutic hypothermia protocols currently used for treatment of infants with

BOX 15.4 Indications for Dialysis

- Hyperkalemia
- Hyponatremia
- Acidosis
- Hypocalcemia
- Hyperphosphatemia
- Volume overload
- Uremic symptoms
- Inability to provide adequate nutrition

perinatal asphyxia may have a beneficial effect in reducing the incidence of neonatal AKI.[28]

Medical Management

In the case of established oliguric AKI, a urinary catheter should be placed to exclude lower urinary tract obstruction. If there is no improvement in urine output after bladder drainage, a fluid challenge of 10 to 20 mL/kg should be administered over 1 to 2 hours to exclude prerenal AKI. Consideration should be given to use of vasopressor support such as dopamine to ensure that the infant has a mean arterial pressure adequate to provide renal perfusion. Lack of improvement in urine output and serum creatinine following adequate bladder drainage, fluid resuscitation, and establishment of an adequate mean arterial pressure suggests intrinsic AKI.

The goal of medical management of intrinsic AKI is to provide supportive care until there is spontaneous improvement in renal function. To prevent symptomatic fluid overload, intake should be restricted to insensible losses (500 mL/m^2 per day, or 30 mL/kg per day) plus urine output and other measured losses. Daily to twice-daily weights and careful intake and output measurements are essential to follow volume status. Nephrotoxic medications should be discontinued when possible to reduce the risk of additional renal injury. All medications should be adjusted by dose, interval, or both according to the estimated GFR. Potassium and phosphorus should be restricted in those neonates with hyperkalemia, hyperphosphatemia, oliguria, and/or rapidly worsening renal function. Metabolic acidosis may require treatment with intravenous or oral sodium bicarbonate. Loop diuretics may prove helpful in augmenting the urinary flow rate but should be withheld if there is no response or in the case of anuria.

Renal Replacement Therapy

Renal replacement therapy is rarely needed in neonates with AKI but should be considered if maximum medical management fails to maintain acceptable fluid and electrolyte levels. The indications for the initiation of renal replacement therapy include hyperkalemia, hyponatremia with symptomatic volume overload, acidosis, hypocalcemia, hyperphosphatemia, uremic symptoms, and an inability to provide adequate nutrition because of the need for fluid restriction (Box 15.4). The two purposes of renal replacement therapy are ultrafiltration (removal of water) and dialysis (removal of solutes). In general, only neonates greater than 1.5 to 2 kg in size may be considered for renal replacement therapies because of limited ability to place and maintain dialysis access in smaller infants.

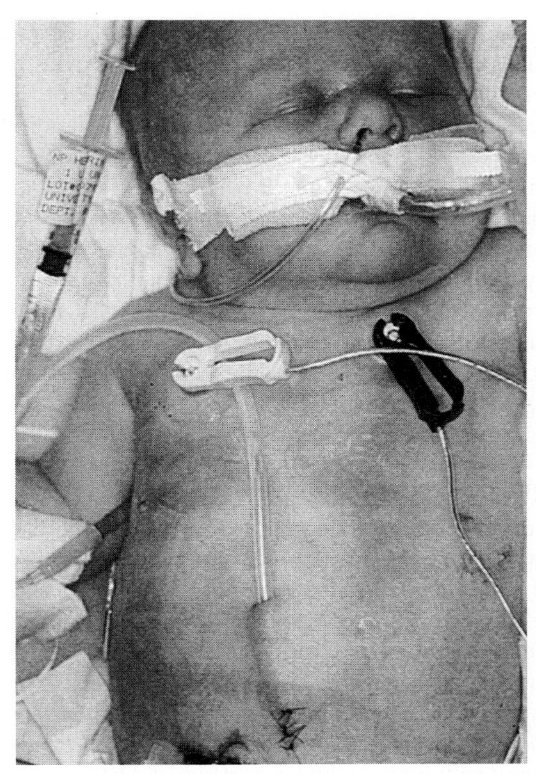

Fig. 15.4 Critically ill infant with acute kidney injury undergoing treatment with peritoneal dialysis. (Courtesy Julie H. Corder, PNP, Cleveland Clinic Children's Hospital, Cleveland, Ohio.)

Peritoneal dialysis is the most commonly used renal replacement modality in the neonatal population because it is technically less difficult and does not require vascular access or anticoagulation. For this procedure, hyperosmolar dialysate is repeatedly infused into and drained out of the peritoneal cavity through a surgically placed catheter, accomplishing ultrafiltration and dialysis (Fig. 15.4). Cycle length, volume of dialysate infused ("dwell volume"), and the osmolar concentration of the dialysate can be varied to accomplish the goals of therapy. Contraindications to peritoneal dialysis include recent abdominal surgery, necrotizing enterocolitis, pleuroperitoneal leakage, and presence of a ventriculoperitoneal shunt.

Continuous renal replacement therapy (CRRT) is becoming a more frequently used therapeutic modality in neonates and infants with AKI.[29] For this procedure, the patient's blood is continuously circulated through a pump-driven extracorporeal circuit containing a highly permeable hemofilter. CRRT can be employed in conjunction with ECMO by putting the CRRT circuit in line with the ECMO circuit. The chief advantage of CRRT is the ability to carefully control fluid removal, which makes this modality especially useful in the neonate with hemodynamic instability. The main disadvantages are the need to achieve and maintain central vascular access and the need for continuous anticoagulation.

Intermittent hemodialysis is a less commonly used but technically feasible mode of renal replacement therapy in the neonatal population. Hemodialysis involves intermittent 3- to 4-hour treatments in which fluid and solutes are rapidly removed from the infant using an extracorporeal dialyzer, with clearance achieved by the use of countercurrent dialysate. The chief advantage of hemodialysis is the ability to rapidly remove solutes, a characteristic that makes this modality the therapy of choice in neonatal hyperammonemia. The main disadvantages are the requirement for central vascular access, usually a double lumen 7 French catheter, and the hemodynamic instability and osmolar shifts that may occur with rapid solute and fluid shifts.

Providing adequate renal replacement therapy may be limited by the challenges of placing and/or maintaining intravascular or peritoneal dialysis access in the very small preterm neonate. If dialysis access cannot be established, care of the infant with AKI is limited to maximal supportive medical management, with meticulous attention to fluid, electrolyte, and acid-base balance.

Prognosis

Research has demonstrated that AKI is not just a marker of severity of illness in neonates but is also independently associated with poor outcomes. A recent large multicenter retrospective study demonstrated that the presence of AKI was independently associated with increased mortality in neonates, (10% vs. 1%) as well as increased length of hospital stay (median 23 vs. 19 days).[25] In addition, infants with higher stages of AKI had higher mortality rates and lengths of hospitalization when compared with infants with lower stages of AKI.

In the past, AKI was felt to be a completely reversible syndrome in neonates, with the idea that serum creatinine returning to baseline indicated no further renal risk. However, observational studies have demonstrated high rates of CKD in survivors of neonatal AKI.[30] The risk of CKD in survivors of neonatal AKI may be compounded by the risks of prematurity and low birth weight, both of which are associated with CKD because of associated inadequate nephron development.[31] Long-term nephrology follow-up care is important in neonates with a history of AKI to monitor for evidence of CKD, including proteinuria, hypertension, and gradual increase in serum creatinine over time. Special attention should be given to those infants with a history of AKI stages 2 and 3, treatment with dialysis, significant prematurity, intrauterine growth restriction, or underlying renal anomalies. Early identification of CKD allows implementation of strategies to slow the loss of kidney function, including healthy lifestyle, good hydration, optimal management of hypertension, reduction of proteinuria, and avoidance of nephrotoxin exposure.

HYPERTENSION

Incidence and Definition

The incidence of hypertension in neonates is estimated to be approximately 1% to 2% and is most often seen in infants with a concurrent condition such as chronic lung disease, renal disease, or a history of umbilical arterial catheterization.[32] Identification of elevated blood pressure in neonates can be difficult because of variations in blood pressure measurement techniques, normal changes in blood pressure with gestational age and weight, and other factors that affect blood pressure readings, including level of wakefulness, feeding, crying, and pain.

CASE 15.4

A 2-month-old former 1100-g 28 weeks' gestation male infant with bronchopulmonary dysplasia (BPD) is noted to have a blood pressure of 110/70 mm Hg. Review of the blood pressures over the previous week show gradual increase in values from 80s/50s to the current level. There is no evidence of volume overload, and the infant does not appear to be in pain or agitated during blood pressure measurement. There is a history of umbilical artery catheterization at birth for 1 week without known complication. Serum electrolyte levels are normal, and creatinine concentration is 0.4 mg/dL. Renal ultrasonography with Doppler reveals no abnormality. The infant is treated with oral amlodipine, with normalization of blood pressures within 1 week. By 12 months of age, the infant is successfully weaned off all antihypertensive therapy and maintains blood pressures within the normal range for age.

The definition of neonatal hypertension is sustained blood pressure above the 95th percentile for infants of similar size, gestational age, and postnatal age. Useful data on normal infant blood pressures were published by Zubrow and colleagues, who prospectively measured blood pressure in nearly 700 infants, showing that blood pressure increased with gestational age, postconceptual age, and birth weight (Fig. 15.5).[33] Based on these data and synthesis of several other studies, a practical table of systolic, diastolic, and mean arterial blood pressure values was created and may be useful in defining normal and elevated blood pressures in neonates greater than 2 weeks of age from 26 to 44 weeks postconceptual age (Table 15.4).[32]

EDITORIAL COMMENT: Despite the prevalence of blood pressure disorders in the neonatal intensive care unit (NICU), there remains no standard definition of hypotension or hypertension in the neonatal period. Additionally, there is clear evidence that different NICUs, and even different clinicians within the same NICU, define and treat blood pressure disorders in completely different ways.

Causes

The causes of neonatal hypertension are varied and are outlined in Box 15.5. Renovascular disease is the most frequent etiology and accounts for 80% to 90% of all neonatal hypertension. Renal artery thromboembolism related to umbilical artery catheterization is the most likely cause of renovascular disease. Less common causes of neonatal renovascular hypertension include congenital renal artery stenosis, fibromuscular dysplasia, midaortic coarctation, and renovascular compression by tumors.

Other causes of neonatal hypertension include renal conditions such as AKI, autosomal recessive PKD, and obstructive uropathy. The most significant nonrenal cause of neonatal hypertension is BPD. Although the mechanism by which BPD is associated with hypertension is not clearly defined, the severity of the blood pressure elevation appears to correlate with the severity of the lung disease.[34] Less common causes of neonatal

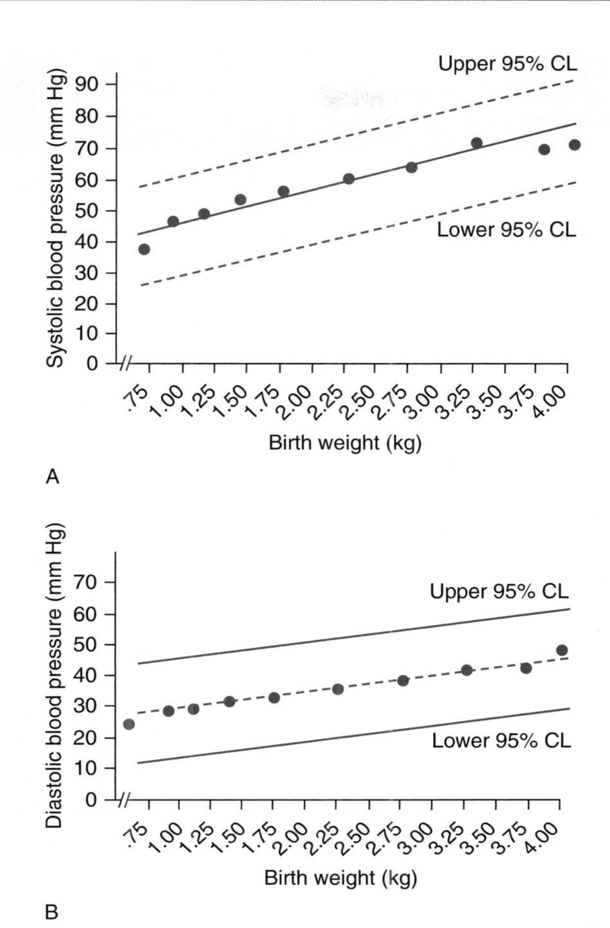

Fig. 15.5 Linear relationship between mean systolic (A) and diastolic (B) blood pressure and birth weight on day 1 of life. *CL,* Confidence limit. (From Zubrow AB, Hulman S. Determinants of blood pressure in infants admitted to neonatal intensive care units: a prospective multicenter study. Philadelphia Neonatal Blood Pressure Study Group. *J Perinatol.* 1995;15:470.)

hypertension include endocrine disorders, coarctation of the aorta, intraventricular hemorrhage, history of abdominal wall closure, tumors, treatment with ECMO, seizures, pain, and drug withdrawal. Medications such as corticosteroids, vasopressors, caffeine, theophylline, and bronchodilators have been associated with elevated blood pressures in neonates.

Clinical Presentation

The majority of neonates with hypertension are asymptomatic, as elevated blood pressures are typically noted in routine monitoring. If present, symptoms of neonatal hypertension are often nonspecific, including poor feeding, irritability, and lethargy. Marked blood pressure elevation may lead to tachypnea, cyanosis, apnea, impaired perfusion, vasomotor instability, congestive heart failure, and hepatosplenomegaly. Neurologic symptoms such as tremors, hypertonicity, hypotonicity, opisthotonos, asymmetric reflexes, hemiparesis, seizures, apnea, or coma may also occur. The renal effects of hypertension may include AKI and sodium wasting related to pressure natriuresis.

Evaluation

The first step is to determine whether the elevated blood pressure persists when the infant is quiet and relaxed. A standardized protocol for accurate blood pressure measurement in neonates is shown in Box 15.6.[32] Blood pressures are preferably measured in the upper arm, as leg blood pressure

TABLE 15.4 Post-Conceptual Age 50Th Percentile 95Th Percentile 99Th Percentile

44 Weeks			
SBP	88	105	110
DBP	50	68	73
MAP	63	80	85
42 Weeks			
SBP	85	98	102
DBP	50	65	70
MAP	62	76	81
40 Weeks			
SBP	80	95	100
DBP	50	65	70
MAP	60	75	80
38 Weeks			
SBP	77	92	97
DBP	50	65	70
MAP	59	74	79
36 Weeks			
SBP	72	87	92
DBP	50	65	70
MAP	57	72	77
34 Weeks			
SBP	70	85	90
DBP	40	55	60
MAP	50	65	70
32 Weeks			
SBP	68	83	88
DBP	40	55	60
MAP	49	64	69
30 Weeks			
SBP	65	80	85
DBP	40	55	60
MAP	48	63	68
28 Weeks			
SBP	60	75	80
DBP	38	50	54
MAP	45	58	63
26 Weeks			
SBP	55	72	77
DBP	30	50	56
MAP	38	57	63

SBP, systolic blood pressure; *DSP,* diastolic blood pressure; *MAP,* mean arterial pressure.

BOX 15.5 Causes of Neonatal Hypertension

Renovascular Disease
- Renal artery thrombosis
- Renal artery stenosis

Congenital Renal Malformations
- Polycystic kidney disease
- Hydronephrosis

Renal Parenchymal Disease
- Acute tubular necrosis

Coarctation of the Aorta

Other
- Endocrine disorders
- Bronchopulmonary dysplasia
- Drug exposure: cocaine, methadone, corticosteroids, aminophylline
- Abdominal wall closure
- Extracorporeal membrane oxygenation

measurements tend to overestimate the true blood pressure. History should focus on prenatal medication exposures, presence or history of an umbilical artery catheter, and treatment with medications that raise blood pressure. Blood pressure trends since birth should be reviewed to establish the onset and severity of hypertension. A complete physical examination should include four extremity blood pressure measurements to assess for aortic coarctation. The infant should be examined carefully for signs of volume overload, including rales, cardiac gallop, or peripheral edema. The abdomen should be carefully inspected for presence of abdominal or flank masses or renal bruits. Ambiguous genitalia in a hypertensive infant should raise the suspicion of congenital adrenal hyperplasia. Initial laboratory studies should include a urinalysis and determinations of serum electrolytes, blood urea nitrogen, creatinine, and calcium. Other diagnostic studies, including renin, aldosterone, cortisol, thyroid function tests, and catecholamines, can be considered based on the clinical scenario and results of screening studies.

Ultrasonography of the kidneys with a Doppler flow study of the aorta and renal arteries should be performed to exclude a renal artery or aortic thrombus or structural anomalies of the urinary tract. Absence of a defined thrombus does not, however, rule out renovascular hypertension, as the majority of thrombi are very small and not detectable by ultrasonography. CT, magnetic resonance angiography, and angiography may be considered in more difficult cases, although their use may be limited in the very small infant. Echocardiography should be performed to exclude aortic coarctation and evaluate the left ventricle.

Treatment

The first approach to the treatment of neonatal hypertension is to correct all iatrogenic causes of blood pressure elevation,

BOX 15.6 Protocol for Blood Pressure Measurement Using an Oscillometric Device

- Wait at least 1.5 hours after a meal or medical intervention.
- Place infant in prone or supine position.
- Use appropriately sized blood pressure cuff.
- Place cuff on right upper arm.
- Leave infant undisturbed for 15 minutes after cuff placement.
- Ensure that infant is asleep or in quiet awake state.
- Take three successive blood pressure readings at 2-minute intervals.

including improper measurement technique, vasopressor administration, volume overload, narcotic withdrawal, and inadequately controlled pain. If blood pressures remain elevated above the 99th percentile, treatment with an intravenous or oral antihypertensive agent is indicated to prevent adverse effects on the kidneys, heart, and central nervous system.

Neonates with signs and symptoms of a hypertensive emergency such as cardiopulmonary failure, acute neurologic dysfunction, and AKI are best treated with a continuous intravenous infusion of an antihypertensive agent such as nicardipine, esmolol, or labetalol (Table 15.5). Careful monitoring using an arterial line is recommended in this situation. The chief advantage of a continuous infusion is the ability to quickly increase or decrease the rate of infusion to achieve the desired blood pressure. The goal of therapy is a gradual decrease in blood pressure to minimize injury to the brain, heart, and kidneys. Blood pressure should not be lowered below the 95th percentile for at least 24 to 48 hours to avoid the possibility of cerebral and optic disc ischemia.

Intermittent administration of intravenous agents such as hydralazine or labetalol may be considered in hypertensive infants with mild to moderate hypertension in whom oral agents cannot be used because of gastrointestinal dysfunction (Table 15.5).

Oral antihypertensive agents are best used in infants with less severe hypertension or in those whose acute hypertension has been controlled with intravenous infusions and who are ready to switch to chronic oral therapy (Table 15.6). Calcium channel blockers such as isradipine and amlodipine are first-choice agents. ACE inhibitors such as captopril may be useful but are not recommended for infants less than 44 weeks' postconceptional age because they may impair the final stages of nephron development. If ACE inhibitors are used, careful attention to urine output and the levels of serum creatinine and potassium is recommended, as neonates may be extremely sensitive to the reduction in renal blood flow associated with these agents. Diuretics such as chlorothiazide may be useful agents in infants with chronic lung disease.

When renovascular hypertension is suspected, the umbilical artery catheter should be removed as soon as possible. If a large thrombus is identified, systemic heparinization may be considered to prevent extension of the clot. If the hypertension cannot be controlled medically or massive aortic thrombosis results in major complications, thrombolysis with urokinase,

TABLE 15.5 Intravenous Antihypertensive Medications

Drug	Dose	Interval	Action
Esmolol	100–500 mcg/kg/min	Continuous infusion	Beta-blocker
Hydralazine	0.15–0.6 mg/kg/dose	Every 4–6 hr	Vasodilator
Labetalol	0.2–1.0 mg/kg/dose	Every 4–6 hr	Alpha- and beta-blocker
	0.25–3.0 mg/kg/hr	Continuous infusion	
Nicardipine	1–4 mcg/kg/min	Continuous infusion	Calcium channel blocker
Sodium nitroprusside	0.5–10.0 mcg/kg/min	Continuous infusion	Vasodilator

TABLE 15.6 Oral Antihypertensive Medications

Drug	Dose	Interval	Class
Amlodipine	0.05–0.3 mg/kg/dose	Daily to BID	Calcium channel blocker
Captopril	0.01–0.5 mg/kg/dose	TID	Angiotensin-converting enzyme inhibitor
Chlorothiazide	5–15 mg/kg/dose	BID	Distal tubule diuretic
Clonidine	5–10 mcg/kg/day	TID	Alpha-agonist
Enalapril	0.04–0.3 mg/kg/dose	Daily to BID	Angiotensin-converting enzyme inhibitor
Furosemide	1–2 mg/kg/dose	Daily to TID	Loop diuretic
Isradipine	0.05–0.15 mg/kg/dose	QID	Calcium channel blocker
Labetalol	0.5–1.0 mg/kg/dose	BID to TID	Alpha and beta blocker
Propranolol	0.5–1.0 mg/kg/dose	TID	Beta blocker

BID, Twice daily; *QID,* four times daily; *TID,* three times daily.

streptokinase, or tissue plasminogen activator may be considered. If severe hypertension persists, surgical thrombectomy or nephrectomy may be contemplated.

Prognosis

Most neonates with hypertension presumed to be caused by umbilical artery catheters or BPD experience improvement in their blood pressures and do not typically require antihypertensive medications beyond 12 months of age. Infants may require periodic increases in their antihypertensive medication doses following discharge because of rapid growth, but over time, antihypertensive agents may be weaned by maintaining a stable medication dose as the infant grows in size. On the other hand, infants with hypertension related to renal disease or another secondary cause will most likely have hypertension that persists into childhood.

Long-term studies of children and adolescents with a history of neonatal hypertension are needed. There is growing evidence that neonates born before completion of nephrogenesis at 36 weeks' gestation may be at increased risk for development of hypertension and CKD in adolescence or adulthood.[31]

NEPHROCALCINOSIS

NC, defined as calcium salt deposition in the renal interstitium, is a well-known complication in the neonatal population, occurring in 7% to 41% of hospitalized premature infants.[35] Infants at highest risk appear to be those with lower gestational age and birth weight, often in combination with severe respiratory disease. NC is usually discovered incidentally on abdominal imaging studies, although infants with NC may present with microscopic or gross hematuria, granular material in the diaper, or UTI.

CASE 15.5

A 4-month-old infant with bronchopulmonary dysplasia (BPD) who had been born prematurely at 25 weeks was incidentally noted to have medullary nephrocalcinosis (NC) on an abdominal ultrasound study. She had required furosemide and corticosteroid administration to treat her lung disease. Urinalysis revealed hematuria (1+) with 10 to 15 red blood cells per high-power field. Urine culture yielded no growth. Spot urine calcium-to-creatinine ratio was elevated at 1.65. Furosemide was discontinued and chlorothiazide initiated to reduce urinary calcium excretion. Corticosteroids were tapered and discontinued over the next 2 months. Urine calcium-to-creatinine ratio decreased to 0.8, and serial ultrasound examinations showed gradual resolution of NC. When the infant was 8 months of age, chlorothiazide was discontinued, and at 1 year of age, a follow-up renal ultrasound study yielded normal findings.

Neonatal NC is multifactorial in etiology and develops as the consequence of an imbalance between stone-promoting and stone-inhibiting factors.[35] The immature renal tubular cells and the lower GFR of preterm infants render them more susceptible to crystal formation and aggregation. Hypercalciuria (excessive urinary calcium excretion) is a common risk factor and may result from chronic treatment with loop diuretics, increased calcium intake from total parenteral nutrition (TPN), or vitamin D supplementation. Subcutaneous fat necrosis following birth trauma is a rare but serious cause of hypercalciuria. Other risk factors for NC include hypocitraturia (low urinary citrate excretion), which is a common finding in patients with persistent metabolic acidosis, which often occurs in ill preterm infants. Uncommon genetic conditions associated with an increased risk of NC include primary hyperoxaluria, distal renal tubular acidosis, Bartter syndrome, Williams syndrome, and idiopathic infantile hypercalcemia.

Routine ultrasonographic screening should be considered for all infants who receive long-term loop diuretics for chronic lung or heart disease. In those with documented NC, loop diuretics should be discontinued, if possible. Thiazide diuretics such as chlorothiazide may be substituted, as they tend to reduce urinary calcium excretion, although serum calcium must be monitored closely to avoid hypercalcemia. Agents that increase urinary calcium excretion such as glucocorticoids, xanthine derivatives, and any sodium-containing supplements should be minimized or discontinued if possible. Administration of calcium and phosphorus in TPN as well as vitamin D supplementation should be reduced if excessive. A high urinary flow rate should be maintained to reduce the probability of urinary crystallization. Metabolic acidosis, if present, should be treated with potassium citrate. The goal of therapy should be the maintenance of the spot urinary calcium-to-creatinine ratio less than 0.8 for infants less than 7 months of age.[35]

The usual outcome for infants with neonatal NC without an underlying genetic defect is spontaneous resolution over the first 2 years of life. Serial renal ultrasonography is needed to confirm resolution of NC. There is concern that neonatal NC may increase risk for impairment in kidney function later in life, particularly in premature infants who are inherently at increased risk of CKD. Although results are conflicting whether NC affects renal growth and function, a recent case series demonstrated evidence of tubular dysfunction and shorter kidney length in the first year of life of infants with NC.[36] Long-term nephrology follow-up care of premature infants with NC is recommended.

RENOVASCULAR THROMBOSIS

CASE 15.6

A 36-week-male infant was born to a 28-year-old woman with poorly controlled type 1 diabetes mellitus; delivery was complicated by perinatal asphyxia and placental abruption. An umbilical venous catheter was placed for access immediately after birth. On day 2 of life, the infant developed macroscopic hematuria. Physical examination revealed normal blood pressure and a left-sided flank mass. Laboratory work revealed platelet count of 75,000 and a serum creatinine of 1.0 mg/dL. Renal ultrasound with Doppler showed an enlarged, echogenic left kidney with impaired venous flow.

Renal Vascular Thrombosis

Thromboembolic complications are rare but serious events in the NICU. The neonatal kidney is particularly vulnerable to thrombosis because of its relatively low blood flow, small vessel diameter, and enhanced renal vasoconstriction. Hypoxia, volume depletion, hypotension, and infection can further disturb the balance between procoagulant and anticoagulant factors and increase the risk of thromboembolism. Both venous and arterial thrombosis may occur in the neonate, although renal vein thromboses (RVT) are more common. Risk factors for RVT include prematurity, maternal diabetes mellitus, congenital heart disease, polycythemia, hypertonic dehydration, acute blood loss, perinatal asphyxia, in utero death of a twin, sepsis, RDS, and prolonged central venous cannulation.[37] A subset of neonates with RVT have an inherited thrombophilia including deficiencies of protein C, protein S or antithrombin, factor V Leiden mutation, or prothrombin gene mutation.

Thrombosis begins in the small renal veins and propagates toward the main renal vein, ultimately reaching the inferior vena cava. Thrombosis is usually unilateral (70%) but may be bilateral or extend into the inferior vena cava, and is associated with adrenal infarction in a minority of patients.

The classic clinical triad of symptoms in RVT includes a flank mass, macroscopic hematuria, and thrombocytopenia, although all elements of the triad are present in fewer than 25% of infants with RVT. Additional signs may include oliguric AKI, hypertension, vomiting, lethargy, anorexia, fever, and shock. Ultrasonography in the acute phase reveals enlarged and echogenic kidneys with loss of corticomedullary differentiation. A Doppler study may reveal resistance or absence of blood flow in the main renal vein and collateral vessels. Uptake may be absent or severely diminished on a radionuclide scan. Follow-up ultrasonography may show gradual decrease in kidney size, suggestive of renal atrophy.

Initial evaluation after identification of a thrombosis should include baseline testing including a CBC, prothrombin time, activated partial thromboplastin time, and fibrinogen. Maternal blood may be tested for lupus anticoagulant and anticardiolipin antibody. Testing for an inherited prothrombotic state should be conducted in neonates with thrombosis, which is clinically significant, recurrent, or spontaneous. Testing is best deferred until after resolution of the acute event.

There are no evidence-based guidelines for management of neonatal RVT, although expert opinion guidelines suggest need for a multidisciplinary team including neonatology, nephrology, radiology, and hematology. If the thrombosis appears to be catheter associated, the catheter should be removed. Supportive medical treatment consists of correction of fluid and electrolyte imbalances as well as supportive treatment of AKI, possibly including dialysis. Anticoagulation (unfractionated heparin or low-molecular-weight heparin) may be employed to prevent the extension of thrombosis, although the benefits of anticoagulation should be weighed against the risks of hemorrhagic events, including intraventricular hemorrhage. Thrombolytic therapies such as recombinant tissue plasminogen activator or urokinase should be reserved for cases of critical compromise of kidney function, as seen in bilateral renal vein thrombosis. Surgical thrombectomy is considered in patients with thrombosis of the inferior vena cava, and nephrectomy may be necessary in infants with severe refractory hypertension.

Although the perinatal mortality rate in infants with RVT has decreased progressively during the past decades, the prognosis for the affected kidney is poor, with progressive atrophy in up to 70% of kidneys.[37] Long-term complications include hypertension in 20% of patients, CKD, and end-stage kidney disease in a minority of patients with a history of bilateral thrombosis.

CONGENITAL KIDNEY DISEASE

CASE 15.7

A 2100-g male infant was delivered at 32 weeks after oligohydramnios had been noted in the third trimester. Apgar scores were 8 at 1 minute and 9 at 5 minutes. Physical examination yielded normal findings, including absence of abdominal masses. The infant fed poorly and showed decreased activity. Laboratory evaluation revealed a rising serum creatinine level, which reached 4.5 mg/dL on day 6 of life. Renal ultrasonography demonstrated absence of the right kidney and a small, hyperechoic left kidney with several small cortical cysts.

The infant's diagnosis was chronic kidney disease (CKD) because of right renal agenesis and left renal dysplasia. A peritoneal dialysis catheter was placed and dialysis initiated. The infant's parents were trained by the nephrology team to perform home dialysis and administer supplemental nasogastric feedings and medications for management of CKD. The infant received home peritoneal dialysis until 2 years of age, when he received a kidney transplant from his mother.

With improved understanding of the molecular and genetic basis of disease, it is now understood that identical single-gene defects can produce disease phenotypes that were previously considered to be distinct. This understanding has led to use of the term CAKUT to refer to the spectrum of urinary tract malformations. CAKUT includes conditions as diverse as renal agenesis, hypoplasia, dysplasia, hydronephrosis, ureterocele, VUR, and posterior urethral valves. CAKUT occurs in 1 in 200 births and accounts for up to 30% of prenatally detected birth defects.[38,39] According to the North American Pediatric Renal Trials and Collaborative Studies, CAKUT is responsible for approximately 36% of ESRD in children worldwide, although only a minority of kidney failure occurs in the neonatal period.

Renal Agenesis

Renal agenesis describes the complete absence of formation of a kidney without the presence of rudimentary tissue. This absence results from failure of the ureteric bud to form or elongate during fetal renal development. The genes controlling ureteric bud induction involve GDNF/Ret signaling interactions along with several critical transcription factors such as PAX2 and Eya1, and many of these genes have been confirmed to cause renal agenesis as well as other CAKUT phenotypes (Table 15.1).[5] Renal agenesis occurs in approximately 1 in 2000 births, although estimates vary because of clinically silent unilateral disease.[40] Bilateral renal agenesis is uniformly fatal because of pulmonary hypoplasia resulting from the oligohydramnios sequence (Potter syndrome), but unilateral agenesis is often asymptomatic.

Evaluation of suspected renal agenesis should exclude other conditions that result in an apparent solitary kidney such as an ectopic kidney or regressed MCDK. The evaluation should assess the structure and function of the solitary kidney to confirm normal function and appropriate compensatory hypertrophy that may be present at birth. Absence of compensatory hypertrophy may herald hypoplasia or dysplasia of the remaining kidney, which alters treatment and prognosis of the condition. A CAKUT phenotype can be identified in the contralateral kidney 30% to 40% of the time following detection of apparent unilateral disease.[40] There is no consensus whether investigation of the contralateral kidney with VCUG needs to be undertaken in all cases of unilateral renal agenesis or only if hydronephrosis is present or following a clinically meaningful event such as a UTI.

Unilateral renal agenesis may be isolated or part of a larger syndrome involving cardiac, genital, gastrointestinal, and skeletal structures, including VACTERL (vertebral defects, anal atresia, cardiac defects, tracheoesophageal fistula, renal anomalies, and limb abnormalities) association, caudal regression syndrome, branchio-oto-renal syndrome, and multiple chromosomal defects. Extrarenal anomalies are found in approximately 30% of patients with unilateral renal agenesis.[40]

Renal Hypoplasia and Dysplasia

Renal dysplasia describes the failure of kidney tissue to differentiate normally, resulting in primitive and disorganized tubular structures, interstitial fibrosis, and cyst formation. In contrast, renal hypoplasia describes normally formed kidneys that are smaller than normal, although dysplasia and hypoplasia commonly occur together. Bilateral renal hypodysplasia is the most common cause of pediatric ESRD worldwide.[41]

There is no single genotype for renal dysplasia, as it can result from disruption of the development of any normal renal structures; thus, any of the identified genes for ureteric bud initiation, branching morphogenesis, epithelial-mesenchymal transformation, and nephron patterning can cause dysplasia (Table 15.1).[5,38] Moreover, urinary tract obstruction can lead to renal dysplasia through increased pressure and the backflow of urine.

The function of dysplastic kidneys is variable; infants with unilateral dysplasia can remain asymptomatic into adulthood, whereas infants with bilateral dysplasia may have complete renal failure in the first week of life. Evaluation of infants with renal dysplasia should focus on the function of both kidneys because of the increased prevalence of CAKUT conditions in the contralateral kidney. Similar to renal agenesis, the clinician should maintain a high suspicion for the coexistence of associated extrarenal anomalies. There is no specific treatment for infants with renal dysplasia; supportive care should focus on treatment of complications of CKD and strategies to slow the progression of renal fibrosis.

Multicystic Dysplastic Kidney

An MCDK represents the most severe form of renal dysplasia. These nonfunctional kidneys consist of multiple large, noncommunicating cysts separated by tissue lacking any normal renal architecture. MCDK can be identified as a unilateral abdominal mass in the neonatal period, although because of its characteristic sonographic appearance, it is usually identified prenatally. MCDK occurs in 1 in 4000 births,[42] usually as a sporadic event. Theories for the pathogenesis for multicystic dysplasia include early urinary obstruction, failure of normal ureteric bud signaling, and teratogenic exposures.[42] There is no genetic association that differentiates MCDK from other forms of renal dysplasia.

Evaluation of infants with an MCDK is similar to that of unilateral renal agenesis, because there is an increased frequency of CAKUT anomalies in the contralateral kidney. Urinary obstruction must be considered in infants with MCDK, as markedly dilated renal calyces can have a similar appearance to MCDK. The primary sonographic difference between the two conditions is that in obstructed kidneys there is communication between the hypoechoic structures, whereas in MCDK the cysts have no communication with each other. If ultrasound is not sufficient to differentiate between these conditions, a MAG-3 renal scan should be performed; any renal uptake of tracer excludes MCDK. Postnatally, an MCDK is expected to become atretic and involute over time, after which time the kidney will no longer be visible by routine imaging. Historically, children with MCDK routinely underwent nephrectomy, as they were considered to have an increased rate of developing Wilms tumor and hypertension, but this is no longer considered standard practice.

Polycystic Kidney Disease

Although the name implies a close clinical relationship to MCDK, these two conditions are entirely different. PKD is a condition in which there is progressive development of diffuse cysts in kidneys that contain no dysplastic tissue. Both autosomal dominant (ADPKD) and autosomal recessive (ARPKD) forms exist, with ARPKD being far less prevalent but presenting more often in neonates because of its more severe phenotype.

ADPKD is the most common inherited genetic kidney disease and is present in approximately 1 in 800 births.[42] Infants with ADPKD may have several macrocysts noted on either prenatal or postnatal ultrasound, but usually are asymptomatic in the newborn period and into childhood. Progressive cyst development occurs into adulthood, and complications include hematuria, flank pain, hypertension, and CKD. ADPKD can also cause cyst development in the liver, pancreas, or lungs as well as aneurysms of the cerebral arteries.[42]

ARPKD often has a much more severe neonatal presentation, but it can range from an asymptomatic condition to complete renal failure with fatal pulmonary hypoplasia. Severe forms of ARPKD are typically identified on prenatal ultrasound as bilaterally enlarged and echogenic kidneys. The microcysts of ARPKD may not be evident on ultrasound, and absence of sonographically visible cysts does not exclude the diagnosis. Even in newborns without significant renal insufficiency, ARPKD often presents with severe hypertension.[42] Liver involvement includes cystic dilatation of the biliary tree (Caroli disease) and congenital hepatic fibrosis, which may progress to cholestasis, cholangitis, and liver failure over time.

The evaluation and treatment of patients with presumed ARPKD begin with review of prenatal ultrasonography to assess for oligohydramnios, reduced or absent bladder filling, and pulmonary hypoplasia. Delivery room resuscitation and high-level ventilatory support should be anticipated. Even with modern intensive care, up to 30% of ARPKD patients do not survive the perinatal period.[43] After initial stabilization, management of renal dysfunction, volume status, hypertension, and nutritional support become the focus. There remains no disease-modifying treatment available, so therapy in the neonatal period is entirely supportive based on identified renal, pulmonary, cardiovascular, and hepatic dysfunction.

HYDRONEPHROSIS

CASE 15.8

At 20 weeks' gestation, screening ultrasonography reveals moderate bilateral hydronephrosis in a male fetus. Serial ultrasound studies show persistence of the hydronephrosis, development of bilateral hydroureter, and a large bladder with a thickened wall. The infant is delivered at 35 weeks' gestation. A bladder catheter is placed immediately to secure adequate bladder drainage. Renal ultrasonography shows moderate bilateral hydronephrosis and hydroureter and a trabeculated bladder. Voiding cystourethrography (VCUG) confirms the diagnosis of posterior urethral valves as well as the presence of bilateral grade III vesicoureteral reflux (VUR). The infant undergoes primary valve ablation to relieve the urinary tract obstruction. Antibiotic prophylaxis is administered to prevent urinary tract infection (UTI). Serum creatinine concentration is 1.6 mg/dL at hospital discharge and 1.1 mg/dL at 12 months of age, which confirms chronic kidney disease (CKD) and suggests a high likelihood of developing end-stage renal disease (ESRD) in childhood.

Hydronephrosis describes any dilatation of the renal pelvicalyceal system without identifying its cause. Antenatal hydronephrosis is the most common fetal abnormality detected on prenatal ultrasound, occurring in 1% to 4% of all pregnancies.[44] Hydronephrosis has a limited differential diagnosis that includes urinary tract obstruction, VUR, or benign physiologic dilatation without long-term consequence.

Antenatal hydronephrosis is graded based on the degree of dilation of the renal pelvis, involvement of the calyces, and if there is associated thinning of the renal cortex. The severity of postnatal pathology is associated with the degree of pelvicalyceal dilation and the presence of hydroureter or oligohydramnios. Postnatal ultrasound is recommended for all babies with antenatal hydronephrosis. Whenever possible, this postnatal imaging should be delayed for at least 14 days to allow the development of adequate urine flow and improve the examination sensitivity. However, imaging should be performed in the first days after birth when obstruction is suspected or severe antenatal hydronephrosis is present.

The evaluation of infants with hydronephrosis is based on the severity and the suspected cause. In up to 80% of neonates with hydronephrosis, no pathologic cause is identified, and the condition is called transient, or physiologic, hydronephrosis.[44] Transient hydronephrosis is most common with mild and moderate hydronephrosis. Infants with mild hydronephrosis may not require definitive diagnostic testing, and expectant surveillance with serial ultrasonography may be all that is required.

If hydronephrosis is severe or associated with UTI, further evaluation is indicated. When urinary tract obstruction is suspected, a MAG-3 renal scan is typically performed. VCUG is often performed to assess for VUR or posterior urethral valves

For patients with mild to moderate hydronephrosis, variability exists in the practice of further radiologic evaluation and prophylactic antibiotic use. Some clinicians routinely use prophylactic antibiotics and obtain further imaging studies, while others only prescribe suppressive therapy and obtain a VCUG after the first UTI.

Ureteropelvic Junction Obstruction

Ureteropelvic junction (UPJ) obstruction is defined as impeded urine flow from the renal pelvis into the proximal ureter. This may occur from a developmental anomaly causing a stricture at the UPJ or from external compression by an accessory renal vessel. UPJ obstruction is the most common cause of pathological congenital hydronephrosis, occurring in about 1 in 1000 births, with bilateral involvement in up to 40% of cases.[44,45] It should be suspected when moderate or severe hydronephrosis is detected without associated hydroureter, and a MAG-3 renal scan is needed for diagnosis.

The spectrum of clinical disease ranges from mild hydronephrosis with spontaneous resolution to complete nonfunction of the affected kidney. In cases of mild disease, conservative observation over time is possible. However, surgical correction is indicated when the obstruction is bilateral or if renal functional impairment develops.[45] UTI is rare with UPJ obstruction and, if present, should prompt evaluation for coexisting VUR.

Ureterovesical Junction Obstruction

UVJ obstruction occurs when urine flow is impeded from the distal ureter into the bladder. It is the second most common cause of congenital hydronephrosis and should be suspected when hydroureter accompanies hydronephrosis, especially if a dilated, tortuous megaureter is present.[44] This disorder results from abnormal ureteral development and also may spontaneously resolve in mild cases. UTI is more common in this condition than with UPJ obstruction.

Evaluation should include a VCUG to exclude VUR, but the diagnosis of UVJ obstruction is confirmed with a MAG-3 diuretic renal scan. Spontaneous resolution can occur in mild cases, and conservative management is possible. If renal impairment develops, however, surgical correction may be indicated.

Posterior Urethral Valves

Posterior urethral valves are membranous folds of tissue in the proximal urethra that can obstruct urine outflow from the bladder. This condition occurs exclusively in boys and represents the most common cause of lower urinary tract obstruction, with an incidence of 1 in 5000 births.[46] Because of a high rate of associated renal dysplasia and bladder dysfunction, this condition accounts for up to 17% of ESRD in children.[46] It also confers significant perinatal morbidity and mortality when associated with severe oligohydramnios and pulmonary hypoplasia.

Posterior urethral valves are usually detected prenatally based on ultrasound findings of bilateral hydroureteronephrosis with a dilated bladder in a male fetus. Postnatal presentation is also possible and should be suspected in males with a weak urinary stream and a palpable bladder. Postnatal ultrasound may show the characteristic "keyhole" sign made by the bladder and dilated proximal urethra, but definitive diagnosis is made by VCUG.

Neonatal treatment of posterior urethral valves is centered on securing adequate drainage of the kidneys. When posterior urethral valves are suspected, an indwelling urinary catheter should be placed in the immediate postnatal period. Surgical correction by valve ablation is nearly always required.

Vesicoureteral Reflux

VUR, the most common form of CAKUT, is defined as retrograde flow of urine into the upper urinary tract. Primary VUR occurs because of an abnormal UVJ or short intravesicular ureter, but secondary VUR may develop from a dysfunctional or neurogenic bladder. Although antenatal hydronephrosis may lead to detection of VUR, it is more commonly found after evaluation of a UTI. VUR is diagnosed by VCUG and is found in approximately 30% of neonates presenting with a UTI.[47]

VUR severity is divided into five grades based on the level of reflux and the associated absence (low grade, I–II) or presence (high grade, III–V) of dilation of the renal pelvis or ureter. Most VUR is mild and resolves over time, although higher grades may predispose patients to develop UTI and renal scarring, leading to reflux nephropathy, which is the fourth most common cause of ESRD in children.[48] Treatment with prophylactic antibiotics reduces the rate of UTI but does not alter the rate of renal scarring, leading to variability in treatment patterns.[48] In general, patients with lower-grade reflux and the absence of frequent UTI may be monitored without prophylaxis, whereas high-grade reflux or frequent UTI typically require antibiotic suppression. Very high-grade (grade V) reflux, breakthrough UTI while receiving prophylaxis, or associated renal impairment may necessitate surgical correction.

16

Hematologic Problems

John Letterio, Sanjay Ahuja

RED BLOOD CELLS

Fetal Erythropoiesis and Changes in Erythropoiesis After Birth

Rapid growth during fetal development demands a brisk pace for red blood cell production, and this capacity must expand with the increase in blood volume, which is proportionate to the weight of the fetus. Blood volumes average 80 mL/kg of fetal body weight at term, but the ratio is larger in the preterm fetus (~90 mL/kg). The rapid pace of erythropoiesis is reflected by a rise in hematocrit throughout gestation, from a mean of 40% at 28 weeks of gestation to 50% at term.

Hematopoiesis during mammalian embryonic development proceeds from the yolk sac blood island to the aorta-gonad-mesonephros (AGM) region, the fetal liver, and subsequently the fetal bone marrow, and is tightly regulated by the stromal cells in each of these unique areas that make up the hematopoietic niche[1,2] (Fig. 16.1). Moreover, there are likely distinct myeloid-erythroid progenitors in the early yolk sac niche that may exist transiently and contribute to the unique regulation of the beta-globin locus in the mammalian embryo.[3] The control of red blood cell production and progression of fetal erythropoiesis from yolk sac to liver (in utero) to bone marrow at birth is also in part orchestrated by Kruppel-like factors (KLFs) that control cell differentiation and embryonic development. KLF1 (erythroid KLF) is essential during both embryonic and adult erythropoiesis. KLF2 is a positive regulator of the mouse and human embryonic beta-globin genes. KLF1 and KLF2 have highly homologous zinc finger DNA-binding domains and have overlapping roles in embryonic erythropoiesis.[4] The ontogeny of fetal erythropoiesis has been reviewed elsewhere.[5]

Fetal erythropoiesis also occurs during chronic bone marrow failure and recovery from marrow suppression. Fetal erythrocytes have hemoglobin F, with more G-gamma than A-gamma chains, i antigen, large mean corpuscular volume, characteristic enzyme levels, low carbonic anhydrase, low hemoglobin A_2, and short life span. Many of these fetal characteristics are present in the red blood cells of patients with temporary or chronic hematopoietic stress. Chronic fetal erythropoiesis is seen in patients with constitutional aplastic anemia, such as Fanconi anemia or Diamond-Blackfan anemia. Thus fetal erythropoiesis occurs during hematopoietic stress, whether chronic or transient, if there is some marrow activity and may be because of expansion of fetal clones.[6]

Several endogenous proteins contribute to the changes in regulation of erythropoiesis after birth, with erythropoietin being the most recognized. Fetal erythropoiesis is regulated by endogenous (fetal) erythropoietin produced in the liver, but in infancy, the main site of production converts to the kidneys. Although the rate of erythropoiesis in the fetus is quite high, serum erythropoietin levels are low, and the erythropoietin response to hypoxia in the fetus and neonate is reduced compared with that in adults. After delivery, erythropoietin levels vary among species, which is probably related to the oxygen transport capacity of the hemoglobin mass. In all mammals, hemoglobin level declines following birth and erythropoiesis nearly ceases, which gives rise to "early anemia." Except in humans, erythropoietin levels increase proportionally with the fall in hemoglobin, but there is a discrepancy between the curves for serum immunoreactive erythropoietin and for erythropoiesis-stimulating factors. The latter include other stimulatory factors in addition to erythropoietin. These other factors work in concert with erythropoietin to control erythropoiesis and probably contribute to enhanced erythropoiesis during periods of rapid growth, which is unlikely to be attributable to the same molecular controls that enhance erythropoiesis during periods of stress or hypoxia. For example, it is known that erythropoietin acts in concert with general growth-promoting factors, particularly growth hormone (GH) and the insulin-like growth factors (IGF-I and IGF-II). The erythropoietin and GH/IGF systems are both activated by hypoxia and share similar receptors and pathways. Recent studies indicate that human fetal and infant growth is stimulated by GH, IGF-I, and IGF-II. Erythropoietin, GH, and IGFs are expressed early in fetal life. IGF-I levels are low in the fetus and increase slowly following birth except in preterm infants, in whom the levels decline. The physiology of erythropoietin during mammalian development has been reviewed elsewhere.[7]

The low level of erythroid production noted earlier persists for over a month following birth, during which time the hematocrit gradually declines. Late in the second or third month of life, the hematocrit approaches 30%. This is commensurate with a rise in serum erythropoietin levels, which prompts a resumption of erythropoiesis and leads to a rise

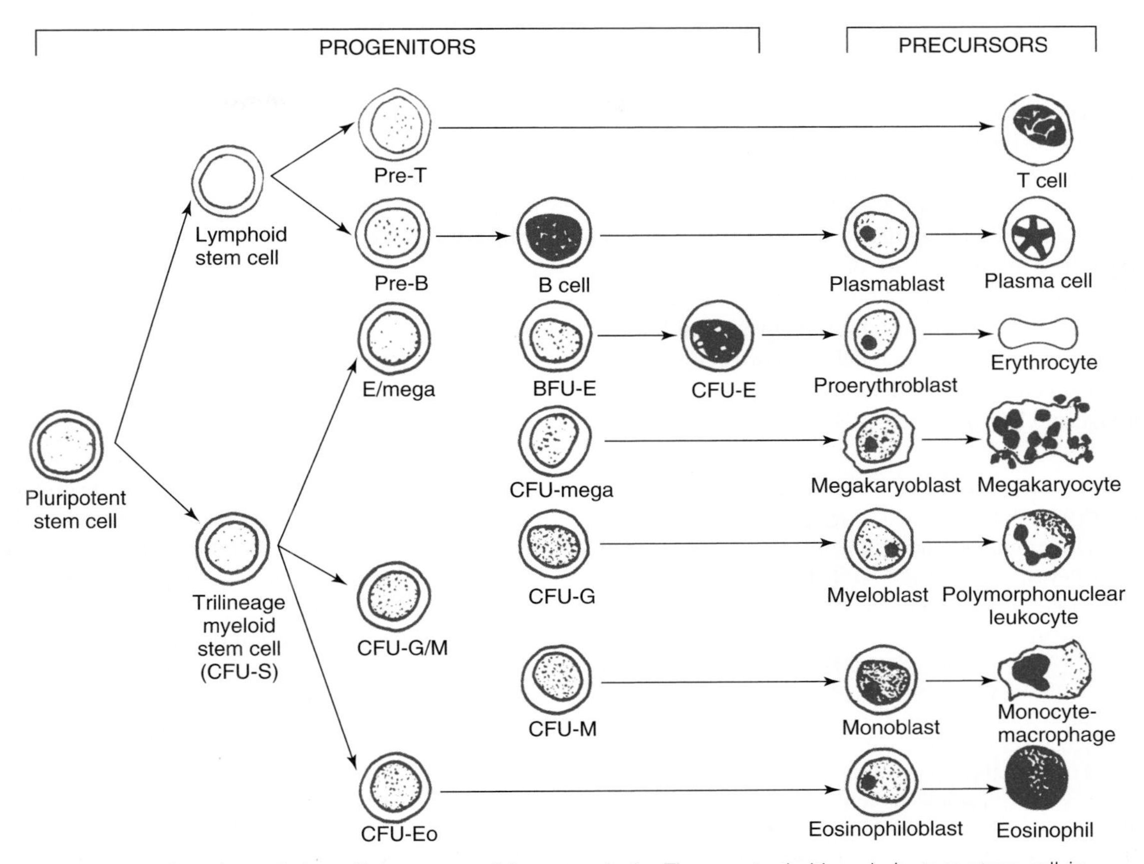

Fig. 16.1 Overview of the cellular stages of hematopoiesis. The most primitive pluripotent stem cell is shown at the far left. As hematopoietic progenitor cells differentiate, they become committed to a single lineage. This diagram does not emphasize the large increase in the number of cells (amplification) that occurs in the progenitor and precursor compartments. *BFU,* Burst-forming unit; *CFU,* colony-forming unit; *E,* erythrocyte; *Eo,* eosinophil; *G,* granulocyte; *M,* macrophage; *mega,* megakaryocyte; *S,* stem cell. (From Lipton JW, Nathan DG. The anatomy and physiology of hematopoiesis. In Nathan DG, Oski FA, eds. *Hematology of Infancy and Childhood.* 3rd ed. Philadelphia, PA: Saunders; 1987.)

in red blood cell mass. This rise in red blood cell mass keeps pace with rapid overall growth and blood volume, and the hematocrit rises relatively little as a consequence.

Erythropoietin and Neuroprotection in the Neonate

One other aspect of the erythropoietin system that is important to the fetus and newborn deserves mention here. Erythropoietin is a pleiotropic neuroprotective cytokine, and recent studies have shed light on the biological basis of its efficacy in the damaged developing brain. Coordinated expression of erythropoietin ligand and receptor expression occur during central nervous system development to promote neural cell survival. Studies of fetal hypoxia-ischemia in rat models have demonstrated that prenatal third-trimester global hypoxia-ischemia disrupts the developmentally regulated expression of neural cell erythropoietin signaling and predisposes neural cells to death. Furthermore, exposure of the neonate to exogenous sources of recombinant erythropoietin can restore the mismatch of erythropoietin ligand and receptor levels and enhance neural cell survival. The data generated by these studies suggest the potential utility of neonatal recombinant erythropoietin when administered in the days immediately after a global prenatal hypoxic-ischemic insult as a means to rescue neural cells and present a novel clinically relevant paradigm in which the benefits of erythropoietin in the context of a stress are linked to the induction of signaling pathways in both erythroid and nonerythroid lineages.[8,9]

Placental Transfusion and Distribution of Blood at Birth

The effect of early and late umbilical cord clamping on neonatal hematocrit has been well studied.[10] Delayed cord clamping has been shown to be associated with a higher hematocrit in very low-birth-weight infants, which suggests effective placental transfusion.[11] Several analyses have confirmed that delaying cord clamping (by at least 30 seconds) increases average blood volume across the full range of gestational ages studied.[12] On average, the infant will gain roughly 14 mL/kg of blood during this first 30 seconds, which leads to a blood volume of 89 mL/kg. This process has been termed *placental transfusion.* It occurs because of the continued circulation of blood through the umbilical arteries and veins, and leads to a net shift of blood from the placenta to the newborn infant. At birth, the partition of blood volume between the infant and the fetal placental vasculature is nearly 2:1 (75 mL/kg body weight in the infant and 40 mL/kg in the placenta). If the umbilical cord is not clamped quickly, a major shift in blood can lead to significant effects on blood volume, hematocrit, and hemoglobin concentration during the first days of life. Infants exposed to a significant delay in umbilical cord clamping may experience excessive placental transfusion, with attendant decreases in plasma volume, increased hematocrit, and elevated blood viscosity. Regardless of the extent of placental transfusion, postnatal adjustments of blood volume and hematocrit begin within 15 minutes after birth and continue for several hours. A controlled trial has suggested that delayed cord clamping in very preterm infants may reduce the incidence of intraventricular hemorrhage and late-onset sepsis.[13]

EDITORIAL COMMENT: Delayed cord clamping has continued to show benefits and little, if any, risk in preterm infants.[14,15] The benefits of delayed cord clamping in preterm infants include increased blood volume,[12,16] improved circulatory and respiratory function, reduced need for blood transfusion, improved cerebral oxygenation, and reduced intraventricular hemorrhage and sepsis.[13,17] The cord blood of extremely preterm infants is a rich source of hematopoietic progenitor cells such as hematopoietic stem cells, endothelial cell precursors, mesenchymal progenitors, and stem cells of multipotent-pluripotent lineage; hence the merit of delayed cord clamping has been magnified. Tolosa et al referred to this aspect of delayed cord clamping as "realizing mankind's first stem cell transfer" and proposed that "it should be encouraged in normal births."[18] The extra endowment of progenitor cells resulting from delayed cord clamping has the potential to both increase red blood cell production and boost host immune defenses through production of leukocytes.

There has been a shift in thinking to explore milking of the umbilical cord as an alternative to delayed cord clamping, which may provide the same benefits without the need to delay resuscitation.

Properties of Fetal Hemoglobin and the Switch to Adult Hemoglobin

The different types of human hemoglobin consist of various combinations of the embryonic, fetal, and adult hemoglobin subunits that are present at distinct times during development. This orderly transition from one form of hemoglobin to another represents a major paradigm of developmental biology but remains poorly understood. Studies have pointed to a competition between subunits for more favorable partners with stronger subunit interactions so that the protein products of gene expression can themselves play a role in the developmental process because of their intrinsic properties.[19] Fetal hemoglobin, or Hb F (two alpha-globin chains and two gamma-globin chains [$\alpha_2\gamma_2$]), is the main hemoglobin synthesized up to birth, at which point it makes up more than 80% of the hemoglobin in circulating red blood cells. However, Hb F subsequently declines, and adult hemoglobin, Hb A ($\alpha_2\beta_2$), becomes predominant.

The main reason for this shift is the transition from synthesis of mainly gamma chains during fetal development to mainly beta chains during late gestation, with a concomitant gradual shift from Hb F to Hb A beginning at 34 weeks' gestation. Several studies have indicated that expression of the Hb F subunit gamma-globin might also be regulated posttranscriptionally. One recently identified mechanism for posttranscription regulation of gene expression is through the production of micro-RNAs. These micro-RNAs are approximately 22 nucleotides in length and can specifically target messenger RNAs (mRNAs) for selected genes, thus acting as disease modifiers as well as molecules that control gene expression during development and in response to environmental stimuli. A study comparing micro-RNA expression in reticulocytes from cord blood and adult blood revealed several micro-RNAs that were preferentially expressed in adults, among them micro-RNA-96, which appears to directly suppress gamma-globin expression and thus contributes to control of Hb F production and its suppression during the switch to postnatal erythropoiesis.[20]

Although new hemoglobin produced during postnatal life is essentially all Hb A, there are exceptions to this rule. Perhaps the most well-known is the persistence of Hb F in patients with sickle cell disease (SCD) and the contribution of Hb F to amelioration of disease severity in these individuals (see later discussion). Hb F expression can be increased during periods of stress erythropoiesis, and in the infant recovering from anemia of prematurity, there is a transient phase in the recovery of erythropoiesis during which Hb F is the predominant hemoglobin synthesized.

Functional Differences of Specific Hemoglobins

The major physiologic function of hemoglobin is to bind oxygen in the lungs and deliver it to the tissues. This function is regulated and/or made efficient by endogenous heterotropic effectors.[21,22]

Hb A is the major oxygen-binding tetrameric protein found in the blood. It is one of the best-recognized proteins in the human body because of its uniquely bright red color, and its color changes in diseases such as anemia, hypoxia, and cyanide and carbon monoxide poisoning. Hemoglobin has drawn the attention of physicians and physiologists since ancient times. Modern quantitative analysis of the structure and function of hemoglobin started in the late 1800s and early 1900s. Important observations of the hemoglobin allostery have been attributed to Christian Bohr (who reported in 1903 that its oxygen-binding process was sigmoidal or cooperative) and to Bohr, Hasselbalch, and Krogh, who reported in 1904 that the position of the oxygen-binding curve of the blood was sensitive to changes in Pco_2 (and H^+ or pH), known as the *Bohr effect*.[23] These observations regarding the allosteric behaviors of hemoglobin are reviewed elsewhere.[24]

It is widely recognized that the most important functional difference between Hb F and Hb A is their different oxygen-binding properties. The higher oxygen affinity of Hb F is an advantage to the fetus because of the site of oxygen uptake, the placenta, where the umbilical venous Po_2 is just 35 to 40 mm Hg, and represents the highest Po_2 in all the fetal circulation. Because the oxygen dissociation curve is "shifted" to the left (because of higher affinity), there is a capacity to maintain a higher O_2 content, but this capacity is no longer needed after birth because the lungs provide an environment with a significantly higher oxygen tension (typically >75 mm Hg) in the pulmonary capillaries. More importantly, the persistence of Hb F is a disadvantage to the newborn because the release of oxygen in the capillary bed depends on a much lower Po_2 for efficient oxygen delivery and maintenance of tissue metabolism, which is in contrast to the dynamics of O_2 release by Hb A. This difference has been shown in clinical investigations to influence morbidity in newborns with cardiopulmonary disease. Studies evaluating the impact of exchange transfusion in extremely premature infants demonstrated a link between improved survival and substantial replacement of Hb F by Hb A, despite the absence of a significant change in hematocrit. This effect is often achieved as a consequence of frequent phlebotomies and multiple small transfusions of packed red blood cells in very low-birth-weight infants.

Hemoglobinopathies

Globin gene mutations are a rare but important cause of cyanosis. Crowley et al identified a missense mutation in the fetal G gamma-globin gene (*HBG2*) in a father and daughter with transient neonatal cyanosis and anemia. This newly recognized mutation modifies the ligand-binding pocket of fetal hemoglobin. The mechanisms described include a diminutive effect of the relatively large side chain of methionine on both the affinity of oxygen for binding to the mutant hemoglobin subunit and the rate at which it does so. In addition, the mutant methionine is converted to aspartic acid posttranslationally, probably through oxidative mechanisms. The presence of this polar amino acid in the heme pocket is predicted to enhance hemoglobin denaturation, causing anemia.[25]

Methemoglobinemia. Methemoglobinemia arises from the production of nonfunctional hemoglobin containing oxidized Fe^{3+}, which results in reduced oxygen supply to the tissues and manifests as cyanosis in the patient. It can develop by three distinct mechanisms: genetic mutation resulting in the presence of abnormal hemoglobin, a deficiency of the methemoglobin reductase enzyme, and toxin-induced oxidation of hemoglobin. The normal hemoglobin fold forms a pocket to bind heme and stabilize the complex of heme with molecular oxygen. This process prevents spontaneous oxidation of the Fe^{2+} ion chelated by the heme pyrroles and the globin histidines. In the abnormal M forms of hemoglobin (Hb M), amino acid substitution in or near the heme pocket creates a propensity to form methemoglobin instead of oxyhemoglobin in the presence of molecular oxygen. Under normal conditions, hemoglobin is continually oxidized, but significant accumulation of methemoglobin is prevented by the action of a group of methemoglobin reductase enzymes. In the autosomal recessive form of methemoglobinemia, there is a deficiency of one of these reductase enzymes, which allows accumulation of oxidized Fe^{3+} in methemoglobin. Oxidizing drugs and other toxic chemicals may greatly enhance the normal spontaneous rate of methemoglobin production. If levels of methemoglobin exceed 70% of total hemoglobin, vascular collapse occurs, resulting in coma and death. Under these conditions, if the source of toxicity can be eliminated, methemoglobin levels will return to normal. Disorders of oxidized hemoglobin are relatively easily diagnosed and, in most cases, except when congenitally defective Hb M is present, can be treated successfully.[26]

> **EDITORIAL COMMENT:** Inhaled nitric oxide (iNO) is often used as a therapy for persistent pulmonary hypertension of the newborn and oxidizes hemoglobin to methemoglobin; consequently, many centers monitor methemoglobin levels in babies on this therapy. The risk appears to be dose dependent, however, and monitoring may not be necessary when levels are kept less than 20 parts per million.

ANEMIA

Neonatal anemia is a condition with a diverse etiologic spectrum. To reach an accurate diagnosis, the pediatrician must have some knowledge of the more common causes of low hemoglobin concentrations and hematocrit in the neonate. Proper history taking, physical examination, and interpretation of diagnostic test results can narrow the focus and aid in establishing an accurate diagnosis and in directing the appropriate therapeutic interventions.[27]

Hemorrhagic Anemias

Hemorrhagic anemia in a newborn is often heralded by some features of the history or clinical findings that allow time to anticipate and prepare for treatment of the infant. The fetus may lose blood through a variety of routes. Hemorrhage commonly occurs through the placenta into the mother's circulation and may be detected most readily through a Kleihauer-Betke test performed on the mother's blood. For monozygotic twins, there is an additional risk that one fetus may hemorrhage through the placental vascular anastomosis into the other twin (see the section on twin-to-twin transfusion syndrome later in this chapter). The fetus may also bleed through the placenta into the birth canal. In many cases of placental abruption, the vaginal blood contains a mixture of fetal and maternal blood. The fetus may lose a large volume of blood into the fetal placental circulation at the time of birth (see also Chapter 2). All of the latter circumstances have the same effect as hemorrhage.

Before delivery, internal hemorrhage may occur, with the most common type being intraventricular hemorrhage. The true incidence of intracranial hemorrhage (ICH) is not certain, but in cases of alloimmune thrombocytopenia in which there is severe thrombocytopenia, ICH may be seen in as many as 20% of cases. Administration of intravenous gamma-globulin (IVIG) and/or corticosteroids to the mother during a subsequent pregnancy with an affected fetus is widely practiced to increase the fetal platelet count and decrease the risk of ICH (see later discussion).[28] Internal hemorrhage can also result from forces incurred around the time of delivery. Important common types of hemorrhage secondary to birth-related injuries are subgaleal hematomas, hepatic subcapsular and mediastinal hematomas, intracerebral and cerebellar hemorrhage, and hematomas in fractured limbs. Adrenal hemorrhage is more common in neonates than in children or adults. The incidence of detected cases ranges from 1.7 to 2.1 per 1000 births. Because adrenal bleeding may remain asymptomatic, the real incidence is probably higher. In published series, the most common clinical feature in infants with adrenal hemorrhage was jaundice, which was observed in 67.6% of cases in at least one series. Thus it has been suggested that in cases of hyperbilirubinemia of unknown cause, adrenal hemorrhage should be kept in mind.[29]

For hemorrhages that are associated with the birth process, the occurrence is highest in difficult term deliveries, particularly in infants who are large for gestational age and require multiple applications of vacuum to assist delivery. Splenic rupture is uncommon but may lead to catastrophic intraabdominal hemorrhage in infants with hemophilia and in babies in whom intrauterine splenomegaly develops as a result of erythroblastosis or other causes. Extensive trauma to the perineum in babies born through breech deliveries can lead to hypovolemia and anemia, and these symptoms are typically exaggerated in the preterm infant.

In the newborn, the clinical presentation and symptoms associated with fetal hemorrhage are directly related to the interval between hemorrhage and delivery, as well as to the extent of hemorrhage. When the bleed occurs only shortly before birth, there is little time for hemodilution; thus these babies will not be anemic initially and will show few if any signs that would indicate hypovolemia or anemia. The hematocrit will fall during the first hour after delivery, but a rise in reticulocyte count may not be seen until the anemia has been present for several days.

When approaching the treatment of hemorrhagic anemia presenting in the newborn period, one needs first to consider any attendant cardiorespiratory effects of blood loss that are present. Because of the capacity for rapid transport of fluid across the placenta and a limitless reservoir for volume replacement, a hemorrhage that occurs sufficiently far in advance of delivery will likely manifest only the consequences of decreased oxygen-carrying capacity from the anemia. This capacity for rapid replacement of volume loss via the placenta is an important safety net for the fetus who might not otherwise tolerate intermittent hypoxemia during the contractions associated with labor. For any infant known to have chronic in utero anemia, volume expansion must be approached carefully. The infant in this situation is often anemic but has normal intravascular volume. Consequently, additional volume may lead to heart failure secondary to volume overload. For symptomatic infants with chronic anemia, partial exchange transfusion with packed red blood cells can be performed to achieve a desired hematocrit and avoid volume fluctuation and severe volume shifts. The amount to be exchanged depends on both the baby's blood, the severity of the anemia, and the hematocrit of the packed red blood cells, but an exchange of between 30 and 50 mL/kg body weight may be required.

When hemorrhage occurs acutely during delivery, the hematocrit will not fully reflect the degree of blood loss because there has been little hemodilution. In this situation, one will need to aggressively manage shock, paying close attention to the hemodynamic and cardiorespiratory parameters. Measures of metabolic acidosis, capillary filling time, and vital signs are important to monitor because they will guide the approach and extent of fluid resuscitation. Acute situations may include placenta previa, vasa previa, abruption, or blood loss from the cut umbilical cord. In such cases, timely volume replacement with blood is preferable because this rapidly enhances oxygen delivery to tissues, which is not the case when crystalloid solutions are used. Anticipation of the need for resuscitation can help decrease the time required to initiate transfusion. Most labor and delivery units have type O Rh-negative uncrossed red blood cells available.[26] The classic approach to shock in the newborn is to transfuse 10 mL/kg of blood over 5 to 10 minutes and to repeat infusions until there are signs of adequate circulation.

Twin-to-Twin Transfusion Syndrome

Twin-to-twin transfusion syndrome (TTTS) is a complication that may occur in monochorionic twins and that may originate in either imbalance or abnormality of the single placenta serving two twins. It is a serious complication in 10% to 20% of monozygous twin gestations with an overall incidence (i.e., including those in which it is not a serious complication) of 4% to 35% in the United States.[30,31] The diagnosis is well established in overt clinical forms through the association of polyuric polyhydramnios and oliguric oligohydramnios. TTTS is a progressive disease in which sudden deterioration in clinical status can occur, leading to the death of a twin. Up to 30% of survivors have abnormal neurologic development because of the combination of profound antenatal insult and complications of severe prematurity. Newer treatment options have improved the outcomes.[32]

TTTS results from an unbalanced blood supply through placental anastomoses in monochorionic twins. These anastomoses may be arterial to arterial, but arterial to venous are believed to be responsible for a majority of the cases presenting clinically. TTTS induces growth restriction, renal tubular dysgenesis, and oliguria in the donor and visceromegaly and polyuria in the recipient. Studies have shown a potentially important role of the renin-angiotensin system with up-regulation in the donor twin, whereas in recipients, renin expression was virtually absent, possibly because it was down-regulated by hypervolemia.[33] In the donor, congestion and hemorrhagic infarction were accompanied by severe glomerular and arterial lesions resembling those observed in polycythemia- or hypertension-induced microangiopathy. Thus fetal hypertension in the recipient twin in TTTS might be partly mediated by the transfer through the placental vascular shunts of circulating renin produced by the donor.

The degree of transfusion from one twin to the other and the time course of the transfusion may be highly variable. It may begin as early as the second trimester and therefore be long-standing at the time of delivery. In the most severe cases in which the transfusion is of long duration, the donor is substantially anemic and exhibits significantly increased erythropoiesis that can even be present in the dermis ("blueberry muffin baby"); the donor also becomes progressively small for gestational age and develops oligohydramnios. Simultaneously, the recipient twin continues to grow normally and becomes polycythemic; in extreme cases, this progresses to polyhydramnios and potentially to hydrops fetalis. If the growth-restricted twin dies in utero, the risk exists for embolization through vascular anastomoses to the surviving twin as a consequence of intravascular coagulation in the dying twin. Embolization in the surviving twin will have major consequences, often affecting vital organs including the brain, gastrointestinal tract, and kidneys. Postpartum management of live-born twins affected by this syndrome will be quite complicated, even when the pediatrician is prepared well in advance of delivery. The polycythemic twin will need reduction of the hematocrit, whereas the treatment of the anemic donor is more straightforward. If either of the newborn twins demonstrates evidence of cardiomyopathy, the infant would be intolerant of blood volume shifts and may be particularly sensitive to blood volume expansion, in which instance a partial exchange transfusion is again the preferred approach.

The best treatment in cases of TTTS presenting before 26 weeks of gestation is fetoscopic laser ablation of the intertwin anastomoses on the chorionic plate.[34–36]

EDITORIAL COMMENT: In twin-to-twin transfusion syndrome (TTTS), the likelihood of perinatal survival of at least one twin was not found to vary with severity as classified by Quintero stage (stage I, 92%; stage II, 93%; stage III, 88%; stage IV, 92%).[37,38] However, dual twin survival did vary by stage (stage I, 79%; stage II, 76%; stage III, 59%; stage IV, 68%; $p < 0.01$), primarily because stage III TTTS was associated with decreased donor twin survival. Sequential selective laser photocoagulation of communicating vessels in pregnancies with TTTS was associated with higher dual survival and donor twin survival rates compared with a nonsequential technique. Overall survival of one or both twins was 91%, and dual twin survival was 72%.

Nonhemorrhagic Anemias

Hyperbilirubinemia is far more common and more severe in neonates with hemolytic anemia than in older children. The bilirubin level may increase rapidly in the first hours after birth, so identification of the underlying cause is important. To diagnose the cause of hemolysis, obtain information about any family history of anemia or neonatal jaundice, and examine both the baby and the blood smear. Clues to the appropriate diagnostic tests are often present in these smears, suggested by morphologic abnormalities of the red blood cells. It is recommended to perform a direct antiglobulin test (DAT, or direct Coombs test) because the majority of hemolytic episodes are a consequence of maternal antibodies that cross the placenta in late gestation and then react with paternal antigen expressed on the infant's erythrocytes. These maternal immunoglobulin G (IgG) alloantibodies against paternal antigen are responsible for most cases of hemolytic disease of the newborn. If the DAT result is negative but hyperbilirubinemia persists and the hematocrit is declining, a more thorough evaluation is required. This typically does not include a bone marrow examination, which is reserved for cases in which anemia is not associated with hemolysis and in which there is evidence suggesting a primary disorder of erythropoiesis.

Hemolytic Anemias

Maternal Antibodies. Fetal-neonatal alloimmune disease is the most common cause of severe hemolytic anemia in an otherwise healthy newborn. Of these disorders, Rh disease remains the most common cause of severe anemia. Anemia varies from mild to severe, the DAT result is strongly positive, and the reticulocyte count is almost uniformly elevated. Antenatal assessment should include maternal screening and frequent surveillance of fetal well-being. In sensitized pregnancies, vigilance in pursuing these evaluations is essential if one is to define the appropriate time for intervention with premature delivery or intrauterine transfusions.

Hyperbilirubinemia. Hyperbilirubinemia is a problem in the majority of cases of Rh disease, and in patients with the most severe degree of hemolysis, the elevated bilirubin level cannot be managed by phototherapy alone and ultimately requires IVIG and/or exchange transfusion. For patients with Rh sensitization and intrapartum complications, correction of anemia can minimize cardiorespiratory distress and is thus an important part of resuscitation in this group of patients. The most extreme cases of Rh sensitization are associated with hydrops fetalis in utero. Antenatal therapies have been implemented to prevent this severe manifestation of alloimmunization, including intrauterine transfusions. Treated infants are born with only mild to moderate anemia, with all of their red blood cells derived from the intrauterine transfusions. In these infants, the DAT finding may often be negative, but the result of the indirect antiglobulin test is strongly positive. Quite frequently, the consequence of intrauterine transfusion is that the newborn will have no reticulocytosis despite moderate anemia, and with the majority of the infant's red blood cells derived from intrauterine transfusions with Rh-negative blood, there is no hemolysis. These infants should be watched closely over the first several months because a late episode of hemolysis and anemia may arise when the donor erythrocytes eventually decline in number. As erythropoiesis begins to accelerate, these infants produce their own Rh-positive blood cells, which are susceptible to attack by residual maternal antibodies. In such infants, the DAT result may remain strongly positive for months, and they will require supplemental folic acid to keep pace with the demands of increased erythropoiesis.

> **EDITORIAL COMMENT:** It is truly remarkable that after the discovery of the blood groups in the 1940s, the virtual elimination of erythroblastosis with anti-D globulin took a mere 30 years, and this is one of the more notable accomplishments in modern medicine. Anti-D, a polyclonal immunoglobulin G, is purified from the plasma of D-alloimmunized individuals. It is routinely and effectively used to prevent hemolytic disease of the fetus and newborn caused by the antibody response to the D antigen on fetal red blood cells. This therapy has effectively reduced the number of cases of Rh isoimmunization from 13% to less than 1% and the mortality rate from one in four to less than 5%. The residual cases are few and far between and have been attributed mainly to failed maternal prophylaxis caused by improper timing or dosage of immunoglobulin anti-D therapy and by immunization during pregnancy resulting from an early occult fetomaternal hemorrhage (at <28 weeks' gestation). With erythroblastosis, the late-onset anemia may be either hemolytic or hyporegenerative.

Alloimmune Disease. Alloimmune disease may also occur as a consequence of other blood group incompatibilities (anti-c, anti-e, and anti-C in the Rh system and anti-Kell). In alloimmune anemia of the newborn, the level of hemolysis caused by the presence of antibodies to antigens of the Kell blood group system is less than that caused by antibodies to the D antigen of the Rh blood group system, and the numbers of reticulocytes and normoblasts in the baby's circulation are inappropriately low for the degree of anemia. These findings suggest that sensitization to Kell antigens results in suppression of fetal erythropoiesis as well as hemolysis. Vaughan et al compared the ex vivo growth of Kell-positive and Kell-negative hematopoietic progenitor cells from cord blood in the presence of human monoclonal anti-Kell and anti-D antibodies and serum from women with anti-Kell antibodies.[39] The growth of Kell-positive erythroid progenitor cells (erythroid burst-forming units and colony-forming units) from cord blood was markedly inhibited by monoclonal IgG and IgM anti-Kell antibodies in a dose-dependent fashion (range of concentrations: 0.2% to 20%), but monoclonal anti-D antibodies had no effect. The growth of these types of cells from Kell-negative cord blood was not affected by either type of antibody. Neither monoclonal anti-Kell antibodies nor monoclonal anti-D antibodies inhibited the growth of granulocyte or megakaryocyte progenitor cells from cord blood. Serum from 22 women with anti-Kell antibodies inhibited the growth of Kell-positive erythroid burst-forming units and colony-forming units but not of Kell-negative erythroid burst-forming units and colony-forming units ($P < .001$ for the difference between groups). The maternal anti-Kell antibodies had no inhibitory effects on granulocyte-macrophage or megakaryocyte progenitor cells from cord blood. These data indicate that anti-Kell antibodies specifically inhibit the growth of Kell-positive erythroid burst-forming units and colony-forming units, a finding that supports the hypothesis that these antibodies cause fetal anemia by suppressing erythropoiesis at the progenitor cell level.

A third form of alloimmune disease is caused by ABO incompatibility. This is perhaps one of the most frequent causes of hyperbilirubinemia in the newborn but is rarely responsible for a significant hemolytic anemia. The peripheral blood smear of patients with ABO incompatibility shows microspherocytes, and in most cases, the mother is type O, whereas the baby is either type A or type B. The elevation in serum bilirubin concentration typically resolves within 1 to 2 weeks, and it less common for this form of alloimmune hemolytic disease to result in a drop in hemoglobin level or hematocrit sufficient to require transfusion in the absence of other complicating factors such as infection. Clinical disease rarely occurs in group A mothers with group B babies or in group B mothers with group A babies.

Congenital Infections

Congenital infections may be associated with hemolytic anemias and have most often been observed in the setting of TORCH infections (*to*xoplasmosis, *r*ubella, *c*ytomegalovirus infections, *h*erpes simplex) as well as syphilis.[40,41] The association of hemolytic anemia with cytomegalovirus infection is well described, and cytomegalovirus infection has been documented as a cause of autoimmune hemolytic anemia in the setting of vertically acquired neonatal infection with human immunodeficiency virus (HIV).[42] Parvovirus B19 has an affinity for erythroid progenitors and produces severe erythroid hypoplasia, with severe infection during fetal development resulting in hydrops fetalis or congenital anemia. Diagnosis is based on examination of bone marrow and virologic studies. Much is known of the pathophysiology of the virus, and studies are in progress to develop a vaccine to prevent this widespread infection. Bacterial infections can precipitate a hemolytic episode, particularly in individuals with glucose-6-phosphate dehydrogenase (G6PD) deficiency, and thus this diagnosis should be considered in the setting of sepsis and severe hemolysis in the neonate.[43]

Enzymopathies

Specific erythrocyte glycolytic enzyme defects can be the cause of hemolytic syndromes in the neonate.[44] Two of the most commonly observed enzymopathies are described in the following sections.

Glucose-6-Phosphate Dehydrogenase Deficiency. G6PD deficiency is the most common human enzyme defect and is present in more than 400 million people worldwide.[45] As with SCD, the global distribution of G6PD deficiency is remarkably similar to that of malaria, which lends support to the hypothesis that these red blood cell disorders confer protection against malaria. G6PD deficiency is an X-linked genetic defect caused by mutations in the *G6PD* gene, which lead to functional variants with many biochemical and clinical phenotypes. Significant deficiency occurs almost exclusively in males. About 140 mutations have been described; most are single-base changes leading to amino acid substitutions. The most common *G6PD* mutation in North America is the *G6PD-A* variant, present in approximately 10% of

African Americans. Term infants are rarely symptomatic. The most frequent clinical manifestations of G6PD deficiency are neonatal jaundice and acute hemolytic anemia, which are usually triggered by an exogenous agent. Jaundice in the neonate with G6PD deficiency may occur without any known oxidant exposure. In contrast to *G6PD-A*, *G6PD-Canton*, a variant common in South China, is commonly associated with significant neonatal jaundice. Some *G6PD* variants cause chronic hemolysis, which leads to congenital nonspherocytic hemolytic anemia. The most effective management of G6PD deficiency is to minimize the risk of hemolysis by avoiding known oxidative stressors.

G6PD is the rate-limiting enzyme in the hexose monophosphate shunt pathway. This pathway is principally important for the production of reduced glutathione, and this antioxidant has a vital role in protecting the red blood cell membrane from oxidant damage. G6PD deficiency is common worldwide, with certain molecular variants associated with neonatal hemolysis and hyperbilirubinemia. A case recently reported in the literature described a novel missense mutation in a white neonate with chronic nonspherocytic hemolytic anemia caused by a class I G6PD deficiency.[46] The missense mutation in exon 8 of the *G6PD* gene (c.827C>T p.Pro276Leu) was associated with severe elevation in serum bilirubin level, which peaked on day 5 at 24 mg/dL with a conjugated bilirubin level of 17 mg/dL. Jaundice resolved within 4 weeks. A detailed workup failed to reveal other specific factors contributing to cholestasis. Severe hemolytic disease of the newborn may cause cholestasis, even in the absence of associated primary hepatobiliary disease. The diagnosis of G6PD-deficient hemolytic anemia should be suspected in male infants with evidence of acute hemolytic anemia and a negative result on Coombs test/DAT. Because the reticulocyte has higher levels of G6PD, screening tests for G6PD activity performed on the heels of a hemolytic episode are less reliable and should be repeated 2 to 3 months after an acute hemolytic episode in conjunction with family studies.

> **EDITORIAL COMMENT:** With the role of glucose-6-phosphate dehydrogenase (G6PD) in severe hyperbilirubinemia and kernicterus, it has been suggested that routine screening for the enzymopathy may be indicated. Although screening tests are available, there is currently no national consensus on the issue. Studies have been suggested by Watchko et al to evaluate whether newborn screening for G6PD deficiency will increase knowledge and ultimately decrease the risk of severe hyperbilirubinemia.
> Watchko JF, Kaplan M, Stark AR, et al. Should we screen newborns for glucose-6-phosphate dehydrogenase deficiency in the United States? *J Perinatol.* 2013;33:499-504.

Pyruvate Kinase Deficiency. Pyruvate kinase deficiency is a rare cause of neonatal hemolytic jaundice, with a prevalence estimated at 1 case per 20,000 live births in the United States, but with a higher prevalence in the Amish communities in Pennsylvania and Ohio. One report described four neonates with pyruvate kinase deficiency born in a small community of individuals practicing polygamy.[47] All four had early, severe hemolytic jaundice. Pyruvate kinase deficiency should be considered in neonates with early hemolytic, Coombs test–negative, nonspherocytic jaundice, particularly in communities with considerable consanguinity. Such cases should be recognized early and managed aggressively to prevent kernicterus. (See also Chapter 12.)

Defects of the Red Blood Cell Membrane

Inherited abnormalities of one of the proteins of the red blood cell membrane may be associated with neonatal hemolysis and jaundice. Hereditary spherocytosis is an autosomal dominant condition and the most common of this class of disorders. Most cases of spherocytosis result from decreased production of spectrin. Hereditary spherocytosis, including the very mild or subclinical forms, is the most common cause of nonimmune hemolytic anemia among people of Northern European ancestry, with a prevalence of approximately 1 in 2000. However, very mild forms of the disease may be much more common. Hereditary spherocytosis is inherited in a dominant fashion in 75% of cases; the remaining are truly recessive cases and de novo mutations.[48] A negative family history does not rule out the diagnosis because new mutations are quite common. Diagnosis may be aided by the evaluation of a peripheral blood smear in infants suspected of one of these disorders of the red blood cell membrane.

Other Congenital Anemias

Congenital Dyserythropoietic Anemias

Congenital dyserythropoietic anemias (CDAs) are rare hereditary disorders characterized by ineffective erythropoiesis and by distinct morphologic abnormalities of erythroblasts in the bone marrow. Although historically, these disorders have been largely diagnosed through identification of characteristic morphologic aberrations, the recent discovery of underlying etiologic genetic abnormalities has established the usefulness of molecular diagnostic approaches that might serve as rapid tools for the identification of these conditions. The first CDA partly accounted for genetically has been CDA I, for which the responsible gene *CDAN1*, encoding codanin-1, was discovered in 2002. Genetic defects linked to CDA II (*SEC23B*) and a previously unrecognized CDA (*KLF1*) have been identified. *SEC23B* encodes SEC23B, which is a component of the coated vesicles transiting from the endoplasmic reticulum to the *cis* compartment of the Golgi apparatus. *KLF1* encodes the erythroid transcription factor KLF1, and the recently identified mutation leads to major ultrastructural abnormalities, the persistence of embryonic and fetal hemoglobins, and the absence of some red blood cell membrane proteins. The current understanding of the various CDAs, including genotype-phenotype relationships, has recently been reviewed elsewhere.[49]

Deficiencies of Red Blood Cell Production

Among the anemias that present in the newborn period, those resulting from inadequate production are rare but, when present, may point to one of the rare congenital disorders affecting red blood cell production. These congenital defects of erythropoiesis exhibit a very low prevalence ranging from 4 to 7 per million live births and include Blackfan-Diamond anemia and Fanconi anemia, which are described in the following sections.

Blackfan-Diamond Syndrome. Blackfan-Diamond syndrome (also called *congenital hypoplastic anemia*) is the most common congenital disorder of red blood cell production in the neonate.[50] Infants with Blackfan-Diamond syndrome are often small for gestational age and may have other anomalies (including renal abnormalities) that must be considered when pursuing this diagnosis. Blackfan-Diamond anemia may result in severe fetal anemia requiring transfusion. Although autosomal dominant inheritance of Blackfan-Diamond syndrome is considered uncommon, it has been described[51]; the onset of anemia characteristically occurs within the first year of life, with 10% of cases presenting at birth. Affected infants exhibit variable degrees of anemia, with normal circulating white blood cell and platelet counts. Hydrops fetalis has been reported in rare cases. Among women with this disorder, a percentage are at risk for having an infant with substantial anemia in both the fetal and perinatal periods. Because the penetrance of the disorder is variable, pregnant women with a history of Blackfan-Diamond anemia should be considered at risk. Recommendations for the prenatal management of Blackfan-Diamond syndrome include prepregnancy counseling for parents with Blackfan-Diamond syndrome, detailed and serial fetal ultrasound and echocardiographic studies, cordocentesis if there are signs of anemia, consideration of in utero transfusion, and planned early delivery if the fetus is affected.[51]

Fanconi Anemia. Fanconi anemia is a rare chromosomal instability disorder associated with a variety of developmental abnormalities, bone marrow failure, and predisposition to leukemia and other cancers.[52] The Fanconi anemia gene family is a recently identified addition to the group of genes coding for the complex network of proteins that respond to and repair certain types of DNA damage in the human genome, but little is known about the regulation of this novel group of genes at the DNA level.[53] A homozygous missense mutation in the *RAD51C* gene has been described in a consanguineous family with multiple severe congenital abnormalities characteristic of Fanconi anemia.[54] *RAD51C* is a member of the RAD51-like gene family involved in homologous recombination-mediated DNA repair. The mutation results in loss of *RAD51* focus formation in response to DNA damage and in increased cellular sensitivity to the DNA interstrand cross-linking agent mitomycin C and the topoisomerase-I inhibitor camptothecin. Fanconi anemia generally affects children and results in bone marrow failure requiring blood or marrow transplantation for survival. A unique feature of the condition is the long waiting period, often many years, between genetic diagnosis and treatment, which presents a significant challenge to the family and requires a strong, supportive multidisciplinary approach to care.[55]

Pearson Syndrome. Rare but significant causes of anemia in the newborn are those related to mitochondrial cytopathies. Most notable among these, the Pearson syndrome is typically diagnosed during infancy and is characterized by refractory sideroblastic anemia with vacuolization of marrow progenitor cells and exocrine pancreatic dysfunction. In cases presenting in the early neonatal period, clinicopathologic features include severe macrocytic aregenerative anemia. Bone marrow aspiration typically reveals sideroblastic anemia and vacuolization of erythroblastic precursors. The diagnosis may be confirmed by genetic analysis revealing a deletion in mitochondrial DNA. Newborns with this disorder will require chronic transfusions. Although rarely diagnosed in newborns, Pearson syndrome should be suspected in the presence of macrocytic aregenerative anemia and diagnosis requires a bone marrow aspirate followed by a genetic analysis from a blood sample.[56,57]

Anemia Secondary to Hemoglobinopathies

Hemoglobinopathies arise from mutations in the globin genes, with the most common hemoglobinopathies resulting from mutations in the beta-globin gene. These are typically clinically silent at birth because of the persistence of Hb F but manifest as the expression switches from gamma- to beta-chain production.

Thalassemias

Mutations in the beta-globin gene that lead to a decrease in production are referred to as *beta-thalassemias*. The beta-thalassemias resulting from large structural deletions of the beta-globin gene cluster are a rare familial cause of microcytic anemia and hyperbilirubinemia.[58] Although blood cell counts are normal at birth, this disorder can be detected by demonstrating the absence of Hb A on electrophoresis. In most states, umbilical cord blood is routinely screened to identify infants with thalassemia and other hemoglobin disorders (including SCD; see later discussion) before they become symptomatic.

Alpha-thalassemia is one of the most common human genetic disorders and is found extremely frequently in populations in Southeast Asia and southern China, and the expanding populations of Southeast Asian immigrants in the United States, Canada, the United Kingdom, and Europe mean that this disorder is no longer rare in these countries.[59] Couples in which both partners carry (alpha zero) α^0-thalassemia traits have a 25% risk of producing a fetus affected by homozygous alpha-thalassemia or hemoglobin Barts (Hb Barts) disease, with severe fetal anemia in utero, hydrops fetalis, and stillbirth or early neonatal death, as well as various maternal morbidities.

The alpha-thalassemias present a different, greater challenge than beta-thalassemia to the neonatologist and pediatrician. The alpha-thalassemias are characterized by the decrease or complete suppression of alpha-globin polypeptide chains, with reduced or absent synthesis of one to all four alpha-globin genes. In the fetus, a complete deficiency of chain synthesis results in an absence of Hb F and the production of Hb Barts. Hb Barts is composed of tetrads of the gamma-globin chain (γ_4) and exhibits a profoundly abnormal oxygen dissociation curve reflecting the reduced capacity to off-load oxygen at the tissue capillary bed. The gene cluster, which codes for and controls the production of these polypeptides, maps near the telomere of the short arm of chromosome 16 within a G+C-rich and early-replicating DNA region. The genes expressed during the embryonic stage (zeta) or fetal and adult stage (alpha-2 and alpha-1) can be modified by point mutations that affect either the processing-translation of mRNA or make the polypeptide chains extremely unstable. Much more frequent are the deletions of variable size (from ~3 kilobases to >100 kilobases) that remove one or both alpha genes in *cis* or even the whole gene cluster. Deletions of a single gene are the result of unequal pairing during meiosis, followed by reciprocal recombination. These unequal crossovers, which produce also alpha-gene triplications and quadruplications, are made possible by the high degree of homology of the two alpha genes and of their flanking sequences.

The interaction of the different alpha-thalassemia determinants results in three phenotypes: alpha-thalassemic trait, clinically silent and presenting with only limited alterations of hematologic parameters; Hb H disease, characterized by the development of a hemolytic anemia of variable degree; and Hb Barts hydrops fetalis syndrome (lethal), a consequence of compromised oxygen delivery to tissues. The diagnosis of alpha-thalassemia caused by deletions is based on electrophoretic analysis of genomic DNA digested with restriction enzymes and hybridized with specific molecular probes. Recently, polymerase chain reaction (PCR)–based strategies have replaced Southern blot analysis. Hemoglobin H disease, a mutation of three alpha-globin genes, is more severe than previously recognized. Anemia, hypersplenism, hemosiderosis, growth failure, and osteoporosis are commonly noted as the patient ages. Infants with one or two functional alpha-globin genes have microcytosis at birth (mean corpuscular volume is <95) and an elevated percentage of Hb Barts on electrophoresis. Alpha-thalassemia major is usually fatal in utero. Surviving newborns who did not undergo intrauterine transfusion often have congenital anomalies and neurocognitive injury. Serious maternal complications often accompany pregnancy. Doppler ultrasonography with intrauterine transfusion ameliorates these complications. The high incidence in selected populations mandates population screening and prenatal diagnosis of couples at risk. Universal newborn screening has been adopted in several regions with DNA confirmatory testing using the methods noted earlier.[60,61]

Sickle Cell Anemia

Sickle cell disease (SCD) is caused by a single-point mutation in the beta-globin gene that causes the hydrophilic amino acid glutamic acid to be replaced with the hydrophobic amino acid valine at the sixth position. SCD is an autosomal recessive genetic blood disorder with incomplete dominance, characterized by red blood cells that assume an abnormal, rigid, sickle shape.[62] Sickling decreases the cells' flexibility and carries a risk of various complications. The introduction of newborn screening in the United States has had a significant impact on morbidity and mortality from SCD. Historically, the failure to achieve early identification of SCD resulted in a high rate of mortality because of the susceptibility of these patients to overwhelming infection, particularly with encapsulated organisms. Penicillin prophylaxis and the introduction of the pneumococcal vaccine have had an additional impact on the risk of sepsis and mortality in this population.[63] Inheritance of the sickle gene with a thalassemia variant, such as beta-thalassemia, can alter the presentation, in part by increasing the relative concentration of Hb S.

Anemia of Prematurity

Anemia of prematurity is thought to be principally a direct consequence of delivery before placental iron transport and fetal erythropoiesis are complete and is exaggerated by various factors, including blood losses associated with phlebotomy to obtain samples for laboratory testing, low plasma levels of erythropoietin as a result of both diminished production and accelerated catabolism, rapid body growth and the need for commensurate increases in red blood cell volume and mass, and disorders causing red blood cell losses as a result of bleeding and/or hemolysis. Blood losses resulting from the phlebotomy required for frequent laboratory studies can be a frequent cause of anemia of prematurity, despite advances in blood conservation with microsampling methods. The sick preterm infant receiving ventilatory assistance may have more than 5 mL of blood per day withdrawn for laboratory studies. At this rate, an 800-g infant would lose his or her entire blood volume for laboratory studies in approximately 13 days. Large infants are less affected because of their greater blood volumes.

Rapid somatic growth of the preterm and very low-birth-weight infant also contributes substantially to anemia of prematurity. Very low-birth-weight infants will typically more than double their body weight and blood volume by the time they are ready for discharge from the nursery. In addition to the factors mentioned earlier, possibly the most significant contributing factor to this process is the prolonged cessation of erythropoietin production. As noted previously, reactivation of erythropoietin production in the infant kidney appears to be determined more by a biologic clock than by a response to stress. Indeed, there is no erythropoietin response to even severe anemia until the infant reaches a corrected gestational age of about 34 to 36 weeks. After this time, the erythropoietin system will respond when the hematocrit declines into the range of 25% to 30%. The reticulocyte count will typically rise within 1 week after the increase in erythropoietin production. Because transfusion during this critical period suppresses the release of endogenous erythropoietin, it can delay the recovery from anemia of prematurity, particularly in the seriously ill preterm requiring multiple transfusions, in whom recovery may not be observed until an even later corrected gestational age. Ultimately, it is the tissue oxygen tension that stimulates erythropoietin release, and recipients of multiple transfusions in whom Hb F has largely been replaced by Hb A will be less likely to achieve a low enough tissue oxygenation to stimulate timely or early erythropoietin release.

The treatment for anemia of prematurity has evolved substantially. Because placental iron transport is incomplete in the preterm infant, these babies require supplemental iron to mount an effective erythroid response. Iron stores are largely acquired during the last month of intrauterine life; thus term infants are born with large iron stores. The combination of a lack of these iron stores and a rapid rate of growth (and concomitant increase in blood volume) during the first 6 months of life place the preterm infant at significant risk of anemia of prematurity. Most infants with a birth weight of less than 1000 g are given multiple red blood cell transfusions within the first few weeks of life. Red blood cell transfusions have typically been the mainstay of therapy for anemia of prematurity; recombinant human erythropoietin (rHuEPO) is largely unused because of the view that it fails to substantially diminish red blood cell transfusion needs despite exerting substantial erythropoietic effects on neonatal marrow.[64]

Multiple randomized, controlled trials have shown that treatment of extremely preterm infants with rHuEPO during the period when their endogenous erythropoietin system is inactive stimulates erythropoiesis, maintains a higher hematocrit, and reduces the need for transfusions. Reticulocytosis appears about 1 week after the start of treatment. The main population thought to benefit are those infants born before 30 weeks of gestation, with the smallest, least mature in this group exhibiting the greatest benefit.

Treatment is usually started after the infant has tolerated the introduction of enteral feedings. Large multicenter trials have demonstrated that administration of rHuEPO plus iron supplementation cannot prevent early transfusions, particularly in very low-birth-weight newborns and in infants with severe neonatal diseases. However, this approach may be effective in preventing late transfusions. Doses of 100 U/kg body weight given 5 days per week or 250 U/kg given three times per week are equally effective, and there is no evidence that larger doses are more effective. Current treatment of anemia of prematurity should focus on efforts to minimize factors that reduce erythrocyte mass (phlebotomies, noninvasive procedures) and promote factors that increase it (placental transfusion, adequate nutritional support).[65]

EDITORIAL COMMENT: Extremely low-birth-weight preterm infants often develop anemia of prematurity from frequent and excessive blood draws, a process referred to by Ed Bell as "gradual exsanguination."[66,67] The hypoproliferative anemia is marked by inadequate production of erythropoietin. rHuEPO has been available since 1990, but trials looking at reduction of red blood cell transfusions with rHuEPO achieved limited success. There has been a focus recently on autologous transfusion, blood-sparing technologies, and limitation in the number of donors. Treatment of anemia of prematurity includes red blood cell transfusions, which are given to preterm infants based on indications and guidelines (hematocrit and hemoglobin levels, ventilation and oxygen needs, apneas and bradycardias, poor weight gain) that are relatively nonspecific.

The need for transfusions can be reduced by limiting phlebotomy losses, providing good nutrition, and using standard guidelines for transfusion based on hemoglobin level or hematocrit. What those guidelines should be is not clear. Analysis of data for the Premature Infants in Need of Transfusion (PINT) trial, which compared management according to restrictive and liberal transfusion guidelines in infants weighing less than 1000 g and used a composite primary outcome of death before home discharge or survival with either severe retinopathy, bronchopulmonary dysplasia, or brain injury on cranial ultrasonography, revealed no statistically significant differences between groups in any secondary outcome.[68] The investigators concluded that in extremely low-birth-weight infants, maintaining a higher hemoglobin level results in more infants receiving transfusions but gives little evidence of benefit. Data on the impact of transfusion practices on long-term outcome are very limited and inconclusive. Until further evidence surfaces, the tendency will probably be to adopt more liberal indications for transfusion. Many centers continue to use the Shannon criteria,[69–71] which call for transfusion in infants if any of the following conditions are met: (1) a requirement for more than 35% inspired oxygen on continuous positive airway pressure (CPAP) or positive pressure ventilation with a mean airway pressure of more than 6 cm H_2O; (2) a requirement for less than 35% inspired oxygen on CPAP or positive pressure ventilation with a mean airway pressure of less than 6 cm H_2O, significant apnea and bradycardia, tachycardia (>180 beats per minute) or a respiratory rate of more than 80 breaths per minute, weight gain of less than 10 g/day over 4 days, or sepsis; or (3) a hematocrit of less than 20%.

The Neonatal Research Network has recently completed active recruitment for the Transfusion of Prematures Trial, with the objective "to determine whether higher hemoglobin thresholds for transfusing ELBW infants resulting in higher hemoglobin levels lead to improvement in the primary outcome of survival and rates of neurodevelopmental impairment at 22 to 26 months of age, using standardized assessments by the Bayley Scales of Infant Development."

POLYCYTHEMIA

Several conditions are associated with polycythemia in utero. These include chronic hypoxia as a result of maternal toxemia and placental insufficiency, placental insufficiency with postmaturity syndrome, pregnancy at high altitudes, pregnancy in a diabetic woman, and trisomy 21. In most instances, newborns who have clinically significant polycythemia have a preexisting high hematocrit in utero as a result of one of the causes listed previously, which is then exaggerated by excessive placental transfusion at delivery. Conversely, early cord clamping and reduced placental transfusion can lead to a normal hematocrit in an infant who developed polycythemia in utero.

The complications of polycythemia are a consequence of the rise in blood viscosity that occurs as the hematocrit rises, which compromises circulation to a variety of tissues and organs. The clinical manifestations are distinct in each organ system. Skin manifestations include plethora and delayed capillary filling. Renal symptoms include proteinuria and hematuria, and in extreme conditions, renal disease can be indistinguishable from renal vein thrombosis. Babies with polycythemia are at increased risk of necrotizing enterocolitis

(NEC). The central nervous system manifestations of polycythemia may be mild, including poor feeding, irritability, and an abnormal cry; more concerning cases are those manifesting apnea, seizures, and cerebral infarction.[73]

The diagnosis of polycythemia is not based solely on hematocrit because there is no precise hematocrit at which symptoms appear in all infants. This is partly attributed to the fact that other factors affect viscosity in addition to hematocrit. Although symptoms are more common when the venous hematocrit exceeds 66%, signs of organ dysfunction may develop in some infants with lower hematocrits. Polycythemia should be confirmed by measuring the venous blood hematocrit because capillary values correlate poorly with the central venous hematocrit (capillary hematocrits are generally higher). The treatment for the symptomatic neonate can involve either intravenous hydration or a partial exchange transfusion in which blood is replaced with a plasma substitute. Isotonic saline, plasma, and a mixture of saline and albumin have all been used with equal efficacy. The goal for the hematocrit is 50%. To achieve this through exchange, the following formula is typically used: $V = [(HCT_1 - HCT_D) \times \text{body weight (kg)} \times 90\ \text{mL}]/HCT_1$, where V = the exchange volume, HCT_1 is the baby's hematocrit, and HCT_D is the desired hematocrit. The hematocrit should be monitored carefully after this procedure because it will ultimately rise, and if the HCT_D is not reached with the initial volume exchange, it may rise again to a concerning level.

The greatest dilemma is that posed by the asymptomatic newborn with polycythemia. The incidence of neurologic handicaps is increased in children who had untreated neonatal polycythemia.[74,75] However, partial exchange transfusion does not improve long-term outcomes.[76]

ERYTHROCYTE TRANSFUSION IN THE FETUS AND NEWBORN

Packed red blood cell transfusions are often administered to patients in the neonatal intensive care unit (NICU). Infants who have significant cardiopulmonary disease are transfused when they become anemic because it is thought that a higher oxygen-carrying capacity improves their tolerance of cardiorespiratory distress.[77] Current blood transfusion guidelines are useful in establishing parameters for transfusion, but it is essential that physicians also modify the application of these guidelines based on their own perceptions and assessments in identifying patients in need of a packed red blood cell transfusion. In an evaluation of the influence of caregiver perception and assessment on transfusion practices, neonates who underwent transfusion based on caregivers' perceptions rather than adherence to strict guidelines were more likely to be receiving noninvasive ventilatory support and were more symptomatic. Neonates who improved after transfusion had a lower pretransfusion hematocrit and were more symptomatic compared with the group that did not show clinical improvement. In this study, tachycardia was the most sensitive predictor of benefit from packed red blood cell transfusion.[78]

Extremely low-birth-weight infants are the most heavily transfused, yet the indications for transfusion do continue to represent an area of controversy. A very important concept to which one should always adhere is that there is no single critical hematocrit that always requires transfusion. In reality, there will be a range of critical hematocrits at which transfusion may be required even for an individual patient, and these different thresholds are values that are influenced by the severity of illness. Several studies have suggested an association between red blood cell transfusion and NEC in premature neonates.[79,80] Withholding feeds during transfusion has never been clearly demonstrated to be beneficial but may have a protective effect against the development of NEC. In a retrospective case-control study of premature low-birth-weight infants (<32 weeks' gestation and <2500 g) who developed NEC over a 6-year period (25 infants with NEC and 25 controls who never developed NEC), more infants in the NEC group received transfusions in the 48 to 72 hours preceding diagnosis (56% vs. 20% within 48 hours [P = .019] and 64% vs. 24% within 72 hours [P = .01]). The total number of transfusions and age of red blood cells were not different in the two groups. The same investigators implemented a policy of withholding feeds during transfusion, and this practice was associated with a decrease in the incidence of NEC from 5.3% to 1.3% (P = .047). These data support the recognized association of NEC with the administration of red blood cell transfusions in the 48 to 72 hours preceding presentation of NEC and provide a rationale for exercising caution in feeding around the time of packed red blood cell transfusions in the neonate, although the literature is mixed and association does not equal causation.

The risk-to-benefit ratio of blood transfusions for preterm infants will continue to be defined by ongoing experience. Although use of a more restrictive transfusion threshold for hemoglobin level or hematocrit or both may decrease the number of blood transfusions in preterm infants, the impact of such an approach on long-term outcomes must be defined.[81,82]

WHITE BLOOD CELLS

Mature white blood cells are derived from pluripotent hematopoietic stem cells. In early development, hematopoietic stem cells emerge separately from the yolk sac, chorioallantoic placenta, and AGM region.[83] Following the initial erythropoietic stage, myeloid progenitor cells can be found in the yolk sac during the third to fourth week of gestation.[84] From the yolk sac, these progenitor cells sequentially migrate to the liver, thymus, and spleen and eventually take up permanent residence in the bone marrow at the 11th to 12th week of gestation.[85] Hematopoietic stem cells with self-renewal capacity give rise to pluripotent progenitors that progress to common lymphoid or common myeloid progenitors.[86,87] Common lymphoid progenitors differentiate into natural killer (NK) cells, B lymphocytes, T lymphocytes, and immature lymphoid dendritic cells. Common myeloid progenitors differentiate into granulocytes (neutrophils, eosinophils, and basophils), monocytes, and immature myeloid dendritic cells. Monocytes give rise to tissue macrophages.[87]

The systems mediating innate immunity have qualitative and quantitative deficiencies that affect the newborn's response to infections. For example, neonatal neutrophils ingest and kill bacteria as efficiently as their adult counterparts, but adhesion and subsequent migration of these cells to sites of infection are impaired. The migratory defect of neonatal neutrophils is exacerbated by limited production of the chemoattractant C5a and low generation of C3b, which is necessary for opsonization and phagocytosis. Neutrophil storage pools are rapidly exhausted in the face of serious infection, and the capacity to replenish those stores is limited in the neonate. Acquired immunity in the newborn is affected by qualitative and quantitative deficiencies in lymphoid lineage as well. Cell-mediated killing by NK and cytotoxic T cells is diminished, which leaves the newborn vulnerable to certain viral and intracellular pathogens.[87,88] The newborn infant produces primarily IgM, and little IgG and IgA, in response to antigenic challenge. Neonatal T and B cells are predominately of a naive phenotype. Because the lymphocyte maturation process is directed largely by cytokines and the capacity of neonatal cells to produce key cytokines such as interleukin-4 and IFNγ interferon-gamma is limited, the acquisition of adult-type functional capabilities is delayed in vivo.

Despite encountering a pathogen-rich environment at the time of birth, most newborn infants do not become ill. The relative immunodeficiency of the neonate has been viewed by some as an adaptive mechanism to optimize survival by balancing the conflicting immunologic requirements of life in utero with those of the external environment.[88]

NEUTROPHIL DISEASES

Neutropenia

The neutrophil counts in an infant vary by birth weight and postpartum age. For term and near-term infants, values published by Manroe et al are considered appropriate.[89] An absolute neutrophil count (ANC) of 1800 to 5500/μL is seen at birth, and ANC increases by threefold to fivefold over the next 12 to 18 hours of life. By 24 hours of life, the ANC begins to fall, decreasing steadily to 1800 to 7200/μL at 5 days; from then it falls to and remains at 1800 to 5400/μL through 28 days of age. Studies by Mouzinho et al show that normal preterm very low-birth-weight neonates have leukocyte reference ranges that differ significantly from those of older neonates (neutrophil counts have lower minimum values in the former group).[90,91] Publications recommend using the Mouzinho et al chart for infants of less than 1500 g birth weight and the Manroe et al chart for larger infants (see also Appendix C).[90,91] Studies suggest that neonates with neutrophil counts above 1000/μL are not likely to be at high risk of acquiring a nosocomial infection. Counts below 500/μL (particularly when they remain below 500/μL for many days) are associated with an increased risk for developing a nosocomial infection. Persistent counts between 500 and 1000/μL may pose some intermediate risk.[90,91]

BOX 16.1 Causes of Neutropenia in the Neonate

Increased Neutrophil Destruction or Utilization

Immune
- Alloimmune/isoimmune neutropenia
- Autoimmune neutropenia in the mother

Nonimmune
- Maternal preeclampsia
- Infection: bacterial, viral
- Periventricular hemorrhage
- Asphyxia
- Metabolic disorders

Reduced Neutrophil Production
- Infants of hypertensive mothers
- Donors of twin-to-twin transfusion
- Nutritional factors
- Kostmann disease (severe congenital agranulocytosis)
- Pure white cell aplasia
- Barth syndrome
- Reticular dysgenesis
- Hyperimmunoglobulin M syndrome
- Shwachman-Diamond syndrome
- Dyskeratosis congenita

Mixed Causes
- Drugs
- TORCH infections (*t*oxoplasmosis, *o*ther, *r*ubella, *c*ytomegalovirus, *h*erpes simplex)

Excessive Neutrophil Margination
- Pseudoneutropenia
- Endotoxin-induced margination

Causes of Neonatal Neutropenia

Box 16.1 lists the most common causes of neutropenia in newborns. In general, neutropenia can be caused by either decreased neutrophil production or increased destruction.

Neutropenia Secondary to Increased Neutrophil Destruction

Alloimmune Neonatal Neutropenia. In alloimmune neonatal neutropenia (ANN), the mother becomes immunized to a father's neutrophil antigen that is expressed on the fetal neutrophils. Subsequently, IgG antibodies directed against fetal neutrophil antigen cross the placenta and destroy the fetal granulocytes. The severity of neutropenia is influenced by the titer and subclass of the maternal IgG neutrophil antibodies, the phagocytic activity of the infant's reticuloendothelial system, and the capacity of the infant's marrow to compensate for the shortened survival of antibody-coated neutrophils.[92,93] Antineutrophil antibodies have been found in as many as 20% of surveyed pregnant and postpartum women, but studies have documented ANN in 0.2% to 2% of consecutively sampled newborns.[92–97] A wide variety of antigenic targets have been identified, including human neutrophil alloantigen (HNA) groups HNA-1, HNA-2, and HNA-3 as well as NC1, SH, SAR, LAN, LEA, and CN1.[92–95,98] The role of human leukocyte antigen (HLA) is controversial.[99] Despite all the available data, in nearly half of cases, the antigens cannot be recognized.[94,95] Symptomatic infants can manifest delayed separation of the umbilical cord, skin infections, otitis media, or pneumonia within the first 2 weeks of life. Although most infections are mild, overwhelming sepsis is known to occur and is associated with a mortality rate as high as 5% in infants with ANN. When neutropenia is prolonged (>7 days), severe (ANC of <500/μL), or associated with serious infections, ANN can be treated with subcutaneous recombinant human granulocyte colony-stimulating factor (rG-CSF). The use of growth factor in this setting is discussed later in the chapter. Fortunately, in the majority of cases, the disorder is self-limiting and resolves over a period of weeks to a few months as levels of the transplacentally acquired maternal antibody diminish.[92–95]

Autoimmune Neutropenia of Infancy. Autoimmune neutropenia of infancy (AIN) is a disorder caused by increased peripheral destruction of neutrophils as a result of antibodies in the infant's blood that are directed against the infant's own neutrophils. It is analogous to immune thrombocytopenic purpura or autoimmune hemolytic anemia. Primary AIN, which is not associated with other diseases such as systemic lupus erythematosus, is often observed in infants and has an incidence of 1 in 100,000.[93,100] A large number of children with primary AIN show the presence of antibodies specific to HNA-1a or HNA-1b. Less frequently, the antineutrophil autoantibodies recognize adhesion glycoproteins of the CD11/CD18 (HNA-4a, HNA-4b) complex, the CD35 molecule (CR1), and FcγRIIb.[101–103] The origin of these autoantibodies is not known. The mechanism proposed includes molecular mimicry of microbial antigens, modification of endogenous antigens as a result of drug exposure, increased or otherwise abnormal expression of HLA antigens, or loss of suppressor activity against self-reactive lymphocyte clones. There have been reported associations with parvovirus B19 infection and exposure to beta-lactam antibiotics.[104–106] AIN is usually diagnosed during the first few months of life (3–8 months).[101]

Diagnosis of AIN in premature twins has been reported, which suggests that sensitization can occur even in utero.[107] Although there is significant neutropenia at presentation (500–1000/μL), the clinical course is usually benign with mild infections.[101,103,108] Severe infectious complications (pneumonia, sepsis, meningitis) are seen in about 12% of these patients.[93,103] AIN resolves spontaneously by the age of 2 or 3 years in 95% of cases.[101,103,108] Therefore most cases require no specific therapy. The usefulness of antibiotic prophylaxis must be assessed on a case-by-case basis. Administration of rG-CSF is currently the first-line therapy to achieve remission of the neutropenia. Treatment with IVIG is effective in less than 50% of cases, and the benefit lasts less than 2 weeks. Steroids have limited effect in immune-mediated neutropenia.[103,109]

Neonatal Autoimmune Neutropenia. Neonatal autoimmune neutropenia is seen when mothers with autoimmune disease transfer their neutrophil autoantibodies passively to the fetus. Most often, the mother and the infant are neutropenic. The infant's neutropenia is transient and asymptomatic. The recovery process takes a few weeks to a few months and depends on the time it takes to clear IgG antibodies.[94–96]

Neutropenia in Neonates With Sepsis. Neonates have immature granulopoiesis. This frequently results in neutropenia after sepsis, which is likely secondary to exhaustion of the storage and proliferative pools of the bone marrow. Neutropenic septic neonates have a higher mortality rate than nonneutropenic septic neonates.[110–112] Whether growth factor or granulocyte infusions should be used in such a setting remains controversial (see later discussion). Neutropenia commonly occurs in neonates who have NEC as well. In this instance, neutropenia results from increased use and/or destruction in tissues, margination attributed to endotoxinemia, and increased mobilization of neutrophils into the peritoneum.

Neutropenia Secondary to Decreased Neutrophil Production

Severe Congenital Neutropenia. Severe congenital neutropenia is a genetically heterogeneous bone marrow failure syndrome characterized by maturation arrest of myelopoiesis at the promyelocyte-myelocyte stage. Estimated frequency is approximately 1 to 2 cases per million with equal male-female distribution. Severe congenital neutropenia follows an autosomal dominant or autosomal recessive pattern of inheritance. About 60% of cases are attributable to mutations in the gene for neutrophil elastase (*ELA2*).[113] Less commonly, mutations in *HAX1, G6PC3,* and other genes cause this disorder. From early infancy, patients who have severe congenital neutropenia experience bacterial infections. Omphalitis, beginning directly after birth, may be the first symptom; however, otitis media, pneumonitis and infections of the upper respiratory tract, and abscesses of the skin or liver are also common and can lead to the diagnosis of severe congenital neutropenia. Patients with the disorder have severe chronic neutropenia with ANCs continuously below 200/μL; in many cases, peripheral blood neutrophils are completely absent. Peripheral monocytosis or eosinophilia may be present. The bone marrow usually shows a maturation arrest of neutrophil precursors at an early stage (promyelocyte-myelocyte level) with few cells of the neutrophilic series beyond the promyelocyte stage. The use of rG-CSF remains first-line treatment for most patients with severe congenital neutropenia. Transplantation of hematopoietic cells from an HLA-identical sibling is beneficial for patients who are refractory to rG-CSF therapy. Patients who have severe congenital neutropenia are at risk of leukemic transformation, and those who develop myelodysplasia or leukemia should proceed urgently to hematopoietic stem cell transplantation.[91,113]

Shwachman-Diamond Syndrome. Shwachman-Diamond syndrome is an autosomal recessive marrow failure syndrome associated with exocrine pancreatic insufficiency and predisposition to leukemia. Approximately 90% of patients meeting clinical criteria for the diagnosis of Shwachman-Diamond syndrome harbor mutations in the *SBDS* gene (Shwachman-Bodian-Diamond syndrome) that maps to the 7q11 centromeric region of chromosome 7.[114,115] The initial symptoms typically are diarrhea and failure to thrive beginning in early infancy, and it is truly rare for the disease to present in the neonatal period. Growth failure and metaphyseal chondrodysplasia associated with dwarfism are seen in some patients. The most common hematologic abnormality, affecting 88% to 100% of patients with Shwachman-Diamond syndrome, is neutropenia. Patients with Shwachman-Diamond syndrome are susceptible to recurrent bacterial, viral, and fungal infections, in particular, otitis media, sinusitis, mouth sores, bronchopneumonia, septicemia, osteomyelitis, and skin infections.[115] The illness may progress to bone marrow hypoplasia or dysplasia, leading to moderate thrombocytopenia and anemia. For treatment, rG-CSF has been used. The only definitive therapy for marrow failure, myelodysplasia, or leukemia is hematopoietic cell transplantation.[114,115]

Neutropenia in Neonates With Hypertensive Mothers. Infants born to mothers who have pregnancy-induced hypertension (PIH) or HELLP syndrome (*h*emolysis, *e*levated *l*iver enzymes, and *l*ow *p*latelet count) are observed to have neutropenia in 40% to 50% of cases, with the most severe neutropenia in the very low-birth-weight infants.[91] This type of neutropenia is the result of placental production of an inhibitor of myelopoiesis. It can be severe with blood neutrophil counts below 500/μL. With no specific treatment, this variety of neutropenia generally resolves in about 72 hours and almost always resolves by the fifth day after birth. Whether a risk of sepsis is associated with neutropenia in infants born to mothers with preeclampsia remains a topic of discussions.[116,117]

Neutropenia in Donor Twins. Neutropenia occurs in the donor twin (the twin who becomes anemic) in twin-to-twin transfusion. It is usually transient. Because the myelopoiesis shifts toward erythropoiesis, neutrophil production decreases, which results in neutropenia. No left shift is present.[118]

Neutropenia in Neonates With Rh Hemolytic Disease. The neutropenia in neonates with Rh hemolytic disease is likely caused by a shift of myelopoiesis toward erythropoiesis, which diminishes neutrophil production. It is usually transient.

Neutropenia Secondary to Mixed Causes

Drugs. Drugs can cause neutropenia through suppressive effects on progenitors, changes in marrow extracellular matrix, development of autoantibodies, and other mechanisms[91]. Ganciclovir has been strongly associated with neutropenia, and cessation of therapy may be necessary[119]. Other drugs used in the NICU that have been implicated in causes of neutropenia include beta-lactam antibiotics, thiazide diuretics, and ranitidine.[106,120–122]

Infection. Intrauterine cytomegalovirus and rubella virus infections can be associated with neutropenia or pancytopenia. Neutropenia in this instance is likely secondary to splenomegaly; however, there might be an element of decreased production as well.[91,123]

Pseudoneutropenia

Artifactual neutropenia has been described that is caused by ethylenediaminetetraacetic acid–induced neutrophil agglutination in vitro. The condition can be diagnosed by the presence of neutrophil clumps on peripheral smears.[121]

Evaluation of the Neonate With Neutropenia

Neutropenia in the NICU requires little diagnostic evaluation if the cause is clear (e.g., NEC, sepsis, maternal PIH). However, if neutropenia persists more than 3 to 5 days, particularly if the count is less than 500/μL, additional evaluation is needed. Helpful findings on physical examination include characteristic dysmorphic features such as skeletal dysplasia, radial or thumb hypoplasia (congenital bone marrow failure syndromes), hepatosplenomegaly (TORCH syndrome, storage disorders), and skin or hair pigmentary abnormalities (Chédiak-Higashi syndrome). A complete blood count, including microscopic examination of the peripheral blood smear to determine neutrophil morphology, can be useful in identifying congenital neutropenia syndromes. The immature-to-total (I/T) neutrophil ratio can be helpful in differentiating defects in production from destruction of neutrophils. The I/T ratio can be calculated as follows:

$$(\text{Bands} + \text{metamyelocytes} + \text{myelocytes}) / (\text{segmented neutrophils} + \text{bands} + \text{metamyelocytes} + \text{myelocytes})$$

A normal or low I/T ratio in the presence of severe neutropenia suggests that the neutropenia is attributed to decreased production. A very high I/T ratio suggests increased neutrophil production, which implies increased peripheral destruction or tissue recruitment of neutrophils.[91] It is also useful to obtain a complete blood count for the infant's mother. If maternal blood neutrophil concentration is normal, maternal neutrophil antigen typing and antineutrophil antibody screening should be pursued at a reference laboratory highly skilled in detection of neonatal alloimmune neutropenia. A bone marrow study is useful in patients with severe and prolonged neutropenia who were not born to mothers with PIH and in whom alloimmune and maternal autoimmune neutropenia have been excluded.[90]

Management of Neonatal Neutropenia

In ill neutropenic neonates, sepsis should be suspected and antibiotic therapy initiated. If the neutropenia is severe and prolonged, reverse isolation procedures might be useful. Accepted treatment options for symptomatic neonatal neutropenia are discussed subsequently.

Treatment

Recombinant Granulocyte and Granulocyte-Macrophage Colony-Stimulating Factors. The availability of recombinant myeloid growth factors has provided new strategies in the management of neonatal neutropenia. rG-CSF is structurally identical to the natural human G-CSF and increases the number of circulating neutrophils by stimulating the release of neutrophils from the bone marrow, inducing myeloid proliferation, and reducing neutrophil apoptosis.

Both rG-CSF and recombinant granulocyte-macrophage colony-stimulating factor (rGM-CSF) have been administered as treatment for neonates with neutropenia with varying degrees of success. Calhoun et al have outlined consistent approaches to procedures and practices in neonatal hematology,[124] including one for the use of rG-CSF.

The decision regarding whether to administer rG-CSF to any given neutropenic patient in the NICU must be individualized with consideration of the risks and benefits. The U.S. Food and Drug Administration (FDA) has approved the use of rG-CSF as long-term treatment to reduce the incidence and duration of sequelae of neutropenia (e.g., fever, infections, oropharyngeal ulcers) in symptomatic patients with congenital neutropenia, cyclic neutropenia, or idiopathic neutropenia. The varieties of severe chronic neutropenia for which rG-CSF administration has been best studied are Kostmann syndrome, Shwachman-Diamond syndrome, Barth syndrome, and cyclic hematopoiesis. At this time, it is not clear whether chronic idiopathic neutropenia or neonatal alloimmune neutropenia fit under the FDA indication of severe chronic neutropenia because although these disorders can be very severe, they are self-limited, and the duration rarely exceeds 6 months. Moreover, administration of rG-CSF to patients with these latter neutropenic disorders has not been tested in randomized placebo-controlled trials.[124] However, these patients generally derive considerable benefit from rG-CSF treatment.[125–127] In addition to increasing circulating neutrophil numbers by stimulating the release of neutrophils from the bone marrow, rG-CSF down-regulates antigen expression, which makes the neutrophils less vulnerable to circulating antibodies. The majority of neonates with either idiopathic or alloimmune forms of neutropenia will respond to doses of 5 to 10 μg/kg given subcutaneously at intervals ranging from every day to less than once per week, as needed, to bring the blood neutrophil concentration to levels above 500 to 1000/μL.[124] It is recommended that rG-CSF be used with caution in patients who have immune-mediated neutropenias caused by antibodies against HNA-2a (NB1), because it has been shown to increase the expression of HNA-2a in healthy adult volunteers. In one case of a neonate who had ANN caused by anti–HNA-2a antibodies, the response was delayed and was achieved only with an unusually high dose.[128] rG-CSF has also been used successfully in patients with neutropenia caused by maternal PIH.[129]

Several studies evaluated the role of rG-CSF therapy in septic neutropenic neonates.[112,130–134] These were followed by two meta-analyses that examined the efficacy and safety of treatment with hemopoietic colony-stimulating factors (rG-CSF or rGM-CSF) in newborn infants with suspected or proven systemic infection. In a meta-analysis by Bernstein et al,[135] rG-CSF recipients were found to have a lower mortality than did controls. However, when the nonrandomized studies were excluded, the analysis did not remain statistically adequate. More importantly, neutropenia was not defined consistently in the studies reviewed, and therefore the significant reduction in mortality noted when rG-CSF was given to neonates with neutropenia requires further confirmation. A meta-analysis by Carr et al examined the effect of adjuvant G-CSF or GM-CSF treatment on 14- and 28-day overall mortality in neonates with suspected or documented sepsis.[136] A combination of five studies (n = 194) in the 28-day mortality analysis showed a reduction in all-cause mortality in treated infants (relative risk: 0.51; 95% confidence interval [CI]: 0.27–0.98). When results from three studies (n = 97) that were limited to neutropenic infants with systemic infection were analyzed, 14- and 28-day overall mortality was found to be reduced by rG-CSF therapy (relative risk: 0.34; 95% CI: 0.12–0.92). Current evidence suggests the need for a multicenter randomized clinical trial demonstrating the clinical efficacy of rG-CSF before this therapy can be universally recommended in the NICU.[137]

> **EDITORIAL COMMENT:** Neonates have a high risk of sepsis if they are either neutropenic or have low concentrations of immunoglobulin. Carr et al reported that early postnatal prophylaxis with granulocyte-macrophage colony-stimulating factor corrects neutropenia but does not reduce sepsis or improve survival and short-term outcomes in extremely preterm neonates.[138] A meta-analysis as well as previously reported prophylactic trials showed no survival benefit.[136]
>
> Although administration of granulocyte colony-stimulating factor and granulocyte-macrophage colony-stimulating factor can raise white blood cell counts, this does not translate into fewer infections. Nor is there conclusive evidence that, in the face of proven sepsis, these cytokines effectively stimulate release of neutrophils and improve outcome. The role of neutrophil transfusions and intravenous immunoglobulin for neutropenic septic babies is still being evaluated.

Intravenous Immunoglobulin. IVIG has been used with success in both ANN and AIN, with a response rate of about 50%.[93–95] However, because of the lack of a titratable dose-response effect and the possibility that IVIG may itself induce neutropenia, this treatment has been used less often than rG-CSF in patients who have immune neutropenia.[93–95]

Granulocyte Transfusions. Current evidence does not show a clear beneficial role for granulocyte transfusion in neonates. Calhoun et al recommend using granulocyte infusions for patients who have early-onset sepsis and shock,[124] are undergoing mechanical ventilation and receiving infusions of pressors, have a blood neutrophil concentration well below 1000/μL with a left shift, and have already received IVIG. A systemic review by Mohan et al found no significant difference in "all-cause mortality during hospital stay" in infants with sepsis and neutropenia who received granulocyte transfusions and those who received placebo or no granulocyte transfusion.[139] Adequately powered multicenter trials of granulocyte transfusion are needed to clarify its role in the treatment of neonates with sepsis and neutropenia.

Neutrophilia

Neutrophilia (defined as >7000 white blood cells/μL in term infants and >13,000 white blood cells/μL in premature infants) typically is a nonspecific response to a stressor.[140] The most common cause of neonatal neutrophilia is infection (Box 16.2). Birth asphyxia and other causes of acute or chronic hypoxia can induce the marrow to prematurely release

BOX 16.2 Conditions Associated With Neutrophilia in the Neonate

- Infection
- Birth asphyxia
- Other causes of acute or chronic hypoxia (pneumothorax, meconium aspiration)
- Hemolytic disease
- Seizures
- Leukemoid reaction
- Neonatal leukemia and transient myeloproliferative disorder
- Congenital anomalies (tetralogy of Fallot)
- Leukocyte adhesion deficiency

immature myeloid and erythroid cells into the circulation, although infection can be a cause of birth depression itself. Nucleated erythrocytes are registered by electronic cell counters as leukocytes, so it is important to correct for the presence of nucleated red blood cells when interpreting the white blood cell count. Neonatal granulocytosis caused by intrinsic disorders of the marrow is rare. Neonatal leukemia and the transient myeloproliferative disorder seen in infants with trisomy 21 are usually associated with large numbers of circulating immature myeloid cells and with hepatosplenomegaly. The diagnosis is established by bone marrow examination, which should include cytogenetic analysis of unstimulated bone marrow.

Neutrophil Functional Defects

Neutrophil functional defects are uncommon disorders that rarely present in the newborn. Because neonates have inherent functional defects in their polymorphonuclear neutrophils and monocytes and also have a higher rate of infections than older infants and children, the clinical manifestations characteristic of dysfunctional phagocytosis may be obscured by the already higher infection rates in neonates. Therefore it is necessary to have a relatively low threshold for specific evaluation of these conditions. Diagnostic evaluation may be difficult because of the limited volume of blood that can be taken from the neonate for diagnostic studies.[140] For all of these reasons, it is difficult to identify the rare infant in whom infection is as a result of an inherited defect in neutrophil function.

EOSINOPHILIA

Eosinophilia (most frequently defined as >700 eosinophils/μL) is common in hospitalized neonates of all gestational ages, but there are significant differences in patterns of incidence and severity based on gestational age, with increased incidence and greater severity of eosinophilia in the more immature infants.[141,142] Eosinophilia in neonates has been attributed to a variety of causes (Box 16.3).

When evaluating the infant with eosinophilia, it is helpful to consider the potential differences in etiology for those who are ill versus those who are well.[143] In the latter group, infection should be strongly considered, especially if the complete blood count was obtained because of clinical suspicion of infection. An evaluation for sepsis is appropriate if

BOX 16.3 Conditions Associated With Eosinophilia in the Neonate

Hematologic disorders
- Hypereosinophilic syndrome
- Eosinophilic leukemoid reaction
- Eosinophilic leukemia
- Thrombocytopenia–absent radius syndrome
- Congenital neutropenia with eosinophilia

Infection
- Bacterial
- Viral
- Fungal

Necrotizing enterocolitis

Immune deficiency disorders
- Congenital immune deficiency syndromes
- Hyperimmunoglobulin E

Familial eosinophilia

Establishment of an anabolic state

Drug reactions
- L-Tryptophan
- Ceftriaxone

Congenital immunodeficiency syndromes
- Hyperimmunoglobulin E
- Omenn syndrome

Cow milk allergy

Miscellaneous
- Congenital heart disease
- Chronic lung disease

risk factors or predictors are present, such as neutropenia, thrombocytopenia, coagulation dysfunction, hypotension, or respiratory distress. An evaluation for NEC is appropriate if signs consistent with gastrointestinal dysfunction are present. If the neonate with eosinophilia is well, close monitoring for 48 hours is suggested. If the eosinophilia persists, then a search for a specific cause of the eosinophilia should be undertaken.[143]

CHRONIC GRANULOMATOUS DISEASE

Chronic granulomatous disease (CDG) is the most common inherited disorder of leukocyte function. CDG has an X-linked or autosomal recessive inheritance pattern involving defects in genes encoding phox proteins, which are the subunits of phagocyte-reduced nicotinamide adenine dinucleotide phosphate oxidase (NADPH oxidase). This results in failure to produce superoxide anion and downstream antimicrobial oxidant metabolites and to activate antimicrobial proteases. Affected patients are susceptible to severe, life-threatening bacterial and fungal infections (such as pneumonia caused by *Aspergillus* or liver abscess caused by *Staphylococcus aureus*) and excessive inflammation characterized by granulomatous enteritis and genitourinary obstruction. Early diagnosis of CGD and rapid treatment of infections are important. The diagnosis of CGD requires demonstration of defective NADPH oxidase activity in neutrophils. The most common diagnostic assays are the nitroblue tetrazolium dye reduction test (a measure of superoxide anion release) and flow cytometry evaluating dihydrorhodamine 123 fluorescence (a measure of intracellular hydrogen peroxide). Infection prophylaxis and interferon-gamma administrations have significantly improved the natural history of CGD. Currently, the only cure is allogeneic hematopoietic cell transplantation, although controversy remains as to which patients with CGD should receive a transplant.[144]

Leukocyte Adhesion Deficiency

Leukocyte adhesion deficiency (LAD) exists in two forms. LAD-1 (Mac-1 deficiency) is attributed to deficiency or dysfunction of leukocyte integrins, and LAD-2 is attributed to congenital deficiency of selectin function. It is a rare disorder that can present in the neonatal period with severe infections, delayed separation of the umbilical stump, and leukocytosis. Diagnosis is made by flow cytometry (absence of CD11b/CD18 on blood phagocytic cells in LAD-1 and absence of sialylated CD15 leukocyte antigens in LAD-2).[140,145]

Chédiak-Higashi Syndrome

Chédiak-Higashi syndrome is a rare autosomal recessive disorder caused by mutations in the *LYST* (or *CHS1*) gene. The Chédiak-Higashi syndrome gene affects the synthesis and/or maintenance of storage-secretory granules in various types of cells. Lysosomes of leukocytes and fibroblasts, dense bodies of platelets, azurophilic granules of neutrophils, and melanosomes of melanocytes are generally larger in size and irregular in morphology. Chédiak–Higashi syndrome manifests as recurrent pyogenic infections, oculocutaneous albinism, and giant intracellular granules in blood leukocytes.[140,145]

NEONATAL IMMUNE DEFICIENCIES OF LYMPHOCYTE LINEAGE (T CELL, B CELL, NATURAL KILLER CELL)

When possible, it is ideal for healthcare professionals to be able to differentiate between immune immaturity and a true primary immunodeficiency that may present during the neonatal period. Late identification of a primary immune deficiency can result in delayed diagnosis and treatment, which in turn may affect the outcome of the disease. Examples of specific T-cell and B-cell disorders that are recognizable during early infancy are presented in Table 16.1. Selected deficiencies are discussed in the following sections.

Humoral Immune Deficiencies

Antibody deficiencies are often unrecognized during the neonatal period because of the protective effect of passively acquired maternal antibodies. In premature neonates, deficiency secondary to immaturity, as opposed to primary antibody deficiency, makes the diagnosis even more difficult. As the levels of maternal antibodies decline, humoral deficiency in the neonate becomes apparent and can be diagnosed as early as 6 months of age (earlier in the preterm infant).

X-Linked Agammaglobulinemia

X-linked agammaglobulinemia is a defect in B-cell development caused by mutations in a cytoplasmic tyrosine kinase called *Btk* that plays a pivotal role in B-cell development. Patients have a profound hypogammaglobulinemia and markedly reduced numbers or absence of B cells (no CD19- or CD20-bearing cells).[140] Onset of recurrent bacterial infections is seen in the first 24 months of life. Overwhelming enteroviral sepsis and paralytic ileus following administration of live polio vaccine have been observed in neonates with X-linked agammaglobulinemia. Treatment is with immunoglobulin replacement.[146]

Hyperimmunoglobulin M Syndromes

Hyperimmunoglobulin M syndromes are a heterogeneous group of genetic disorders causing primary immunodeficiency in which defective immunoglobulin class-switch recombination leads to deficiency of IgG, IgA, and IgE with preserved or elevated levels of IgM. The most common form of hyperimmunoglobulin M syndrome, accounting for at least 70% of cases of class switch recombination defects, is caused by mutations in the gene encoding the CD40 ligand (*CD40LG*). Clinical problems occur early in life with a

TABLE 16.1 Most Common Immune Deficiencies Encountered in Neonates

Type	Disorder	Clinical Features
Humoral immune deficiencies	X-linked agammaglobulinemia	Upper respiratory infections
	Hyperimmunoglobulin M syndrome	
	Transient hypogammaglobulinemia of infancy	
Predominantly cellular immune deficiencies	Neonatal human immunodeficiency virus infection	
Combined immune deficiencies	Severe combined immunodeficiency	
	Omenn syndrome	
Combined immune deficiency associated with other syndromes	Wiskott-Aldrich syndrome	Eczema, thrombocytopenia, recurrent infections
	DiGeorge syndrome	Characteristic facial features, hypocalcemia, microdeletion of chromosome 22
	Ataxia-telangiectasia	Recurrent infections

median age at diagnosis of younger than 12 months. Two-thirds of infants have neutropenia with associated perirectal abscesses and oral ulcers. Patients have increased susceptibility to *Pneumocystis* and other opportunistic organisms (e.g., chronic cryptosporidial infection leading to persistent diarrhea and failure to thrive). The mainstay of treatment for these forms of hyperimmunoglobulin M syndrome is immunoglobulin replacement therapy.[147]

Transient Hypogammaglobulinemia of Infancy

Transient hypogammaglobulinemia of infancy is a common and heterogeneous immune deficiency with indistinct pathophysiology presenting with a delay in maturation of immunoglobulin production in an infant as maternal antibodies disappear. This diagnosis encompasses cases in which serum concentrations of one or more of the three major immunoglobulin classes is more than 2 standard deviations below normal for age in at least two specimens obtained during infancy, and the disorder lacks features consistent with other forms of primary immunodeficiency. In transient hypogammaglobulinemia of infancy, there is an extended period of hypogammaglobulinemia, which usually resolves by 30 to 40 months of life. Infants usually remain asymptomatic or develop recurrent sinopulmonary infections, but severe or life-threatening infections are rare.[148]

Predominantly Cellular Immune Deficiencies

Neonatal HIV infection is discussed in Infectious Disease, Chapter 13.

Combined Immune Deficiencies

T-cell and combined immune deficiencies commonly manifest initially during the neonatal period (secondary to a lack of maternally acquired immunity and a vital T-cell role in immune response). Patients experience severe infections including opportunistic infections (*Pneumocystis jiroveci* [*Pneumocystis carinii*] pneumonia, infection with *Mycobacterium* species, fungal infections), viral infections, and graft-versus-host disease (caused by either maternally derived T cells or transfusions with nonirradiated blood products). Some combined immunodeficiencies present as a part of a syndrome that also includes altered function of other organ systems (Wiskott-Aldrich syndrome, DiGeorge syndrome, etc.).

Severe Combined Immunodeficiency

Severe combined immunodeficiency (SCID) designates a genetically heterogeneous group of syndromes that have in common a profound disturbance of both T and B cells. At least 15 different molecular defects have now been identified, all of which lead to early death in the absence of therapy.[149,150] The affected genes encode cell surface receptors and other activation signaling molecules (IL2RG, JAK3, IL7R, CD45, CD3 components, FOXN1), T-cell and B-cell antigen receptor gene recombinases (RAG1, RAG2, Artemis, DNA ligase 4), and purine pathway enzymes (adenosine deaminase, purine nucleoside phosphorylase).[150] Typical symptoms of SCID are noted from birth and include recurrent severe infections, chronic diarrhea, and failure to thrive. However, infants may appear normal at birth and have no family history of immunodeficiency. Therefore infants with severe T-cell deficiencies may not be identified until life-threatening infections occur. Physical examination may reveal thrush and absence of lymphoid tissue. Hypogammaglobulinemia is often present, and T cells are often absent. B-cell and NK cell pattern varies, which results in various SCID phenotypes.[145]

Hematopoietic stem cell transplantation and enzyme replacement (in the case of adenosine deaminase deficiency) have made this previously fatal set of diseases treatable.[150]

If the diagnosis is made early in the first months of life before the onset of serious infections, the long-term prognosis for infants with SCID may be markedly improved (better survival, less morbidity, and lower treatment costs than when SCID is recognized only after the onset of serious infections). Administration of attenuated vaccines that are recommended in early infancy and that can cause serious infection in infants with T-cell lymphopenia should be avoided.

Molecular identification of SCID gene mutations now enables early diagnosis in affected families. Infants with SCID identified because of a family history can undergo prenatal mutation diagnosis and be treated early in life.[150]

Universal newborn screening for SCID has become an important public health goal. As a potential screening tool, a test of T-cell receptor gene excision circles (TRECs) was chosen by some researchers. This test is performed on DNA from the dried blood spots collected for screening newborns. It can identify any infant with profound T-cell lymphopenia and not just infants with SCID. In a study by Routes et al, TREC assay by real-time quantitative PCR was performed on newborn screening cards for newborn infants. Seventeen of 64,397 infants older than 37 weeks' gestation screened using the TREC assay (approximately 0.026%) had TREC values below the cutoff limit (<25 TRECs/μL blood).[151] Eleven infants subsequently underwent a confirmatory flow cytometry screening test, which confirmed the presence of T-cell lymphopenia in eight infants. The ongoing trials of SCID screening will need to answer questions on optimal screening protocols and the costs of treatment and screening that would provide appropriate information for policy makers deciding among competing healthcare priorities.[152]

EDITORIAL COMMENT: One interesting and unexpected discovery after implementation of newborn screening for SCID is the early diagnosis of chromosome 22q11.2 deletion syndrome (22q11.2DS), which is the most common cause of DiGeorge syndrome. A retrospective chart review of patients with 22q11.2DS at the Children's Hospital of Philadelphia found 11 newborns with a positive newborn screen for SCID. The early diagnosis led to significant associated findings that may not have been recognized and treated in a timely manner without the newborn screen. Accordingly, a neonate with a positive newborn screen for SCID but who does not have SCID should be evaluated for 22q11.2DS.

Barry JC, Crowley TB, Jyonouchi S. et al. Identification of 22q11.2 deletion syndrome via newborn screening for severe combined immunodeficiency. *J Clin Immunol.* 2017;37(5):476-485.

Omenn Syndrome

Omenn syndrome is an autosomal recessive combined immunodeficiency characterized by infiltration of the skin and gastrointestinal tract by activated oligoclonal T lymphocytes. In contrast with other forms of SCID, the total number of circulating T lymphocytes in Omenn syndrome is normal, and they show activated phenotype. However, their proliferative response to in vitro stimulation by mitogens and antigens is markedly decreased. In contrast, B cells are usually undetectable both in peripheral blood and in lymphoid tissues, and hypogammaglobulinemia results. A remarkable hypereosinophilia and increased IgE serum levels are observed. T-cell repertoire in Omenn syndrome is highly restricted as well.[153] The most common causes of Omenn syndrome are hypomorphic mutations of the recombination-activating genes. Mutations of the Artemis (*DCLRE1*), *IL7RA, RMRP, IL2RG,* and *CHD7* genes may also result in the Omenn syndrome phenotype.[154] Patients with Omenn syndrome develop early-onset, generalized, exudative erythrodermia associated with lymphadenopathy, and hepatosplenomegaly. The loss of protein through the skin (and often also as a result of chronic diarrhea) results in hypoproteinemia and generalized edema. In addition, alopecia is a frequent finding. Many of the clinical features of Omenn syndrome are reminiscent of acute graft-versus-host disease. Because of their unique susceptibility to severe infections, patients with Omenn syndrome inevitably die early in life unless treated with hematopoietic stem cell transplantation.[153]

Combined Immune Deficiencies Associated With Other Syndromes

Wiskott-Aldrich Syndrome

Wiskott-Aldrich syndrome is discussed later in the section on thrombocytopenia caused by reduced platelet production.

DiGeorge Syndrome

DiGeorge syndrome is caused by a hemizygous deletion of chromosome band 22q11.2. It is extremely common, with nearly 1 in 3000 children affected.[155] Patients display characteristic facies (hypertelorism, short philtrum, low-set ears), cardiac defects, parathyroid hormone deficiency, and immune deficiency. Approximately 20% of patients have no evidence of diminished T-cell numbers, and fewer than 1% have true thymic aplasia requiring transplantation.[155]

Based on clinical and immunologic profiles, partial and complete DiGeorge syndrome have been distinguished. In the complete form of DiGeorge syndrome, the thymus is absent. Therefore T cells are absent or markedly decreased in number, and B cells (although present) make few antibodies. Complete DiGeorge syndrome is usually fatal unless treated with thymus transplantation.[155] In partial DiGeorge syndrome, T-cell numbers correlate with the amount of thymus tissue present. T-cell proliferative responses, as well as immunoglobulin levels, are usually normal. However, IgA deficiency, impaired responses to vaccines, and frank hypogammaglobulinemia have been described. Clinical studies show that most patients do not demonstrate a susceptibility to opportunistic infections.[155]

Ataxia-Telangiectasia

Ataxia-telangiectasia is an autosomal recessive disorder that is characterized by early-onset progressive cerebellar ataxia, oculocutaneous telangiectasia, immunodeficiency, and lymphoid tumors.[145,156] Various other abnormalities are also associated with this disorder, including the absence or rudimentary appearance of a thymus, progressive apraxia of eye movements, insulin-resistant diabetes, and clinical and cellular radiosensitivity (higher incidence of malignancies). The gene that is mutated in ataxia-telangiectasia (*ATM*) has been localized to chromosome band 11q22-23.[156]

Immunodeficiency is seen in approximately 70% of patients with ataxia-telangiectasia. T- and B-cell numbers are normal. T cells bearing the gamma-delta form of the T-cell receptor constitute up to 50% of T cells (normal: 1%–5%), and T-cell function is impaired. A varying degree of humoral deficiency (IgA, IgG) is common. Patients usually have bronchopulmonary infections at presentation.[156]

NEONATAL THROMBOCYTOPENIA

Neonatal thrombocytopenia is the most common hematologic problem in the neonate. A normal platelet count in healthy newborn infants irrespective of gestational age is considered to be 150 × 10^9/L and above.[157–162] Some 1% to 5% of newborns show thrombocytopenia at birth, and 0.1% to 0.5% have severe thrombocytopenia (<50 × 10^9 platelets/L). In contrast, 22% to 35% of all infants admitted to the NICU develop thrombocytopenia, the rate of which increases as gestation age decreases.[158] Christensen et al observed that 73% of extremely low-birth-weight neonates had one or more platelet counts below 150 × 10^9/L, and 38% of them had a severely low count.[163]

Causes of thrombocytopenia can be classified into those leading to increased platelet destruction (including consumption), those resulting in decreased platelet production, and those involving both.[162,164] Box 16.4 lists the most common causes of thrombocytopenia in neonates.

Classification can also be based on whether the thrombocytopenia was caused by maternal factors.[162,164] Cause can be predicted by the timing of the onset of thrombocytopenia and its natural history.[157–159] For instance, thrombocytopenia presenting during fetal life is most commonly caused by an alloimmune reaction, congenital infection, or aneuploidy, whereas thrombocytopenia presenting within 72 hours of birth (early-onset neonatal thrombocytopenia) mostly affects preterm neonates born after pregnancies characterized by impaired placental function. Neonatal alloimmune or autoimmune thrombocytopenia is common as well. Finally, thrombocytopenia presenting in infants in the NICU after the first 72 hours of life (late-onset neonatal thrombocytopenia) can result from late-onset sepsis or NEC.[157–159] When the cause is being sought, the gestational age of the infant is important as well. In one study of extremely low-birth-weight infants, more than 60% of cases of thrombocytopenia were as a result of infection, disseminated intravascular coagulation, or NEC, and 10% were not explained.[163]

BOX 16.4 Causes of Thrombocytopenia in the Neonate

Increased Platelet Destruction or Consumption
- Alloimmune neonatal thrombocytopenia
- Autoimmune neonatal thrombocytopenia
- Sepsis
- Birth trauma
- Acidosis/hypoxia
- Disseminated intravascular coagulation
- Thrombosis
- Kasabach-Merritt syndrome
- Malignancies (leukemia, etc.)
- Cyanotic heart disease

Decreased Platelet Production
- Thrombocytopenia–absent radius syndrome
- Congenital amegakaryocytic thrombocytopenia
- Amegakaryocytic thrombocytopenia and radioulnar synostosis
- X-linked macrothrombocytopenia as a result of *GATA1* mutation
- Fanconi anemia
- Wiskott-Aldrich syndrome
- Bernard-Soulier syndrome
- MYH9-related thrombocytopenias
- Chromosomal abnormalities
- Preeclampsia

Mixed Causes
- Maternal medications
- Intrauterine growth restriction
- TORCH infections (*t*oxoplasmosis, *o*ther, *r*ubella, *c*ytomegalovirus, *h*erpes simplex)
- Rh disease

Despite our growing knowledge of neonatal thrombocytopenia, the cause cannot be identified in a significant number of patients.

Thrombocytopenia as a Result of Increased Platelet Destruction

Neonatal Alloimmune Thrombocytopenia

Neonatal alloimmune thrombocytopenia (NAIT) is the platelet equivalent of Rh disease. Human platelet antigens (HPAs) are uniquely expressed on platelets, and 16 HPAs have been identified, although fetomaternal incompatibility between only three (HPA-1a, HPA-5b, and HPA-15b) cause 95% of cases in Caucasian populations. Fetomaternal incompatibility for HPA-1a is the most common and is responsible for 75% of cases in white populations.[165] In NAIT, the mother is HPA-1a negative and the father is HPA-1a positive, as is the fetus. When the mother is exposed to fetal platelets, anti–HPA-1a antibodies are generated. These antibodies traverse the placenta via the neonatal Fc receptor, as does all maternal IgG, and cause fetal thrombocytopenia.[166] Because of its frequency and severity, NAIT is the most important cause of severe fetal-neonatal thrombocytopenia.

HPA-1a incompatibility occurs in 1 in 350 pregnancies, although thrombocytopenia develops in only 1 in 1000 to 1 in 1500 pregnancies. The ability of an HPA-1a–negative woman to form anti–HPA-1a is class II restricted and is controlled by the *HLA-DRB3*0101* allele so that HLA-DRB3*0101–positive women are 140 times more likely to make anti–HPA-1a than HLA-DRB3*0101–negative women.[167] NAIT is usually suspected in neonates with bleeding or severe, unexplained, and/or isolated postnatal thrombocytopenia. Three criteria distinguish cases of NAIT from other causes of unexplained thrombocytopenia[168]:

1. severe thrombocytopenia (platelet count of $<50 \times 10^9/L$)
2. ICH associated with one or more of the following:
   - Apgar score at 1 min of more than 5
   - birth weight of more than 2200 g
   - documented antenatal or postnatal bleeding
3. no additional nonhemorrhagic neonatal medical problems

Thrombocytopenia is often extremely severe (platelet count of $<20 \times 10^9/L$) and begins early in gestation. It may result in major bleeding, particularly ICH. Although the incidence of ICH is difficult to ascertain precisely, large series report ICH in 10% to 20% of pregnancies in which NAIT is present.[158] It is reported that 80% of ICH events associated with NAIT occur in utero, with 14% occurring before 20 weeks and a further 28% occurring before 30 weeks.[169] Overall, two-thirds of infants with NAIT-associated ICH develop neurodevelopmental problems, approximately half of which are severe (e.g., severe cerebral palsy and/or sensory impairment).[165] The course of NAIT in otherwise well neonates is variable, with thrombocytopenia resolving in most cases within 1 week without long-term sequelae.

Considerable advances have been made in the clinical and laboratory diagnosis of NAIT and its postnatal and antenatal management. Detailed laboratory investigations are required to confirmation the diagnosis and should be performed by an experienced reference laboratory.

Current consensus is that screening should be performed for HPA-1, HPA-3, and HPA-5 in all cases of potential NAIT and for HPA-4 as well if the patient is of Asian descent. HPA-9 and HPA-15 are the next most commonly involved in antigen incompatibilities. For testing to confirm NAIT, analysis must reveal both a platelet antigen incompatibility between the parents and a maternal antibody directed against that antigen.

Because of the morbidity and mortality associated with NAIT, this disorder requires expert management with close collaboration between fetal medicine specialists, hematologists, and neonatologists.

The mainstay of postnatal management of affected neonates is prompt random-donor platelet transfusion.[170] If promptly available, matched (antigen-negative) platelets are preferred. The latter are platelets from donors negative for HPA-1a or HPA-5b (which are compatible in >90% of NAIT cases, can be given in larger increments, and have a longer half-life). Concentrated maternal platelets can also be used; however, their processing takes at least 12 to 48 hours.

Platelet transfusion is recommended in well term neonates if the count is less than $30 \times 10^9/L$ unless an ICH is diagnosed, in which case a threshold of 100 × 10^9/L is used. A higher count, for example, 50 × 10^9/L, may be selected in cases of prematurity, birth asphyxia, or another condition predisposing to ICH.[166]

IVIG can also be infused (effective in at least 75% of cases).[171] The IVIG dose is 0.8–1 g/kg/day for 1 to 3 days depending on response. Some centers administer steroids with IVIG.[166] However, with these therapies, platelet count increase is slow (requiring about 48–72 hours), and therefore platelet transfusion may still be needed. Head ultrasonography is strongly recommended for a thrombocytopenic neonate via NAIT. If NAIT is complicated by even asymptomatic ICH, the target platelet count is higher—more than 100 × 10^9/L—and management of the next affected pregnancy will be more intensive and start earlier. NAIT often resolves within 2 to 4 weeks.[166,171]

Another important aspect of NAIT care is antenatal management of subsequent pregnancies. If the previously affected sibling had an ICH, the next affected fetus will have early, severe thrombocytopenia and in utero ICH, which may be ameliorated by effective treatment.[166] Radder et al performed a literature search for ICH cases in untreated NAIT pregnancies. The recurrence rate of ICH in the subsequent offspring of women with a history of NAIT with ICH was 72% (CI: 46%–98%) when fetal deaths were not included and 79% (CI: 61%–97%) when they were included.[172] The risk of ICH after a previous occurrence of NAIT without ICH was estimated to be 7% (CI: 0.5%–13%). The lack of laboratory parameters predictive of severe disease remains one of the major barriers to optimizing antenatal management of NAIT and is an important area for future research.[171] Antenatal treatment intensity depends on the occurrence of ICH and severity of thrombocytopenia in the previous sibling. Maternally administered therapy (maternal IVIG, steroids) should be the first-line approach. This recommendation is based on data describing the effectiveness and safety of maternal treatment in contrast to the toxicity of serial administration of fetal bovine serum to deliver weekly fetal platelet transfusions. Different centers currently have different strategies based on their own experience and results of published studies.[167,171]

Neonatal Autoimmune Thrombocytopenia

Neonatal autoimmune thrombocytopenia is mediated by the transplacental passage of maternal antiplatelet antibodies. Unlike in NAIT, in this case the antibody responsible binds both maternal and fetal platelets and causes thrombocytopenia in the mother and the neonate.[164] In most instances, the underlying maternal disease is idiopathic thrombocytopenic purpura, but other disorders (e.g., systemic lupus erythematosus) can also produce this syndrome. Maternal platelet autoantibodies occur in 1 to 2 in 1000 pregnancies; however, they are much less likely to cause a clinical problem than NAIT. Thrombocytopenia occurs in only 10% of neonates whose mothers have autoantibodies, and the incidence of ICH is 1% or less. Maternal disease severity and/or platelet count during pregnancy and the occurrence of severe thrombocytopenia in a previous neonate are the most useful indicators of the likelihood that significant fetal and neonatal thrombocytopenia will complicate the current pregnancy.[161,173,174] The platelet count should be determined at birth for neonates of mothers with autoimmune disease. In neonates with normal platelet counts (>150 × 10^9/L), no further action is necessary. In those with thrombocytopenia, a platelet count should be repeated after 2 to 3 days because platelet counts are often at a nadir at this time before rising spontaneously by day 7 in most cases.[158] In a small number of cases, thrombocytopenia may persist for several weeks. In this situation, when the thrombocytopenia is severe (platelet count of <30 × 10^9/L), treatment with IVIG (2 g/kg over 2–5 days) may be useful.[175]

Disseminated Intravascular Coagulation

Disseminated intravascular coagulation (DIC) complicates several disease processes (bacterial or viral sepsis, respiratory distress syndrome, meconium aspiration, asphyxia). Thrombocytopenia is a consistent and very early finding in neonates with DIC.[161] Prolonged prothrombin times (PTs) and partial thromboplastin times, increased levels of fibrin degradation products, increased D-dimer levels, and depletion of fibrinogen are other abnormal laboratory findings usually seen in neonates with DIC. Successful treatment of neonatal DIC depends on the diagnosis and treatment of the underlying disorder. Treatment of the hemostatic abnormalities in neonates with DIC is not clearly established and depends on the clinical manifestations.[161] Platelets, fresh frozen plasma, and cryoprecipitate are commonly used, with the goal of reducing significant bleeding.

Kasabach-Merritt Syndrome

Kasabach-Merritt syndrome typically presents in the neonatal period with profound thrombocytopenia together with microangiopathic anemia, DIC, and an enlarging vascular lesion. Hemangiomas are usually cutaneous, but in 20%, there is visceral involvement (e.g., in the liver). Thrombocytopenia in Kasabach-Merritt syndrome is mainly as a result of the trapping of platelets on the endothelium of the hemangioma. Usually it is severe, but it is exacerbated in some cases by the development of DIC. Review of the blood film often, although not always, reveals red blood cell fragmentation, which can help in the diagnosis of difficult cases. When treatment is required, administration of steroids followed by interferon and/or vincristine is effective in over 50% of cases, although the mortality is 20% to 30%.[176]

Necrotizing Enterocolitis

NEC frequently causes thrombocytopenia in neonates. In fact, probably 80% to 90% of patients with NEC develop thrombocytopenia (platelet count of <150 × 10^9/L) as part of the presentation, and many have platelets counts in the range of 30 to 60 × 10^9/L. Platelet destruction seems to be the primary mechanism.[161]

Thrombosis

Thrombosis can cause thrombocytopenia in a neonate when platelet uptake in the thrombus is more rapid than platelet production. If thrombocytopenia is severe, it can be treated by platelet transfusions until the underlying cause of the platelet destruction is removed.[157,161]

Thrombocytopenia as a Result of Decreased Platelet Production

Bernard-Soulier Syndrome

Bernard-Soulier syndrome is an autosomal recessive disorder caused by qualitative or quantitative defects in the glycoprotein Ib-IX-V complex. Bernard-Soulier syndrome may present in the neonatal period, although bleeding is not usually severe in neonates. A diagnosis of Bernard-Soulier syndrome is suggested when there is mild to moderate thrombocytopenia together with giant platelets. Treatment by platelet transfusion is effective but should be reserved for cases of life-threatening hemorrhage.[177]

Wiskott-Aldrich Syndrome

Wiskott-Aldrich syndrome, caused by mutations in the Wiskott-Aldrich syndrome gene, is a complex and diverse disorder with X-linked inheritance.[178] Affected boys exhibit microthrombocytopenia with hemorrhagic diathesis in early childhood and variable degrees of eczema, combined immunodeficiency, and increased risk of autoimmunity and lymphoid malignancies. The numbers of T and B lymphocytes decline over the years, and in vitro proliferation of T lymphocytes to specific antigens is reduced. IgA and IgE serum levels are often increased, which reflects immune dysregulation. Unless hematologic and immune reconstitution by hematopoietic stem cell transplantation or gene therapy is achieved, patients with classic Wiskott-Aldrich syndrome tend to develop autoimmune disorders and lymphoma or other malignancies that lead to an early death.[178]

Fanconi Anemia

Fanconi anemia is an autosomal recessive disease characterized by aplastic anemia and congenital abnormalities (absent radii, absent or malformed thumbs, microcephaly, hypogonadism, hypertelorism, gastrointestinal malformations, renal-ureteral malformations, café au lait spots). Hypersensitivity to DNA cross-linking agents like diepoxybutane is often used as a diagnostic test.[179] At birth, the blood count is usually normal, and macrocytosis is often the first detected abnormality. This is typically followed by thrombocytopenia and anemia that progresses to pancytopenia. The majority of patients develop progressive bone marrow failure or acute myelogenous leukemia, which are diagnosed with peak frequencies at the ages of 7 and 10 to 15 years, respectively.[180] Of subjects registered between 1982 and 1992 in the International Fanconi Anemia Registry, several showed hematologic abnormalities during the neonatal period.[179]

Thrombocytopenia–Absent Radius Syndrome

Thrombocytopenia–absent radius (TAR) syndrome is characterized by bilateral absence of the radii with the presence of both thumbs and thrombocytopenia. Thrombocytopenia may be congenital or may develop within the first few weeks to months of life. Patients usually show severe symptomatic thrombocytopenia in the first week of life with increased mortality as a result of ICH when the platelet count is less than 20 $\times 10^9$/L. With increasing age, the recurrence of thrombocytopenic episodes decreases, and platelet count can improve to near-normal levels. Leukocytosis and eosinophilia may precede thrombocytopenia. Typically, patients have bilateral aplasia of the radii, but abnormalities involving the lower extremities have also been described. Unlike in Fanconi anemia, thumbs are present bilaterally. Cardiac and facial anomalies, as well as hypoplasia of the cerebellar vermis and corpus callosum, may be present. Symptomatic allergy to cow's milk is present in 47% of individuals with TAR syndrome. Treatment is based on provision of platelet support when needed.[181,182]

Congenital Amegakaryocytic Thrombocytopenia

Congenital amegakaryocytic thrombocytopenia (CAMT) is an autosomal recessive disorder caused by mutations in the thrombopoietin receptor c-Mpl. It presents at birth with severe thrombocytopenia (platelet count of $<50 \times 10^9$/L) with platelets that are of normal size and granularity. Importantly, phenotypic findings in CAMT are usually limited to those related to thrombocytopenia, including cutaneous and ICHs before or after birth. Several patients have been described with clinical features of CAMT who also exhibited growth or developmental delay, strabismus, or central nervous system abnormalities, including cerebellar malformations and cortical dysplasia.[182–184] Reduction or absence of megakaryocytes is seen in the bone marrow with evolution of hypocellular or aplastic bone marrows later in the course. Measurement of plasma thrombopoietin levels is a useful diagnostic assay in the evaluation of congenital thrombocytopenia; however, this assay is not widely available.[183] In children in whom the diagnosis is suspected based on clinical findings, CAMT can be confirmed by identification of homozygous or compound heterozygous mutations in the thrombopoietin receptor c-Mpl. Supportive care for patients with CAMT consists primarily of platelet transfusions. Novel therapies such as CRISPR-Cas9 gene editing of primary hematopoietic stem cells are being developed to rescue the mutant mpl function.[185] Currently, the only definitive treatment available for the long-term management of patients with CAMT is hematopoietic stem cell transplantation.[182–184]

Amegakaryocytic Thrombocytopenia and Radioulnar Synostosis

Amegakaryocytic thrombocytopenia and radioulnar synostosis is an autosomal dominant disorder associated with *HOXA11* mutation with features that include CAMT, aplastic anemia, proximal radioulnar synostosis, clinodactyly, syndactyly, hip dysplasia, and sensorineural hearing loss.[186] Symptomatic thrombocytopenia with bruising and bleeding is present from birth, necessitating ultimate correction by stem cell transplantation.[187]

MYH9-Related Inherited Thrombocytopenia

MYH9-related inherited thrombocytopenia (MYH9-related disease) is one of the most frequent forms of inherited thrombocytopenia. It is transmitted in an autosomal dominant fashion and derives from mutations of *MYH9,* the gene for the heavy chain of nonmuscle myosin IIA. Patients have congenital macrothrombocytopenia with mild bleeding tendency and may develop kidney dysfunction, deafness, and cataracts later in life. The term *MYH9-related disease* encompasses four autosomal dominant thrombocytopenias that were previously described as distinct disorders: namely, May-Hegglin anomaly, Sebastian syndrome, Fechtner syndrome, and Epstein syndrome. Thrombocytopenia is usually mild and derives from complex defects of megakaryocyte maturation and platelet formation. Usually the presence of giant platelets in peripheral blood raises the suspicion of MYH9-related disease, and a simple immunofluorescence test showing the distribution of nonmuscle myosin heavy chain IIA within neutrophils on blood films confirms the diagnosis. Characteristic Döhle-like bodies are identified in the cytoplasm of neutrophil granulocytes in 42% to 84% of patients.[188]

X-Linked Macrothrombocytopenia

X-linked macrothrombocytopenia caused by mutation in *GATA1* is a recently described isolated X-linked macrothrombocytopenia without anemia (but with some dyserythropoietic features). In this disorder, immature platelets are released into the circulation that have hyperplastic endoplasmic reticulum and a disturbed glycoprotein Ib-V-IX complex with weakened function. The disorder may present with severe thrombocytopenia and profound bleeding at birth.[189,190]

Chromosomal Abnormalities

Infants with chromosomal abnormalities (trisomies of chromosomes 13, 18, or 21; Turner syndrome) can have neonatal thrombocytopenia in addition to the characteristic physical features of these disorders. Although, historically, trisomy 21 has been associated mostly with other hematologic disorders, such as polycythemia, transient myeloproliferative disorder, and acute leukemia, isolated neonatal thrombocytopenia is a frequent finding. The thrombocytopenia is usually mild to moderate and transient, with resolution at 2 to 3 weeks of life. Therefore an extensive evaluation of mild to moderate thrombocytopenia in neonates with Down syndrome is not suggested.[161]

Pregnancy-Induced Hypertension

PIH is a common cause of thrombocytopenia in neonates, but the pathogenesis of the condition is unclear. Possibly, it is the kinetic result of decreased platelet production. Of all infants born to women with PIH, preterm babies are at highest risk of developing thrombocytopenia. The thrombocytopenia presents at birth or in the first few days of life, reaches a nadir on days 2 to 4, and resolves by days 7 to 10.[161]

Thrombocytopenia as a Result of Mixed Causes

Infection

Intrauterine cytomegalovirus infection and rubella can be associated with neutropenia or pancytopenia. Thrombocytopenia is most likely secondary to splenomegaly; however, an element of decreased production might be associated as well.[123]

Intrauterine Growth Restriction

Thrombocytopenia is particularly common in preterm infants who are small for gestational age, but it is relatively uncommon in term infants who are small for gestational age. The cause of the thrombocytopenia is not known. The pathogenesis may involve accelerated platelet removal from the blood or decreased platelet production related to a failure to compensate by increasing production of thrombopoietin.[161]

Evaluation of the Neonate With Thrombocytopenia

The first step in evaluating a neonate with thrombocytopenia is to classify the thrombocytopenia into one of the categories discussed previously. This involves consideration of the infant's age (early versus late thrombocytopenia), the severity of the thrombocytopenia, the presence of dysmorphic features, the clinical condition (sick versus not sick), and the medications used. In determining the cause of thrombocytopenia in an affected neonate, it is important first to consider conditions that could be life-threatening (e.g., infections, DIC, NEC, thrombosis) or that have significant implications for further pregnancies (e.g., alloimmune or autoimmune thrombocytopenia, genetic disorders). If any of these entities is suspected, appropriate diagnostic testing should be conducted (e.g., bacterial or viral cultures, assays for antiplatelet antibodies, chromosome analysis). Once these conditions have been ruled out, other causes of thrombocytopenia (generally more benign) should be considered. Several tests have been used for indirect evaluation of the mechanisms causing thrombocytopenia. Two of them (mean platelet volume and time between transfusions) are easily available to the clinician caring for a thrombocytopenic neonate. A high mean platelet volume usually suggests increased platelet production, presumably as a compensation for accelerated platelet destruction. In cases in which the cause is clearly defined, no further evaluation is necessary unless the thrombocytopenia is especially severe or more prolonged than is expected given the cause identified. A bone marrow evaluation may be warranted in a patient with prolonged and severe thrombocytopenia of unclear cause despite extensive evaluation.[161]

Platelet Transfusion Guidelines

Until data from controlled trials become available, decisions about platelet transfusion in neonates will be based on consensus guidelines.[124] Patients qualifying for a platelet transfusion should initially receive 10 to 15 mL/kg of cytomegalovirus-negative standard platelet suspension, prepared from a fresh unit of whole blood or by platelet pheresis. No volume-reducing processing is routinely recommended because of the risk of platelet loss, clumping, and dysfunction because of the additional handling.[124]

The decision to administer a prophylactic platelet transfusion should be made on the basis of many factors, including the platelet count, the mechanism responsible for the thrombocytopenia, the medications administered, and the condition

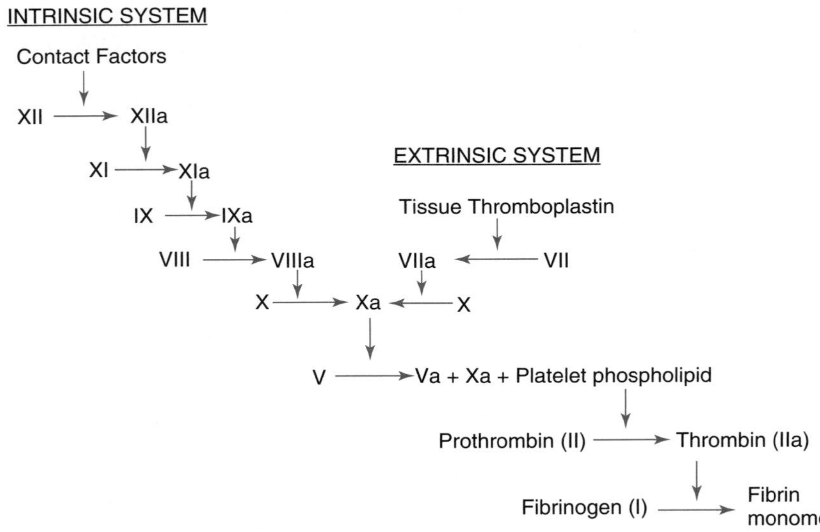

INTRINSIC SYSTEM

Contact Factors

XII → XIIa

XI → XIa

IX → IXa

VIII → VIIIa

EXTRINSIC SYSTEM

Tissue Thromboplastin

VIIa ← VII

X → Xa ← X

V → Va + Xa + Platelet phospholipid

Prothrombin (II) → Thrombin (IIa)

Fibrinogen (I) → Fibrin monomer

Fig. 16.2 Overview of the coagulant proteins of the intrinsic system (upper left) and extrinsic system (upper right), which both feed into the common pathway (bottom).

of the patient. Usually such decisions are institution-driven, "best-guess" estimates. For patients in the first week of life at greatest risk of hemorrhage (e.g., extremely preterm neonates in unstable condition), administration of prophylactic platelet transfusions at trigger thresholds of up to 50×10^9/L is generally considered to represent acceptable and safe clinical practice. Platelet transfusions in neonates with platelet counts of more than 50×10^9/L should be reserved for patients with active major bleeding, such as new or extending intraventricular hemorrhage or pulmonary, gastrointestinal, or renal hemorrhage.[158,191]

Infants who are being treated with medications known to induce platelet dysfunction (e.g., indomethacin, aspirin, or nitric oxide) should probably be maintained at higher platelet counts than neonates who are not receiving such medications. The same applies to neonates receiving anticoagulants (heparin or low-molecular-weight heparin [LMWH]) or thrombolytic agents (e.g., tissue plasminogen activator [TPA]), whose risk of bleeding is significantly higher in the presence of thrombocytopenia.[124] As discussed earlier, special consideration should be given to the transfusion of HPA-1b–negative platelets, or platelets obtained from the mother, to neonates with alloimmune thrombocytopenia.

COAGULATION SYSTEM IN THE NEONATE

The human hemostatic system starts developing in utero and continues to develop well into childhood. This system can be thought of as having discrete fluid phase (circulating proteins), cellular (platelets), and vascular (vessel wall) compartments. Although this approach is useful in classifying specific disorders, the component parts of the hemostatic system are functionally and biochemically interrelated. The functional levels of many of the procoagulants, coagulation inhibitors, and fibrinolytic components in the neonate differ from those in the adult. The component functions reach adult levels by 6 months of age. The pioneering work of Dr. Maureen Andrew in the 1980s elucidated the unique aspects of the neonatal and fetal coagulation system (Fig. 16.2). The term *developmental hemostasis* was used for the first time to describe her work. Even though neonates have different functional levels of all the coagulation components compared with adults, they rarely have problems with bleeding or thrombosis. The differences in prothrombotic and antithrombotic components are uniquely balanced in the neonate, which creates a normal physiologic state. Table 16.2 presents the reference ranges for coagulation test values for healthy full-term neonates and healthy preterm babies.

A number of bleeding and clotting disorders can present in the neonatal period. The following sections briefly review the presentation, workup, and initial management of common inherited bleeding and clotting disorders.

Initial Laboratory Evaluation of the Neonate With Bleeding

About 15% to 30% of patients with inherited bleeding disorders have bleeding symptoms in the neonatal period.[192] Evaluation of a bleeding neonate always begins with taking a detailed maternal and family history. It is important to obtain details about the mother's state of health during pregnancy and labor, including infections, maternal autoimmune disease, and platelet count. Other details about the labor and delivery itself, such as prolonged time between rupture of membranes and delivery, fetal distress, and chorioamnionitis, are also important. Next, history taking for the infant should focus on confirming administration of vitamin K. A detailed family history focusing on the types and severity of any bleeding symptoms, as well as the sex of the affected members, gives valuable information on the type and inheritance pattern of a possible bleeding disorder. However, a third of new cases of severe hemophilia represent new mutations, and therefore no family history of such disorders is present.

TABLE 16.2 Normal Values for Coagulation Tests in Healthy Full-Term and Premature Infants

Coagulation Test	Full-Term Infant	Premature Infant	Older Child
Platelets (per μL)	150,000–400,000	150,000–400,000	150,000–400,000
Prothrombin time (sec)	10.1–15.9	10.6–16.2	10.6–11.4
Partial thromboplastin time (sec)	31.3–54.5	27.5–79.4	24–36
Thrombin clotting time (sec)	19–28.3	19.2–30.4	19.8–31.2
Fibrinogen (mg/dL)	167–399	150–373	170–405
Fibrin degradation products (μg/mL)	<10	<10	<10
Factor VIII (U/mL)	0.50–1.78	0.50–2.13	0.59–1.42
Factor IX (U/mL)	0.15–0.91	0.19–0.65	0.47–1.04
von Willebrand factor (U/ml)	0.50–2.87	0.78–2.10	0.60–1.20

Modified from Cantor AB. Developmental hemostasis: relevance to newborns and infants. In Orkin SH, Fisher D, Look AT, et al, eds. *Nathan and Oski's Hematology of Infancy and* Childhood. 7th ed. Philadelphia, PA: Saunders; 2009.

Examination of the neonate should quickly differentiate between a well-appearing baby and a sick one. A sick infant may have medical conditions contributing to hemorrhage. Findings of birth trauma, evidence of bruises and petechiae, and presence of flank masses suggestive of renal vein thrombosis should be sought. Hepatosplenomegaly in a sick neonate may suggest disseminated intrauterine infection. The most common cause of bleeding in healthy infants is thrombocytopenia secondary to transplacental passage of a maternal antiplatelet antibody, sepsis, vitamin K deficiency, or congenital coagulation factor deficiencies. In an otherwise well infant, bleeding from a circumcision site, oozing from the umbilicus, bleeding into the scalp, large cephalohematomas, or ICH may point to coagulation factor deficiencies such as hemophilia or von Willebrand disease (VWD), or disorders of platelet numbers such as NAIT. NAIT is the most common cause of severe thrombocytopenia in a well infant, occurring in approximately 1 in 1000 to 2000 births. A detailed description of the causes and investigation of thrombocytopenic bleeding can be found elsewhere in this chapter.

Blood volume in a neonate is low, and hence a small blood loss, even for investigative blood draws, can impact the hematocrit. Judicious use of laboratory tests for screening for underlying bleeding disorders requires partnership with a hematologist specializing in coagulation disorders. If the history and physical examination are not suggestive of a specific disorder, a panel of screening tests should be ordered. These include a complete blood count with review of the peripheral smear, including platelet number and morphology, PT, activated partial thromboplastin time (APTT), and thrombin time (TT). The results must be compared with the expected normal ranges based on the gestational age of the infant as mentioned previously. Reference ranges for PT and APTT in healthy term newborns and preterm infants are given in Table 16.2. The PT and APTT measure the overall function of proteins in the coagulation cascade. The PT measures the activities of factors I (fibrinogen), II (prothrombin), V, VII, and X. PT is generally prolonged when the functional activities of one of these factors goes below 30%. The most common cause of isolated prolongation of PT is factor VII deficiency. The APTT measures the functional activities of the factors in the intrinsic arm of the coagulation cascade: namely, VIII, IX, XI, XII, prekallikrein, and high-molecular-weight kininogen. It also measures the functional activities of factors I (fibrinogen), II (prothrombin), and V. Deficiency of any of these factors results in the prolongation of the APTT. The sensitivity and reproducibility of the APTT, unlike those of the PT, depend strongly on the specific reagents used. With most reagents, the APTT is not prolonged unless the factor VIII level is less than 35% (0.35 U/mL). Deficiencies of factor XII, prekallikrein, and high-molecular-weight kininogen result in prolongation of APTT but no clinical bleeding symptoms. Isolated prolongation of the APTT in the neonate is likely because of deficiency of factor VIII, IX, or XI, if contamination with heparin is ruled out. For a child with mild bleeding, if hemophilia is suspected, factor VIII and IX assays should be performed regardless of the APTT value. The APTT is somewhat less sensitive to vitamin K deficiency than the PT. The TT measures the thrombin-induced conversion of fibrinogen to fibrin and hence is useful for investigating the clotting function of fibrinogen in a variety of fibrinogen disorders.

A number of pitfalls exist in performing and interpreting tests such as the PT and APTT. Caution should be taken when sending blood for coagulation testing. The blood sample must be from free-flowing blood without any air bubbles present. Particular attention should be paid to keeping the 1:10 ratio of the anticoagulant sodium citrate to plasma by filling the tube up to the appropriate mark. Specialized microcollection tubes (1 mL) in the neonatal unit help avoid wastage. Drawing blood from an indwelling catheter may result in contamination of the sample with heparin and other fluids, which then leads to spurious prolongation of clotting times. In neonates with polycythemia (hematocrit of >55%), the amount of citrate can be reduced to maintain the 1:10 ratio of citrate to plasma. This is particularly helpful in neonates with cyanotic congenital heart disease who have very high hematocrit values. If the sample is suspected of being contaminated with heparin, measuring TT and reptilase time

TABLE 16.3 Conditions Associated With Bleeding and Normal Platelet Count

Diagnosis	Appearance	PT	APTT	Other Useful Tests
Hemorrhagic disease of the newborn	Well	↑	↑	Fibrinogen, fibrin degradation products
Hepatic disease	Sick	↑	↑	Albumin, fibrinogen, fibrin degradation products, liver function tests
von Willebrand disease*	Well	Normal	Normal or ↑	Bleeding time (see text)
Hemophilia	Well	Normal	↑	Mixing tests, factor VIII and IX assays
Factor XIII deficiency	Well	Normal	Normal	Urea clot solubility
Disorders of platelet function*	Well	Normal	Normal	Bleeding time, platelet aggregometry

Some patients with these disorders show mild to moderate thrombocytopenia (see text for details).
APTT, Activated partial thromboplastin time; *PT*, prothrombin time.

helps differentiate between prolongation of APTT as a result of heparin and prolongation because of other causes. A 1:1 mixing study of the sample with prolonged APTT can also be performed by adding normal plasma to the specimen. If the prolonged APTT corrects, the cause is not heparin contamination.

Other coagulation tests include closure time measured by platelet function analyzer, platelet aggregation test, urea clot solubility, and other coagulation factor assays. These tests are not useful as screening tests in the neonate and should not be performed unless there is a strong suspicion of a specific disorder. These tests are described in the discussions of the individual bleeding disorders to which they are relevant.

Bleeding in a neonate with thrombocytopenia is discussed in a different section of this chapter.

BLEEDING IN NEONATES WITH NORMAL PLATELET COUNTS

The disorders considered in the differential diagnosis of bleeding in a neonate with a normal platelet count can be broadly classified based on whether the infant appears well or sick. These various disorders are discussed in the following sections. The clinical and laboratory features of these disorders are summarized in Table 16.3.

Hemorrhagic Disease of the Newborn (Vitamin K Deficiency)

Hemorrhagic disease of the newborn (HDN) is defined as hemorrhage from multiple sites on days 1 to 5 in an otherwise healthy infant. It was first described by Townsend in 1894.[193] Vitamin K acts on the precursors of factors II, VII, IX, and X (vitamin K–dependent factors) to generate active procoagulants. Its biochemical function involves creating calcium-binding sites in these proteins by carboxylating specific glutamic acid residues. Levels of the vitamin K–dependent factors are physiologically low in newborns.[194] It is a common practice to routinely administer parenteral vitamin K after birth. As a result, HDN is a rare condition.

The clinical manifestations of HDN can be of three different types based on the timing and type of bleeding complications. Classic HDN is defined as bleeding on days 2 to 7 of life in breast-fed, healthy, full-term infants.[195] The bleeding manifestation is usually in the form of oozing from the umbilicus, bleeding from circumcision and puncture sites, ICH, and gastrointestinal hemorrhage. Causes include poor placental transfer of vitamin K,[196] marginal vitamin K content in breast milk (<20 µg/L), inadequate milk intake, and a sterile gut. Vitamin K deficiency bleeding (VKDB) rarely occurs in formula-fed infants because commercially available formulas are supplemented with vitamin K.[197] In the absence of vitamin K prophylaxis, the incidence of VKDB ranges from 0.25% to 1.7%.[198] The incidence depends on the population studied, the supplemental formula used, and the prevalence of breast feeding in the community. Early HDN develops in the first 24 hours of life and is linked to maternal use of specific medications that interfere with vitamin K stores or function, such as some anticonvulsants. Bleeding can be in the form of ICH, gastrointestinal bleeding, or cephalohematomas. Late HDN occurs between weeks 2 and 8 of life and is linked to disorders that compromise ongoing vitamin K supply, such as cystic fibrosis, alpha-1 antitrypsin deficiency, biliary atresia, and celiac disease. Infants with these disorders are at risk of development of late vitamin K deficiency weeks to months after receiving parenteral vitamin K at birth.

Results of screening laboratory tests reveal a normal platelet count and an abnormal PT and APTT. The PT is often markedly prolonged compared with the APTT. Levels of fibrinogen and fibrin degradation products as well as TT are normal. Other tests that can aid in the diagnosis are specific factor assays, measurement of the levels of decarboxylated forms of vitamin K–dependent factors, assay of protein induced by vitamin K antagonists, and direct measurement of vitamin K levels.

All newborns suspected of having HDN should be treated with vitamin K without waiting for the results of laboratory tests. For hemorrhages that are not life-threatening, parenteral vitamin K can be used to rapidly correct the bleeding diathesis. Vitamin K works within a few hours because it generates active procoagulants from the precursors with no requirement for new protein synthesis. Infants with VKDB should be given vitamin K either subcutaneously or intravenously, depending on the situation. Vitamin K should not be given intramuscularly to infants with VKDB because large hematomas may form at the site of the injection. Intravenous vitamin K should be administered slowly, and a test dose should be given because it may induce an anaphylactoid reaction. For infants with major or life-threatening hemorrhage, fresh frozen plasma should be administered to stop bleeding and increase levels of vitamin K–dependent proteins. Prothrombin complex concentrates, if available, can also be used to treat life-threatening hemorrhages.

A number of special considerations apply to the high-risk newborn. Vitamin K production by bacteria in the gut is reduced by illnesses that require that enteral feedings be delayed or interrupted. Treatment with broad-spectrum antibiotics also decreases vitamin K synthesis. For these reasons, it is highly recommended that vitamin K be administered weekly to infants who are not breast fed and to those who are being treated with parenteral antibiotics.

EDITORIAL COMMENT: A growing number of parents are refusing to permit vitamin K administration to their newborns according to a survey of newborn nurseries in the United States. The parents cited a number of different reasons for the refusal, from stating that it was unnecessary to safety concerns. Healthcare professionals will need to develop appropriate strategies to discuss and address parental concerns but also may encounter an increased incidence of hemorrhagic disease of the newborn (HDN).

Loyal J, Taylor JA, Phillipi CA, et al. Refusal of vitamin K by parents of newborns: a survey of the Better Outcomes through Research for Newborns Network. *Acad Pediatr.* 2017;17(4):368-373.

Liver Disease

Coagulopathy associated with liver disease in newborns is a result of failure of the hepatic synthetic function. There is generalized impairment of hepatic synthesis of proteins, including the coagulation proteins. In a newborn, the problem may be exacerbated because of the already existing physiologic immaturity of the coagulation system. Common causes of liver dysfunction in newborns are total parenteral nutrition, hypoxia, shock, fetal hydrops, and viral hepatitis. Rarely, genetic diseases such as alpha-1 antitrypsin deficiency, galactosemia, and tyrosinemia are responsible for the liver impairment.

Laboratory abnormalities induced by acute liver disease include prolongation of the PT and low plasma concentrations of several coagulation proteins, including fibrinogen. Fibrinogen is present at adult levels in newborns and may be a useful marker. The diagnosis is also supported by a low serum albumin level and by abnormal results on liver function studies. Secondary effects of liver disease on platelet number and function also occur in newborns. Secondary vitamin K deficiency may occur as a result of impaired absorption from the small intestine, particularly in infants with intrahepatic and extrahepatic biliary atresia. Supplemental vitamin K should be administered to these infants. Severe bleeding is best treated by infusion of fresh frozen plasma. Cryoprecipitate is indicated for patients with severely reduced fibrinogen levels. Patients with clinical bleeding may benefit temporarily from replacement of coagulation proteins using fresh frozen plasma, cryoprecipitate, or exchange transfusion. Without recovery of hepatic function, however, replacement therapy is futile. Hence the overall goal should be to identify and reverse the underlying condition.

Hereditary Coagulation Factor Deficiencies

A number of hereditary coagulation factor deficiencies can present in the neonatal period. Deficiencies of factors VIII and IX are common and have an X-linked inheritance pattern, whereas deficiencies of factors II, V, VII, XI, and XII, prekallikrein, and high-molecular-weight kininogen are autosomally inherited disorders and are rare, with consanguinity present in many affected families. Rarely, combined deficiencies of factors II, VII, and IX and/or factors V and VIII present in the neonatal period.[199] Only the common inherited coagulation factor deficiencies such as the hemophilias and VWD are described here. A detailed discussion of the rarer forms of coagulation factor deficiencies can be found in Nathan and Oski's *Hematology of Infancy and Childhood.*

The Hemophilias

Hemophilia A and hemophilia B are X-linked bleeding disorders caused by congenital deficiencies of proteins in the intrinsic coagulation cascade. Hemophilia A (or classic hemophilia) is as a result of a deficiency of factor VIII and accounts for 85% of cases. Hemophilia B (Christmas disease) results from absent or decreased factor IX activity and is responsible for the remaining 15% of cases. Hemophilia A and hemophilia B are clinically indistinguishable. The percentage of factor VIII or IX coagulant activity is used to classify the hemophilias as severe (<1%), moderate (1%–5%), or mild (5%–15%). Severe factor VIII deficiency is the most common inherited bleeding disorder manifesting in the neonatal period. Although a positive family history is helpful in making the diagnosis, new mutations account for about one-third of all cases of factor VIII deficiency. The bleeding symptoms in infants with hemophilia range from mild to catastrophic. Large cohort studies have shown that approximately 10% of children with hemophilia have clinical symptoms in the neonatal period.[200] Approximately 50% of patients with severe hemophilia bleed excessively following circumcision. Other cases present with severe visceral or ICH after difficult vaginal deliveries. These infants may be acutely ill from hypovolemia or local hemorrhage into vital organs.

The only abnormality in laboratory test results is prolongation of the APTT (up to 100 seconds in severe cases (APTT can be as high as 100 seconds)). The PT and the platelet count are normal. Specific assays for factors VIII and IX quickly confirm the diagnosis, but these are not available in all laboratories. When hemophilia is suspected in a male infant with a prolonged APTT and factor assays are not immediately available, other studies are helpful. The PTT should be repeated using a 50:50 mix of patient and normal plasma. In hemophilia, the PTT corrects to normal. Even small clinical laboratories often have a stock of factor VIII–deficient plasma. If the PTT corrects with normal plasma, the mixing study is repeated with this factor VIII–deficient plasma. If the PTT

TABLE 16.4 Products Used in the Treatment of Neonatal Coagulopathies

Product	Contents	Usual Dose	Indications
Fresh frozen plasma	All factors	10–20 mL/kg	Disseminated intravascular coagulation (DIC), protein C deficiency, liver disease
Cryoprecipitate	Factor VIII, factor XIII, von Willebrand factor, fibrinogen	1 bag (~250 mg fibrinogen, 80–120 U factor VIII)	Factor XIII deficiency, DIC, liver disease, factor VIII deficiency, von Willebrand disease
Factor VIII concentrates	Factor VIII	25–50 U/kg	Factor VIII deficiency
Factor IX concentrates	Factor IX	50–120 U/kg	Factor IX deficiency
Vitamin K		1–2 mg	Vitamin K deficiency
Platelet concentrates	Platelets	1–2 U/5 kg	Thrombocytopenic bleeding

corrects to normal, hemophilia A is excluded, and hemophilia B is the likely diagnosis. If the PTT does not correct to normal, factor VIII deficiency is the presumptive diagnosis.

Recombinant concentrates of factor VIII or factor IX (produced in vitro using recombinant DNA technology) have been the mainstay for treating bleeding in patients with hemophilia. In the early 1980s, use of lyophilized concentrates was associated with a high incidence of transfusion-transmitted HIV infection. Routine heating of factor concentrates in the manufacturing process has apparently eliminated this problem. The dose of factor VIII or IX used to treat hemorrhagic complications depends on the severity of the bleeding. Life-threatening hemorrhages in infants with hemophilia A should be treated with an initial dose of factor VIII concentrate of 50 U/kg followed either by a continuous infusion of 8 to 10 U/hr or by boluses of 50 U/kg every 8 hours. Infants with hemophilia B who have severe bleeding are given a bolus of 100 to 120 U/kg of factor IX concentrate followed either by a continuous infusion starting at 5 U/kg/hr or by bolus doses given every 12 hours. Lower dosages are recommended for less severe bleeding.[201] The presence of inhibitors is rare in neonates. The duration of replacement therapy is based on the location and extent of the bleeding and on the clinical response of the patient. Less severe hemorrhages (such as those that typically follow circumcision) often resolve after application of pressure to the wound or may require a single bolus dose of 10 to 25 U/kg of factor VIII concentrate or 15 to 30 U/kg of factor IX concentrate. Replacement therapy is not indicated for infants with hemophilia who are not bleeding unless they require surgery. Cryoprecipitate contains factor VIII but not factor IX and can therefore be used to treat bleeding complications in hemophilia A. One unit of cryoprecipitate per 5 kg of body weight increases the factor VIII level by about 40%. The Medical and Scientific Advisory Committee of the National Hemophilia Foundation recommends against the use of cryoprecipitate because it is not a virally inactivated product. Several advances in hemophilia therapy such as extension of half-life of factor products, and introduction of novel nonfactor therapies, have been made. However, because of lack of data, use in the neonatal population is not yet recommended by the FDA.[202] Recommended dosages of factor concentrates and cryoprecipitate are presented in Table 16.4.

Von Willebrand Disease

Although von Willebrand Disease (VWD) is probably the most common inherited bleeding disorder, it is rarely diagnosed in the nursery. Von Willebrand factor is the product of an autosomal gene, and the common form of VWD is transmitted as a dominant condition. Von Willebrand factor plays a central role in hemostasis by promoting platelet adherence to the vascular endothelium, a reaction mediated through a specific receptor on the platelet called *glycoprotein Ib.* Von Willebrand factor is stored in platelet granules and is also released from the endothelial cell lining of the injured vessel. Von Willebrand factor circulates as high-, intermediate-, and low-molecular-weight complexes called *multimers.* In addition to playing a role in platelet adherence, von Willebrand factor associates with and stabilizes factor VIII. This, in turn, delivers factor VIII to sites of vascular injury. Although there is extraordinary clinical heterogeneity in the common, autosomal dominant type of VWD, hemorrhage typically occurs in the skin and mucosal surfaces. Screening tests usually reveal a normal PT and platelet count, although some patients have mild thrombocytopenia. The APTT is either normal or mildly prolonged, depending on the amount of factor VIII activity. Plasma concentrations of von Willebrand factor are increased in neonates. Therefore laboratory testing of affected adults in the family is a good initial step in evaluating infants suspected of having VWD. The results may be used to determine the best test (or tests) for the infant. However, even this approach has pitfalls, particularly because pregnancy markedly alters VWF levels, which renders evaluation of the mother unreliable. Some plasma-derived factor VIII concentrates are manufactured so that they also contain von Willebrand factor. These products are an excellent treatment for bleeding complications in neonates with VWD. A recombinant form of von Willebrand factor recently available; however, it is not approved for use in children and neonates.[203] Cryoprecipitate is another effective therapy for treating hemorrhage in infants with a family history of VWD. Circumcision should not be performed if a parent has VWD. In the absence of significant bleeding, laboratory workup of infants with a family history of VWD should be deferred until after 6 months of age.

The autosomal recessive form of VWD (type III VWD) is a much rarer and more severe condition. Affected infants have a severe bleeding disorder caused by a combination of profoundly abnormal platelet function and low factor VIII levels, and they require regular treatment with an appropriate von Willebrand factor–containing concentrate.

Disorders of Platelet Function

Inherited disorders of platelet function are rare. In general, they present with petechiae, purpura, and bleeding from puncture sites, a circumcision site, and umbilical cord separation. Because these disorders are uncommon and are often inherited as autosomal recessive conditions, a history of consanguinity is especially important. The PT and APTT values are normal. In some disorders (e.g., gray platelet syndrome, Bernard-Soulier syndrome), there is mild thrombocytopenia, and the platelets are morphologically abnormal. Careful examination of the blood smear is therefore indicated whenever an inherited disorder of platelet function is suspected. In certain diseases (e.g., Glanzmann thrombasthenia), both the platelet count and platelet appearance are normal. A hallmark of inherited disorders of platelet function is marked prolongation of the bleeding time. Studies of platelet aggregation in response to various stimuli, antibody staining for antigens expressed on the surface of the platelets, electron microscopy, and molecular analysis are all useful in selected cases. Transfusions of platelet concentrates are given for severe bleeding.

THROMBOSIS

Despite prolongation of the PT and APTT well beyond the normal adult range, many experts in neonatal hematology believe that neonates are better viewed as being in a "hypercoagulable" state.[204] Indeed, thrombotic complications are more common in the neonatal period than at any other time during the first two decades of life and are receiving increased attention as more high-risk patients survive invasive medical interventions. Why newborns experience a relatively high incidence of thrombosis is unknown; however, increased blood viscosity resulting from a high hematocrit at birth may play an important role. Polycythemia may partially account for why infants of diabetic mothers are at high risk of thrombosis. In addition, the levels of protein C, a vitamin K–dependent serine protease, are low at birth. Preterm infants with respiratory distress syndrome have very low levels of antithrombin, increasing their risk of thromboembolic complications.[205]

Although thrombosis is a serious complication in high-risk infants, this problem has received relatively limited attention until recently. Investigators at McMaster University estimated that the incidence of clinically apparent thrombotic episodes was 2.4 per 1000 admissions to the NICU based on a multicenter survey of 97 cases.[206] Ninety percent of cases in their series were associated with the use of indwelling catheters. Twenty-one infants had renal vein thrombosis, 39 had right atrial thrombosis or other major venous thromboses, and 33 had arterial thrombosis. Because severe thrombosis is relatively uncommon in neonates, almost no data from controlled trials are available addressing the efficacy of thrombolytic or anticoagulant therapies.

Thrombosis Associated With Indwelling Catheters

Thromboembolic complications have been associated with the use of venous and arterial catheters. Autopsy studies reveal that 20% to 65% of infants who die with an umbilical venous catheter have an associated thrombus. Use of appropriate technique and proper placement of umbilical venous catheters can decrease but not eliminate the risk of a thrombus and its possible complications, such as portal vein thrombosis with portal hypertension, splenomegaly, gastric and esophageal varices, and hepatic necrosis. The incidence of asymptomatic clot formation in the aorta is also high. A number of studies have shown that continuous infusion of heparin at a rate of 0.5 to 3.5 U/kg/hr improves catheter patency, reduces the rate of thrombus formation, and decreases the incidence of hypertension.[207] It is uncertain whether higher dosages of heparin provide any additional benefit, and the evidence linking heparin use to intraventricular hemorrhage is weak.[208] Damping of the arterial pressure wave tracing is a frequent early sign of catheter thrombosis. Blanching or cyanosis of a "downstream" anatomic area suggests obstruction. The involved segment may include only the tip of a toe, or it may encompass an entire extremity or even half of the body.

Ultrasonography is a useful, noninvasive initial test and may be followed by arteriography in severe cases.[209] Contrast-enhanced angiography is considered the gold standard for diagnosis of arterial thrombosis. The sensitivity and specificity of Doppler ultrasonography for diagnosis of venous and arterial thrombosis are unknown.

Management of severe thrombosis should be individualized. Systemic heparinization, treatment with fibrinolytic agents, and thrombectomy have all been used.[206,209] In infants without evidence of major vessel obstruction, catheter removal is often followed by resolution of symptoms.

Renal Vein Thrombosis

Renal vein thrombosis in infants occurs most commonly (80% of cases) in the first month and usually in the first week of life. There is no sex predilection, and the left and right sides are equally affected. About 24% of infants have bilateral renal vein thrombosis. The clinical triad of flank mass, hematuria, and mild thrombocytopenia (average platelet counts of 100 $\times 10^9$/L) is the classical presentation of renal vein thrombosis in the neonatal period. Proteinuria and impaired kidney function are also seen. If the inferior vena cava is involved, cold, cyanotic, and edematous lower limbs can be noted. Doppler ultrasonography is the test of choice for diagnosis. Treatment depends on the extent and severity of involvement. Supportive care alone is sufficient for unilateral renal vein thrombosis with no uremia or extension into the inferior vena cava. However, heparin therapy is usually indicated in infants with unilateral renal vein thrombosis with inferior vena cava extension or bilateral renal vein thrombosis because the risk of pulmonary embolism and renal failure increases. In cases of bilateral renal vein thrombosis with evidence of renal failure, thrombolytic therapy must be considered. More than 85% of children survive with adequate renal function. Long-term morbidity data are lacking, however.

Protein C Deficiency

Severe protein C deficiency is a recessive disorder associated with catastrophic thrombosis and necrosis of dependent tissues, consumption of coagulation factors, and DIC.[210,211] A history of consanguinity or thrombotic disease in multiple adult relatives may be elicited. Infants with severe protein C deficiency are severely ill with purpura fulminans-diffuse tissue infarction with secondary hemorrhage, particularly in the skin. The PT and PTT are prolonged, the platelet count and fibrinogen level are reduced, and the level of fibrin degradation products is elevated. An important diagnostic clue that helps distinguish protein C deficiency from DIC is its propensity to be associated with prominent areas of segmental tissue infarction. Although the diagnosis is strongly supported by the demonstration of profoundly reduced levels of protein C, Manco-Johnson et al observed transient reductions in some infants that later improved.[212] Their data emphasize the importance of parental blood studies and serial testing to confirm the diagnosis. Treatment may initially include exchange transfusions, infusions of fresh frozen plasma at 10 to 20 mL/kg every 6 to 12 hours to raise the protein C level and replenish consumed coagulation factors, and heparinization.[213] A protein C concentrate (Ceprotin) has been approved by the FDA for use in the treatment of congenital protein C deficiency. The dose of Ceprotin for acute thrombotic episodes and short-term prophylaxis is 100 to 120 IU/kg in neonates with subsequent doses of 60 to 80 IU/kg every 6 hours and maintenance doses of 45 to 60 IU/kg every 6 to 12 hours.[214] Warfarin is preferred for long-term management, with a target international normalized ratio of 2.5 to 4.5.[213]

Factor V Leiden

A missense mutation in the factor V gene was first associated with resistance to the action of activated protein C in adults with venous thrombosis. This allele encodes a molecule called *factor V Leiden* that is relatively insensitive to inactivation by protein C and is most prevalent in Northern European populations. Individuals who are heterozygous for the factor V Leiden mutation show a five- to tenfold increase in the incidence of venous thrombosis as young adults, and homozygotes are at very high risk. Pediatric patients with thrombosis have been shown to have a higher than expected incidence of factor V Leiden mutation.[215,216]

Evaluation of Infants With Thrombosis

In general, thrombosis appears to be both underdiagnosed and undertreated in neonates. Symptoms and signs are highly variable and depend on the location and severity of the thrombotic process. Not only do a high percentage of infants with thrombosis have indwelling catheters, but thrombosis often occurs in the context of systemic infection. A constellation of hematuria, abdominal mass, and thrombocytopenia is observed in many infants with renal vein thrombosis. Although the PT, APTT, and platelet count all should be measured, the values of these indicators are frequently unremarkable in infants with thrombosis. The mother should be screened for the presence of antiphospholipid antibodies (lupus anticoagulant) because these may be associated with neonatal thrombosis. In addition, studies should be performed to exclude hereditary conditions, including factor V Leiden mutation, prothrombin gene mutation, and deficiencies of antithrombin III, protein C, and protein S. With the exception of DNA analysis for factor V Leiden mutation and prothrombin gene mutation, all of these tests may be unreliable in the setting of acute thrombosis. For this reason, it is suggested that parents be screened initially, with follow-up testing of the infant as indicated. Although contrast angiography is the most definitive modality for demonstrating thrombi, Doppler ultrasonography is preferred by most clinicians because it can be performed at the bedside.[217] Prospective studies have not been reported comparing the sensitivity of contrast angiography and Doppler ultrasonography in infants with thrombosis. It is imperative to use imaging studies to evaluate clinically significant thrombotic events because this aids in therapeutic decision-making and provides a baseline for clinical follow-up. Infants should not be exposed to the risks of systemic anticoagulant therapy unless thrombosis is well documented.

Anticoagulant and Fibrinolytic Therapy

The paucity of data from controlled studies and the clinical heterogeneity seen in newborns with thrombosis preclude definitive recommendations regarding which infants are likely to benefit from anticoagulant and fibrinolytic treatment and which agents, doses, and schedule should be used. The following discussion describes the guidelines and therapeutic agents for such therapy. The Children's Thrombophilia Network (1-800-NO-CLOTS) offers telephone advice on management of infants and children with thrombosis. Although this service is very helpful, its optimal use is in combination with on-site pediatric hematology consultation. To exclude ICH and hemorrhagic infarction, central nervous system imaging should be performed before systemic anticoagulant or thrombolytic therapy is administered in the NICU.

Heparin is the mainstay of anticoagulant therapy for infants with acute thrombosis. McDonald and Hathaway studied the use of continuous heparin infusions in 15 infants with significant thrombosis.[218] They achieved plasma heparin levels in the therapeutic range at dosages of 16 to 27 U/kg/hr and found that infants who had large thrombi showed the most rapid clearance. Because of the very wide range of normal APTT values, the authors followed micro–whole blood clotting times to monitor heparin effects. The recommendation is that heparin therapy begin with a loading dose of 75 U/kg followed by a continuous infusion at 28 U/kg/hr. Heparin treatment should be continued for at least 7 days in infants with significant thrombosis.

The advantages of LMWH products include a longer plasma half-life than standard heparin, which permits subcutaneous dosing and less variability in anticoagulant effects in different patients. Given the difficulties in administering and monitoring heparin therapy in neonates, LMWH drugs appear to offer considerable theoretic advantages over standard heparin in managing thrombosis in the NICU. There are important differences in the biochemical mechanisms of action of standard heparin and LMWH (enoxaparin sodium [Lovenox]). In particular, although heparin markedly accelerates the rate of thrombin inactivation through its ability to form a stable ternary complex that includes antithrombin III and thrombin, the major anticoagulant effect of LMWH occurs through antithrombin III–mediated destruction of activated factor X. The APTT is therefore not a useful test for measuring the anticoagulant effects of LMWH, which can be monitored by following anti-factor Xa levels. Studies have begun to elucidate optimal dosing for neonates. In a series that included seven infants and 18 older children, Massicotte et al found that infants required higher doses of enoxaparin per kilogram to achieve therapeutic anti–factor Xa levels than older children.[219] In a much larger study examining 147 courses of enoxaparin in pediatric patients, the same group reported clinical resolution of thromboembolic events in 84% of patients.[220]

Warfarin is a competitive inhibitor of vitamin K and therefore depresses the levels of active procoagulant factors II, VII, IX, and X and of the anticoagulant proteins C and S. Warfarin is not an appropriate treatment for acute thrombosis, but warfarin administration may be instituted later and used as long-term therapy in some infants with ongoing hypercoagulable disorders. There is little published experience in the use of warfarin in neonates, and dosing is problematic given the rapid growth and dietary changes that occur during the first few months of life. Advances in antithrombotic therapy have been made in the adult population with the FDA approval of direct oral anticoagulants (DOACs). Data on the use of DOACs is, however, lacking in the pediatric and neonatal population.[221]

The fibrinolytic agents urokinase and TPA are used in the acute management of certain types of vascular occlusion in adults.[222] TPA is the most commonly used thrombolytic agent in neonates. The administration of TPA to 23 neonates with venous thrombosis, most of whom were treated for renal vein, atrial, or vena cava thrombosis, resulted in complete clot lysis in 56%, partial lysis in 35%, and no lysis in 9%. Major hemorrhagic complications occurred in three infants (13%), two of whom had ICH. Both infants experiencing ICH were thrombocytopenic.[223–225] An absolute contraindication to the use of TPA in neonates is the presence of ICH or active bleeding from any site. A platelet count above 100,000/μL and fibrinogen level above 100 mg/dL is highly recommended during TPA therapy. Laboratory responses include a decrease in the fibrinogen level and an increase in the D-dimer level. A hematologist with experience in the management of neonatal thrombosis should be consulted when fibrinolytic treatment is considered.

CASE 16.1

You are called to evaluate a 2-day-old full-term male infant who was noted to have continued oozing from the circumcision site. The nurse provides results for a complete blood count and coagulation studies, which reveal a normal platelet count of 220 x 10^9/L, a prothrombin time (PT) of 12.9 seconds (normal for age), and an activated partial thromboplastin time (APTT) of 72 seconds (prolonged).

What is your initial approach?

The first goal is to determine whether the baby is a well-appearing or sick-appearing infant. In a sick-appearing infant, disseminated intravascular coagulation (DIC) or sepsis can cause bleeding. Usually the platelet count is abnormally low in such cases. If the baby appears ill, a sepsis workup should be performed, and parenteral antibiotic therapy should be initiated. The platelet count, as mentioned earlier, is normal in this case. Investigation of bleeding in a well-appearing infant always includes obtaining a detailed family and maternal history. Maternal infection, prolonged period between rupture of the placental membranes and delivery, and maternal idiopathic thrombocytopenic purpura all predispose to bleeding in the neonate. A detailed family history should focus on the type and severity of bleeding in family members with particular emphasis on the sex of the family members affected. This information gives important clues to the inheritance pattern of the bleeding disorders under investigation. If only male members on the maternal side are affected, the diagnosis is most likely one of the hemophilias. If both sexes are affected in the family, one should think of von Willebrand disease (VWD), keeping in mind the autosomal inheritance pattern. Finally, administration of vitamin K should be confirmed in any neonate with bleeding symptoms. Although physical examination may not contribute much to the diagnosis of a bleeding disorder, it is required for completeness.

The baby appears well except for bleeding from the circumcision site. The remainder of the physical examination is unremarkable. Family history is negative for any bleeding symptoms in any of the family members.

What should be done next?

About 15% to 30% of patients with an inherited bleeding disorder come to medical attention in the neonatal period. Moreover, 30% of cases of newly diagnosed hemophilia are caused by a new mutation in patients with no family history of bleeding. In a case such as this, an isolated prolongation of the APTT is suggestive of hemophilia. Ideally, factor VIII and IX assays will be performed to quickly confirm the diagnosis. However, factor assays are not available in all centers and at all times. The APTT test should be repeated using a 50:50 mix of patient and normal plasma. In hemophilia, the APTT corrects to normal. Even small clinical laboratories often have a stock of factor VIII–deficient plasma. If the APTT corrects when the specimen is mixed with normal plasma, the mixing study is repeated with the factor VIII–deficient plasma. If the APTT corrects to normal, hemophilia A is excluded, and hemophilia B is the likely diagnosis. If the APTT does not correct to normal, factor VIII deficiency is the presumptive diagnosis.

The baby's APTT corrected to normal when a 50:50 mix of patient and normal plasma was tested. The APTT did not correct to normal when factor VIII–deficient plasma was used, which confirms a diagnosis of factor VIII deficiency, or hemophilia A.

What should be done now?

The baby's diagnosis is severe hemophilia A with a factor VIII level of less than 1%. Infusion of recombinant factor VIII concentrate at a dose of 50 U/kg will raise the plasma factor VIII level by 100% and stop the bleeding from the circumcision site. The baby may need additional smaller doses of the recombinant factor over the next day or two if the oozing from the circumcision site continues.

The mother should be checked to determine if she is a carrier of hemophilia by measuring factor levels and possibly performing genetic mutation analysis. If the mother is a carrier of hemophilia A, there is a 25% chance that she will have a male child in subsequent pregnancies who is affected. If the mother is not a carrier, the baby is deemed to have a new mutation that caused hemophilia.

CASE 16.2

You are called to evaluate a 12-hour-old infant who was noted to have a petechial rash soon after delivery. A complete blood count is obtained, which reveals a platelet count of 8×10^9/L.

What is your initial approach?

The baby should be examined. The first goal is to determine whether there is clinical evidence of severe pathology (i.e., does the baby look sick?). Thrombocytopenic bleeding may be the first sign of sepsis or NEC. Maternal fever, rupture of the placental membranes a prolonged time before delivery, and premature birth all predispose to invasive infection. If the baby appears ill, a sepsis workup should be performed, and parenteral antibiotic therapy should be initiated. Physical examination may disclose other abnormalities that suggest the correct diagnosis. Babies with thrombocytopenia caused by congenital viral infections often show microcephaly and hepatosplenomegaly. Radial and ulnar aplasia or hypoplasia suggests a primary defect in platelet production (e.g., Fanconi anemia or thrombocytopenia–absent radius [TAR] syndrome).

The baby weighs 3450 g, and vaginal delivery was uncomplicated. She appears well except for scattered petechiae and bruising from heel-stick and venipuncture sites. The remaining results of the complete blood count are unremarkable (white blood cell count: 10,000/μL with a normal differential; hemoglobin level: 17.2 g/dL).

What should be done next?

Factitious thrombocytopenia should always be considered, but it is unlikely in this case because of the presence of clinical signs. The blood smear should be examined for normal-appearing red and white blood cells and for giant platelets, which, if present, suggest an increased rate of peripheral platelet destruction with the marrow attempting to compensate by releasing young platelets into the circulation. The mother's platelet count should be checked, and she should be questioned regarding medication use and any history of idiopathic thrombocytopenia purpura, lupus, or other collagen-vascular disorder. Maternal thrombocytopenia is an important clue that suggests transplacental transmission of maternal antiplatelet immunoglobin G (IgG) autoantibodies. This is a common cause of neonatal thrombocytopenia in babies who appear well.

The baby's blood smear reveals giant platelets and marked thrombocytopenia, but findings are otherwise normal. The mother's platelet count is normal, and there is no history suggesting maternal autoimmune disease.

What is the most likely diagnosis and what should be done?

The most likely diagnosis is neonatal alloimmune thrombocytopenia (NAIT). Detailed laboratory investigations are required for confirmation of the diagnosis and should be performed by an experienced reference laboratory. Current consensus is that both parents should be screened for human platelet antigens ([HPAs]; HPA-1, HPA-3, and HPA-5) in all cases of potential NAIT and for HPA-4 as well if the patient is of Asian descent. HPA-9 and HPA-15 are the next most commonly involved in antigen incompatibilities. For testing to confirm NAIT, results must reveal both a platelet antigen incompatibility between the parents and maternal antibody directed against that antigen.

The baby's platelet count should be measured at least daily for the first few days of life, and she should be observed for signs of active hemorrhage.

While discussing the probable diagnosis with the parents, you are called urgently to the nursery because the baby has developed worsening petechiae and gross hematuria. Her vital sign values are stable.

What should be done next?

The baby now has evidence of significant active hemorrhage and should receive a random-donor platelet transfusion promptly. If readily available, matched (antigen-negative) platelets are preferred. The latter are platelets from donors negative for HPA-1. They can be given in larger increments and have a longer half-life. Concentrated washed irradiated maternal platelets can be used as well; however, their processing takes at least 12 to 48 hours.

The baby's platelet count increases, and she stops bleeding after she is transfused with HPA-1–negative platelets. The mother is HPA-1 negative. The parents are interested in having other children and are concerned about the risk of recurrence.

What do you tell them?

The risk of severe neonatal hemorrhage in subsequent pregnancies is high. The mother should be followed as a "high-risk" patient. If the previously affected sibling had an intracranial hemorrhage (ICH), the next affected fetus will have early, severe thrombocytopenia and in utero ICH unless effective treatment is instituted. Recent data indicate that the administration of intravenous gamma-globulin (IVIG) to the mother before delivery decreases the incidence of neonatal thrombocytopenia.

CASE 16.3

You are asked to evaluate a newborn who appears pale shortly after birth and reportedly has a low blood capillary venous hematocrit.

What is your initial approach?

An important first step is to obtain an accurate history of both the prenatal course and the delivery. This should be accompanied by a thorough examination of the newborn that looks for signs of bleeding as well as for organomegaly (increased size of the liver and spleen, in particular).

You learn that this baby boy was born at 39 weeks' gestation and weighs 3700 g. All routine prenatal screening yielded negative results, and the prenatal course was uneventful. The mother is a 28-year-old white female, now gravida 3 para 3, who failed to report for the majority of her routine visits to her obstetrician leading up to this delivery. Her other two children were also term deliveries, and there was no report of problems in the newborn period. You are told that the mother is group O, Rh negative, that her antibody screen results are negative, and that she did not receive anti-Rh globulin. The delivery was reportedly without complications, and the baby had Apgar scores of 8 and 9 with normal vital sign values at birth. A venous specimen obtained at 25 minutes of age showed a hematocrit of 37%, and the test was repeated because of the increase in pallor. Examination shows no petechiae, bruising, or evidence of bleeding, and no splenomegaly or hepatomegaly.

What should be done next?

Continued

CASE 16.3—cont'd

A thorough review of the available laboratory results is necessary to determine the appropriate tests and the next steps needed to confirm the diagnosis.

A hematocrit of venous blood obtained at 45 minutes was 30%.

What do you consider in your differential diagnosis, and what should be done?

A decline in the hematocrit in the newborn period should raise a concern for hemolytic disease. An important consideration is Rh disease, given the maternal blood type and the mother's failure to follow up with her obstetrician during the latter part of gestation. ABO incompatibility and isoimmune disease should also be considered. The quickest way to determine whether these might be a real concern is to perform a direct antiglobulin test (DAT) (Coombs test), the results of which will invariably be strongly positive in Rh disease. The absence of organomegaly in this instance argues against this possibility; however, it cannot be ruled out on the basis of examination alone, and accurate diagnosis will depend on the results of blood typing on both mother and infant.

You request the tests mentioned. The results of the direct antiglobulin test are negative, the baby's blood type is group O, Rh(D) positive. The reticulocyte count is 138,000/μL (4%), and the platelet count is 300 x 10^9/L, with a normal white blood cell count and differential.

What is the diagnosis? What should be done?

For the reasons discussed earlier (negative result on DAT, absence of splenomegaly, lack of elevated reticulocyte count), this is not a case of Rh disease. It is also clearly not ABO incompatibility, because mother and infant are both blood group O. The negative DAT result also rules out other isoimmune disorders. One could consider glucose-6-phosphate dehydrogenase (G6PD) deficiency because this is a male infant, but G6PD deficiency is most common in the African American population, which makes it less likely in this instance. A hint in this case is the low reticulocyte count. This provides a clue that the anemia has an onset and cause that are more acute in nature and could indeed be caused by blood loss, despite the lack of any physical evidence on examination of the baby.

What do you tell the physician requesting the consultation?

The most likely cause, and greatest concern, is that transplacental blood loss occurred. This would place the mother at significant risk of being sensitized to the Rh(D) antigen. This risk is further heightened because she did not receive hyperimmune anti-Rh globulin during pregnancy, but in the setting of a significant bleed, even the standard dose may fail to provide sufficient protection from sensitization of the mother to the Rh(D) antigen. In this case, because the mother and infant share the blood group antigen O, the mother's risk of becoming sensitized to D antigen is even greater. You should instruct the obstetrician to order a Kleihauer-Betke test on the mother's blood immediately to look for fetal cells. If increased numbers of fetal cells are present, a larger dose of hyperimmune globulin must be given to the mother. One can establish an estimated blood loss based on the baby's blood volume and hematocrit at birth.

17

Neonatal Brain Disorders

Terrie Eleanor Inder, Lillian G. Matthews

BRAIN DEVELOPMENT IN THE FETUS AND THE NEWBORN

Maturation of the brain is defined through descriptions of sequential and overlapping developmental processes, beginning with conception and involving continual interactions of the gene environment. Beginning during gestation and following trimester-specific stages of development of the embryo and fetus, anatomic, biochemical, and physiologic processes occur: neural induction followed by neuronogenesis, programmed cell death and neuroblast migration, formation of axons and dendrites, continuous energy generation to provide membrane excitability, synaptogenesis, neurotransmitter biosynthesis, and myelination of axons. These prenatal time periods are fundamental for brain development. However, postnatal processes of programmed cell death, continued synaptogenesis, and neurotransmitter maturation highlight important brain maturational events needed for continued preservation of appropriate structure and function.[1] Regional differences in the rate of maturation of the nervous system also must be recognized. Different brain structures do not express equivalent function at specific times during the development of the fetus, premature infant, and full-term neonate. Table 17.1 summarizes the major prenatal developmental sequences in brain maturation that occur in the cerebrum and cerebellum, and lists representative disorders at each stage. Both volume and gyral-sulcal complexity increase during prenatal development, with prominent changes in the last 3 months of gestation (Fig. 17.1),[2] reflecting major molecular and histologic maturational changes during the formation of maturing cortical-subcortical cellular connections.

NEUROLOGICAL EXAMINATION OF THE PRETERM AND TERM BORN INFANT

A systematic approach to the neurological examination of the newborn is an important first step in the diagnostic evaluation. Observation is critical in each domain of the neurological examination of the newborn. It is important to remember that the neurologic system is derived from ectoderm, and thus one should pay particular attention to the examination of the skin. Outgrowths such as encephaloceles, cutaneous lesions such as port-wine stains, and the presence of sacral dimples or sinuses should be sought as clues to underlying neurologic dysfunction. Additionally, head circumference should be measured with a tape measure. The normal term infant's head circumference is approximately 35 cm and is reflective of the underlying intracranial volume. Macrocephaly and microcephaly can be indications of underlying metabolic, genetic, or infectious processes.

Mental Status

Timing of the examination is a careful consideration in the newborn. One of the best times to examine a baby is between feeds to avoid distress from hunger, or after a feed, although the baby may be too sleepy to obtain an optimal examination. Observation of the newborn's spontaneous eye opening, movements of the face and extremities, and response to stimulation are essential for the mental status examination. Arousal is defined by the duration of eye opening and spontaneous movements. Before 28 weeks' gestation, the newborn states of wakefulness and sleep can be difficult to distinguish. As the newborn matures toward term equivalency, there is increasing duration, frequency, and quality of alertness. With regard to defining mental state, an irritable infant is one who is agitated and cries with minimal stimulation and is unable to be soothed. Lethargic infants cannot maintain an alert state. Stuporous or comatose infants can be minimally aroused, or not aroused at all.

Cranial Nerves

Cranial nerves (CN) II and III can be tested by the pupillary reflex, which appears consistently at 32 to 35 weeks' gestation. A 28-week infant will blink to light shone into the eyes. Beginning at 34 weeks of gestation, an infant will be able to fix and follow on an object with an increasing arc, reaching a full 180-degree arc at term equivalency. Spontaneous roving eye movements are common at 32 weeks' gestation, as are dysconjugate eye movements in the term infant when not fixing on an object. Facial sensation (CN V) can be tested with pinprick and by observing facial grimace or change in sucking. Facial symmetry and movement should be observed in both the quiet state and during active movement (such as crying). Hearing (CN VIII) can be tested with a bell, keeping in mind that a ringing bell within an isolette can be quite loud and generate 90 dB. The newborn may have a very subtle response to auditory stimulus and respond with only a blink. To test CN V, VII, and XII, the newborn can be observed sucking on a pacifier. This can also be used to evaluate CN IX and X, which are tested when the baby swallows.

TABLE 17.1 **Major Stages of Central Nervous System Development**

Stage	Peak Time of Occurrence	Major Morphologic Events in Cerebrum	Major Morphologic Events in Cerebellum	Main Corresponding Disorders[a]
Uterine implantation	1 wk			
Separation of three layers	2 wk	Formation of neural plate		Enterogenous cysts and fistulae
Dorsal induction Neurulation	3–4 wk	Formation of neural tube, neural crest, and derivatives Closure of anterior (day 24) and posterior (day 29) neuropores	Paired alar plates	Anencephaly, encephalocele, craniorachischisis, spina bifida, meningocele
Caudal neural tube formation	4–7 wk	Canalization and regressive differentiation of cord	Rhombic lips (day 35), cerebellar plates	Diastematomyelia, Dandy-Walker syndrome, cerebellar hypoplasia
Ventral induction	5–6 wk	Forebrain and face (cranial neural crest) Cleavage of prosencephalon into cerebral vesicles (day 33), optic placodes (day 26), olfactory placodes, diencephalon	Fusion of cerebellar plates	Holoprosencephaly, median cleft face syndrome
Neuronal and glial proliferation	8–16 wk	Cellular proliferation in ventricular and subventricular zone (interkinetic migration) Early differentiation of neuroblasts and glioblasts	Migration of Purkinje cells (9–10 wk) Migration of external granular layer (10–11 wk)	Microcephaly, megalencephaly
Migration	12–20 wk	Radial migration and accessory pathways (e.g., corpus ganglio-thalamicum) Formation of corpus callosum	Elaboration of the dendritic tree of Purkinje cells (16–25 wk)	Lissencephaly-pachygyria (types I and II), Zellweger syndrome, glial heterotopia, microgyria (some forms), agenesis of corpus callosum
Organization[b]	24 wk to postnatal	Late migration (to 5 mo) Alignment, orientation, and layering of cortical neurons Synaptogenesis Glial proliferation-differentiation well into postnatal life	Monolayer of Purkinje cells (16–28 wk) Migration of granules to form internal granular layer (to postnatal life)	Minor cortical dysplasias, dendritic and synaptic abnormalities, microgyria (some forms)
Myelination	24 wk to 2 yr postnatally			Dysmyelination, clastic insults

[a]Disorders do not necessarily correspond to abnormal development. They may also result from secondary destruction or disorganization.
[b]Programmed cellular death takes place throughout the second half of pregnancy and the first year of extrauterine life.
Modified from Aicardi J, Bax M, Gillberg C, et al. *Diseases of the Nervous System in Childhood.* 2nd ed. New York, NY: MacKeith Press; 1998

Motor Examination

Observation of the resting posture can reveal the symmetry and maturity of the passive tone. It is important to keep the head midline to avoid asymmetries in tone related to the asymmetric tonic neck reflex. Flexor tone tends to develop first in the lower extremities and proceed cephalad. A 28-week infant will lie with minimally flexed limbs and have minimal resistance to passive movement of all extremities. In contrast, at 32 weeks, the newborn develops flexor tone at the hips and knees, with some resistance to manipulation of the lower extremities. This progression correlates with increasing myelination of the subcortical motor pathways originating in the brainstem. By 36 weeks, the infant develops flexion at the elbows, and by term, the infant is flexed in all extremities. The quality as well as the quantity of the infant's movements mature greatly between 28 weeks and term equivalent. For example, the 28-week infant will have writhing movements of the extremities, but by term, the movements are best described as large-amplitude, swatting-like movements. Abnormalities in the motor characteristics may include such things as a 28-week infant with jerky movements or a term infant with choreoathetoid movements.

Sensory Examination

In the newborn, the examination is limited to touch and pinprick. Particular emphasis should be placed on dermatomal evaluation of the lower extremities, especially in the sacral region in a child with a neural tube defect. Assessment of sensation can be made by using the sharp end of a cotton applicator on the face and observing the facial grimace or change in state of the infant.

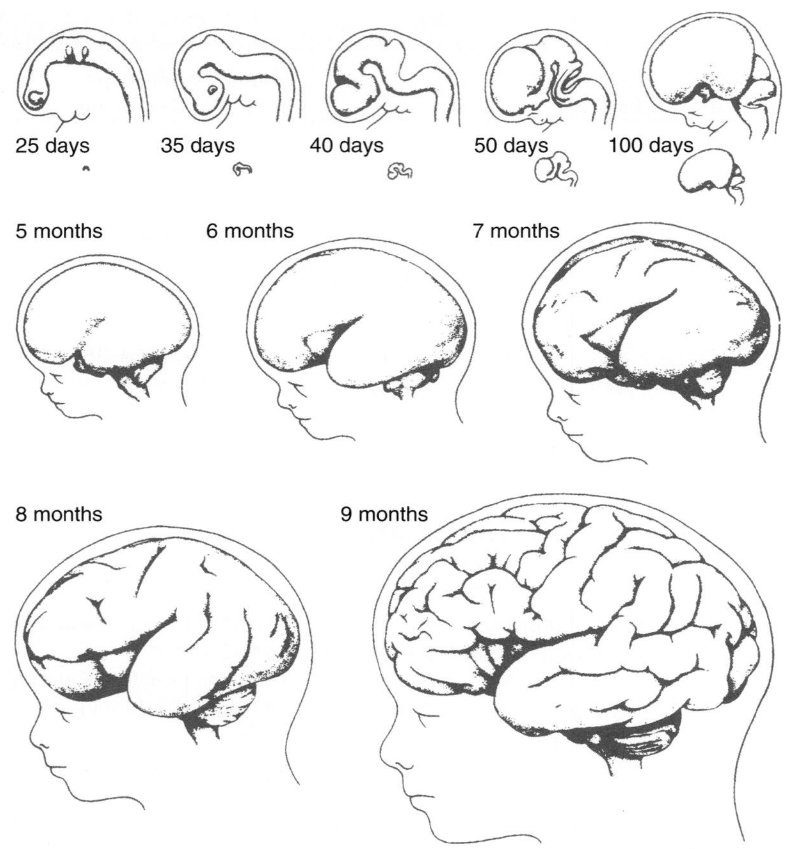

Fig. 17.1 Gyral development in the human brain from 25 days to 9 months. Note the prominent increase in volume and gyral complexity in the last 3 months of gestation. (From Cowan WM. The development of the brain. *Sci Am.* 1997;241:113-133.)

Reflexes

Reflexes can be easily elicited in the biceps, brachioradialis, knees, and ankles. Cross-adductor responses and unsustained clonus are not uncommon in the newborn. Many child neurologists agree that the plantar response is not helpful, as many factors may elicit flexor or extensor responses inadvertently.

Primitive Reflexes

A full Moro reflex consists of bilateral hand opening with upper extremity extension and abduction, followed by anterior flexion of the upper extremities, then an audible cry. This is best elicited by dropping the head in relation to the body into the examiner's hands. The asymmetric tonic neck reflex is elicited by rotating the head to one side, with subsequent elbow extension to the side the head is turned and elbow flexion on the side of the occiput. The palmar grasp reflex is elicited by stimulating the palm with an object. The palmar grasp is present at 28 weeks' gestation, strong at 32 weeks, and is strong enough at 37 weeks' gestation to lift the baby off the bed. This reflex disappears at 2 months of age with the development of a voluntary grasp. To test the placing reflex, the infant is held under the axilla in an upright position, and the dorsal aspect of the foot is brushed against a tabletop. The infant's hip and knee will flex, and the infant will appear to take a step. This reflex is useful if asymmetry is present.

BRAIN INJURY IN THE PRETERM INFANT

Intraventricular Hemorrhage

Neonatal germinal matrix hemorrhage/intraventricular hemorrhage (GMH/IVH) is the most common form of intracranial hemorrhage in preterm infants and an important cause of long-term morbidities among survivors of neonatal intensive care. In its least severe form, the hemorrhage may be restricted to the germinal matrix area or subependyma. However, frequently, the hemorrhage extends beyond the germinal matrix into the cerebral ventricles, following rupture of the GMH into the ventricular space.

Incidence

GMH/IVH is a neurological disorder that occurs most frequently among preterm infants.[3] Its incidence decreases as gestational age and birth weight increase.[4] Because of improvements in perinatal and neonatal care, the incidence of GMH/IVH has decreased over the past several decades but to a lesser extent than the decline in neonatal mortality.[5,6] In the 1970 to 1980s, GMH/IVH was noted in 45% of very low-birth-weight (VLBW) infants and in greater than 60% of those with birth weight of 750 g or less. By the mid-1990s, it had decreased further to 24% of VLBW infants.[7,8] Since that time, however, the incidence has become static, remaining about 25% among all VLBW infants based on

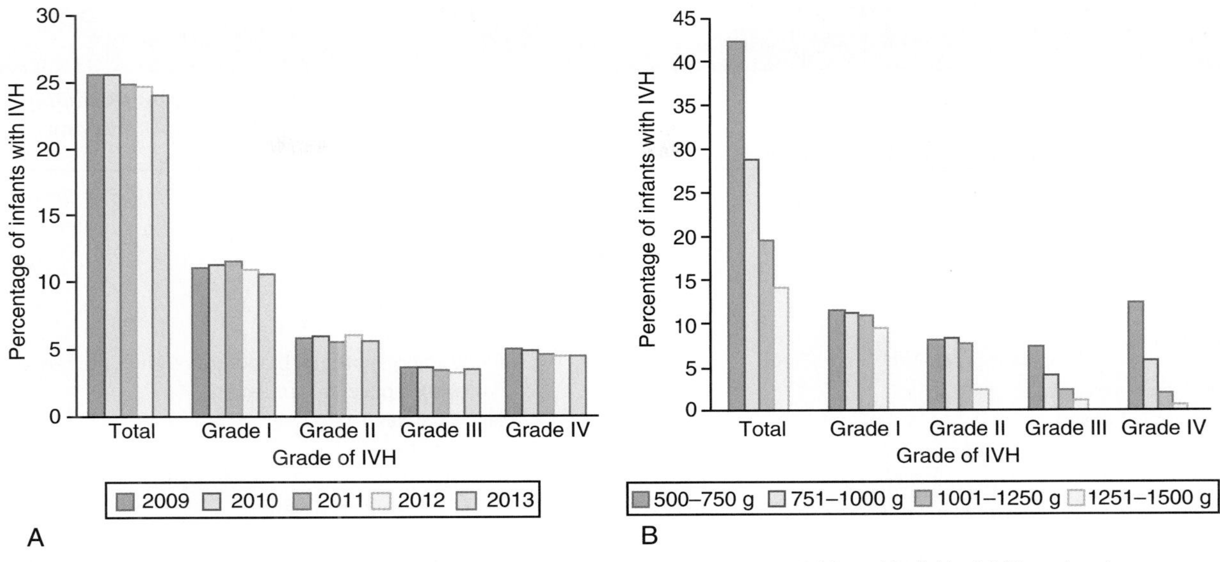

Fig. 17.2 (A) The incidence of all grades of intraventricular hemorrhage *(IVH),* and individual IVH grades, in the Vermont Oxford Network database from 2009 to 2013, stratified by year. (B) The incidence of all grades of IVH, and individual IVH grades, in the Vermont Oxford Network database from 2009 to 2013, stratified by birth weight.

data from the Vermont Oxford database (Fig. 17.2).[9,10] The more severe hemorrhages, grades III and IV, occur in 12% to 17% of extremely low-birth-weight (ELBW) infants[5] and in as high as 20% of those with birth weight of 750 g or less.[4] These severe hemorrhages occur in 17% to 28% of those with gestational age 22 to 26 weeks and in 9% to 14% of those 27 to 32 weeks' gestation.[11]

Pathogenesis

The pathogenesis of GMH/IVH is complex and involves multiple risk factors and disorders that may cause biochemical, inflammatory, and hemodynamic alterations, predisposing to the development of hemorrhage. The origin of hemorrhage is the germinal matrix, a prominent structure in the preterm brain in the second and early third trimesters that undergoes involution beginning at 24 to 26 weeks. The germinal matrix structure contains neuronal precursor cells before 20 weeks of gestation. As development progresses, the differentiating glioblasts give rise to oligodendroglial cells, which are important to myelination. The germinal matrix is supplied by a complex vascular network but is a low blood flow structure.[12,13] The origin of the hemorrhage appears to be from the endothelial lined vessels of the matrix, in particular, vessels in communication with the venous circulation, including capillary-venule junctions and small venules.[14,15] The susceptibility of the thin-walled germinal matrix capillaries to rupture may be because of their large diameter, which offers lesser resistance to changes in intravascular pressure,[16] to immature endothelial cell tight junctions, and to lower levels of structurally stabilizing proteins such as fibronectin and collagen in the extracellular matrix.

Among the clinical risk factors associated with IVH are lower gestational age, lack of antenatal corticosteroids, clinical chorioamnionitis, male sex,[18] significant delivery room resuscitation, mechanical ventilation,[21] and hypotension requiring multiple inotropes.[17,22] Table 17.2 lists cerebrovascular factors and alterations in cerebral hemodynamics that may result from a variety of antenatal and postnatal conditions that are thought to be associated with the pathogenesis of GMH/IVH.

Clinical Manifestations and Diagnosis

GMH/IVH is usually detected in the first 4 to 5 days of life, with approximately 40% to 50% occurring in the first day of life and up to 90% within the first 72 hours.[23–25] Approximately 20% of early-onset hemorrhage may evolve to become more severe, with the maximum extent typically seen within the first week of life.[26] The majority of hemorrhages, in particular smaller ones, are asymptomatic and are only detected by routine cranial ultrasound (CUS). However, larger GMH/IVH may present with sudden clinical deterioration, especially when there is significant blood loss. Other clinical manifestations include anemia; seizures; tense, full, and/or bulging fontanels; split and wide sutures; apnea and bradycardia with desaturation episodes; poor perfusion; hypotension; severe metabolic acidosis; increase in oxygen requirement; and increase in ventilator support.

Imaging studies will establish the diagnosis of GMH/IVH. The current standard approach to diagnosis is the use of cranial ultrasonography. The procedure can be performed at the bedside, thus avoiding the risks of transporting the infant for either a computed tomography (CT) scan or magnetic resonance imaging (MRI) procedure. Table 17.3 shows the grading of GMH/IVH, based on Papile criteria from CT scanning[27] still employed by clinicians and researchers for CUS findings. Volpe proposed a modification to the grading system for CUS findings. This newer, modified grading system takes into consideration the location of hemorrhage and the amount of blood detected in the ventricles. Examples of CUS findings are shown in Fig. 17.3.

TABLE 17.2 Factors That Influence Pathogenesis of Germinal Matrix Hemorrhage/ Intraventricular Hemorrhage

	Factors in the Pathogenesis of GMH/IVH	Antenatal and Postnatal Conditions Leading to Vascular and Hemodynamic Alterations, Increasing Risks for GMH/IVH
Intravascular	Increased Cerebral Blood Flow	Systemic hypertension in presence of a pressure-passive circulation Rapid volume expansion Hypercarbia Reduced hematocrit Hypoglycemia
	Fluctuating Cerebral Blood Flow	Fluctuating systemic blood pressure in presence of a pressure-passive circulation Hypercarbia Hypovolemia Hypotension Patent ductus arteriosus High FiO_2
	Decreased Cerebral Blood Flow (Resulting in Reperfusion Injury)	Systemic hypotension in presence of a pressure-passive circulation Asphyxia
	Increased Cerebral Venous Pressure	Asphyxia Venous anatomic arrangement Prolonged labor and vaginal delivery (some conflicting reports) Respiratory management (high peak inspiratory pressure, tracheal suctioning, pneumothorax)
Vascular	Immature Vasculature Undergoing remodeling and involution Simple endothelial-lined vessels without collagen or muscle Immature tight junctions	Preterm birth and low birth weight
	Large diameter of germinal matrix vessels relative to cortical vessels	Conditions associated with $\downarrow PaO_2$, $\uparrow PaCO_2$, $\downarrow pH$
	Vulnerability to hypoxemia-ischemia as located in vascular border zone	Hypoxia-ischemia reperfusion
	Vessel endothelial damage	Inflammation/infection Hypotension/shock Oxygen therapy, hyperoxia, generation of oxygen-reactive species and other free radicals
Extravascular	Deficient vascular and extracellular matrix support	Preterm birth and low birth weight
	Excessive fibrinolytic activity	Low factor XIII levels (conflicting reports of significance)

GMH/IVH, Germinal matrix hemorrhage/intraventricular hemorrhage.

Complications and Neuropathological Associations of Germinal Matrix Hemorrhage/Intraventricular Hemorrhage

GMH/IVH may be associated with destruction of the germinal matrix, periventricular hemorrhagic infarction, ventriculomegaly or hydrocephalus, white matter injury, and loss of cerebellar volume, each of which may have implications on the prognosis for the infant. During the second trimester, the ganglionic eminence and subventricular zone, which are part of and immediately associated with the germinal matrix, respectively, are rich locations for neuronal and glial proliferation.[28] Therefore destruction of the germinal matrix during this vulnerable period leads to a reduction in proliferation and migration of neuronal and glial precursor cells, which in turn is thought to impact brain growth and potentially the developmental outcome of these infants.[29]

Periventricular hemorrhagic infarction (PVHI) can be seen as large echodensities on CUS within the parenchyma adjacent to the GMH/IVH. Papile initially described this as extension of the IVH into the parenchyma. However, subsequent study has indicated that although PVHI is strongly associated with IVH, it is not an extension of the IVH; rather,

TABLE 17.3 Cranial Ultrasound Findings and Grades of Hemorrhages

Papile Criteria	Description	Volpe Criteria	Description
Grade I	Hemorrhage limited to the germinal matrix; may be unilateral or bilateral	Grade I	Blood in the germinal matrix area with or without minimal intraventricular hemorrhage (less than 10% of the ventricular space with blood)
Grade II	Blood noted within the ventricular system but not distending it	Grade II	Intraventricular hemorrhage with blood occupying 10%–50% of the ventricular space (sagittal view)
Grade III	Blood in ventricles with distension or dilation of the ventricles	Grade III	Intraventricular hemorrhage with blood occupying greater than 50% of the ventricles with or without periventricular echodensities
Grade IV	Intraventricular hemorrhage with parenchymal extension	Separate notation of other findings	Periventricular hemorrhagic infarction Cystic periventricular leukomalacia

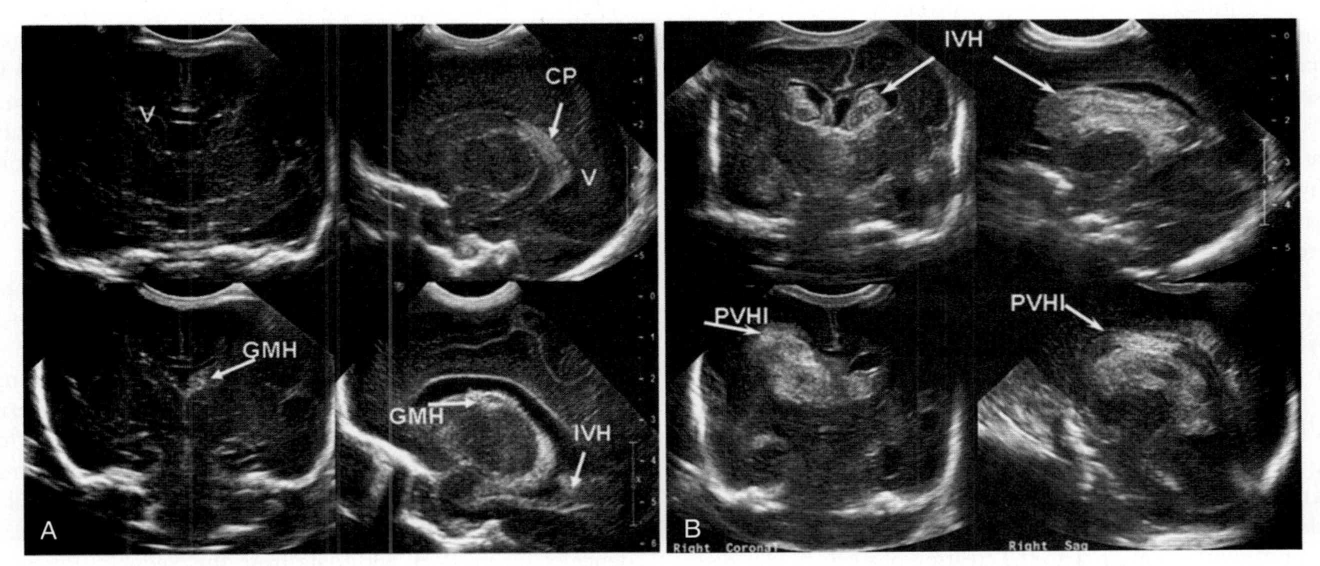

Fig. 17.3 (A) The top panel shows coronal (left) and sagittal (right) views from a normal preterm brain (*V*, ventricle; *CP*, choroids plexus). The bottom panel (left) shows a coronal view with a left germinal matrix hemorrhage *(GMH)* or grade I. On the right is a sagittal section showing blood in the lateral ventricle (intraventricular hemorrhage [*IVH*]) and filling less than 50% of the ventricular space; grade II germinal matrix hemorrhage/intraventricular hemorrhage. (B) The top panel on the left shows a coronal view of bilateral hemorrhage *(IVH)* in the anterior ventricles and almost filling the ventricles. On the right is a sagittal view of the hemorrhage or blood cast (IVH) filling and distending the lateral ventricle; grade III hemorrhage. The bottom panel shows on the left a coronal view of hemorrhage with parenchymal involvement (see *arrows*) representing periventricular hemorrhagic infarction *(PVHI)*.

it occurs because of obstruction of venous drainage leading to a venous hemorrhagic infarct.[30,31] The area of infarction evolves into tissue loss such that a porencephalic cyst may be noted on later follow-up CUS.

About 2 to 3 weeks after detection of GMH/IVH, some infants may present with increasing head circumference, separation of sutures, full and tense fontanelles, and sunsetting appearance. A repeat CUS in the presence of these manifestations of increased intracranial pressure will reveal prominence and enlargement of the cerebral ventricles (ventriculomegaly) and thus a diagnosis of *posthemorrhagic hydrocephalus* (PHH). PHH results from disturbance in cerebrospinal fluid (CSF) dynamics because of (1) the obstruction of the CSF pathway by blood clots, in the posterior fossa cisterns, aqueduct of Sylvius, or foramen of Monroe; and (2) postinflammatory changes in the arachnoid villi, which may impair CSF absorption. Obstruction and delayed absorption of CSF leads to progressive increase in ventricular size.[32] Among those with GMH/IVH who survive for more than 14 days, 50% will develop ventricular dilation, which will progress in half of these infants.[33] In 62% of those with progressive ventricular dilation, spontaneous arrest occurs, whereas the remaining 38% will require nonsurgical or surgical treatment. Surgical intervention to relieve the increase in intracranial pressure and ameliorate-associated clinical manifestations will be necessary for rapidly increasing head size, frequent apnea and bradycardia, and the need for increasing ventilatory support.

Studies have demonstrated that GMH/IVH is associated with reductions in cerebellar volume.[34–36] This is thought to occur secondary to (1) a direct toxic effect of hemosiderin on the surface of the cerebellum, impairing the proliferation of the external granular layer; and (2) the loss of cortical neuronal inputs, leading to underdevelopment of the contralateral cerebellum from the site of the cortical injury (a maturation-distinctive form of diaschisis).[37,38]

Management of Germinal Matrix Hemorrhage/ Intraventricular Hemorrhage

The treatment of GMH/IVH is primarily supportive. Management strategies include initiation of mechanical ventilation or increase in ventilatory support and/or administration of oxygen to maintain optimal levels of $PaCO_2$ and PaO_2, treatment of hypotension with slow volume expansion and cautious use of pressors if unresponsive to volume expansion, blood transfusion to correct anemia from blood loss, correction of metabolic acidosis, anticonvulsant therapy for seizures, and administration of fresh frozen plasma, platelets, and other products if there is associated coagulopathy. Progression or evolution of GMH/IVH is monitored by serial CUSs, especially when needed for decision making and parental counseling in the face of rapid clinical deterioration.

During early posthemorrhagic hydrocephalus, interventions such as diuretics and intraventricular fibrinolytic therapy have been trialed; however, both were shown to have no benefit in small, randomized trials.[39] The infants must be monitored with frequent CUSs, which will provide data on the alterations in the ventricular size. If there is increasing ventriculomegaly and raised intracranial pressure, the management is then directed at drainage of the CSF fluid to reduce the ventricular size, either by serial lumbar puncture or surgical intervention with the creation of a ventricular reservoir, or drainage of CSF by ventriculostomy. The optimum timing of intervention is unclear; however, retrospective data suggests that earlier intervention with serial therapeutic lumbar punctures may avoid the need for surgical intervention and improve neurodevelopmental outcome.[40,41] Ventriculoperitoneal shunt is the definitive surgical treatment when there is continued progression of ventriculomegaly accompanied by increase in intracranial pressure. Shunt obstruction, malfunction, and infection can complicate shunt placement and long-term function. Endoscopic third ventriculostomy with choroid plexus cauterization may avoid the necessity for a shunt among those requiring surgical intervention; however, although the data has been encouraging for its use to treat hydrocephalus because of alternate etiologies, to date, it has been less successful for the management of PHH in preterm infants, and ventriculoperitoneal shunt remains the gold standard.

Prognosis and Long-Term Outcomes

In severe GMH/IVH, sudden deterioration may be observed with no response to any attempt at escalation of support. Mortality in severe GMH/IVH, especially with associated periventricular hemorrhagic infarction, is 40%.[42] Among those who survive for weeks after detection of hemorrhage and with complicating progressive and persistent ventricular dilation, death occurs in 18%.[33] In ELBW infants, after excluding deaths because of extreme immaturity, 7% to 9% of the deaths are attributed to hemorrhage.

Some 40% of ELBW infants who survive following a grade III or IV GMH/IVH have moderate–severe neurosensory impairments. This includes cerebral palsy, which occurs in 30% of survivors, severe neurodevelopmental impairment (developmental quotients two standard deviations below the mean) in 15% to 20%, bilateral deafness in 8%, and blindness in 2%.[43,44] Among infants with lower grades of IVH (grade I and II), there is reported to be a twofold increase in the risk for neurodevelopmental impairment and a 2.6-fold increase in the risk of cerebral palsy compared with those children of similar birth weight but normal CUS.[45] An alternate large cohort study of infants less than 29 weeks' gestation reported that 20% of those with grade I or II IVH had moderate to severe neurosensory impairment, with 10% having cerebral palsy and 8% having a severe neurodevelopmental impairment (developmental quotients two standard deviations below the mean).[44]

Prevention

Several studies have addressed prevention from the antenatal through the postnatal period. Antenatal prevention is directed toward prevention of preterm birth through use of tocolytics, the treatment of maternal complications (bleeding, chorioamnionitis, conditions that may predispose to preterm delivery), intrapartum fetal surveillance, and preference for epidural anesthesia, controlled vaginal delivery, and administration of antenatal steroids. Antenatal steroids in particular have been repeatedly shown to significantly reduce the incidence of severe IVH, with data from the Neonatal Research Network finding the odds ratio for a severe IVH following a complete course of antenatal steroids was 0.39 (95% confidence interval [CI]: 0.27–0.57).[46,47]

Postnatal preventive strategies include supportive measures such as resuscitative measures as indicated at delivery with a goal of preventing hyperoxia, maintenance of optimal oxygenation and acid-base balance, gentle ventilation to prevent pneumothoraces and other air-leak syndromes, minimizing abrupt hemodynamic alterations, including slow volume expansion for low blood pressure and judicious use of inotropic agents (noting the risks associated with sudden changes in systemic pressures in the presence of a pressure passive cerebral circulation), and careful surfactant administration to improve respiratory status and oxygenation. Studies of pharmacologic agents such as pancuronium, ethamsylate, vitamin E, and phenobarbital do not demonstrate clear benefit. Indomethacin, a prostaglandin H synthase inhibitor, inhibits generation of oxygen-free radicals, promotes maturation of the germinal matrix, stabilizes cerebral blood flow, and attenuates the hyperemic response to hypoxia and hypercapnia. Indomethacin has been shown to reduce the incidence of severe IVH, but despite this, its use has not been associated with an improvement in neurodevelopmental outcome.[48,49]

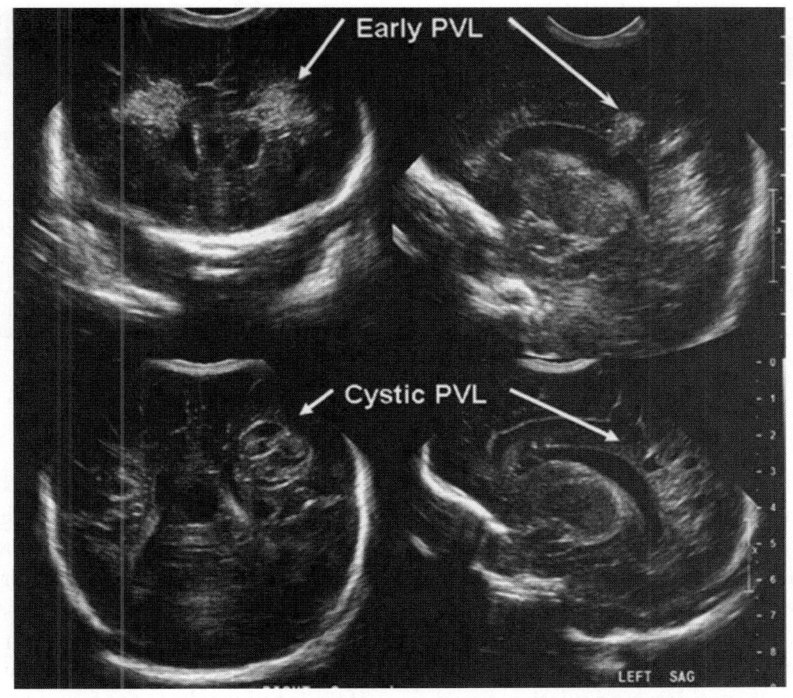

Fig. 17.4 The top panel shows the coronal and sagittal views of early periventricular leukomalacia *(PVL)*, which appears echodense, as indicated by the arrows. A week later on the same child, the echodense areas have turned into multiples cysts in the periventricular area (cystic periventricular leukomalacia).

Additionally, administration of indomethacin has been associated with increased risk of renal insufficiency, ileal perforation, and chronic lung disease.

EDITORIAL COMMENT: As quality improvement projects have been implemented in neonatal intensive care units (NICUs) across the globe, some have created care bundles aimed at reducing intraventricular hemorrhage (IVH). At Swedish Medical Center in Seattle, a meticulous care bundle was created including education of NICU staff, improving antenatal corticosteroid and magnesium for neuroprotection, delayed cord clamping and preventing delivery room hypothermia, and a protocol to maintain midline head positioning in the neonate from birth to 72 hours. Additionally, there was minimal handling and stimulation, no daily weights, and slow infusion of boluses in the first 72 hours. Despite improved compliance in most bundle components, IVH rates did not decrease and, in fact, increased, showing the difficulty in decreasing a condition with such a complex and multifactorial etiology.

(Nervik T, Moore L, Ryan A, et al. Reducing Intraventricular Hemorrhage Using a Care Bundle website. https://media.vtoxford.org/meetings/AMQC/Handouts2015/LearningFair/swedish_reducingintraventricularhemorrhage.pdf. Accessed August 28, 2018.)

Periventricular Leukomalacia

Periventricular leukomalacia (PVL) is a form of white matter injury that is commonly associated with GMH/IVH. It occurs in the periventricular arterial border zones.[31] Although the exact mechanism of injury is not fully defined, it is thought to occur secondary to ischemia and/or inflammation, with associated glial activation and damage of the preoligodendrocytes.

PVL may be either focal or diffuse. The classic description of focal PVL consists of macroscopic areas of necrosis. These initially appear as echodense lesions in the periventricular area with or without blood in the ventricles. After several weeks, these echodense areas can become cystic, and are referred to as cystic PVL (see Fig. 17.4). Cystic PVL occurs in less than 5% of VLBW infants and represents the minority of PVL.[28] More commonly, focal PVL consists of microscopic areas of necrosis and is termed *noncystic PVL*. Diffuse PVL is characterized by a loss of preoligodendrocytes rather than areas of necrosis. It leads to hypomyelination, and is associated with ventriculomegaly because of decreased cerebral tissue volume. CUS has limited use in identifying noncystic and diffuse PVL, with MRI being a superior neuroimaging modality to screen for these types of injury. MRI findings among these infants include abnormalities on diffusion-weighted imaging (DWI) and diffuse signal abnormalities.[50–52]

NEONATAL ENCEPHALOPATHY AND BRAIN INJURY IN THE TERM INFANT

Neonatal encephalopathy occurs in 2 to 5 per 1000 live births and is principally related to hypoxic-ischemic injury to the newborn brain in the peripartum period. In the last decade, there have been significant advances in neuroprotection that have been successful in reducing the risk of death and disability in infants who have suffered from a potential

TABLE 17.4 Estimates of Frequency of Maternal and Fetal Factors in Term Encephalopathic Populations

		Frequency in General Population	Frequency in HIE population
Antepartum/maternal	Hypothyroidism	0.5%	3%
	Obesity	10%–25%	15%–50%
	Diabetes (particularly pregestational)	0.5%–2%	5%–20%
	Fetal growth restriction <5%	5%	10%–15%
	Hypertension	3%–5%	5%–15%
	Clinical chorioamnionitis	1%–4%	5%–10%

Note: variability related to population reported.
HIE, Hypoxic-ischemic encephalopathy.

hypoxic-ischemic cerebral injury. The advent of therapeutic hypothermia has led to a major focus on the early clinical recognition of infants who may benefit from such therapies.

It is important to recognize that not all neonatal encephalopathies are related to hypoxic-ischemic disease. Antepartum and postpartum disorders (e.g., infectious, metabolic, dysgenetic) may lead to neonatal encephalopathies,[53,54] as discussed later in this chapter. In one large population-based observational study, the prevalence of moderate to severe encephalopathy was 1.64 per 1000 live term births, and the prevalence of "birth asphyxia" was 0.86 per 1000 live term births.[55] Fully 56% of all cases of newborn encephalopathy were related to hypoxic-ischemic injury that occurred during the intrapartum period. These findings are consistent with a more recent large cohort study of 4,165 singleton term infants with any one of the following: seizures, stupor, coma, Apgar score at 5 minutes less than 3, and/or receiving hypothermia therapy.[56] In this study, 15% of the infants experienced a clinically recognized sentinel event, such as antenatal hemorrhage (presumably, often placental abruption), uterine rupture, or cord prolapse, all of which are capable of compromising oxygen supply. Almost one-half of the infants displayed umbilical cord blood gas acidemia and/or fetal bradycardia. Of note, signs of inflammation were also not uncommon, with 27% of mothers displaying elevated maternal temperature in labor and 11% clinical chorioamnionitis. However, the contributing role of chorioamnionitis varies in different studies.[57] Although intrapartum sentinel events provide clear evidence of a hypoxic-ischemic insult, in three studies of neonatal encephalopathy sentinel, intrapartum events were only identified in 8% to 25% of infants.[20,22,58,59]

In a referral sample of 500 term infants with neonatal encephalopathy evaluated for therapeutic hypothermia, 48 (9%) had a sentinel birth event.[60] Thus it can be challenging to confirm a hypoxic-ischemic etiology for the infant with neonatal encephalopathy and/or the need for resuscitation because only 10% to 20% of such infants may have a clinical history of a major risk factor, whereas approximately 50% or more may have a constellation of risk factors, including maternal history, cord acidemia, and need for resuscitation that supports this as an etiology for their neurological syndrome.[19]

Additionally, although obvious, hypoxic-ischemic injury may affect the infant's brain during the antepartum and postnatal periods, albeit less commonly than the intrapartum period. On the basis of earlier work,[61] approximately 20% of hypoxic-ischemic injury recognized in the newborn period was said to be related primarily to antepartum insults. These data should be interpreted with the awareness that assessment of timing of insults to the fetus in these reports generally were based on imprecise methods, and the variability of findings is considerable.

Antepartum factors also appear to be of some importance in the risk for neonatal encephalopathy related to peripartum events. Such factors may *predispose* to intrapartum hypoxia-ischemia during the stresses of labor and delivery, especially through threats to placental flow. Maternal and fetal factors (Table 17.4) may include maternal diabetes, preeclampsia, placental vasculopathy, intrauterine growth restriction, and twin gestation that may compromise fetal cerebral perfusion. In one series, such factors were present in approximately one-third of cases of intrapartum asphyxia.[62] Indeed, "perinatal asphyxia" was identified in 27% of infants of diabetic mothers, and its occurrence correlated closely with diabetic vasculopathy (nephropathy) and presumed placental vascular insufficiency.[63] In a more recent cohort of infants that received therapeutic hypothermia (n = 98), the frequency of pregestational diabetes and preeclampsia were significantly higher (three- to fivefold) in women with infants requiring cooling.[59]

Although the importance of intrauterine hypoxic-ischemic injury, especially intrapartum asphyxia with or without antepartum predisposing factors, in the genesis of the clinical syndrome of neonatal hypoxic-ischemic encephalopathy (HIE) is apparent, most infants who experience intrapartum hypoxic-ischemic insults do *not* exhibit overt neonatal neurological features *or* subsequent neurological evidence of brain injury.[61,64] The severity and duration of the hypoxic-ischemic insult is obviously critical. Studies have demonstrated a relationship between the severity and duration of intrapartum hypoxia, assessed by the use of fetal acid-base studies, the subsequent occurrence of a neonatal neurological syndrome, and later neurological deficits.[65] Current data suggest that approximately 10% of all term deliveries require some

TABLE 17.5 Standardized Neurological Evaluations of the Term Infant With Neonatal Encephalopathy

Scoring System	Purpose/Utility	Number of Elements	Elements	EEG Necessary?
Sarnat	Prognosis applied in first 7 days	14	Alertness, tone, posture, reflexes: myoclonus, suck, Moro, oculovestibular, tonic neck, pupils, heart rate, secretions, GI motility, seizures, EEG	Yes
Modified Sarnat	Prognosis applied in first 7 days	5	Alertness, tone, suck, Moro, seizures	No
Thompson	Prognosis applied in first 7 days	6	Alertness, tone, respiratory status, reflexes, seizure, feeding method	No
NICHD	Selection in first 6 hours of life of moderate-severe NE for hypothermia	9	Alertness, spontaneous activity, posture, tone, suck, Moro, pupils, heart rate, respirations	No
Siben	Defining mild, moderate and severe NE in first 6 hours of life	10	Alertness, spontaneous activity, posture, tone, suck, Moro, pupils, heart rate, respirations, seizures	No

EEG, Electroencephalography; *GI,* gastrointestinal; *NE,* neonatal encephalopathy; *NICHD,* National Institute of Child Health and Human Development.

resuscitation, with 1% requiring extensive resuscitation.[66,67] Of the latter, only 1 to 3 per 1000 will develop signs of evolving encephalopathy consistent with HIE.[68,69]

Earlier in this chapter, we reviewed the neurological examination of the newborn. However, the evaluation of an infant who required resuscitation following delivery and may meet criteria for the administration of therapeutic hypothermia poses a special challenge to the neonatologist and neonatal neurologist. To improve interobserver reliability, standardized scores have been developed and have proven useful in large-scale clinical research studies (see later) (Table 17.5).[70,71]

The initial neurological examination classification systems developed evaluated infants over the first week of life to define the severity of their encephalopathy for prognostication. The first of these scorings systems was that developed by Sarnat and based on serial examinations of 21 term born infants over the first few weeks of life.[72] This scoring system was then simplified and referred to as the Modified Sarnat Scoring System.

The next scoring system developed for prognostication in neonatal encephalopathy was the Thompson Encephalopathy Score, developed in 1997 (Table 17.5).[70] This scoring system was simpler to apply and did not require electroencephalograph (EEG) to increase its widespread applicability. The initial evaluation showed a good correlation between the maximal score in the first 7 days of life and neurodevelopmental outcome at 18 months in 44 infants with neonatal HIE. Note that both the Sarnat and Thompson scoring systems aimed to define neonatal neurological signs during the first week of life to improve the prediction of subsequent neurological deficits.

However, as the era of neuroprotection emerged, it became apparent that a standardized neonatal neurological examination tool to be applied in the first few hours of life would be necessary to define eligibility for randomized controlled trials, such as therapeutic hypothermia. For some of the latter trials, the modified Sarnat and Thompson scales were utilized. For the largest North American study, a new scoring system was developed, that is, the National Institute of Child Health and Human Development (NICHD) Neonatal Encephalopathy Scoring System (Table 17.5).[73] The aim of this scoring system was to identify infants with moderate–severe encephalopathy who were eligible for entry into the trial within the first 6 hours of life. There was recognition that the examination could evolve and usually worsen consistent with secondary energy failure over the 24 hours of life.

To further refine the NICHD scoring system by the addition of a *mild encephalopathy* grouping, the HIE Score of the Iberoamerican Society of Neonatology was developed in 2016 and involved the assessment of 10 clinical aspects that could be undertaken from immediately after delivery room resuscitation (Table 17.5).[74] The recognition of mild encephalopathy is of great relevance, as it is recognized that at least 40% of hypoxic-ischemic cerebral injury presents as mild disease. It remains the only current published scoring system to include the evaluation of all three grades of neonatal encephalopathy in the first 6 hours of life. It is important to note that there has been no systematic investigation for the utility in application of any of the scoring systems in relationship to their inter- and intraobserver reliability and/or their validity to the evaluation of all infants requiring resuscitation who may benefit from therapeutic hypothermia.

NEUROLOGICAL INVESTIGATIONS IN TERM NEONATAL ENCEPHALOPATHY

The EEG changes in HIE may provide valuable information concerning the severity of the injury. Most commonly, the initial alteration is voltage suppression and a decrease in the frequency (i.e., slowing) into the delta and low theta ranges. Within approximately 1 day and often less, an excessively discontinuous pattern appears, characterized by periods of greater voltage suppression interspersed with bursts, usually asynchronous, of sharp and slow waves. Some infants exhibit multifocal or focal sharp waves or spikes at this time, often with a degree of periodicity. Over the next day or so, the excessively discontinuous pattern may become very prominent, with more severe voltage suppression and fewer bursts, now characterized by spikes and slow waves. This burst-suppression pattern can be of ominous significance, particularly if it persists after 24 hours of life. Continuous monitoring of conventional EEG with portable equipment has been found to be particularly useful in the identification of seizure activity.

Amplitude-integrated EEG (aEEG), an increasingly common method for continuous monitoring of electrical activity in the newborn, has been of considerable value in the assessment of the encephalopathic term newborn. The most useful tracings for detection of severe encephalopathy have been continuous low-voltage, flat, and burst-suppression tracings. Positive predictive values for an unfavorable outcome with such tracings in the first hours of life are 80% to 90%. Of infants with these marked background abnormalities, 10% to 50% may normalize within 24 hours. Rapid recovery is associated with a favorable outcome in 60% of cases.[75,76] However, with the evolution of hypothermia therapy, the predictive value of early aEEG has changed, and infants have been shown to have a normal neurological outcome if the aEEG background voltage activity recovers by 48 hours. In a recent meta-analysis of 520 infants treated with therapeutic hypothermia for moderate or severe HIE, the authors found that (1) a persistent severely abnormal aEEG background at 48 hours of age or beyond predicted an adverse outcome (positive predictive value of 85% and diagnostic odds ratio of 67 at 48 hours); and (2) at 6 hours of age, the aEEG background in hypothermia-treated infants had a good sensitivity of 96% (95% CI: 89%–97%) but low specificity at 39% (95% CI: 32%–45%).[77]

Patterns of Brain Injury in the Encephalopathic Term Infant

The patterns of injury in the term newborn have been delineated on both neuropathology and MRI. In this chapter, we briefly review neuropathological classification, as proposed by Volpe,[3] which is also well visualized on MR imaging.[78] The injury types discussed include the broad spectrum of patterns observed following neonatal hypoxic-ischemic injury: selective neuronal injuries, parasagittal cerebral injury, white matter injury, and focal and multifocal ischemic brain necrosis. Although these lesions are discussed as separate discrete entities, overlap between them is common.

Selective Neuronal Injury

The selective vulnerability of specific neuronal populations appears to be because of such factors as their high energy demand and glutamate distribution.[79] Four different patterns of selective neuronal injuries are seen and reflect the severity, duration, and nature of the insult.

The first form is that of diffuse neuronal injury with widespread injury in the cerebral cortex, basal ganglia, hippocampus, brainstem, and cerebellum. Injury of this magnitude can result from a severe near-total perinatal ischemic insult, such as total placental abruption, cord prolapse, or prolonged and severe total vascular interruption. This lesion is often referred to as global, total, or diffuse injury on MRI. In a recent study of patterns of brain injury in term infants following perinatal sentinel events, thalamic and basal ganglia injury was widespread, with 50% displaying cortical and brain stem injury and 25% displaying hippocampal injury.[60]

The second form is cerebral-deep nuclear neuronal injury, which combines neuronal damage in the deep nuclear gray matter with injury in the cerebral cortex, usually the parasagittal areas of the perirolandic cortex (Fig. 17.5). This is referred to on imaging studies as *deep nuclear gray matter* or *basal nuclei predominant* pattern. Areas of the deep nuclear gray matter that are more vulnerable include the putamen and the ventrolateral thalamus. This pattern accounts for over one-third of term infants following hypoxic-ischemic insults,[80–82] and is recognized most commonly after an acute near-total hypoxic-ischemic insult. With an increasing duration of hypoxia-ischemia, the distribution of cortical injury expands (Fig. 17.5).

The third form is deep nuclear gray matter-brain stem that often results from an "abrupt-severe" insult. This pattern of neuronal injury only seems to affect the deep gray matter without other cerebral neuronal involvement. Affected areas include the basal ganglia, thalamus, and the tegmentum of the brainstem.[83,84] This pattern of brain injury is rare in imaging studies of neonatal encephalopathy in the term born infant (<5%). The presence of intact myelination signal within the posterior limb of the internal capsule (PLIC) has been shown to be of prognostic significance and is frequently altered in significant deep nuclear gray matter/thalamic injury.

The final, least common form of selective neuronal injury is pontosubicular necrosis with injury to the neurons of the ventral pons and the subiculum of the hippocampi.[85] Etiologies for this injury are more diverse and include hypoxia, acute ischemia, hypocapnia, hyperoxemia, and hypoglycemia.[86–89] This pattern is more commonly seen in the premature infant, often associated with PVL.

Parasagittal Cerebral Injury (Neuronal and White Matter)

Parasagittal cerebral injury is unique to the term infant, occurring over the cerebral cortex and the underlying subcortical white matter of the parasagittal regions. It was first reported in 1977 by Volpe and Pasternak.[90] Parietal-occipital regions are the most commonly affected. Injury is usually bilateral in distribution and results from mild to moderate

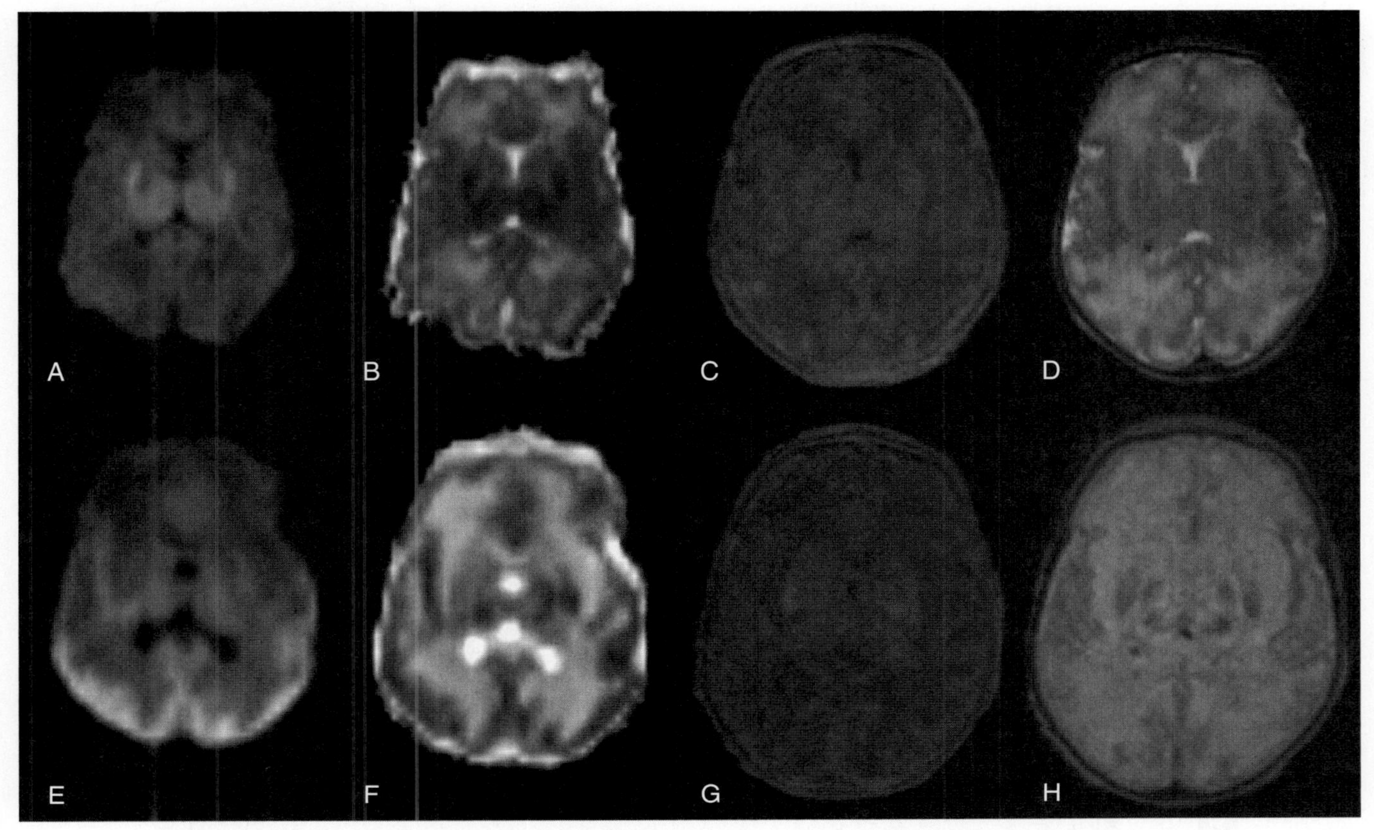

Fig. 17.5 Deep nuclear and cerebral injury. A 35 weeks' gestation infant with history of placental abruption for several hours before hospital admission. Apgars 1^{1}, 3^{5}, 7^{10}. Magnetic resonance imaging on day 1 for diffusion-weighted imaging (A), apparent diffusion coefficient map (B), T1-weighted (C), and T2-weighted imaging (D) reveal isolated thalamic and deep nuclear gray matter injury that is most apparent on the diffusion imaging. At day 10, there is now evolution with more prominent T1- and T2-weighted signal changes in the deep nuclear gray matter and thalamus (G, H), but also prominent restriction in the cortical ribbon on diffusion-weighted (E) and apparent diffusion coefficient (F) imaging, suggesting a secondary neuronal degeneration.

hypoperfusion in this "watershed" region between the anterior, middle, and posterior cerebral circulation. This lesion is often referred to as a *watershed injury* or *border-zone injury* in MRI studies. Watershed cortical infarcts have been well recognized in the term infant, occurring in between 30% to 45% of published series, dependent on the enrollment criteria, and commonly involve the underlying white matter (Table 17.6).

White Matter Injury

Damage to the white matter dorsal and lateral to the external angles of the lateral ventricle has been well described in the premature infant but is also seen in the term infant following hypoxic-ischemic injury. In one series of term encephalopathic infants, white matter injury of presumed hypoxic-ischemic origin was identified in 23% of infants.[91] Lower gestational age at birth was associated with an increasing severity of white matter injury, suggesting a role for brain maturation.[91] It is also important to note that preterm infants display a pattern of cerebral injury, with both neuronal and white matter lesions. In a study of 55 infants with median gestation of 35 weeks who presented with low Apgar score and the need for major resuscitation, basal ganglia injury occurred in 75%, white matter injury in 89%, and cortical injury in 58%.[92] Brainstem injury was seen in infants with severe diffuse injury.

Ischemic Perinatal Stroke

The incidence of ischemic perinatal stroke ranges from 1/2300 to 1/5000 live births[93–96] and is now recognized as the second most common etiology for term encephalopathy, predominantly because of neonatal seizures. Arterial lesions, usually unilateral, most commonly involve the middle cerebral artery, with the left cerebral hemisphere being more frequently affected than the right. Venous thrombosis most commonly affects the superior sagittal sinus. This pattern of injury, increasingly recognized by MRI, is the "focal or multifocal" pattern of injury. Data suggest that strokes (arterial or venous) are also associated with neonatal encephalopathy in the term newborn.[97–99] In an observational study of 62 newborns with focal or multifocal stroke, 36 had stroke alone, and 26 had stroke with a concurrent pattern of nonfocal hypoxia-ischemia. Multiple risk factors for hypoxia-ischemia occurred in most newborns in both groups.[100]

TABLE 17.6 **Characteristics and Magnetic Resonance Imaging Findings From Studies on Term Encephalopathy**

STUDY	Cowan 2003[97]	Miller 2005[144]	Okereafor 2008[60]	Chau 2009[120]	Steinman 2009[150]	Rutherford 2010[156]	Vermont Oxford 2011[119]	Cheong 2009[159]	Martinez-Biarge [147,149]
Inclusion criteria	Either fetal heart rate monitoring abnormalities and/or cord pH <7.1 and/or delayed respiration and/or 5-min Apgar score <7 and/or multiorgan failure.	One of: Apgar score ≤5 at 5 minutes, and/or pH <7.1, BD >10	Acute sentinel event—umbilical cord prolapse (19%), uterine rupture (23%), placental abruption (46%)	Neonatal encephalopathy and one of fetal distress, cord acidemia and/or 5-min Apgar score ≤5	One of: Apgar score ≤5 at 5 minutes, and/or pH <7.0, BD >10	Neonatal encephalopathy and abnormal EEG and cord pH <7.0 and/or delayed respiration and/or 10-min Apgar score <5	Seizures or stupor/coma or hypothermia or Apgar score at 5 minutes <3	Two of: Apgar score ≤5 and/or need for mechanical ventilation at 10 minutes, and/or pH <7.0, BD >12	Term NE and MRI in first 6 weeks; Apgar score ≤5 at 5 minutes, and/or pH <7.1; fetal distress
Number of infants	245	173	48	48	64	67 nonhypothermia	1074	61 nonhypothermia	425
Day of MRI scan (range)	14 days of birth	6 days (1–24)	10 days	72 hours	14 days of life	8 days (2–30)	7 days	6 days (3–8)	10 days (2–42)
Normal	16%	30%		33%	40%	20%	18%	13%	See cortical
Basal Ganglia-Thalamus injury	80%	25%	75% any injury 65% mod-severe	31%	33%	80% any injury 58% mod-severe	30%	36% mod-severe	41%
Cortical Injury	10%	45%	58%	36%	45%	63%	15%	28%	44% (n = 186) normal or white matter/cortical
White Matter Injury	5%	Not recorded	Not recorded	21%	15%	84% any 13% severe	25%	23%	See cortical
Other diagnosis	4%	None noted	None noted	Arterial infarction in 10%		4%	2%		11% from total of 555

BD, Base deficit; *EEG*, electroencephalography; *MRI*, magnetic resonance imaging; *NE*, neonatal encephalopathy.

TABLE 17.7 Neuroimaging in 1421 Term Infants With Neonatal Encephalopathy in the Vermont Oxford Neonatal Encephalopathy Registry (2006–2008)

		Ultrasound	CT Scan	MRI
Number of infants		729 (51%)	477 (34%)	1074 (75%)
Mean (SD) age (days) at first examination		3.1 (4.4)	3.2 (3.5)	7.3 (8.7)
Abnormal		232 (32%)	271 (57%)	717 (67%)
Hemorrhage	IVH/SE	56 (8%)	59 (12%)	79 (7%)
	Extraaxial	24 (3%)	165 (35%)	212 (20%)
	Parenchymal	37 (5%)	57 (12%)	105 (10%)
Deep nuclear gray matter injury		70 (10%)	50 (10%)	309 (29%)
White matter injury		16 (2%)	15 (3%)	271 (25%)

CT, Computed axial tomography; *IVH/SE,* intraventricular hemorrhage/subependymal; *MRI,* magnetic resonance imaging; *SD,* standard deviation.

Evolution of Neuropathology

The unique patterns of injury in the term-born infant brain reflect selective vulnerabilities combined with the nature and severity of the insult. This vulnerability reflects developmentally regulated biochemical processes that mature at different rates in specific anatomical brain structures (e.g., expression of glutamate receptor subunits, antioxidant enzymes, and nitric oxide synthase) that render neurons particularly vulnerable.[101–103] The neuropathology following a cerebral insult evolves over a period of days to weeks. Initial extensive injuries may be accompanied by hemorrhages, especially in the cerebellum and the choroid plexus.[103] By 3 to 5 days after initial injury, the subacute phase is characterized by "reactive processes" targeting parenchymal clean up and repair: vascular proliferation with endothelial hypertrophy, activation and proliferation of resident microglia, and macrophage influx. A severe insult may result in total infarction with damage to all cellular elements. The proliferation of astrocytes in response to the neuronal loss (i.e., gliosis) is usually not prominent until a week or more following the injury. In the chronic phase, weeks to months after the insult, small collapsed glial scars or calcification are observed, with larger parenchymal cysts observed following severe injuries.[103] In this chronic stage, "ulegyria" and "multicystic encephalomalacia" are observed following severe hypoxic-ischemic injury in the term newborn.[103]

Major Neuroimaging Modalities

Cranial Ultrasound

CUS relies on the reflection of ultrasound waves from tissue to provide images. CUS can be performed at the bedside with minimal risk to the patient. It is performed through an open fontanelle, and thus its use is restricted to the first 6 months of life. It remains the most commonly used neuroimaging modality in the neonatal intensive care unit (NICU) setting. CUS is sensitive to blood products, ventricular size, gross brain malformations, and cystic changes in the brain parenchyma. It is less sensitive to smaller and more subtle anomalies within the brain, including noncystic white matter abnormalities and minor cerebral dysgenesis. It is a very useful screening evaluation in the term infant with encephalopathy, identifying cerebral dysgenesis in approximately 2% to 4% of infants that had been diagnosed with hypoxic-ischemic injury. It can also be used to identify established prenatal severe HIE on the first day of life.[104]

Computed Axial Tomography

Computed tomography (CT) scanning is based on the passing of an x-ray beam (ionizing radiation) through a sample at a series of different angles. Based on the attenuation of these beams, an image can be constructed. CT scanning has several advantages, including providing a quantitative measure, high sensitivity for the detection of acute blood products and bone abnormalities, short examination time, and wide availability. However, MRI appears to be more sensitive, particularly for injury to the deep nuclear gray matter and white matter. This is demonstrated in the results from the Vermont Oxford Neonatal Encephalopathy Registry from 2006 to 2008 (Table 17.7). There are also increasing concerns regarding the impact of radiation exposure from CT on the developing brain because of the risk of future malignancy and later cognitive impairments.[105] Until further data are available, CT should be restricted to select settings in which the information obtained is clearly of benefit to the patient and cannot be readily obtained using some other modality.

Magnetic Resonance Imaging

MRI provides the highest sensitivity to both anatomical and functional detail. It does, however, have some drawbacks compared with other imaging modalities, particularly in the neonatal period. Unlike CUS, patients must typically be transported from the NICU to a radiology suite for MR imaging, which may pose some risk to the patient. Some facilities sedate infants/children for MR imaging, which also carries risk, although this practice is not routinely required for MR imaging in the newborn period. MR imaging sessions typically take longer than CT or CUS, and the infant/child is less readily able to be accessed in the event of an emergency such as displacement of an endotracheal tube. Finally, MR scanners are much more expensive than CUS or CT scanners to install and maintain. Despite these issues, MR is in widespread use because of superior neurodiagnostic information.

Conventional images. Conventional images include T1- (short repetition and short echo times) and T2-weighted images (long repetition times and long echo times). These sequences offer superiority in differentiating cortical gray matter from cerebral white matter and myelinated from unmyelinated white matter when compared with ultrasound and CT. Injury will appear hypointense on T1-weighted and hyperintense in T2-weighted images in the acute phase (first few days), then hyperintense on T1-weighted and hypointense on T2-weighted later within the first week. T1-weighted hyperintensity may persist for weeks, whereas T2-weighted hypointensity transitions to hyperintensity over that interval. Conventional images alone can lack sensitivity to injury in the acute phase (<4 days).

Diffusion-weighted imaging. DWI measures the random diffusion of water through brain tissue. This diffusion of water in tissue is referred to as apparent diffusion, thus the term apparent diffusion coefficient (ADC), the quantitative measure of tissue diffusivity. More recently, the term mean diffusivity has been utilized. Brain tissue following ischemic injury will experience a decrease in water diffusion compared with healthy adjacent tissue. Following neonatal ischemic brain injury, ADC values can decrease slowly as compared with adult stroke, with up to 30% of infants having "normal" appearing DWI in the first 12 to 24 hours.[106] "Pseudonormalization" of the ADC occurs by 7 to 10 days, a time when injury should be apparent on conventional MRI. Secondary alterations in cerebral regions, such as Wallerian degeneration in axonal pathways following a primary neuronal injury, can alter the representation of these "acute" changes. For example, restriction in the PLIC or corpus callosum may become noticeable on days 6 to 10.[107–109] Thus one must take care in the interpretation of the timing of the insult based solely on ADC restriction, but also consider the pattern of restriction.

Magnetic resonance spectroscopy. MR spectroscopy is based on the ability of the same nuclei in various molecules to demonstrate different resonant frequencies because of different electron densities. The most commonly applied nucleus is the 1H proton (^{1}H-MRS). The signal is expressed in parts per million (ppm) and can detect N-acetylasparate (NAA), creatine + phosphocreatine (Cr), choline (Cho), myo-inositol (mI), glutamine (Gln), glutamate (Glu), glucose (G), taurine (Tau), and lactate (Lac). NAA (a free amino acid) is present in large quantities in the developing brain, both in neuronal tissue and developing oligodendrocytes, making it a great indicator of intact central nervous tissue.[110] Multiple studies have used NAA ratios (NAA/Cr and NAA/Cho) to assess the degree of brain injury both in animal models and human infants.[111–113] ^{1}H-MRS detects this presence of lactate, a doublet peak at 1.3 ppm that is upright at 288 s and inverted at 144 s echo time, and is a useful marker for tissue injury.

Magnetic resonance angiography/magnetic resonance venography. MR angiography and venography are noninvasive techniques used to delineate arterial and venous supply and topography while avoiding catheterization and contrast administration.[114–116] However, in the newborn, there are limitations with small caliber vessels and slow cerebral flow compared with children and adults, making flow voids more frequent.[117]

The Patterns of Neuroimaging Abnormalities Found in Newborn Encephalopathy

There is wide variation in current clinical practice for the use of neuroimaging modalities in the term infant with encephalopathy. We have used the term *neonatal encephalopathy*, in preference to HIE, as suggested by current research and clinical leaders[118] and to recognize the clinical syndrome in the infant that is often being evaluated. There are still a significant number of infants with neonatal encephalopathy who do not undergo any neuroimaging evaluation to define the nature and/or severity of brain injury.

Within the Vermont Oxford Network Neonatal Encephalopathy Registry from 2006 to 2008, 88,527 infants were screened from 70 centers. Of these, 82% underwent some form of neuroimaging evaluation, the type and timing of which is shown in Table 17.7.[119] Approximately one-third of infants received a CT scan, one-half received a CUS, and three-quarters received MRI. The major abnormality detected on CT scanning was extraaxial blood. MRI had higher detection rates for deep nuclear gray matter and white matter injury. To more accurately compare these imaging modalities, a subset of infants received both a CT scan and MRI. White matter injury was 10 times and deep nuclear gray matter injury three times more likely to be diagnosed with MRI than CT scans in the same infants. In one study, comparing CT and DWI for detection of patterns of brain injury in term newborns with neonatal encephalopathy, diffusion MRI was still the most sensitive technique, particularly for cortical injury and focal-multifocal lesions.[120] Thus although the American Academy of Neurology recommendations for MRI as the neuroimaging modality for neonatal encephalopathy in the term infant have been present for close to a decade,[121] a translational gap remains.

With the wider use of MRI, the recognition of different patterns of injury has become established. It is worth noting that the interpretation of the MRI literature in neonatal encephalopathy is limited by two major weaknesses: (1) the exact timing of the insult is generally not known; and (2) more importantly, there is little to no data on the neuropathological correlate of the MRI pattern. However, two main patterns are often distinguished on MRI:

1. A basal-ganglia-thalamus pattern predominantly affecting bilaterally the central gray nuclei and perirolandic cortex. This pattern of injury is consistent with the selective neuronal necrosis described above and has been associated with a partial neonatal insult, with near-total insult. Basal ganglia involvement can also occur in other mechanisms of brain injury, particularly if the injury is severe. The presence of brainstem and/or cerebellar involvement with basal ganglia injury may suggest an isolated profound event. Basal ganglia injury is reported in 25%–80% of cases (Table 17.6). This variation may relate to (1) selection bias in the patient

populations, (2) subjective differences in the reporting or interpretation of signal abnormalities in the basal ganglia and thalamus, and (3) the use, including timing, of DWI.
2. The watershed or border-zone predominant pattern of injury affects mainly the white matter and, in more severely affected infants, the overlying cortex in the vascular watershed zones (anterior-middle cerebral artery and posterior-middle cerebral artery).[122] The lesions can be unilateral or bilateral and predominantly posterior and/or anterior. Although loss of the cortical ribbon, and therefore the gray-white matter differentiation, can be seen on conventional MRI, DWI highlights the abnormalities and is especially helpful in making an early diagnosis. A repeat MRI may show cystic evolution, but more often, atrophy and gliotic changes will be recognized. This pattern of injury is typically thought to be seen following "partial insult."[123] The frequency of this lesion has varied between studies (25%–60%) and may reflect enrollment criteria and/or the utility, including timing, of DWI.

When either of these patterns of injury become extreme, a total injury pattern results. Additionally, there are infants with lesions restricted to the periventricular white matter not dissimilar from the so-called punctate white matter lesions described in preterm infants; these can be distinguished as a separate pattern of injury, although less common than the patterns outlined above.

Clinical Interpretation of Magnetic Resonance Imaging in the Term Encephalopathic Infant

The aim in undertaking neurologic imaging of a sick term infant with encephalopathy is to enhance the information obtained from the history and examination to aid the physician in answering the following questions: What is the nature and extent of brain injury? What was the likely etiology of the injury? When did the injury occur? Are there ways to intervene other than supportive care that could impact on outcome? What is the prognosis for this patient?

Conventional Imaging

In the first 48 hours following injury, there may be no visible changes on conventional MR imaging. If MRI abnormalities are present at this time, T1-weighted images will appear hypointense or display no abnormalities, whereas T2-weighted images may be hyperintense. The hyperintensity in affected areas on T2-weighted images evolves into hypointensity by 6 to 10 days of life, whereas the T1-weighted imaging will become hyperintense.[78,106] Acutely affected infants may only demonstrate diffuse edema of the cortical tissue on conventional images. This increase in water content of the brain tissue causes the cortex to become iso-intense with adjacent white matter, making differentiation of the border between the two tissues difficult. Areas of involvement vary according to the nature and severity of the insult. Mild hypoxic-ischemic injuries that are because of an acute total lesion or a partial lesion with terminal total insult will commonly involve the bilateral putamen, the ventrolateral nucleus of the thalamus. If the lesion resulted from total loss of all perfusion, then there is likely to be brainstem and/or cerebellar involvement. Affected areas include the basal ganglia, the thalamus, and the tegmentum of the brainstem. More severe injuries or prolonged insults of a partial (less common) and/or partial with total insult pattern will also include diffuse areas of the deep and superficial gray matter along with diffuse white matter involvement. Chronically, this will evolve into a picture of multicystic encephalopathy.

Diffusion-Weighted Imaging/Diffusion Tensor Imaging

In contrast to conventional MRI, diffusion imaging is sensitive to acute cerebral injury. The evolution in diffusion over time in HIE infants has been described with basal ganglia injury in the early postnatal period.[109] In the first 12 to 24 hours, some infants may have no visible changes on diffusion imaging.[106] The pattern of the early predominance of the ventrolateral nucleus of the thalami (first 48 hours) becomes more evident in the putamen, corticospinal tracts, and the perirolandic cortex by 3 to5 days of life. Subcortical white matter and white matter pathways such as the corpus callosum and the cingulum may show involvement early, or this may appear as a secondary change by 7 days after injury. Clues to the timing and extent of brain injury can therefore be elucidated by DWI within the first 4 days of life. Although the changes in diffusion can be detected as early as 6 hours after injury, the most significant change in diffusion occurs between 2 to4 days after the insult.[106,124] These diffusion changes correlate not only with later conventional imaging but also with neurodevelopmental outcome.[125] If DWI shows involvement of the PLIC with an ADC of 0.74 or less, poor neurodevelopmental outcome is highly likely.[126] The presence of Wallerian degeneration in the PLIC on DWI is also a strong predictor for hemiplegia in infants with perinatal cerebral infarcts.[127,128]

Measuring anisotropy (fractional anisotropy [FA]) with diffusion tensor imaging gives additional information on severity and timing of injury. Anisotropy decreases with both severe and moderate white matter and basal ganglia injury during the first week of life, whereas ADC decreases only for severe injury. Anisotropy (FA) values continue to decrease during the second week of life and do not undergo pseudonormalization like ADC values. In the mild and moderate HIE population, FA has been shown to correlate with short-term neurodevelopmental outcome.[129]

Magnetic Resonance Spectroscopy

The in vivo assessment of metabolites was first described in neonates by Groendaal et al. who observed higher lactate and lower NAA values in the basal ganglia in infants with poor outcome at 3 months following encephalopathy.[111] Since this observation, studies have looked at both metabolite ratios (Lac/Cho, Lac/Cr, NAA/Cho) and absolute levels (Lac, NAA), and correlated them with outcome. The abnormal rise in lactate and fall in NAA are most significant within the first week after injury, with lactate being detected within 24 hours following injury, whereas NAA starts to decrease after 48 hours.[113] An elevated Lac/Cho ratio early in the first week and a fall in NAA/Cho later in the first week have been shown to be most predictive for neurodevelopmental outcomes.[128,130–136] These metabolite levels can remain abnormal for long periods of time. Elevated lactate levels are seen for months after injury and thus do not always indicate acute injury. The persistence of lactate signifies a worse prognosis.[132] A study in 81 term infants who underwent conventional, DWI, and MR spectroscopic measurements in the basal ganglia on imaging at a median of day 4 showed that the addition of quantitative measures of ADC and/or lactate-N-acetyl aspartate ratio improved the predictive power of conventional imaging.[128] In a meta-analysis of 32 studies grouping 806 newborns with neonatal encephalopathy, the ratio of lactate over NAA in the deep gray matter had strong diagnostic accuracy,[137] with a pooled sensitivity of 82% and specificity of 92%. Although this measure was useful for death or profound disability, more detailed anatomical imaging may assist in refining prognostic information.

Evaluation of the Timing of Cerebral Injury

MRI can provide mutual information from conventional imaging, DWI, and MR spectroscopy that can inform timing. However, information regarding the likely timing is best obtained with early imaging (first 48–72 hours of life) with further follow-up imaging at 7 to 14 days of life. If the insult were in the immediate perinatal period, early imaging in the first 24 to 48 hours would show no changes in conventional imaging, no (day 1) to mild restriction in diffusion imaging, and an elevated lactate, but no alteration in N-acetyl aspartate on MR spectroscopy. By day 4 to 5, diffusion imaging remains restricted with the evolution of early conventional imaging changes, and lactate remains elevated. By day 7 to 14, diffusion normalizes in the region of primary injury but may have secondary restriction in areas of Wallerian degeneration. Conventional imaging will reveal signal abnormality to confirm the nature and extent of injury, whereas spectroscopy will show a reduction in N-acetyl aspartate, with lactate potentially persisting or resolving. Thus an infant who suffered an insult associated with decreased fetal movements 48 hours before delivery would display a pattern for day 4 imaging findings at day 2. It is important to note that imaging studies with the predominant MRI studies obtained after day 7 can discern the absence of chronic findings, such as cystic changes and atrophy, but are not able to discern the acute or subacute nature of an insult.

There are few imaging studies that have attempted to undertake MRI in the first 24 hours of life to define the timing and evolution of injury. Although some of these studies have tended to have "a priori" inclusion of infants with sentinel acute events,[42] they nonetheless suggest a predominance of intrapartum injuries. However, it is also important that clinicians recall that fetal stillbirth rates in the third trimester remain higher than neonatal encephalopathy by a factor of threefold,[138] suggesting that injury and death can occur outside the setting of labor. Thus research into the timing of cerebral injury remains critical to our understanding of the pathway to neonatal encephalopathy. Although MRI studies support that the period around the time of birth accounts for greater than 75% of the causative period, studies have not systematically investigated the extent to which injury may have occurred over 24 hours before delivery. This area is worthy of greater investigation and may be more plausible as NICUs acquire access to MRI scanners within their nursery setting, combined with investigation of the placenta.

Section Conclusions—Patterns of Neuroimaging Abnormalities

- Neuroimaging in the neonatal period should be obtained on all term-born infants with evidence of encephalopathy, with a gap in current clinical practice.
- MRI is the neuroimaging modality of choice and can be utilized within the first 14 days of life to define the pattern of cerebral injury. Two key patterns are defined, including basal ganglia predominant or watershed. Involvement of the brainstem and/or cerebellum should be carefully noted. Experienced neuroradiological interpretation of MRI is critical to confirm the diagnosis. The etiology of a potential ischemic cerebral insult cannot be determined by neuroimaging.
- The timing of an ischemic cerebral insult can be suggested by MRI obtained in the first 4 days of life with a combination of diffusion, conventional, and spectroscopic imaging.
- Imaging obtained later than 7 days can define patterns of injury, and longer time intervals can help define the potential timing of a cerebral insult, such as weeks or months rather than days.

NEURODEVELOPMENTAL CORRELATES OF NEUROIMAGING PATTERNS

It is now accepted that identifying the predominant pattern of brain injury is the strongest predictor of neurodevelopmental outcome for a term newborn with encephalopathy. It is important to note that most studies relating patterns of injury to neurodevelopmental outcome undertook imaging after day 7 of life. Conventional images provide a robust measure of the nature and severity of injury when done a week following the initial insult, correlating well with neurodevelopmental outcome.[61,137,139] However, conventional MRI in the first 4 days may underestimate the total extent of the injury.

Studies have demonstrated that the extent of brain injury on MRI is an important predictor of neurodevelopmental outcome in newborns with HIE.[82,140–149] Additionally, the predominant pattern of brain injury on MRI is more strongly associated with long-term outcome than the severity of injury in any given region.[141,143,147]

Several studies have divided patterns of injury into either watershed predominant or deep nuclear gray matter predominant with long-term follow-up. Deep nuclear gray matter (basal ganglia, thalamus) predominance is associated with more intensive need for resuscitation, more severe encephalopathy, increased seizure burden, and worse neurodevelopmental outcome as far out as 5 years of age.[82,144,145] The basal nuclei pattern and abnormal signal intensity in the PLIC on MRI are both predictive of severely impaired motor and cognitive functions,[141–144] the latter a particularly powerful prognostic indicator for poor neurodevelopmental outcome, correctly predicting outcome in 92% of infants with stage II HIE.[141]

Although the motor and cognitive deficits following the basal nuclei pattern of injury are often evident during the first years of life, the cognitive deficits following the watershed pattern may appear later after 2 years of age.[144] Importantly, cognitive deficits at 4 years of age are more strongly related to the severity of watershed injuries than the severity of injury in the deep nuclear gray matter.[150] Most recently, Martinez-Biarge et al reported findings on a large cohort of term infants with encephalopathy collected over a 15-year period.[147] Neuroimaging markers in the newborn period were clearly demonstrated for death (brainstem lesion) and cerebral palsy (basal ganglia and thalamus injury). A previous report on the same cohort[149] reported associations between basal ganglia and thalamic lesions and other clinically relevant outcomes, including feeding, speech and language, vision, and intellect, as well as the risk of epilepsy, demonstrating the spectrum of disabilities that children with perinatal brain injury suffer.

HYPOTHERMIA AND PATTERNS OF BRAIN INJURY

Systemic hypothermia reduces the risk of death and/or disability in term-born infants with HIE with a number needed to treat of eight.[73,151–155] In the TOBY (TOtal Body hYpothermia) trial, total body cooling therapy was associated with less injury in the basal ganglia, thalami, and PLIC in the second week of life.[156] In another study of total body cooling, systemic hypothermia down to 33° to 34°C reduced cortical injury.[157] In an experimental study of 42 newborn piglets, optimal neuroprotection by delayed hypothermia was found to occur at different temperatures in the cortical and deep gray matter.[158] Whether a cooling protocol could be tailored to provide more optimal brain protection to a particular pattern of brain injury is an important question for future research. Importantly, therapeutic hypothermia does not affect the predictive value of conventional MRI for subsequent neurological impairment.[157,159] However, further studies are needed to define the optimal timing of brain imaging for newborns treated with hypothermia.

EDITORIAL COMMENT: In June 2014, the Committee on Fetus and Newborn of the American Academy of Pediatrics published a clinical report, "Hypothermia and Neonatal Encephalopathy." They recommended that infants offered hypothermia should meet inclusion criteria outlined in published clinical trials, that the treatment should be done in centers capable of providing comprehensive clinical care, and that cooling infants who do not meet inclusion criteria should only be done in a research setting with informed parental consent. (Papile L, Baley J, Benitz W, et al, *Pediatrics.* 2014;133:1146-1150.)

NEONATAL SEIZURES

Neonatal seizures remain one of the few neurologic emergencies, and may indicate significant dysfunction or damage to the immature nervous system both on a remote and on an acute basis.[160–166] Advances in neurophysiologic monitoring of the high-risk infant have spurred the development of an integrated classification of both clinical and electrographic criteria for diagnosis of seizures.[167] Synchronized video EEG-polygraphic techniques as well as computer-assisted analyses allow the clinician to better characterize suspicious clinical behaviors that may or may not be associated with coincident surface-generated electrographic seizures. Nonetheless, because of the reliance on detecting suspicious clinical behaviors, recognition of neonatal seizures is still hampered by both overestimation and underestimation of their occurrence.

Clinical criteria for suspected seizures may not easily distinguish seizure activity from either normal or pathologic nonepileptic behavior; coincident EEG is needed to best define the diagnosis. Subclinical EEG seizures may also occur that escape detection by clinical observation alone. Conversely, EEG criteria may not adequately recognize ictal patterns that originate from subcortical brain regions, but no universal classification based on clinical criteria can distinguish subcortical seizures from nonepileptic paroxysmal activity, although there is speculation regarding electroclinical disassociation. Certain clinically apparent seizures originate in subcortical structures and only intermittently propagate to the cortical surface where EEG electrodes can readily record electrographic seizures. One pragmatic approach to the diagnosis and management of neonatal seizures is therefore based on the documentation of seizures by surface-recorded EEG studies. A therapeutic end point for the use of antiepileptic medications can be more practically achieved using EEG documentation because clinical signs may be absent, minimal, or nonepileptic in origin.

ELBW infants with clinical seizures are at increased risk of an adverse neurodevelopmental outcome, independent of multiple confounding factors.

Seizure Detection: Clinical Versus Electroencephalographic Criteria

Neonates are unable to sustain generalized tonic followed by clonic seizures as observed in older patients, although separately occurring generalized tonic and clonic events do appear, even in the same neonate. Most seizures are brief and subtle, and consequently are expressed as clinical behaviors that are unusual to recognize. Five clinical categories of neonatal seizures have been described.[3] Several caveats should be mentioned before these five clinical categories are reviewed.[168] First, the clinician should be suspicious of any abnormal repetitive stereotypic behavior that could represent a possible seizure. Second, certain behaviors, such as orbital and buccolingual movements, tonic posturing, and myoclonus, can be associated with either normal neonatal sleep behaviors or nonepileptic pathologic behaviors. Third, clinical events may have only an inconsistent relationship to coincident electrographic seizures.

Subtle or Fragmentary Seizures

Subtle or fragmentary seizures constitute the most frequently observed clinical group of seizure-like phenomena and may be characterized by repetitive facial activity, unusual bicycling or pedaling movements, momentary fixation of gaze, or autonomic dysfunction. Specific autonomic signs such as apnea are rarely seen in isolation but usually occur in the context of other seizure phenomena in the same neonate. Even though these clinical expressions appear unimpressive, they may reflect significant brain dysfunction or injury. An inconsistent relationship between specific subtle behaviors and EEG seizures has been documented using synchronized video EEG-polygraphic recordings, which emphasizes the need for further classification.[169] It is generally considered standard practice to require that suspicious clinical behaviors occurring in close temporal proximity to EEG seizure patterns be considered indicative of seizure.

Clonic Seizures

Clonic seizures are characterized by rhythmic movements of muscle groups in a focal or multifocal distribution. Rapid followed by slow movement phases distinguish clonic movements from the symmetric to-and-fro movements of nonepileptic tremulousness or jitteriness.[170,171] Whereas gentle flexion of the extremity can suppress tremors, this is not possible with clonic seizure activity. The clonic event may involve any muscle group of the face, limbs, or torso. Focal clonic seizures may be associated with localized brain injury, but they can also accompany generalized cerebral disturbances.[172,173] Following seizures, newborns may also have a transient period of paresis or paralysis, called *Todd's phenomenon.*

Tonic Seizures

Tonic seizures are characterized by sustained flexion or extension of either axial or appendicular muscle groups, such as decerebration or dystonic posturing. Focal head or eye turning or tonic flexion or extension of an extremity exemplifies tonic seizures. Although some tonic behaviors are coincident with EEG seizures, there is a high false-positive correlation, with tonic behavior occurring in the absence of concurrent electrical seizure activity.

Myoclonic Seizures

Myoclonic movements are rapid, isolated jerks involving the midline musculature or a single extremity, either in a generalized or multifocal fashion. Unlike the movements in clonic seizures, which show fast and slow phases, myoclonic movements lack a two-phase movement. Healthy preterm and term infants may demonstrate abundant myoclonic movements during either sleep or wakefulness.[170,171] However, sick neonates may also exhibit myoclonus, which is either verified as seizure activity by EEG or determined to be a manifestation of nonepileptic abnormal motor activity.[174]

Electroencephalographic Seizure Criteria

EEG remains an invaluable tool for the assessment of both ictal and interictal cerebral activity, as expressed on surface recordings. Although an EEG finding is rarely pathognomonic for a particular disease, important information about the presence and severity of a brain disorder with or without seizures can be gained from careful visual interpretation.[175] Major EEG background rhythm disturbances in the absence of seizures carry major prognostic implications for compromised outcome. Specific interictal EEG abnormalities on serial EEG recordings offer invaluable information to the clinician regarding the presence, severity, and persistence of an encephalopathic state in the neonate.

Interictal Electroencephalograph Patterns

Background EEG abnormalities have prognostic significance for both preterm and full-term infants.[176,177] Such patterns include burst suppression, electrocerebral inactivity, low-voltage invariant, and persistent multifocal sharp wave abnormalities. Other interictal EEG abnormalities, such as disparity in the maturity of EEG and polygraphic activities, also have prognostic importance but require greater skill in visual analysis to identify.[175]

Ictal Electroencephalograph Patterns

Ictal EEG patterns in the newborn are composed of repetitive waveforms of a certain minimum duration and similar morphology that evolve in response to frequency, amplitude, and electric field. The electroencephalographer can readily identify seizures that are at least 10 seconds in duration.[178] Four categories of ictal patterns have traditionally been described: focal ictal patterns with normal background, focal ictal patterns with abnormal background, focal monorhythmic periodic patterns of various frequencies, and multifocal ictal patterns.

Neonatal encephalopathies should be characterized in functional terms based on both interictal and ictal abnormalities and on severity and persistence over time.[179] The persistence of abnormal patterns in serial studies is more significantly correlated with neurologic sequelae, although EEG patterns rarely denote a particular disease state. Brain lesions documented on neuroimaging or postmortem examination may have had an electrographic signature on EEG studies on an acute, subacute, or chronic basis. Therefore EEG patterns must be analyzed in the context of history, clinical findings, laboratory information, and neuroimaging.

Clinical Correlates of Neonatal Seizures

Neonatal seizures are not disease specific and may be caused by a number of medical conditions. Establishing a specific reason for seizures in any infant is helpful both for treatment and for prediction of neurologic outcome. Neonates with an encephalopathy or brain disorder may or may not have seizures, and they commonly come to attention because of a variety of disturbances.[175]

Asphyxia

Postasphyxial encephalopathy, the principal disorder during which neonatal seizures may occur, can also be accompanied by hypoglycemia, hypocalcemia, cerebrovascular accidents, or intraparenchymal hemorrhage. These latter conditions, individually or in combination, can contribute to seizures.

Most neonates experience asphyxia either before or during parturition. In only 10% of affected neonates does asphyxia result from postnatal causes. Intrauterine factors leading to asphyxia before or during labor and delivery compromise gas exchange or glucose movement across the placenta. These factors may be maternal (e.g., toxemia) or uteroplacental (e.g., placental abruption or cord compression) in origin. However, other maternal conditions, such as antepartum trauma or infection, not only are associated with acquired brain insults from asphyxia but also may contribute to the formation of congenital malformations during early pregnancy, as detected by fetal ultrasonography or cranial imaging of the infant immediately after birth. Respiratory distress syndrome, pulmonary hypertension of the newborn, and severe right-to-left cardiac shunts associated with congenital heart disease are other major causes of postnatal asphyxia in a newborn who may also experience seizures. Therefore the events that lead to asphyxia must be considered in the context of the findings of the maternal, placental, and neonatal examinations, as well as the corroborative laboratory results. Adverse events during labor and delivery may reflect longer-standing maternal, placental, or cord disorders that contribute to postnatal seizures, hypotonia, or coma. HIE, including neonatal seizures, develops in only 45% of infants who experience asphyxia at the time of birth.[180] Similarly, meconium staining of skin, placental tissue, or cord tissue can occur in asymptomatic infants with or without intrauterine insults. Distribution of meconium-laden macrophages throughout the placental amnion generally indicates fetal distress in the antepartum period.[181] Placental weights lower than the 10th or higher than the 90th percentile, altered placental villous morphology, lymphocytic infiltration, and erythroblastic proliferation in the villi indicate longer-term stress to the fetus, whether or not seizures occur during the period immediately after birth in a neonate who is neurologically depressed. In neonates with EEG-confirmed seizures, the odds that antepartum placental lesions would be identified increased by a factor of 12 as postconceptual age increased by 15 weeks.[182] Other findings on neurologic examination, such as hypertonia, joint contractures without profoundly depressed consciousness, seizures within the first hours after delivery, growth restriction, and neuroimaging evidence of encephalomalacia, separately or collectively point to the antepartum period as the time when brain injury occurred.

Hypoglycemia

Low blood glucose levels can result in seizures, either in association with asphyxia or as a separate metabolic consequence of the hypoglycemia. Infants of diabetic or toxemic mothers, those born as one of multiple-gestation siblings, and, less commonly, those with metabolic diseases, may also have hypoglycemia.

Hypocalcemia

Whereas hypoglycemia may be associated with seizures in neonates with asphyxia, hypocalcemia may be seen in the context of trauma, hemolytic disease, or metabolic disease. Hypomagnesemia may also occur in infants with hypocalcemia. Rarely, a form of hypocalcemia may be caused by congenital hypoparathyroidism or may occur with delayed onset in an infant who received a high-phosphate infant formula. Congenital cardiac lesions have been found in some infants with seizures caused by hypocalcemia or hypomagnesemia.[183]

Cerebrovascular Lesions

Intracranial hemorrhage as well as ischemic cerebrovascular lesions can occur as a result of asphyxia, trauma, or infection, or in association with developmental or congenital lesions. Intraventricular hemorrhage in the preterm infant who also has seizures has already been discussed.[184] However, full-term infants with seizures may also have intraventricular hemorrhage, usually arising within the choroid plexus or thalamus. Intracranial hemorrhage at other sites (e.g., subdural space, subarachnoid space, or into the parenchyma) can also be associated with seizures that occur together with, or independently of, postasphyxial encephalopathy.

Arterial and venous infarctions have been noted in neonates with seizures.[172,173] Cerebral infarctions can occur during the antepartum, intrapartum, or neonatal periods from diverse causes such as persistent pulmonary hypertension, polycythemia, and hypertensive encephalopathy. When isolated seizures occur in neonates with no accompanying encephalopathy, the cause can be timed to the antepartum period.[185]

Infection

Central nervous system (CNS) infection acquired in utero or postnatally may give rise to neonatal seizures. Congenital infections that are usually associated with a severe encephalitis are also accompanied by seizures and major interictal EEG background disturbances. For instance, neonatal herpes encephalitis is associated with severe ictal and interictal EEG pattern abnormalities consisting of multifocal seizures as well as multifocal periodic discharges.[186] Acquired in utero or postnatal bacterial infections caused by *Escherichia coli* or group B streptococci may result in neonatal seizures. *Listeria monocytogenes* and mycoplasma infections can also produce areas of lymphocytic infiltration and resultant encephalomalacia.

Central Nervous System Malformations

Brain lesions that result from either genetic or acquired defects during early fetal brain development also contribute to neonatal seizures. Such lesions include microgyria, heterotopia, and lissencephaly. Other dysgenic CNS conditions, such as holoprosencephaly, schizencephaly, and congenital hydrocephalus, may also be associated with neonatal seizures.

Inborn Errors of Metabolism

Inherited biochemical defects are relatively rare causes of neonatal seizures.[166] Peculiar body odors, intractable seizures that occur later in the newborn period, and persistently elevated lactate, pyruvate, ammonia, or amino acid levels in the blood may reflect inherited biochemical disorders rather than transient postasphyxial insults. Neonates with metabolic disease may also have otherwise normal prenatal and delivery histories. The emergence of food intolerance, increasing lethargy, and late onset of seizures may be the only indication of an inborn error of metabolism. Certain conditions are responsive to supplementation or dietary alteration; for example, vitamin B_6 dependency is a rare form of metabolic disturbance that can lead to intractable seizures, which are unresponsive to conventional antiepileptic medication.[187] Glucose transporter deficiency syndromes are suspected when CSF levels of glucose are low, and some patients may respond to the ketogenic diet regimen.[188]

Neonatal Epileptic Syndromes

Few clinical situations involving neonatal seizures represent a chronic epilepsy syndrome. Most seizures in newborns reflect transient disturbances that resolve over days (e.g., asphyxia, metabolic-toxic conditions, infections). Rarely, a newborn has an ongoing epileptic condition that is independent of, but perhaps is triggered by, adverse events during fetal or neonatal life. A rare form of familial neonatal seizures has been described with an autosomal dominant inheritance pattern.[189] The diagnosis requires careful exclusion of acquired causes. In two pedigrees, the genetic defect for this condition was assigned to two genetic loci on chromosome 20. Although most newborns with the disorder respond promptly to antiepileptic drug treatment and develop in an age-appropriate manner, some children experience delay at older ages. A defect in potassium-dependent channel kinetics has been described.

Other rare epileptic states include progressive syndromes associated with severe myoclonic seizures and progressive developmental delay. These children have been described as having an early infantile epileptic encephalopathy (Ohtahara syndrome) and usually have severe brain dysgenesis.

Treatment of Neonatal Seizures

Before antiepileptic medications are administered, an acute rapid infusion of glucose or other electrolytes such as calcium or magnesium should be considered. Low magnesium level and altered sodium metabolism are less common causes of neonatal seizures and do not require antiepileptic medications.[166]

Questions persist with respect to when, how, and for how long to administer antiepileptic medications to neonates who experience seizures. Some believe that neonates should undergo treatment only when the clinical signs of seizure are recognized and that brief electrographic seizures need not be treated. Others argue that this practice may be potentially harmful because undetected repetitive or continuous electrographic seizures may adversely affect the metabolism and cellular integrity of the immature brain. Consensus is lacking on the need for treatment when clinical seizure phenomena are minimal or absent.[168]

Major antiepileptic drug classes have been used to treat neonatal seizures. Phenobarbital is the most commonly used antiepileptic medication, with a recommended loading dose of 20 mg/kg and a maintenance dosage of 3 to 5 mg/kg/day. Half-life of the drug is long, 40 to 200 hours.

Phenytoin is the second most commonly used medication for the treatment of seizures. A loading dose of phenytoin is 15 to 20 mg/kg and a maintenance dosage is 4 to 8 mg/kg/day. Maintenance doses may be given intravenously or orally; however, oral absorption can be erratic.[190]

Some clinicians prefer to use benzodiazepines for the acute treatment of seizures, particularly when phenobarbital or phenytoin is no longer effective. Lorazepam is one choice in this class of medication, and the recommended intravenous dose is 0.1 mg/kg.[190] Other benzodiazepines such as diazepam or midazolam, which vary in half-life, have also been used. Benzodiazepines are not typically used for maintenance therapy because of the potential for tolerance and side effects.

For refractory seizures, new agents are available that have been used with some success as adjuvant therapy. Levetiracetam is the most common of these new agents, but its safety and efficacy data in neonates are limited. The small studies that have been done suggest that it prevents neurodegeneration better than other agents. Dosing begins at 10 mg/kg every 24 hours and can be increased to a maximum of 60 mg/kg/day. Mild sedation is the only side effect that has been observed.[191,192]

Free or unbound drug fractions have been suggested to affect the efficacy and potential toxicity of antiepileptic drugs in pediatric populations, including the neonatal population. Binding of drugs can be altered significantly in neonates with seizures, particularly in sick neonates with metabolic dysfunction. Biochemical alterations may cause toxic side effects by increasing the free fraction of the drug, which readily affects cardiovascular or respiratory function. Regular monitoring of serum drug levels (free and total), along with assessment of seizure control, may improve the titration of antiepileptic drugs.[193]

The decision to maintain or discontinue antiepileptic drug treatment is fraught with uncertainty.[166] Practice varies widely, with discontinuation of long-term therapy occurring from 1 week to 12 months after the last seizure. Because there is the potential for antiepileptic medications to damage the developing nervous system, prompt discontinuation in the late neonatal period or early infancy is recommended. This is especially true for infants who show no demonstrable brain lesions on cranial imaging, infants who exhibit appropriate findings on neurologic examination, and those who express normal interictal EEG background patterns.[3]

Despite the urgent need to establish the cause of a seizure, several unique aspects of neonatal seizures impede prompt diagnosis and treatment. There are a number of etiologic possibilities for neonatal seizures, and the efficacy of conventional antiepileptic drugs in controlling seizures remains controversial. Neonatal seizures can reflect either acute or remote disease processes or can result from a series of insults that began in the antepartum period and extend to include events during the intrapartum or postnatal periods. This knowledge of the acute or chronic causes of neonatal seizures will alter the clinician's choice of an antiepileptic treatment in the future. Neurorescue protective therapy such as hypothermia can be helpful, as can combinations of drugs that prevent seizures from arising in immature neuronal pathways that are injured, namely, phenobarbital and levetiracetam.

EDITORIAL COMMENT: Seizures occur in approximately 1 to 5 per 1000 live births and are often associated with serious underlying brain injury such as hypoxia-ischemia, stroke, hemorrhage, metabolic disturbances, and infection. Several age-specific factors particular to the developing brain influence seizure generation, response to medications, and impact of seizures on brain structure and function. Neonatal seizures because of acute brain injury are associated with high rates of death, disability, and epilepsy. Amplitude-integrated electroencephalograph (EEG) is a convenient and useful bedside tool to detect seizure activity, but continuous video electroencephalogram is the gold standard for detecting seizures.

(Bashir RA, Espinoza L, Vayalthrikkovil S, et al. Implementation of a neurocritical care program: improved seizure detection and decreased antiseizure medication at discharge in neonates with hypoxic-ischemic encephalopathy. *Pediatr Neurol.* 2016;64:38-43.)

HYPOTONIA IN THE TERM INFANT—NEUROMUSCULAR DISORDERS

Evaluation of tone in the newborn infant requires considerable experience and perseverance by the clinician.[194] The earlier section on clinical examination techniques discussed evaluation of the motor system and evaluation of the infant with altered tone, principally hypotonia and, less commonly, hypertonia. Clearly, the approach to the diagnosis of hypotonia requires an understanding of the neuroanatomic locations in the neuroaxis that may be responsible for producing low tone in the neonate. Such locations include the cerebrum, spinal cord, peripheral nerve, and neuromuscular junction or muscle. The clinical approach to hypotonia in the neonate is summarized in Table 17.8.

Most hypotonic neonates have disorders of the cerebrum. In these situations, hypotonia is usually not accompanied by profound weakness, and other signs of brain dysfunction, such as lethargy, swallowing difficulties, and abnormal primitive reflexes, are present. Hypotonia can be one prominent clinical manifestation of HIE (as discussed previously) or of other acute forms of neonatal disease with metabolic or infectious causes. Other cerebral causes of hypotonia are congenital infections and genetic diseases, including inherited disorders of metabolism involving glucose, amino acids, fatty acids, or peroxisomal pathways.

Peripheral causes of neonatal hypotonia also usually result in greater degrees of weakness, often including respiratory and swallowing difficulties. In cases of hypotonia associated with anterior horn cell disease (i.e., progressive spinal muscular atrophy), infants are alert, and their behavior is otherwise normal. In other clinical situations, such as neonatal myotonic dystrophy or Prader-Willi syndrome, there may be a mixture of central and peripheral involvement in motor pathways, causing hypotonia as well as other disorders of cerebral or systemic function.[195]

Neonatal myasthenia gravis should be considered in neonates who are the offspring of myasthenic mothers and who have hypotonia located at the neuromuscular junction. These infants exhibit cranial nerve deficits such as facial diparesis, ptosis, and ophthalmoplegia, as well as respiratory depression.[196] Exogenous causes of hypotonia include the administration of drugs to the mother, such as inappropriate systemic or local injections of anesthetics that pass to the infant through the placental circulation or are introduced directly into the infant's scalp at the time of administration of paracervical or pudendal blocks. These medications may cause a characteristic syndrome of hypotonia, respiratory depression, and seizures during the first day of life. Administration of magnesium or aminoglycoside may result in transient neuromuscular dysfunction leading to profound weakness and hypotonia.

Connective tissue abnormalities also may be associated with low tone, particularly those involving mesenchymal tissue, such as in Marfan syndrome and Ehlers-Danlos syndrome.

Myopathies associated with either specific muscular dystrophies or congenital myopathies can present with neonatal hypotonia and are generally accompanied by some degree of weakness or decrease in muscle bulk. A mixture of lower and upper motor neuron diseases is noted in certain congenital muscular dystrophies, as well as in mitochondrial myopathies.

EDITORIAL COMMENT: Neonatal hypotonia is a common problem in the neonatal intensive care unit. The genetic differential diagnosis is broad, encompassing primary muscular dystrophies, chromosome abnormalities, neuropathies, and inborn errors of metabolism in addition to maternal drug effects such as magnesium sulfate.

Because many disorders present similar clinical manifestations, the differentiation of the causes of neonatal hypotonia is difficult. Many genetic causes have been identified using next-generation sequencing, which provides the advantage of speed and diagnostic specificity without invasive procedures.

TABLE 17.8 Approach to Diagnosis of Hypotonia

		CLINICAL FEATURES						LABORATORY AIDS			
Anatomic Site	**Pathogenesis**	**Alertness**	**Cry**	**Eye Movements**	**Tongue Fasciculation**	**Deep Tendon Reflexes**	**Muscle Bulk**	**Electro-myography**	**Muscle Biopsy**	**Muscle Enzyme (CPK)[a]**	**Neostigmine**
Cerebral	Malformation Hemorrhage Hypoxia-ischemia Metabolic disorder Infection Drugs	Poor	Poor	Occasionally abnormal	No	Normal or increased	Normal	Normal	Normal	Normal	Negative
Spinal cord	Injury	Good	Normal	Normal	No	Decreased or increased	Normal	Normal	Normal	Normal	Negative
Anterior horn cell	Spinal muscular atrophy (Werdnig-Hoffmann disease)	Good	Normal or weak	Normal	Yes	Absent	Decreased	Neurogenic pattern	Neuro-genic group	Normal	Negative
Neuro-muscular junction	Neonatal myasthenia gravis	Good	Weak	Abnormal	No	Normal	Normal	± Normal	Normal	Normal	Negative
Muscle	Congenital myopathy	Good	Good	Normal	No	Decreased or normal	Decreased	Myopathic pattern	Myop-athic change	Normal or elevated	Positive

[a]*CPK*, Creatine phosphokinase.

18

Neonatal Imaging

Sheila C. Berlin, Mariana L. Meyers

Imaging provides anatomic and functional information critical to the care of the high-risk neonate. An expanding selection of imaging tools offers safe and timely diagnostic procedures for infants both before and after birth. Advances such as fetal magnetic resonance imaging (MRI) and point-of-care ultrasound provide new opportunities to impact patient care earlier in the disease process. This chapter reviews imaging modalities key to the evaluation of the critically ill neonate, including both commonly performed radiographic and sonographic exams as well as more complex imaging techniques. Following an introduction to imaging by modality, the chapter will review the imaging approach to common medical and surgical conditions of the high-risk neonate.

IMAGING MODALITIES

Radiography, Fluoroscopy, and Computed Tomography

Radiography of the chest and abdomen comprises the vast majority of imaging performed in the immediate postnatal period. Digital radiography, a widely available and relatively inexpensive diagnostic examination, can be performed at the bedside with minimal disruption to a fragile patient. Because a large number of portable radiographs may be performed in critically ill neonates, attention has been drawn to the potential cancer risk from cumulative doses of ionizing radiation from these exams. The radiation dose of a portable chest radiograph is approximately 0.02 mSv; this is a very small fraction of the 3 mSv of annual natural background radiation to which the average individual is exposed. Commonly performed fluoroscopy procedures in the newborn, such as an upper gastrointestinal series (UGI), contrast enema, or voiding cystourethrogram, can be performed at doses between 0.5 and 2.0 mSv. Computed tomography (CT) is also performed at low-radiation doses; most head and body CT scans can be performed at a dose less than 2 mSv. Current literature indicates that the risk of a future cancer from low-dose radiation (below 100 mSv for serial exams) is "too low to be detectable and likely nonexistent."[1] In the absence of data confirming a causal relationship between low-dose radiation from medical imaging and cancer, parents and providers should be reassured that the benefits of a medically necessary examination far exceed any potential future cancer risk.[2] Current recommendations endorse limiting radiation exposure to doses that are "as low as reasonably achievable"[3] by using patient size-based tube current and tube voltage, attention to patient positioning, artifact removal, and beam collimation.

Short scan times allow nearly all newborns to undergo CT scans of the brain and body without the need for sedation. Iodine-based intravenous contrast may be administered to evaluate for cardiovascular abnormalities, neoplasm, or infectious disease. In the absence of known renal failure, neonates show no increased risk for renal toxicity after receiving iodinated intravenous contrast material.[4] A distinct disadvantage of CT imaging is the lack of portability. Because CT equipment requires room shielding and a relatively large footprint and is highly sensitive to small fluctuations in temperature and humidity, patients must travel to the radiology CT suite for imaging.

Ultrasound

Following radiography, sonography is the most common imaging examination performed in the neonate. Ultrasound is particularly suitable for newborns because of its low cost, accessibility, portability, lack of ionizing radiation, and absence of known health risks. There is no need for patient sedation, and operators can easily capture both static and cine images that include characterization of flow dynamics with color and spectral Doppler. High-quality sonographic images are far more dependent on operator skill than any other imaging modality. Knowledge of both normal and abnormal anatomy, identification of optimal windows, and appropriate selection of ultrasound probes of varying frequencies are critical to obtaining diagnostic images. Small handheld ultrasound devices now offer rapid, real-time options for acute point-of-care diagnostic images performed by neonatologists.[5,6] The role of lung ultrasound has increased in some centers where trained neonatologists use bedside sonography to diagnose respiratory distress syndrome, transient tachypnea of the newborn, neonatal pneumonia, pneumothorax, and atelectasis.[7] Because sound waves travel poorly through air and calcified structures, sonographic evaluation is limited if obscured by gas-filled bowel, aerated lung, or overlying bone. Another disadvantage of ultrasound is the relatively low spatial resolution relative to CT and MRI.

Magnetic Resonance Imaging

MRI can provide vital detailed information that ultrasound and CT cannot—particularly in the diagnosis of traumatic or anoxic brain injury and congenital anomalies. Gadolinium-based intravenous contrast may be used without risk of renal toxicity in the absence of known renal failure.[4] Despite scan times that may exceed 30 minutes, the majority of infants under 3 months of age can be scanned without sedation using the "feed and swaddle" technique.[8] Because MR scanners require housing in a carefully shielded and monitored physical space, MR scanning in the most fragile infants is infrequent. New dedicated infant-sized MR scanners designed to be housed in the neonatal intensive care unit (NICU) may offer a solution to the risks of infection and injury while minimizing the disruption of care for critically ill neonates and their families.[9]

Fetal Magnetic Resonance Imaging

Over the past 20 years, there have been numerous developments in fetal and perinatal management. Although ultrasound remains the screening modality of choice in the prenatal period, fetal MRI has become a valuable adjunct to evaluate the fetus requiring additional diagnostic imaging. Advantages of MRI such as high soft tissue contrast, large field of view, and high resolution can help exclude or confirm diagnoses suggested by ultrasound.[10,11] Quantitative MRI analysis provides measurements of structural volumes in the fetus. In congenital diaphragmatic hernia (CDH), congenital pulmonary airway malformation (CPAM), and other processes associated with pulmonary hypoplasia, calculating the total lung volume is helpful to determine prognosis, assess for in utero fetoscopic endoluminal tracheal occlusion treatment, provide parental counseling, and plan a safe delivery.[12,13,14,15,16,17,18] In cases of cervical masses or severe micrognathia, MRI can visualize the airway for patency and contribute to planning a safe delivery. Some centers perform ex utero intrapartum treatment (EXIT) procedures when there is high risk of airway obstruction or a repairable malformation that puts the infant at high risk of respiratory insufficiency at birth.

Fetal MRI has become integral to both identifying at-risk infants who may benefit from in utero intervention as well as preparing for optimal perinatal management.

Scintigraphy

Nuclear medicine contributes to the care of newborns with congenital anomalies, infection, and neoplasm. Radiopharmaceuticals, otherwise known as "tracers," are nonallergenic and have shown no toxic effects. The radiation dose for most exams is between 0.6 to 5.5 mSv, in the range of CT imaging. Though most studies require that the patient remain still for a relatively long period of time, most neonates can be imaged without sedation.[19] As with CT and ultrasound, these exams require patient transport to the nuclear medicine suite of the radiology department.

CHEST

Evaluating a Normal Chest

The chest radiograph is the most commonly performed imaging examination in the critically ill neonate. Portable chest radiographs are obtained using an anteroposterior (AP) projection in the supine infant. The arms should be extended away from the body or above the head and the torso immobilized. With proper positioning, the radiograph should demonstrate symmetry of the clavicles and ribs and a midline superior mediastinum (Fig. 18.1). A rotation-distorted image may obscure or mimic cardiac and pulmonary pathology.

Familiarity with the normal appearance of the newborn chest radiograph improves recognition of pathologic changes. Normal lungs appear primarily radiolucent and symmetric in volume. The pulmonary vessels are seen as branching, linear shadows that taper in size as they extend from the hilum to the lung periphery. Normally collapsed, the pleural space is visualized only when it is distended from fluid, air, or pleural thickening. The heart borders should be distinct, and the diaphragm should be outlined clearly against aerated lung. The normal thymus is visible on the chest radiograph of most newborns. Extremely variable in size and shape, it is composed of two asymmetric lobes and may therefore have an asymmetric appearance in chest radiography. The "wavy" undulations of the lateral borders often silhouette a portion of the heart and can give the appearance of cardiomegaly.

Catheters, Tubes, and Lines

Positioning of life support devices should be documented on all radiographs. The endotracheal tube (ETT) tip should overlie in the trachea between the medial ends of the clavicles and the carina. Intubation of the right mainstem bronchus is the most common site of tube malposition and may result in volume loss in the right upper lobe and left lung (Fig. 18.2). The enteric tube should terminate in the stomach body, beyond the gastroesophageal junction.

Umbilical catheters are easily identified by their characteristic paths (Fig. 18.3). The umbilical venous catheter (UVC) courses superiorly and gradually posteriorly within the umbilical vein to intersect the left portal vein, continuing through the ductus venosus, left or middle hepatic vein, and then into the inferior vena cava (IVC). Its tip should be directed superiorly, ending at the right atrial (RA)/IVC junction. Malposition

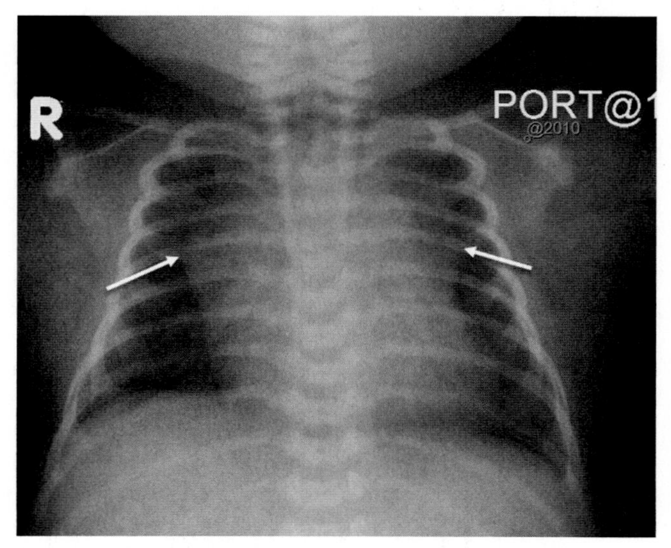

Fig. 18.1 Normal anteroposterior chest radiograph. Wavy appearance of the normal thymic borders *(arrows)*.

of the UVC within the liver is the most common complication and may result in portal vein thrombosis or portal hypertension. The umbilical arterial catheter (UAC) courses inferiorly to the junction of the umbilical artery and internal iliac artery before turning superiorly into the common iliac artery and aorta. The tip of the UAC should terminate below the ductus arteriosus and above or below the visceral arteries; in a "high position," the tip ends between T6 and T10, and in a "low position," the tip ends between L3 and L5.

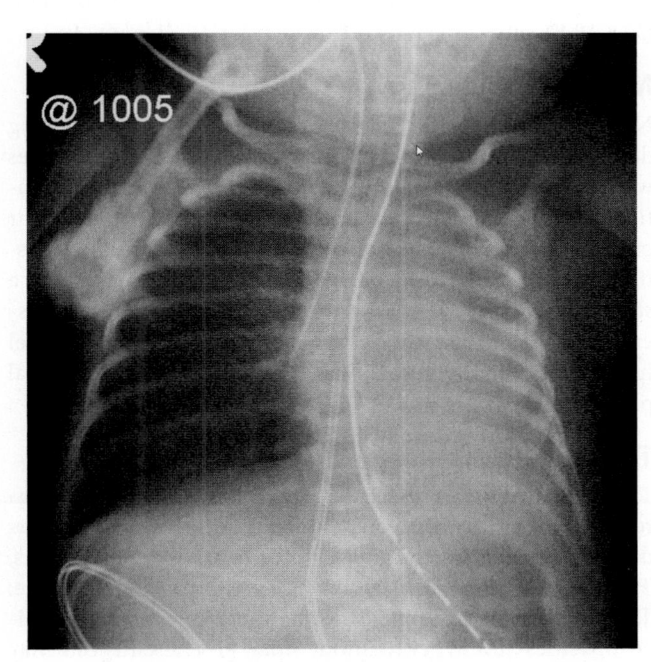

Fig. 18.2 Malposition of the endotracheal tube. Anteroposterior chest radiograph shows the tip of the endotracheal tube in the right main bronchus with left lung atelectasis.

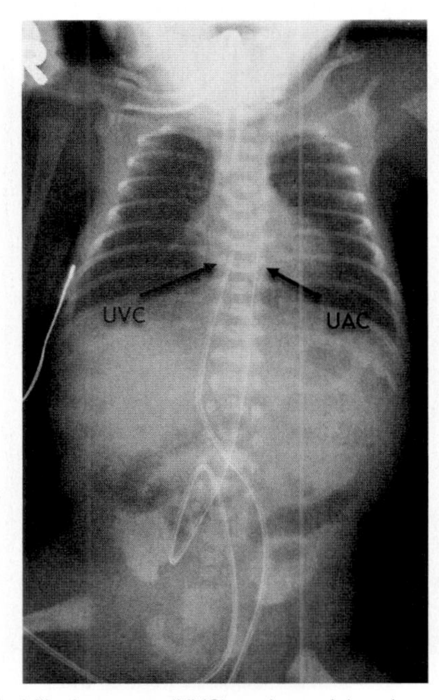

Fig. 18.3 Umbilical venous (UVC) and arterial catheter (UAC) positions on chest/abdominopelvic radiograph.

The position of percutaneously placed catheters, including peripheral inserted central venous catheters (PICC lines), central venous catheters, and extracorporeal membrane oxygenation (ECMO) catheters, must also be documented. The tip of an upper-extremity PICC line or central venous catheter should lie within the superior vena cava (SVC) or at the RA/SVC junction. A lower-extremity PICC line should end between the 9th and 12th ribs. An ECMO circuit may use a venous and an arterial catheter or a dual lumen veno-venous catheter. The venous catheter is inserted through the right internal jugular vein and ends in the RA. The arterial catheter is inserted into the common carotid artery and ends near the origin of the innominate artery.

Respiratory Distress Syndrome

Respiratory distress syndrome (RDS) from surfactant deficiency is the most common cause of respiratory distress and a leading cause of morbidity in the premature infant.

The typical radiographic appearance of RDS reflects generalized alveolar collapse and shows a finely granular or ground-glass pattern with diminished lung volumes. The severity of radiographic disease is variable and usually correlates with the severity of clinical disease. Mild radiographic disease is characterized by a finely granular pattern that allows visualization of normal vessels (Fig. 18.4), whereas severe disease results in silhouetting of the heart borders and diaphragm. Air bronchograms may be seen with severe disease because of air in the bronchi visualized against a background of alveolar collapse. The distribution of disease is usually diffuse and symmetric; however, patchy or asymmetric disease may be seen. The radiographic changes associated with RDS are often seen immediately after birth but can also develop over the first 6 to 12 hours of life. The radiographic abnormalities related to uncomplicated RDS should resolve by the time the neonate is 3 to 4 days of age. New diffuse worsening of bilateral opacities in the lungs may be seen with pulmonary

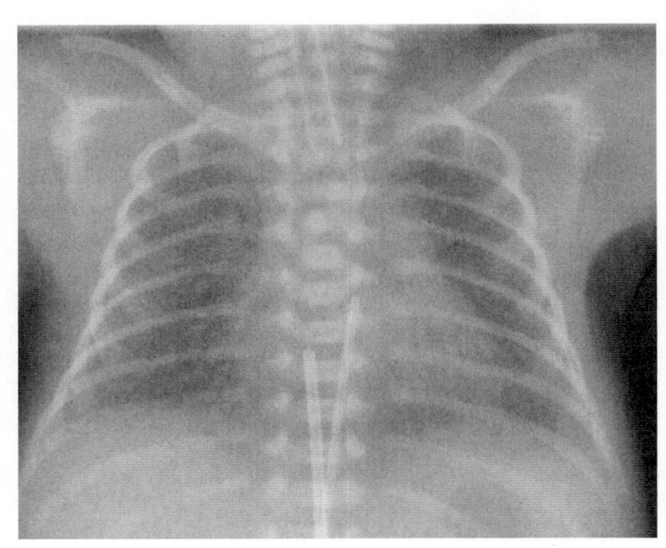

Fig. 18.4 Respiratory distress syndrome. Anteroposterior chest radiograph shows fine granular opacity overlies both lungs.

edema or pulmonary hemorrhage. The acute appearance of focal parenchymal opacity suggests atelectasis.

Complications can result from the high distending pressures of mechanical ventilation that may be required in the treatment of RDS. Alveolar rupture from overdistention may result in pulmonary interstitial emphysema (PIE). PIE may be diffuse or localized and appears as linear meandering lucencies from interstitial air coursing along the bronchovascular sheaths (Fig. 18.5). Interstitial air may result in a larger focal air collection and create a discrete parenchymal pseudocyst. Interstitial air can dissect into the mediastinum or the pleural space, resulting in a pneumomediastinum or pneumothorax. Radiographic signs of pneumomediastinum include lateral displacement of the mediastinal pleura, a continuous diaphragm, and superior elevation of the thymus (Fig. 18.6A,B). Radiographic findings of pneumothorax include increased lucency, identification of the visceral pleural line, and increased sharpness of the adjacent mediastinal border or hemidiaphragm. Lateral decubitus or cross-table lateral radiographs can be useful in the detection of pneumothoraces (Fig. 18.7). Large pneumothoraces can produce tension, resulting in contralateral shift of mediastinal structures and depression or eversion of the ipsilateral hemidiaphragm (Fig. 18.8).

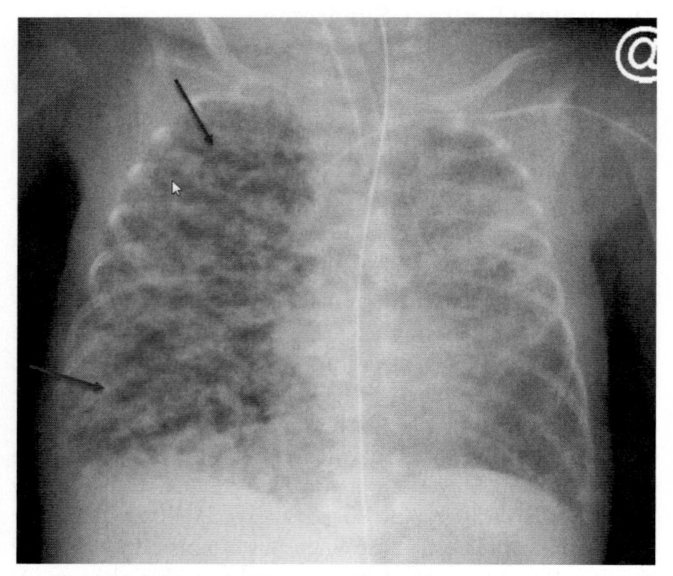

Fig. 18.5 Pulmonary interstitial emphysema. Anteroposterior chest radiograph shows meandering radiolucencies throughout the right lung *(arrows)*.

Neonatal Pneumonia

Neonatal pneumonias may be acquired in utero, during delivery, or after birth. Infection typically disseminates widely throughout the lungs because of incomplete formation of the interlobar fissures at this age. Diffuse granular or ground-glass opacities are often seen and may be indistinguishable from RDS. Alternatively, coarse nodularity or a streaky, hazy appearance of the lungs may be seen. The presence of pleural fluid should raise the suspicion of bacterial infection because effusions are uncommon in RDS or viral pneumonia.[20]

Transient Tachypnea of the Newborn

Transient tachypnea of the newborn (TTN) results from retained lung fluid that may be associated with precipitous delivery or cesarean section. Typically a clinical diagnosis, TTN has a varied and nonspecific radiographic appearance. The radiograph may appear normal or show streaky, perihilar opacities and hyperinflation. Small pleural effusions may also be seen (Fig. 18.9). A normal heart size helps distinguish retained fluid from pulmonary edema or heart failure. The radiographic and clinical findings of TTN usually resolve within the first 24 to 48 hours of life.

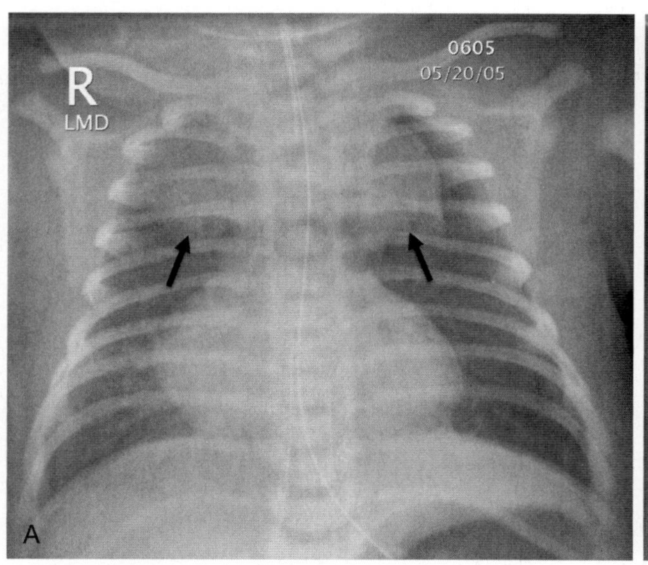

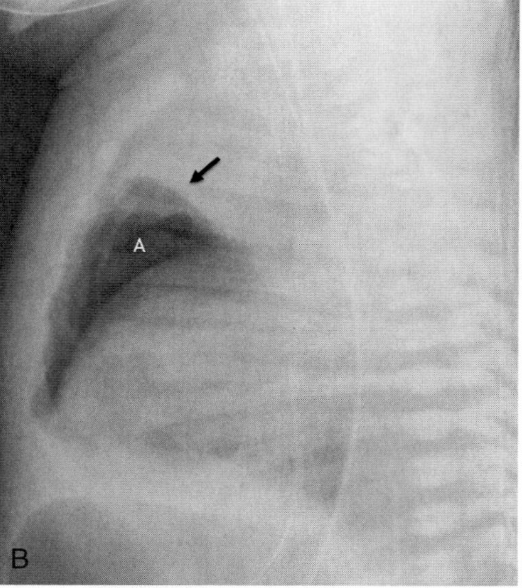

Fig. 18.6 Pneumomediastinum. Anteroposterior chest radiograph (A) shows superior displacement of the thymus *(arrows)*. Lateral radiograph (B) of the chest demonstrates air *(A)* in the mediastinum uplifting the thymus *(arrow)*.

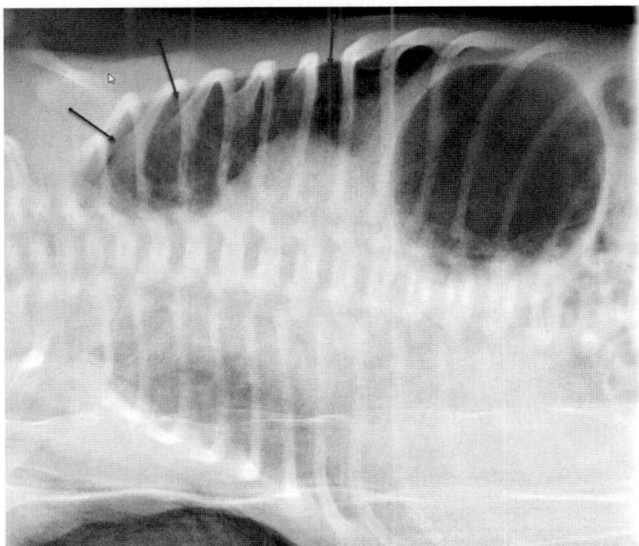

Fig. 18.7 Pneumothorax. Decubitus view of the chest shows radiolucency outlining the left lung.

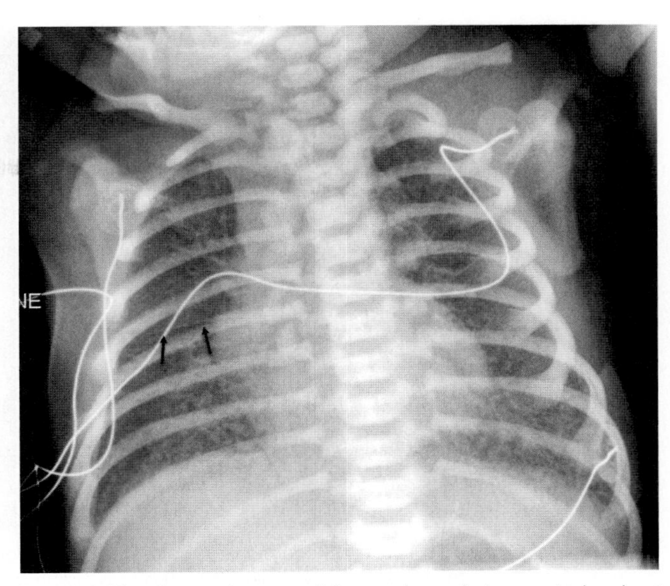

Fig. 18.9 Transient tachypnea of the newborn. Anteroposterior chest radiograph shows bilateral symmetric interstitial fluid and pleural fluid *(arrows)*. Normal heart size.

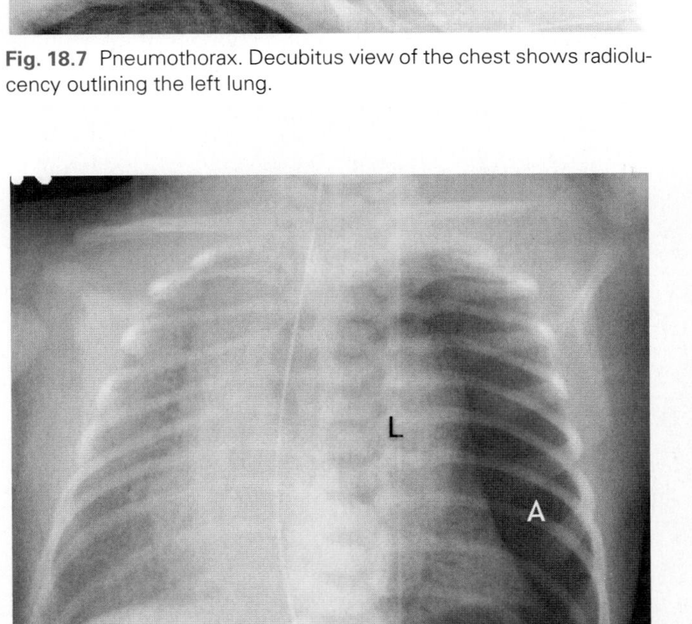

Fig. 18.8 Tension pneumothorax. Air *(A)* fills the left pleural space and causes compressive atelectasis of the left lung (L) and midline shift rightward.

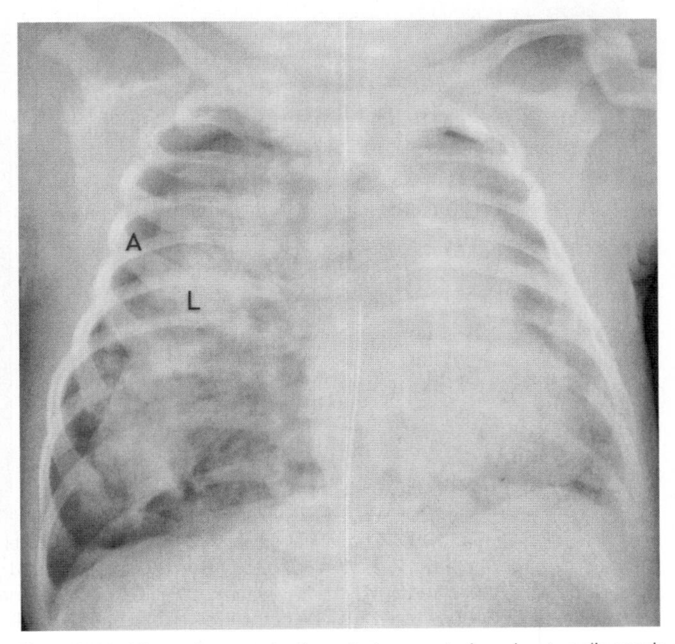

Fig. 18.10 Meconium aspiration. Anteroposterior chest radiograph demonstrates coarse, patchy asymmetric alveolar opacity throughout both lungs. Right pneumothorax *(A)* outlines the right lung *(L)*.

Meconium Aspiration Syndrome

Fetal aspiration of meconium causes obstruction of small airways with associated atelectasis and air trapping. Radiographic findings of meconium aspiration syndrome present in the first few hours of life and include coarse, patchy, or nodular opacities; segmental hyperinflation; and possible pleural effusion. The distribution of disease is bilateral and often asymmetric. Complications include chemical pneumonitis, surfactant inactivation, pulmonary hypertension, and air-leak phenomena such as pneumothorax and pneumomediastinum (Fig. 18.10).

Pulmonary Hemorrhage

In intubated patients, the diagnosis of pulmonary hemorrhage is usually established by detecting blood in the endotracheal tube. The radiographic appearance of pulmonary hemorrhage is variable and nonspecific: small amounts of hemorrhage may not be visible, but more extensive hemorrhage results in focal or diffuse ground-glass opacities. Findings may mimic pneumonia or pulmonary edema. The radiographic changes from a single episode of pulmonary hemorrhage are usually transient, resolving within 24 to 48 hours. More recently, bedside ultrasound has been used to diagnose pulmonary hemorrhage.[21]

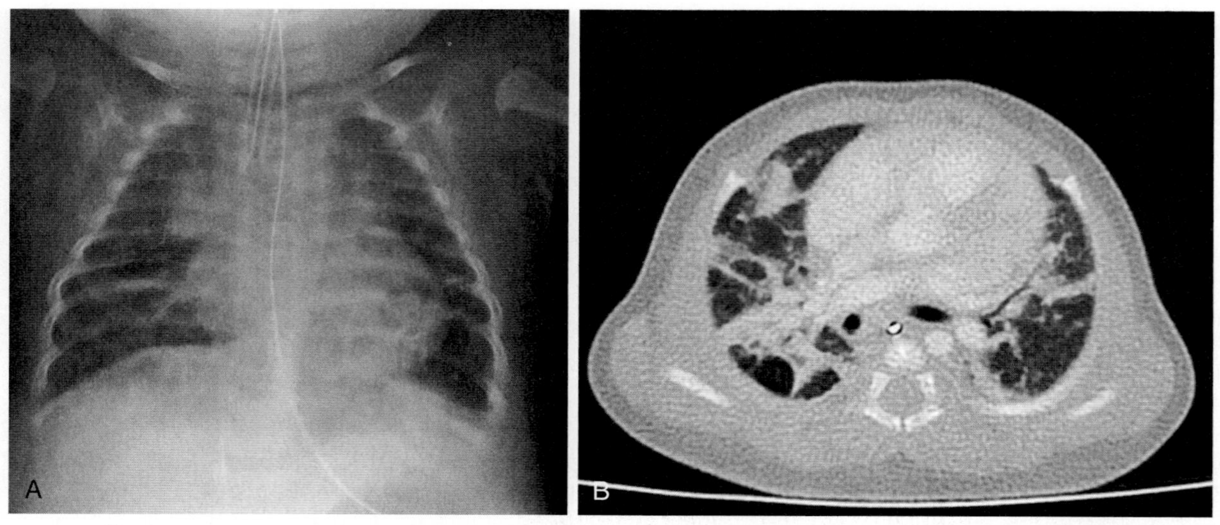

Fig. 18.11 Bronchopulmonary dysplasia. (A) Anteroposterior chest radiograph shows diffuse, coarse parenchymal opacities. (B) Axial computed tomography shows bilateral fibrosis and air trapping.

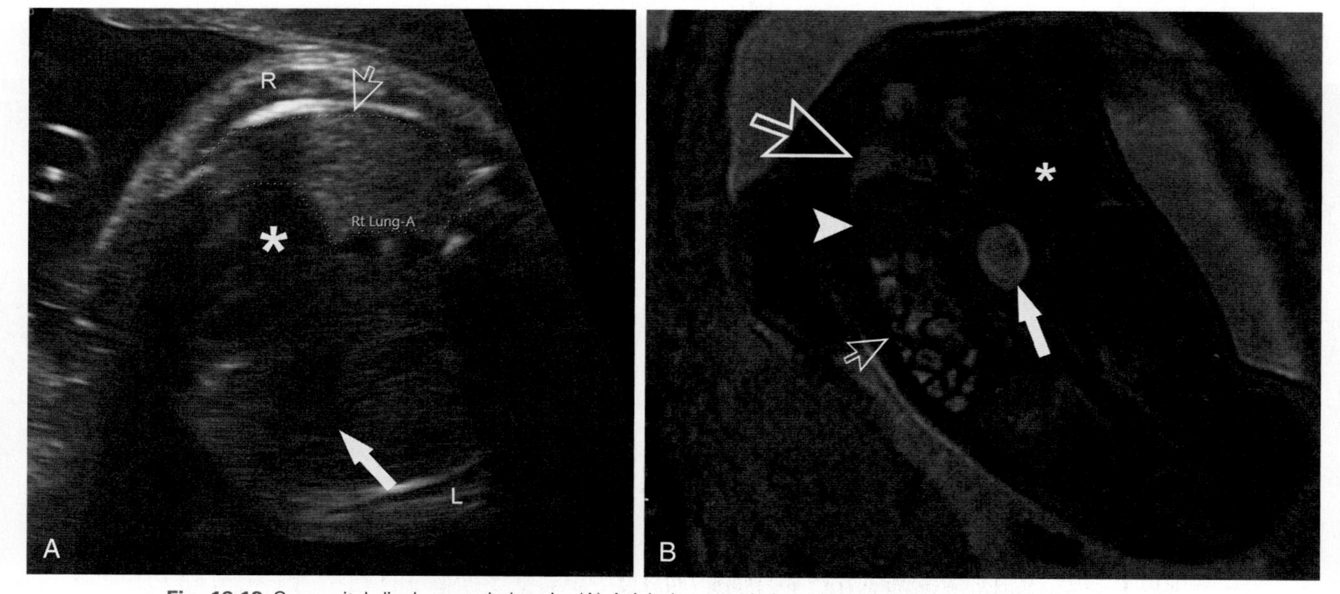

Fig. 18.12 Congenital diaphragmatic hernia. (A) Axial ultrasound shows herniated organs in the left chest with the heart (*) displaced to the right chest *(open arrow)*. R, right, L, left. The stomach *(white solid arrow)* is partially obscured by rib-shadowing artifact. (B) Coronal fetal magnetic resonance imaging through the chest better depicts the herniated left lobe of the liver *(arrowhead)*, fluid-filled small bowel loops *(small open arrow)*, and stomach *(solid arrow)* adjacent to the very hypoplastic lung *(large open arrow)*. The heart (*) is displaced to the right hemothorax.

Bronchopulmonary Dysplasia

Classic chest radiograph findings of bronchopulmonary dysplasia include: hyperinflation; asymmetric, coarse, and patchy opacities; and cystic emphysematous changes.[22] CT findings range from near-normal to disordered lung architecture with hyperlucent areas, linear and subpleural opacities, and bullae typical of chronic lung disease (Fig. 18.11A,B).[23–25]

Congenital Diaphragmatic Hernia

CDH is a complex, life-threatening lesion caused by defective fusion of the pleuroperitoneal folds during embryologic development. Bowel and solid organs may herniate through the foramen of Bochdalek into the hemithorax. Though more common on the left, hernias may occur on the right side or bilaterally. The role of prenatal imaging is instrumental in delivery and perinatal planning. Quantitative measurements of the lungs and thorax can help predict the risk of neonatal pulmonary insufficiency and need for EXIT procedure or immediate perinatal intubation. The size of the main right and left pulmonary arteries are assessed using the McGoon index to help predict the risk of postnatal pulmonary hypertension.[26] MRI provides the most detailed assessment of the herniated organs and provides valuable prognostic information in patients where a lobe or the entire liver is in the thorax (Fig. 18.12A,B).

At birth, fluid-filled bowel appears as nonspecific opacity over the ipsilateral hemithorax. Within the first 24 to 48 hours of life, air fills bowel loops in the thorax, and a paucity of bowel loops is apparent in the abdomen. The ipsilateral lung is almost universally hypoplastic, and there is usually contralateral mediastinal shift, resulting in contralateral lung hypoplasia (Fig. 18.13).

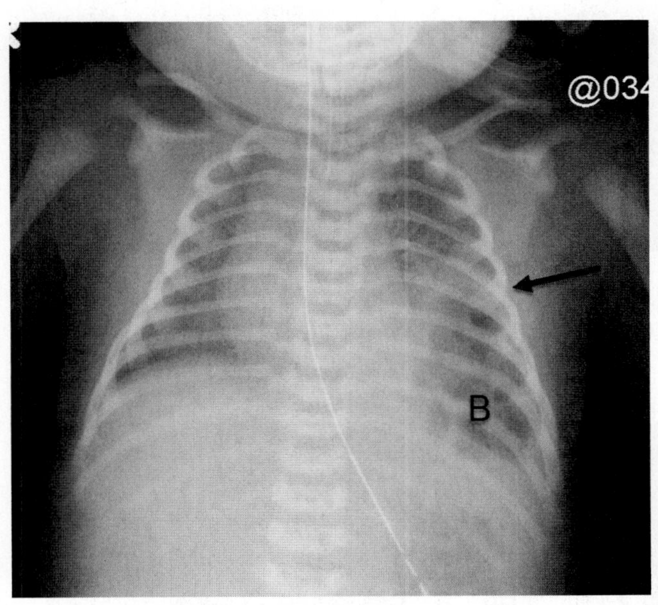

Fig. 18.13 Congenital diaphragmatic hernia. Anteroposterior radiograph shows gas-filled bowel *(B)* in the lower left hemithorax with preserved aeration of the left lung above the superior margin of the hernia *(arrow)*.

Congenital Pulmonary Airway Malformations and Bronchopulmonary Sequestration

CPAMs are a group of congenital, hamartomatous cystic and noncystic lung masses characterized by overgrowth of the primary bronchioles and a proximal communication with a defective bronchial tree.[27] Bronchopulmonary sequestration is a lesion containing bronchial and pulmonary tissue without communicating with the tracheobronchial tree or pulmonary arteries. They can be extralobar (extrapleural) or intralobar (intrapleural), and either supradiaphragmatic or infradiaphragmatic. These lesions will appear mostly solid in imaging, and the systemic feeding vessel is frequently identified on prenatal ultrasound and MRI (Fig. 18.14A,B).

Prenatal sonography and fetal MR classifies CPAMs primarily based on the presence of macrocysts, microcysts, or solid tissue (Fig. 18.15A,B). The CPAM volume ratio is calculated to predict the risk of hydrops in the setting of the pulmonary lesion; prenatal ultrasound and fetal MRI provide similar metrics.[28] MRI can confirm or exclude the presence of a systemic vessel arising from the aorta in the setting of a "hybrid" lesion.

At birth, chest radiography may show a range of findings from a large single or multiple air-filled cystic structures to solid lesions that resemble consolidation. CT angiography (CTA) provides the most detailed anatomic evaluation of the lung parenchymal and vascular anatomy of these lesions in the postnatal period.

Congenital Lobar Overinflation

Congenital lobar overinflation (CLO) is a condition characterized by progressive overinflation of one or more pulmonary lobes. CLO most commonly affects the left upper lobe,

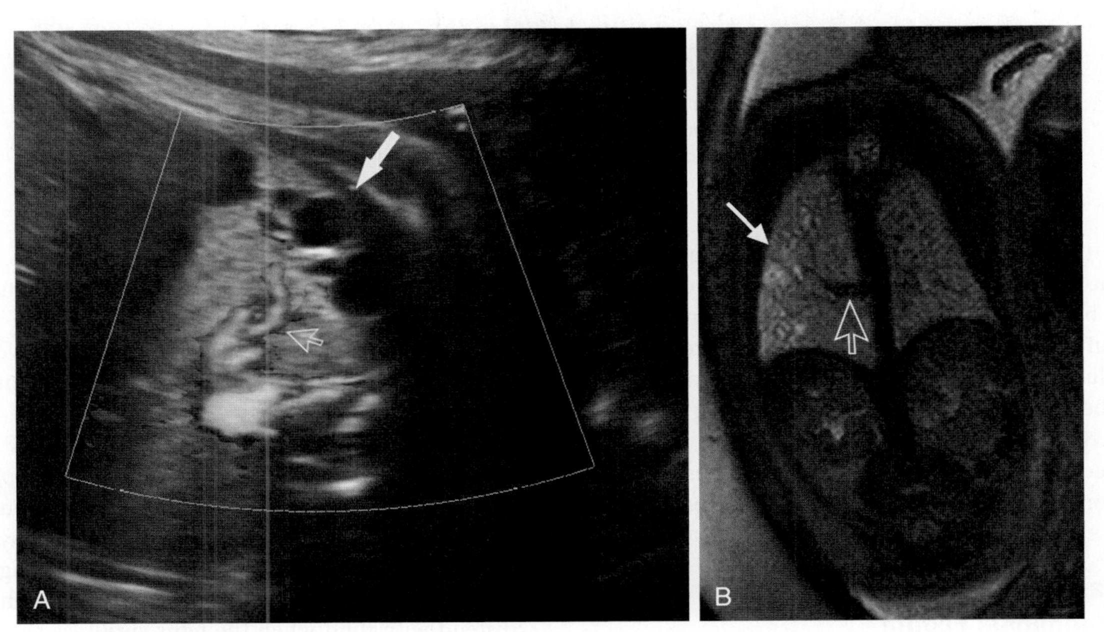

Fig. 18.14 Bronchopulmonary sequestration. (A) Axial ultrasound with Doppler image shows cystic and solid lesion *(solid arrow)* in the chest with a systemic vessel *(open arrow)* arising from the aorta. (B) Coronal magnetic resonance imaging image shows mixed solid and cystic lesion *(solid arrow)* and the systemic vessel arising from the aorta *(open arrow)*.

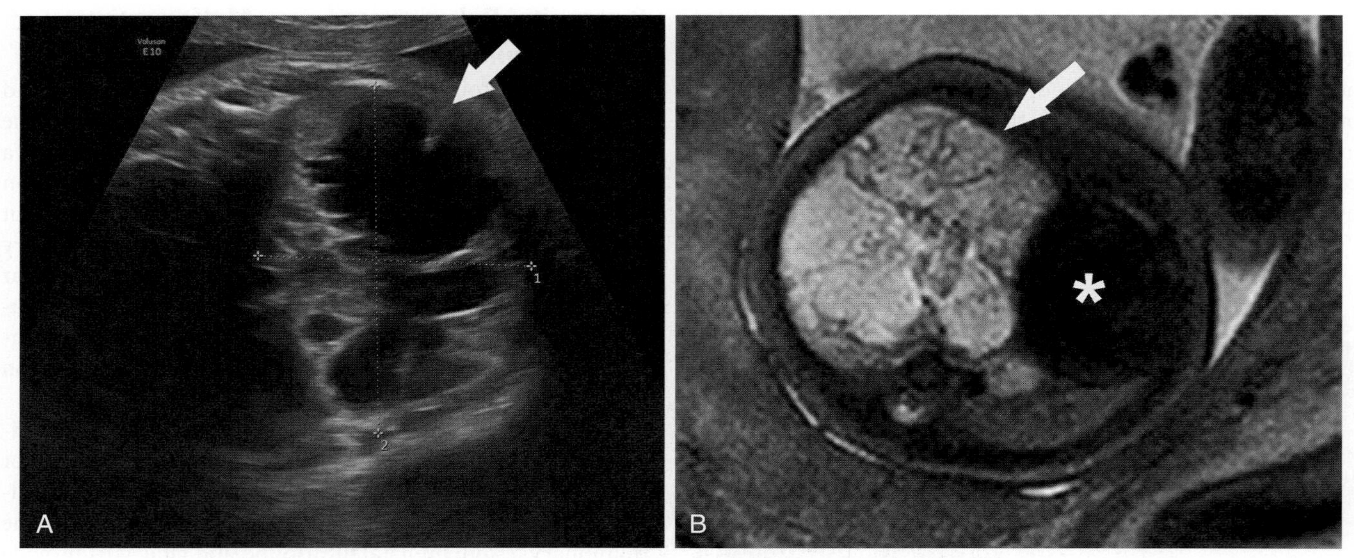

Fig. 18.15 Congenital pulmonary airway malformation. (A) Axial fetal sonographic image shows a lesion with cystic spaces divided by thick septations in half of the thorax *(arrow)*. (B) Axial fetal magnetic resonance imaging image shows the right-sided lesion containing septations and hyperintense fluid *(arrow)*. Leftward displacement of the heart (*).

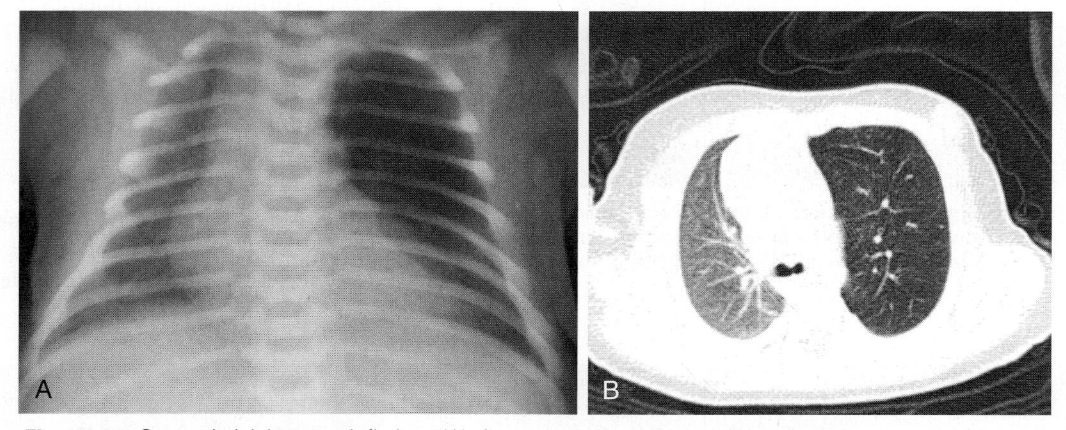

Fig. 18.16 Congenital lobar overinflation. (A) Anteroposterior chest radiograph demonstrates abnormal lucency of the left upper lobe and rightward mediastinal shift. (B) Axial chest computed tomography shows marked overinflation of the left upper lobe with attenuated vascular markings, contralateral mediastinal shift, and compression of the normal left lung.

followed by the right middle lobe and the right upper lobe. At birth, the involved lobe may appear opaque on a chest radiograph because of retained lung fluid. When the fluid clears, imaging demonstrates progressively increased volume, hyperlucency, and attenuated vascular markings of the involved lobe with compression of the remaining ipsilateral lung and mediastinal shift (Fig. 18.16A,B).[27] CT characterizes the precise lobar involvement and excludes extrinsic bronchial compression such as vascular anomalies or mediastinal masses.

Esophageal Atresia and Tracheoesophageal Fistula

The pairing of the terms *esophageal atresia* and *tracheoesophageal fistula (TEF)* describes a disorder in formation and separation of the primitive foregut, specifically abnormal separation of the bronchial tree and esophagus. A spectrum of malformations is noted, ranging from esophageal atresia (with or without a proximal or distal TEF) to a TEF without esophageal atresia. The most common type, involving proximal esophageal atresia with a distal TEF, accounts for more than 80% of cases.

The findings of esophageal atresia and TEF are difficult to identify with prenatal imaging. With esophageal atresia, there is polyhydramnios because of interruption of the swallowing-voiding cycle, and the stomach may be small or not fluid filled. In conjunction with static images, dynamic MRI cine images may show the proximal esophageal pouch distend with fluid when the fetus swallows and decompress when the fluid is expelled by the oral cavity because of downstream obstruction. If there is a fistulous communication with the airway, then the fluid may trickle into the airway

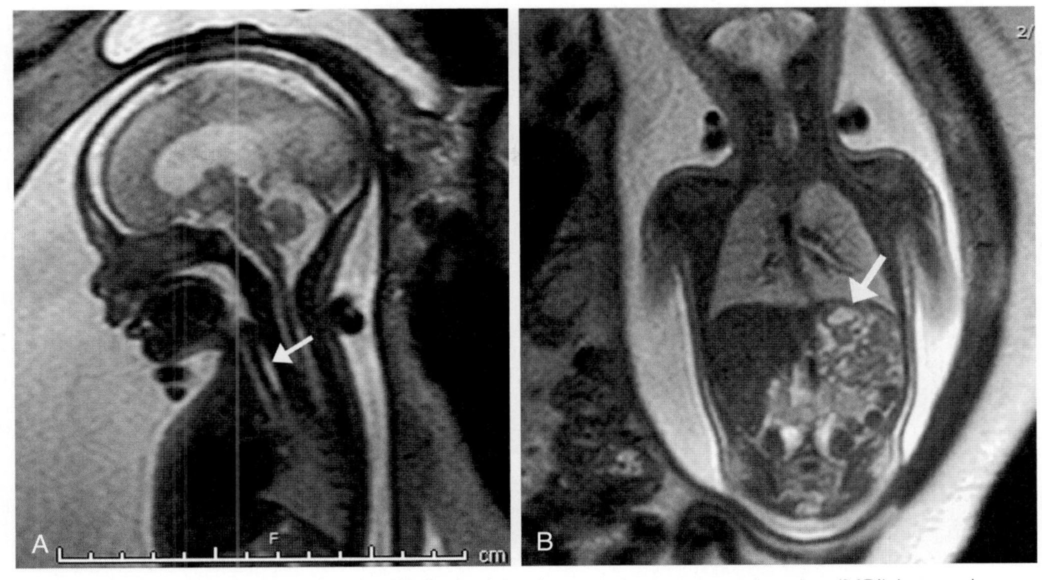

Fig. 18.17 Tracheoesophageal fistula. (A) Sagittal fetal magnetic resonance imaging (MRI) image demonstrating the fluid-filled esophageal pouch *(arrow)*, which distended and collapsed on real-time imaging (not shown). (B) Coronal fetal MRI image in the same fetus shows minimally fluid-filled stomach *(arrow)* associated with esophageal atresia. There was associated polyhydramnios.

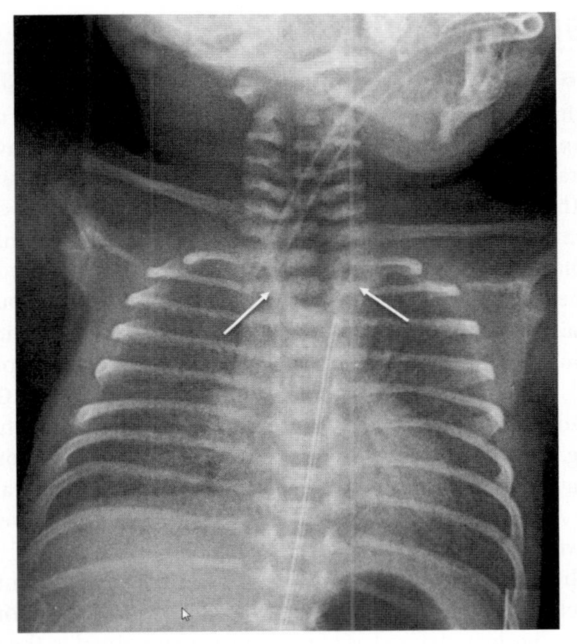

Fig. 18.18 Esophageal atresia with distal fistula. Anteroposterior chest radiograph demonstrates a blind-ending esophageal pouch *(arrows)* in this intubated patient.

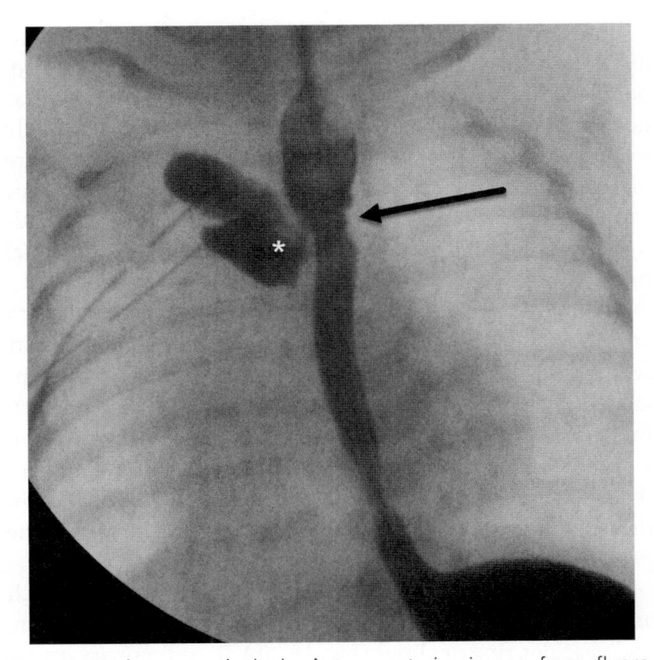

Fig. 18.19 Anastomotic leak. Anteroposterior image from fluoroscopic contrast swallow shows a contained bilobed leak *(asterisk)* along the right side of the esophageal anastomosis *(arrow)*.

and explain the lack of visualization of the blind pouch (Fig. 18.17A,B). When esophageal atresia with or without TEF is suspected prenatally, it is important to evaluate the thoracic, abdominal organs, and skeletal structures, including the spine, to rule out VACTERL syndrome (vertebral defects, anal atresia, cardiac defects, TEF, renal anomalies, and limb abnormalities).

After birth, a blind-ending, air-filled proximal esophageal pouch is noted on a chest radiograph (Fig. 18.18) in patients with esophageal atresia. The presence of a distal fistula is supported by air in the gastrointestinal tract. An esophagram can be performed to evaluate for a fistulous tract. Postoperative esophagram is performed to evaluate for anastomotic leak or stricture (Fig. 18.19).

Heart

Cardiac disease in infants is usually congenital in origin. Chest radiography rarely leads to a specific diagnosis and is primarily used to exclude pulmonary conditions as a cause of

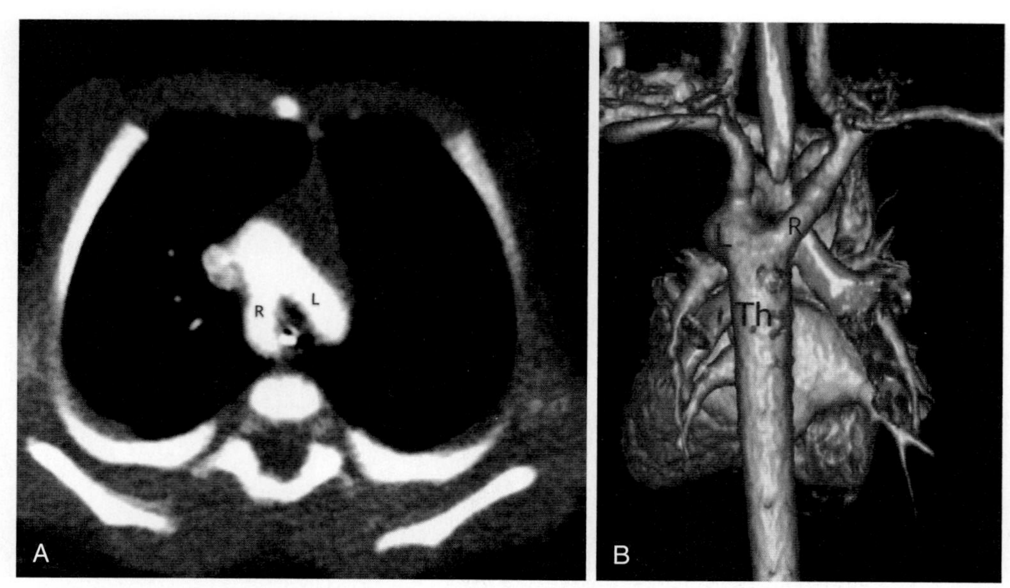

Fig. 18.20 Double aortic arch. (A) Axial image from CT angiogram shows the right *(R)* and *(L)* aortic arches encircling the trachea and esophagus. (B) Three-dimensional reconstruction shows posterior view of the right *(R)* and left *(L)* arches and the thoracic aorta *(Th)*.

respiratory distress. Echocardiography is the primary modality for evaluation of cardiac anatomy and function. Targeted, point-of-care neonatal echocardiography, also known as neonatologist-performed echocardiography, is increasingly recognized in the care of the sick newborn and premature infants.[6] CTA and cardiac MRI (CMRI) complement echocardiography with high spatial and contrast resolution multiplanar images as well as providing additional functional information.

Radiography is useful in diagnosing increased pulmonary arterial vascularity associated with large left-to-right shunts seen in infants with patent ductus arteriosus, ventricular septal defect, atrial septal defect, and endocardial cushion defect. Increased pulmonary arterial vascularity becomes visible on a chest x-ray when the ratio of left-to-right shunt is greater than 3:1. Increased branching linear shadows will be seen in the perihilar region, and vascular markings will be seen in the periphery of the lung fields.

CTA is particularly useful in evaluation of aortic arch anomalies (coarctation of the aorta, interrupted aortic arch, and vascular ring or sling) (Fig. 18.20A,B), pulmonary artery anomalies (pulmonary artery stenosis and aortopulmonary collaterals), anomalies of pulmonary venous return (anomalous pulmonary venous return and pulmonary vein stenosis), coronary artery anomalies, extracardiac anatomy (pericardial masses, airway compression, and parenchymal disease), and postoperative evaluation after surgery.[29] Indications for CMRI include: cardiac chamber volume, mass, and functional analysis; cardiac morphologic analysis in complex congenital heart disease; soft tissue characterization of cardiac masses and tumors; hemodynamic analysis of pulmonary to systemic blood flow, ejection fraction, and valvular stenosis and regurgitation; and postoperative assessment.[29]

ABDOMEN

Evaluation of the Normal Abdominal Radiograph

Plain film abdominal radiography is a frequently performed examination in the high-risk neonate suspected of having intra-abdominal pathology. The examination is obtained in the AP projection with the infant supine. If there is concern for free air, a cross-table lateral view (with the infant supine) or a lateral decubitus view (with the infant turned on either their right or left side) will identify smaller amounts of air than the AP view. Air is seen in the stomach within minutes of birth, within most of the small bowel by 3 hours, and within most of the large bowel by 8 to 9 hours. Gas-filled normal bowel loops should appear polygonal in shape (Fig. 18.21). Gas-filled loops of bowel that are conspicuously located in the central abdomen suggest the presence of ascites. A paucity of bowel gas may relate to fluid-filled bowel or bowel obstruction.

Intestinal obstruction is the most common abdominal emergency in the newborn period. Neonatal obstruction is typically characterized as high, occurring proximal to the distal ileum, or low, involving the distal ileum or colon.[30] The clinical presentation of infants with high and low intestinal obstruction may overlap with symptoms of abdominal distention, vomiting, and poor feeding. Low obstructions are often characterized by failure to pass meconium. An abdominal radiograph is the initial imaging examination of choice to distinguish between high and low intestinal obstructions. The distinction between high and low intestinal obstruction dictates the type of imaging that the infant may need. With a high obstruction, the UGI series is the examination of choice. Infants with a suspected low obstruction are typically evaluated with a water-soluble contrast enema.[31]

High Intestinal Obstruction

Midgut malrotation

Midgut malrotation is the most critical etiology of upper intestinal obstruction. Most infants with malrotation present with bilious vomiting; up to 75% of patients present in the first month of life.[32] Bilious vomiting in an infant should be considered a potential surgical emergency, and in the absence of another defined cause, a UGI series should be performed.

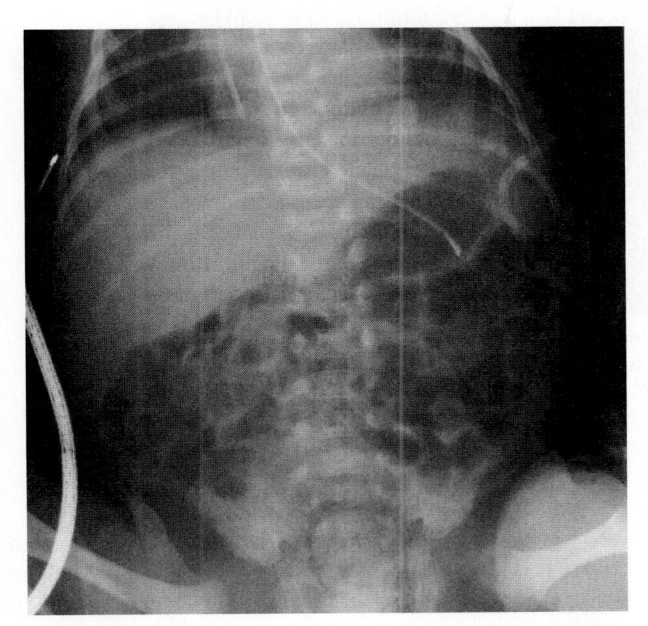

Fig. 18.21 Normal abdominal radiograph shows polygonal pattern of gas-filled bowel in the abdomen and pelvis.

The diagnosis of midgut malrotation by imaging is challenging and the findings variable.[6,32] The abdominal radiographic findings may be normal in infants with malrotation. A high obstruction pattern may be seen in the setting of abnormal peritoneal attachments (Ladd bands) or midgut volvulus. Dilatation of multiple bowel loops may indicate volvulus-induced ischemia. On a UGI exam, the third portion of the duodenum courses posteriorly in the retroperitoneum, crossing the midline to reach the duodenal-jejunal junction (DJJ). This junction is normally located to the left of midline and at the level of the pyloric channel. An abnormal course of the duodenum and abnormal location of the DJJ is diagnostic of midgut malrotation (Fig. 18.22A,B). The wrapping of the superior mesenteric artery around the superior mesenteric vein, known as the "whirlpool sign," is specific for the diagnosis of midgut volvulus.[33,34]

Duodenal Atresia

Duodenal atresia is the most common congenital small bowel obstruction accurately diagnosed prenatally. A "double bubble" representing the fluid-filled obstructed stomach and dilated duodenum is noted (Fig. 18.23A,B). Meconium will still be produced by the distal small bowel and visualized as hyperintense T1-weighted signal on fetal MRI.

Because the majority of cases occur distal to the ampulla, infants often present with bilious vomiting. Approximately two-thirds of patients have associated anomalies of the heart or genitourinary or gastrointestinal tracts. Nearly 40% have Down syndrome. Early abdominal radiographs confirm the "double bubble" sign (Fig. 18.24). These findings are diagnostic for duodenal atresia; when present, no further study is necessary.[30]

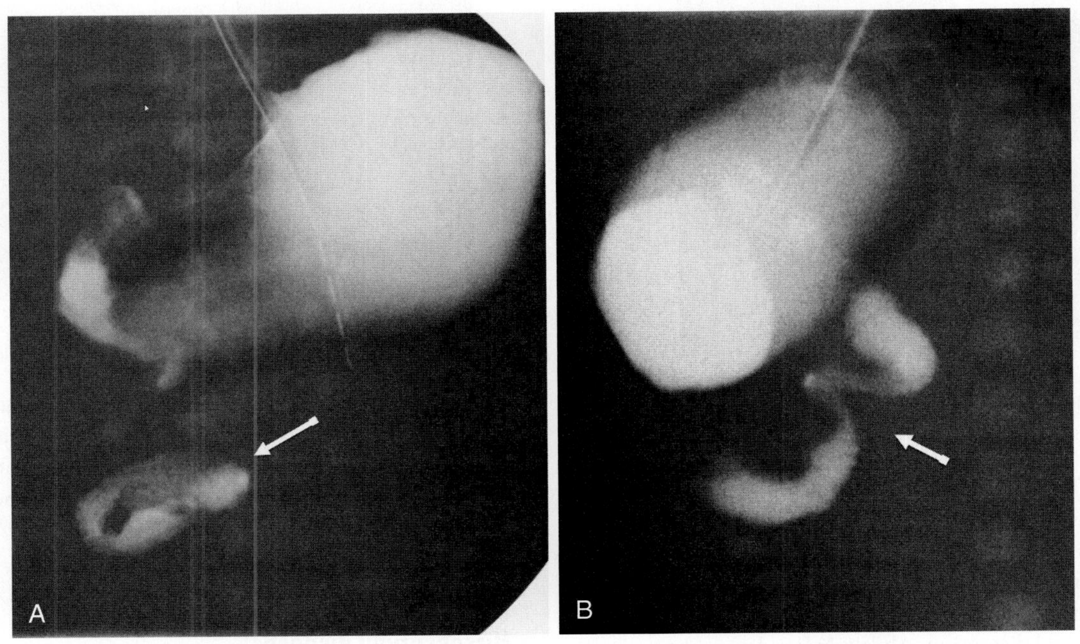

Fig. 18.22 Malrotation and midgut volvulus. (A) Anteroposterior and lateral (B) views from an upper gastrointestinal series demonstrates a "corkscrew" appearance of the duodenum with the duodenal-jejunal junction to the right of midline *(arrow)*.

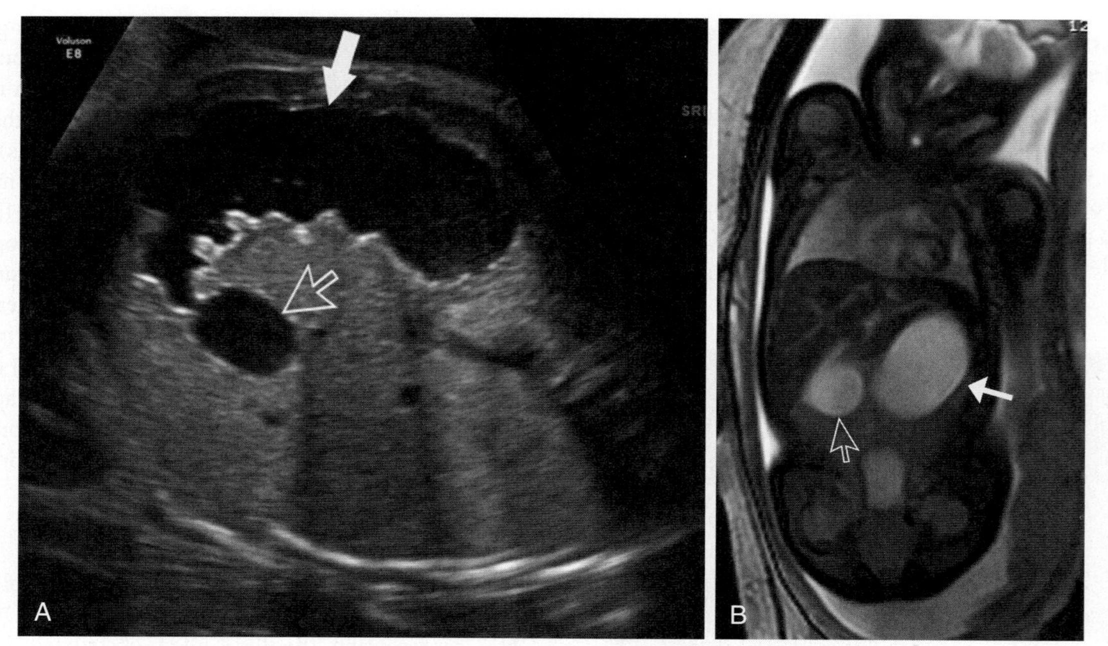

Fig. 18.23 Duodenal atresia. (A) Fetal ultrasound image through the abdomen shows the dilated stomach *(solid arrow)* and the obstructed duodenal bulb *(open arrow)* representing the typical "double bubble" sign. (B) Coronal fetal magnetic resonance imaging (MRI) image shows the large fluid-filled stomach *(solid arrow)* and the dilated duodenal bulb *(open arrow)*.

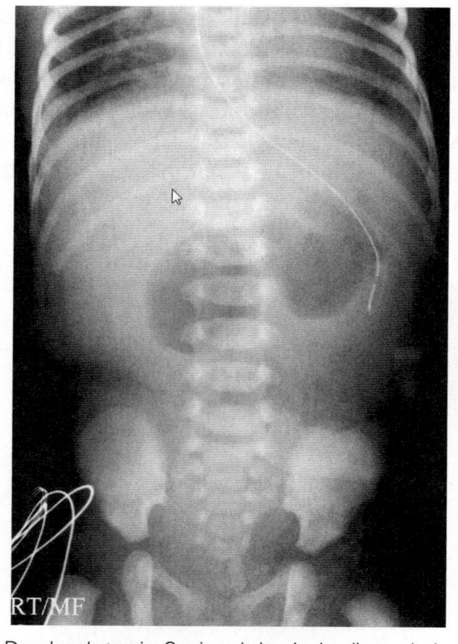

Fig. 18.24 Duodenal atresia. Supine abdominal radiograph demonstrates a "double bubble" comprised of the stomach and dilated duodenum.

Jejunal Atresia

Jejunal atresia results from an ischemic injury to the developing small intestine. The injury may result from a primary vascular accident or a mechanical obstruction, such as an in utero volvulus. Newborns with jejunal atresia present with bilious emesis and abdominal distention. Abdominal radiographs typically demonstrate dilated small bowel loops that may contain air-fluid levels. A "triple bubble" sign may be seen, characterized

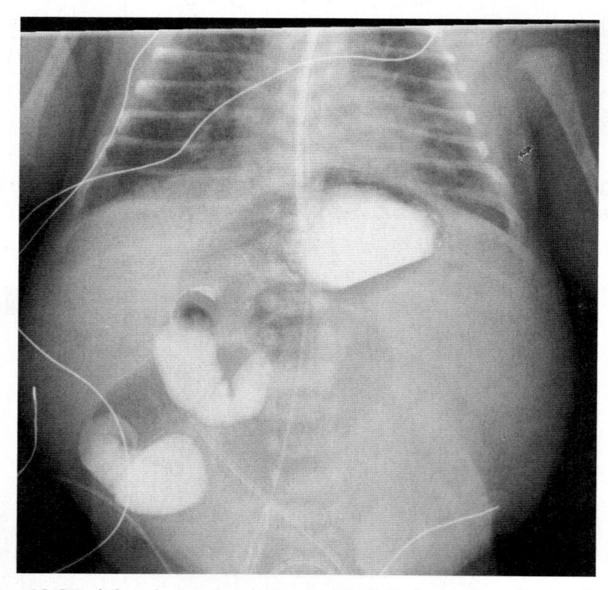

Fig. 18.25 Jejunal atresia. Anteroposterior view of abdomen from an upper gastrointestinal series shows dilated proximal small bowel.

by dilation of the stomach, duodenum, and proximal jejunum. UGI will show obstruction in the proximal jejunum (Fig. 18.25). Because there may be additional sites of atresia in these patients, contrast enema is usually performed before surgical repair to define the anatomy of the distal bowel.[30]

Low Intestinal Obstruction

Hirschsprung disease

Hirschsprung disease (HD) is characterized by the absence of distal enteric ganglion cells. Abdominal radiographic findings

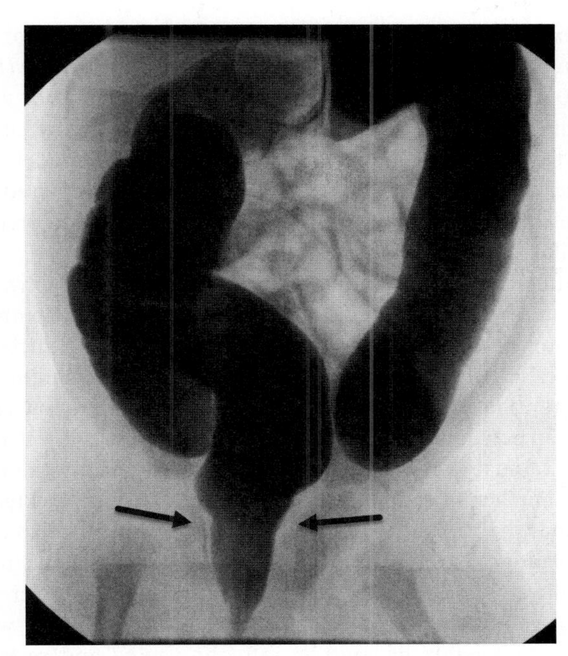

Fig. 18.26 Hirschsprung disease. Anteroposterior view from a water-soluble contrast enema showing the transition *(arrows)* from normal colon to the narrowed distal aganglionic segment.

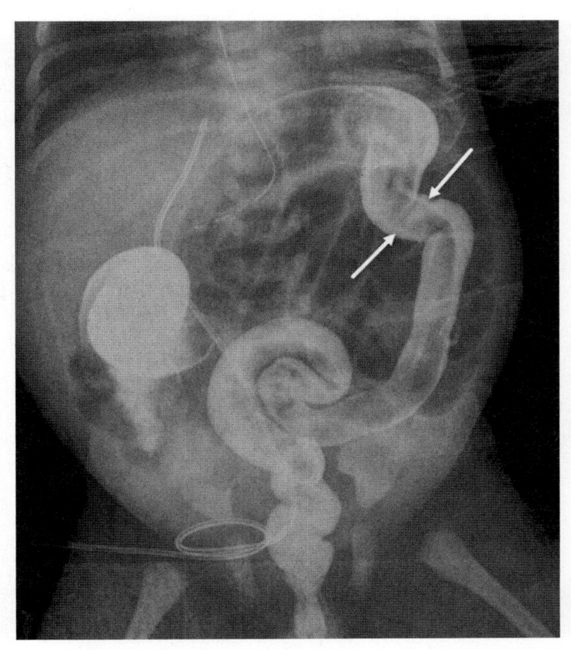

Fig. 18.27 Small left colon syndrome. (Anteroposterior view from a water-soluble contrast enema shows a smaller-caliber left colon and a tubular filling defect representing a meconium plug *(arrows)*.)

in HD are usually nonspecific, with variable dilation of bowel and frequent absence of air in the rectum.

Although there are some published reports where prenatal diagnosis of Hirschsprung disease was correctly made, the in utero diagnosis remains very difficult.[35,36]

Postnatally, the diagnostic imaging examination of choice in patients with suspected HD is a water-soluble contrast enema. A contrast enema may also be therapeutic because the water-soluble contrast promotes the passage of meconium. A small, soft catheter should be used without inflation of a catheter balloon so as not to obscure a transition zone. A discrete transition zone between normal, dilated proximal colon and the contracted aganglionic distal segment may be seen on the AP or lateral views (Fig. 18.26). The transition zone is most commonly located in the rectosigmoid region. Tubular filling defects may be noted in the colon, representing meconium or stool. The affected aganglionic segment always includes the rectum and extends proximally to involve a variable length of colon without skip areas. Although contrast enema is diagnostic in the majority of patients, the transition point identified by imaging does not always correlate with the pathologic extent of aganglionic colon.[37]

Approximately 5% of patients have total colonic aganglionosis and demonstrate a diffusely small-caliber colon (microcolon) without a transition zone. As some infants have a normal contrast enema, a rectal biopsy should be performed in patients where there is a high clinical suspicion for HD.

Functional Immaturity of the Colon

Functional immaturity of the colon, also known as *meconium plug syndrome* or *small left colon syndrome*, is a benign transient functional obstruction of the colon seen in the newborn period. Functional immaturity of the colon is the most common diagnosis in newborns who fail to pass meconium in the first 48 hours.[30] Abdominal radiography shows a low bowel obstruction with or without air-fluid levels. Water-soluble contrast enema shows tubular filling defects representing meconium plugs. The caliber of the colon is variable; it may be normal in its entirety, or there may be a dilated proximal colon with a small-caliber left colon distal to the level of the splenic flexure and a normal caliber rectum (Fig. 18.27). The contrast enema often accelerates evacuation of retained meconium plugs and resolves the obstruction.

Meconium Ileus

Meconium inspissation in the distal ileum results in meconium ileus and is the earliest clinical manifestation of cystic fibrosis.[30] The abnormally thick meconium in these infants results in a distal small bowel obstruction. Meconium ileus may be complicated by in utero volvulus or perforation with peritonitis. Abdominal radiography demonstrates multiple dilated small bowel loops, often without air fluid levels. A "soap bubble" appearance of rounded foci of gas may be noted in the right side of the abdomen. Calcified meconium resulting from meconium peritonitis can be seen in the abdomen and scrotum. Water-soluble contrast enema should be performed in infants suspected of having meconium ileus. The enema typically demonstrates a microcolon (Fig. 18.28) and may also have a therapeutic effect in disrupting the inspissated meconium.

Ileal Atresia

Ileal atresia may be caused by a vascular accident similar to jejunal atresia, or may result from other gastrointestinal anomalies such as meconium ileus. Abdominal radiographs in neonates with ileal atresia usually show a low intestinal

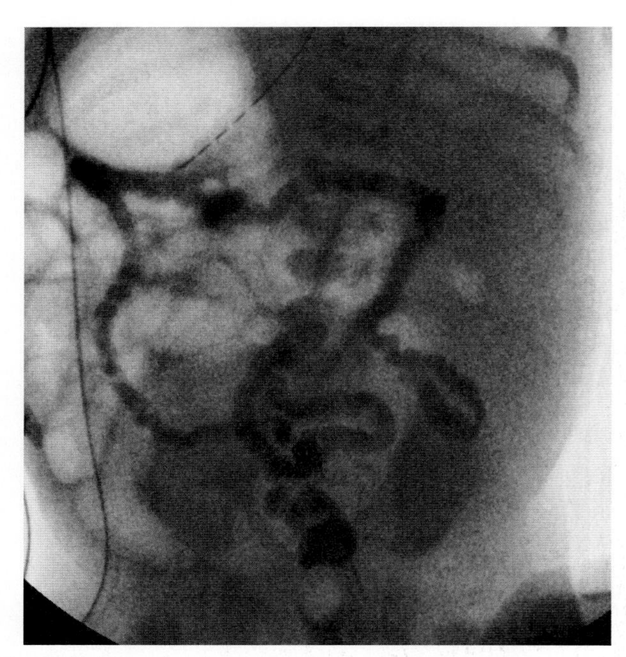

Fig. 18.28 Meconium ileus. Anteroposterior view from a water-soluble contrast enema demonstrates a diminutive caliber of the microcolon.

obstruction pattern. Contrast enema demonstrates an unused microcolon and may be diagnostic if reflux of contrast into the distal ileum demonstrates the level of the atresia.

Anorectal Malformation

Anorectal malformations (ARM) represent a spectrum of abnormalities ranging from a rectoperineal fistula to very complex malformations such as a persistent cloaca and cloacal exstrophy. A persistent cloaca represents a fusion of the rectum, vagina, and urinary tract to create a common channel (or cloaca). This common channel may end in the perineum with one or more perineal openings. The type of cloaca is categorized by the length of the common channel that can be measured endoscopically. The length of the common channel can vary from 1 to 10 cm, and the longer the common channel (>3 cm), the higher the chance for poor bowel control, neurogenic bladder, and reproductive abnormalities.[38,39]

There is always a component of obstruction in a cloacal malformation because of the common drainage. Fetal MRI exquisitely details the anatomy of the cloaca or urogenital sinus. It is common to see a fluid-filled bladder, a fluid-filled uterus posterior to the bladder, and an abnormally positioned rectum that tapers toward the vagina. The most common Müllerian duct anomaly associated with cloaca is a didelphys uterus; the duplicated vagina, uterine horns, and fallopian tubes all may appear dilated and fluid filled. Urine may flow from the bladder to the common channel, reflux into the vagina, and then pass through the fallopian tubes into the peritoneum (Fig. 18.29A,B). Visualization of the anal opening is infrequently identified prenatally.[40]

In the infant with an ARM, imaging plays a significant role in treatment planning.[41] After birth, radiographs of the chest, spine, and pelvis may show osseous anomalies and distal bowel obstruction. Pelvic radiographs showing the sacrum are extremely important, because congenital anomalies of the sacrum, such as partial hypoplasia or scimitar deformity (Fig. 18.30), can be associated with a presacral mass and/or with a Currarino triad (anorectal malformation, presacral mass, and sacral hypoplasia/aplasia). In 1995, a new model was described to assess the risk of bowel incontinence based on sacral anatomy; this "sacral ratio" is currently used to predict the likelihood of incontinence.[42]

After birth, fluoroscopic cloacogram (colostography/fistulography) can provide the anatomic detail of the communication between the different pelvic structures. A metallic marker is placed on the perineum to allow measurements between the end of the rectum and the perineum for surgical reconstructive planning. Subsequently, contrast is injected at high manual pressure via the colostomy to opacify the rectum. Further injection will cause reflux of contrast extending into the vagina (in females) and less frequently also into the bladder via the fistulous connection. These patients usually have a bladder catheter, and some surgeons prefer the initial contrast injection to be made into the bladder with subsequent reflux of contrast into the vagina and rectum. Otherwise, contrast injection through the vesicostomy tube can be performed immediately after the distal colostogram. Together, these images demonstrate all structures connected by the common channel (Fig. 18.29C).[43] In male patients, a voiding cystourethrogram (VCUG) has been reported to be as accurate as distal colostogram in the evaluation of ARM.[44]

High-resolution MRI of the pelvis can help define the level of the rectal pouch as well as the size, morphology, and degree of development of the sphincteric muscles before surgical repair.[45] Pelvic MRI also helps in the identification of associated Müllerian duct anomalies, sacral anomalies, and presacral masses.

Necrotizing Enterocolitis

Necrotizing enterocolitis (NEC), seen predominantly in premature infants, is the most common acquired gastrointestinal emergency in the NICU. Infants usually present with abdominal distention, abdominal tenderness, feeding disturbance, and guaiac-positive stools.

Abdominal radiography plays an important role in the diagnosis of NEC. Early radiographic findings of NEC are nonspecific and include bowel dilation and rounded or elongated loops. Focal or asymmetric fixed bowel dilation may be seen. As the disease progresses, intramural gas, specific for pneumatosis intestinalis, is seen.

Radiographically, pneumatosis intestinalis appears as a "bubbly" pattern or as curvilinear lucencies (Fig. 18.31). Pneumatosis is most commonly seen in the right lower quadrant. Intramural gas may extend into the veins of the bowel wall and then into the portal venous system. Portal venous gas is seen in the porta hepatis as branching, linear lucencies overlying the liver (Fig. 18.32) and is typically a later finding in more severe cases of NEC.

Once the diagnosis of NEC is established, serial imaging is performed to evaluate for the complication of bowel perforation. A cross-table lateral radiograph or left lateral decubitus radiograph of the abdomen (left side down) is performed

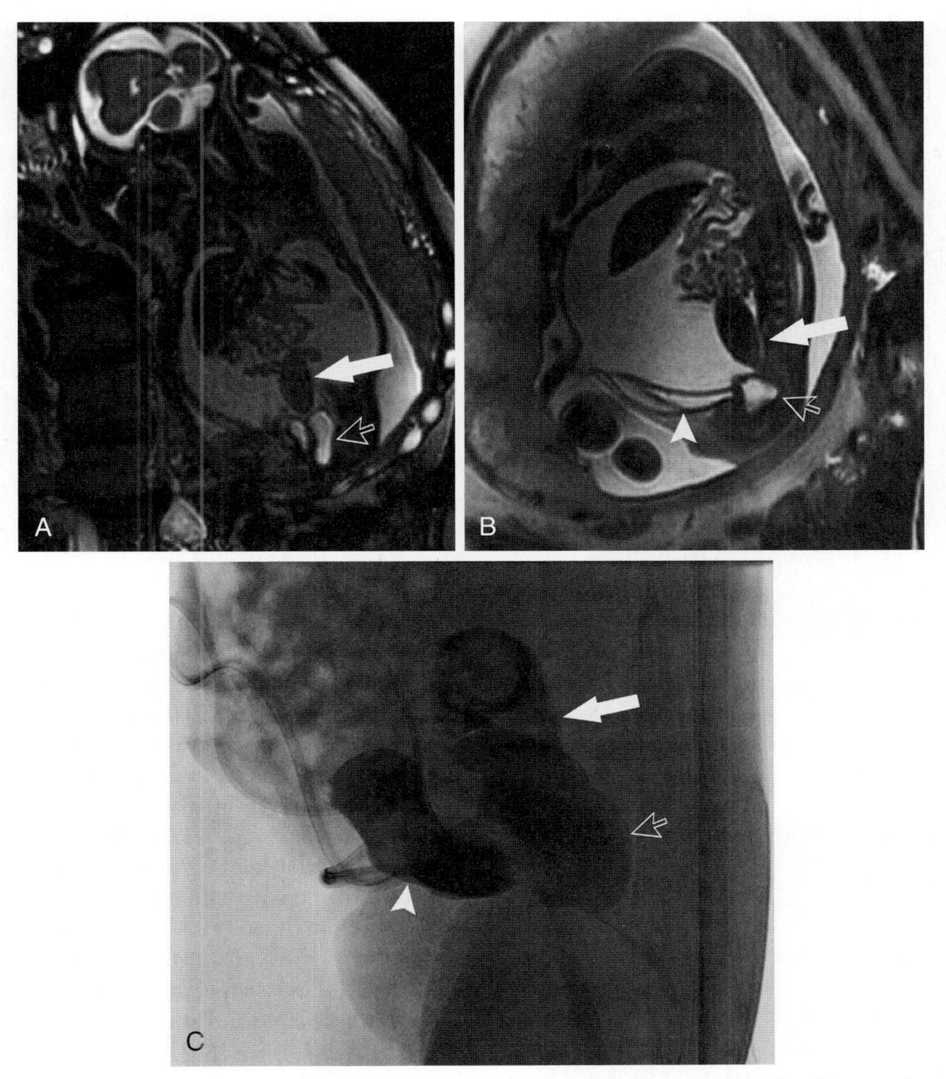

Fig. 18.29 Cloacal anomaly. (A) Coronal and (B) sagittal fetal magnetic resonance imaging images show the tapering rectum *(solid arrows)* inserting in between the duplicated vagina *(open arrows)* of a didelphys uterus. The partially fluid-filled bladder is noted on the sagittal view *(arrowhead)*. (C) Postnatal cloacogram with contrast injection through the distal colostomy *(solid arrow)* with reflux into the duplicated vagina *(open arrow)*. Contrast was simultaneously injected through the suprapubic catheter, opacifying the bladder *(arrowhead)*.

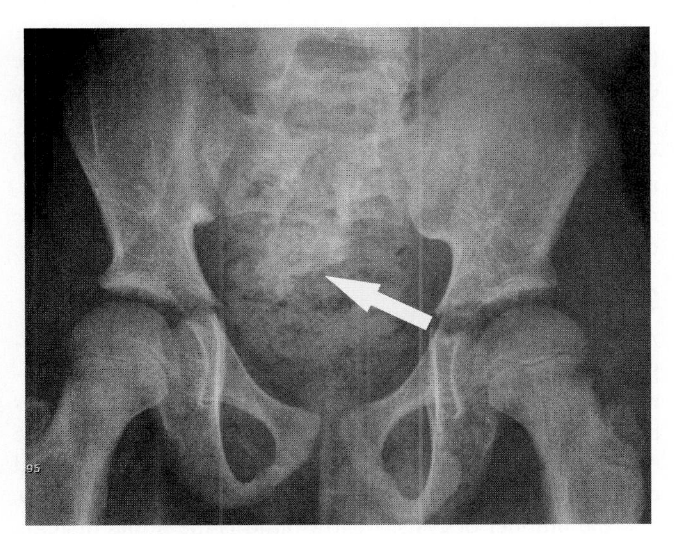

Fig. 18.30 Cloacal malformation. Anteroposterior radiograph of the pelvis demonstrating hypoplasia of the sacrum *(arrow)* with scimitar-like-shaped lower sacrum and absent coccyx.

to assess for free intraperitoneal air. Free air collects in the least dependent portion of the abdomen and is seen as extraluminal lucency adjacent to bowel loops or solid organs just beneath the abdominal wall (Fig. 18.33).

Sonography has been used in the evaluation of NEC.[46] Pneumatosis intestinalis is seen as fixed hyperechoic foci in a thickened, ill-defined bowel wall that has abnormal vascularity. Portal venous gas is seen as intraluminal echogenic foci within the liver. The presence of focal peritoneal fluid collections or free peritoneal fluid containing internal echoes correlates with bowel perforation and abscess formation or peritonitis.

A delayed complication of NEC is bowel stricture, representing the sequela of necrotic areas of bowel wall. Strictures occur in 20% to 30% of survivors of NEC. Strictures may be single or multiple and are usually located in the colon at the level of the splenic flexure. Water-soluble contrast enema is useful for identifying these sites of focal narrowing.

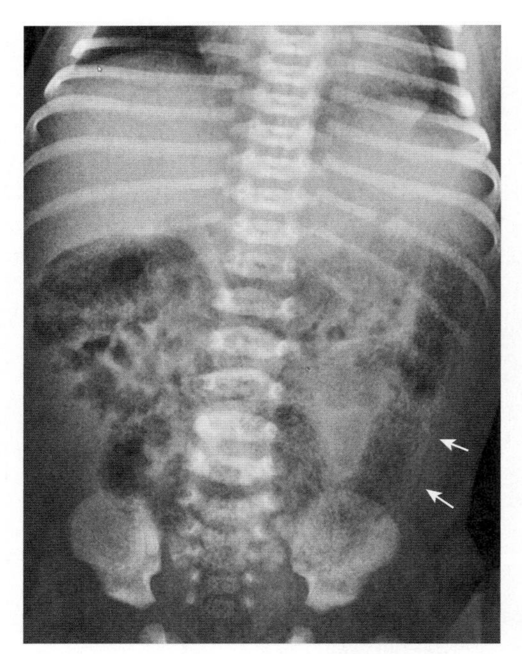

Fig. 18.31 Necrotizing enterocolitis. Anteroposterior radiograph of the abdomen shows pneumatosis intestinalis with mottled radiolucency over the entire colon and curvilinear radiolucency along the descending colon *(arrows)*.

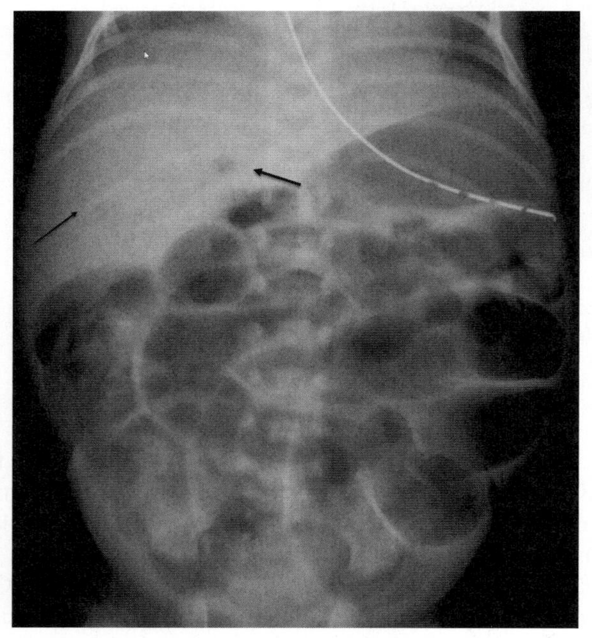

Fig. 18.32 Portal venous gas. Anteroposterior radiograph of the abdomen shows air in the branching portal venous system *(arrows)*.

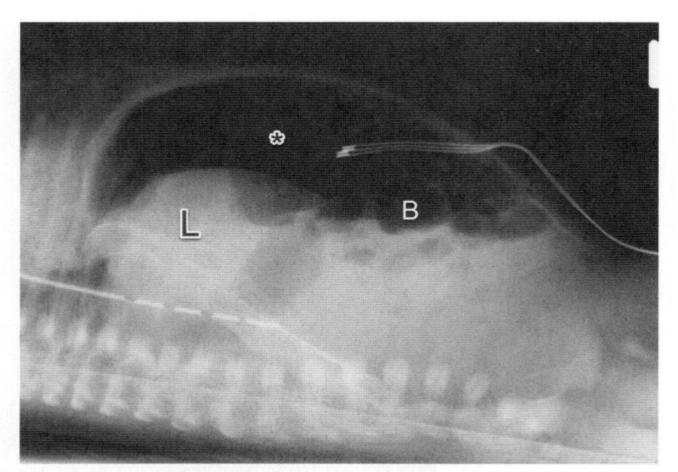

Fig. 18.33 Pneumoperitoneum from necrotizing enterocolitis. Anteroposterior radiograph of the abdomen shows free intraperitoneal air (*) outlining the liver *(L)* and bowel *(B)*.

Hepatobiliary Tract

Biliary Atresia

A frequent clinical challenge is differentiating biliary atresia from idiopathic neonatal hepatitis (INH), as both present with conjugated hyperbilirubinemia. The principal difference between the two entities is patency of the biliary tree in infants with INH. Biliary atresia is associated with other abnormalities, including choledochal cyst, polysplenia, preduodenal portal vein, cardiac and pulmonary malformations, azygous continuation of the IVC, and malrotation.[47–49] Sonography is the initial imaging examination in children with neonatal jaundice, as it can identify alternative etiologies such as choledochal cyst, biliary sludge, and cholelithiasis. The most specific sonographic finding for biliary atresia is the triangular cord sign.[49] This thickening of the anterior wall of the right portal vein represents the fibrous remnant of the bile duct within the hepatic hilum. The gallbladder is not identified in approximately 80% of patients with biliary atresia, and is usually small with an abnormal shape and abnormal wall in the remainder.[50] When the gallbladder is present, sonography performed before and after oral feeding can help differentiate biliary atresia from INH. In biliary atresia, the gallbladder is not affected by oral feeding, whereas contraction of the gallbladder is typically seen in INH.[49]

Hepatobiliary scintigraphy is a highly sensitive examination used to distinguish biliary atresia from other causes of neonatal jaundice.[48] The infant is pretreated with phenobarbital to enhance hepatocellular function and improve specificity. Gastrointestinal excretion of the administered isotope excludes biliary atresia, whereas lack of excretion of isotope by 24 hours is highly suggestive of the condition. Hepatobiliary scintigraphy has 97% sensitivity, 82% specificity, and 91% accuracy in the diagnosis of biliary atresia.[19] Definitive diagnosis requires percutaneous or intraoperative transhepatic cholangiography.

Choledochal Cyst

A choledochal cyst represents cystic dilation of the extrahepatic or intrahepatic biliary tree and is a rare cause of neonatal cholestatic jaundice.[51] Biliary atresia should always be excluded in these infants, given the association of these entities and similar clinical presentations.[49] Choledochal cysts are classified on the basis of their location, morphology, and the number of cysts.[52] Ultrasound is the initial imaging method used to evaluate the size and location of the cyst and

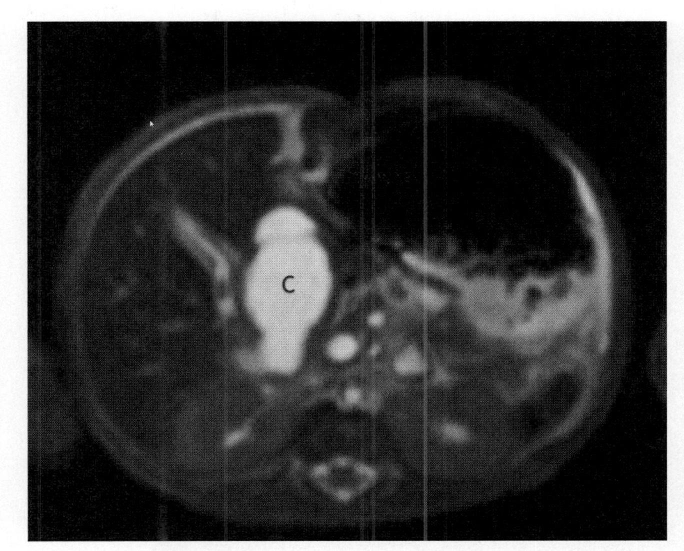

Fig. 18.34 Choledochal cyst. T2-weighted axial image through the upper abdomen shows bright signal in the fluid-filled choledochal cyst *(C)*.

to evaluate for additional cystic changes of the biliary tree. The sonographic appearance includes a focal, rounded, thin-walled cyst or fusiform dilation of the common bile duct, or cystic segments of the intrahepatic biliary tree. MR cholangiography is now the gold standard for the evaluation of choledochal cysts, as these images confirm the biliary origin of the cyst and assist with preoperative planning (Fig. 18.34).

Liver Tumors

The most symptomatic hepatic tumor in the neonatal period, infantile hepatic hemangioendothelioma (IHHE), is diagnosed in the first 6 months of life in over 80% of patients. The prenatal diagnosis is highly accurate, as prenatal and postnatal images show similar findings. At sonography, IHHE appears as a complex lesion with solid and complex fluid components and dilated hepatic vasculature; some contain flow in large anechoic vascular spaces, and others can show a peripheral ring of vascular flow (Fig. 18.35A). IHHE is best evaluated with MRI, where flow voids may be seen in a heterogeneous lesion, which enhances centripetally following gadolinium administration (Fig. 18.35B,C).

URINARY TRACT

Sonography is the initial imaging examination used in the evaluation of urinary tract abnormalities both before and following birth. Fetal MR may prove helpful in better characterization of genitourinary abnormalities, specifically in cases of bladder outlet obstruction and severe oligo-anhydramnios[53] because of its large field of view, higher image resolution, and better visualization of the renal parenchyma.

Postnatal MR urography may be used to evaluate complex renal and urinary tract anatomy and suspected urinary tract obstruction; gadolinium-enhanced MR urography allows for functional evaluation that includes an estimation of differential renal function,[54] although in many centers, a Tc-99m mercaptoacetyltriglycine (MAG3) nuclear medicine study is performed in place of the functional MR urography.

Obstructive Uropathy

Small amounts of fluid may be seen in the renal pelvis of normal infants. The Urinary Tract Dilatation (UTD) Classification System—developed by consensus among urology, nephrology, and radiology societies—standardizes the description of the severity of both fetal and postnatal collecting system dilatation. In the absence of calyceal dilatation, an AP renal pelvic dimension (APRPD) of less than 10 mm is considered normal.[55] An abnormal UTD score is based on the findings of an APRPD of greater than 10 mm, calyceal dilatation, ureteral dilatation, and parenchymal thinning.[55] The most common cause of urinary tract obstruction and flank mass in infants is ureteropelvic junction (UPJ) obstruction.[56] UPJ obstruction is commonly identified on prenatal imaging, but infants may also present after birth with a palpable abdominal mass.

The sonographic findings include a dilated intrarenal collecting system without hydroureter (Fig. 18.36). Renal scintigraphy MAG3 is required to quantify the degree of obstruction and evaluate renal function. Scintigraphic MAG3 findings in UPJ obstruction include progressive increase in radionuclide activity within the renal collecting system and delayed excretion. Because UPJ obstruction may be associated with vesicoureteral reflux in the contralateral kidney, the imaging evaluation of infants with the condition should include a VCUG.

Posterior urethral valves are the most common cause of lower urinary tract obstruction and the leading cause of end-stage renal disease in boys. The urethral valves represent obstructive folds or urethral tissue at the level of the prostatic urethra.[57,58]

Prenatal ultrasound will demonstrate severe oligo- or anhydramnios because of bladder outlet obstruction. An enlarged, thick-walled bladder with dilatation of the posterior urethra forms the pathognomonic typical "keyhole" appearance (Fig. 18.37A,B). Dilatation of the bladder, posterior urethra, and ureters and pelvocaliceal systems may also be seen with the prune-belly syndrome. MR adds value in evaluation of the renal parenchymal cortical thinning, abnormal signal intensity, and tiny cortical cysts in keeping with renal cortical dysplasia (Fig.18.37C).[53,59–63]

Postnatally, VCUG confirms the diagnosis with demonstration of a dilated posterior urethra, diminution of the urethral caliber distal to the valves, and possible vesicoureteral reflux (Fig. 18.38).[57] A MAG3 nuclear medicine study is obtained to evaluate the remaining renal split function to aid the management and treatment of these patients.

Renal cortical dysplasia is a different entity than multicystic dysplastic kidney (MCDK). With renal dysplasia, tiny cortical cysts appear as a beaded ring of cyst in the renal cortex, and a central collecting system is usually present with a small amount of fluid, with or without hydroureter (Fig. 18.39). These findings are associated with poor renal function upon birth and, in certain cases, need for peritoneal dialysis, depending on the degree of renal damage. In contrast, MCDK

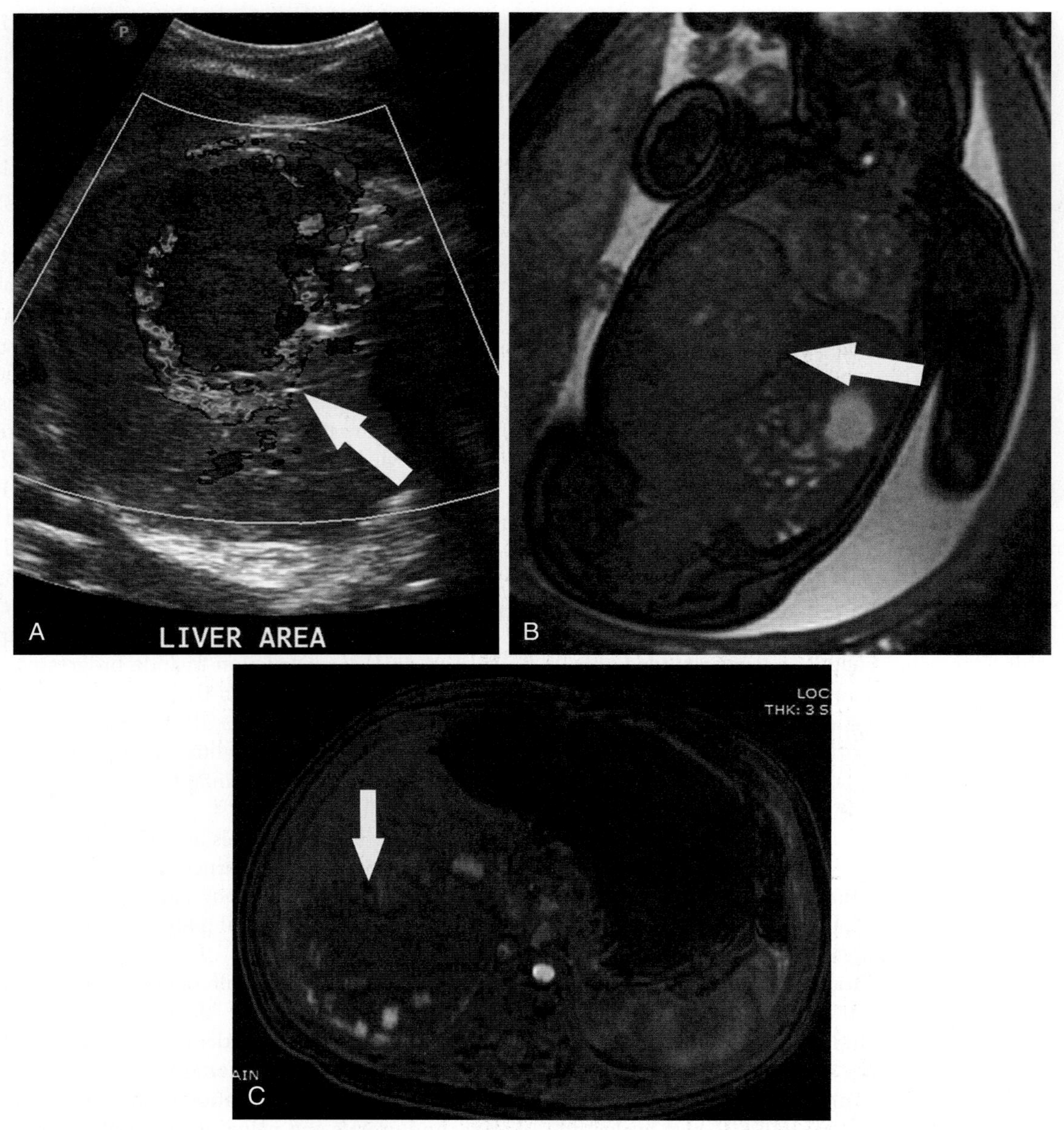

Fig. 18.35 Congenital hepatic hemangioendothelioma. (A) Ultrasound image with color Doppler shows the ring of high vascularity surrounding the lesion *(arrow)*. (B) Coronal fetal magnetic resonance imaging (MRI) shows the large mass *(arrow)*, hyperintense and well distinguished from the liver parenchyma and internal vessels. (C) Postnatal axial MRI image demonstrating the typical centripetal enhancement of these type of lesions *(arrow)*.

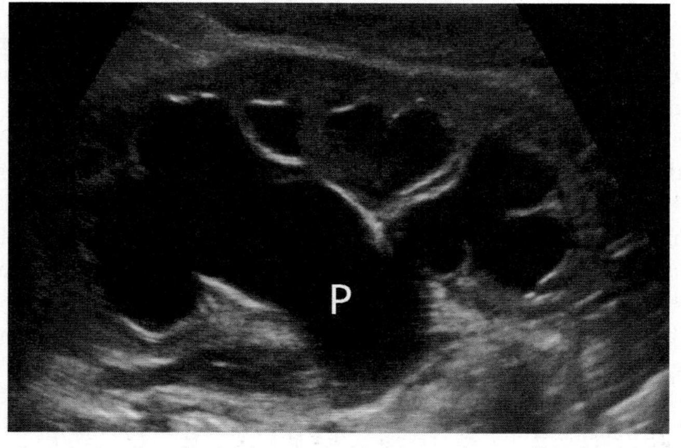

Fig. 18.36 Ureteropelvic junction obstruction. Sagittal sonographic image shows dilatation of the renal pelvis *(P)* and calyces.

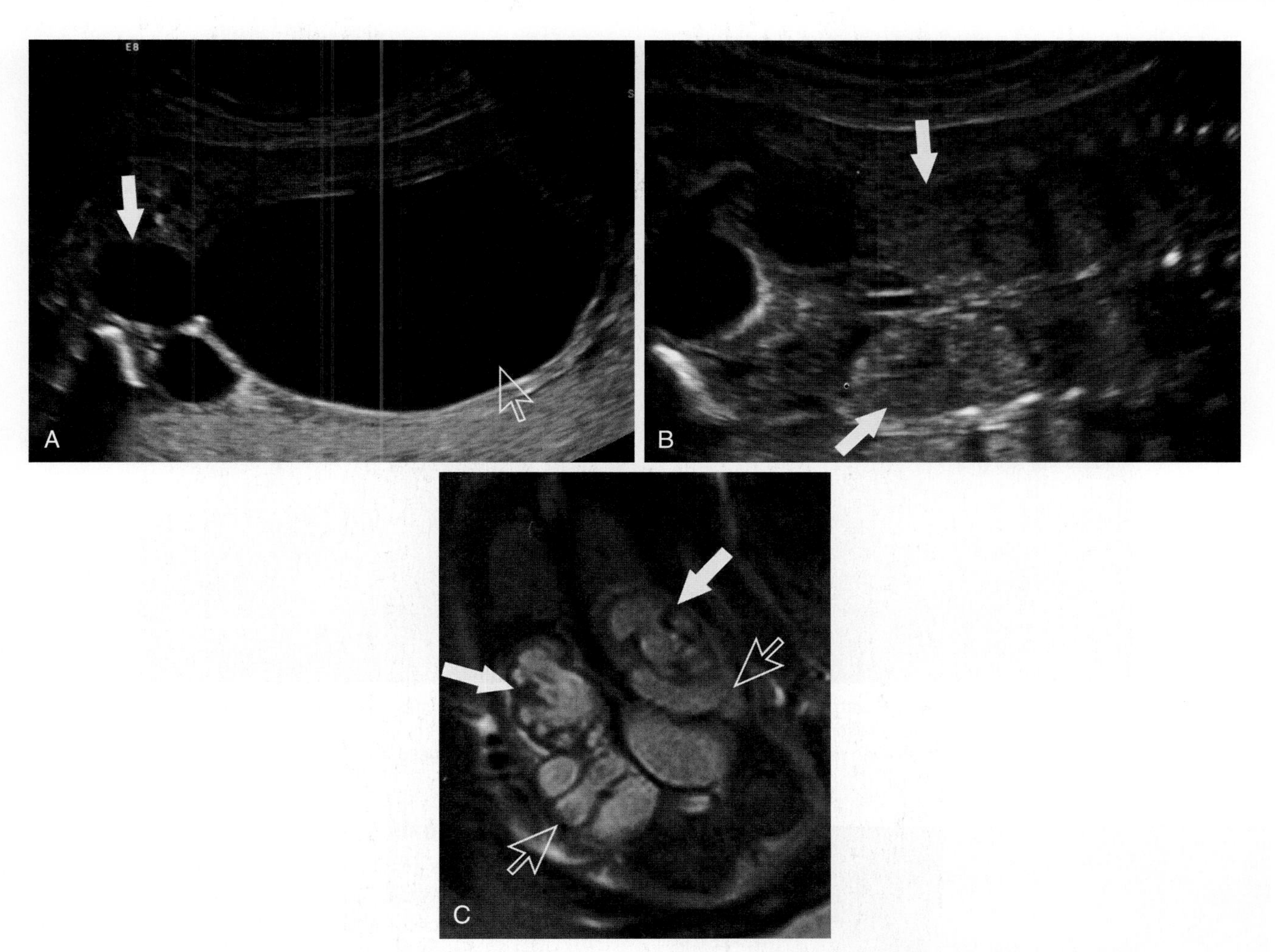

Fig. 18.37 Posterior urethral valves. (A) Fetal ultrasound images demonstrating the massive bladder *(open arrow)* and dilatation of the posterior urethra *(solid arrow)*; and (B) increased echogenicity of both kidneys *(arrows)*. (C) Coronal fetal magnetic resonance imaging shows hydronephrosis *(solid arrows)* and marked hydroureters *(open arrows)*.

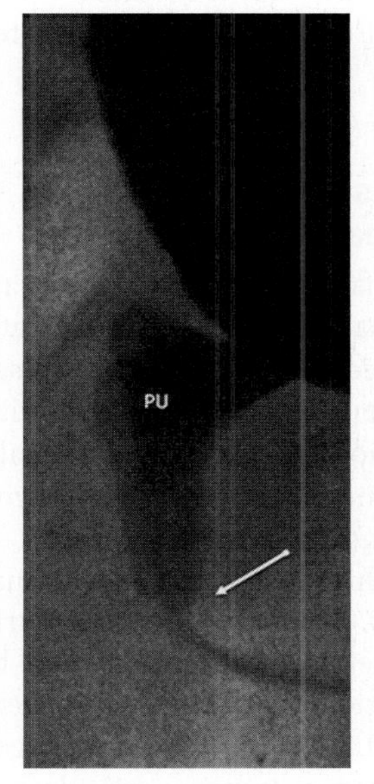

Fig. 18.38 Posterior urethral valves. Voiding cystourethrogram shows dilatation of the posterior urethra *(PU)* with attenuation of the urinary stream distal to the obstructing valves *(arrow)*.

is secondary to an aberrant embryologic process with lack of communication between the ureter and renal mesenchyme. It presents with a nonfunctioning kidney replaced by noncommunicating cysts of varying sizes (Fig. 18.40), and the renal pelvis or ureter are never seen.

Autosomal Recessive Polycystic Kidney Disease

Autosomal recessive polycystic kidney disease (ARPKD) is an inherited disorder characterized by nephromegaly, microscopic or macroscopic cystic dilation of the renal collecting system, and periportal hepatic fibrosis. The diagnosis may be confirmed prenatally with fetal ultrasound and MR (Fig. 18.41B). Infants with ARPKD typically present with large palpable abdominal masses or renal insufficiency. The characteristic sonographic appearance is that of symmetric markedly enlarged, hyperechoic kidneys (Fig. 18.41A) High-resolution sonographic equipment may also allow visualization of tiny macroscopic cystic structures.[64]

Renal Vein Thrombosis

Renal vein thrombosis (RVT) in neonates is frequently associated with hemoconcentration caused by dehydration, sepsis,

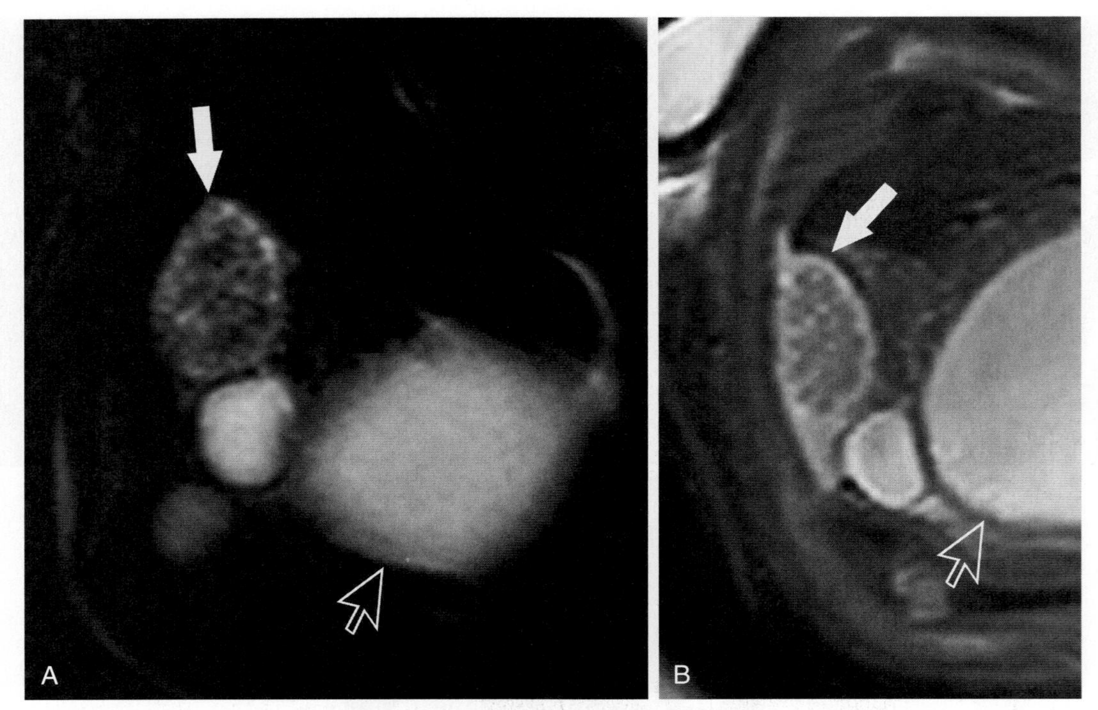

Fig. 18.39 Renal dysplasia with posterior urethral valves. (A) Sagittal fetal magnetic resonance urography and (B) T2-weighted magnetic resonance imaging images show multiple tiny cysts primarily in the renal cortex *(solid arrows)* consistent with renal cystic dysplasia. The large bladder is partially visualized *(open arrows)*.

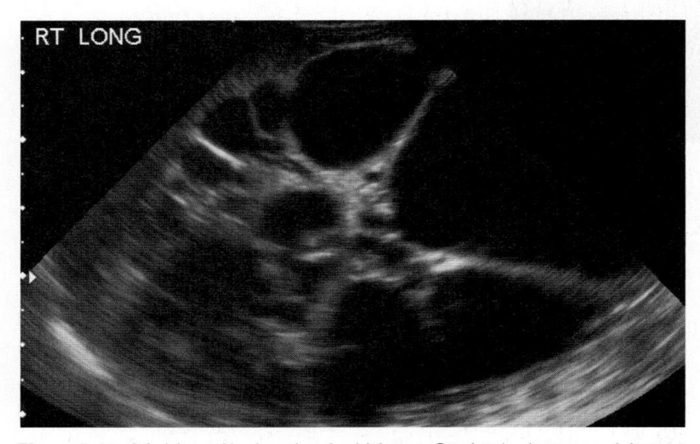

Fig. 18.40 Multicystic dysplastic kidney. Sagittal ultrasound image shows replacement of the kidney by numerous noncommunicating cysts of varying sizes.

or maternal diabetes mellitus. In these cases, RVT is thought to begin in the small intrarenal veins and progress to the hilum; thrombus within the main renal vein may not be present.[65,66] RVT may also be seen in infants who develop IVC thrombi associated with an indwelling catheter. The clinical presentation of RVT includes a palpable mass, renal insufficiency, hematuria, or hypertension. Acutely, the involved kidney is enlarged with diffuse increase in parenchymal echogenicity and loss of corticomedullary differentiation. Over the next several weeks, the renal parenchymal echogenicity of the involved kidney becomes heterogeneous, and renal size decreases. Doppler examination may show diminished perfusion and high-resistance arterial flow with reversal of diastolic flow (Fig. 18.42).

Nephrocalcinosis

Nephrocalcinosis results from the deposition of calcium in the renal parenchyma, most commonly in the medullary pyramids and most commonly related to furosemide therapy.

Initial sonographic findings include increased echogenicity without acoustic shadowing in the normally hypoechoic renal pyramids (Fig. 18.43). In the first few days of life, the normal neonatal kidney may also demonstrate transient increased echogenicity of the medullary pyramids. This finding is usually diffuse and bilateral and resolves within 10 days.[67]

Adrenal Glands

Adrenal hemorrhage

Adrenal hemorrhage is the most common cause of a neonatal adrenal mass. Conditions associated with adrenal hemorrhage include perinatal asphyxia, sepsis, coagulation disorders, hypotension, and surgery. Although unilateral involvement is more common, the clinical manifestation of adrenal insufficiency is typically seen only when there is diffuse, bilateral gland involvement.

The sonographic appearance of adrenal hemorrhage is that of an oval or triangular suprarenal structure of variable echogenicity, depending on the age of the bleed (Fig. 18.44). Adrenal calcifications may develop weeks to months after the hemorrhage. Large adrenal hemorrhages may be difficult to differentiate from a tumor, particularly if calcification is already present. In such cases, follow-up sonographic images show a gradual decrease in size over 1 to 2 weeks.

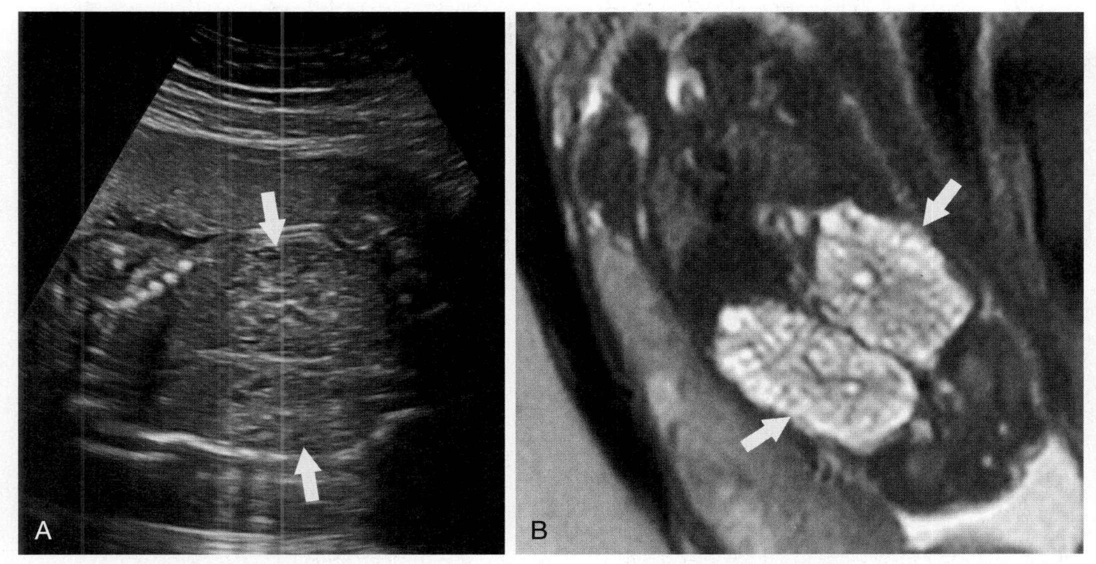

Fig. 18.41 Autosomal recessive polycystic kidney disease. (A) Coronal fetal ultrasound; and (B) fetal magnetic resonance imaging images of the abdomen showing multiple cortical and medullary cysts in very enlarged kidneys *(arrows)*. Note the lack of fluid surrounding the fetus.

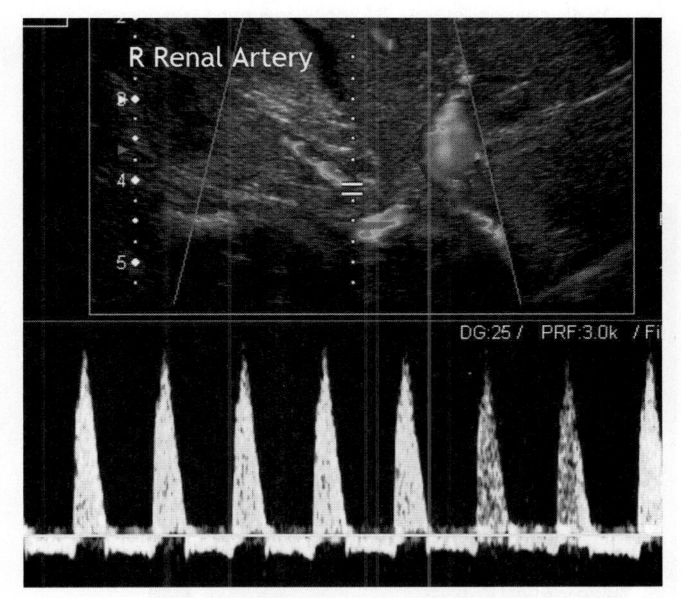

Fig. 18.42 Renal vein thrombosis. Duplex Doppler with spectral analysis shows a high-resistance waveform of the renal artery and reversal of diastolic flow.

Neuroblastoma

Neuroblastoma is the most common neonatal neoplasm and may present in the prenatal or neonatal period. Sonography is the initial imaging examination of choice and demonstrates a solid suprarenal mass that may contain cystic components.[56] CT or MRI offers more precise characterization of the organ of origin and are required for staging (Fig. 18.45). MRI can be useful to assess intraspinal extension.[68] Iodine 123 (^{123}I) metaiodobenzylguanidine (MIBG) functional imaging shows uptake in 90% of tumors and is used to identify both the primary tumor and sites of metastatic disease (Fig. 18.46A,B).[69] ^{99m}Tc-methylene diphosphonate bone scan identifies sites of cortical bone metastases; however, recent work suggests that it does not affect disease staging or management compared with MIBG scintigraphy and cross-sectional imaging in MIBG-avid tumors.[70] ^{18}Fluorine-fluorodeoxy-glucose positron emission tomography CT may be helpful in the evaluation of tumors that fail to or only weakly accumulate ^{123}I-MIBG.[69,71]

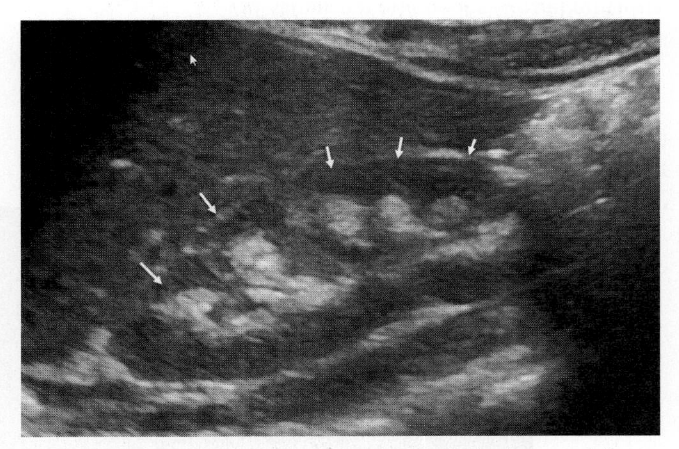

Fig. 18.43 Medullary nephrocalcinosis. Sagittal ultrasound image through the kidney shows echogenic medullary pyramids *(arrows)*.

Central Nervous System

Sonography is the primary means of evaluating intracranial and neck pathology in the critically ill infant. Although the most frequent indication for cranial ultrasound is to screen for germinal matrix hemorrhage (GMH) in premature infants, ultrasound is also used to screen for congenital anomalies. Fetal and postnatal MRI offers more detailed characterization of central nervous system anomalies identified or suggested with screening ultrasound. Conventional images are obtained with a high-frequency transducer using the

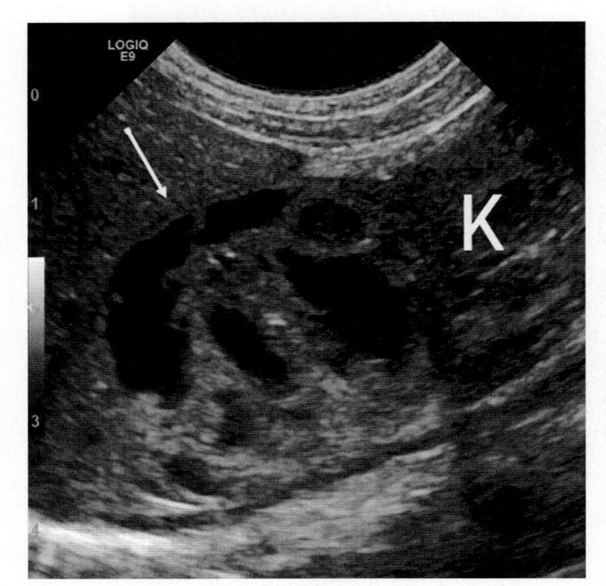

Fig. 18.44 Adrenal hemorrhage. Sagittal ultrasound image through the kidney shows a well-circumscribed complex cystic structure *(arrow)* superior to the kidney *(K)*.

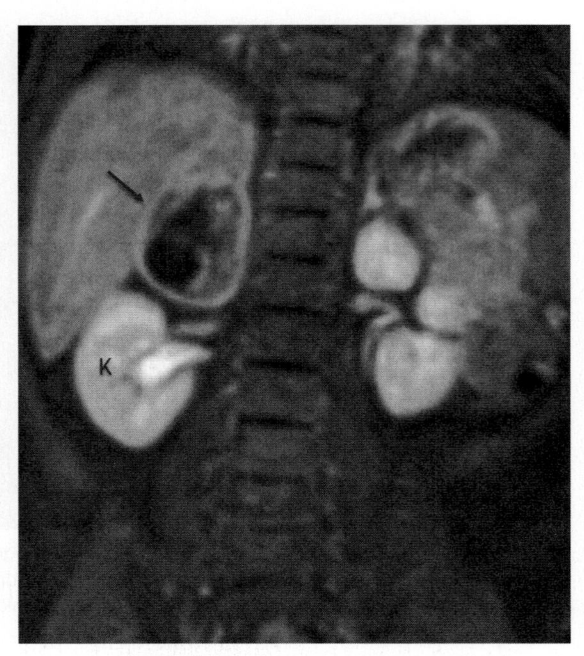

Fig. 18.45 Neuroblastoma. Coronal magnetic resonance image shows the complex solid and cystic mass *(arrow)* superior to and separate from the right kidney *(K)*.

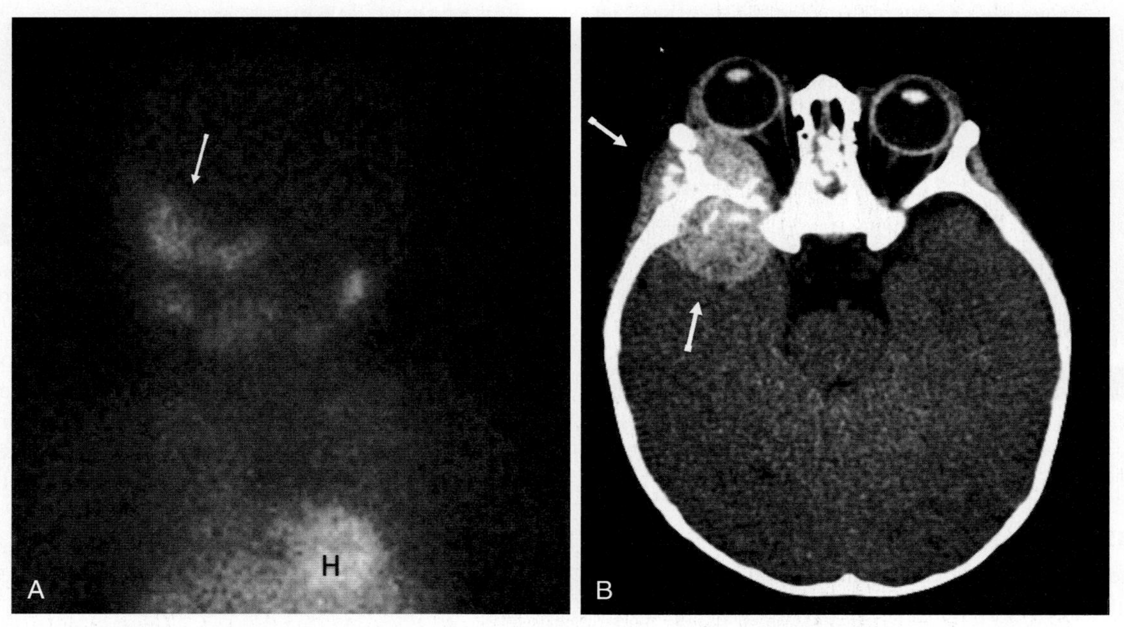

Fig. 18.46 Neuroblastoma metastases. (A) Iodine 123 metaiodobenzylguanidine shows abnormal activity in the region of orbital metastases *(arrow)*. Normal activity in the heart *(H)* and salivary glands. (B) Axial computed tomography images through the orbits show an enhancing mass with calcifications.

anterior fontanelle as a sonographic window. Supplemental images obtained using the lambdoid (posterior), mastoid, and temporal (lateral) fontanelles improve detection of findings in the posterior fossa (Fig. 18.47).[72] Doppler ultrasound offers effective screening of large intracranial arteries and veins for sinovenous thrombosis and vascular malformations (Fig. 18.48A,B).

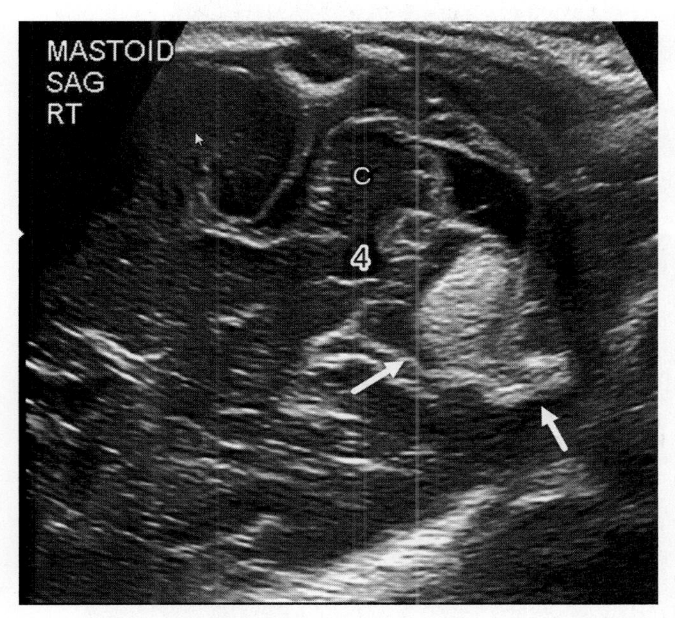

Fig. 18.47 Cerebellar hemorrhage. Axial sonographic image using the mastoid fontanelle as a window shows a focal hemorrhage in the left cerebellar hemisphere *(arrows)*. Fourth ventricle *(4)* and normal contralateral cerebellar hemisphere *(c)*.

Germinal Matrix Hemorrhage

GMH is seen primarily in premature infants with a gestational age of less than 32 weeks or a birth weight of less than 1500 g. The site of origin for GMH is the caudothalamic groove, an area bordered by the ventricular surface of the caudate nucleus and the thalamus. This extremely vascular area is composed of fragile thin-walled blood vessels with little surrounding connective tissue. Conditions associated with increased intracranial blood flow in the premature infant may result in intracranial hemorrhage

The traditional classification system for GMH is based on the presence of subependymal and intraventricular hemorrhage, ventriculomegaly, and parenchymal abnormalities. Grade 1 is subependymal hemorrhage only (Fig. 18.49A); grade 2 is subependymal and intraventricular hemorrhage (Fig. 18.49B); grade 3 is subependymal and intraventricular hemorrhage and ventriculomegaly (Fig. 18.49C); and grade 4 is subependymal and intraventricular hemorrhage, ventriculomegaly, and periventricular hemorrhagic infarction (Fig. 18.49D). Periventricular infarcts are thought to be caused by compression of the periventricular veins by the subependymal hemorrhage. GMH can be seen in isolation or associated with other intracranial abnormalities (Fig. 18.50).

Periventricular Leukomalacia

Periventricular leukomalacia (PVL) represents infarction of deep white matter adjacent to the trigones and frontal horns of the lateral ventricles in the watershed zone of premature infants. Approximately half of infants with PVL also have intraventricular hemorrhage. Cranial ultrasound performed soon after the infarction is most often normal. The earliest

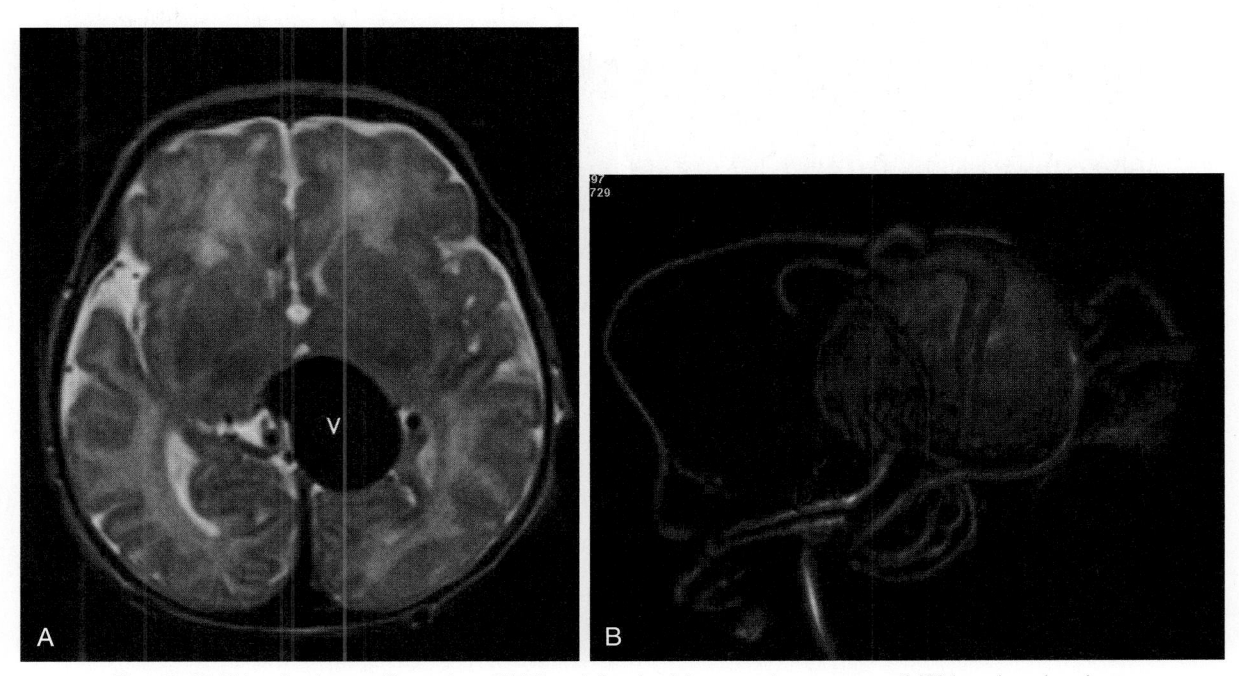

Fig. 18.48 Vein of galen malformation. (A) T2-weighted axial magnetic resonance (MR) imaging showing a large dark flow void in the dilated vein of Galen (V). (B) Three-dimensional image from MR angiogram shows the posterior circulation supplying the malformation.

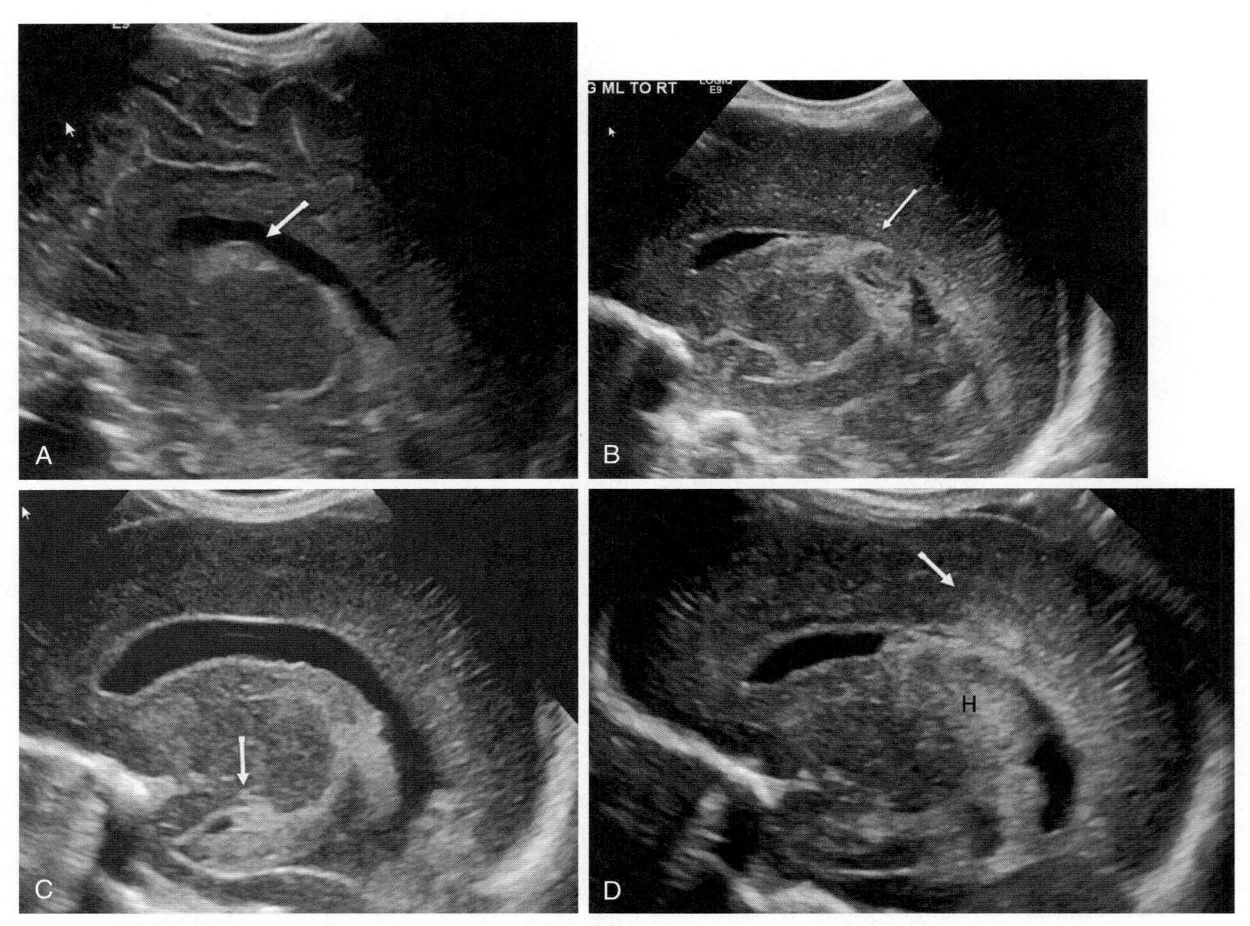

Fig. 18.49 Germinal matrix hemorrhage. (A) Grade 1: Subependymal focus of increased echogenicity *(arrow)*. (B) Grade 2: Extension of subependymal echoes *(arrow)* into the normal sized lateral ventricle. (C) Grade 3: Intraventricular hemorrhage (IVH) *(arrow)* with lateral ventricular dilatation. (D) Grade 4: IVH (H refers to hemorrhage) with associated increased echogenicity of the periventricular white matter *(arrow)*.

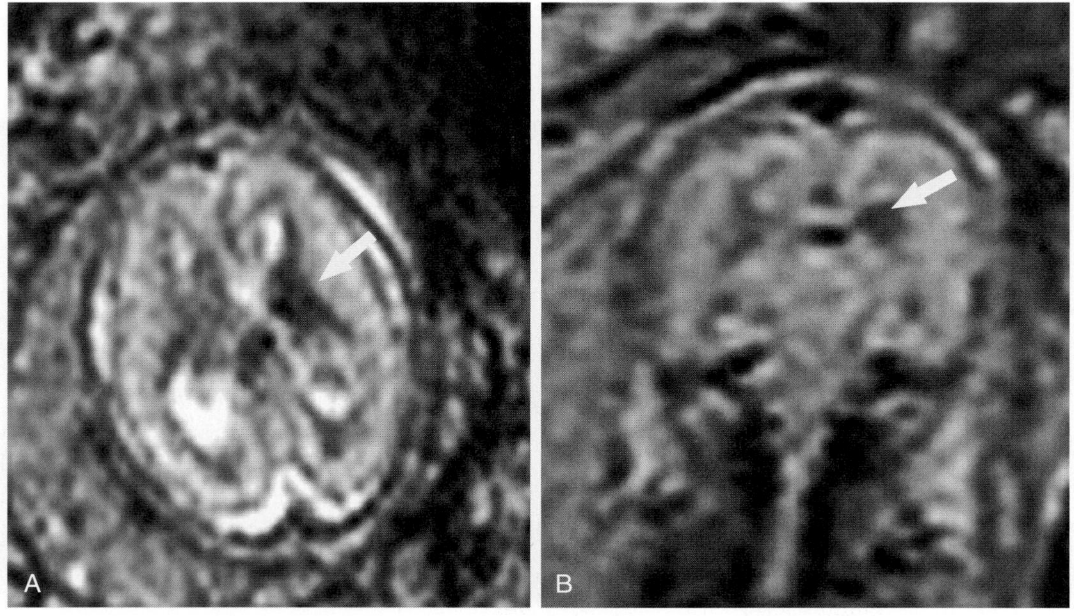

Fig. 18.50 Germinal matrix hemorrhage. (A) Axial and (B) coronal fetal echo-planar images demonstrating blooming artifact (dark signal) in the left germinal matrix consistent with grade I germinal matrix hemorrhage *(white arrows)*.

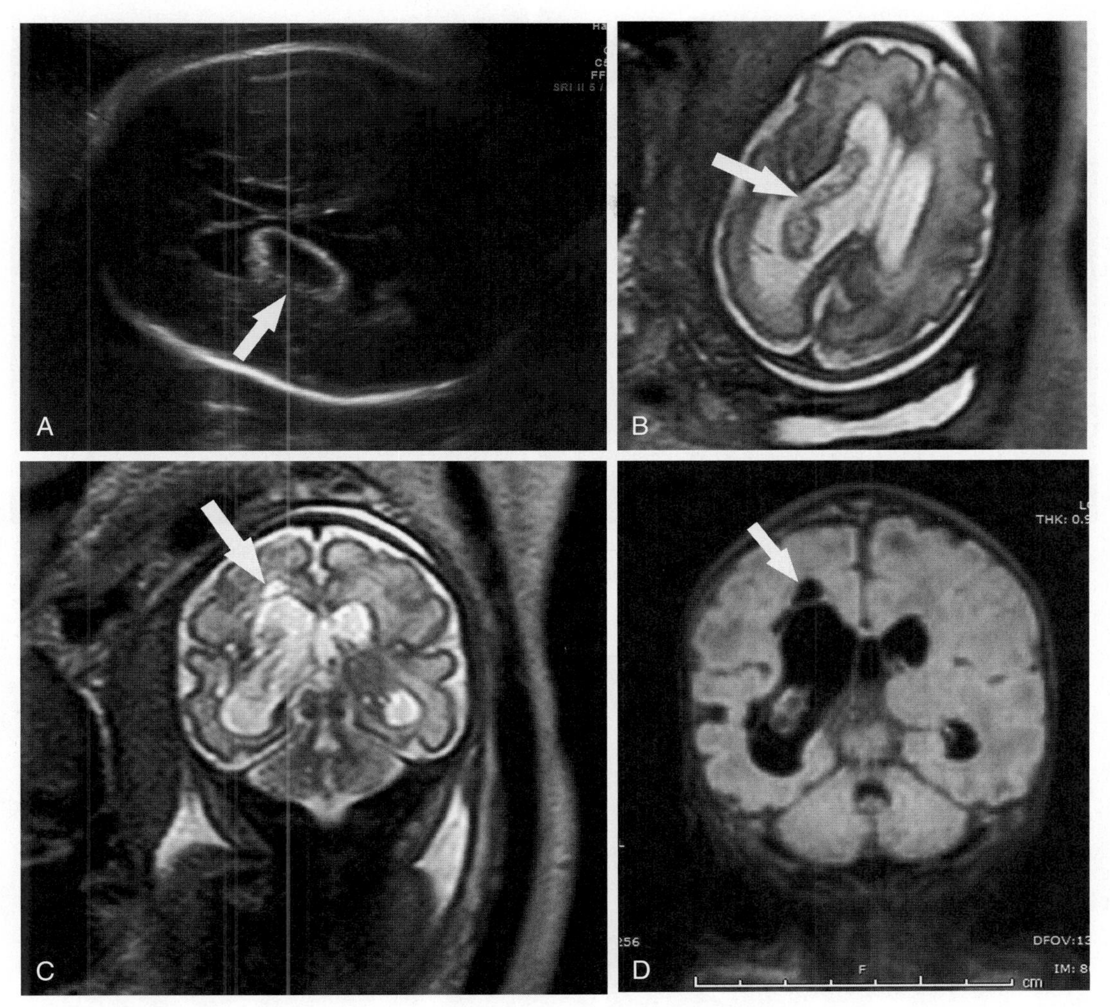

Fig. 18.51 Periventricular leukomalacia. (A) Axial fetal ultrasound through the brain shows enlargement of the right choroid plexus *(solid arrow)*. (B) Axial fetal magnetic resonance imaging shows blood products within the choroid plexus *(solid arrow)*. (C) Coronal T2-weighted, and (D) coronal FLAIR images show cystic lesions in the periventricular region *(arrows)* consistent with periventricular leukomalacia.

sonographic abnormality is increased periventricular echogenicity. With progression of disease, cavitation occurs, resulting in parenchymal cystic areas (Figs. 18.50 and 18.51, A–D). These areas may communicate with the ipsilateral lateral ventricle.[73] MRI is the most sensitive imaging modality for the assessment of PVL.[74] Peritrigonal areas of hyperintensity are seen on T2-weighted images. The corpus callosum is often thinned or atrophic. In addition, irregularity of the lateral ventricular contour and asymmetric ventricular enlargement may be noted.

Hypoxic-Ischemic Encephalopathy in Term Infants

Neonatal hypoxic-ischemic encephalopathy (HIE) is a condition that may result in severe neurologic deficit. Cranial ultrasound may appear normal or show diffuse cerebral edema. MR with special techniques like diffusion-weighted imaging (DWI) play a central role in diagnosis.[75] DWI may show cytotoxic edema of hypoxic injury during the acute phase before signal intensity changes are evident on conventional T1- or T2-weighted images. Cytotoxic edema appears as high signal–restricted diffusion on DWI and low signal on corresponding diffusion coefficient mapping (Fig. 18.52A,B). Diffusion restriction on DWI often predicts a poor outcome.

Congenital Central Nervous System Anomalies

Because of its superior contrast resolution and soft tissue characterization, fetal and postnatal MR plays a primary role in the evaluation of congenital anomalies of the brain and spine. MR is the imaging modality that best characterizes intracranial anomalies. Fetal MRI detects additional CNS abnormalities compared with ultrasound alone, changing the diagnosis in 32% of cases of ultrasound-detected abnormalities, changing counseling in 50%, and altering patient management in 19%.[76] (Fig. 18.53A–D).

Spinal dysraphism occurs early in gestation when normal closure of the neural tube fails. Sonography alone can diagnose the majority of neural tube defects; however, fetal

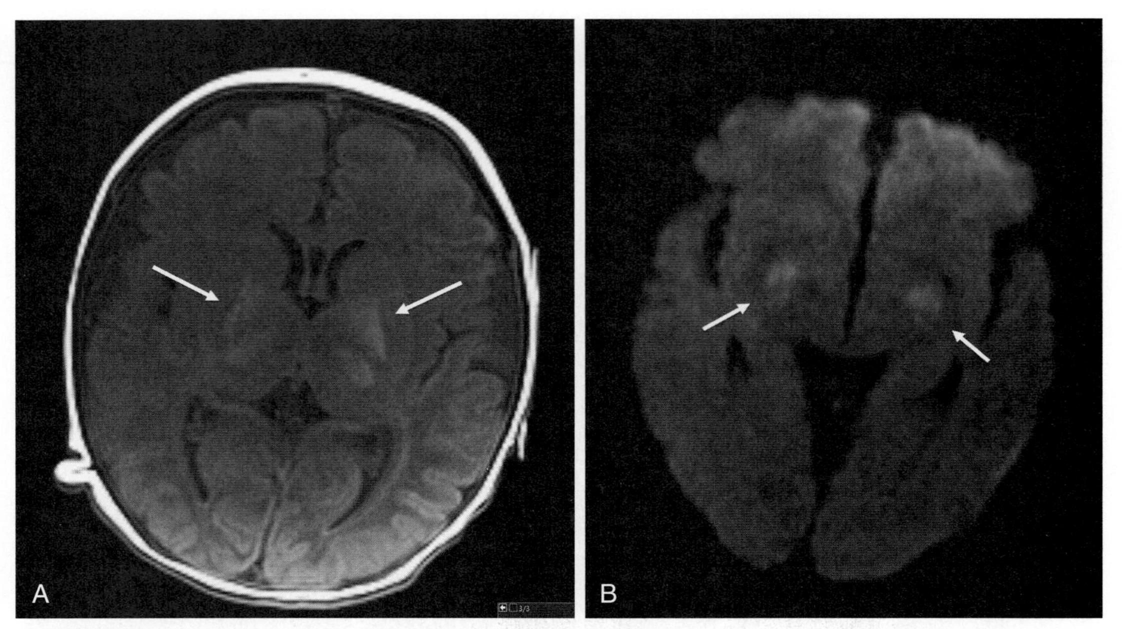

Fig. 18.52 Hypoxic-ischemic encephalopathy. (A) Axial T1-weighted magnetic resonance (MR); and (B) axial diffusion–weighted MR images show bright signal in the basal ganglia and thalami *(arrows)* in keeping with subacute hypoxic-ischemic change.

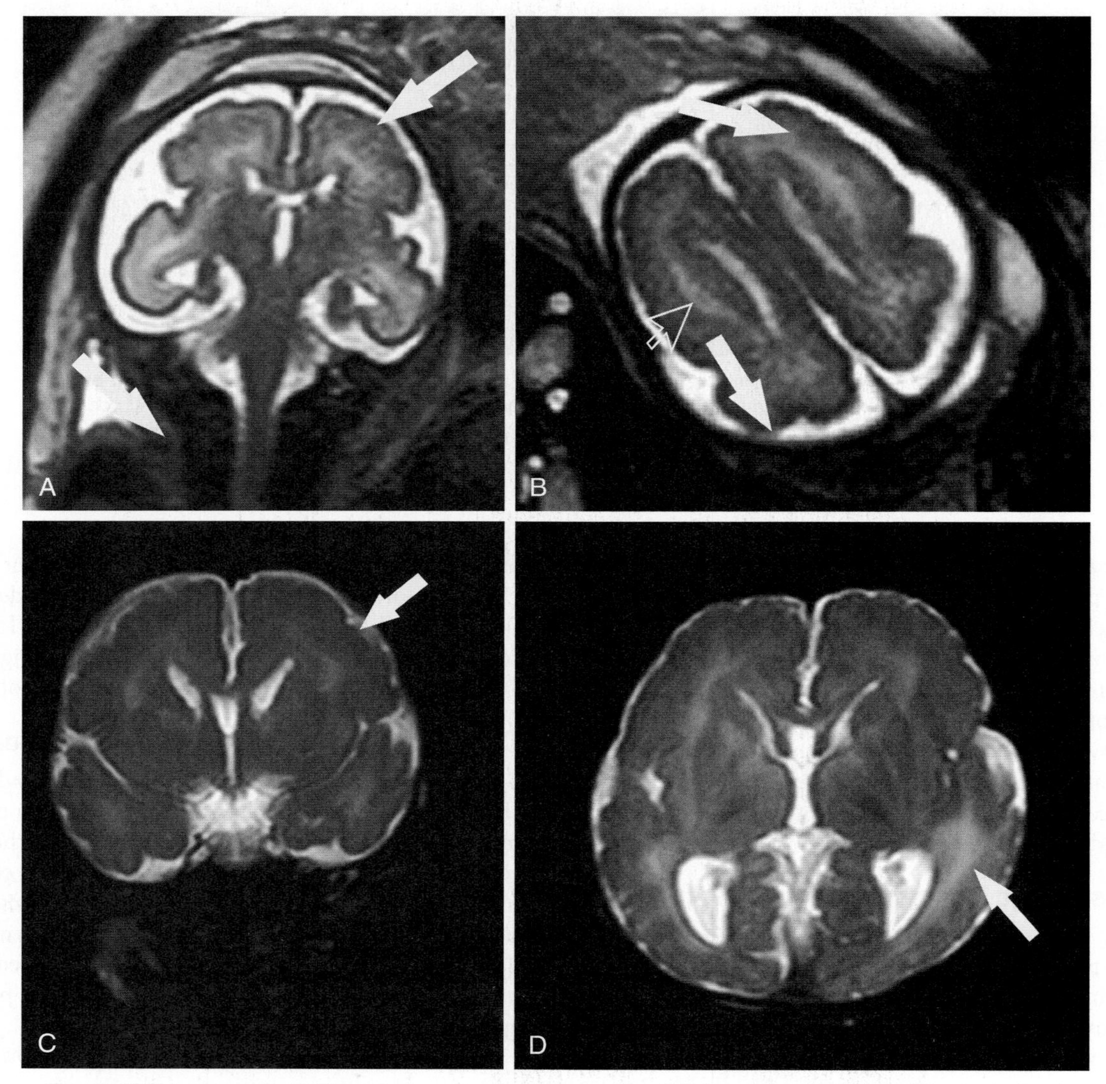

Fig. 18.53 Polymicrogyria. (A,B) Fetal magnetic resonance imaging (MRI) showing thickening of the cortical and subcortical region suggesting cortical malformations *(solid arrows)*. Abnormal white matter signal is also noted *(open arrow)*. (C,D) Comparison postnatal MRI show bilateral perisylvian polymicrogyria extending to the frontal lobes *(solid arrow)*. Immature myelination is seen corresponding to abnormal white matter seen prenatally (*arrow* on D).

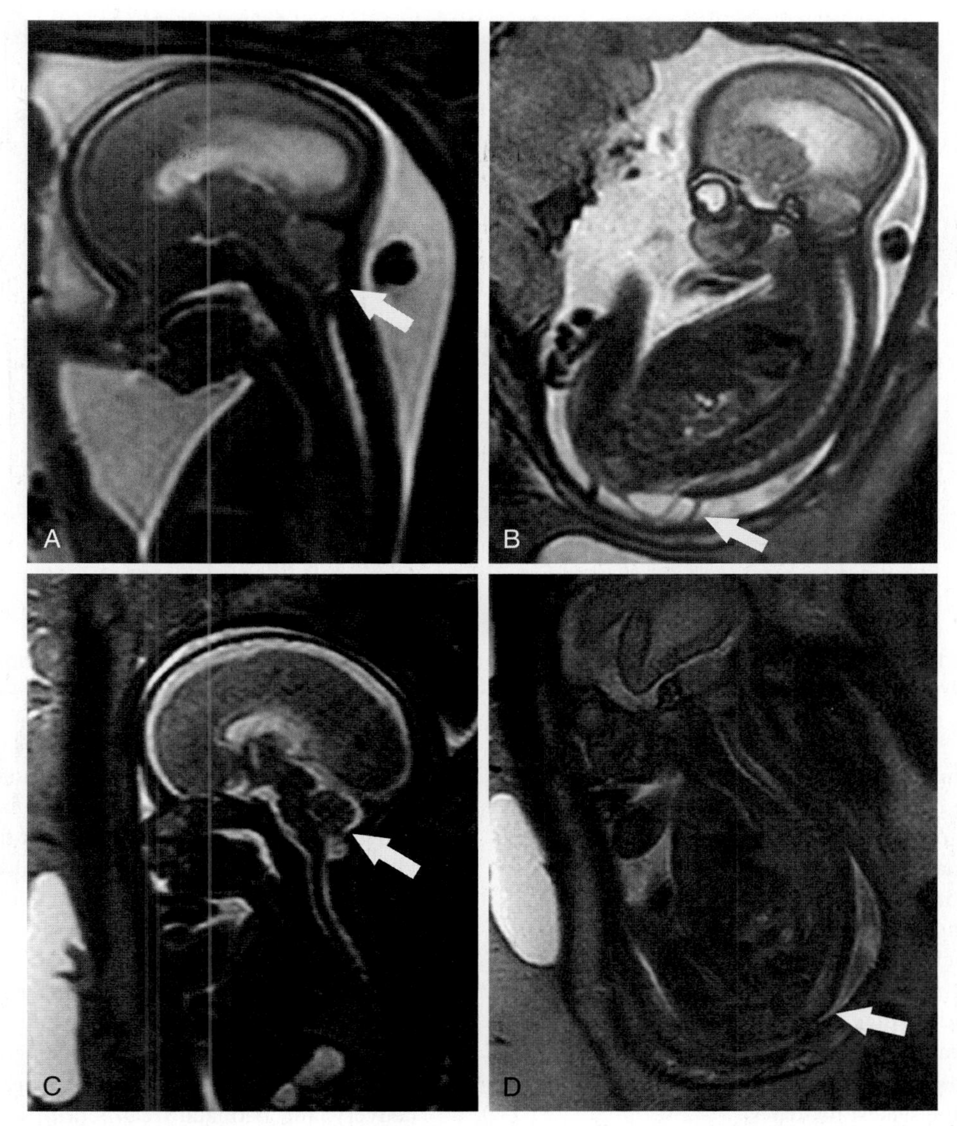

Fig. 18.54 Myelomeningocele. (A) Sagittal fetal magnetic resonance imaging (MRI) shows herniation of the hindbrain with crowding of the posterior fossa and lack of cerebrospinal fluid (CSF) *(arrow)*. (B) Sagittal fetal MRI spine shows an open posterior spinal dysraphism *(arrow)*. After in utero open myelomeningocele repair, the images show (C) repositioning of the hindbrain and restoration of the CSF in the posterior fossa *(arrow)*; and (D) dark T2 line over the myelomeningocele after closure *(arrow)*.

MRI is increasingly used for the evaluation of hindbrain herniation and evaluation of the fetal brain and spinal cord anatomy—especially before in utero intervention.[77] Fetal MR distinguishes between an open or closed (skin-covered) dysraphism, visualizes the ventricular system and accurately measures its size, evaluates the degree of hindbrain herniation, and assesses for additional intracranial malformations of cortical migration or myelination (Fig. 18.54A–D). Yet fetal three-dimensional ultrasound is more accurate at depicting the level of the spinal dysraphism than fetal MRI.

For those infants suspected of occult spinal dysraphism after birth, sonographic examination using a high-frequency linear transducer is the primary screening tool. Terminal positioning of the conus medullaris at or below the L2-3 disc space confirms a tethered cord (Fig. 18.55A). MRI is typically performed in all abnormal cases to better evaluate for associated abnormalities (Fig. 18.55B).

FUTURE DIRECTIONS

The use of diagnostic imaging in the high-risk neonate continues to evolve with advances in both imaging technology and novel options for clinical management of these patients. The increasing use of fetal MRI will facilitate earlier diagnoses as well as targeted in utero and postnatal treatment. MRI evaluation of the newborn continues to progress with the design of faster sequences and increased use of functional imaging. In the near future, smaller MR scanners will allow imaging of critically ill patients to be performed within the NICU. Novel MR sequences will provide options for rapid

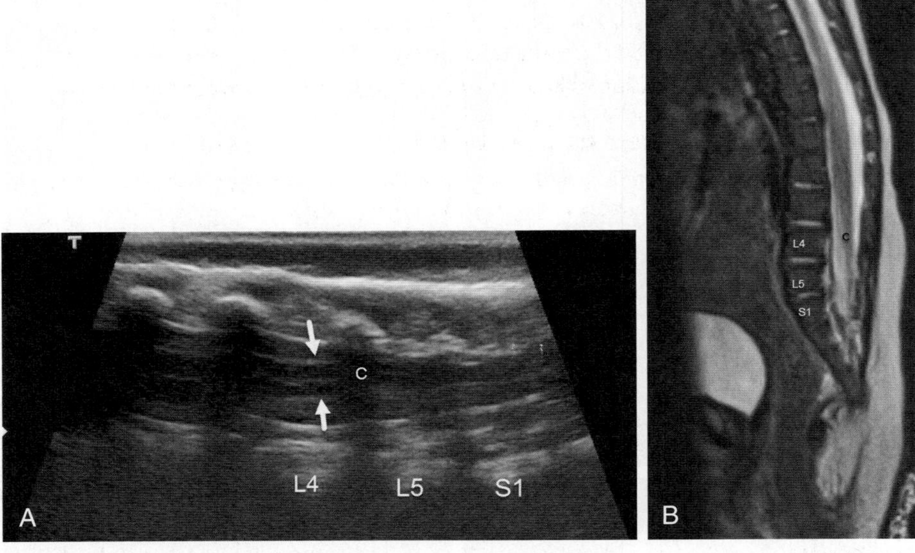

Fig. 18.55 Tethered cord. (A) Sagittal ultrasound image shows the low position of the conus medullaris *(arrows)* below L4. (B) Sagittal magnetic resonance imaging of the spine confirms a tethered cord. C indicates cord.

screening with reduced motion artifact. New postprocessing techniques like iterative reconstruction will continue to decrease doses of ionizing radiation for infants needing a CT scan. The availability of higher-frequency transducers and advancements in duplex and color Doppler technology are improving vascular anatomic imaging and the ability to visualize lower velocities of blood flow in smaller vessels. The use of handheld ultrasound technology will grow, providing point-of-care providers diagnostic information in minutes. These collective advances promise not only to improve image quality and safety but also to accelerate the delivery of diagnostic imaging for the sickest neonates.

KEY POINTS

- Radiography remains the most widely used imaging modality in the newborn; cumulative radiation doses from serial neonatal radiographs are considered low-dose radiation.
- The risk of a future cancer from low-dose radiation used in neonatal imaging is considered too low to be detectable and may be nonexistent.
- Fluoroscopy remains the imaging modality of choice for diagnosis of intestinal malrotation, bowel obstructions, and gastrointestinal and urinary tract fistulae.
- Ultrasound, the second most widely used imaging modality in newborns, offers quick, portable, and dynamic cine imaging of the neonatal brain, abdominal solid organs, urinary tract, and vasculature.
- MR imaging is increasingly performed prenatally for congenital neurologic, thoracic, and abdominal malformations. It not only aids in the diagnosis of ultrasound suspected pathology but also guides prenatal therapy, delivery, and neonatal treatment. It is specifically helpful in cases of intracranial abnormalities. Postnatal MR is most widely used for follow-up of these malformations, early detection of hypoxic-ischemic change, and cardiac disease.
- CT, usually performed without sedation, is indicated for newborns with lesions not fully characterized with radiography and ultrasound. CT also offers diagnostic imaging for infants with congenital heart disease involving the aortic arch, pulmonary vascularity, or coronary arteries.

19

The Outcome of Neonatal Intensive Care

Deanne Wilson-Costello, Allison H. Payne

Technical advances and aggressive improvements in perinatal care have been primarily responsible for the improved survival of high-risk neonates (Fig. 19.1, Tables 19.1 and 19.2) Despite marked improvements in survival, there has been minimal progress in decreasing morbidities. A major concern persists that neonatal intensive care can result in an increase in the number of permanently handicapped children. Because perinatal interventions can impact later growth and development, long-term follow-up is essential to ensure that newer therapies that demonstrate dramatic and immediate positive effects are not associated with adverse long-term outcomes. In recognition of the importance of these long-term outcomes, many modern prospective randomized interventional trials have extended their primary outcome to school age, with the goal being absence of harm and normal long-term neurodevelopment.

EDITORIAL COMMENT: Although there has been tremendous progress in neonatology over the last century, there has also been a history of errors in neonatology and babies who were injured when given therapies designed to help them. It is for this reason that one of the forefathers of neonatology, Bill Silverman, exhorted clinicians to "teach thy tongue to say I do not know and thou shalt progress." At the same time, it must be acknowledged how difficult it is for researchers to design trials with questions that will only be answered 10 years later. Additionally, as noted above, over a period of a decade, there has only been a 4% increase in survival without any neurodevelopmental impairment in babies born between 23 and 25 weeks' gestation. (Younge N, Goldstein RF, Bann CM, et al. Survival and neurodevelopmental outcomes among periviable infants. *N Engl J Med.* 2017;376:617-628.)

The initial follow-up studies of preterm infants in the early 1970s described a decrease in unfavorable neurodevelopmental sequelae compared with the era before neonatal intensive care. Despite the continued decrease in mortality rates, the incidence of neurosensory and developmental handicaps initially remained constant in the 1980s; however, morbidity increased in the 1990s following a further decrease in mortality, which was associated with antenatal steroid and surfactant therapies introduced in the early 1990s. These treatments resulted in the survival of high-risk infants who previously would have died. Furthermore, postnatal steroid therapy, which was widely used to prevent or treat bronchopulmonary dysplasia, resulted in higher rates of cerebral palsy (CP).[1–3] The absolute number of both healthy and neurologically impaired children in the population thus increased in the 1990s.[3] Additional morbidity resulted from increased infection, necrotizing enterocolitis, and poor physical growth in infants of extremely low birth weight (<1 kg) and short gestation (<26 weeks).[3–5]

Since 2000, the outcomes of children with a birth weight of less than 1 kg have improved; this improvement has resulted from a significant decrease in nosocomial infections and intraventricular hemorrhage, together with a decrease in the use of postnatal steroid therapy.[6]

When outcome results are evaluated, considerable variation is noted in the results cited in different reports. One reason is that selection of patients by birth weight does not guarantee a homogeneous group, and populations studied in one center may differ considerably from those studied in another center. There are several causes for these differences. One of the most important factors is the pattern of referral to the neonatal intensive care unit (NICU). Units that receive admissions from numerous outlying hospitals have a selected population that may contain a disproportionate number of the sickest babies or may include only those infants deemed well enough to transport. In addition, patients treated in an "inborn" unit have the advantage of consistent and, presumably, good obstetric care coupled with the opportunity for immediate postnatal resuscitation and management. Inadequate resuscitation at birth and prolonged hypoxia and acidemia, together with the cold stress associated with transport that may be seen in referred patients, influence not only the outcome in the period immediately after birth but also the type and frequency of developmental sequelae. Other factors that may influence outcome include (1) the socioeconomic profile of the parents, (2) the proportion of infants with intrauterine growth restriction, (3) the incidence of extreme prematurity, (4) a selective admission policy, (5) a selective treatment policy, and (6) changes in therapy during the study period.

The major clinical outcomes that are important to preterm infants and their families are not only survival, but survival accompanied by normal long-term neurodevelopment.

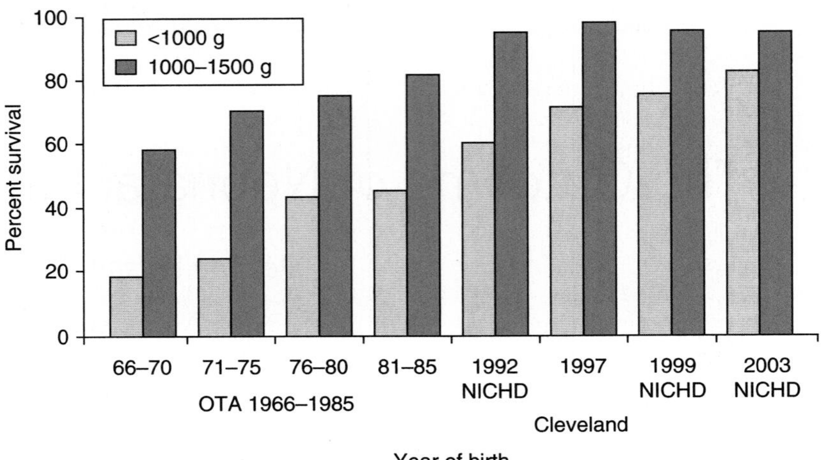

Fig. 19.1 Trends in Survival. Improvement in survival of low-birth-weight infants. Note that the figure stops in 2003 because of the fact that more recent outcomes research has focused more on gestational age as opposed to weight. *NICHD,* National Institute of Child Health and Human Development; *OTA,* Office of Technology Assessment. (Data for 1966 to 1985 from U.S. Congress, Office of Technology Assessment (OTA): *Neonatal Intensive Care for Low-Birthweight Infants: Cost and Effectiveness.* Health Technology Case Study 38. Washington, DC: U.S. Congress; 1987; data for 1992, 1999, and 2003 from Stevenson DK, Wright LL, Lemons JA, et al. Very low birth weight outcomes of the National Institute of Child Health and Human Development (NICHD) Neonatal Research Network, January 1993 through December 1994. *Am J Obstet Gynecol* 1998;179:1632; Fanaroff AA, Stoll BJ, Wright LL, et al; NICHD Neonatal Research Network: Trends in neonatal morbidity and mortality for very low birthweight infants. *Am J Obstet Gynecol* 2007;196[2]:147, e1; data for 1997 from Rainbow Babies and Children's Hospital, Cleveland, Ohio.)

TABLE 19.1 Survival and Neurodevelopmental Impairment According to Gestational Age

Gestational Age (wk)	Survival (%)	NDI (%)	Survival Without NDI (%)
22	5	80	1
23	26	65	9
24	56	50	28
25	76	39	46

NDI, Neurodevelopmental impairment.
Modified from Tyson JE, Parikh NA, Langer J, et al for the National Institute of Child Health and Human Development Neonatal Research Network. Intensive care for extreme prematurity—moving beyond gestational age. *N Engl J Med* 2008;358:1672.

TABLE 19.2 Outcome Variables at 23 to 25 Months' Corrected Age

	24–26 Weeks	27–31 Weeks	32–34 Weeks
Total followed (*n*)	450	2264	885
Cerebral palsy	7%	4%	1%
Deafness	1%	0.6%	0.5%
Blindness	0.7%	0.3%	1%
Subnormal development[a]	50%	41%	36%
Moderate/severe neuromotor or sensory disability[b]	6%	3%	1%

[a]Ages and Stages Questionnaire score <2 standard deviations below mean
[b]Cerebral palsy with Gross Motor Function Classification System (GMFCS) level 3–5 and /or bilateral deafness and or bilateral blindness
Modified from Pierrat V, Marchand-Martin L, Arnaud C, et al. Neurodevelopmental outcome at 2 years for preterm children born at 22 to 34 weeks' gestation in France in 2011: EPIPAGE-2 cohort study. *BMJ.* 2017;358:j3448.

These goals are not easily attainable; however, the landscape has improved over the past two decades, and there are now more intact survivors who attend mainstream schools and ultimately live independently. How to preserve brain function and permit normal brain development ex utero remain enormous challenges. The period between 20 and 32 weeks after conception is one of rapid brain growth and development. Illness, hemorrhage, ischemia, and metabolic disturbances such as hypoglycemia, hyperbilirubinemia, undernutrition, and infection during this time may compromise neurodevelopment. Indeed, events leading to the premature birth such as chorioamnionitis may have stimulated the release of cytokines that in turn injure the developing brain. Scores of publications continue to demonstrate a myriad of cognitive (mental), behavioral, and functional problems in the most immature babies compared with their term peers.

EDITORIAL COMMENT: Follow-up of graduates from the intensive care unit has shed the orphan role it had for so long, and outpatient neonatology clinics are now a genuine and legitimate component of neonatology. Minimizing harm and maximizing the opportunity for long-term neurodevelopment are the desired outcome.

Measures of outcomes of neonatal care include the rate of mortality before and after discharge from the neonatal intensive care nursery, rate of rehospitalizations, and incidence of chronic medical conditions such as asthma and growth failure.

According to the Centers for Disease Control and Prevention (CDC), the mortality rate for US preterm infants was 3.46% in 2013, a survival rate of more than 96%. In 2016, the CDC reported a 9.8% prematurity rate up from 9.6% in 2015.

Survival is proportional to the gestational age, and there is marked variability in outcome and interventions by country and even within countries. The survival at 22 weeks' gestational age ranges from 40% in Japan, 20% in Sweden, to less than 5% in parts of Europe where no effort is made to care for infants at this gestational age. About 40% of infants will survive at 23 weeks' gestation, but even though approximately 70% of infants survive at 24 weeks' gestation, few survive without major morbidity defined as one or more of necrotizing enterocolitis, infection, bronchopulmonary dysplasia, severe periventricular haemorrhage, periventricular leukomalacia, or retinopathy of prematurity stage 3 or greater.

At 25 weeks and 26 weeks, 81% and 87% of infants survive, respectively, with approximately one-fifth who do so free of major morbidity. From 27 weeks on, survival is 94%, and half of them survive free of major morbidity.[7] Observing the long-term follow-up of these infants is essential, and the impression is that long-term neurodevelopmental outcome is improving for at least some gestational age groups. Norman's data[8] from Sweden including 1196 extremely preterm infants, revealed that 1-year survival among live-born infants increased from 70% during 2004 to 2007 to 77% during 2014 to 2016, and survival without any major morbidity increased from 32% to 38%, respectively.

Neurodevelopmental sequelae include subnormal and borderline cognitive function and neurosensory deficits such as CP, deafness, and blindness. These sequelae have traditionally been used as outcome measures.[7] Other outcomes include functional abilities and the ability to perform the activities of daily living.[8–10] Additional measures involve special healthcare requirements such as the need for technologic aids, frequent physician visits and medications for chronic conditions, occupational and physical therapy, and special education and counseling.[8] Other measures may include impact on the family, quality of life,[11] and cost of care.

EDITORIAL COMMENT: Preterm subjects, even excluding those with severe disabilities, compared with term controls, are at increased risk of exhibiting problems related to executive dysfunction. Among adolescents born preterm, severe brain injury on neonatal ultrasound and lower maternal education are the most consistent factors associated with poor outcomes and problems with executive function.

Regional outcome studies provide the most accurate data because they include all infants born in a region rather than hospital-based results. Such studies have rarely been undertaken in the United States, although they have been performed in Canada, the United Kingdom, and Australia.[1] Results may also be reported from multigroup studies or randomized controlled trials of various therapies[12–14] (Box 19.1).

EDITORIAL COMMENT: International studies are helpful but must be interpreted with caution. A study examining neonatal survival rates among several countries found that the variation in survival rates at 22 to 23 weeks' gestation decreased significantly when stillbirths were added to the denominator. Data may be collected, interpreted, and analyzed differently in different parts of the world. (Smith LK, Morisaki N, Morken N, et al. An international comparison of death classification at 22 to 25 weeks' gestational age. *Pediatrics*. 2018;142[1]:e20173324.)

BOX 19.1 Measures of Very Low-Birth-Weight Outcome

Survival
- To discharge
- After discharge

Medical morbidity
- Rehospitalization
- Chronic lung disease
- Growth failure

Neurodevelopmental outcome
- Motor dysfunction (cerebral palsy)
- Mental retardation
- Seizures
- Vision problems
- Hearing disorders
- Behavioral problems
- School-age outcomes

Functional outcomes
- Health or illness
- Activity and skills of daily living
- Ambulation
- Need for technologic aids (gastric tube, oxygen)
- Need for special services

Quality of life

Impact on family

Cost of care

The risk of neurodevelopmental problems increases as birth weight and gestational age decrease. Additional risk factors include the occurrence of neonatal seizures; severe periventricular hemorrhage[15]; periventricular leukomalacia[16]; bronchopulmonary dysplasia, defined as an oxygen requirement at 36 weeks' postconceptional age; and severe intrauterine or neonatal growth failure, specifically a subnormal head circumference (≤2 standard deviations [SDs] from the mean) at discharge. Children born to mothers who have a low educational level or live in poverty demonstrate the additional detrimental effects of the environment. Among term-born children, risk factors for later neurologic and developmental sequelae also include perinatal asphyxia, neonatal seizures, an abnormal neurologic finding at discharge, and persistent pulmonary hypertension requiring prolonged ventilator therapy, nitric oxide therapy, or extracorporeal membrane oxygenation.[17] Children born with multiple major malformations also constitute a group that generally has a poor developmental outcome (Box 19.2). Over the past decade, evidence has emerged that children who experience critical illness in the newborn period, regardless of the underlying diagnosis, are at risk for memory impairment and academic problems, even with normal intelligence.[18]

IMPORTANCE OF FOLLOW-UP FOR HIGH-RISK INFANTS

Follow-up clinics should be an integral part of every NICU. Specialized care for problems of growth, sequelae of bronchopulmonary dysplasia, and adaptation is best provided within the setting of a neonatal follow-up program. This care should initially be provided by the neonatal department and then gradually transferred to developmental and educational specialists. The initial continuity of care is important to the family, who will find reassurance in the fact that the same people who were responsible for the life-saving decisions early in the infant's life are continuing to assume responsibility for the child's adaptation into home life. There is also a moral obligation to maintain this contact. Furthermore, even if the neonatologist does not continue the follow-up for an extended period, he or she will benefit greatly by maintaining contact with the nursery graduates and recognizing the sequelae of the early neonatal interventions.

When growth and neurodevelopmental outcomes are assessed, it is important to correct the child's age to account for the preterm birth. This should be done at least until the child is 3 years of age. For extremely immature infants (i.e., those born at 23–25 weeks' gestation), such age correction may be necessary until at least 5 years of age. Although the concept of correction for prematurity is most important during the early childhood years, evidence suggests that this correction continues well into school age, as standardized test scores for cognition and development continue to show improvement throughout school years.

BOX 19.2 Factors Affecting Outcomes for the Very Low-Birth-Weight Infant

- Birth weight <750 g or <26 weeks' gestation
- Periventricular hemorrhage (grade III or IV)
- Periventricular leukomalacia or other echodense lesions
- Persistent ventricular dilatation
- Neonatal seizures
- Chronic lung disease
- Neonatal meningitis
- Subnormal head circumference
- Poverty or parental deprivation
- Congenital malformations
- Outborn status (born at a center without a tertiary care neonatal intensive care unit)

MINOR TRANSIENT PROBLEMS

The first few months after the neonate's discharge can be considered a period of convalescence for the infant and parents as well. Many infants have minor problems specifically related to being born preterm, but these may be seen as major problems to their parents. These problems include anemia of prematurity, umbilical and inguinal hernias, relatively large, dolichocephalic, "preemie-shaped" heads, and subtle behavioral differences. Most healthy preterm infants are discharged home at 36 to 37 weeks' gestational age (or when they weigh about 1.9 kg). At this age, they still tend to sleep most of the day, waking only for feedings; to feed slowly and not always to demonstrate hunger; to sometimes be jittery; and to have "preemie" vocalizations, which include grunts and a relatively high-pitched cry. It is important to introduce parents of children recovering from neonatal illness to the concept of developmental milestones, as these children have often been secluded from contact with other children and developmentally restricted by medical issues.

TRANSIENT NEUROLOGIC ABNORMALITY

There is a very high incidence of transient neurologic abnormality during the first year of life, ranging from 20% to 40% among preterm infants, with a peak incidence of transient dystonia occurring at 7 months' corrected age.[19] These include abnormalities of muscle tone such as hypotonia or hypertonia. Such abnormalities present as poor head control at 40 weeks' corrected age (the expected term date), poor back support at 4 to 8 months, and sometimes a slight increase in the tone of the upper extremities. Because there is normally some degree of hypertonia during the first 3 months after term, it is difficult to diagnose the early developing spasticity related to CP. Children in whom CP later develops show hypotonia (poor head control and back support) initially and only later manifest spasticity of the extremities combined with truncal hypotonia. Spasticity during the first 3 to 4 months of life is an indicator of poor prognosis. Mild hypertonia or hypotonia persisting at 8 months usually resolves by the second year of life. Persistence of primitive reflexes beyond 4 months' corrected age might be a sign of early CP. Major neurologic handicap presents during the first 6 to 8 months after term in about

10% of newborns in the most high-risk categories; however, 90% of high-risk newborns will be or become neurologically normal after the first year of life. Although most cases of mild hypotonia or hypertonia detected at 8 months usually resolve, they may indicate later subtle neurologic dysfunction.[20]

PERSISTENT NEUROLOGIC SEQUELAE

Major neurologic handicap can usually be defined during the latter part of the first year of life or even earlier if severe. It is usually classified as CP (spastic diplegia, spastic quadriplegia, or spastic hemiplegia or paresis), hydrocephalus (with or without accompanying CP or sensory deficits), blindness (usually caused by retinopathy of prematurity), or deafness. Blindness currently occurs very rarely because laser treatment or cryotherapy for severe retinopathy of prematurity may prevent the progression of this disease. CP is an umbrella term encompassing a group of nonprogressive, noncontagious motor conditions that cause physical disability in human development, chiefly in the various areas of body movement. The neurologic symptoms of spastic CP include increased tone with velocity-dependent increased resistance to passive movement, pathologic reflexes such as hyperreflexia or pyramidal signs like the Babinski response, and abnormal patterns of movement and posture characterized in the lower limbs by equines foot, crouch gait, internal rotation, and hip adduction. In the upper limbs, the typical posture is arm flexion with fisted hands, adducted thumbs, and poorly coordinated finger movements. Symptoms of bilateral spastic CP include motor deficit with contractures, impaired normal gait, cognitive problems (seen less often in preterm than term children), visual problems such as blindness or strabismus, and epilepsy in the most severe cases. Although the vast majority of affected children have spastic CP, extrapyramidal forms, such as ataxic, dystonic, or dyskinetic CP, are increasing and may present with poor coordination, global hypotonia, or abnormal movements.

EDITORIAL COMMENT: Most healthcare providers are familiar with the relatively high risk of cerebral palsy in preterm infants. Nonetheless, as the vast majority of births are at term, numerically it is term and late preterm infants who account for the majority of cases of cerebral palsy despite their significantly lower risk. In an extensive review on cerebral palsy, Shepherd found that magnesium sulfate for women at risk of preterm birth for fetal neuroprotection can prevent cerebral palsy. Also, prophylactic antibiotics for women in preterm labor with intact membranes, and immediate rather than deferred birth of preterm babies with suspected fetal compromise, may increase the risk of cerebral palsy. (Shepherd E. Antenatal and intrapartum interventions for preventing cerebral palsy: an overview of Cochrane systematic reviews. *Cochrane Database Syst Rev.* 2017;8:CD012.)

Because CP is a central motor disorder with an incidence that is inversely related to gestational age, it is often used as a marker of neonatal outcome. The developmental and intellectual outcomes differ according to the severity of CP. For example, children with spastic quadriplegia usually have severe intellectual disability, whereas children with spastic diplegia or hemiplegia may have relatively intact mental functioning. Mental functioning is not always measurable in these children until after 2 to 3 years of age. In recognition of the fact that the severity of CP greatly affects the functional outcomes, there has been increased emphasis on functional assessments such as the Gross Motor Function Classification System, which defines motor function according to self-initiated movement with emphasis on sitting, walking, and mobility using a five-level classification system in which criteria meaningful to daily living distinguish the levels.[21]

Isolated motor disorders, such as developmental coordination disorder, which affects approximately one-third of preterm children, are more common than CP. By definition, these children have no neurosensory impairment and demonstrate intact cognitive function. They display a variety of fine and gross motor delays resulting in difficulties with common motor tasks such as manipulating pencils or silverware, pedaling a bicycle, or performing routine motor tasks of daily living.

PHYSICAL SEQUELAE AND CHRONIC DISEASE

A variety of common problems of prematurity often continue after NICU discharge. Anemia of prematurity is common, necessitating the monitoring of hemoglobin levels and reticulocyte counts, which typically rise by 3 to 6 months. Apnea of prematurity, resulting from immature regulation of breathing, may recur in infants who develop upper respiratory infections or require anesthesia for surgical procedures such as inguinal hernia repair.

Chronic diseases of prematurity, mainly chronic lung disease (bronchopulmonary dysplasia), gradually resolve during infancy, although children with bronchopulmonary dysplasia have higher rates of recurrent respiratory infections and asthma during childhood. Some may require weaning from home oxygen or withdrawal of discharge medications such as diuretics or bronchodilators. Scars from various neonatal surgical procedures (tracheotomy, thoracocentesis, Broviac lines, shunt procedures) tend to fade gradually and appear less significant as the child grows. There is, however, a high rate of rehospitalization, especially for those children of extremely low birth weight who have bronchopulmonary dysplasia or neurologic sequelae. Fifty percent of children with chronic lung disease may be hospitalized in the first year after discharge. Many hospitalizations that occur in winter have been because of respiratory syncytial virus infections. These may be minimized with respiratory syncytial virus immunization. Children with neurologic sequelae such as CP or hydrocephalus also have a higher rate of rehospitalization for shunt complications, orthopedic correction of spasticity, and eye surgery for strabismus.

PHYSICAL GROWTH

Premature infants typically require 110 to 130 kcal/kg/day to maintain growth, but may require more with increased work of breathing. Intrauterine and/or neonatal growth restriction is present in many very low-birth-weight neonates who require intensive care and a prolonged hospitalization. For infants born at a size appropriate for gestational age, poor neonatal growth may be related to a number of factors such as inadequate nutrition during the neonatal period, increased caloric requirements associated with breathing in chronic lung disease, poor feeding in neurologically impaired children, and/or the lack of parental care or an optimal environment for growth in the nursery and at home. As these conditions gradually resolve, and when an optimal home environment is provided, catch-up of growth may occur during childhood. However, many of these infants still remain subnormal in weight and height in their third year. Growth attainment after discharge is a very good measure of physical, neurologic, and environmental well-being. To promote optimal catch-up growth, neonatal nutrition needs to be maximized and sufficient calories provided during the recovery phase. This is especially important because catch-up of head circumference in both appropriate-for-gestational age and small-for-gestational age infants may occur during the first 6 to 12 months after term.

The prognosis for catch-up growth is less optimal in infants born small for gestational age after intrauterine growth failure because their initial period of growth failure occurred relatively early in gestation and extended for a longer time during the critical perinatal period of growth.

Predictors of poor catch-up growth include severe intrauterine growth failure, severe neonatal complications including bronchopulmonary dysplasia following prolonged ventilator and oxygen dependence, necrotizing enterocolitis requiring surgery, and neurologic impairment such as CP. Neurologically impaired children may also show failure to thrive after the neonatal discharge. The genetic potential for growth, as measured by midparental height, also plays a role in the potential for catch-up growth.[22] Studies on the prediction of catch-up growth from birth to adulthood suggest that catch-up in height extends into school age but is difficult to predict with great accuracy.[23] During later years of adolescence and young adulthood, emerging data raises questions about the relationship between early catch-up growth and increased risk of obesity, cardiac disease, and hypertension among former preterm born children.[24]

Use of increased-calorie formulas providing 22 calories per ounce and increased calcium might enhance growth during the first few months after discharge home; however, there are no reported studies of the longer-term effect of such formulas on growth to the second year of life and thereafter.

Extremely low-birth-weight infants with chronic lung disease (bronchopulmonary dysplasia) who can feed orally may be discharged home with oxygen supplementation when they are in stable condition. These infants need close follow-up with pediatric pulmonary specialists or neonatologists with expertise and interest in pulmonary follow-up care. As the infant is gradually weaned from oxygen, close attention needs to be paid to optimizing growth with the use of increased-calorie formulas and to the gradual weaning of any medications the child might be receiving such as diuretics or antireflux medication. Such children also require respiratory syncytial virus immunization in winter.

Most neurologic or physical problems resolve or become permanent during the first year of life. Furthermore, during the second year of life, the environmental effects of parental education and social class begin to influence the outcome measures. Clinical follow-up is essential for all high-risk infants during this period. After the first year, the new problems that become evident may include subtle motor, visuomotor, and behavioral difficulties. These are best diagnosed and treated in an educational rather than a medical setting.

It is important to pay attention to the mother's and father's well-being, their support systems, and their ability to care for the infant. Maternal depression is fairly prevalent following the birth of preterm and/or chronically ill infants.

FOLLOW-UP—WHO, WHAT, HOW, AND WHEN

Infants at highest risk should be followed. These include infants who had severe asphyxia complicated by seizures or signs of brain edema, periventricular or other intracranial injury, meningitis, or multisystem congenital malformations; infants who required ventilatory assistance; and those born with very low birth weights (especially those weighing <1 kg) or at 23 to 25 weeks' gestation.[25]

Growth (weight, height, and head circumference), neurologic development, psychomotor development, ophthalmologic status, vision, and hearing should all be examined on a regular basis.

TIMING OF FOLLOW-UP VISITS

The initial follow-up visit should be no more than 7 to 10 days after the neonatal discharge. This is essential to evaluate how the infant is adapting to the home environment. This visit usually occurs around the time of the expected date of delivery. For infants with complex medical needs, multidisciplinary follow-up clinics have merged primary pediatric care with neurodevelopmental follow-up, creating a "medical home" for children with sequelae of prematurity. A clinic visit at 4 months' corrected age is important to document problems of inadequate catch-up growth and severe neurologic abnormality that might require intervention or physical therapy. Because many of the active medical issues have resolved, this visit offers the opportunity to direct families toward emerging developmental and behavioral issues.

Eight months' corrected age is a good time to identify the presence of developing CP or other neurologic abnormality. It is also an excellent time for the first developmental assessment (preferably using the Bayley Scales of Infant Development). At this age, infants show very little outward stranger anxiety and are most cooperative. Although behavioral patterns are becoming established, early cognitive skills are still very dependent on motor function.

The Bayley score attained at 8 to 12 months' corrected age tends to decrease by the second year (partly as a function of the test and partly because of the increased effect of the environment) and is not of great prognostic significance. However, low scores (<80) are predictive of poor later functioning, as is CP. By 18 to 24 months' corrected age, most transient neurologic findings have resolved, and the neurologically abnormal child may show adaptation to neurologic sequelae. Furthermore, most of the potential catch-up growth has been achieved, although catch-up growth may occur into the adolescent years. During the second year of life, the mental scale of the Bayley scales provides some assessment of the child's cognitive performance, although these scales have very poor prognostic validity for IQ measurement at school age.[26,27] Cognitive function is not easily measured before 1 year of age because the test is based mainly on motor function. Children who have a Mental Development Index (MDI) score of less than 70 at 18 to 24 months' corrected age and do not have CP may have higher IQ scores on testing at school age, although they tend to have poorer school functioning than children who have a normal MDI score (>70) at 18 to 24 months of age.

Beyond the age of 3 years, other tests may be performed. These tests further validate the child's mental abilities. Language may also be measurable at this age. From 4 years of age, more subtle neurologic, visuomotor, and behavioral difficulties are measurable. These difficulties affect school performance even in children who have normal intelligence.[26,28]

NEUROSENSORY AND DEVELOPMENTAL ASSESSMENT

Neurodevelopmental handicap is usually defined in children who have a neurologic abnormality or a developmental quotient or IQ of less than 80. Some researchers include only a subnormal IQ (<70), whereas others include all children with an IQ less than 1 SD from the norm (IQ <85). Neurologic abnormality is usually classified by neurologic diagnosis, which can include hypotonia or hypertonia, CP (spastic diplegia or quadriplegia), hydrocephalus, blindness, or deafness.

The neurologic examination during infancy is best based on changes in muscle tone that occur during the first year of life. The scale developed by Amiel-Tison measures the progressive increase in active muscle tone (head control, back support, sitting, standing, and walking) together with the concomitant decrease in passive muscle tone that occurs during infancy.[29] Furthermore, it documents visual and auditory responses and some primitive reflexes. This method gives a qualitative assessment of neurologic integrity, which is defined as normal, suspect, or abnormal during the first year after term. The Amiel-Tison method of evaluation extends into early childhood.[29]

Short-term outcome studies of preterm infants who sustained a neonatal grade IV intraventricular hemorrhage (also known as *periventricular hemorrhagic infarction*) have reported a high rate of CP ranging from 40% to 85%; however, there has been no consensus regarding cognitive outcome, with normal cognition noted in 20% to 79%.[30] Roze et al prospectively collected a cohort of preterm infants with periventricular hemorrhagic infarction to determine motor,[31] cognitive, and behavioral outcome at school age and to identify cerebral risk factors for adverse outcome. Of 38 infants, 15 (39%) died. Twenty-one of the 23 survivors were included in the follow-up. The investigators concluded that the majority of surviving preterm children with periventricular hemorrhagic infarction had CP with limited functional impairment at school age. Intelligence was within 1 SD of the norm of preterm children without lesions in 60% to 80% of the children. Verbal memory, in particular, was affected. Behavioral and executive function problems occurred slightly more than in preterm infants without lesions. The functional outcome at school age of preterm children with periventricular hemorrhagic infarction is better than previously thought. Papile notes, "Roze et al's study points out one of the major shortcomings of infant neurodevelopmental testing. Because successful completion of many test items relies heavily on motor function, the scores achieved by preterm infants with motor impairment such as CP underestimate their true ability and may lead to an unduly pessimistic view regarding their ultimate outcome."[32]

EDITORIAL COMMENT: Morbidity and mortality data are often used to guide decision making for critically ill neonates both antenatally and in the neonatal intensive care unit (NICU). Although parents want honesty and truthfulness, it is important to recognize the danger of being overly pessimistic. This issue is discussed further in the "Ethics" chapter (see Chapter 20), with the goal being "for parents to feel like they have agency and ability and are good parents, before birth, at birth, and after, either in the NICU or until the death of their child." (Haward MF, Gaucher N, Payot A, Robson K, Janvier A. Personalized decision making: practical recommendations for antenatal counseling for fragile neonates. *Clin Perinatol.* 2017;44[2]:429-445.)

Psychomotor Developmental Tests

The Bayley Scales of Infant Development are the recognized standard for measuring infant development and may be used between early infancy and 42 months of age. Separate motor and mental scales each yield a developmental index with a mean of 100. The scales were revised and restandardized in 1993 and more recently in 2006. In the first year, motor skills are weighted heavily, even in the mental scale, but by the second year, cognitive functions, including speech and behavior, may be more reliably measured. The 2006 edition of the test has three scales that measure cognitive, language, and motor development as well as two scales that measure social-emotional development and adaptive behavior as reported by a parent. It is not clear that infant tests measure the same constructs as intelligence tests that are administered to older children. Infant tests are seen as a description of current functioning and thus tend not to be predictive. Generally, infant tests performed on very low-birth-weight children have overestimated the degree of intellectual impairment detected at school age.

In the preschool years and into adolescence, the following tests are often used both clinically and for research:

- The *Stanford-Binet Intelligence Scale* is used from age 2 years into the elementary school years. It provides a measure of intelligence that is highly correlated with school performance.
- The *Wechsler scales* (Wechsler Preschool and Primary Scale of Intelligence—Third Edition for preschoolers and Wechsler Intelligence Scale for Children—Fourth Edition for ages 6 to 16 years) yield verbal, performance, and full-scale scores with means of 100.
- The *Kaufman Assessment Battery for Children* is used between the ages of 3 and 10 years. Like the Stanford-Binet and Wechsler tests, it has a number of subscales to assess various components of intelligence.
- The *McCarthy Scales of Children's Abilities* provide measures of cognitive, perceptual-performance, and quantitative abilities in children between ages 2.5 and 8 years as well as a composite score (comparable to an IQ) and measures of motor and memory functions. However, this test has not been restandardized since 1972, and it is likely that the norms are outdated.
- The *Denver Developmental Screening Test* is used as a clinical screening tool in the first 6 years. It is not highly sensitive and fails to identify a significant number of at-risk children. Because it is not a quantitative assessment, it is rarely used for research to document outcomes in specific high-risk populations.
- The *Ages and Stages Questionnaire* provides a reliable developmental and social-emotional screening for children from birth to age 6 years. It has been designed to pinpoint developmental progress and catch delays, paving the way for interventions.

Visual Testing

An ophthalmologic examination should be performed on all high-risk infants before discharge. Infants younger than 30 to 32 weeks' gestation should have been followed with serial examinations in the nursery for signs of developing retinopathy of prematurity. Those who have residual findings at discharge or who have undergone laser therapy or cryotherapy should be followed by an ophthalmologist until the abnormal findings resolve. All children should undergo a repeat eye examination between 12 and 24 months of age. Infants of extremely low birth weight or gestational age who have had severe retinopathy of prematurity might require correction with glasses during infancy or early childhood.

Hearing

Hearing should be screened before the infant's discharge from the NICU. This may be done by measuring base-of-brain evoked responses or otoacoustic emissions. Hearing should be reexamined between 12 and 24 months of age, because the most common cause of hearing loss is upper respiratory tract and middle ear infections, which may occur during the first 2 years of life.

EARLY INTERVENTION

Early environmental enrichment with close attention to the family's needs may improve the developmental outcome of all children, including infants with normal birth weight as well as low birth weight and low gestational age, and especially of children in disadvantaged homes.[33] Studies of early intervention have, however, shown a decrease in beneficial effects after discontinuation of the intervention or with advancing age of the child. Initial home visits during early childhood by experienced nurses are also important for surveillance of the child's growth and medical needs, for education concerning preterm behavior and development, and for support of the mother. Such home visits can gradually be phased out as the mother becomes more confident and when the child becomes enrolled in an educational enrichment program, if available.

POINTS TO REMEMBER

1. Correct for gestational age (preterm birth) until at least 3 years of age.
2. Do not emphasize to the parents the many abnormalities observed during the 3-month postdischarge period of convalescence because most are transient and have little prognostic significance.
3. Be available, be honest, be optimistic. After the initial diagnosis of abnormality is made, most children show improvement, restitution, and growth.
4. The majority of high-risk children do well.
5. In some cases, the diagnosis of CP, hydrocephalus, or blindness is made during the first year of life. Early intervention and supportive psychological help that can be facilitated by the follow-up clinic are essential.
6. Except when a severe neurologic or sensory disorder persists, ultimate development depends on multiple factors including parental education, social class, the child's genetic potential, and the environment. For children of extremely low birth weight and short gestation, neonatal risk factors tend to predominate.[3]
7. The functional capacity attained is more important than the medical diagnosis of abnormality.

EARLY CHILDHOOD OUTCOMES

A summary of some outcome variables for extremely immature and low-birth-weight infants is presented in Fig. 19.2. The importance of early identification of developmental deficits to plan and establish early appropriate interventions should be emphasized. Developmental outcomes of children are influenced by many risk factors, including social, genetic, and biologic ones.

SCHOOL-AGE OUTCOMES

A summary of rates of school problems among 8-year-old very preterm versus term-born children from the nationwide EPIPAGE follow-up cohort in France is presented in

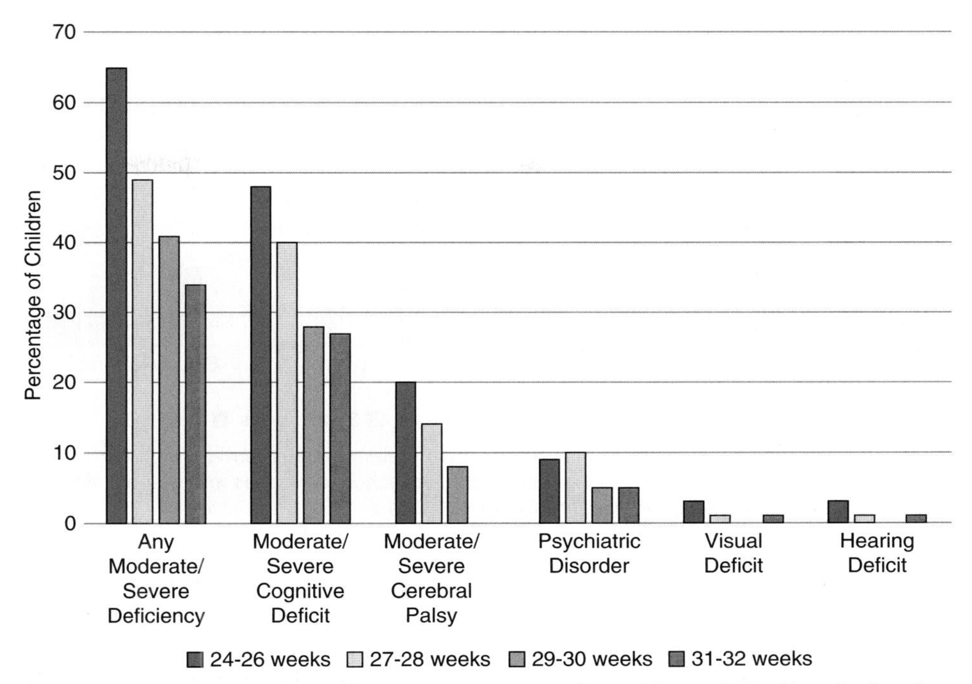

Fig. 19.2 Percentage of 8-year-old children born very preterm from 1997 to 1998 with major impairments. (From Marret S, Marchand-Martin L, Picaud JC, et al. Brain injury in very preterm children and neurosensory and cognitive disabilities during childhood: the EPIPAGE cohort study. *PLoS One* 2013;8(5):e62683.)

Fig. 19.3. At school age, children are required to conform to formal learning in a classroom. Many have difficulty in this regard because of attention and other neuropsychologic deficits, including poor memory, visuomotor and fine and gross motor function, and difficulty with spatial concepts and executive function.[34,35] Children who were born preterm are often also shy and withdrawn and have social difficulties as well as behavioral problems, including attention-deficit/hyperactivity disorder (ADHD) and symptoms of depression or anxiety.[36]

EDITORIAL COMMENT: The EPICure study began as an ongoing longitudinal evaluation of extremely premature infants born in the United Kingdom and the Republic of Ireland between March and December 1995. The initial cohort consisted of the 308 children who were 20 to 25 weeks' gestational age at birth and survived beyond the first year after birth. Among extremely preterm children in mainstream schools, 105 (57%) had special educational needs, and 103 (55%) required special educational needs resource provision. The investigators concluded that survivors of extremely preterm birth remain at high risk of learning impairments and poor academic attainment in middle childhood. Papile noted, "The high prevalence of intellectual and learning difficulties suggests that a disruption/delay of global brain development rather than a specific lesion may be the underlying cause."[32]. Given changes in care since the original EPICure study, EPICure 2 began in 2006 and found slightly better outcomes for babies born at 24 and 25 weeks as well as a higher percentage of babies who do not have problems at follow-up. (Moore TM, Hennessy EM, Myles J, et al. Neurological and developmental outcome in extremely preterm children born in England in 1995 and 2006: the EPICure studies. *BMJ*. 2012; 345:e7961.)

Taylor et al reviewed the topic of mathematics deficiencies in children with very low birth weight or very preterm birth.[37] They noted that children with birth weights of less than 1.5 kg and those with a gestational age of less than 32 weeks have more mathematics disabilities or deficiencies and higher rates of mathematics learning disabilities than normal-birth-weight, term-born children. They commented, "Mathematics disabilities or deficiencies are found even in children without global disorders in cognition or neurosensory status even when IQ is controlled, and they are associated with other learning problems and weaknesses in perceptual motor abilities and executive function. Factors related to poorer mathematics outcomes include lower birth weight and gestational age, neonatal complications, and possible abnormalities in brain structure." Little is known about mathematics disabilities or deficiencies. Thus, although the outcomes have improved overall, there is no room for complacency. Understanding the mechanisms of injury may help provide the solutions because neuroplasticity is known to permit the neonatal brain to move a given function to a different location as a consequence of normal experience or brain damage.

A variety of behavioral problems are common among preterm survivors at school age, including attention and hyperactivity disorders, emotional difficulties and socialization issues. Rates of ADHD range from 25% for preterm children to 7% for term-born children.[38] Poor cognition may contribute to attention deficits or vice versa. Reports based on screening assessments have suggested that autism may be more prevalent among preterm children. Internalization problems such as depression, anxiety, and poor adaptive

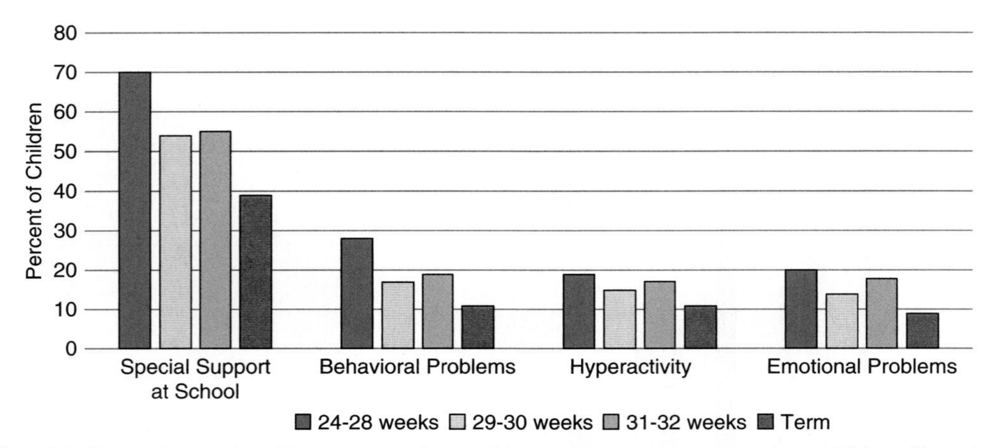

Fig. 19.3 Rates of school problems among 8-year-old very preterm versus term-born children (From Larroque B, Ancel PY, Marchand-Martin L, et al. Special care and school difficulties in 8-year-old very preterm children: the EPIPAGE cohort study. *PLoS One* 2011;6(7):e21361.)

skills have all been associated with prematurity, resulting in socialization and peer relationship difficulties. Motor delays may compromise playground skills, causing peer victimization and rejection. Immature behavioral patterns leading to parental overprotection may yield poor socioemotional adjustment.

YOUNG ADULT OUTCOMES

The initial survivors of the early years of neonatal intensive care in the 1970s are now adults. The results, to date, reveal that although these individuals may have a lower IQ on formal testing and fewer attend college than normal-birth-weight, term-born controls, they function fairly well and, with few exceptions, are satisfied with their health-related quality of life, which, when studied, is similar to that of controls.[39] Very low-birth-weight young adults also demonstrate less risk-taking behavior than normal-birth-weight controls, including alcohol use, drug abuse, and delinquent activities. Rates of ADHD tend to decrease during young adulthood, although symptoms of depression and withdrawal have been reported in women.[39]

Overwhelming evidence is accumulating that the neurodevelopmental consequences of extremely preterm birth extend far beyond the confines of CP (a static lesion) and intellectual delay. Problems in attention, executive function, memory, spatial skills, fine and gross motor function, speech and language, visual integration, and mathematics, together with behavioral disorders, are common. *Executive function* refers to a collection of processes that are responsible for purposeful, goal-directed behavior, such as planning, setting goals, initiating, using problem-solving strategies, and monitoring thoughts and behavior. Executive functioning is important for a child's intellectual development, behavior, emotional control, and social interaction. Luu et al evaluated executive and memory function in 337 adolescents born preterm compared with those in term-born controls at 16 years.[40] After adolescents with neurosensory disabilities and those with an IQ of less than 70 were excluded, adolescents born preterm, compared with term controls, were found to show deficits in executive function on tasks of verbal fluency, inhibition, cognitive flexibility, planning and organization, and working memory as well as verbal and visuospatial memory. The presence of these deficits was associated with severe brain injury as detected by neonatal ultrasonography and lower maternal educational level. This implies that providing a more stimulating and enriched home environment may be of some benefit in averting executive function deficits.

Preliminary long-term follow-up data suggest that preterm and low-birth-weight children have a higher incidence of hypertension, visceral obesity, asthma, and perturbations in glucose-insulin homeostasis, including type 2 diabetes. Speculation exists regarding the relationship between these noncommunicable disorders and possible alteration in genetic programming caused by events such as intrauterine growth restriction, premature interruption of pregnancy with change in redox state, nutritional and pharmacologic protocols used in the nursery, and postdischarge maximization of catch-up growth. Unfortunately, a limited understanding of the mechanisms underlying these possible programming effects exists because premature birth, neonatal intensive care, and survival of extremely immature babies is a historically recent and uniquely human phenomenon.

The reference list for this chapter can be found online at www.expertconsult.com.

20

Ethical Issues

Jennifer McGuirl, Peter D. Murray, Jonathan M. Fanaroff

The mortality rate of imperiled newborns has decreased since the inception of neonatology as a specialty.[1] Neonatologists are now able to save smaller and sicker infants, yet this decrease in mortality has not seen a concomitant decrease in severe morbidity such as impaired neurodevelopmental outcome.[2] The lack of a decrease in morbidity is most apparent in those infants born extremely preterm or on the edge of viability, for purposes of this chapter defined as 22 to 25 weeks' gestation.[2] The ever-present question in caring for imperiled newborns, particularly those for whom survival is either unlikely or associated with significant morbidity, is what factors should be taken into account when pursuing shared decision making on their behalf.

Central to any decision-making framework in clinical medicine is a basic understanding of the foundational principles of biomedical ethics. Originally described by the landmark text *Principles of Biomedical Ethics* in 1977, the foundational principles include respect for autonomy, beneficence, justice, and nonmaleficence.[3] Understanding that infants are members of the human species, it follows then that they are deserving of having the principles of biomedical ethics applied to their care in the same way that an adult would. The principle of autonomy protects the decisions of the competent individual as they apply to their own health care, in turn ensuring one's self-governance of themselves.[3] The classic example of respect for autonomy in medicine is the well-informed Jehovah's Witness refusing a blood transfusion that may be life-saving. Infants in the neonatal intensive care unit (NICU) are special in that they themselves cannot make decisions on their behalf. Pervasive in pediatrics is the understanding that, as long as decision makers do not have material conflicts of interests (such as a parent suspected of child abuse refusing to allow withdrawal of life-sustaining measures out of a fear of a homicide charge after the patient dies), their choices ought to be respected.[4] The decisions of a parent as they pertain to their child should rarely be challenged with a court order except for cases where the intention of the parent is outside of the realm of what a reasonable person would do.[4]

The principle of beneficence ("do good") refers to possible obligations in a broad sense that contribute to the overall benefit of a person and are typically thought of as a positive action.[3] In this sense, a positive action means the actual performance of an act meant to benefit another. Beneficent actions are not always obligatory; that is to say, just because something may benefit someone else, that action may not always have to be performed. For example, when the outcome of resuscitation is nebulous at best, we defer to the parents for guidance on their wishes, thus respecting their autonomy. When the outcomes of resuscitation are reasonably known to be favorable (a well-grown 32 weeks' gestation fetus, for example, who needs to be delivered given maternal health problems), we then act in a way such as to maximize benefit to the infant and will resuscitate. This holds true even if the parents object to the resuscitation. Similarly, a life-saving blood transfusion in an emergent situation for the infant of a Jehovah's Witness parent will be given such as to maximize the benefit of the infant. This is not to say that every possible action to benefit an infant must be undertaken; there are discretionary constraints.[3]

In contrast to the principle of beneficence and a positive action, the principle of nonmaleficence may be thought of as a negative action. We are obligated to not harm the infants under our care and should therefore intentionally avoid harmful actions. That being said, many of the treatments we prescribe and the procedures we perform are, indeed, harmful. How are we justified in harming our patients then? As long as there is a reasonable expectation of benefit from a painful procedure (inserting a chest tube to evacuate a pneumothorax in an otherwise healthy preterm infant, for example), it is justified, even when considering the principle of nonmaleficence. The same act of inserting a chest tube into the thorax of an infant with no chance of survival would be viewed as a violation of the principle of nonmaleficence, given the benefits of treatment are highly likely to not outweigh the burdens. The principle of nonmaleficence often relies on language that is imprecise in its meaning, such as the word *futility.* Although physicians strive to avoid providing care they deem nonbeneficial, thus avoiding violation of the principle of nonmaleficence, such care is often provided at the request of family.[5]

The principle of justice is, perhaps, the hardest of all of the principles to grasp as it pertains to neonates. Justice can be thought of in a formal sense; that is to say equals, must be treated equally. For example, imagine two women are both at 22 weeks and 6 days' gestation. Woman A presents to hospital X where a policy against resuscitation of infants less than 23 weeks is in place. Woman B presents to hospital Y that has no such policy, and resuscitation is offered and provided as long as the parents are well informed of the possible outcomes of resuscitation. Although it is within the realm of reasonable that hospital X has such a policy against resuscitation, such monumental decisions should not be left to lottery. In this case, hospital X may want to suggest transfer to hospital Y if the parents desire an attempt of resuscitation after being well informed of the possible outcomes.

WHAT/WHO DEFINES THE LIMITS OF VIABILITY, AND MUST ALL THESE INFANTS BORN AT THE LIMITS OF VIABILITY BE RESUSCITATED?

Continued improvement in neonatal care has shifted the limits of viability to younger, more immature gestational ages. In 2014, an executive summary of a workshop conducted by the National Institutes for Child health and Human Development (NICHD), the Society for Maternal-Fetal Medicine, the American Academy of Pediatrics (AAP), and the American College of Obstetricians and Gynecologists (ACOG) that focused on periviable birth (defined as birth period from 20 0/7–25 6/7 weeks' gestation) was published. This is a critical period of gestation during which brief pregnancy prolongation can significantly alter the potential for survival and long-term complications. This consensus group encouraged more intensive treatment at younger gestational ages than previously recommended, adding significantly to the ongoing debate about specific gestational age–based recommendations.[6]

Currently in 2018, 23 weeks' gestation remains the accepted lower limit of viability, although this threshold continues to be the focus of intense deliberation. There are many institutions where medical professionals are initiating resuscitation and providing neonatal intensive care for fetuses born at 22 weeks' gestation, whereas others strictly adhere to this gestational age range for no or limited options for intervention. The gray zone time period of periviability most often quoted is between 22 to 25 weeks' gestation; it is a gestational age spectrum during which optimal treatment options are unclear, and treatments offered vary based on provider and/or parental preference. The outer thresholds of less than 22 weeks and greater than 25 completed weeks' gestation represent points at which treatment variation is limited, and so, too, are parental authority and provider preference. It has been generally accepted that fetuses less than 22 weeks' gestation receive comfort care only and no intensive treatment, and that infants born after 25 weeks' gestation generally receive intensive treatment, providing there are no anomalies or conditions inconsistent with survival. Advances in obstetric management of preterm and periviable pregnancies and significant enhancements in neonatal treatments over the past 30 years have resulted in lowering of the threshold for potential survival to 22 to 23 weeks' gestation, and raised concerns about what is appropriate practice at the upper end of the periviability threshold at 25 weeks' gestation.

These parameters have been established based primarily on morbidity and mortality statistics collected by various neonatal research networks throughout North America, Europe, and Australasia. Consensus guidelines have been promulgated by a variety of perinatal organizations, including the National Institutes of Health, ACOG, AAP, British Association of Perinatal Medicine, World Association of Perinatal Medicine, and the Nuffield Council on Bioethics in the United Kingdom. The NICHD neonatal research network reports survival rates of 6% at 22, 26% at 23, 55% at 24, and 72% at 25 weeks' gestation, respectively.[7] Morbidity rates that encompass mild, moderate, and severe neurodevelopmental impairment are reported as: 100% at 22, 92% at 23, and 91% at 24 weeks' gestation, respectively.[7] Survival data and neurodevelopmental outcomes reported by the Vermont Oxford Neonatal Network, a consortium of NICUs across the United States and including neonatal units worldwide, are similar.[8] A systematic review of guidelines for the management of extremely premature deliveries published in 2015 by Guillén et al concluded that there continues to be wide variation in treatment recommendations (comfort care, parental wishes, individualized care, or active care), particularly between 23 and 24 weeks' gestation, although there is general agreement across highly developed countries in the world and among international professional organizations that comfort care is appropriate at 22 weeks' gestation, with active care more commonly recommended at 25 weeks of gestation.[9] It is of interest that at 23 weeks' gestation, these guidelines emphasize comfort care, deferring fully to parental wishes, individualized care (allows for physician assessment at the time of birth, informing the treatment options), or offer no recommendation. In contrast, at 24 weeks' gestation, these guidelines focus recommendations on following parental wishes, individualizing care or active care; several guidelines offer no specific recommendations. AAP and ACOG guidelines are in

CASE 20.1

A 38-year-old G4P0 woman presents at the hospital in active labor with premature rupture of membranes at 22 4/7 weeks' gestation. The fetus is a product of in vitro fertilization, which is the fifth cycle this couple has gone through. It is a female, singleton pregnancy with an estimated fetal weight of 500 g. The woman has received good prenatal care, and all fetal ultrasounds have been normal. The woman's labor is progressing, and she is expected to deliver in the next 48 hours. The neonatal and obstetric teams meet with the woman and her husband to discuss the plan of care for the woman and the fetus.

Thought questions:

1. What/who defines the limits of viability, and must all these infants born at the limits of viability be resuscitated?
2. What delivery options should be offered to the woman? Should she be offered prenatal steroids? Should she be offered a monitored delivery? Is it appropriate to offer a cesarean section for a fetal indication?
3. Who should make decisions regarding forgoing resuscitation or treatment of an infant in the periviable period? What ethical principles can be applied?

agreement, recommending that care be individualized across the period of 22 through 25 weeks' gestation. The American Heart Association neonatal resuscitation guidelines supports comfort care at 22 weeks, deferring to parental wishes at 23 and 24 weeks' gestation, and providing active care at 25 weeks of gestation.

Some clinicians argue that the data on which these recommendations are based are biased. The potential for bias may be because of the reporting of older birth cohorts born during the 1980s and early 1990s. These studies offer true longitudinal information in terms of outcomes into adulthood, but are not reflective of the outcomes for the beneficiaries of advances in obstetric and neonatal practices that have occurred since 1990. In addition, some health, cognitive, and neurologic morbidities have remained relatively static, whereas others have improved. Although survival rates have increased for infants born between 22 and 25 weeks' gestation and there have been some shifts in the severity of disability experienced by these extremely preterm survivors to more moderate and mild neurodevelopmental impairment, on the whole, overall impairment rates have remained stable since the mid-1990s, when use of antenatal corticosteroid therapy and postnatal exogenous surfactant administration became standard practice. Reduction in severe morbidity has been greatest among infants born at or greater than 25 weeks' gestation. Other clinicians make the case that if one creates an arbitrary cutoff line at 23 weeks' gestation for active care and doesn't attempt to resuscitate fetuses at 22 weeks' gestation, then a self-fulfilling prophecy is sustained, and there will be no further improvements in survival or developmental outcomes. There are data to support this. Data from Japan where active care is provided to fetuses at 22 weeks' gestation demonstrate lower mortality rates of 64% before hospital discharge for this group of infants.[10] An important caveat is that many of the infants in the Japanese studies were lost to follow-up, so better outcome data is needed to more accurately assess the impact of active intervention at this gestation. In conjunction with increased survival, the study investigators reported an increase in the number of infants with cerebral palsy, indicating that improved survival does not necessarily equate to better outcomes.[10]

Tyson and colleagues reported that gestational age alone does not independently predict outcomes for these extremely immature fetuses; other characteristics such as weight, sex, administration of antenatal steroids, and whether the infant is a multiple or a singleton are also important predictors and should be considered when counseling a family.[11] Although we have outcome data in terms of numbers of children who have died or who experience a particular outcome, there are significant variations in outcomes influenced by myriad sociodemographic and management practices that confound our ability effectively predict an individual child's expected outcome. This makes antenatal counseling and discussions about treatment decisions for the periviable fetus very challenging. A 2015 report in the *New England Journal of Medicine* shows significant between-hospital variation in the treatment of neonates at the edge of viability. Practice variations and differences in available resources likely account for some of the discrepancies in outcomes, adding further complexity to antenatal counseling.[12] One example cited a range of active treatments of infants born at 22 weeks' gestation from 7.7% to 100%, depending on the birth hospital.[12] There is much less interhospital variation in active treatment of infants born at or greater than 25 weeks' gestation, but the authors still report differences in outcomes, so these outcome differences are not solely attributable to differences in treatment decisions between hospitals.[12]

A framework centered on probability-based thresholds has been proposed by Tyson and colleagues as a strategy to help families and clinicians approach decision making when outcomes are variable or unclear.[13] The model proposes that when the probability of survival without profound impairment is 10% or less and the probability of death or profound impairment (developmental score <50 or physical impairments that limit voluntary control of movement and involve all areas of motor function) is 90% or greater, intensive care should not be offered; instead, we should support families through the process of comfort care for their infant. For fetuses for whom the expected outcome would be a 10% to 20% chance of survival without profound impairment and an 80% to 90% chance of death or profound impairment, comfort care is an acceptable choice, although parental wishes for treatment can be honored with an understanding that treatment should be considered experimental. As the probability of survival without profound impairment increases and the odds of the combined outcome of death or survival with profound disability decreases, intensive care becomes optional or automatic (mandatory). The continuum for which intensive care would be optional encompasses the probability of survival without profound impairment ranging from 20% to 65%, with a concurrent probability of death or profound impairment of 35% to 80%. Fetuses for whom intensive care would be deemed mandatory are those whose unimpaired survival ranges from 65% to 100%, and risk of death or profound impairment is less than 35%. Using this framework provides clinicians and families with a means for incorporating changing outcomes associated with advances in treatment.

The fetus in case 1 is estimated to be 22 4/7 weeks' gestation, 500 g, female, and a singleton. The pregnancy is a product of in vitro fertilization; consequently, the estimated gestational age is likely accurate. When the infant's characteristics of female gender, 22 weeks' gestation, singleton pregnancy are put into the NICHD calculator, the results predict a 91% chance of death or moderate to severe neurodevelopmental impairment if antenatal steroids have been given before delivery. Without antenatal steroid administration, the death or moderate to severe disability rate rises to 95%. It is clear that when counseling families of periviable fetuses, the information shared and recommendations offered are in part guided by the available outcome data that is utilized.

WHAT DELIVERY OPTIONS SHOULD BE OFFERED TO THE WOMAN? SHOULD SHE BE OFFERED PRENATAL STEROIDS? SHOULD SHE BE OFFERED A MONITORED DELIVERY? IS IT APPROPRIATE TO OFFER A CESAREAN SECTION FOR A FETAL INDICATION?

In case 1, after sufficient discussion with the family, it is ethically justifiable to withhold obstetric interventions and aggressive neonatal resuscitation. If such a decision is made by the family, antenatal steroids should not be given, but if there is lack of clarity and the family is unsure of how they want to proceed, then the antenatal steroids should be administered. Universally, antenatal steroid administration improves neonatal outcomes and carries minimal risk to the fetus and the pregnant woman in most circumstances. Yet it should be understood that just because steroids are given, neither the parents nor the physician are obligated to offer/initiate other intensive treatment measures. The administration of antenatal corticosteroids is not ethically mandatory, but treatment with antenatal steroids should be offered if the parents are unsure about how they want to proceed, while making it clear that choosing to give antenatal steroids does not obligate the fetus, once born, to a course of intensive treatment. If the decision is made not to proceed with further obstetrical inventions and neonatal resuscitation, then a plan for comfort care should be created.

Discussions regarding a monitored delivery and cesarean section for fetal indications are more controversial primarily because these interventions can contribute to increased maternal risk with unclear fetal benefit. Intrapartum continuous electronic fetal heart rate monitoring is used to alert the obstetrician of a fetus potentially exposed to an intrapartum hypoxic insult and thus requiring emergent delivery to improve perinatal outcome.[14] In the case of periviable neonates, it is unclear what to do with the information monitoring provides. If a family requests intrapartum fetal monitoring, it is important to discuss what their expectations and goals are and the possible responses to a change in the fetal status in the context of monitoring that is difficult to evaluate because of the fetal immaturity. Again, it is important to discuss that the use of continuous intrapartum monitoring does not commit the pregnant woman to a cesarean section for a concerning category III tracing indicating fetal distress.

Cesarean sections for a category III tracing, indicating fetal distress in infants born in the periviable period, are not routinely offered. The evidence supports that there is no benefit to an operative delivery in infants in the periviable period; an operative delivery does not improve perinatal or neonatal outcomes.[15] The potential risks and the benefits to both fetus and the pregnant woman must be considered, and the physician has the right to refuse to perform a cesarean section for solely fetal indications if she/he feels it would cause short- or long-term harm to the pregnant woman with no proven benefit to the fetus.[15] In this case, with an infant at 22 4/7 weeks' gestation, it would be reasonable and ethically permissible to offer antenatal steroids, but if the parents choose to administer antenatal steroids, there is not then an obligation to offer a monitored delivery or a cesarean section for fetal indications. The benefit to the fetus is ambiguous, and the risks to the pregnant woman and the future childbearing are significant.

WHO SHOULD MAKE DECISIONS REGARDING FORGOING RESUSCITATION OR TREATMENT OF AN INFANT IN THE PERIVIABLE PERIOD? WHAT ETHICAL PRINCIPLES CAN BE APPLIED?

When an individual is unable to make autonomous decisions, a surrogate decision maker is designated. In the case of neonates, this is most often presumed to be the infant's parents. Typically the surrogate decision maker is encouraged to make decisions for the individual based on what the individual would have wanted, a concept known as substitute judgment. However, for newborns, there is no way to know what they would have wanted, and so the surrogate decision maker is expected to decide based on the best interests of their baby. The best-interest standard is based on the principles of beneficence and nonmaleficence. Recall, beneficence means "acts of mercy, kindness, and charity."[3] The principle of beneficence "refers to a statement of moral obligation to act for the benefit of others."[3] The principle of nonmaleficence is the obligation to do no harm.[3] Although the best interest standard is based on beneficence and nonmaleficence, it is often still hard to determine what is or is not going to be in the infant's best interest. It is a subjective concept that reminds us to place the child at the center of our discussions. It involves a full assessment of benefits versus burdens of the proposed treatment. Quality of life (QOL), although controversial, is often a leading contributor to the equation, and some question of whether consideration of an infant's QOL in isolation or within the context of the family structure should be considered.[15]

The majority of physicians will defer decisions regarding resuscitation in infants in the periviable period to the parents. The outcomes in these infants in the periviable period are uncertain, and the risk/benefit ratio of such treatment choices might be best evaluated by the parents once a clear and detailed explanation of what is known by the physicians is communicated to them.[15] This gives the parents the opportunity to interpret the information in the context of their own moral values and to make a decision that is in the best interest of their child.

It is often debated whether the best interest of the child should be evaluated in isolation, excluding the family's interests, or if such considerations truly play a role in what is ultimately in the best interest of these imperiled infants. Chiswick and others believe that the best interest of the infants is inextricably linked to that of their parents/families and deserves considerable weight.[16] It is a false assumption to believe that we can force families to only focus on the interests of the child; it is inevitable that families are going to bring in the interests of the family, siblings, and partners. Allowing families to include their interests as well as the infants' in decisions regarding treatments at the margins of viability is ethically justifiable. Their decisions should be respected unless they demonstrate a lack of regard for the infant's life.[17]

Although the primary decision makers for infants are considered to be their parents, a model of shared decision making between parents/guardians and physicians is recommended. Shared decision making is a more comprehensive approach and involves both the physician and the parents. Each play an essential role in the decision-making process. Physicians bring their expertise in medical knowledge and their experience with similar cases, whereas the parents can help elucidate their values and preferences.[18] Shared decision making is a continuum during which the physician may explain the available medical options or may make recommendations and patients/parents may be either completely passive or active in the decision-making process.[18] Such a model for decision making is advocated for because it supports the respect for persons' self-determination and enhances patients' well-being.

It is important to identify and evaluate factors that influence decision making: the patient, patient sociodemographics, provider perspectives, and institutional guidelines.[19] Patients and providers bring personal experiences, values, and preferences to every encounter. In addition to the clinical situation, there is the balance of maternal and fetal well-being as described previously. Patient preference carries significant weight. Often, pregnant women and their families express a preference to "do everything" or "do nothing." The phrase "do everything" is an amorphous term, unclear in its meaning unless time is taken to explore with parents what the phrase means to them. Individual views about hope versus pessimism affect both parents and providers. Providers can have strongly held beliefs that influence their willingness to offer some interventions. Education and socioeconomic status should not influence decision making. Although each pregnancy is cherished, often pregnancies achieved through assisted reproductive technologies are considered more precious. This perspective may alter parental preferences and the decisions made. Institutional policies may also influence care options and decision making. Hospital policies may be based on established professional practice parameters or internal consensus guidelines and are often subject to significant variation.

Thus selective resuscitation in the gray zone of viability should be based on the infant's best interest, inclusive of the family's values, and guided by the physician. For infants at the margins of viability, outcomes are uncertain and ambiguous. Some may consider the potential harms acceptable in relation to the benefit, and others may feel that the potential harms are too great and the benefit too uncertain. The treatment choices regarding resuscitation should be explained to the parents, and a model of shared decision making should be used. The physician should provide recommendations allowing them to share the decisional responsibility.[15] Some families may want an active role in the decision-making process, and others may prefer a more passive role. Whatever their desired level of involvement is, it should be respected.[15] The parental level of involvement is often influenced by religious and cultural beliefs; these, too, should be respected.

Finally, there is the concept of parental authority, which is intended to replace autonomy. Infants in the NICU do not have capacity and cannot make autonomous choices. Therefore it is generally accepted that in most circumstances, parents have the right to speak on their child's behalf. This is often referred to as parental autonomy, although this is a misnomer because one person cannot have "self-rule" over another.[20] A more appropriate term is *parental authority*, which includes the authority to consent to medical and surgical treatments and presumably the authority to refuse treatments on the infant's behalf.[20] Decision making based on parental authority is contingent on disclosure of all information necessary to make an informed decision.[21] It is important to note that this right to refusal is not without limitations, which is different than the autonomy granted to a competent adult. This parental right to refusal for treatment of the infant is constrained, or counterbalanced, by what is deemed to be in the infant's best interest. The AAP Committee on Bioethics clarifies this concept, stating: "Our social system generally grants patients and families wide discretion in making their own decisions about health care and continuing, limiting, declining or discontinuing treatment, whether life-sustaining or otherwise. Medical professionals should seek to override family wishes only when those views clearly conflict with the interests of the child."[22]

For the infant at 22 4/7 weeks' gestation, in this scenario, the parents should be counseled regarding the extremely low chance for survival (<10%) and extremely high probability of death or profound disability (>90%) if the infant were to survive, based on national and international results. Although comfort care is an appropriate and well-supported course of action when this fetus is born, should the family wish individualized or active care, despite recommendations for comfort care at this gestation, there should be a thorough discussion about the extremely low likelihood of survival with neonatal intensive care and the universal health and developmental sequelae experienced by the few survivors at this gestation. Within a framework of individualized care, a trial of therapy in the delivery room could be offered based on parental wishes. More aggressive treatment should not be recommended or encouraged. If the infant appears more mature at the time of birth, an individualized approach can be initiated in the delivery room, predicated on discussions with the family regarding their wishes related to a trial of therapy. A trial of therapy does not obligate families or neonatal care providers to a continuing or aggressive course of care. If the infant does not respond to treatment, the goals of care should be reassessed and care redirected to comfort care and support for the family through the death of their infant. Again, parental requests for comfort care should be honored and encouraged. Both withholding (not escalating) and withdrawing (deescalating) treatment are ethically and morally permissible, although in reality, caregivers and families may find it more difficult to withdraw treatment than to withhold or not escalate therapy.

Counseling and treating pregnant women who deliver at the margins of viability and their infants is not easy. Three main ethical principles guide how we proceed. As discussed, these include the best-interest standard, parental authority, and shared decision making.

There are some who will argue that justice should be part of the equation. Justice, assuring fairness and equity in the care delivered, although implicitly understood, is not often applied while making treatment decisions. Cost considerations are less acute when considering neonatal intensive care. On the basis of quality-adjusted life years, a measure of the efficacy of treatment for a particular disease state or chronic health condition, neonatal intensive care for extremely preterm infants is much more cost effective compared with adults at the end of their life. In addition, most extremely premature neonates who die do so in the first days to weeks of life, thereby constraining expenditures and resource use (90% of the neonatal healthcare costs being spent on survivors).[23] The justice principle is also rarely applicable to neonates because our society currently has not limited access to neonatal intensive care and its associated resources to this most vulnerable population of newborn infants. Although there have been theoretical discussions about resource allocation during times of limited resources and rising costs, this argument is rarely used during healthcare decisions and is not something likely to be applied at present when it comes to care of the infant at the margins of viability.

In conclusion, although advances in neonatal care have led to increased survival at decreasing gestational age, the global disability rates have essentially remained unchanged.[24] In the end, some babies who may have survived will receive comfort care and die, whereas others will receive active treatment and survive with severe impairments. As healthcare providers working with families and infants born at the margins of viability, we have to accept uncertainty.[24] Thus we must live with and accept that two infants both at 22 4/7 weeks' gestation born on the same day may not be managed exactly the same.[24] For fetuses at the upper margin of periviability, shared decision making requires a greater focus on assessing parental wishes and beliefs (values) in conjunction with an individualized approach to care that should incorporate the most current available survival and outcome data for infants born during the 25th week of pregnancy. Increasingly, recommendations during the 25th week of gestation encourage active care, although honoring parental wishes and individualized care (trial of therapy initiated in the delivery room based on the assessed infant's degree of development and physiologic activity) are also accepted approaches to care at birth. There are no current guidelines that recommend comfort care as a routine or recommended option at 25 weeks' gestation, although approximately 20% of guidelines offer no recommendations.[9]

APPENDIX A.1

Drugs Used for Emergency and Cardiac Indications in Newborns

Jacquelyn D. McClary, Jaime Marasch

APPENDIX A.1 Table 1

Agent	Dosage	Comments
Adenosine (Adenocard)	50 μg/kg rapid IV (over 1–2 sec) followed immediately by a rapid NS flush of 5–10 mL. Increase dose every 2 min by 50-μg/kg increments if no response; max dose 250 μg/kg	Facial flushing, irritability, and transient arrhythmias (asystole) may occur. Apnea in a premature infant has been reported. Monitor electrocardiograph (ECG) and blood pressure continuously during administration.
Alprostadil (prostaglandin E_1)	Starting dose: 0.05–0.1 μg/kg/min continuous IV infusion Maintenance dose: after response titrate down to lowest effective dose, which may be as low as 0.01 μg/kg/min	May cause apnea, fever, hypotension, and flushing. Administration via a large vein is preferred; may administer via UAC near the ductus arteriosus.
Amiodarone	Loading dose: 5 mg/kg IV over 60 min Maintenance dose: 7–15 μg/kg/min continuous IV infusion	Monitor ECG and blood pressure continuously for bradycardia and hypotension. Administration into central line preferred to minimize risk of extravasation.
Atropine	0.01–0.03 mg/kg IV push over 1 min or IM and repeat every 10–15 min prn to max total dose of 0.04 mg/kg; may be given via endotracheal tube	Administer rapidly and undiluted.
Calcium chloride 10% (27 mg elemental Ca^{2+} per mL)	20–70 mg/kg (0.2–0.7 mL/kg), 5–20 mg/kg elemental calcium IV over 10–60 min	Dilute with compatible solution to a final concentration of 20 mg/mL. Stop infusion if HR <100. Extravasation may lead to tissue necrosis. Administration via central line is preferred.
Calcium gluconate 10% (9.3 mg elemental Ca^{2+} per mL)	Emergency dose: 100–200 mg/kg (1–2 mL/kg), 10–20 mg/kg elemental calcium IV over 10–60 min Maintenance dose in IV fluids: 200–800 mg/kg/day (20–80 mg/kg/day elemental calcium)	Dilute with compatible solution to a final concentration of 50 mg/mL. Stop infusion if HR <100. Extravasation may lead to tissue necrosis. Administration via central line is preferred.
Digoxin	Loading dose: divided into 3 doses over 24 h administered IV over 15–30 min or PO PMA ≤29 wk: 15 μg/kg IV or 20 μg/kg PO PMA 30–36 wk: 20 μg/kg IV or 25 μg/kg PO PMA 37–48 wk: 30 μg/kg IV or 40 μg/kg PO PMA ≥49 wk: 40 μg/kg IV or 50 μg/kg PO Maintenance dose: PMA ≤29 wk: 4 μg/kg IV or 5 μg/kg PO q24h PMA 30–36 wk: 5 μg/kg IV or 6 μg/kg PO q24h PMA 37–48 wk: 4 μg/kg IV or 5 μg/kg PO q12h PMA ≥49 wk: 5 μg/kg IV or 6 μg/kg PO q12h	Use loading dose only if treating arrhythmias or acute heart failure. Avoid hypokalemia, hypomagnesemia, hypocalcemia, and hypercalcemia. Assess renal function. Monitor HR and heart rhythm. Follow serum drug concentrations with a target range of 1–2 ng/mL.

Continued

APPENDIX A.1 **Table 1—cont'd**

Agent	Dosage	Comments
Dobutamine	2–25 μg/kg/min continuous IV infusion	Tachycardia may occur at high dosages. Hypotension risk increases in hypovolemic patients. Administer via large vein. Tissue ischemia with extravasation; inject phentolamine into affected area as soon as possible.
Dopamine	2–20 μg/kg/min continuous IV infusion "Renal dose": 2–5 μg/kg/min Cardiac stimulation: 5–15 μg/kg/min Vasoconstriction: >5 μg/kg/min	Pharmacologic effect is dose dependent. Administer via large vein. Extravasation may lead to necrosis; inject phentolamine into affected area as soon as possible.
Epinephrine	Emergency dose: 0.01–0.03 mg/kg using the 0.1 mg/mL concentration IV push followed by 1 mL NS; 0.05–0.1 mg/kg ET followed by positive pressure ventilations Continuous IV infusion: 0.02–1 μg/kg/min	Monitor HR and blood pressure continuously. Infiltration may cause tissue necrosis; inject phentolamine into affected area as soon as possible. Correct acidosis if possible before administration.
Esmolol (Brevibloc)	Supraventricular tachycardia: 100 μg/kg/min continuous IV infusion; increase by 50–100 μg/kg/min every 5 min; usual max 200 μg/kg/min Postoperative hypertension: 50 μg/kg/min continuous IV infusion; increase by 25–50 μg/kg/min every 5 min; usual max 200 μg/kg/min	Monitor ECG continuously. May cause hypotension at doses >300 mcg/kg/min.
Hydralazine (Apresoline)	0.1–0.5 mg/kg/dose IV or IM q6–8h; increase gradually to max 2 mg/kg/dose q6h 0.25–1 mg/kg/dose PO q6-8h, approximately twice the IV dose	Administration with a beta-blocker may increase antihypertensive effect and decrease the hydralazine dose required.
Ibuprofen lysine (NeoProfen)	First dose: 10 mg/kg IV over 15 min Second and third doses (starting 24 h after first dose): 5 mg/kg IV over 15 min q24h	Monitor urine output and signs of bleeding. Avoid administration if anuria or urine output <0.6 mL/kg/h develops before the second or third dose.
Indomethacin (Indocin)	3 doses given IV over 20–30 min q12–24h Age at first dose determines dosing regimen: <48 h: 0.2/0.1/0.1 mg/kg 2–7 days: 0.2/0.2/0.2 mg/kg >7 days: 0.2/0.25/0.25 mg/kg Prolonged treatment option: 0.2 mg/kg q24h for 5–7 days	Monitor urine output, electrolytes, blood urea nitrogen, creatinine, and platelet count. Monitor for signs of bleeding. If anuria or severe oliguria develop, delay subsequent doses.
Isoproterenol (Isuprel)	0.05–0.5 μg/kg/min continuous IV infusion; max dose 2 μg/kg/min	May cause arrhythmias and hypoxemia. Correct acidosis before starting therapy.
Lidocaine	Bolus dose: 0.5–1 mg/kg IV push over 5 min; may repeat every 10 min to a max of 5 mg/kg Continuous IV infusion: 10–50 μg/kg/min	May cause CNS toxicity—monitor for seizures, apnea, respiratory depression. High dosages may cause bradycardia, heart block, hypotension—monitor ECG, HR, and blood pressure continuously. Contraindicated in heart block.
Milrinone (Primacor)	Loading dose: 75 μg/kg over 60 min Continuous IV infusion: 0.25–0.75 μg/kg/min	Loading dose optional based on status of patient. Correct hypovolemia before initiation of therapy. Blood pressure may decrease 5%–9% after loading dose and HR may increase 5%–10%.

APPENDIX A.1 **Table 1—cont'd**

Agent	Dosage	Comments
Naloxone (Narcan)	0.1 mg/kg IV push repeated every 2–3 min until opioid effect reversed; may need to repeat doses every 20–60 min; may be given IM, SC, or ET, but not recommended because of unpredictable absorption and delayed onset of action	Not recommended as part of the initial resuscitation of newborns with respiratory depression.
Neostigmine (Prostigmin)	0.03–0.07 mg/kg slow IV push; max total dose 0.07 mg/kg	Give in addition to atropine 0.02 mg/kg to reverse neuromuscular blockade.
Nicardipine (Cardene)	0.5 μg/kg/min continuous IV infusion; titrate up to 2 μg/kg/min	Monitor blood pressure, HR, and heart rhythm continuously. May take up to 2 days to see final effect of dose. Protect from light.
Procainamide (Pronestyl)	Bolus dose: 7–10 mg/kg IV over 60 min Continuous IV infusion: 20–80 μg/kg/min	Monitor for hypotension (increased with rapid infusion), bradycardia, arrhythmias. Monitor serum levels, especially in patients with hepatic or renal impairment, or those receiving high dosages. Monitor CBC regularly for neutropenia and thrombocytopenia. Contraindicated in patients with torsades de pointes and complete heart block.
Propranolol (Inderal)	0.01 mg/kg/dose IV push over 10 min q6h; titrate up to max 0.15 mg/kg/dose q6h 0.25 mg/kg/dose PO q6h; titrate up to max 3.5 mg/kg/dose q6h	Monitor ECG continuously during acute treatment of arrhythmias. Monitor blood glucose for hypoglycemia. Monitor blood pressure.
Sodium nitroprusside (Nipride)	0.25–0.5 μg/kg/min continuous IV infusion; titrate up every 20 min. Usual maintenance dose is <2 μg/kg/min Hypertensive crisis: doses up to 10 μg/kg/min can be used for no longer than 10 min	Monitor HR and intraarterial blood pressure continuously. May produce severe hypotension and cyanide/thiocyanate toxicity; increased risk of toxicity with prolonged treatment, high dosages, and renal or hepatic impairment. Protect from light.

CBC, Complete blood count; *ET,* endotracheal; *HR,* heart rate; *IM,* intramuscular; *IV,* intravenous; *NS,* normal saline; *PMA,* postmenstrual age; *PO,* oral; *UAC,* umbilical arterial catheter.

A.2 APPENDIX

Drug Dosing Table

Jaime Marasch, Jacquelyn D. McClary

APPENDIX A.2 Table 1

Medication (Trade Name)/Route of Administration	Mechanism of Action/Dosing	Important Adverse Events	Special Considerations
Acetaminophen (Tylenol) IV/PO/PR	Inhibits prostaglandin synthesis in central nervous system. Peripherally blocks pain impulse generation. Inhibits hypothalamic thermal regulating center. IV: GA ≥32 wk: 12.5 mg/kg q6h PO: 10–15 mg/kg q4–6h. PR: 15–20 mg/kg q6–8h PDA: 15 mg/kg PO q6h Max dose 50–75 mg/kg/day depending on indication and PMA	Liver toxicity in overdose (acute or chronic)	Rectal administration results in prolonged, variable absorption. Elimination prolonged in patients with liver dysfunction.
Acyclovir (Zovirax) IV	Inhibits DNA synthesis and viral replication by incorporation into viral DNA. IV: PMA <30 wk: 20 mg/kg q12h; PMA 30–36 wk: 20 mg/kg q8h; PMA ≥36 wk: 20/kg q6h	Renal dysfunction, neutropenia, phlebitis	Maintain proper hydration, monitor renal function. Consider prolonging dosing interval in infants with significant renal impairment.
Adenosine (Adenocard) IV	Slows AV conduction, thereby interrupting reentry pathway and restoring normal sinus rhythm. IV: 50 µg/kg initially; increase in 50-µg/kg increments and repeat every 2 min to max dose of 250 µg/kg	Momentary complete heart block after administration, bronchoconstriction in patients with reactive airway disease	Administer over 1–2 seconds and as close to IV insertion site as possible; follow immediately with NS flush. Contraindicated in patients with second- or third-degree heart block. Methylxanthines diminish effect of adenosine.
Albuterol (Proventil, Ventolin) Neb/MDI	Beta-2 agonist that relaxes bronchial smooth muscle. Nebulizer: 2.5 mg q2–6h MDI: 2 actuations q2–6h	Tachycardia, hypokalemia with continuous administration	Not recommended for the treatment of bronchiolitis.
Alprostadil (prostaglandin E_1) (Prostin VR) IV	Prostaglandin E_1 analog that produces direct vasodilation of vascular and ductus arteriosus smooth muscle. IV: 0.05–0.1 µg/kg/min via continuous infusion; maintenance doses may be as low as 0.01 µg/kg/min	Hypotension, flushing, bradycardia, fever, apnea	Apnea occurs in ~10%–12% of neonates and typically appears within the first hour of infusion.

Continued

APPENDIX A.2 **Table 1—cont'd**

Medication (Trade Name)/Route of Administration	Mechanism of Action/Dosing	Important Adverse Events	Special Considerations
Amikacin (Amikin) IV/IM	Inhibits bacterial protein synthesis by inhibiting 30S ribosomal subunit. • PMA ≤29 wk: 0–7 days old: 18 mg/kg q48h; 8–28 days old: 15 mg/kg q36h; ≥29 days old: 15 mg/kg q24h • PMA 30–34 wk: 0–7 days old: 18 mg/kg q36h; ≥8 days old: 15 mg/kg q24h • PMA ≥35 wk: 15 mg/kg q24h	Nephrotoxic, ototoxic, additive neuromuscular blockade with neuromuscular blocking agents	Monitor serum concentrations. Therapeutic peak serum concentration is 20 to 30 μg/mL. Therapeutic trough serum concentration is 2–5 μg/mL. Should not be concurrently administered in same IV line with penicillin-containing compounds. Synergistic antibacterial action in combination with beta-lactam antibiotics.
Amiodarone (Cordarone, Pacerone) IV/PO	Inhibits adrenergic stimulation, prolongs action potential and refractory period in myocardial tissue, decreases AV conduction and sinus node function. IV: 5 mg/kg loading dose followed by maintenance infusion of 7–15 μg/kg/min PO: 5–10 mg/kg q12h	Hypotension, bradycardia, AV block, pneumonitis, pulmonary fibrosis, liver injury, hyperthyroidism, hypothyroidism	Consider switching to PO therapy within 24 to 48 hours of IV therapy
Amphotericin B (Amphocin, Fungizone) Amphotericin B lipid complex (Abelcet) Amphotericin B liposome (AmBisome) IV	Binds to fungal ergosterol, compromising fungal cell wall integrity, ultimately causing cell death. Amphotericin B: 1–1.5 mg/kg q24h over 2–6 hours Amphotericin B lipid complex: 2.5–5 mg/kg q24h over 2 hours Amphotericin B liposome: 2.5–7 mg/kg q24h over 2 hours	Hypomagnesemia, hypokalemia nephrotoxicity, fever, chills, thrombocytopenia, phlebitis	Monitor renal function, electrolytes. Hold conventional dose for 2–5 days if serum creatinine increases >0.4 mg/dL from baseline. Do not flush or mix with saline solutions.
Ampicillin (Omnipen, Polycillin, Principen) IV/IM	Inhibits bacterial cell wall synthesis by binding to specific penicillin-binding proteins. Causes cell wall death resulting in bacteriocidal activity. • PMA ≤29 wk: 0–28 days old: 50–100 mg/kg q12h; >28 days old: 50–100 mg/kg q8h • PMA 30–36 wk: 0–14 days old: 50–100 mg/kg q12h; >14 days old: 50–100 mg/kg q8h • PMA 37–44 wk: 0–7 days old: 50–100 mg/kg q12h; >7 days old: 50–100 mg/kg q8h • PMA ≥45 wk: 50–100 mg/kg q6h	CNS excitation or seizure activity with very large doses	For GBS bacteremia, use dose of 200 mg/kg/day divided every 8–12 hours. For GBS meningitis, use dose of 300–400 mg/kg/day divided every 6–8 hours.
Atropine IV/IM/ET/PO	Competitively inhibits actions of acetylcholine in secretory glands, smooth muscle, and CNS. IV/IM: 0.01–0.03 mg/kg over 1 min; may repeat every 10–15 min (max cumulative dose 0.04 mg/kg) ET: 0.01–0.03 mg/kg followed by 1 mL NS PO: 0.02 mg/kg q4–6h; increase gradually to max 0.09 mg/kg/dose	Tachycardia, arrhythmias, urinary retention, decreased GI motility	Administer rapidly and undiluted. For premedication for intubation, give IV and before other premedications. May give IV formulation orally.

APPENDIX A.2 **Table 1—cont'd**

Medication (Trade Name)/Route of Administration	Mechanism of Action/Dosing	Important Adverse Events	Special Considerations
Azithromycin (Zithromax) IV/PO	Inhibits bacterial protein synthesis by binding to 50S ribosomal subunit. Chlamydial conjunctivitis/pneumonia: 20 mg/kg IV/PO q24h ×3 days All other infections: 10 mg/kg IV/PO q24h ×5 days	Diarrhea, rash, blood in stool	IV dosing not well studied in pediatric patients.
Aztreonam (Azactam) IV/IM	Inhibits bacterial cell wall synthesis and causes cell wall destruction by binding to penicillin-binding proteins. • PMA ≤29 wk: 0–28 days old: 30 mg/kg q12h; >28 days old: 30 mg/kg q8h • PMA 30–36 wk: 0–14 days old: 30 mg/kg q12h; >14 days old: 30 mg/kg q8h • PMA 37–44 wk: 0–7 days old: 30 mg/kg q12h; >7 days old: 30 mg/kg q8h • PMA ≥45 wk: 30 mg/kg q6h	Hypoglycemia, eosinophilia, elevated transaminases, phlebitis	Contains L-arginine. Provide adequate glucose to avoid hypoglycemia.
Beractant (Survanta) Intratracheally (IT)	Modified bovine pulmonary surfactant analog. Replaces deficient or ineffective endogenous lung surfactant. IT: 4 mL/kg divided into 4 aliquots administered as soon as possible after birth; repeat up to 3 additional doses within 48 h of life if needed, no more frequently than q6–12h	Reflux of surfactant up ETT, decreased oxygenation, bradycardia	For IT administration only. Suspension should be at room temperature before administering. Do not artificially warm. Swirl suspension; do not shake or filter suspension. Do not warm and return to refrigerator more than once. Monitor heart rate and oxygen saturation during administration.
Bumetanide (Bumex) IV/IM/PO	Inhibits chloride and sodium reabsorption in ascending loop of Henle and proximal renal tubule, causing increased excretion of water and electrolytes. IV/IM/PO: 0.005–0.05 mg/kg q12–24h	Hyponatremia, hypokalemia, hypochloremic alkalosis	Higher dosages required with abnormal renal function or congestive heart failure. May displace bilirubin at high dosages or with long duration of therapy. May administer the IV formulation orally.
Caffeine citrate (Cafcit) IV/PO	Stimulates central inspiratory drive and improves skeletal muscle contraction. Loading dose: 20 mg/kg Maintenance dose: 5–10 mg/kg q24h	Tachycardia, cardiac dysrhythmias, restlessness, GI disturbances, gastroesophageal reflux	Therapeutic trough serum concentration range is 5–25 μg/mL; toxicity is associated with serum concentrations of >40–50 μg/mL. Monitoring serum concentrations not typically necessary at recommended dosages.

Continued

APPENDIX A.2 **Table 1—cont'd**

Medication (Trade Name)/Route of Administration	Mechanism of Action/Dosing	Important Adverse Events	Special Considerations
Calfactant (Infasurf) Intratracheally (IT)	Natural surfactant extracted from calf lung. Replaces deficient or ineffective endogenous lung surfactant. IT: 3 mL/kg divided into 2 aliquots administered as soon as possible after birth; repeat up to a total of 3 doses if needed, no more frequently than q12h	Reflux of surfactant up ETT, decreased oxygenation, bradycardia	For IT administration only. Warming of suspension is not necessary. Do not artificially warm. Swirl suspension; do not shake or filter suspension. Do not warm and return to refrigerator more than once. Monitor heart rate and oxygen saturation during administration.
Captopril (Capoten) PO	Competitively inhibits angiotensin-converting enzyme. Initial dose: 0.01–0.05 mg/kg q8–12h; adjust dose based on response. Max dose: 0.5 mg/kg q6–24h	Decreased cerebral or renal blood flow, hyperkalemia	Monitor blood pressure and renal function. Onset of action is 15 min, and peak effect is 30–90 min after dosing.
Caspofungin (Cancidas) IV	Inhibits synthesis of essential cell wall component in susceptible fungi. IV: 25 mg/m^2 q24h	Thrombophlebitis, hypercalcemia, hypokalemia, increased liver enzymes	Monitor electrolytes and hepatic transaminases. Do not dilute in dextrose-containing solutions. Usage in neonates should be limited to salvage therapy.
Cefazolin (Ancef, Kefzol) IV/IM	Inhibits bacterial cell wall synthesis by binding to penicillin-binding proteins. • PMA ≤29 wk: 0–28 days old: 25 mg/kg q12h; >28 days old: 25 mg/kg q8h • PMA 30–36 wk: 0–14 days old: 25 mg/kg q12h; >14 days old: 25 mg/kg q8h • PMA 37–44 wk: 0–7 days old: 25 mg/kg q12h; >7 days old: 25 mg/kg q8h • PMA ≥45 wk: 25 mg/kg q6h	Phlebitis, eosinophilia	Poor CNS penetration. Often used for perioperative infection prophylaxis.
Cefepime (Maxipime) IV/IM	Inhibits bacterial cell wall synthesis by binding to penicillin-binding proteins. IV/IM: 50 mg/kg q12h	Eosinophilia, rash, elevated hepatic transaminases	Widely distributed in body tissues and fluids, including CNS.
Cefotaxime (Claforan) IV/IM	Inhibits bacterial cell wall synthesis by binding to penicillin-binding proteins. <7 days old: 50 mg/kg q12h; GA <32 wk, ≥7 days old: 50 mg/kg q8h; GA ≥32 wk, ≥7 days old: 50 mg/kg q6h	Leukopenia, granulocytopenia, eosinophilia, phlebitis, rash	Widely distributed in CSF and other tissues.
Cefoxitin (Mefoxin) IV/IM	Inhibits bacterial cell wall synthesis by binding to penicillin-binding proteins. IV: 90–100 mg/kg/day divided q8h	Eosinophilia, elevated hepatic transaminases	Use often limited to skin, intraabdominal, and urinary tract infections.

APPENDIX A.2 Table 1—cont'd

Medication (Trade Name)/Route of Administration	Mechanism of Action/Dosing	Important Adverse Events	Special Considerations
Ceftazidime (Fortaz) IV/IM	Inhibits bacterial cell wall synthesis by binding to penicillin-binding proteins. • PMA ≤29 wk: 0–28 days old: 50 mg/kg q12h; >28 days old: 50 mg/kg q8h • PMA 30–36 wk: 0–14 days old: 50 mg/kg q12h; >14 days old: 50 mg/kg q8h • PMA 37–44 wk: 0–7 days old: 50 mg/kg q12h; >7 days old: 50 mg/kg q8h • PMA ≥45 wk: 50 mg/kg q8h	Eosinophilia, rash, elevated hepatic transaminases, positive Coombs test	Widely distributed in body tissues and fluids. Synergistic with aminoglycosides.
Ceftriaxone (Rocephin) IV/IM	Inhibits bacterial cell wall synthesis by binding to penicillin-binding proteins. Sepsis: 50 mg/kg q24h Meningitis: 100 mg/kg q24h	Increased bleeding time, leukopenia, eosinophilia, transient gallbladder precipitations	Displaces bilirubin from albumin-binding sites—not recommended for use in neonates with hyperbilirubinemia. Contraindicated with concurrent administration of calcium-containing solutions.
Chlorothiazide (Diuril) IV/PO	Inhibits sodium and chloride reabsorption in distal renal tubules, causing increased excretion of sodium, chloride, potassium, bicarbonate, magnesium, phosphate, and water. IV: 5–10 mg/kg q12h PO: 10–20 mg/kg q12h	Hypochloremic metabolic alkalosis, hypercalcemia, hypokalemia, hyponatremia, hyperglycemia	Synergistic effect with loop diuretics (e.g., furosemide). Monitor serum electrolytes, urine output, and blood pressure closely.
Cholecalciferol (vitamin D_3, D-Vi-Sol) PO	Stimulate or support skeletal growth. Supplementation: 200–400 U q24h Vitamin D deficiency: 1000 U q24h	Signs of toxicity attributed to hypercalcemia (vomiting, irritability, nephrocalcinosis)	Monitor 25-hydroxyvitamin D concentrations, particularly in neonates receiving higher dosages. Monitor calcium and phosphorous levels.
Clindamycin (Cleocin) IV/IM/PO	Inhibits bacterial protein synthesis by reversibly binding to 50S ribosome subunit. • PMA ≤29 wk: 0–28 days old: 5–7.5 mg/kg q12h; >28 days old: 5–7.5 mg/kg q8h • PMA 30–36 wk: 0–14 days old: 5–7.5 mg/kg q12h; >14 days old: 5–7.5 mg/kg q8h • PMA 37–44 wk: 0–7 days old: 5–7.5 mg/kg q12h; >7 days old: 5–7.5 mg/kg q8h • PMA ≥45 wk: 5–7.5 mg/kg q6h	*Clostridium difficile*–associated diarrhea, pseudomembranous colitis, phlebitis	Increase dosing interval in the presence of significant liver dysfunction.
Dexamethasone (Decadron) IV/IM/PO	Decreases inflammation by suppressing proinflammatory mediators. Facilitation of ventilator weaning: 0.01–0.075 mg/kg q12h; follow 10-day DART trial protocol Airway edema: 0.25–0.5 mg/kg q8h for 3 doses; max dose: 1.5 mg/kg/day	Hypertension, hyperglycemia, GI bleeding or perforation, growth inhibition	Administration with indomethacin or ibuprofen significantly increases the risk of GI perforation.

Continued

APPENDIX A.2 **Table 1—cont'd**

Medication (Trade Name)/Route of Administration	Mechanism of Action/Dosing	Important Adverse Events	Special Considerations
Diazoxide (Proglycem) PO	Inhibits insulin release from pancreas. PO: 2–5 mg/kg q8h	Sodium and fluid retention, pulmonary hypertension, cardiac failure	Alcohol content of oral suspension is 7.25%; GI upset and abdominal distension are common.
Digoxin (Lanoxin) IV/PO	Inhibits Na-K ATPase pump and ultimately promotes increased calcium influx within myocardial cells, resulting in increased myocardial contractility. See Appendix A.1 for dosing.	Atrial and ventricular arrhythmias, avoid extravasation	Hypokalemia, hypomagnesemia, hypermagnesemia, and hypercalcemia predispose patients to digoxin toxicity. Follow serum drug concentrations with target range of 1–2 ng/mL. Closely monitor heart rate and rhythm.
Dobutamine IV	Reversibly binds to and stimulates beta-1-adrenergic receptor, causing increased contractility and heart rate. Continuous IV infusion: 2–25 μg/kg/min	Hypotension in setting of hypovolemia, tachycardia, arrhythmias, phlebitis	Correct hypovolemia before initiation of therapy if possible. Use phentolamine for treatment of extravasation.
Dopamine IV	Stimulates α- and β-adrenergic and dopaminergic receptors, which results in cardiac stimulation, increased renal blood flow, and vasoconstriction. Continuous IV infusion: 2–20 μg/kg/min	Hypertension, tachycardia, arrhythmias, phlebitis	Pharmacologic effect is dose dependent. Use phentolamine for treatment of extravasation.
Enalaprilat/Enalapril (Vasotec) IV/PO	Exerts blood pressure and cardiac effects through competitive inhibition of angiotensin-converting enzyme. Enalaprilat (IV): 0.005–0.01 mg/kg q8-24h Enalapril (PO): 0.04–0.15 mg/kg q6–24h	Hypotension, renal dysfunction, hyperkalemia	Monitor blood pressure and renal function. Begin at low doses q24h and titrate up based on response.
Enoxaparin (Lovenox) SC	Potentiates antithrombin III activity and inactivates anticoagulation factor Xa. Thrombosis treatment: term: 1.7 mg/kg q12h; preterm: 2 mg/kg q12h Prophylaxis: 0.75 mg/kg q12h	Intracranial hemorrhage, GI bleeding, hematoma at injection site	Monitor anti–factor Xa levels 4 h after a dose; target range is 0.5–1 U/mL for treatment and 0.1–0.4 U/mL for prophylaxis. Therapeutic dosages in preterm neonates are widely variable. Renally cleared; reduced dosages required in renal dysfunction. Call 1-800-NOCLOTS for dosing assistance.
Epinephrine (Adrenalin) IV/ET	Stimulates alpha- and beta-adrenergic receptors, which results in cardiac stimulation and dilation of skeletal muscle vasculature. IV: 0.01–0.03 mg/kg/dose q3–5min followed by 1 mL NS Continuous IV infusion: 0.03–1 μg/kg/min ET: 0.05–0.1 mg/kg followed by positive pressure ventilations	Hypertension, tachycardia, arrhythmias, phlebitis, renal vascular ischemia, hyperglycemia	For IV push and ET doses, use 0.1 mg/mL solution. Correct acidosis before administration if possible. Use phentolamine for treatment of extravasation.

APPENDIX A.2 **Table 1—cont'd**

Medication (Trade Name)/Route of Administration	Mechanism of Action/Dosing	Important Adverse Events	Special Considerations
Epoetin alfa (Epogen, Procrit) IV/SC	Synthetic analog of erythropoietin that stimulates erythropoiesis. IV/SC: 400–500 U/kg 3 times per week	Neutropenia	Subcutaneous route preferred. Concurrent administration of iron supplementation should be initiated.
Erythromycin (Eryped, E.E.S.) IV/PO	Inhibits bacterial protein synthesis by reversibly binding to the 50S ribosome subunit. PO erythromycin ethylsuccinate: Infection: 10–12.5 mg/kg q6h Gastric motility: 10 mg/kg q6h × 48 hr, then 4 mg/kg q6h IV erythromycin lactobionate: 5–10 mg/kg q6h	Bradycardia and hypotension during IV administration, phlebitis, diarrhea, abdominal pain	Administer PO with feeds to reduce GI side effects and increase absorption.
Esmolol (Brevibloc) IV	Competitively blocks response to beta-1-adrenergic stimulation with minimal effect on beta-2-adrenergic receptors. Supraventricular tachycardia: 100 μg/kg/min continuous IV infusion; increase by 50–100 μg/kg/min every 5 min to usual max 200 μg/kg/min Postoperative hypertension: 50 μg/kg/min continuous IV infusion; increase by 25–50 μg/kg/min every 5 min to usual max 200 μg/kg/min	Hypotension (most common with doses >300 mcg/kg/min), phlebitis	.
Famotidine (Pepcid) IV/PO	Competitively inhibits histamine receptors in gastric parietal cells, which results in inhibition of gastric acid secretion. PO: 0.5–1 mg/kg q24h IV: 0.25–0.5 mg/kg q24h	Late-onset bacterial or fungal sepsis	
Fentanyl (Sublimaze) IV	Binds with opioid stereospecific receptors in CNS to decrease pain. IV push: 0.5–4 μg/kg q2–4h Continuous IV infusion: 0.5–5 μg/kg/hr	Respiratory depression, chest wall rigidity, urinary retention	Patients treated with continuous infusions for ≥5 days may experience signs of withdrawal. Effects reversed by naloxone. Approximately 100 times more potent than morphine.
Ferrous sulfate (Fer-In-Sol) PO	Repletes diminished iron stores and is incorporated into hemoglobin. Routine supplementation: 2–4 mg/kg/day divided q12–24h Patients receiving erythropoietin: 6 mg/kg/day divided q12–24h	Constipation, discolored stool	Infants who have received multiple recent blood transfusions are at risk of iron overload—monitor ferritin levels to determine if supplementation is needed.

Continued

APPENDIX A.2 **Table 1—cont'd**

Medication (Trade Name)/Route of Administration	Mechanism of Action/Dosing	Important Adverse Events	Special Considerations
Fluconazole (Diflucan) IV/PO	Interferes with fungal cytochrome P-450 activity and decreases ergosterol synthesis, which ultimately inhibits cell membrane formation. Invasive Candidiasis Treatment: Loading dose (IV/PO): 25 mg/kg Maintenance dose (IV/PO): • PMA ≤29 wk: 0–14 days old: 12 mg/kg q48h; >14 days old: 12 mg/kg q24h • PMA ≥30 wk: 0–7 days old: 12 mg/kg q48h; >7 days old: 12 mg/kg q24h Invasive Candidiasis Prophylaxis: (IV/PO) 6 mg/kg twice weekly for 6 weeks Thrush: 6 mg/kg PO × 1 dose, then 3 mg/kg PO q24h	Increased liver enzymes	Extend dosing interval in setting of renal dysfunction with serum creatinine >1.3 mg/dL. Prophylaxis indicated in intensive care units with high incidence of *Candida* infections.
Flumazenil (Romazicon) IV/IN/PR	Antagonizes effect of benzodiazepines on GABA/benzodiazepine receptors. IV: 5–10 μg/kg over 15 s; repeat q45s to max cumulative dose of 50 μg/kg or 1 mg (whichever is smaller) IN: 20 μg/kg per nostril PR: 15–30 μg/kg; may repeat within 15–20 min	Hypotension, seizures	Seizures most common in patients receiving benzodiazepines for long-term sedation.
Fosphenytoin (Cerebyx) IV/IM	Phenytoin prodrug. Increases efflux or decreases influx of sodium ions across cell membranes in motor cortex, which results in neuronal membrane stabilization. Dosing expressed in phenytoin equivalents (PE): Fosphenytoin 1 mg PE = phenytoin 1 mg Loading dose: 15–20 mg PE/kg Maintenance dose: 2–4 mg PE/kg q12h	Hypotension, arrhythmias, venous irritation	Administer 1–2 mg PE/kg/min. Displaces bilirubin from protein-binding sites. Target total serum phenytoin levels are 10–20 μg/mL.
Furosemide (Lasix) IV/IM/PO	Inhibits chloride and sodium reabsorption in ascending loop of Henle and proximal and distal renal tubules, which causes increased excretion of water and electrolytes. IV: 1–2 mg/kg/dose q6–48h PO: 1–4 mg/kg/dose q6–48h	Hypochloremic alkalosis, hyponatremia, hypokalemia, hypercalciuria and renal calculi, ototoxicity	Monitor electrolytes and renal function closely. Risk of ototoxicity increased in neonates also receiving aminoglycosides.
Ganciclovir (Cytovene) IV	Competes for incorporation into viral DNA and interferes with viral DNA chain elongation, which results in inhibition of viral replication. Acute infection: 6 mg/kg IV q12h Chronic suppression: 30–40 mg/kg PO q8h	Thrombocytopenia, anemia, neutropenia	Treat acute infections for minimum of 6 wk. Monitor complete blood count every 2–3 days for first 3 weeks, then weekly if infant's condition is stable. Decrease dose by half for neutropenia (<500 cells/mm^3). Discontinue if neutropenia does not resolve.

APPENDIX A.2 **Table 1—cont'd**

Medication (Trade Name)/Route of Administration	Mechanism of Action/Dosing	Important Adverse Events	Special Considerations
Gentamicin IV/IM	Inhibits bacterial protein synthesis by binding to the 30S ribosomal subunit, resulting in a defective bacterial cell membrane. IV: 5 mg/kg q36h	Nephrotoxicity, ototoxicity (increased risk with concurrent use of other nephrotoxic or ototoxic drugs)	Monitor serum trough concentration before third dose if treating for >48 hr. Target trough concentration is <1 µg/mL. Extend dosing interval if trough is >1 µg/mL. Should not be concurrently administered in same IV line with penicillin-containing compounds.
Glucagon IV/IM/SC	Increases hepatic glycogenolysis and gluconeogenesis, which causes increase in blood glucose. 0.02–0.2 mg/kg up to max dose of 1 mg; repeat q20min prn	Tachycardia, GI disturbances rebound, hypoglycemia	Rise in blood glucose lasts about 2 hr.
Heparin IV	Potentiates action of antithrombin III, inactivates thrombin, inhibits conversion of fibrinogen to fibrin. Loading dose: 75 U/kg IV push Maintenance dose: 28 U/kg/h Continuous IV infusion—adjust based on APTT; target range dependent on indication	Hemorrhage, thrombocytopenia	Effects reversible with protamine. Monitor platelet levels closely. Nontherapeutic doses added to TPN or IV fluids to maintain patency of lines (0.5–1 U/mL).
Hyaluronidase (Amphadase, Vitrase) SC	Modifies permeability of connective tissue and increases distribution and absorption of locally injected substances. SC: 150 U as 5 separate injections around extravasation site	Erythema	Administer as soon as possible after extravasation. Not for use with extravasation of vasoactive agents.
Hydralazine (Apresoline) IV/PO	Produces direct vasodilation of arterioles causing decreased systemic vascular resistance. PO: 0.25–1 mg/kg q6–8h IV: 0.1–0.5 mg/kg q6–8h gradually increased to max of 2 mg/kg q6h	Agranulocytosis, hypotension, tachycardia	If used with beta-blocker, expect reduction in hydralazine dose required.
Hydrochlorothiazide (Microzide) PO	Inhibits Na reabsorption in distal renal tubules, which causes increased excretion of water and electrolytes. PO: 1–2 mg/kg q12h	Hypochloremic metabolic alkalosis, hypokalemia, hyperuricemia, hyperglycemia	Has synergistic effect with loop diuretics (e.g., furosemide).
Hydrocortisone (Solu-Cortef) IV/PO	Corticosteroid that decreases inflammation by suppressing migration and decreasing capillary permeability of proinflammatory mediators. Stress dose: 20–30 mg/m^2/day divided q8–12h Physiologic dose: 7–9 mg/m^2/day divided q8–12h	Possible aggravation of fluid retention, pituitary-adrenal axis suppression, hyperglycemia, hypertension, GI perforation (increased risk if given with indomethacin/ibuprofen)	Taper stress dose and physiologic dose based on patient response and condition.

Continued

APPENDIX A.2 **Table 1—cont'd**

Medication (Trade Name)/Route of Administration	Mechanism of Action/Dosing	Important Adverse Events	Special Considerations
Ibuprofen lysine (NeoProfen) IV/PO	Inhibits prostaglandin synthesis by decreasing cyclooxygenase activity. Dose 1: 10 mg/kg Doses 2 and 3 starting 24 h after dose 1: 5 mg/kg q24h	GI perforation, renal impairment, impaired platelet function	Monitor urine output, BUN, and serum creatinine—extend dosing interval if severe oliguria occurs. Verify adequate platelet count before administration. Monitor for signs of bleeding.
Imipenem/cilastatin (Primaxin) IV	Inhibits bacterial cell wall synthesis by binding to penicillin-binding proteins. IV: 20–25 mg/kg q 8–12h	Seizures in patients with meningitis or renal dysfunction, increased platelet count, eosinophilia, elevated liver enzymes, diarrhea	Cilastatin prevents renal metabolism of imipenem but has no antibacterial activity. Restricted to treatment of non-CNS infections. Clearance is directly related to renal function.
Indomethacin (Indocin) IV	Inhibits prostaglandin synthesis by decreasing cyclooxygenase activity. Dose 1: 0.2 mg/kg followed by: • Postnatal age <48 h at time of dose 1: 0.1 mg/kg q12–24h for 2 doses • Postnatal age 2–7 days at time of dose 1: 0.2 mg/kg q12–24h for 2 doses • Postnatal age >7 days at time of dose 1: 0.25 mg/kg q12–24h for 2 doses	Oliguria, anuria, GI perforation, impaired platelet function	Monitor urine output, BUN, and serum creatinine—extend dosing interval if severe oliguria occurs. Verify adequate platelet count before administration. Monitor for signs of bleeding.
Insulin (Humulin R) IV/SC	Regulates metabolism of macronutrients and facilitates glucose transport into muscle, adipose, and other tissues. SC: 0.1–0.2 U/kg q6–12h Continuous IV infusion: 0.01–0.1 U/kg/hr	Hypoglycemia and associated signs and symptoms	Assess blood glucose every 15–30 min after starting infusion and after any changes. To avoid binding of insulin to tubing, fill IV tubing with insulin solution, and wait 20 min before starting infusion.
Intravenous immune globulin (IVIG) (Gamunex, Flebogamma, Carimune NF) IV	Concentrated form of immunoglobulin G antibodies for replacement therapy. Likely decreases hemolysis in newborns with hemolytic disease by blocking Fc receptor sites of reticuloendothelial cells Standard dose: 500–1000 mg/kg, may repeat in 12 hours Neonatal alloimmune thrombocytopenia: 1000 mg/kg q24h ×2 doses	Hypotension, renal dysfunction, phlebitis	Monitor heart rate and blood pressure during infusion. If infusion not well tolerated, decrease in rate may be warranted.
Ipratropium (Atrovent) MDI/Nebulizer	Bronchodilator that blocks acetylcholine action in bronchial smooth muscle. MDI: 2–4 puffs q6–8h Nebulizer: 75–175 μg (0.4–0.9 mL) q6–8h		
Iron dextran (INFed) IV	Replaces iron and allows for transportation of oxygen via hemoglobin. Continuous IV infusion: 0.4–1 mg/kg/day	If given intermittently, delayed infusion reactions (24–48 h after administration), phlebitis	Add to TPN solution and infuse continuously to avoid adverse reactions.

APPENDIX A.2 **Table 1—cont'd**

Medication (Trade Name)/Route of Administration	Mechanism of Action/Dosing	Important Adverse Events	Special Considerations
Lamivudine (3TC, Epivir) PO	Antiretroviral agent that inhibits reverse transcription via viral DNA chain termination. PO: ≥32 weeks: 2 mg/kg q12h ×4 weeks; increase to 4 mg/kg q12h ×2 weeks	Lactic acidosis, elevated hepatic enzymes	Often used in combination with zidovudine and nevirapine for prevention of mother-to-child HIV transmission. Consider consulting infectious disease specialist for specific antiretroviral regimen recommendations. Monitor liver enzymes regularly if long-term treatment required. Consider reducing dose or increasing dosing interval in patients with renal impairment.
Lansoprazole (Prevacid) PO	Inhibits proton pump and leads to decreased gastric acid secretion. PO: 1 mg/kg q24h	Increased transaminases with prolonged therapy	Monitor liver function with prolonged therapy.
Levetiracetam (Keppra) IV/PO	Exact mechanism unknown, but activity may include blocking GABAergic inhibitory transmission and inhibiting voltage-dependent calcium channels. IV/PO: 10 mg/kg q12h; titrated up to max of 30 mg/kg q12h.	Sedation, irritability, GI disturbances	Second-line therapy for seizures refractory to phenobarbital or other anticonvulsants. Consider dosage adjustment in renal impairment. Tapering is recommended upon discontinuation.
Levothyroxine (Synthroid) PO/IV	Replacement therapy for thyroid hormone involved in normal metabolism, development, and growth. PO: 10–14 μg/kg q24h IV: 5–8 μg/kg q24h	Tachycardia, fever, GI disturbances	Adjust PO dose in 12.5-μg increments and always round up. For oral doses, crush tablet and suspend in small amount of sterile water, breast milk, or formula, and use immediately. Do not use IV formulation for PO administration.
Linezolid (Zyvox) IV/PO	Inhibits initiation of bacterial protein synthesis by binding to 50S ribosome subunit. Preterm ≤1 wk of age: PO/IV: 10 mg/kg q12h Full term or preterm >1 wk of age: PO/IV: 10 mg/kg q8h	Elevated transaminases, diarrhea, anemia, thrombocytopenia	Limit use to infections caused by gram-positive organisms that are refractory to treatment with other antibiotics including vancomycin.
Lorazepam (Ativan) IV/PO	Binds to GABA-A receptors, enhancing effects of GABA, which is the major inhibitory neurotransmitter. IV/PO: 0.05–0.1 mg/kg; repeat based on clinical response	Hypotension, respiratory depression, rhythmic myoclonic jerking, phlebitis	Injectable form contains benzyl alcohol, polyethylene glycol, and propylene glycol. Use limited to acute management of seizures refractory to conventional therapy.
Meropenem (Merrem) IV	Inhibits bacterial cell wall synthesis by binding to penicillin-binding proteins. GA <32 wk: 0–14 days old: 20 mg/kg q12h; >14 days old: 20 mg/kg q8h GA ≥32 wk: 20 mg/kg q8h	Thrombocytosis, eosinophilia, phlebitis	Limit use to treatment of severe infections resistant to other antibiotics; use of broad-spectrum antibiotics increases risk of fungal infection and pseudomembranous colitis.

Continued

APPENDIX A.2 **Table 1—cont'd**

Medication (Trade Name)/Route of Administration	Mechanism of Action/Dosing	Important Adverse Events	Special Considerations
Methadone (Dolophine) IV/PO	Binds to opiate receptors in CNS, altering perception of and response to pain. Exhibits NMDA receptor antagonism. IV/PO: 0.05–0.1 mg/kg q6–24h	Respiratory depression, abdominal distension, delayed gastric emptying	Start with lower doses at more frequent intervals and titrate up as needed based on NAS scores. Adjust doses in 10%–20% increments and modify weaning schedule as needed based on withdrawal symptoms. Extend dosing interval first until administration is every 12 hr, then wean dose. Long elimination half-life requires slow weaning.
Metoclopramide (Reglan) IV/PO	Dopamine receptor antagonist that promotes gastric emptying and accelerates intestinal transit time. PO/IV: 0.033–0.1 mg/kg q8h	Extrapyramidal symptoms, dystonic reactions	Extrapyramidal symptoms more likely at higher dosages or with prolonged use.
Metronidazole (Flagyl) IV/PO	Breaks helical structure of DNA, which results in inhibition of protein synthesis and cell death. Loading dose: 15 mg/kg Maintenance dose: • PMA 24–25 wk: 7.5 mg/kg q24h • PMA 26–27 wk: 10 mg/kg q24h • PMA 28–33 wk: 7.5 mg/kg q12h • PMA 34–40 wk: 7.5 mg/kg q8h • PMA >40 wk: 7.5 mg/kg q6h	GI disturbances, neutropenia	
Micafungin (Mycamine) IV	Inhibits synthesis of essential cell wall components of susceptible fungi, which results in osmotic stress and lysis of the fungal cell. IV:10 mg/kg q24h	Hypokalemia, elevated liver enzymes, increased bilirubin, hypertension	
Midazolam (Versed) IV/IM/PO/IN/SL	Binds to r GABA-A receptors, enhancing effects of GABA, the major inhibitory neurotransmitter. IV/IM: 0.05–0.15 mg/kg q2–4h prn Continuous IV infusion: 0.01–0.06 mg/kg/hr, titrated as needed IN/SL: 0.2 mg/kg PO: 0.25 mg/kg	Hypotension, respiratory depression, myoclonus	Used most often for sedation, but can also be used for refractory seizures. Prolonged or repeated use may have detrimental effects on neurodevelopmental outcomes. Respiratory depression more common when administered with narcotics. Preservative-free injection available.
Milrinone (Primacor) IV	Inhibits phosphodiesterase III, which potentiates delivery of calcium to the myocardium and results in a positive inotropic effect. Also causes relaxation of vascular muscle and vasodilation Loading dose: 75 μg/kg over 60 min Continuous IV infusion: 0.25–0.75 μg/kg/min	Thrombocytopenia, arrhythmias, tachycardia, hypotension	Loading dose optional based on status of patient. Correct hypovolemia before initiation. Blood pressure may decrease 5%–9% after loading dose, and heart rate may increase 5%–10%.

APPENDIX A.2 **Table 1—cont'd**

Medication (Trade Name)/Route of Administration	Mechanism of Action/Dosing	Important Adverse Events	Special Considerations
Morphine (Astramorph, Duramorph) IV/IM/SC/PO	Binds to opiate receptors in the CNS, altering perception of and response to pain. Analgesia: IV/IM/SC: 0.05–0.2 mg/kg q4h prn Continuous IV infusion: 10–20 µg/kg/hr, titrated as needed PO: 0.2 mg/kg q4h prn (or 3 times IV dose) Neonatal Abstinence Syndrome: PO: 0.03–0.1 mg/kg q3–4h, increase as needed to control withdrawal	Hypotension, vasodilation, flushing, pruritus, respiratory depression, GI disturbances, urinary retention	Closely monitor respiratory rate, blood pressure, heart rate, oxygen saturation, and bowel sounds. Metabolized to an active metabolite that is renally excreted. Effects reversed by naloxone. When used for NAS, wean 10%–20% daily as tolerated.
Nafcillin IV/IM	Inhibits bacterial cell wall synthesis by binding to penicillin-binding proteins. Sepsis: 25 mg/kg Meningitis: 50 mg/kg • PMA ≤29 wk: 0–28 days old: q12h; >28 days old: q8h • PMA 30–36 wk: 0–14 days old: q12h; >14 days old: q8h • PMA 37–44 wk: 0–7 days old: q12h; >7 days old: q8h • PMA ≥45 wk: q6h	GI disturbances, phlebitis	Increase dosing interval in the presence of hepatic dysfunction.
Naloxone (Narcan) IV/IM/SC	Reverses respiratory depression by competing with and displacing narcotics at CNS opioid receptor sites. IV/IM: 0.1 mg/kg q2–3 min prn		Half-life of naloxone may be shorter than that of opioids; therefore repeating doses every 1–2 h may be necessary. Monitor for signs of acute withdrawal such as excessive crying, convulsions, and hyperactive reflexes.
Neostigmine (Prostigmin) IV	Inhibits hydrolysis of acetylcholine, which facilitates cholinergic activity. IV: 0.03–0.07 mg/kg ×1 dose	Bradycardia, hypotension, respiratory depression, tremors	Use for reversal of nondepolarizing neuromuscular blockade. Administer with 0.02 mg/kg atropine to minimize bradycardia.
Nevirapine (Viramune) PO	Antiretroviral agent that binds to reverse transcriptase and blocks HIV-1 replication. Birth wt 1.5–2 kg: 8 mg/dose Birth wt >2 kg: 12 mg/dose Give three doses in the first wk of life; administer first dose within 48 h of life, second dose 48 h after first, and third dose 96 h after second dose.	GI disturbances, eosinophilia, neutropenia, hepatoxicity, granulocytopenia	Used in combination with other antiretroviral medications for prevention of mother-to-child HIV transmission. Consider consulting infectious disease specialist for specific recommendations on antiretroviral regimen and treatment.
Nystatin (Nystop) PO/Topical	Binds to fungal cell membrane and disrupts the cell structure. Topical: q6h PO: Preterm: 1 mL (100,000 U) divided and applied to each side of mouth q6h Term: 2 mL (200,000 U) divided and applied to each side of mouth q6h	Rash attributed to inactive ingredients in topical product	Continue treatment for 3 days after symptoms resolve.

Continued

APPENDIX A.2 **Table 1—cont'd**

Medication (Trade Name)/Route of Administration	Mechanism of Action/Dosing	Important Adverse Events	Special Considerations
Omeprazole (Prilosec) PO	Inhibits the proton pump, which results in decreased gastric acid secretion. PO: 1 mg/kg q24h	Mild increase in transaminases with prolonged therapy	Monitor liver function with prolonged therapy.
Oxacillin IV/IM	Inhibits bacterial cell wall synthesis by binding to penicillin-binding proteins. Sepsis: 25 mg/kg Meningitis: 50 mg/kg • PMA ≤29 wk: 0–28 days old: q12h; >28 days old: q8h • PMA 30–36 wk: 0–14 days old: q12h; >14 days old: q8h • PMA 37–44 wk: 0–7 days old: q12h; >7 days old: q8h • PMA ≥45 wk: q6h	Thrombocytopenia, leukopenia, eosinophilia, neutropenia, rash, elevated liver enzymes, phlebitis	Poor CSF penetration. Consider extending dosing interval in the presence of poor renal function.
Palivizumab (Synagis) IM	Monoclonal antibody that inhibits respiratory syncytial virus (RSV) replication. IM: 15 mg/kg every month during RSV season Maximum of 5 doses per season	Swelling at injection site, fever	Immunoprophylaxis against RSV infection in high-risk infants; not effective for treatment of RSV disease.
Papaverine IV	Smooth muscle spasmolytic that produces generalized smooth muscle relaxation and vasodilation. Continuous IV infusion: 30 mg per 250 mL arterial catheter solution; infuse at 1 mL/hr	Chronic hepatitis with long-term therapy	Prolongs patency of peripheral arterial catheter. Use with caution in VLBW infants in first days of life attributed to the risk of developing/extending intracranial hemorrhage.
Penicillin G IV/IM	Inhibits bacterial cell wall synthesis by binding to penicillin-binding proteins. Bacteremia: 25,000–50,000 U/kg • PMA ≤29 wk: 0–28 days old: q12h; >28 days old: q8h • PMA 30–36 wk: 0–14 days old: q12h; >14 days old: q8h • PMA 37–44 wk: 0–7 days old: q12h; >7 days old: q8h • PMA ≥45 wk: q6h GBS meningitis: ≤7 days 450,000 U/kg/day divided q8h >7 days 500,000 U/kg/day divided q6h Congenital syphilis: 50,000 U/kg IV q12h ×7 days, then q8h ×3 days	Phlebitis; cardiorespiratory arrest and death if IM form given IV	Use only aqueous penicillin for IV administration. Use procaine or benzathine penicillin for IM administration.
Phenobarbital (Luminal) IV/IM/PO	Inhibits neurotransmission, resulting in depressed CNS activity. Loading dose (IV): 20 mg/kg; repeat 10 mg/kg prn every 20–30 min to total 40 mg/kg Maintenance dose (IV/IM/PO): 3–5 mg/kg q24h	Phlebitis, respiratory depression, sedation, elevated liver enzymes	Begin maintenance dose 12–24 h after loading dose. Target serum concentration is 15–40 μg/mL; increased sedation at concentrations of >40 μg/mL and increased respiratory depression at concentrations of >60 μg/mL.

APPENDIX A.2 **Table 1—cont'd**

Medication (Trade Name)/Route of Administration	Mechanism of Action/Dosing	Important Adverse Events	Special Considerations
Phentolamine SC	Blocks alpha-adrenergic receptors and reverses vasoconstriction caused by vasopressor extravasation. SC: 1–5 mL of 0.5 mg/mL solution		Amount injected into extravasation site depends on size of infiltrate. Use for extravasation of vasoconstrictive agents (dopamine, epinephrine, etc.).
Phenytoin (Dilantin) IV/PO	Stabilizes neuronal membranes and decreases seizure activity by altering sodium ion transport across cell membranes in the motor cortex. Loading dose (IV): 15–20 mg/kg Maintenance dose (IV/PO): 4–8 mg/kg q8–24h	Bradycardia, arrhythmia, and hypotension during intravenous administration; extravasation, nystagmus, vitamin D deficiency	Infuse slowly at maximum rate of 1 mg/kg/min. Do not administer IM. Target total serum concentration is 6–15 μg/mL in first few weeks of life, then 10–20 μg/mL. Target free serum concentration is 1–2 μg/mL. Injectable form contains alcohol and propylene glycol.
Piperacillin/tazobactam (Zosyn) IV	Piperacillin inhibits bacterial cell wall synthesis by binding to penicillin-binding proteins. Tazobactam binds to beta-lactamases and prevents degradation of piperacillin. IV: 100 mg/kg • PMA ≤29 wk: 0–28 days old: q12h; >28 days old: q8h • PMA 30–36 wk: 0–14 days old: q12h; >14 days old: q8h • PMA 37–44 wk: 0–7 days old: q12h; >7 days old: q8h • PMA ≥45 wk: q8h	Leukopenia, neutropenia, hypokalemia	In noninflamed meninges, there is limited CNS penetration.
Poractant alfa (Curosurf) IT	Modified porcine-derived pulmonary surfactant analog. Replaces deficient or ineffective endogenous lung surfactant. Initial dose: 2.5 mL/kg administered as soon as possible after birth Repeat doses: 1.25 mL/kg q12h prn ×2 doses	Reflux of surfactant up ETT, decreased oxygenation, bradycardia	For IT administration only. Suspension should be at room temperature before administering. Do not artificially warm. Swirl suspension; do not shake or filter suspension. Do not warm and return to refrigerator more than once. Monitor heart rate and oxygen saturation during administration.
Propranolol (Inderal) IV/PO	Blocks stimulation of beta-1-and beta-2-adrenergic receptors, which results in decreased heart rate, myocardial contractility, and blood pressure. IV: 0.01 mg/kg q6h; increase prn to max 0.15 mg/kg q6h PO: 0.25–1 mg/kg q6h; increase prn to max 3.5 mg/kg q6h	Bradycardia, bronchospasm, hypoglycemia, hypotension	Rebound tachycardia may occur with abrupt discontinuation.

Continued

APPENDIX A.2 **Table 1—cont'd**

Medication (Trade Name)/Route of Administration	Mechanism of Action/Dosing	Important Adverse Events	Special Considerations
Protamine IV	Combines with heparin to form a complex and negate the anticoagulant activity of both drugs. Dose based on time since last heparin dose: • <30 min: 1 mg per 100 U heparin received • 30–60 min: 0.5–0.75 mg per 100 U heparin received • 60–120 min: 0.375–0.5 mg per 100 U heparin received • >120 min: 0.25–0.375 mg per 100 U heparin received Max dose: 50 mg	Hypotension, bradycardia, bleeding problems with excessive doses, pulmonary hypertension/edema	Infusion rate should not exceed 5 mg/min. Increased risk of severe adverse reactions with high dose, rapid administration, or repeated doses.
Ranitidine (Zantac) IV/PO	Competitively inhibits histamine receptors in gastric parietal cells, which results in inhibition of gastric acid secretion. IV, term: 1.5 mg/kg q8h IV, preterm: 0.5 mg/kg q12h Continuous IV infusion: 0.0625 mg/kg/h PO: 2 mg/kg q8h	Bradycardia (with rapid administration), increased risk of late-onset bacterial or fungal sepsis, pneumonia, and NEC	Oral solution contains 7.5% alcohol. To administer continuously, add to TPN.
Rifampin (Rifadin) IV/PO	Inhibits bacterial RNA synthesis by binding to beta subunit of DNA-dependent RNA polymerase, thereby inhibiting RNA transcription. Staphylococcal infection: IV: 5–10 mg/kg q12h PO: 10–20 mg/kg q24h Meningococcal prophylaxis: 5 mg/kg PO q12h × 2 days Haemophilus influenzae type B: 10 mg/kg PO q24h × 4 days	Extravasation, elevated hepatic transaminases, hyperbilirubinemia, thrombocytopenia	Causes orange-red discoloration of urine, sputum, tears, and other bodily fluids. Do not use as monotherapy attributed to risk of developing resistance.
Rocuronium (Zemuron) IV	Binds to cholinergic receptor sites and blocks neural transmission at myoneural junction. IV: 0.3–1.2 mg/kg over 5–10 s	Increased pulmonary vascular resistance	Must be given with adequate analgesia and sedation. Primarily used before intubation attributed to rapid onset and intermediate duration of action.
Sildenafil (Revatio) IV/PO	Phosphodiesterase type-5 inhibitor that causes vasodilation in the pulmonary vasculature. IV: 0.4 mg/kg over 3 hours, then 1.6 mg/kg/day via continuous infusion PO: 0.5–2 mg/kg q6–12h	Worsening oxygenation, hypotension	Start therapy with lower dosages and titrate slowly based on oxygenation and blood pressure. Pharmacokinetics in neonates is not well defined. Some experts recommend a max dose of 1 mg/kg PO q8h
Sodium bicarbonate IV	Dissociates to provide bicarbonate ion, which neutralizes hydrogen ion and raises blood and urinary pH. Usual dosage: 1–2 mEq/kg	Tissue necrosis with extravasation, hypocalcemia, hypokalemia, hypernatremia	Administer 1–2 mEq/kg over at least 30 min. Maximum concentration used in neonates is 0.5 mEq/mL (4.2%). Do not administer with calcium- or phosphate-containing solutions. Not recommended for use in neonatal resuscitation.

APPENDIX A.2 Table 1—cont'd

Medication (Trade Name)/Route of Administration	Mechanism of Action/Dosing	Important Adverse Events	Special Considerations
Sotalol (Betapace) PO	Blocks stimulation of beta-1-and beta-2-adrenergic receptors, which results in decreased heart rate and AV node conduction. Prolongs refractory period of atrial muscle, ventricular muscle, and AV accessory pathways. PO: 1 mg/kg q12h; increase every 3–5 days until stable rhythm maintained to max dose of 4 mg/kg q12h	Arrhythmias (sinoatrial block, AV block, torsade de pointes, ventricular ectopic activity), QTc prolongation, hypotension, dyspnea	Continuous cardiac monitoring required for at least 3 days at maintenance dose. High dosages increase risk of torsade de pointes.
Spironolactone (Aldactone) PO	Competes for aldosterone receptors in distal renal tubules, increasing sodium, chloride, and water excretion while conserving potassium and hydrogen ions. PO: 1–3 mg/kg q24h	Hyperkalemia, GI upset, rash	Significantly less diuretic effect than thiazide and loop diuretics; use only in combination with other diuretics. May help decrease potassium losses secondary to use of other diuretics.
Tobramycin IV/IM	Inhibits bacterial protein synthesis by binding to the 30S ribosomal subunit, which results in defective bacterial cell membrane. IV: 5 mg/kg q36h	Nephrotoxicity, ototoxicity (increased risk with concurrent use of other nephrotoxic or ototoxic drugs)	Monitor serum trough concentration before third dose if treating for >48 hr. Target trough concentration is <1 μg/mL. Extend dosing interval if trough is >1 μg/mL. Should not be concurrently administered in same IV line with penicillin-containing compounds
Ursodiol (Actigall) PO	Reduces secretion of cholesterol from liver and reabsorption of cholesterol by intestines, which results in decreased cholesterol in bile and bile stones. PO: 15 mg/kg q12h	Abdominal pain, constipation, flatulence, nausea and vomiting	
Valganciclovir (Valcyte) PO	Rapidly metabolized to the active component ganciclovir, which competes for incorporation into viral DNA and interferes with viral DNA chain elongation, which results in inhibition of viral replication. PO: 16 mg/kg q12h	Thrombocytopenia, neutropenia, anemia, leukopenia	Treat acute infections for minimum of 6 wk. Hold dose for ANC of <500 cells/mm^3 until ANC is >750 cells/mm^3. If ANC falls again to <750 cells/mm^3, reduce dose by 50%. If ANC falls to <500 cells/mm^3 again, discontinue drug.
Vancomycin (Vancocin) IV	Inhibits bacterial cell wall synthesis by blocking glycopeptide polymerization. IV:15 mg/kg • PMA ≤29 wk: 0–14 days old: q18h; >14 days old: q12h • PMA 30–36 wk: 0–14 days old: q12h; >14 days old: q8h • PMA 37–44 wk: 0–7 days old: q12h; >7 days old: q8h • PMA ≥45 wk: q6h	Nephrotoxicity and ototoxicity (increased with aminoglycoside therapy), phlebitis, neutropenia	Serum trough concentrations correlate best with both efficacy and toxicity. Target serum trough concentration is 10–15 μg/mL. Concentrations up to 20 μg/mL have been targeted in severe infections.

Continued

APPENDIX A.2 Table 1—cont'd

Medication (Trade Name)/Route of Administration	Mechanism of Action/Dosing	Important Adverse Events	Special Considerations
Vecuronium (Norcuron) IV	Inhibits depolarization by blocking acetylcholine from binding to motor end plate receptors. IV push: 0.1 mg/kg q1–2h Continuous IV infusion: 0.1 mg/kg/h	Bradycardia and hypotension when used with narcotics	Must be given with adequate sedation and analgesia. Provide eye lubrication.
Vitamin A (Aquasol A) IM	Retinol metabolites exhibit potent effects on gene expression and on lung growth and development. IM: 5000 U 3 times per week ×4 wk	Signs and symptoms of toxicity include lethargy, hepatomegaly, edema, bony tenderness, mucocutaneous lesions	Use in premature infants at highest risk of developing chronic lung disease.
Vitamin K (Mephyton, phytonadione) IV/IM	Promotes formation of clotting factors II, VII, IX, and X in the liver. Prophylaxis of hemorrhagic disease: Term: 0.5–1 mg IM Preterm <1000 g: 0.3–0.5 mg IM Treatment of hemorrhagic disease: 1–5 mg slow IV push	Pain and swelling at IM injection site	Administer IV doses very slowly, not to exceed 1 mg/min. Severe reactions have been reported very rarely in adults.
Zidovudine (AZT, Retrovir) IV/PO	Interferes with HIV viral RNA–dependent DNA polymerase, resulting in inhibition of viral replication • GA<30 wk: 2 mg/kg PO q12h ×4 wk, then 3 mg/kg PO q12h ×2 wk OR 1.5 mg/kg IV q12h ×4 wk, then 2.3 mg/kg IV q12h ×2 wk • GA 30–35 wk: 2 mg/kg PO q12h ×2 wk, then 3 mg/kg PO q12h ×2–4 wk OR 1.5 mg/kg IV q12h ×2 wk, then 2.3 mg/kg IV q12h ×2–4 wk • GA ≥35 wk 4 mg/kg PO q12h ×4 wk, OR 3 mg/kg IV q12h ×4 wk	Anemia, neutropenia, thrombocytopenia	Begin within 6–12 h of birth and continue for 4–6 wk. Consider consulting infectious disease specialist for specific antiretroviral regimen recommendations.

ANC, Absolute neutrophil count; *APTT,* activated partial thromboplastin time; *AV,* atrioventricular; *BUN,* blood urea nitrogen; *CNS,* central nervous system; *CSF,* cerebrospinal fluid; *DART,* Dexamethasone: A Randomized Trial; *ET,* endotracheal; *ETT,* endotracheal tube; *GABA,* gamma-aminobutyric acid; *GA,* gestational age; *GBS,* group B beta-hemolytic Streptococcus; *GI,* gastrointestinal; *HIV,* human immunodeficiency virus; *IM,* intramuscular; *IN,* intranasal; *IV,* intravenous; *MDI,* metered dose inhaler; *NAS,* neonatal abstinence syndrome; *NEC,* necrotizing enterocolitis; *NDMA,* *N*-methyl-D-aspartate; *NS,* normal saline; *PDA,* patent ductus arteriosus; *PMA,* postmenstrual age; *PO,* oral; *PR,* per rectum; *SC,* subcutaneous; *SL,* sublingual; *TPN,* total parenteral nutrition; *VLBW,* very low birth weight.

Modified from *Micromedex NeoFax*, Ann Arbor, Michigan, 2017, Truven Health Analytics LLC; and *Lexicomp*, Hudson, Ohio, 2018, Wolters Kluwer Clinical Drug Information, Inc.

B APPENDIX

Drug Compatibility Table

Jacquelyn D. McClary, Jaime Marasch

APPENDIX B Table 1

Name	Dosage	Indications	Side Effects	Compatibility	Considerations
Alprostadil (prostaglandin E_1)	Initial dose: 0.05–0.1 µg/kg/min Maintenance dose: 0.01–0.1 µg/kg/min	Maintain patency of ductus arteriosus	Apnea, hypotension, hyperthermia, flushing, bradycardia, diarrhea, seizures	*Solution:* D_5W, NS *Y-site:* TPN, ampicillin, gentamicin, dopamine, dobutamine, furosemide, fentanyl, vancomycin *Incompatible:* fat emulsion	Give through UAC only if absolutely necessary and if flow is not interrupted by obtaining laboratory specimens. Requires constant, patient IV access.
Dobutamine	2–25 µg/kg/min	Hypoperfusion or hypotension related to myocardial dysfunction	Tachycardia at high dosages, arrhythmia, hypertension, increased myocardial oxygen consumption, infiltration may result in tissue ischemia	*Solution:* D_5W, $D_{10}W$, NS *Y-site:* TPN, fat emulsion, alprostadil, dopamine, epinephrine, fentanyl, gentamicin, morphine, vancomycin, vecuronium *Incompatible:* acyclovir, ampicillin, ibuprofen, indomethacin, sodium bicarbonate	Correct hypovolemia before initiation of treatment. Monitor BP and HR continuously. Pink discoloration of solution is not significant.
Dopamine	2–20 µg/kg/min	Hypotension	Tissue sloughing with infiltration, arrhythmias, increased pulmonary artery pressure	*Solution:* D_5W, $D_{10}W$, NS *Y-site:* TPN, fat emulsion, alprostadil, dobutamine, epinephrine, gentamicin, heparin, midazolam, morphine, vecuronium, vancomycin *Incompatible:* acyclovir, ampicillin, ibuprofen, indomethacin, sodium bicarbonate, Smoflipid	Use 1–5 mL of phentolamine 0.5 mg/mL for extravasation. Monitor BP and HR continuously. Check urine output and peripheral perfusion frequently. Do not use if solution is darker than slightly yellow.

Continued

APPENDIX B **Table 1—cont'd**

Name	Dosage	Indications	Side Effects	Compatibility	Considerations
Epinephrine	0.02–1 μg/kg/min	Asystole, severe bradycardia	Tachycardia, hypertension, arrhythmias, tremors, hyperglycemia, decreased renal and splanchnic blood flow, ischemia, and necrosis of tissue if IV infiltration occurs	*Solution:* D_5W, $D_{10}W$, NS *Y-site:* TPN, dobutamine, dopamine, furosemide, gentamicin, heparin, midazolam, morphine, vecuronium, vancomycin, *Incompatible:* fat emulsion, acyclovir, ampicillin, hyaluronidase, indomethacin phenobarbital, sodium bicarbonate	Use 1–5 mL of phentolamine 0.5 mg/mL for extravasation. Never give through UAC or other artery. Discard if brown or pink color observed. Attempt to correct acidosis before administration.
Milrinone	Loading dose: 75 μg/kg over 60 min (optional) Maintenance dose: 0.25–0.75 μg/kg/min	Low cardiac output	Decreased BP after loading dose, increased HR, arrhythmias, thrombocytopenia	*Solution:* D_5W, NS *Y-site:* TPN, acyclovir, ampicillin, dopamine, gentamicin, midazolam, morphine, sodium bicarbonate vecuronium, vancomycin *Incompatible:* fat emulsion, furosemide	Correct hypovolemia before initiation of therapy. Monitor HR and BP continuously. Monitor fluid and electrolyte changes. Assess renal function regularly. Monitor platelets.
Sodium nitroprusside (Nipride)	Initial dose: 0.25–0.5 μg/kg/min Maintenance dose: usually <2 μg/kg/min	Hypertension, afterload reduction in refractory congestive heart failure	Hypotension, tachycardia, decreased thyroid function, possible cyanide or thiocyanate toxicity with high doses and prolonged treatment, tissue necrosis with extravasation	*Solution:* D_5W, NS *Y-site:* TPN, fat emulsion, heparin, furosemide, gentamicin, midazolam, morphine, dopamine, vecuronium, vancomycin *Incompatible:* acyclovir, ampicillin, hydralazine	Monitor BP and HR continuously. Assess renal and hepatic function daily. Follow cyanide and thiocyanate levels—levels should be <200 ng/mL and <50 μg/mL, respectively. Administer via large vein. Protect from light during administration with opaque material. Discard tubing after 24 h. Slight brownish color is common and not significant.

BP, Blood pressure; *HR,* heart rate; *NS,* nasal solution; *TPN,* total parenteral nutrition; *UAC,* umbilical arterial catheter.

C APPENDIX

Normal Values

Mary Elaine Patrinos

CHEMISTRY VALUES

TABLE C-1 Serum Magnesium, Calcium, Phosphate, and Alkaline Phosphatase in the First Month of Life (Mean ± SD)

Day of life	Magnesium mmol/L	Calcium mmol/L	Phosphate mmol/L	Alkaline Phosphatase IU/L
1	0.85 ± 0.14	2.18 ± 0.27	1.99 ± 0.48	_
2	0.96 ± 0.18	2.24 ± 0.33	1.94 ± 0.56	_
3	1.05 ± 0.13	2.55 ± 0.19	1.49 ± 0.47	_
4	1.09 ± 0.10	2.65 ± 0.17	1.39 ± 0.44	_
5	1.06 ± 0.10	2.72 ± 0.27	1.29 ± 0.37	_
6	1.02 ± 0.12	2.71 ± 0.20	1.30 ± 0.37	_
7	0.98 ± 0.10	2.66 ± 0.16	1.37 ± 0.30	_
14	0.91 ± 0.10	2.57 ± 0.12	1.64 ± 0.38	1,323 ± 639
21	0.89 ± 0.08	2.61 ± 0.16	1.71 ± 0.34	1,359 ± 430
28	0.91 ± 0.10	2.61 ± 0.16	1.74 ± 0.35	1,238 ± 439
Reference range	0.7–1.17	1.8–2.7	1.62–2.52	146–1000

SD, Standard deviation.
Modified from Noone D, Kieran E, Molloy EJ. Serum magnesium in the first week of life in extremely low birth weight infants. *Neonatology* 2012;101:274.

TABLE C-2 Cord Blood Calcium, Phosphate, Magnesium, and Alkaline Phosphatase (23–36 weeks' gestation)

Gestational Age (weeks)	PHOSPHATE (mean ± SD)		CALCIUM (mean ± SD)		MAGNESIUM (mean ± SD)		ALKALINE PHOSPHATASE (mean ± SD)
	mg/dL	mmol/L	mg/dL	mmol/L	mg/dL	mmol/L	units/L
23–27	6.5±0.9	2.1±0.3	10.0±1.0	2.5±0.2	1.9±0.2	0.79±0.07	201±61
28–31	6.3±1.0	2.0±0.3	10.2±1.2	2.6±0.3	1.9±0.3	0.79±0.1	196±68
32–34	6.1±0.8	2.0±0.2	10.5±1.0	2.6±0.2	1.8±0.2	0.76±0.08	174±55
35–36	6.1±1.0	2.0±0.3	10.4±1.1	2.6±0.3	1.8±0.2	0.76±0.09	166±56
>36	5.7±0.7	1.8±0.2	10.9±0.5	2.7±0.1	1.9±0.2	0.77±0.08	159±49

SD, Standard deviation.
Modified from Fenton TR, Lyon AW, Rose MS. Cord blood calcium, phosphate, magnesium, and alkaline phosphatase gestational age-specific reference intervals for preterm infants. *BMC Pediatr.* 2011;11:76.

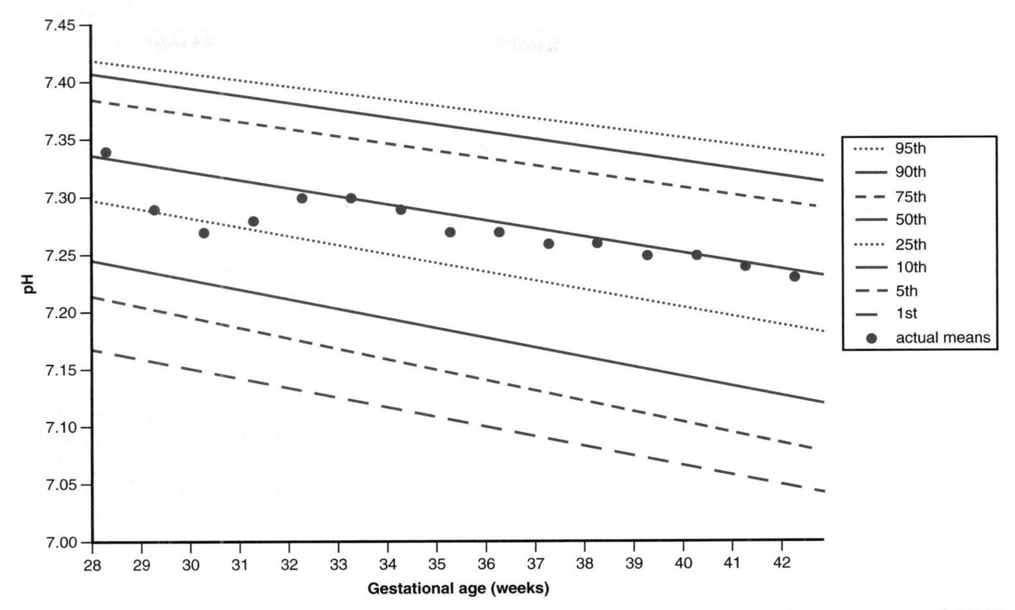

Fig. C.1 Normal reference curve for umbilical cord arterial pH values within the reference group of 46,199 appropriate-for-gestational-age infants born after a noninstrumental vaginal delivery from 28–42 weeks with Apgar score ≥7 at 5 min. (From Skiold B, Petersson G, Ahlberg M, Stephansson O, Johansson S. Population-based reference curve for umbilical cord arterial pH in infants born at 28-42 weeks. *J Perinatol.* 2016;37:254.)

TABLE C-3 Measured Variables in Cord and Whole Venous Blood in Healthy Term Neonates

	CORD BLOOD		2- TO 4-HOUR BLOOD	
	Mean ± SD	**Range**	**Mean ± SD**	**Range**
pH	7.35 ± 0.05	7.19–7.42	7.36 ± 0.04	7.27–7.45
P_{CO_2} (mm Hg)	40 ± 6	24.5–56.7	43 ± 7	30–65
Hct (%)	48 ± 5	37–60	57 ± 5	42–67
Hb (g/L)	1.65 ± 0.16	1.29–2.06	1.90 ± 0.22	0.88–2.3
Na^+ (mmol/L)	138 ± 3	129–144	137 ± 3	130–142
K^+ (mmol/L)	5.3 ± 1.3	3.4–9.9	5.2 ± 0.5	4.4–6.4
Cl^- (mmol/L)	107 ± 4	100–121	111 ± 5	105–125
iCa (mmol/L)	1.15 ± 0.35	0.21–1.5	1.13 ± 0.08	0.9–1.3
iMg (mmol/L)	0.28 ± 0.06	0.09–0.39	0.30 ± 0.05	0.23–0.46
Glucose (mmol/L)	4.16 ± 1.05	0.16–6.66	3.50 ± 0.67	5.11–16.10
Glucose (mg/dL)	75 ± 19	2.9–120	63 ± 12	29–92
Lactate (mmol/L)	4.6 ± 1.9	1.1–9.6	3.9 ± 1.5	1.6–9.8
BUN (mmol/L)	2.14 ± 0.61	1.07–3.57	2.53 ± 0.71	1.43–4.28
BUN (mg/dL)	6.0 ± 1.7	3.0–10.0	7.1 ± 2.0	4–12

Abbreviations: *BUN,* Blood urea nitrogen; *SD,* standard deviation.
From Dollberg S, Bauer R, Lubetzky R, et al. A reappraisal of neonatal blood chemistry reference ranges using the Nova M electrodes. *Am J Perinatol* 2001;18:433.

TABLE C-4 Plasma Ammonia Levels in Preterm Infants of 32 Weeks' or Less Gestational Age

Age (days)	AMMONIA LEVEL*	
	μmol/L	μg/dL
Birth	71 ± 26	121 ± 45
1	69 ± 22	117 ± 37
3	60 ± 19	103 ± 33
7	42 ± 14	72 ± 24
14	42 ± 18	72 ± 30
21	43 ± 16	73 ± 28
28	42 ± 15	72 ± 25
Term infants at birth	45 ± 9	77 ± 16

Modified from Usmanii SS, Cavaliere T, Casatelli J, et al. Plasma ammonia levels in very low birth weight preterm infants. *J Pediatr* 1993;123:798.

TABLE C-5 Liver Function Test Values

Test	Age	Value
Albumin (g/L)	0–5 days (<2.5 kg)	20–36
	0–5 days (>2.5 kg)	26–36
	1–30 days	26–43
	31–182 days	28–46
	183–365 days	28–48
PT (s)	30–36 weeks of gestation	
	1 day	10.6–16.2
	5 days	10.0–15.3
	30 days	10.0–13.6
	90 days	10.0–14.6
	180 days	10.0–15.0
	Full Term	
	1 day	11.6–14.4
	5 days	10.9–13.9
	30 days	10.6–13.1
	90 days	10.8–13.1
	180 days	11.5–13.1
PTT (s)	30–36 weeks of gestation	
	1 day	27.5–79.4
	5 days	26.9–74.1
	30 days	26.9–62.5
	90 days	28.3–50.7
	180 days	21.7–53.3
	Full Term	
	1 day	37.1–48.7
	5 days	34.0–51.2
	30 days	33.0–47.8
	90 days	30.6–43.6
	180 days	31.8–39.2
Ammonia (μmol/L)	1–90 days	42–144
	3–11 mo	34–133
Aspartate aminotransferase (U/L)	0–5 days	35–140
	1–3 yr	20–60
Alanine aminotransferase (U/L)	0–5 days	6–50
	1–30 days	1–25
	31–365 days	3–35
Alkaline phosphatase (U/L)	0–5 days	110–300
	1–30 days	48–406
	31–365 days	82–383
Gamma-glutamyltransferase (U/L)	0–5 days	34–263
	1–182 days	12–132
	183–365 days	1–39

PT, Prothrombin time; *PTT,* partial thromboplastin time.

Modified from Rosenthal P. Assessing liver function and hyperbilirubinemia in the newborn. National Academy of Clinical Biochemistry. *Clin Chem.* 1997;43:228.

TABLE C-6 Reference Intervals for Urine Amino Acid Excretion in Untimed Samples (mmol per mol creatinine)

Amino Acid	0–1 Months (Mean)	1–12 Months (Mean)
Aspartic acid	9–57 (23)	10–69 (26)
Glutamic acid	31–96 (54)	24–102 (50)
Alpha-aminoadipic acid	7–96 (26)	7–110 (29)
Hydroxyproline	11–556 (100)	5–238 (34)
Phosphoethanolamine	13–167 (46)	12–216 (51)
Serine	48–509 (156)	34–329 (51)
Asparagine	15–223 (58)	18–197 (59)
Glycine	127–2042 (510)	133–894 (345)
Glutamine	37–600 (148)	63–446 (168)
Beta-Alanine	2–41 (8)	2–38 (8)
Taurine*	12–1057	10–809
Histidine	23–676 (125)	69–392 (164)
Citrulline	1–18 (5)	2–46 (9)
Threonine	9–337 (56)	12–145 (41)
Alanine	34–358 (109)	27–313 (93)
Beta-aminoisobutyric acid	0–520 (14)	5–258 (36)
Carnosine	3–184 (21)	8–160 (36)
Arginine	0–81 (10)	0–40 (5)
Proline	3–257 (29)	2–90 (14)
1-Methylhistidine	0–78 (7)	0–98 (7)
3-Methylhistidine	5–85 (20)	10–95 (31)
Ethanolamine	33–253 (91)	57–221 (112)
Aminobutyric acid	1–43 (5)	1–58 (7)
Tyrosine	5–74 (19)	12–64 (28)
Valine	3–34 (10)	3–43 (11)
Methionine	2–24 (7)	2–18 (6)
Cystathionine	1–26 (6)	1–11 (4)
Cystine	5–109 (24)	2–42 (10)
Isoleucine	2–37 (8)	2–21 (6)
Leucine	4–84 (17)	4–72 (17)
Hydroxylysine	3–49 (11)	2–50 (9)
Phenylalanine	2–49 (9)	7–42 (17)
Tryptophan	1–46 (8)	3–37 (10)
Ornithine	2–37 (8)	2–19 (6)
Lysine	6–464 (54)	4–80 (18)
No. of subjects (male/female)	20 (11/9)	30 (16/14)

Modified from Venta R. Year-long validation study and reference values for urinary amino acids using a reverse-phase HPLC method. *Clin Chem.* 2001;47:575.

HEMATOLOGIC VALUES

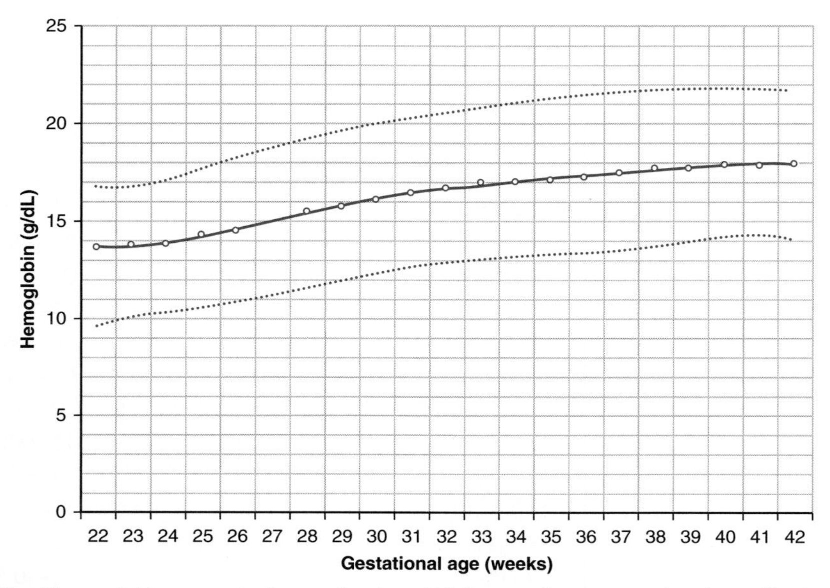

Fig. C.2 Blood hemoglobin concentration on the day of birth according to gestational age. The lower dotted line is the fifth percentile, the solid middle line is the mean, and the upper dotted line is the 95th percentile. (From Henry E, Christensen RD. Reference intervals in neonatal hematology. *Clin Perinatol.* 2015;42:485.)

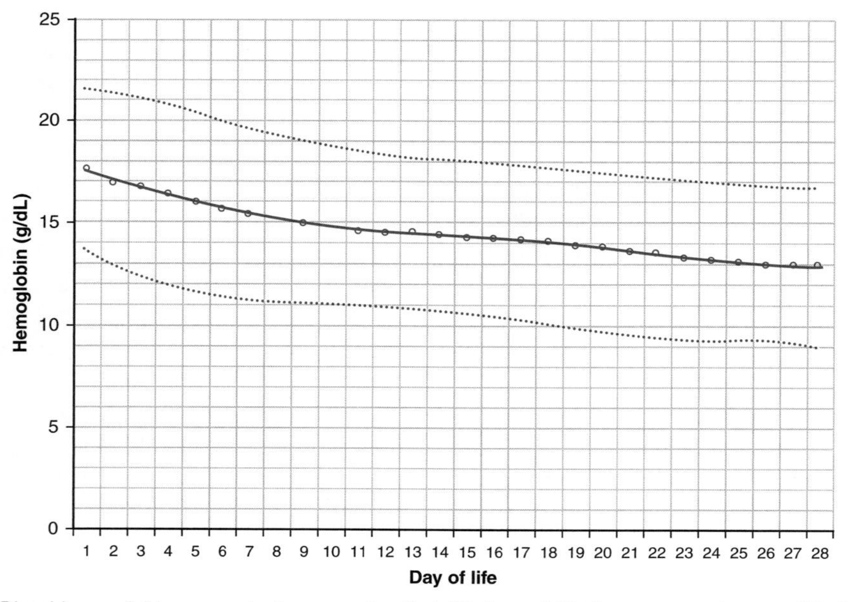

Fig. C.3 Blood hemoglobin concentration over the first 28 days of life for neonates born at 35–42 weeks' gestation. The lower dotted line is the fifth percentile, the solid middle line is the mean, and the upper dotted line is the 95th percentile. (From Henry E, Christensen RD. Reference intervals in neonatal hematology. *Clin Perinatol.* 2015;42:485.)

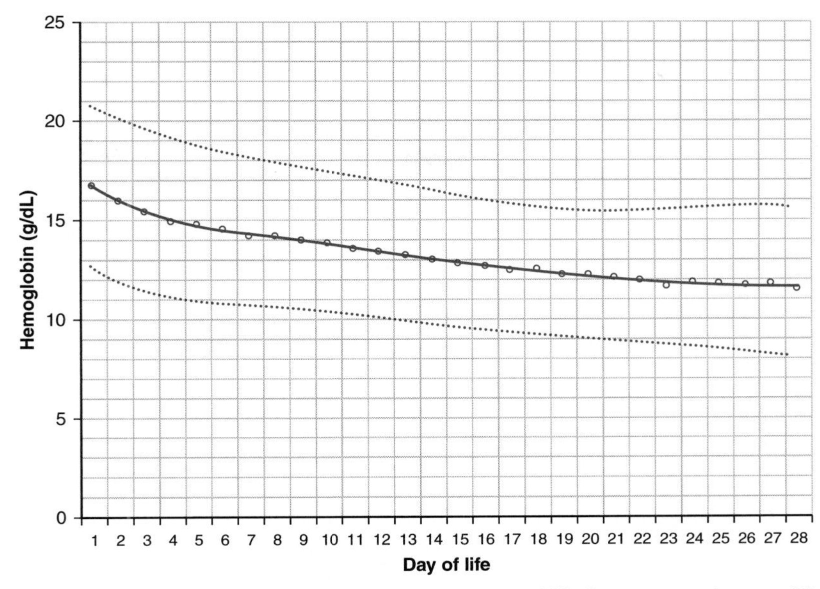

Fig. C.4 Blood hemoglobin concentration over the first 28 days of life for neonates born at 29–34 weeks' gestation. The lower dotted line is the fifth percentile, the solid middle line is the mean, and the upper dotted line is the 95th percentile. (From Henry E, Christensen RD. Reference intervals in neonatal hematology. *Clin Perinatol.* 2015;42:486.)

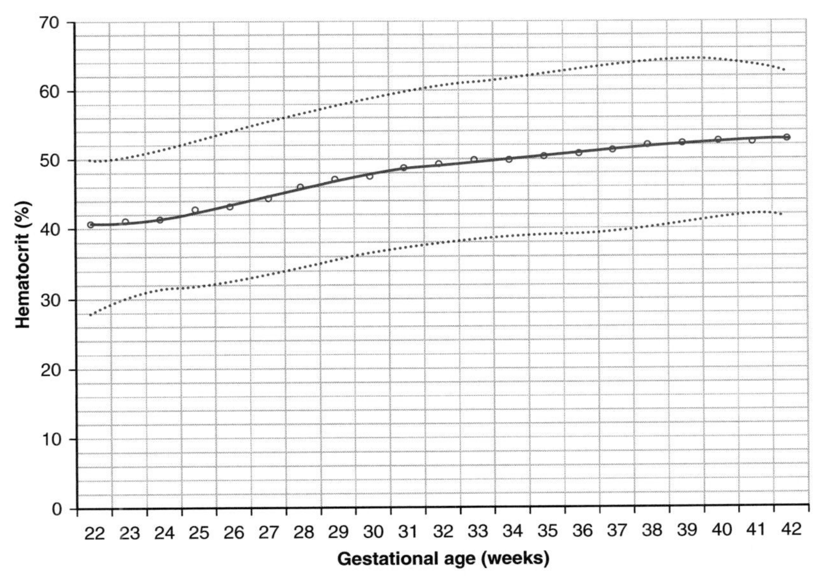

Fig. C.5 Hematocrit on the day of birth according to gestational age. The lower dotted line is the fifth percentile, the solid middle line is the mean, and the upper dotted line is the 95th percentile. (From Henry E, Christensen RD. Reference intervals in neonatal hematology. *Clin Perinatol.* 2015;42:486.)

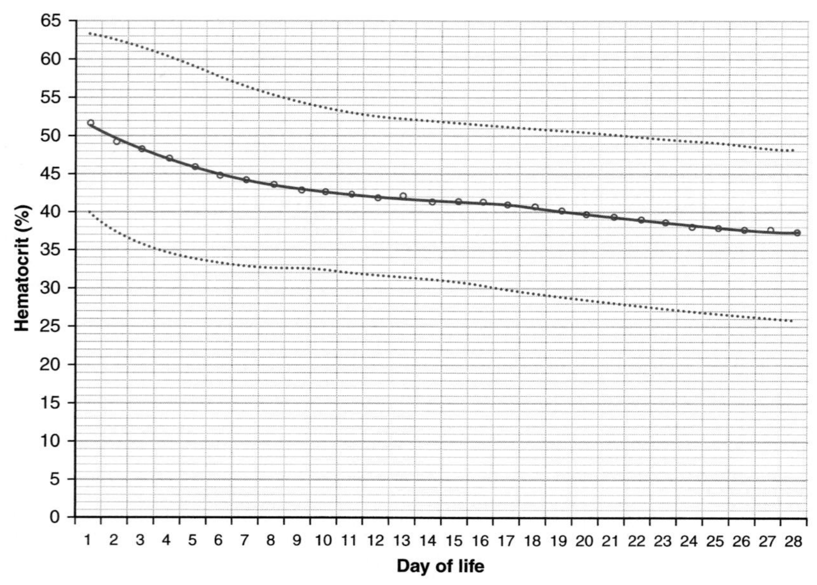

Fig. C.6 Hematocrit over the first 28 days of life for neonates born at 35–42 weeks' gestation. The lower dotted line is the fifth percentile, the solid middle line is the mean, and the upper dotted line is the 95th percentile. (From Henry E, Christensen RD. Reference intervals in neonatal hematology. *Clin Perinatol* 2015;42:487.)

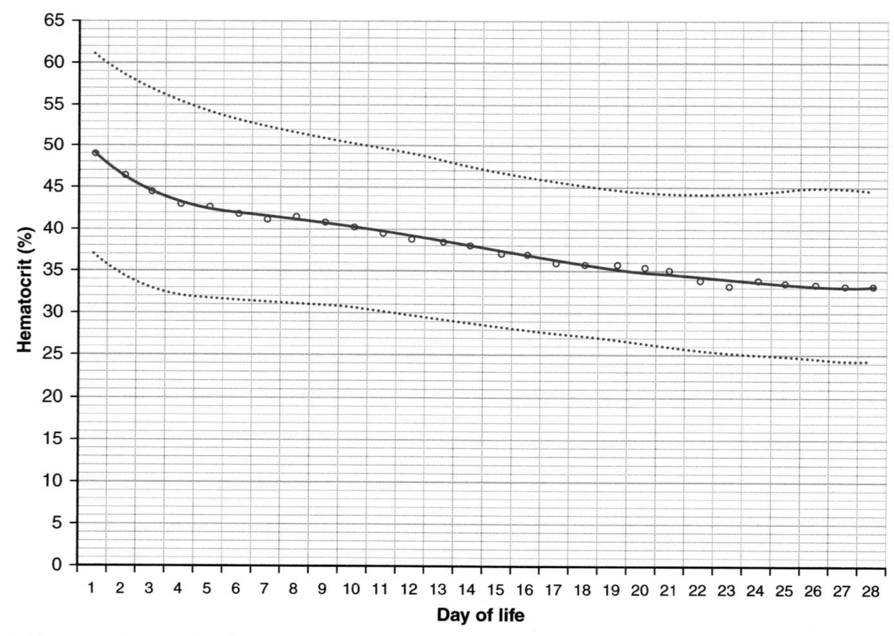

Fig. C.7 Hematocrit over the first 28 days of life for neonates born at 29–34 weeks' gestation. The lower dotted line is the fifth percentile, the solid middle line is the mean, and the upper dotted line is the 95th percentile. (From Henry E, Christensen RD. Reference intervals in neonatal hematology. *Clin Perinatol.* 2015;42:487.)

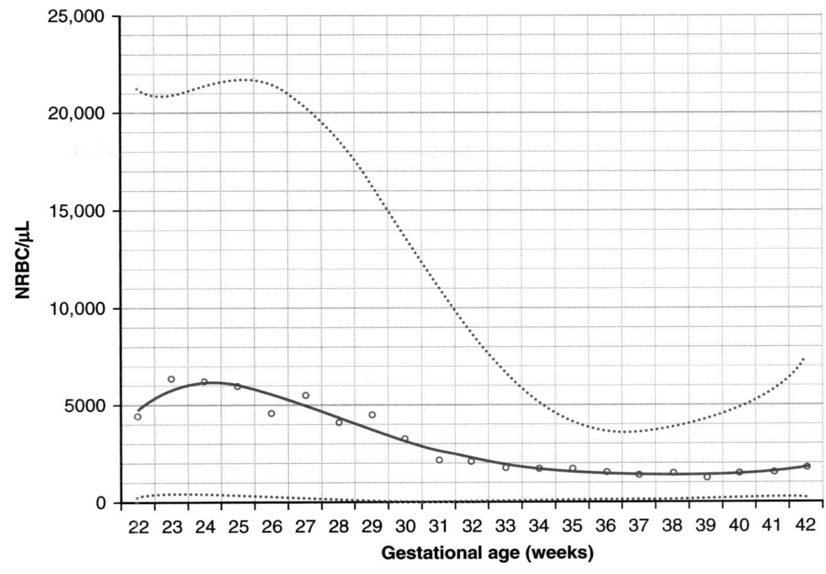

Fig. C.8 Nucleated red blood cell *(NRBC)* levels on the day of birth according to gestational age. The lower dotted line is the fifth percentile, the solid middle line is the mean, and the upper dotted line is the 95th percentile. (From Henry E, Christensen RD. Reference intervals in neonatal hematology. *Clin Perinatol.* 2015;42:489.)

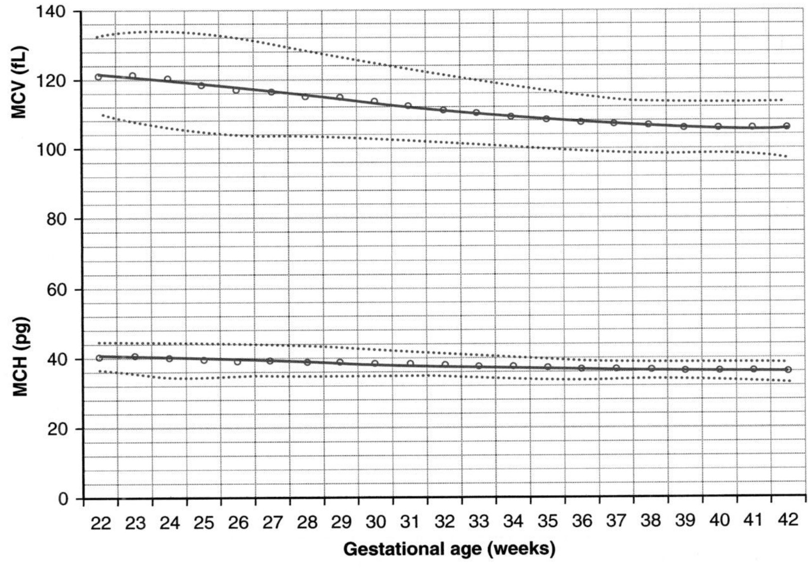

Fig. C.9 Mean corpuscular volume *(MCV)* and mean corpuscular hemoglobin *(MCH)* on the day of birth according to gestational age. For each, the lower dotted line is the fifth percentile, the solid middle line is the mean, and the upper dotted line is the 95th percentile. (From Henry E, Christensen RD. Reference intervals in neonatal hematology. *Clin Perinatol.* 2015;42:488.)

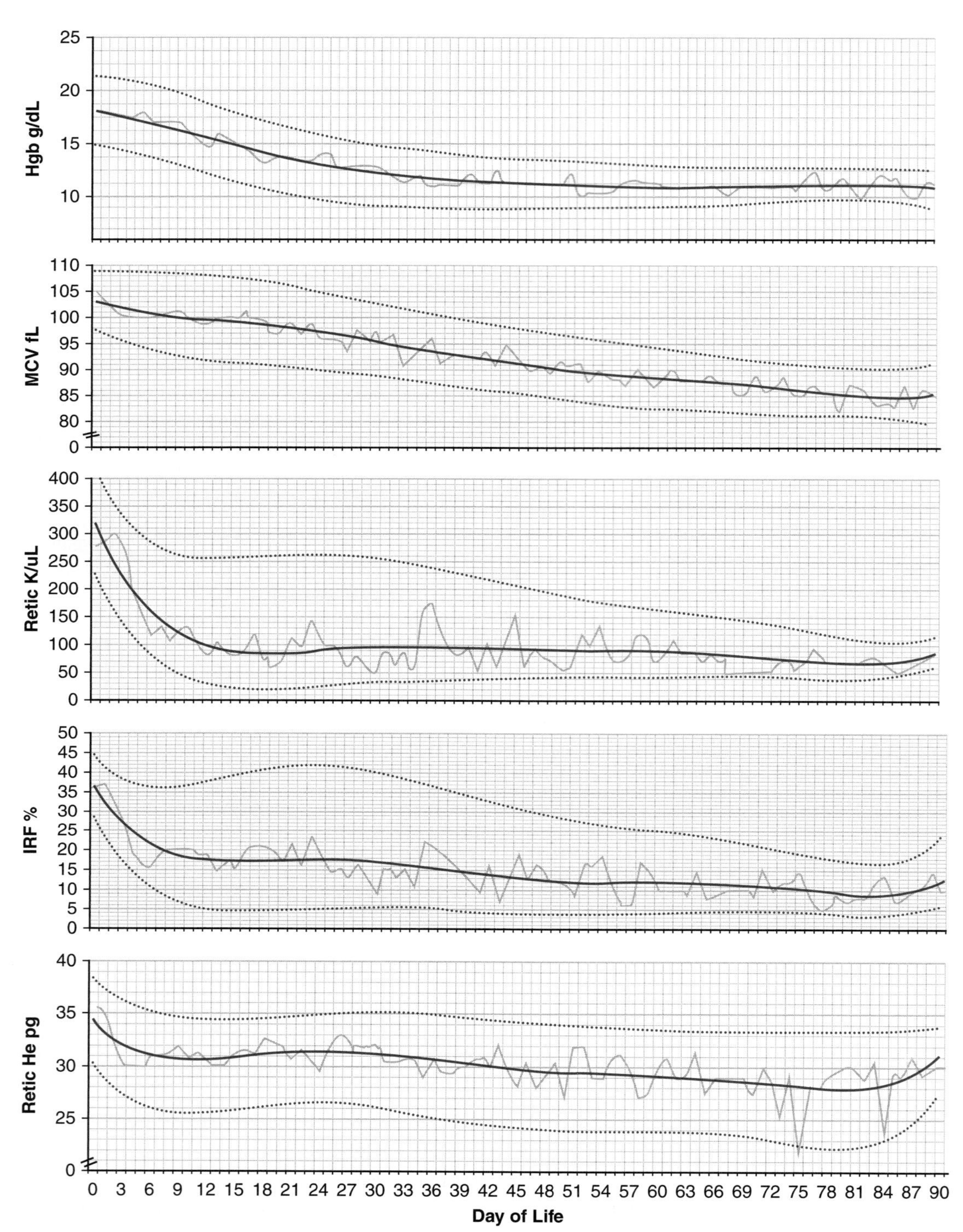

Fig. C.10 Reference intervals are displayed from the day of birth to 90 days for: (1) blood hemoglobin *(Hgb)* concentration ($g dL^{-1}$), (2) erythrocyte mean corpuscular volume *(MCV; fL)*, (3) reticulocytes (Retic × 10^3 per μL blood), (4) immature reticulocyte fraction *(IRF %)*, and (5) reticulocyte hemoglobin content *(RET-He pg)*. The dashed lines show the 10th percentile and 90th percentile values, the solid black line shows the "smoothed" median values, and the light gray solid line shows the actual median values each day. (From Christensen RD, Henry E, Bennett ST, Yaish HM. Reference intervals for reticulocyte parameters of infants during their first 90 days after birth. *J Perinatol.* 2016;36:64.)

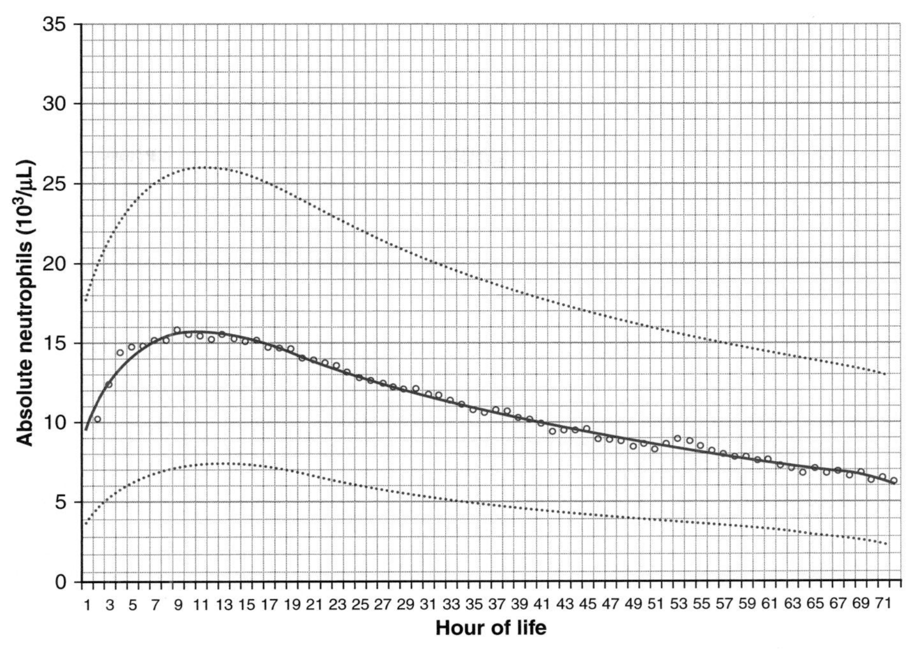

Fig. C.11 Neutrophil levels of neonates ≥36 weeks' gestation during the first 72 hours of life. The lower dotted line is the fifth percentile, the solid middle line is the mean, and the upper dotted line is the 95th percentile. (From Henry E, Christensen RD. Reference intervals in neonatal hematology. *Clin Perinatol* 42:492, 2015.)

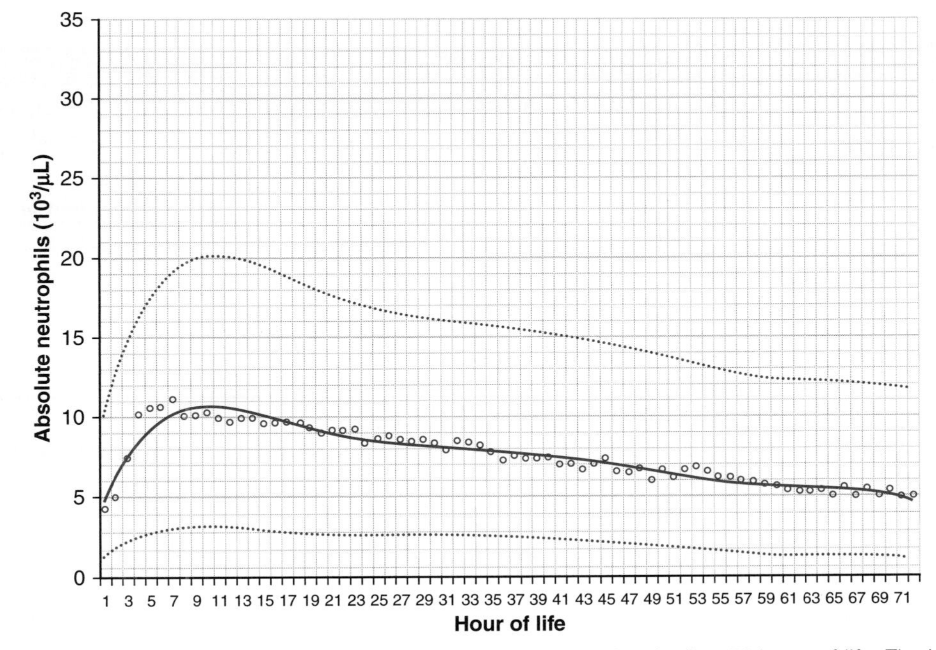

Fig. C.12 Neutrophil levels of neonates 28–36 weeks' gestation during the first 72 hours of life. The lower dotted line is the fifth percentile, the solid middle line is the mean, and the upper dotted line is the 95th percentile. (From Henry E, Christensen RD. Reference intervals in neonatal hematology. *Clin Perinatol.* 2015;42:492.)

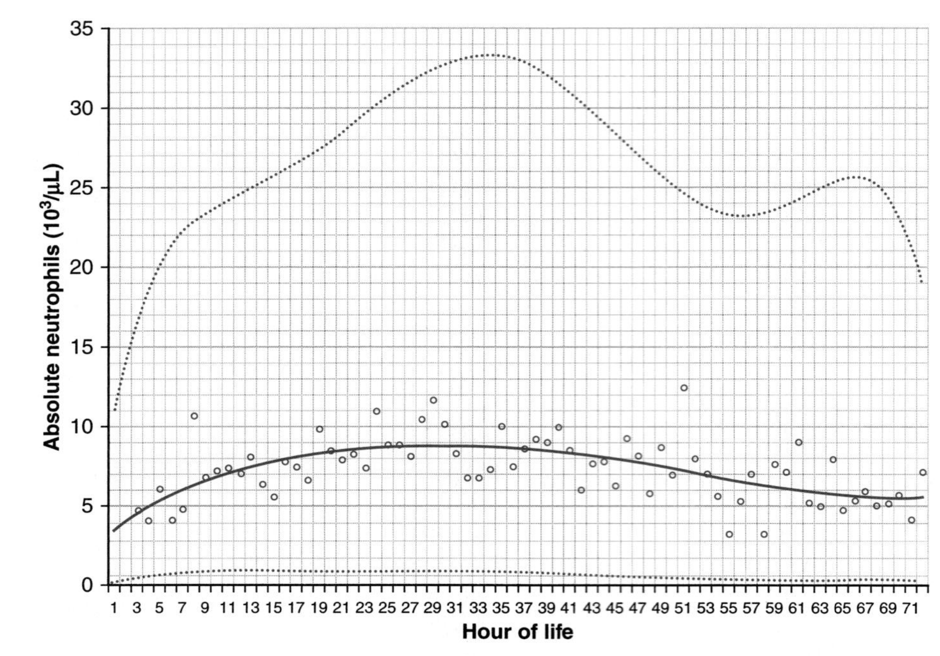

Fig. C.13 Neutrophil levels of neonates <28 weeks' gestation during the first 72 hours of life. The lower dotted line is the fifth percentile, the solid middle line is the mean, and the upper dotted line is the 95th percentile. (From Henry E, Christensen RD. Reference intervals in neonatal hematology. *Clin Perinatol.* 2015;42:493)

TABLE C-7 Reference Intervals for Measurements of "Left Shift"

	FIRST 48 HOURS AFTER BIRTH N = 4808			BEYOND 48 HOURS OF LIFE N = 1654		
Measurement	**Median ± SD**	**5th percentile**	**95th percentile**	**Median ± SD**	**5th percentile**	**95th percentile**
IG%	1.99 ± 1.7	0.5	6.2	1.62 ± 0.7	0.2	4.2
I/T	0.09 ± 0.08	0	0.29	0.12 ± 0.05	0	0.31
IG (cells per μL)	539 ± 270	50	1460	308 ± 70	10	613
Bands (cells per μL)	1303 ± 680	0	3710	702 ± 160	0	1785

IG, Immature granulocyte; *I/T,* immature to total neutrophil ratio; *SD,* standard deviation.
From MacQueen BC, Christensen RD, Yoder BA, et al. Comparing automated vs manual leukocyte differential counts for quantifying the 'left shift' in the blood of neonates. *J Perinatol.* 2016;36(10):845.

CEREBROSPINAL FLUID VALUES

TABLE C-8 Cerebrospinal Fluid Findings in Preterm and Term Infants Hospitalized in the Neonatal Intensive Care Unit

	PRETERM INFANTS (<37 WEEKS)			TERM INFANTS		
	All *n* **= 148**	**≤7 days** *n* **= 66**	**>7 days** *n* **= 82**	**All** *n* **= 170**	**≤7 days** *n* **= 130**	**>7 days** *n* **= 40**
CSF WBC, cells/μL						
All infants						
Median (IQR)	3 (1–6)	3 (1–7)	3 (1–4)	3 (1–6)	3 (1–6)	2 (1–4)
95th percentile	16	18	12	26	23	32
Antibiotic: unexposed						
95th percentile	11	17	10	32	31	53
CSF PROTEIN, mg/dL						
All infants						
Median (IQR)	104 (79–131)	116 (93–138)	93 (69–122)	74 (54–96)	78 (60–100)	57 (42–77)
95th percentile	203	213	203	137	137	158
Antibiotic: unexposed						
95th percentile	195	195	136	136	136	284
CSF GLUCOSE, mg/dL						
All infants						
Median (IQR)	49 (42–62)	53 (43–65)	47 (40–58)	51 (44–57)	50 (44–56)	52 (45–64)
5th percentile	33	33	33	36	35	38
Antibiotic: unexposed						
5th percentile	33	33	35	33	33	33

Studied infants were aged <6 months and underwent LP for evaluation for sepsis. Infants were excluded if there was culture-proven bacterial meningitis, unknown CSF culture results, positive CSF viral PCR, a ventriculoperitoneal shunt present, seizures, bacteremia, or CSF RBC >500 cells/μL.

CSF, Cerebrospinal fluid; *IQR,* interquartile range; *LP,* lumbar puncture; *RBC,* red blood cells; *WBC,* white blood cells.

Modified from Srinivasan L, Shah SS, Padula MA, Abbasi S, McGowan KL, Harris MC. Cerebrospinal fluid reference ranges in term and preterm infants in the neonatal intensive care unit. *J Pediatr.* 2012;161(4):731.

PHYSIOLOGIC PARAMETERS

Growth Charts

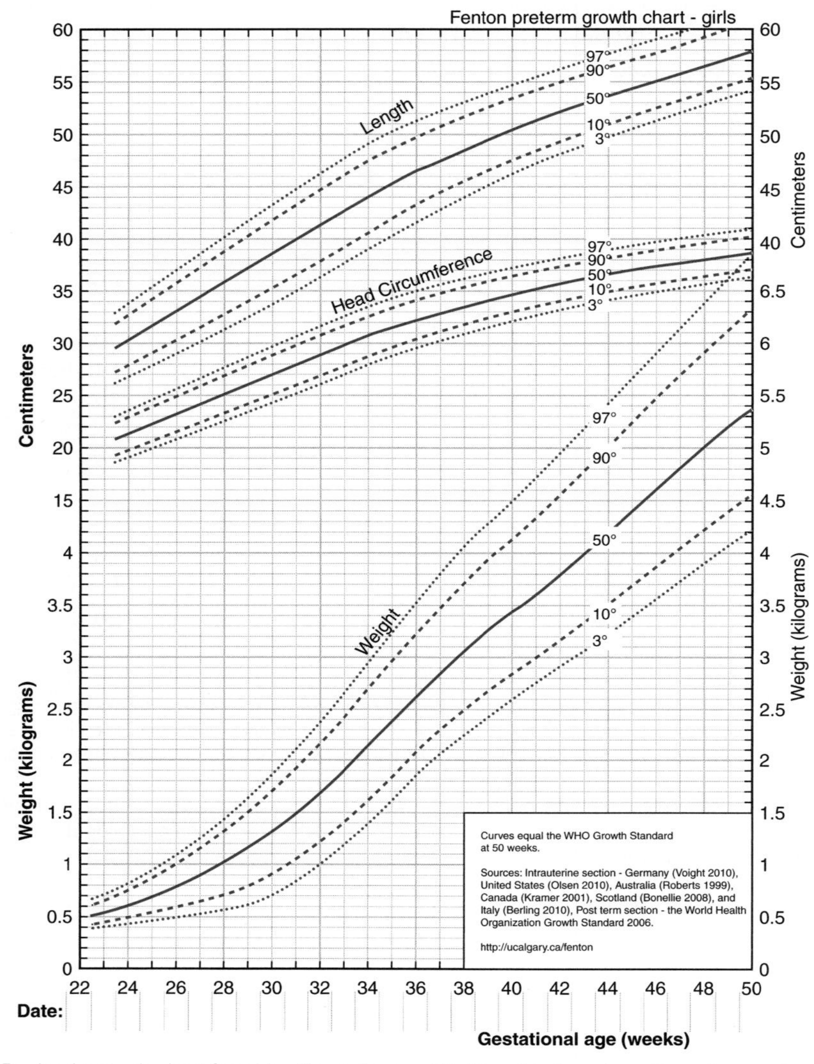

Fig. C.14 Revised growth chart for girls. (From Fenton TR, Kim JH. A systematic review and meta-analysis to revise the Fenton growth chart for preterm infants. *BMC Pediatr.* 2013;13:59.)

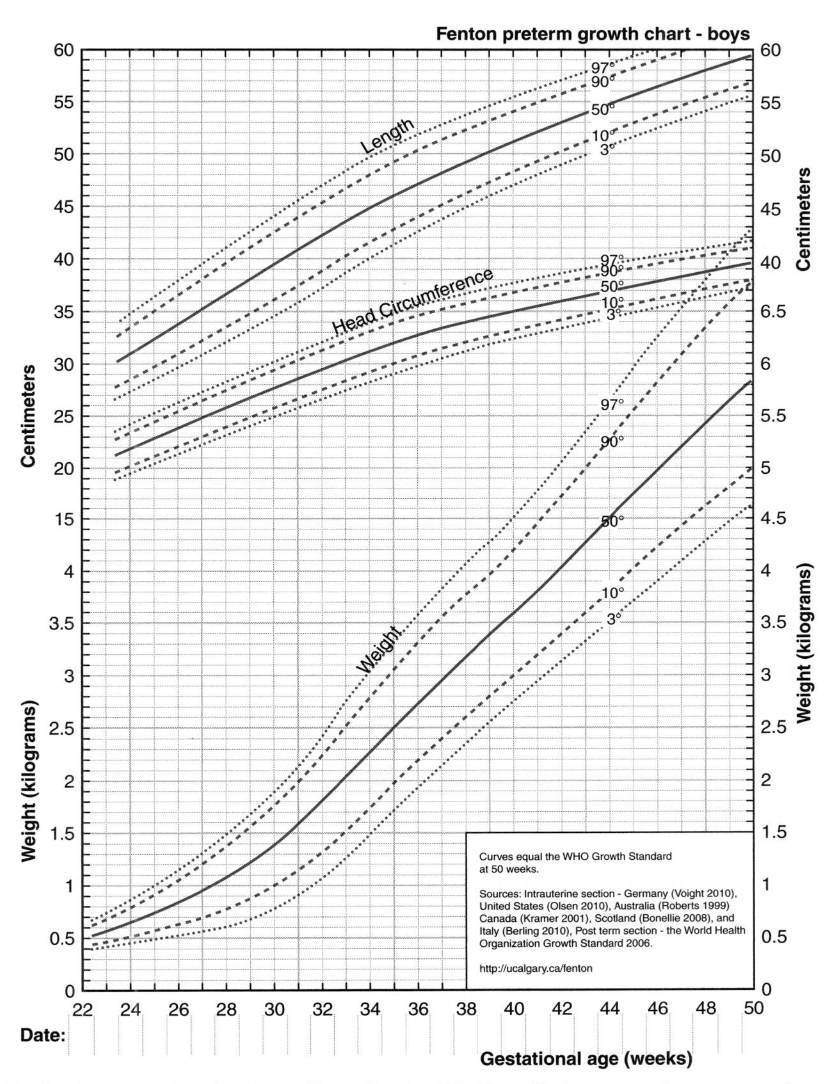

Fig. C.15 Revised growth chart for boys. (From Fenton TR, Kim JH. A systematic review and meta-analysis to revise the Fenton growth chart for preterm infants. *BMC Pediatr.* 2013;13:59.)

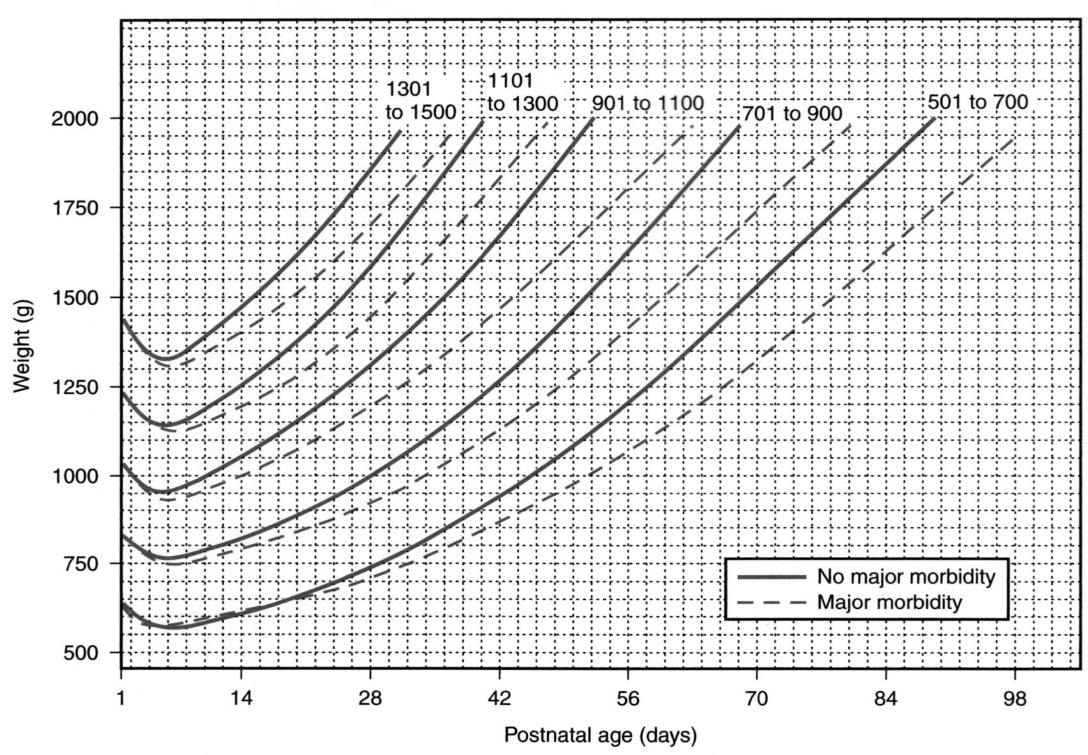

Fig. C.16 Growth curves of infants with major morbidities (dashed lines) and reference infants without major morbidities (solid line) as a function of postnatal age in days. The infants are stratified by 200-g birth-weight intervals. Reference group infants without major morbidities were appropriate size for gestational age and survived to discharge without development of chronic lung disease, severe intraventricular hemorrhage, necrotizing enterocolitis, or late-onset sepsis. (From Ehrenkranz RA, Younes N, Lemons JA, et al. Longitudinal growth of hospitalized very low birth weight infants. *Pediatrics* 1999;104:280.)

TIME OF FIRST VOID AND STOOL

TABLE C-9 **Time of First Void and Stool**

TIME OF FIRST VOID BY 920 FULL-TERM INFANTS				TIME OF PASSAGE OF FIRST STOOL BY 920 FULL-TERM INFANTS			
Time	**No.**	**%**	**Cumulative %**	**Time**	**No.**	**%**	**Cumulative %**
Delivery room	139	15.1	15.1	Delivery room	210	22.8	22.8
Hours				Hours			
1–24	743	80.8	95.9	1–24	674	73.3	96.1
24–48	35	3.8	99.7	24–48	35	3.8	99.9
>48	3	0.3	100.0	>48	1	0.1	100.0
TIME OF FIRST VOID BY 280 PREMATURE INFANTS				**TIME OF PASSAGE OF FIRST STOOL BY 280 PREMATURE INFANTS**			
Time	**No.**	**%**	**Cumulative %**	**Time**	**No.**	**%**	**Cumulative %**
Delivery room	62	22.1	22.1	Delivery room	30	10.7	10.7
Hours				Hours			
1–24	201	71.8	93.9	1–24	191	68.2	78.9
24–48	17	6.1	100.0	24–48	46	16.4	95.3
>48				>48	13	4.7	100.0

Modified from Sherry S, Kramer I. The time of passage of the first stool and first urine by the newborn infant. *J Pediatr.* 1955;46:158; Kramer I, Sherry S. The time of passage of the first stool and urine by the premature infant. *J Pediatr.* 1957;51:353; Clark D. Times of first void and stool in 500 newborns. *Pediatrics* 1977;60:457.

BLOOD PRESSURE

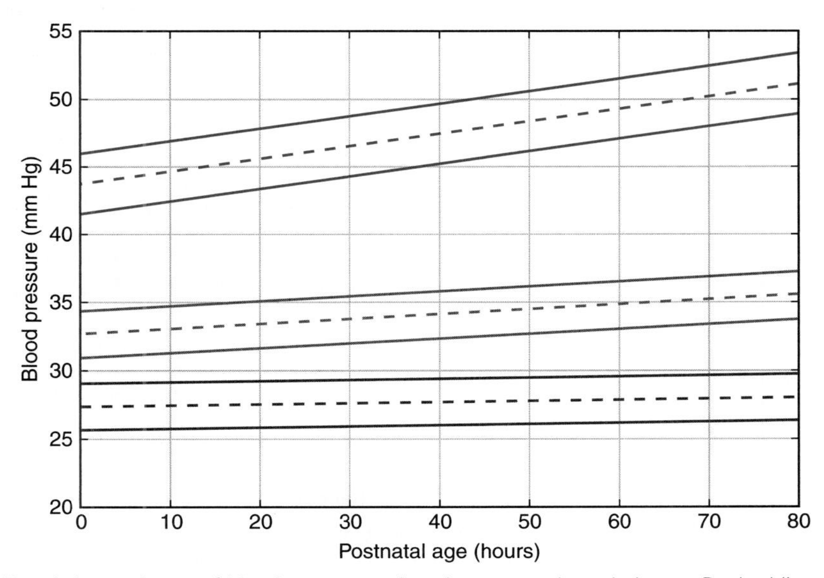

Fig. C.17 Population estimate of blood pressure values by postnatal age in hours. Dashed line represents the blood pressure estimate, whereas solid line represents the boundaries of the 95% confidence interval. *Green*, systolic blood pressure; *light gray*, mean arterial blood pressure; *black*, diastolic blood pressure. (From Vesoulis ZA, El Ters NM, Wallendorf M, Mathur AM. Empirical estimation of the normative blood pressure in infants <28 weeks, gestation using a massive data approach. *J Perinatol.* 2016;36:291.)

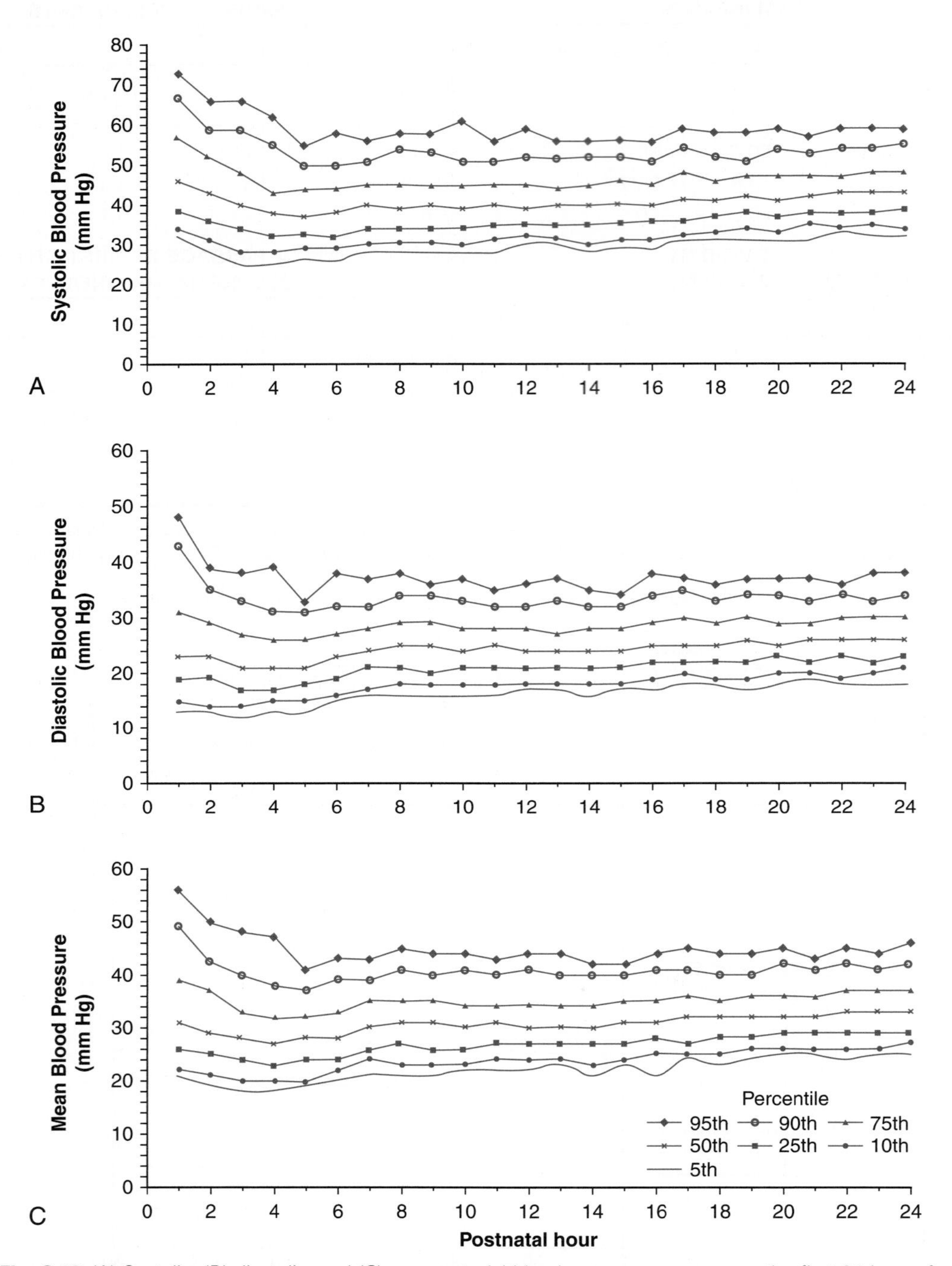

Fig. C.18 (A) Systolic, (B) diastolic, and (C) mean arterial blood pressure curves over the first 24 hours for extremely preterm infants (n = 367). (From Batton B, Li L, Newman S, et al. Evolving blood pressure dynamics for extremely preterm infants. *J Perinatol.* 2014;34[4]:301-305.)

TABLE C-10 Mean Arterial Blood Pressure by Birth Weight

Birth Weight (g)	MAP ± SD		
	Day 3	Day 17	Day 31
501–750	38 ± 8	44 ± 8	46 ± 11
751–1000	43 ± 9	45 ± 7	47 ± 9
1001–1250	43 ± 8	46 ± 9	48 ± 8
1251–1500	45 ± 8	47 ± 8	47 ± 9

MAP, Mean arterial pressure; *SD,* standard deviation.

From Fanaroff AA, Wright E; NICHD Neonatal Research Network. Profiles of mean arterial blood pressure (MAP) for infants weighing 501-1500 grams, *Pediatr Res.* 1990;27:205A.

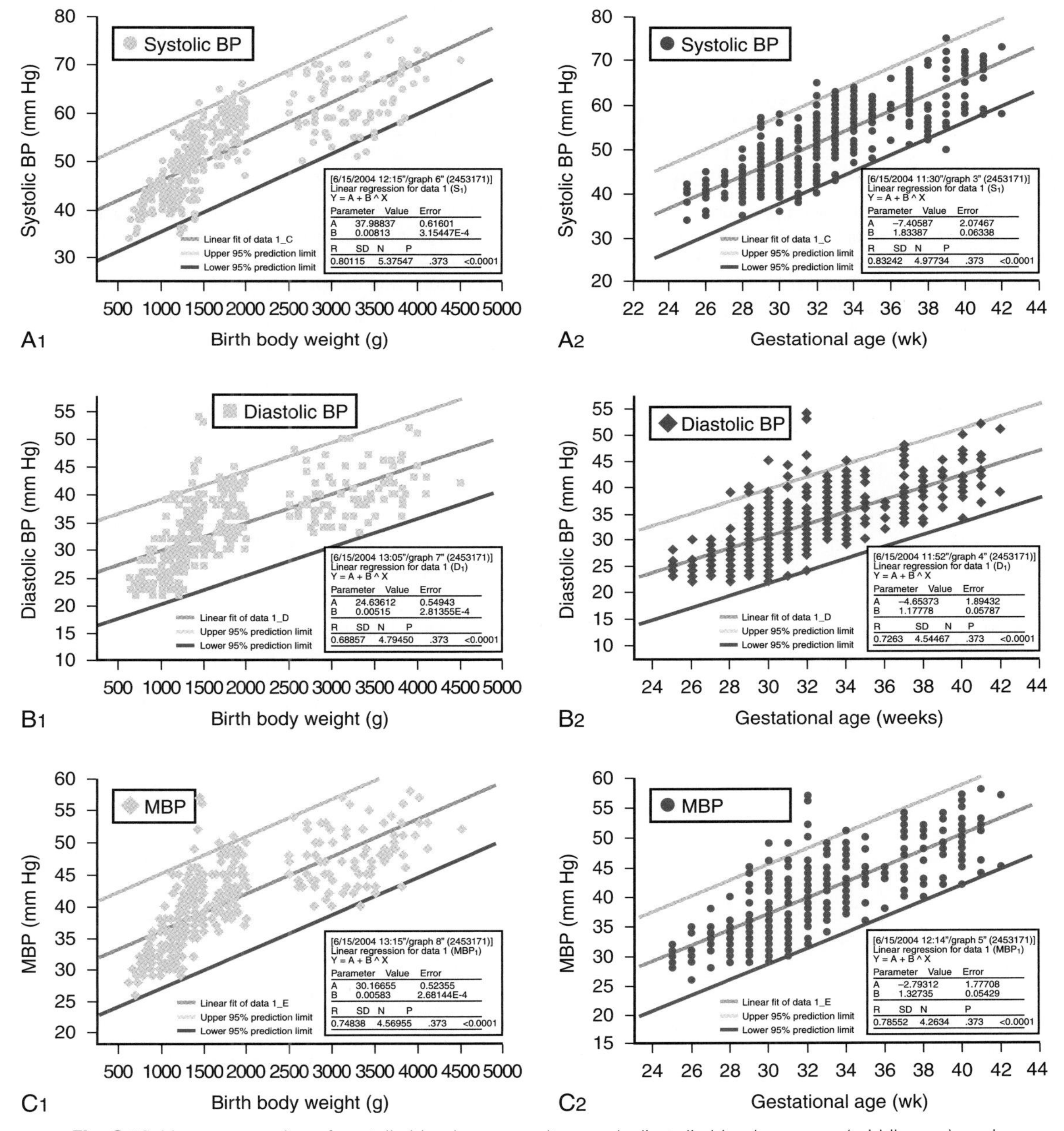

Fig. C.19 Linear regression of systolic blood pressure (top row), diastolic blood pressure (middle row), and mean blood pressure (bottom row) on birth weight (left column) and gestational age (right column) on day 1 of life, with 95% confidence limits (upper and lower solid lines). The 95% confidence limits approximate ±2 standard deviations (SDs) from the mean. *BP,* Blood pressure; *MBP,* mean blood pressure. (From Pejovic B, Peco-Antic A, Marinkoviv-Eri J. Blood pressure in non-critically ill preterm and full-term neonates. *Pediatr Nephrol.* 2007;22:249.)

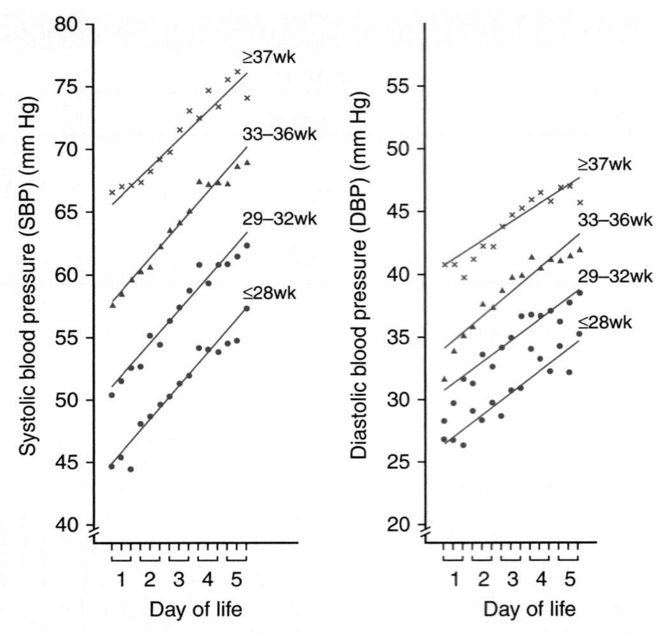

Fig. C.20 Systolic blood pressure and diastolic blood pressure in the first 5 days of life, with each day subdivided into 8-hour periods. Infants are stratified by gestational age into four groups: 28 weeks or less (n = 33), 29 to 32 weeks (n = 73), 33 to 36 weeks (n = 100), and 37 weeks or more (n = 110). (From Zubrow AB, Hulman S, Kushner H, et al. Determinants of blood pressure in infants admitted to neonatal intensive care units: a prospective multicenter study. Philadelphia Neonatal Blood Pressure Study Group. *J Perinatol.* 1995;15:470.)

APPENDIX D

Selected Procedures in Neonatology

Ricardo J. Rodriguez

INTRODUCTION

Procedural skills are an important component of care in the neonatal intensive care unit (NICU). Procedures have inherent risks and can be the source of significant morbidity and mortality if the proper techniques are not applied. Historically, the acquisition of these competencies required that trainees observed a procedure and then attempted to perform it under close supervision. Obviously, although this practice served a laudable purpose, it is fraught with significant limitations, and therefore most training programs abandoned it. The traditional practice of "see one, do one, and teach one" has been put to rest because of the introduction of highly sophisticated simulation laboratories where trainees can learn the proper techniques of most procedures without subjecting patients to potentially painful and harmful unsuccessful attempts. Also, this novel learning modality takes the pressure away from the learner, who can now hone in on the skills and acquire the confidence to perform successfully in a real-life situation at bedside. The introduction of point-of-care ultrasonography is another important advancement in the procedural arena in neonatology. Introduction of a central vascular catheter, or performing a paracentesis under ultrasonographic guidance, is standard in adult and pediatric intensive care units, and that practice is quickly gaining momentum in neonatal units as well.

Before any procedure is performed in a newborn, a thorough and thoughtful consideration of the indications, contraindications, benefits, and potential complications is required. A discussion with the family and obtaining parental informed consent are mandatory, except in emergency situations where a delay may pose a life-threatening risk. Gathering the appropriate clinical information and patient identification, preparation of the supplies, and making sure that all caregivers involved are aware of the procedure to be performed is fundamental. Utilization of checklists and procedural bundles as well as a huddle or "time out" have significantly facilitated these processes and decreased errors.

In this chapter, a few select procedures are discussed; however, the information presented here is meant to provide the reader with only a general overview and should not be considered enough to achieve competence.

UMBILICAL VESSEL CATHETERIZATION

Use of central catheters requires careful consideration of the risks involved (Box D.1). The relatively easy access to the umbilical vessels makes these vessels a very good option for central access in emergency situations. A central catheter inserted into the aorta via an umbilical artery may be required in the management of the sick neonate for monitoring of blood pressure, intermittent blood sampling to check acid–base status, and, while in place, infusion of parenteral fluids and medications.

Umbilical artery catheters must be precisely located. A major objective is to avoid the origin of the renal arteries because a catheter may occlude a renal artery, and catheters in the area may produce thrombosis.[1] Both situations can result in renal infarction. Some prefer to position the catheter in the midthoracic aorta (high); others prefer to locate the catheter tip between L3 and L4 (low). Thrombotic complications are reported with both high and low placement.[2] Resolution of the thrombus or development of collateral circulation generally occurs, even when extensive thrombosis (e.g., aorta distal to renal arteries, common iliac) has been documented.[1,3] Occasionally, a neonatal death is considered a direct consequence of complications related to umbilical vessel catheterization.[4] Hypertension in the neonate following use of high umbilical artery catheters has been described. However, in a prospective study, the incidence of hypertension was similar with low and high catheters.[5]

BOX D.1 Catheter Complications

Hemorrhage
Perforation into
- Peritoneal cavity
- Urachus
- Pericardium

Hepatic laceration
Thrombi and emboli
- Splenic vein thrombus or embolus
- Displacement of thrombus in ductus venosus
- Pulmonary infarction (pulmonary vein thrombus)

Retained broken-off catheter fragment
Calcification of portal vein or umbilical vein

Hemorrhage, either resulting from loose connections or careless use of the stopcocks or occurring at the time of removal, is a major complication of arterial catheters. Another major complication is thrombus formation with release of microemboli into the systemic circulation. It is speculated that the catheter tip can traumatize the vessel wall, which may release tissue thromboplastin and activate intravascular coagulation. Alternatively, the presence of the catheter itself may produce clot formation. More rare complications include intimal flap formation and aneurysmatic dilatation of the abdominal artery. Ultrasonographic examination of the abdominal aorta and its branches is indicated when any of these complications are suspected.

Arterial blood samples may be obtained by multiple arterial punctures (of the radial artery) or an indwelling radial artery cannula as the method of choice or in cases in which umbilical artery catheterization is unsuccessful.[6,7]

In general, umbilical vein catheterization is technically easier. However, it should be avoided except when immediate access to a vein is needed because of an unexpected emergency (e.g., the need for delivery room resuscitation) because complications may be serious and difficult to avoid. An umbilical vein catheter tip may locate in a branch of the portal vein and lead to areas of liver necrosis without perforation of the vein wall following infusions of hypertonic solutions such as sodium bicarbonate and hypertonic glucose. Portal vein thrombosis and aseptic abscess formation have also occurred with and without infection. In addition, spontaneous perforation of the colon after exchange transfusion via an umbilical vein catheter has been reported. Radiographic verification of catheter tip location was not performed in any of these cases; most likely, the catheter tip was in the portal vein, and the cause of perforation was local necrosis of the bowel wall following hemorrhagic infarction as a result of retrograde microemboli or obstructive hemodynamic changes. Air embolism in the portal system has also been observed rarely.

In the first hour or so of life in a normal term infant, or for many hours and occasionally for many days in a sick or preterm infant, an umbilical vein catheter may be passed through the ductus venosus into the inferior vena cava.

Depending on the circumstances and preference of the physician, exchange transfusions can be done using either vessel or both, but not by infusing into the artery.

The umbilical vessel catheter should be removed as soon as possible and a peripheral intravenous line substituted, if necessary. In a nondistressed newborn infant requiring parenteral fluids, under no circumstances should an umbilical vessel catheter be used when a peripheral intravenous line could be started via a scalp vein or an extremity vein. In the extremely low-birth-weight group, in whom parenteral nutrition is essential until enteral feeds are established, common practice is to routinely place percutaneous indwelling central catheters and remove umbilical lines as soon as possible.

TECHNIQUE OF CATHETERIZATION

In the small premature infant, the entire catheterization should be done as an operating room procedure with the infant in an incubator or under a radiant warmer to prevent hypothermia. In the delivery room, a radiant heater should be used.

When not precluded by an emergency (e.g., acute asphyxia), the following protocol should be followed. The operator carefully scrubs hands and arms to the elbows and puts on sterile gloves. A 3.5F or 4F (for infants weighing <1500 g) or a 5F catheter with rounded tip, which has a radiopaque line and end hole (Argyle umbilical artery catheter, Coridien, Mansfield, MA), is attached to a syringe by a three-way stopcock. The system is filled with heparinized saline solution (1 U heparin per milliliter of normal or half-normal saline). (Box D.2 lists the equipment found on the catheterization tray.) Before the procedure is begun, the length of the catheter to be inserted should be marked according to the location desired (Figs. D.1 and D.2). After the umbilical stump and surrounding abdominal wall are carefully prepared with an antiseptic solution, sterile towels are placed around the stump, and a circumcision drape is placed with the hole over the stump. The base of the cord is loosely tied with umbilical tape, with care taken to avoid the skin. The cord stump is then grasped and cut perpendicular to its axis to within approximately 1.5 cm of the abdominal wall with a surgical blade. The exposed vessels are identified—thin-walled oval vein and two smaller thick-walled round arteries with tightly constricted lumens. Occasionally, only one artery is present. The cord is stabilized by grasping the Wharton jelly with one or two Kelly clamps.

The lumen of the vessel to be used is gently dilated with curved Iris dressing forceps or a small obturator (Fig. D.3A,B). The catheter is then inserted and gently advanced. Obstruction at the level of the abdominal wall may be relieved by applying gentle traction on the umbilical cord stump accompanied by steady but gentle pressure for about 30 seconds. During umbilical artery catheterization, obstruction may also occur at the level of the bladder. It may be overcome by application of gentle, steady pressure for 30 seconds. Alternatively, marked resistance may be found where the umbilical artery meets the internal iliac artery (usually at 5 cm). The operator should avoid applying undue pressure to overcome this point of resistance because of the possibility of perforation of the vessel and severe hemorrhage. If continued resistance is met,

BOX D.2 Equipment Found on the Umbilical Catheterization Tray at University Hospitals, Cleveland Medical Center, Cleveland, Ohio

- 2 Iris dressing forceps, 4 inch curved
- 1 Iris dressing forceps, 4 inch straight
- 2 Halsted mosquito forceps, 4 inch curved
- 2 Halsted mosquito forceps, 4 inch straight
- 1 Derf needle holder, 4.75 inches
- 1 Iris scissors, 4.5 inches
- 1 Operating scissors, 5.5 inches
- 1 Medicine cup
- 4 Gauze preparation sponges, 3 × 3 inch
- 1 Huck towel, folded
- 1 Steam chemical integrator

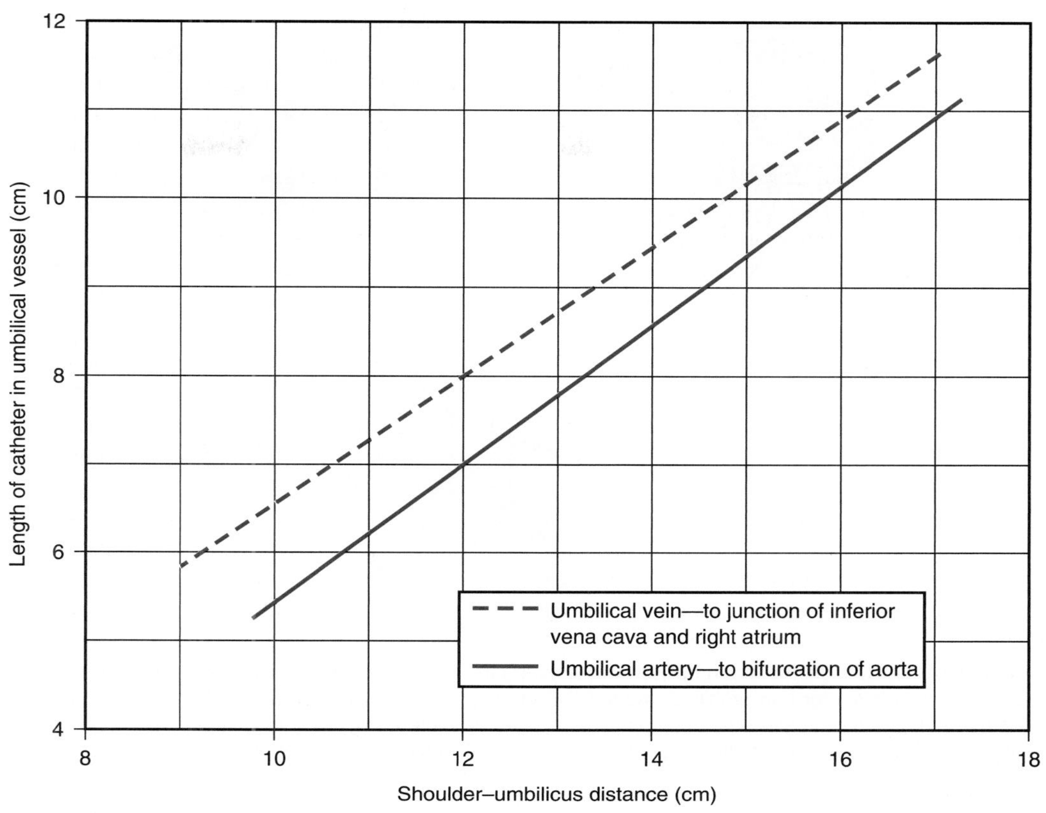

Fig. D.1 Determination of the length of catheter to be inserted for appropriate arterial or venous placement. The length of the catheter read from the diagram is to the umbilical ring; the length of the umbilical cord stump present must be added. The shoulder–umbilicus distance is the perpendicular distance between parallel lines at the level of the umbilicus and through the distal ends of the clavicles. (Modified from Dunn P. Localization of the umbilical catheter by post-mortem measurement. *Arch Dis Child.* 1966;41:69)

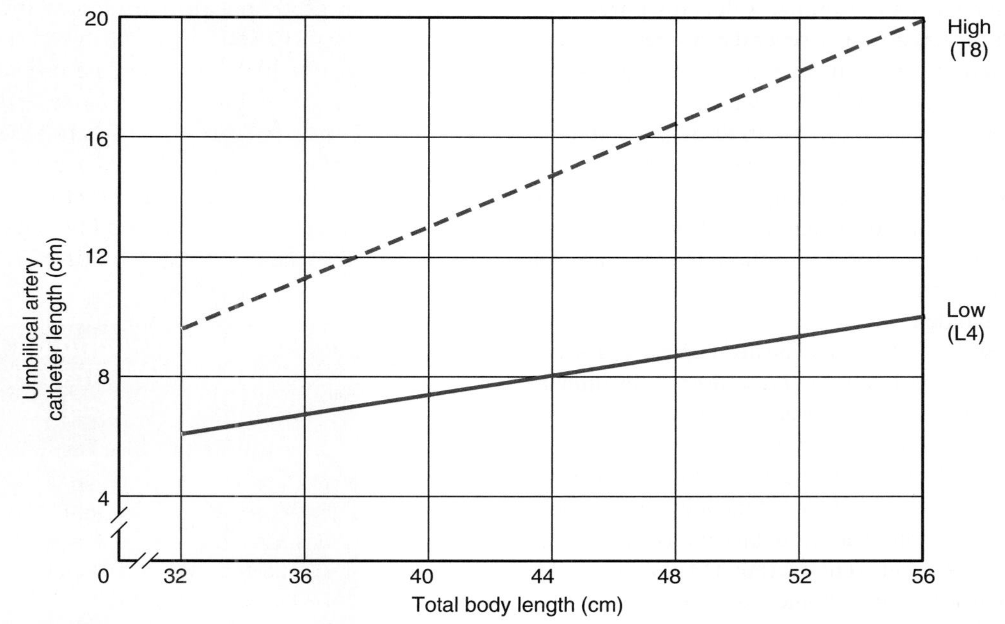

Fig. D.2 Catheter position determined from total body length. (Modified from Rosenfield W, Biagtan J, Schaeffer H, et al. A new graph for insertion of umbilical artery catheters. *J Pediatr.* 1980;96:735.)

the other artery should be used. If at any point during or after the line placement persistent blanching or cyanosis of the ipsilateral or contralateral extremity is observed, the catheter should be promptly removed. Cyanosis involving the toes or part of the foot on the side of the catheter may be relieved by warming the contralateral foot; if this is not successful, the

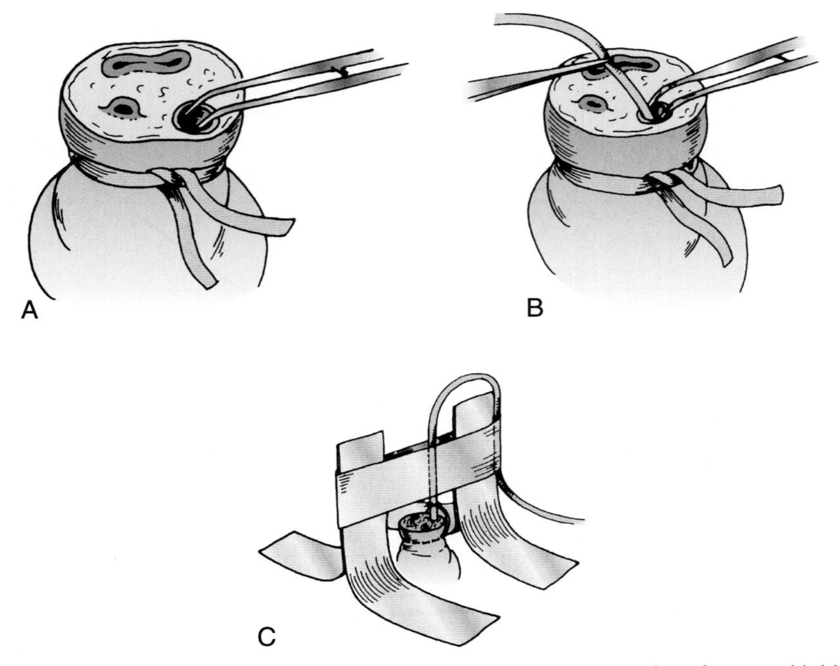

Fig. D.3 (A) Cross-section of the umbilical cord showing tie in place and dilatation of artery with Iris forceps. (B) Insertion of catheter into umbilical artery. (C) Bridge technique used to secure catheter after suturing. A purse string suture is used that incorporates all three vessels. A square knot is tied at the base of the catheter, and a second knot is tied 1 cm above the base. The tape bridge further ensures against the line becoming dislodged.

catheter should be removed. Both lower extremities and buttocks should be carefully watched for alterations in blood supply when an umbilical artery catheter is in place.

If an umbilical vein catheterization is performed, the next site of obstruction after the abdominal wall is the portal system. (The catheter meets resistance several centimeters before the distance marked on the catheter is reached.) The catheter should be withdrawn several centimeters, gently rotated, and reinserted in an attempt to get the tip through the ductus venosus into the inferior vena cava. Gentle application of caudal traction to the umbilical cord stump sometimes facilitates the introduction of an umbilical venous line. Occasionally, it is not possible to get the catheter into the inferior vena cava for anatomic reasons, and vigorous attempts to advance the catheter are to be avoided.

An umbilical vessel catheter should be tied in place with a silk suture around the vessel and catheter and sutured to the umbilical stump or taped to the abdominal wall. Disastrous hemorrhage can occur if the catheter is inadvertently pulled out or the stopcocks are disconnected by the activity of the infant. The position of the catheter must be identified by radiography immediately after insertion. It is important that the umbilical vein catheter tip be at least well into the ductus venosus (Fig. D.4) to protect the portal system from receiving hypertonic solutions.

If the radiograph obtained after umbilical vessel catheterization indicates that the catheter has been inserted too far, it may be gently withdrawn an estimated amount for appropriate placement. If the catheter is not in far enough, it must be completely withdrawn and a new sterile one inserted after the area is appropriately prepared again.

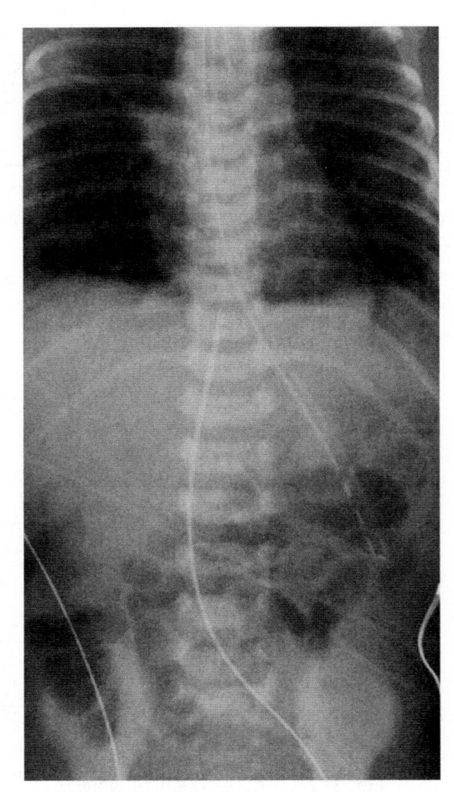

Fig. D.4 Anteroposterior radiographic image showing the preferred location of the umbilical vein catheter tip at the most superior portion of the inferior vena cava, where it receives the hepatic veins and the ductus venosus and is about to empty into the right atrium. (From Oestreich AE. Umbilical vein catheterization—appropriate and inappropriate placement. *Pediatr Radiol.* 2010;40:1941.)

PERIPHERALLY INSERTED CENTRAL CATHETERS

The administration of fluids, parenteral nutrition, and life-sustaining medications are essential aspects of the care of the critically ill or preterm neonatal patient; therefore securing venous access is of paramount importance. Peripherally inserted central catheters (PICC) have been shown to be a valuable alternative to traditional central venous devices and to significantly reduce complications compared with the use of peripheral venous catheters.[8,9] The insertion of these lines at bedside has become a routine procedure in the NICU, and practitioners should familiarize themselves with the techniques required for patient selection, insertion, and maintenance of these devices. Patients who are candidates for a PICC line include those newborns who will require long-term intravenous access for administration of parenteral nutrition, continuous infusion of critical drugs, and maintenance fluids. Once the candidate patient has been identified and parental consent is obtained, the practitioner will proceed to determine the insertion site and the proper-size device. Veins of the upper of lower extremities and scalp have been used successfully. However, lower-extremity lines have been associated with a higher rate of complications in surgical patients. The use of the axillary veins seems to be associated with higher success rates and lower complications compared with other insertion sites.[10] PICC line placement is a sterile procedure, and strict adherence to sterile precautions is mandatory. The use of insertion bundles and the use of checklists have been associated with decreased central line associated bloodstream infections. There are a number of different commercially available devices, and it is preferred that teams become familiarized with as few devices as possible to minimize technical errors. This procedure is ideally performed under ultrasound guidance to facilitate intravenous access; however, this practice has not become the standard of care in neonatal units yet.[11–13.]

EDITORIAL COMMENT: Training the team and strictly following the bundles has dramatically reduced the number of infections related to catheters.

PICCs should be inserted by use of maximal barrier precautions using antiseptic hand wash, sterile gown, gloves, and a large sterile drape. The area of insertion is cleaned with antiseptics, and it is allowed to dry. Nonpharmacologic and pharmacologic pain control and occasionally mild sedation are required to diminish patient discomfort. Careful inspection of the catheter and the introducer for manufacturing imperfections is paramount. Many clinicians prefer to flush the introducer to verify patency and prevent blood stasis within its lumen. The PICC is prepared by filling it with isotonic saline and cutting the catheter to the appropriate length utilizing specially designed guillotines or sharp scissors or scalpel. Care should be taken not to trim the stylet. To avoid that, the stylet is pulled back such that its tip is retracted by approximately half a centimeter from the catheter tip before trimming the catheter. Peel-away sheaths and breakaway needles are common introducer types. Puncture the vein with the introducer needle and observe for blood return. The practitioner will stop advancing the needle as soon as there is blood return, to prevent puncture of the posterior wall of the vein. When using a peel-away sheath, withdraw the needle and then insert the catheter through the introducer to the appropriate premeasured length. The catheter should be advanced carefully without undue force. Once the catheter is properly located in the inferior vena cava or superior vena cava, depending on the access site, blood return should be observed. Then, the stylet should be slowly removed to prevent damage to the catheter. Lastly, the needle introducer is peeled away and the line secured and dressed in place according to the institutional protocols. Catheter placement should be confirmed with an X-ray or ultrasound to visualize the position of tip of the catheter. Ideally, the tip of the line should be in the right atrial/superior vena cava or right atrial/inferior vena cava junction. When obtaining radiographic studies, the position of the extremity in relation to the body should be noted because it will affect the position of the tip of the line.

A PICC line, just like any other vascular access device, has many potential complications (Box D.3). The use of maintenance bundles and the implementation of institutional protocols have been shown to dramatically decrease the incidence of complications. Training of new providers and maintenance of procedural skills of personnel in simulation laboratories are of utmost importance to establish a successful program of vascular access in NICUs. It is critical to evaluate the need for these devices on a daily basis to avoid keeping them in situ when they are no longer required, and hence increase the incidence of complications. As a rule, the need for indwelling lines and tubes should be assessed on a daily basis and removed as soon as they are deemed not essential for patient care.

EDITORIAL COMMENT: Pharande reported a progressive decrease in the late-onset sepsis rate, from 4.3 to 1.6 per 1000 patient days ($P < .001$), and the central line–associated bloodstream infection rate dropped from 25 in 2003 to 5 in 2016 per 1000 central line days ($P = .001$). Hand hygiene compliance rates remained consistent, over 80%. They concluded, "Multifaceted infection control bundle practices with a concerted team effort in the implementation, with continuing education, feedback and reinforcement of best infection control practices, can sustain the gains achieved by infection control for a long period of time."
(Pharande P, Lindrea KB, Smyth J, Evans M, Lui K, Bolisetty S. Trends in late-onset sepsis in a neonatal intensive care unit following implementation of infection control bundle: a 15-year audit. *J Paediatr Child Health.* 2018;54[12]:1314-1320.)

Meticulous sterile techniques, not violating the line, and removing the line sooner rather than later are important aspects of PICC line management and the infection control bundle.

BOX D.3 Complications Associated With Peripherally Inserted Central Catheters

- Catheter dislodgment/break
- Malposition/coiling
- Bleeding—hematomas in insertion site
- Central line associated blood stream infections
- Local infection—phlebitis/cellulitis
- Thrombosis—occlusion
- Pleural/pericardial/peritoneal effusions
- Extravasation of fluids into subcutaneous tissues—chemical burns
- Arrhythmias

LUMBAR PUNCTURE

Lumbar puncture (LP) is usually performed in the NICU to rule out meningitis. Other indications include the evaluation of spinal fluid for inborn errors of the metabolism, refractory seizures, and measurements of catecholamines and amino acids. Also, serial spinal taps have been used to manage communicating posthemorrhagic hydrocephalus in preterm infants. Although a very common procedure, there is still a significant rate of unsuccessful attempts, or the so-called traumatic tap, reaching in some series up to 50%. Several factors have been suggested as the reasons for this observation.[14,15] One interesting factor is that in recent years, there has been a significant decrease in the number of babies who are subjected to this procedure before initiation of antibiotic therapy to rule out sepsis; hence it is more difficult to maintain procedural proficiency. The technique itself is relatively simple, but variations in the way it is performed may account for some of the failure rate. Although pediatric procedure textbooks dictate that withholding local analgesia for this procedure is strongly discouraged, establishing the efficacy of pain relief for neonatal LPs has been difficult. There are also variations in the way the babies are positioned and held, as well as the way the needle and stylet are inserted. For example, the method of early stylet removal entails the removal of the stylet after passage of the spinal needle through the epidermis and subcutaneous tissue and then advancing the needle without the stylet in place into the subarachnoid space. The professed benefit of this method is to allow observation of cerebrospinal fluid (CSF) flow immediately on entering the subarachnoid space and thus to decrease the chance of inserting the needle too deeply. Two studies have reported increased success rate in pediatric LPs with the use of this technique; however, there is no literature in the neonatal population. Differences in the way babies are positioned and held for the procedure vary among practitioners. For example, in comparison to the lateral recumbent position, the vertical sitting position optimizes spinal alignment, lumbar interspinous space width, and subarachnoid space width. The vertical position is also associated with less hypoxemia and hypercarbia than the traditional lateral recumbent position in newborns, and it may increase thecal distension and hydrostatic CSF pressure for effective needle penetration.[16,17] Avoiding excessive flexion of the neck seems to avert some of the problems encountered, especially in the newborn and the preterm infant. Some programs have introduced educational videos for training before hands-on sessions in the simulation laboratory.[18,19] Minimal CSF and thecal displacement by subdural or epidural hematomas are common after failed clinical attempts. The use of ultrasound guided LP in newborns is reserved for those difficult cases but is probably underused; however, this technique can prove invaluable in the care of these neonates. Ultrasound guidance has many advantages, including the ability to evaluate and to directly visualize the thecal sac and conus medullaris in real time before puncture and to verify needle placement, all without exposure to ionizing radiation. Real-time guidance increases not only the success rate but also the safety of diagnostic LP.[20]

Spinal taps are performed under sterile conditions, and commercial kits are available with the supplies required to perform the procedure. The patient is positioned in a sitting position or lateral decubitus, and the head is maintained in a neutral position avoiding compression of the airway. The iliac crests are identified, and a horizontal line between them is followed to the middle of the spinal column, where a space between the third and fourth lumbar spinous processes is identified as the entry site. The overlying skin is cleansed with either a povidone-iodine or a chlorhexidine-based solution employing widening concentric circles, and then the area is draped in aseptic fashion. Once the skin is sterile, local anesthetic can be administered, although the benefits of this practice in newborns have been questioned. Nonpharmacologic techniques can be used successfully. If the needle is positioned properly, it should pass through the following anatomic structures: skin, subcutaneous tissue, supraspinous ligament, interspinous ligaments, ligamentum flavum, epidural space, dura, and finally the subarachnoid space. The classical "popping" sensation occurs when the needle has passed through the ligamentum flavum. The needle should then be advanced slowly until CSF is obtained. If CSF flow is slow, the needle can be rotated 90 degrees because a nerve root may be obstructing the opening. Although not routinely done, an opening pressure can be measured once CSF is obtained if the patient is in the recumbent position. The manometer is connected to the hub of the needle. A measurement can be determined after cessation of the increase of the CSF column. The recorded pressure is determined by identifying the lowest mark of the fluid meniscus at the top of the fluid column. Samples of 1 to 2 cc are placed in sterile tubes for measurement of cell count and differential, protein, and glucose. A sample is obtained for culture and gram stain to help identify pathogenic organisms. Additional CSF samples can be sent for viral cultures, polymerase chain reaction, and metabolic studies.

LP is contraindicated in cerebral herniation, increased intracranial pressure, focal neurologic signs, suspected spinal epidural abscess, coagulopathy, or anticoagulation therapy (Box D.4). A rare complication of LP may occur when the skin is penetrated without use of a stylet and a small plug of epidermal tissue implants within the spinal canal, later growing into a small tumor. There are well-documented cases where these tumors have been discovered years to decades after, and the LP was felt to be the inciting cause. Most of these complications have occurred in children with the proposed reason being that while performing LPs, some practitioners remove the stylet before puncturing the dura. However, this complication has been reported after LP with needles with stylet.[21] In a review of LP success rate among residents, early stylet removal was associated with a greater chance of success in infants younger than 6 weeks, which might suggest an advantage of that technique, although training programs continue to emphasize the practice of not to remove the stylet until well past the dermis.

CHEST TUBES

Pneumothorax is a life-threatening condition that occurs most commonly during the newborn period. Although the reported incidence in term infants with normal lungs is low (1%–2%), it is much higher in preterm infants (6.3%).[22–26] Neonates have a supple chest wall, close proximity of vital structures, and frail lung tissue. Intrapleural air or fluid collections can significantly affect the cardiovascular system by applying indirect compression of the heart and great vessels. This leads to decreased cardiac output and decreased venous return of blood flow to the heart, potentially resulting in clinically significant hypotension. As a result of the newborn's limited respiratory reserve, a rapidly evolving tension pneumothorax can develop into a life-threatening situation. Practitioners in a NICU must be prepared to diagnose and treat air leaks in a timely manner to avoid morbidity and mortality. Decreased air exchange on examination and a positive transillumination of the chest are characteristic. A confirmatory chest X-ray is usually done except during emergencies (Figs. D.5A and D.6A). Historically, straight catheters such as polyethylene feeding tubes, red rubber catheters, and intravenous cannulas were used. In emergency situations, large intravenous cannulas are still used to temporarily drain fluid or a tension pneumothorax to stabilize the patient during resuscitation.

BOX D.4 Indications and Contraindication for Lumbar Puncture in Newborns

Indications
- Rule out meningitis
- Diagnosis of inborn errors of metabolism
- Cerebrospinal fluid drainage for hydrocephalus
- Intrathecal administration of drugs

Contraindications
- Coagulopathy/bleeding
- Increased intracranial pressure
- Epidural abscess
- Focal neurological signs

Later, pigtail catheters were introduced, and they are now widely used because of their safety profile, efficacy, and ease of placement.[24] Furthermore, less force is required to insert a pigtail catheter with the Seldinger technique, as it avoids the use of the force required for the insertion of a conventional chest tube using a trocar and dissection. Several different sites on the chest are usually used for insertion and it varies according to the indication. The second intercostal space on the midclavicular line or the fourth–fifth intercostal spaces at the anterior or middle axillary line are used for evacuation of a pneumothorax, and care is taken to direct the catheter's tip anteriorly.[25] Posteriorly and inferiorly placed catheters are usually reserved for draining pleural effusions. Pharmacologic pain control and sedation are required before placing a thoracostomy tube, as this procedure is very painful. Local anesthesia is also administered if the patient is stable before the insertion of the chest tube. In most situations, the airway is already secured, and patients are on mechanical ventilation, although in spontaneously breathing patients on continuous pressure airway pressure or noninvasive support, endotracheal intubation may not be required before chest tube placement. Once the site of insertion has been determined, the patient is placed

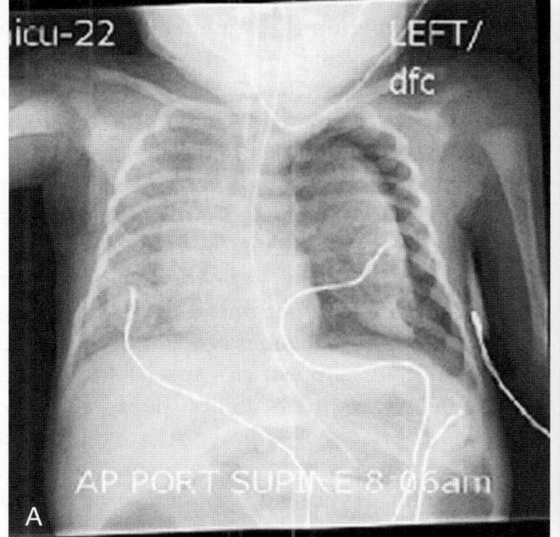

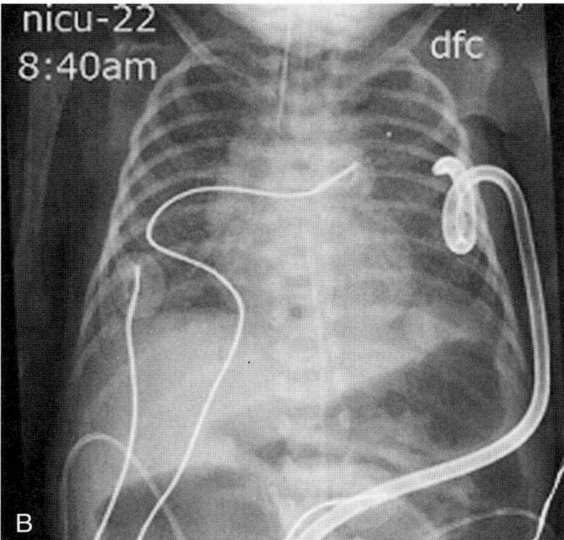

Fig. D.5 Chest x-rays. (A) Left-sided pneumothorax. (B) Resolution after chest tube placed.

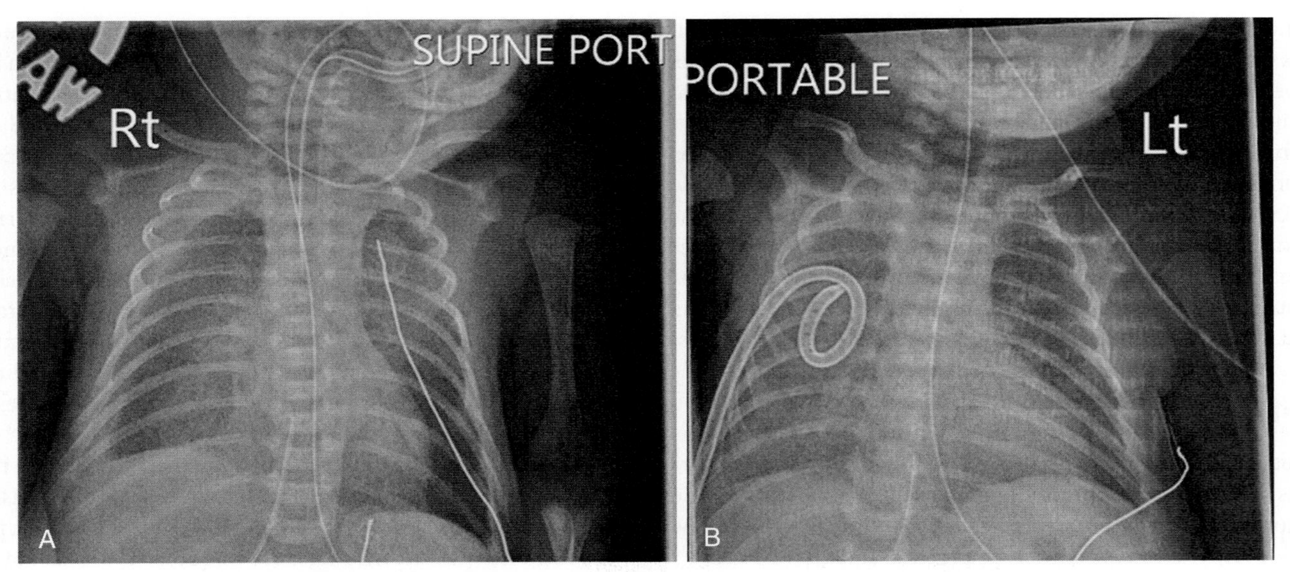

Fig. D.6 Chest x-ray. Pleural effusion (A) before and (B) after chest tube placement.

supine or slightly on his or her side if a posterior tube is to be inserted. Commercial kits are now available that include all of the supplies necessary for the procedure. Currently, pigtail tubes are preferred over straight ones by most practitioners. The insertion site is identified, and the skin is cleaned with an antiseptic solution. A local anesthetic is administered, and a needle introducer attached to a syringe filled with normal saline solution is used to enter the chest cavity. Air bubbles will be aspirated as the needle enters the chest cavity. With a modified Seldinger technique, a wire is then advanced into the needle, and the needle is pulled out of the chest while holding the wire in position. A dilator is then slid over the wire and is introduced slowly to create a path for the catheter. The dilator is replaced with the pigtail, and after all the side holes are in the chest cavity, the guide wire is removed from the chest. The chest tube is attached to a chamber (Neumovac), and negative pressure is applied with wall suction to 10–20 cm H_2O. Air bubbling in the chamber indicates an active air leak. A secure dressing per institutional protocol is applied. A chest X-ray is obtained to verify chest tube position and resolution of the air leak or pleural effusion (Figs. D.5B and D6B). As the patient's condition improves, the tube is placed to water seal, and if no reaccumulation or active leak is identified, the chest tube is removed. There is still significant debate as to whether the chest tube should be clamped before removal. Despite the fact that chest tube placement is a very straightforward procedure, it is not free of potential complications (Box D.5), and it should only be performed by very well-trained individuals. Radiographic evidence of malpositioned pigtail catheters includes persistent or repeated pneumothoraces and atelectasis/infiltrate near the tip of the chest tube.[26]

EXCHANGE TRANSFUSION

Blood exchange transfusion has become a rare event in most developed countries. As a result, many pediatricians and neonatologists may have never performed or even seen one. Blood exchange transfusion was introduced in the late 1940s to decrease the mortality attributable to rhesus hemolytic disease of the newborn and to prevent kernicterus in surviving infants.[27–30] The current indications for exchange transfusion in the neonate are limited to hyperbilirubinemia to avoid the toxic effects of unconjugated bilirubin on the brain, and in some select cases, a single volume exchange transfusion may be performed in patients with polycythemia. The volume of the exchange transfusion is calculated based on the patient's blood volume, which is 100 mL/kg for a preterm and 80 mL/kg for a full-term newborn. Double volume exchange transfusions replace 86% of the neonate's circulating blood volume and are usually done via the umbilical vessels. Partial exchange transfusions for polycythemia can be performed via an umbilical vessel or a peripheral one. The procedure can be performed by a single operator with the currently available push-pull kits equipped with special stopcocks. The blood should be warmed with a blood/fluid warmer to avoid any deleterious effects of hypothermia on the newborn. The actual exchange should be performed slowly in aliquots of 5 to 10 mL/kg body weight with each withdrawal-infusion cycle approximating 3 minutes per cycle, so a complete double volume exchange should be completed in less

BOX D.5 Complications of Chest Tube Placement

- Dislodgement/misplacement
- Obstruction/clogging/kinking
- Lung perforation
- Pericardial and cardiac perforation
- Phrenic nerve palsy
- Horner syndrome
- Diaphragmatic paralysis/laceration
- Chylothorax/hemothorax
- Laceration of abdominal organs

than 2 hours. During the procedure, the patient's vital signs should be recorded and closely monitored, including heart and respiratory rate, oxygen saturation by pulse oximetry, temperature, and blood pressure. The institutional blood bank should participate in the development of policies and procedures for the provision, handling, and transport of blood products to be used. Blood should have a hematocrit between 50% and 60% and be as fresh as possible, cytomegalovirus negative, and irradiated. Complications of this procedure are not very frequent, but they can be life-threatening and may be underestimated because of the decrease in the number of procedures performed and lack of operator experience (Box D.6). Exchange transfusions should only be performed by individuals with subspecialty training and experience with this procedure.

ENDOTRACHEAL INTUBATION

(See also Chapter 10.)

Videolaryngoscopy

Airway management is a key element in the management of the critically ill neonate. A priori identification of the difficult airway is of extreme importance in several clinical scenarios including the delivery room or the patient undergoing a surgical procedure or requiring endotracheal intubation for respiratory support. Anticipating the need for advanced airway management in the difficult-to-intubate patient allows the practitioner to resort to new techniques to effectively deal with such situations. Videolaryngoscopy (VL) entails the use of equipment that provides a view of the larynx without aligning the oral cavity, pharynx, and larynx. The blade of a videolaryngoscope is equipped with a video camera and a light source at its tip, which enables the transmission of an indirect image of the glottis to the operator. These devices generally have a liquid crystal display screen mounted on either the handle of the device or as a separate screen for visualization of the airway, and allow a wider and larger magnified view than with traditional direct laryngoscopy. Furthermore, still images and video can be recorded for teaching purposes. In recent years, VL has become a common procedure in the NICU for the management of the neonatal airway. In a recent randomized trial, novice operators were significantly more successful at airway intubation when their instructors could share their view on a screen. The use of VL devices may result in airway injury, especially if used with improper training and experience. Whether videolaryngoscopy is superior to direct laryngoscopy for the routine endotracheal intubation of newborns remains to be proven in large, randomized, controlled trials.[31,32]

BOX D.6 Complications of Exchange Transfusions

- Hemodynamic instability/arrhythmias
- Hypotension/hypertension
- Infection
- Thrombosis/air embolism
- Hemorrhage/intracranial hemorrhage in preterm infants
- Thrombocytopenia/neutropenia
- Catheter-related complications
- Hypothermia/hyperthermia
- Death

RETINOPATHY OF PREMATURITY SCREENING

Retinopathy of prematurity (ROP) is a retinal vascular disease characterized by abnormal angiogenesis that may result in permanent visual impairment or complete blindness in premature and low-birth-weight infants. Low birth weight and prematurity are strongly associated with an increased risk of the disease. In the Early Treatment for ROP study, 68% of premature infants weighing less than 1251g developed ROP, and severe ROP was observed in 37%. ROP is currently the leading cause of childhood blindness in the world.[33] In 1984, the International Classification of ROP developed a standard framework and nomenclature for examination findings through the definition of parameters such as zone, stage, clock hour extent, and plus disease. Fundus examination with indirect ophthalmoscopy remains the criterion standard for screening and monitoring patients with ROP; however, because of the inherent subjectivity of this technique, there can be significant variation in reported findings, even among experienced screeners.[34] The development of wide-angle retinal imaging devices (e.g., RetCam; Natus Medical, CA, and the ICON, Phoenix Technology Group, CA) has created opportunities for more objective documentation of examination findings. Furthermore, the application of these portable technologies allows for trained practitioners to obtain images that can be evaluated by experts via telemedicine. Studies have suggested that image-based diagnosis may even be superior to ophthalmoscopy in certain situations because it provides the opportunity for careful scrutiny of images to identify morphological features such as presence of zone I disease. However, this technology is unable to reproducibly visualize the far peripheral retina, and may cause variation in the appearance of clinically significant peripheral findings and vascular appearance if not performed properly. The ROP screening guidelines published in 2013 by the American Academy of Pediatrics, American Academy of Ophthalmology, and American Association for Pediatric Ophthalmology and Strabismus support the use of digital imaging for this purpose. New imaging technologies are currently under clinical evaluation, including handheld ocular coherence tomography (OCT) and OCT angiography.[35] These techniques may allow the identification of anatomical precursors of severe ROP, which may lead to novel treatments to prevent retinal detachment and improve visual outcomes. Another promising innovation, computer-assisted image analysis through machine learning, is likely to be incorporated in the armamentarium for screening and diagnosis of ROP in the near future.

BOX D.7 Risk factors for hearing loss in newborns

- Physical findings of syndromes associated with hearing loss, craniofacial malformations
- Abnormal ears, microtia, preauricular tags, dimples
- Family history of hearing loss
- History of congenital infections: CMV, toxoplasmosis, rubella
- Neonatal bacterial meningitis
- Exposure to ototoxic medications: aminoglycosides, furosemide
- Severe hyperbilirubinemia
- Neurometabolic disorders
- Persistent pulmonary hypertension of the newborn: assisted ventilation with hyperventilation to high pH

CMV, Cytomegalovirus.

HEARING SCREEN IN THE NEONATAL INTENSIVE CARE UNIT

Each year, approximately 12,000 infants in the United States are born with permanent hearing loss. The goal of universal newborn hearing screening can help ensure early detection of hearing loss for these infants, which would allow for early intervention.[36] Several risks factors for hearing loss have been identified, and some of them are summarized in Box D.7.

Different techniques for testing are currently used. Otoacoustic emission testing comprises the application of a stimulus into the ear via a microphone. The machine records the response generated by a normal cochlea. Automated auditory brainstem responses records the neural responses coming from the brain stem after a click sound is delivered. This technique evaluates the auditory nerve pathway. All of these tests results are reported as pass or fail. If patients failed an initial screening tests, a referral to an audiology clinic is necessary for a more comprehensive evaluation. Auditory brainstem responses of brainstem auditory-evoked response then performed. This test permits the identification of type of hearing loss (conductive, sensorineural, or mixed) and also helps determine its severity.

For patients who failed their newborn screen, close follow-up is critical to allow for early intervention if congenital hearing loss is confirmed. There are patients who passed their newborn screen but are identified as having hearing loss later in life, when lack of speech development or behavioral issues prompt an audiology evaluation in an infant. These patients represent a different population in terms of the etiology for their hearing deficit.

The reference list for this appendix can be found online at www.expertconsult.com.

APPENDIX E

Conversion Charts

Jonathan M. Fanaroff

TABLE E.1 Conversion of Pounds and Ounces to Grams

Pounds	OUNCES															
	0	1	2	3	4	5	6	7	8	9	10	11	12	13	14	15
0	—	28	57	85	113	142	170	198	227	255	283	312	340	369	397	425
1	454	482	510	539	567	595	624	652	680	709	737	765	794	822	850	879
2	907	936	964	992	1021	1049	1077	1106	1134	1162	1191	1219	1247	1276	1304	1332
3	1361	1389	1417	1446	1474	1503	1531	1559	1588	1616	1644	1673	1701	1729	1758	1786
4	1814	1843	1871	1899	1928	1956	1984	2013	2041	2070	2098	2126	2155	2183	2211	2240
5	2268	2296	2325	2353	2381	2410	2438	2466	2495	2523	2551	2580	2608	2637	2665	2693
6	2722	2750	2778	2807	2835	2863	2892	2920	2948	2977	3005	3033	3062	3090	3118	3147
7	3175	3203	3232	3260	3289	3317	3345	3374	3402	3430	3459	3487	3515	3544	3572	3600
8	3629	3657	3685	3714	3742	3770	3799	3827	3856	3884	3912	3941	3969	3997	4026	4054
9	4082	4111	4139	4167	4196	4224	4252	4281	4309	4337	4366	4394	4423	4451	4479	4508
10	4536	4564	4593	4621	4649	4678	4706	4734	4763	4791	4819	4848	4876	4904	4933	4961
11	4990	5018	5046	5075	5103	5131	5160	5188	5216	5245	5273	5301	5330	5358	5386	5415
12	5443	5471	5500	5528	5557	5585	5613	5642	5670	5698	5727	5755	5783	5812	5840	5868
13	5897	5925	5953	5982	6010	6038	6067	6095	6123	6152	6180	6209	6237	6265	6294	6322
14	6350	6379	6407	6435	6464	6492	6520	6549	6577	6605	6634	6662	6690	6719	6747	6776
15	6804	6832	6860	6889	6917	6945	6973	7002	7030	7059	7087	7115	7144	7172	7201	7228
16	7257	7286	7313	7342	7371	7399	7427	7456	7484	7512	7541	7569	7597	7626	7654	7682
17	7711	7739	7768	7796	7824	7853	7881	7909	7938	7966	7994	8023	8051	8079	8108	8136
18	8165	8192	8221	8249	8278	8306	8335	8363	8391	8420	8448	8476	8504	8533	8561	8590
19	8618	8646	8675	8703	8731	8760	8788	8816	8845	8873	8902	8930	8958	8987	9015	9043
20	9072	9100	9128	9157	9185	9213	9242	9270	9298	9327	9355	9383	9412	9440	9469	9497
21	9525	9554	9582	9610	9639	9667	9695	9724	9752	9780	9809	9837	9865	9894	9922	9950
22	9979	10,007	10,036	10,064	10,092	10,120	10,149	10,177	10,206	10,234	10,262	10,291	10,319	10,347	10,376	10,404

TABLE E.2 Conversion to International System Units

Component	Conventional Unit	×	Conversion Factor	=	International System Unit
Clinical Hematology					
Erythrocytes	per mm^3		1		10^6/L
Hematocrit	%		0.01		(1) volume of RBCs/volume of whole blood
Hemoglobin (mass concentration)	g/dL		10		g/L
Leukocytes	per mm^3		1		10^6/L
Mean corpuscular hemoglobin concentration (MCHC)	g/dL		10		g/L
Mean corpuscular volume (MCV)	μm^3		1		fL
Platelet count	$10^3/mm^3$		1		10^9/L
Reticulocyte count	%		10		10^{-3}
Clinical Chemistry					
Acetone	mg/dL		0.1722		mmol/L
Albumin	g/dL		10		g/L
Aldosterone	ng/dL		27.74		pmol/L
alpha-Fetoprotein	ng/mL		1		μg/L
Ammonia (as nitrogen)	μg/dL		0.7139		μmol/L
Bicarbonate	mEq/L		1		mmol/L
Bilirubin	mg/dL		17.1		μmol/L
Calcium	mg/dL		0.2495		mmol/L
Calcium ion	mEq/L		0.50		mmol/L
Carotenes	μg/dL		0.01836		μmol/L
Ceruloplasmin	mg/dL		10.0		mg/L
Chloride	mEq/L		1		mmol/L
Cholesterol	mg/dL		0.02586		mmol/L
Complement, C3 or C4	mg/dL		0.01		g/L
Copper	μg/dL		0.1574		μmol/L
Cortisol	μg/dL		27.59		nmol/L
Creatine	mg/dL		76.25		μmol/L
Creatinine	mg/dL		88.40		μmol/L
Digoxin	ng/mL		1.281		nmol/L
Epinephrine	pg/mL		5.458		pmol/L
Fatty acids	mg/dL		10.0		mg/L
Ferritin	ng/mL		1		μg/L
Fibrinogen	mg/dL		0.01		g/L
Folate	ng/mL		2.266		nmol/L
Fructose	mg/dL		0.05551		mmol/L
Galactose	mg/dL		0.05551		mmol/L
Gases					
PO_2	mm Hg (= torr)		0.1333		kPa
PCO_2	mm Hg (= torr)		0.1333		kPa
Glucagon	pg/mL		1		ng/L
Glucose	mg/dL		0.05551		mmol/L
Glycerol	mg/dL		0.1086		mmol/L
Growth hormone	ng/mL		1		μg/L
Haptoglobin	mg/dL		0.01		g/L
Hemoglobin	g/dL		10		g/L
Insulin	μg/L		172.2		pmol/L

TABLE E.2 Conversion to International System Units—cont'd

Component	Conventional Unit	×	Conversion Factor	=	International System Unit
	mU/L		7.175		pmol/L
Iron	μg/dL		0.1791		μmol/L
Iron-binding capacity	μg/dL		0.1791		μmol/L
Lactate	mEq/L		1		mmol/L
Lead	μg/dL		0.04826		μmol/L
Lipoproteins	mg/dL		0.02586		mmol/L
Magnesium	mg/dL		0.4114		mmol/L
	mEq/L		0.50		mmol/L
Osmolality	mOsm/kg		1		mmol/kg
Phenobarbital	mg/dL		43.06		μmol/L
Phenytoin	mg/L		3.964		μmol/L
Phosphate	mg/dL		0.3229		mmol/L
Potassium	mEq/L		1		mmol/L
	mg/dL		0.2558		mmol/L
Protein	g/dL		10.0		g/L
Pyruvate	mg/dL		113.6		μmol/L
Sodium ion	mEq/L		1		mmol/L
Steroids					
17-hydroxycorticosteroids	mg/24 hour		2.759		μmol/day
17-ketosteroids	mg/24 hour		3.467		μmol/day
Testosterone	ng/mL		3.467		nmol/L
Theophylline	mg/L		5.550		μmol/L
Thyroid Tests					
Thyroid-stimulating hormone	μU/mL		1		mU/L
Thyroxine (T_4)	μg/dL		12.87		nmol/L
Thyroxine free	ng/dL		12.87		pmol/L
Triiodothyronine (T_3)	ng/dL		0.01536		nmol/L
Transferrin	mg/dL		0.01		g/L
Triglycerides	mg/dL		0.01129		mmol/L
Urea nitrogen	mg/dL		0.3570		mmol/L
Uric acid (urate)	mg/dL		59.48		μmol/L
Vitamin A (retinol)	μg/dL		0.03491		μmol/L
Vitamin B_{12}	pg/mL		0.7378		pmol/L
Vitamin C (ascorbic acid)	mg/dL		56.78		μmol/L
Vitamin D					
Cholecalciferol	μg/mL		2.599		nmol/L
25 OH-cholecalciferol	ng/mL		2.496		nmol/L
Vitamin (Eα-tocopherol)	mg/dL		23.22		μmol/L
D-Xylose	mg/dL		0.06661		mmol/L
Zinc	μg/dL		0.1530		μmol/L
Energy	kcal (kilocalorie)		4.1868		kJ (kilojoule)
Blood Pressure	mm Hg (= torr)		1.333		mbar

RBC, Red blood cell.
Modified from Young DS: Implementation of SI units for clinical laboratory data. Style specifications and conversion tables, *Ann Intern Med* 106:114, 1987.

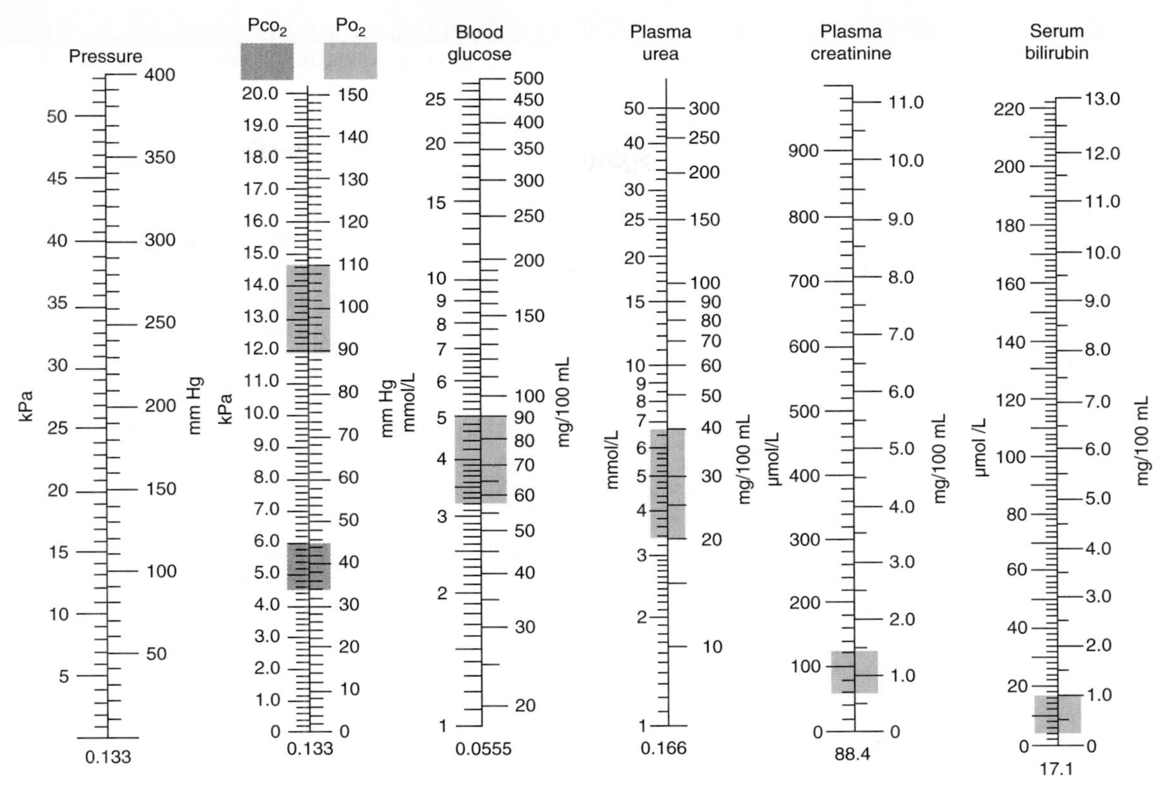

Fig. E.1 Conversion chart for pressure, gases, and selected blood chemistry values. Shading indicates the normal range where appropriate. To convert from an old (conventional) unit *(right side of each scale)* to a new (SI) unit *(left side of each scale),* multiply by the conversion factor at the foot of each column. (Modified from Halliday HL, McClure G, Reid M: *Handbook of neonatal intensive care,* ed 2, Philadelphia, 1985, Saunders.)

INDEX

Note: Page numbers followed by "f" indicate figures and "t" indicate tables.